Cardiac Mechano-Electric Coupling and Arrhythmias

Cardiac Mechano-Electric Coupling and Arrhythmias

SECOND EDITION

Peter Kohl, Frederick Sachs and
Michael R. Franz

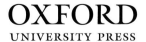

OXFORD

UNIVERSITY PRESS

Great Clarendon Street, Oxford ox2 6dp

Oxford University Press is a department of the University of Oxford.
It furthers the University's objective of excellence in research, scholarship,
and education by publishing worldwide in

Oxford New York

Athens Auckland Bangkok Bogotá Buenos Aires Calcutta
Cape-Town Chennai Dar-es-Salaam Delhi Florence Hong-Kong Istanbul
Karachi Kuala-Lumpur Madrid Melbourne Mexico-City Mumbai
Nairobi Paris São-Paulo Singapore Taipei Tokyo Toronto Warsaw

with associated companies in Berlin Ibadan

Oxford is a registered trade mark of Oxford University Press
in the UK and in certain other countries

Published in the United States
by Oxford University Press Inc., New York

First edition published 2005
Second edition published 2011

British Library Cataloguing in Publication Data

Data available

Library of Congress Cataloguing in Publication Data

ISBN 978-0-19-957016-4

10 9 8 7 6 5 4 3 2 1

Typeset in Minion
by Cenveo Publisher Services, Bangalore, India
Printed in Italy
on acid-free paper by
Lego S.p.A

Foreword I

Why should basic cardiac researchers know about stretch effects on heart rhythm?

Just over 5 years ago, the first edition of this book was published. In it the editors compiled a comprehensive series of well-organized, well-executed and timely chapters covering important aspects of this subject, from the ion channels and proteins involved in the so-called stretch response of the cardiac cell to the response of the human heart. In this second edition, these same editors have developed this by broadening their scope, with a 50% increase in the number of chapters, contributed by the leading experts in the field, and by exploring this subject at even greater depth.

While many of the original basic science chapters are included, with very significant updates, this volume is characterized by the additional inclusion of chapters that address the translation of basic science findings to the electro-mechanical activity of atria and ventricles. These new key chapters are crucial in that they help the basic scientist and the young clinical investigator to understand the concept of mechano-electric coupling (MEC), and approaches towards studying this in ways that are relevant to human health. Furthermore, in this second edition there are more chapters that are directly related to clinical observations, notably in the new Sections V–VIII. These chapters are a must-read for the researcher in that they address the effects of stretch on myocardial function and electrical activity in both normal and diseased hearts.

Personally, I find the chapters in Section VII on MEC as a mechanism involved in therapeutic interventions particularly informative. Collectively, these chapters approach control of the mechanical environment as an anti-arrhythmic intervention. While readers will be aware of the benefits associated with cardiac resynchronization therapy, it is intriguing to see the expanding body of insight related to mechanical modulation of arrhythmogenesis and defibrillation. Equally exciting are observations on mechanical components in the electrocardiogram, the often ignored role of the pericardium, and the host of remodelling events that occur in atrial and ventricular overload, or their partial reversal by cardiac assist devices. The puzzle for the basic scientist is: why? Section VIII forms another unique focus in this book. It consists of well-written chapters by outstanding clinical investigators who review the evidence from clinical trials for MEC, again emphasizing to the reader the effects of stretch on cardiac rhythms and function.

Once again I applaud the editors and contributors for a fine job, which illustrates that the field has made considerable progress in recent years. We are beginning to understand more about 'what stretch has to do with arrhythmias', and how mechanisms at the molecular level relate to clinically relevant phenomena. Perhaps we are even on our way to the development of a new class of anti-arrhythmic drugs.

For basic scientists, physiological and/or clinical relevance should be a key guide for directing research efforts. This book provides a superb compass for fundamental exploration of cardiac MEC.

Penelope A. Boyden
Professor of Pharmacology
Columbia University

Foreword II

Why should clinical cardiologists know about stretch effects on cardiomyocyte electrophysiology?

In normal hearts, electrical activation occurs by an orchestrated sequence of selective channel openings and closures, ultimately delivering a calcium signal to the myofilaments that return the favour by contracting. For cardiologists, arrhythmia most often is viewed in a similar unidirectional manner, i.e. as stemming from disruption of ion channel function with abnormal ion levels occurring at the wrong place and/or the wrong time, stimulating extra contractions and impairing normal intracellular function and homeostasis. However, as one will learn after reading this extraordinary and newly updated book, this process is far from a one-way street. Mechanical forces generated by excited muscle can themselves trigger changes in ion channel function, calcium–myofilament interactions and intercellular communication. These forces may be in the form of dis-coordinated contraction or acute stretch – where one piece of muscle pulls on the other, or where a whole heart is suddenly loaded. It can also ensue from chronic changes in loading such as occur in dilated heart failure, valvular disease, ventricular infarction and hypertrophy.

The mechanisms of what is known as mechano-electric feedback, or coupling, are many, and they are authoritatively presented in Sections I–III of this book. The first section, dedicated to the subcellular mechanisms of cardiac mechano-sensitivity, is followed by one that explains cellular correlates. In the third section, multicellular manifestations of cardiac mechano-electric coupling are reviewed. Together, they are believed to play a major role in numerous clinical heart diseases (see Sections V–VIII). Examples are the reduced threshold of arrhythmia induction that often accompanies excessive chamber enlargement (atrial or ventricular), the adverse effects of dis-coordinate wall motion in patients with heart failure, and the impact of regional loading of pulmonary veins on atrial fibrillation. Treatment of arrhythmia-by targeting ion channelopathies had been a mainstay approach for decades, yet has been rather disappointing – the best we generally have to offer is an insurance policy that shocks you back when needed.

As clinical cardiologists, we pay most attention to controlling electrical abnormalities when they negatively impact heart mechanics. The material presented in this volume will make you think about how it can work the other way. Modifying how mechanics might impact the electrophysiology has been previously more theoretical than practical – but this is changing. Cardiac resynchronization provided a novel way to reduce dis-coordinate motion, and research is yielding surprising insights into how this can improve electrophysiological disease in failing hearts. Ventricular assist devices can profoundly alter chamber loading and with it such mechanical feedback stimulation. The identity of 'stretch-activated channels' has long been mysterious and, in an important way, this has limited progress in the field. However, this too is rapidly changing, with new data revealing putative proteins such as members of the non-selective cation transient receptor potential channel superfamily. This opens up opportunities for targeted translational studies (as highlighted in Section IV), and may even have future potential for novel treatment approaches, such as via selective stretch-channel blockers that maybe particularly relevant in the setting of abnormal mechanics (see Section IX). Better understanding of how wall stretch translates into electrical instability could yield an entirely new class of mechano-sensitive drugs.

This book fills a unique position in the field, bringing together an outstanding group of basic, translational and clinician scientists to explore cardiac mechano-electric coupling phenomena in a broad and comprehensive manner. The chapters are lucid and accessible, and the book impresses by how well it links basic science (Sections I–III), via translational studies (IV) to clinically relevant scenarios (V–VIII) with an outlook towards future developments (IX).

The clinician, in particular, will learn about an area rarely dealt with in traditional medical education, yet one with the potential to profoundly impact how we view arrhthmogenicity and, hopefully, how we can improve our ability to treat it. If you are looking for a place to explore the mechanisms and implications for cardiac mechano-electric responses, you have found it.

David A. Kass
Abraham and Virginia Weiss Professor of Cardiology
Johns Hopkins University

Foreword to the 1st Edition (Reprinted)

Stretching our views of cardiac control

Excitation–contraction coupling (ECC), the transduction of electrical impulses into changes in the rate and mechanical force of muscle contraction, is a fundamental concept essential to both a basic and clinical understanding of the heart. Modulators of ECC, and hence of cardiac muscle performance, include neuro-humoral transmitters such as catecholamines, as well as many other regulators, notably those that affect intracellular Ca handling. This affects the actin–myosin interactions, and adjusts the haemodynamics in accord with changing requirements, on a beat by beat, year by year basis.

The complementary concept that changes in cardiac mechanical function which occur in response to neural and hormonal influences impact back on the excitatory and conductive electrical properties of the heart, i.e. mechano-electric coupling or feedback (MEF), is a less established idea whose role in normal and pathological physiology has become an exciting new chapter in contemporary biology. Mechanisms and pathways whereby mechanical events, changes in tension, force and spatial displacement, alter the heart's electrical properties are now recognized as an important dimension for development of new approaches in therapeutic cardiac control.

The figure provides a simplified, but conceptually useful view of this emerging bi-directional dynamic. While the left-to-right pathway, ECC, appears a familiar element in current therapeutic strategies, the right-to-left pathway, MEF, has only recently begun to be explored as a topic of medical interest. However, while it has become well established that dysfunction in pathways of ECC is important in a number of cardiac pathologies (e.g. in various cardiomyopathies), there are as yet only a few clues for a parallel influence of factors involved in pathways of MEF. This situation appears likely to change, however, as greater attention is given to mechanisms involved in acute and chronic processes of cardiac remodelling.

These include some of the most common forms of heart disease such as dilative failure, atrial fibrillation and post-infarction scarring. Although we now suspect MEF effects are likely to play a role in both electrical and mechanical pathological remodelling, direct evidence for this has remained elusive. Thus while much basic information is becoming available on topics such as how MEF effects may facilitate normal physiological processes, we still have few clues on how they may be applied in prevention or reversal of disease.

This book represents an important step in documenting the elusive yet important role of MEF. Here, assembled in one source, are the current thoughts and findings of many, if not most of the leading investigators in the field. As one reviews the pages that follow, it becomes apparent that progress in MEF research is indeed a topic whose 'time to shine' has arrived and that this volume contributes much to lighting this path. The three editors are among the field's pioneers and their selection of topics has resulted in an excellent summary of much of the world's current thinking. The book continues the momentum established though their leadership in organizing a number of important international symposia on MEF that have addressed many of the field's outstanding questions in forums encompassing most of its working investigators. The synthesis and distillation from these efforts have contributed much to the pages that follow, in providing coverage of important concepts proceeding from basic physiology towards an integrated understanding of cardiac control, and the exploration of new targets of largely unexplored therapeutic potential.

Classical studies on MEF and how it might contribute to well-established events such as the Bainbridge response, or the function of stretch-activated channels, or the fatal phenomenon of *Commotio cordis*, are all discussed. In addition, new approaches by many of today's cutting edge MEF exponents employ a wide range

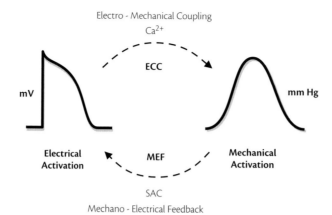

Fig. 1 Simplified conceptual view of the complementarity in coupling between electrical activation of contraction and the influence of mechano-electric feedback (MEF) in cardiac muscle. Electrical activation and excitation–contraction coupling (ECC) is believed to be mediated by convergence of signalling cascade pathways altering cellular Ca^{2+} levels, resulting in activation and alterations in actin–myosin interactions. Pathways by which mechanical influences, changes in tension, length and directional displacement alter cardiac electrical function are believed in many cases to be mediated by stretch-activated ion channels (SAC), which affect intracellular electrical potential and excitation. (Based on a figure provided to the author by Michael R. Franz.)

of molecular, biophysical and genetic tools. Thus, the various sections of the book detail not just the potential impact, influence and implications of MEF, but they also provide clues regarding future directions.

While the core concepts of mechano-electric coupling are covered in the initial sections of the book, there are many interesting additional clinical presentations. Such highlights are likely to be different for each reader. For this observer, chapters that explore chronic as well as the better known acute influences of MEF pertain to atrial fibrillation and perhaps other arrhythmias. Here is a groundwork illustrative of how changes in MEF may determine disease reversibility and refractoriness to various therapies. Other unique and fascinating topics include contributions that deal with how MEF responses vary in different cardiac cell types (e.g. cardiomyocytes versus cardio-fibroblasts), and several that touch on new questions about the sub-membranous cardiac cell structural architecture.

The network of filamentous cytoskeletal proteins has recently been recognized as important in diseases as different as inherited monogenic arrhythmias and rare forms of cardiomyopathy. Yet, we have little idea of how these phenotypes may arise at a cellular or physiological level. Are they parts of the MEF response mediated by alterations in process, such as the organization or anchoring of cell surface receptors and signalling complexes, or even interactions among various ion channel subunits that may be involved? Lastly this reader noted several intriguing new approaches represented in studies that deal with still mysterious topics, such as how changes in trans-cellular electrical and physical

communication influence expression of specific proteins that in turn determine 'who says what to whom' in the close world of *in situ* cardiobiology.

In concluding I'd express the personal view that further discoveries concerning the integration between pathways of cardiac mechanical and electrical control, between ECC and MEF, are likely to provide new clues to the treatment and prevention of many forms of recalcitrant cardiac disease, and especially those causative of life-threatening arrhythmias. Given that bias, it also seems worth suggesting that work on mechano-electro coupling, with all its extensions in man, should be supported nationally and internationally with an elevated level of health priority than has been the case recently. Despite decades of attempts at developing efficacious therapies for disturbances in the heart's electrical system, effective treatment and prevention options are few in number, and either problematic with respect to efficacy and side effects, or increasingly more difficult to justify on a cost-effectiveness, resource utilization basis. The imperative for improvements in arrhythmia therapy is, nevertheless, but one of a number of reasons that speak to a need to expand fundamental and model studies on cardiac control to improve clinical translation and therapy. This book presents an excellent view of how such progress can be successfully achieved, and the potential applications.

Peter M. Spooner
Johns Hopkins Division of Cardiology
Department of Medicine
Baltimore, December 2004

Preface

This second edition of *Cardiac Mechano-Electric Coupling and Arrhythmias* marks the maturation of a key concept in cardiac science: that of the heart as an integrated electro-mechanical organ, in which many interdependent pathways couple electrical and mechanical behaviour. It extends the original concept of mechano-electric feedback (MEF now more broadly referred to as mechano-electric coupling, (MEC), spelled out in 1967 by Kaufmann and Theophile (aka Ravens)[1], who interpreted the effects of stretch on the spontaneous and ectopic automaticity of atrial and ventricular tissue as a manifestation of '*Mechano-elektrische Rückkoppelung*', or MEF. The original feedback concept has served to develop a rationale basis for clinically observed effects of cardiac mechanical stimulation on heart rate and rhythm[2]. As early as 1763, Akenside gave an account of heart rhythm disturbance after a chest impact[3]. His case report involved severe tissue trauma, however, and it was not until 1882 that Riedinger and colleagues highlighted that chest impacts may also induce arrhythmias in the absence of structural damage – a setting termed *Commotio cordis*[4]. In 1915, Bainbridge reported his famous observation of a mechanically induced increase in cardiac beating rate[5], and 5 years later Schott described 'precordial percussion' as an effective means of keeping Stokes-Adams sufferers conscious during periods of complete atrio-ventricular block[6].

The molecular mechanism linking mechanical and electrical activity fits well with stretch-activated ion channels[7], whose pharmacological block was found to be sufficient to terminate mechanically promoted atrial fibrillation[8] as well as ventricular rhythm disturbances[9]. In fact, the majority of acute mechanically induced changes in cardiac electrophysiology can be reproduced, in quantitative computer models, simply by including trans-sarcolemmal stretch-activated ion channels[10]. However, there are many additional coupling mechanisms and modulators, at microscopic and macroscopic levels. These involve changes in calcium handling, auto- and paracrine messenger cascades, homo- and heterotypic cell interactions, as well as spatial and temporal variations in wall stress.

This finds a reflection in the present edition of the book, which has grown in scope and content to reflect the dynamic development this area of research has seen over the past half-decade. Chapters are arranged in nine sections that cover basic, translational and clinical insight into MEC, from pipette to patient. As in the first edition, chapters have been written by internationally established experts who collectively emphasize the multiplicity of signalling pathways and manifestations of MEC, and who identify future targets for research. These include the need to obtain prospective and controlled clinical data, to devise and apply better tools for the exploration of MEC in chronic pathologies, and to identify the physiological role of mechanisms underlying mechanically induced changes in electrical behaviour.

In spite of the above-mentioned complexity, there is universal agreement on two key messages: the heart is exquisitely mechano-sensitive, and this mechano-sensitivity is clinically relevant. We are indebted to our contributors for the insights provided and hope that this compilation will help in addressing identified challenges and bring into practice new approaches to therapy.

We would like to finish by expressing our gratitude to several individuals whose unfaltering effort has been crucial for this project. We are indebted to Naomi Wood (née Jordan) of the Oxford Cardiac Mechano-Electric Feedback Laboratory, for coordinating manuscript handling and review. We thank Marionne Cronin and Priya Sagayaraj for patience and determination through production and, last but not least, Helen Liepman and Susan Crowhurst of Oxford University Press for making it possible to publish this 2nd edition of *Cardiac Mechano-Electric Coupling and Arrhythmias* at 'the Press'.

Peter Kohl
Frederick Sachs
Michael R. Franz

References

1. Kaufmann R, Theophile U. Automatie-fördernde Dehnungseffekte an Purkinjefäden, Papillarmuskeln und Vorhoftrabekeln von Rhesus-Affen. *Pflüg Arch* 1967;**297**:174–189.
2. Kohl P, Hunter P, Noble D. Stretch-induced changes in heart rate and rhythm: clinical observations, experiments and mathematical models. *Prog Biophys Mol Biol* 1999;**71**:91–138.
3. Akenside M. An account of a blow upon the heart, and of its effects. *Phil Trans R Soc (Lond)*, 1763;**53**:353–355.
4. Riedinger F. Über Brusterschütterung. In: *Festschrift zur dritten Saecularfeier der Alma Julia Maximiliana Leipzig*. Verlag von F.C.W. Vogel, Leipzig, 1882, pp. 221–234.
5. Bainbridge FA. The influence of venous filling upon the rate of the heart. *J Physiol* 1915;**50**:65–84.

6. Schott E. Über Ventrikelstillstand (Adams-Stokes'sche Anfälle) nebst Bemerkungen über andersartige Arhythmien passagerer Natur. *Deutsch Arc Klin Med* 1920;**131**:211–229.

7. Sachs F, Sigurdson W, Ruknudin A, Bowman C. Single-channel mechanosensitive currents. *Science* 1991;**253**:800–801.

8. Bode F, Sachs F, Franz MR. Tarantula peptide inhibits atrial fibrillation. *Nature* 2001;**409**:35–36.

9. Hansen DE, Borganelli M, Stacy GP, Taylor LK. Dose-dependent inhibition of stretch-induced arrhythmias by gadolinium in isolated canine ventricles. Evidence for a unique mode of antiarrhythmic action. *Circ Res* 1991;**69**:820–831.

10. Kohl P, Bollensdorff C, Garny A. Mechano-sensitive ion channels in the heart: experimental and theoretical models. *Exp Physiol* 2006;**91**:307–321.

Contents

Contributors   *xvii*

List of abbreviations   *xxv*

BASIC SCIENCE, SECTION I
**Sub-cellular mechanisms
of cardiac mechano-electric
coupling**

1. **Evolutionary origins of stretch-
   activated ion channels**   *3*
   Boris Martinac and Anna Kloda

2. **Stretch-activated channels in the heart**   *11*
   Frederick Sachs

3. **The mechano-gated K$_{2P}$ channel TREK-1
   in the cardiovascular system**   *19*
   Eric Honoré and Amanda Patel

4. **Cell volume-sensitive ion channels and
   transporters in cardiac myocytes**   *27*
   Clive M. Baumgarten, Wu Deng and Frank J. Raucci, Jr

5. **Non-sarcolemmal stretch-
   activated channels**   *35*
   Gentaro Iribe and Peter Kohl

6. **Pacemaker, potassium, calcium, sodium:
   stretch modulation of the voltage-gated
   channels**   *42*
   Catherine E. Morris

7. **Role of caveolae in stretch-sensing:
   implications for mechano-electric coupling**   *50*
   Sarah Calaghan

8. **The membrane/cytoskeleton interface
   and stretch-activated channels**   *57*
   Thomas M. Suchyna and Frederick Sachs

9. **Cardiomyocyte stretch-sensing**   *66*
   Michiel Helmes and Henk Granzier

10. **The response of cardiac muscle
    to stretch: calcium and force**   *74*
    John Jeremy Rice and Donald M. Bers

11. **Stretch effects on second messengers**   *81*
    Jean-Luc Balligand and Chantal Dessy

12. **Functional implications of myocyte
    architecture**   *87*
    Kevin Kit Parker

BASIC SCIENCE, SECTION II
**Cellular manifestations of cardiac
mechano-electric coupling**

13. **Mechanical modulation of pacemaker
    electrophysiology**   *95*
    Patricia J. Cooper and Ursula Ravens

14. **Mechano-electric coupling in working
    cardiomyocytes: diastolic and
    systolic effects**   *103*
    Michael R. Franz

15. **Mechano-sensitivity of pulmonary
    vein cells: implications for atrial
    arrhythmogenesis**   *110*
    Chang Ahn Seol, Won Tae Kim, Jae Boum Youm,
    Yung E. Earm and Chae Hun Leem

16. **Heterogeneity of sarcomere length and function as a cause of arrhythmogenic calcium waves**   117
Henk E.D.J. ter Keurs, Ni Diao, Nathan P. Deis, Mei L. Zhang, Yoshinao Sugai, Guy Price, Yuji Wakayama, Yutaka Kagaya, Yoshinao Shinozaki, Penelope A. Boyden, Masahito Miura and Bruno D.M. Stuyvers

17. **Cellular mechanisms of arrhythmogenic cardiac alternans**   125
Kenneth R. Laurita

18. **Remodelling of gap junctions in ventricular myocardium, effects of cell-to-cell adhesion, mediators of hypertrophy and mechanical forces**   132
André G. Kléber and Jeffrey E. Saffitz

19. **The origin of fibroblasts, extracellular matrix and potential contributions to cardiac mechano-electric coupling**   138
Troy A. Baudino and Thomas K. Borg

20. **Advantages and pitfalls of cell cultures as model systems to study cardiac mechano-electric coupling**   143
Leslie Tung and Susan A. Thompson

BASIC SCIENCE, SECTION III
Multi-cellular manifestations of mechano-electric coupling

21. **Activation sequence of cardiac muscle in simplified experimental models: relevance for cardiac mechano-electric coupling**   153
Vladimir S. Markhasin, Alexander Balakin, Yuri Protsenko and Olga Solovyova

22. **Mechanical triggers and facilitators of ventricular tachy-arrhythmias**   160
T. Alexander Quinn and Peter Kohl

23. **Acute stretch effects on atrial electrophysiology**   168
Michael R. Franz and Frank Bode

24. **Stretch effects on potassium accumulation and alternans in pathological myocardium**   173
Christian Bollensdorff and Max J. Lab

25. **The effects of wall stretch on ventricular conduction and refractoriness in the whole heart**   180
Robert W. Mills, Adam T. Wright, Sanjiv M. Narayan and Andrew D. McCulloch

26. **Mechanical triggers of long-term ventricular electrical remodelling**   187
Darwin Jeyaraj and David S. Rosenbaum

27. **Mechanisms of mechanical pre- and postconditioning**   193
Asger Granfeldt, Rong Jiang, Weiwei Shi and Jakob Vinten-Johansen

TRANSLATIONAL SCIENCE, SECTION IV
Integrated model systems to study specific cases of cardiac MEC and arrhythmias

28. **Mechano-electric coupling in chronic atrial fibrillation**   203
Ulrich Schotten

29. **Mechanically induced pulmonary vein ectopy: insight from animal models**   212
Omer Berenfeld

30. **Regional variation in mechano-electric coupling: the right ventricle**   217
Ed White, David Benoist and Olivier Bernus

31. **Mechanical induction of arrhythmia in the *ex situ* heart: insight into *Commotio cordis***   223
Frank Bode and Michael R. Franz

32. **Arrhythmias in murine models of the mechanically impaired heart**   227
Larissa Fabritz and Paulus Kirchhof

33. **Studying cardiac mechano-sensitivity in man**   234
Flavia Ravelli and Michela Masè

34. **Mathematical models of cardiac structure and function: mechanistic insights from models of heart failure**   241
Vicky Y. Wang, Martyn P. Nash, Ian J. LeGrice, Alistair A. Young, Bruce H. Smaill and Peter J. Hunter

35. **Mathematical models of human atrial mechano-electrical coupling and arrhythmias**   251
Elizabeth M. Cherry

36. **Mathematical models of ventricular mechano-electric coupling and arrhythmia**   258
Natalia A. Trayanova, Viatcheslav Gurev, Jason Constantino and Yuxuan Hu

CLINICAL RELEVANCE, SECTION V
**Pathophysiology of cardiac
mechano-electric coupling:
general aspects**

37. **Load dependence of ventricular
    repolarization**   269
    Peter Taggart and Peter Sutton

38. **Is the U wave in the electrocardiogram a
    mechano-electrical phenomenon?**   274
    Rainer Schimpf and Martin Borggrefe

39. **Mechanical modulation of cardiac
    function: role of the pericardium**   281
    John V. Tyberg

40. **Mechanically induced electrical
    remodelling in human atrium**   290
    Geoffrey Lee, Prashanthan Sanders, Joseph
    B. Morton and Jonathan M. Kalman

41. **Drug effects and atrial fibrillation:
    potential and limitations**   298
    Jurren M. van Opstal, Yuri Blaauw and
    Harry J. G.M. Crijns

42. **Stretch as a mechanism linking short-
    and long-term electrical remodelling
    in the ventricles**   305
    Eugene A. Sosunov, Evgeny P. Anyukhovsky
    and Michael R. Rosen

43. **Volume and pressure overload and
    ventricular arrhythmogenesis**   313
    Michiel J. Janse and Ruben Coronel

44. **Stretch effects on fibrillation dynamics**   318
    Masatoshi Yamazaki and Jèrôme Kalifa

CLINICAL RELEVANCE, SECTION VI
**Pathophysiology of cardiac mechano-
electric coupling: specific cases**

45. ***Commotio Cordis*: sudden death from
    blows to the chest wall**   325
    Mark S. Link

46. **Repolarization changes in the
    synchronously and dyssynchronously
    contracting failing heart**   330
    Takeshi Aiba and Gordon F. Tomaselli

47. **Ventricular arrhythmias in heart
    failure: link to haemodynamic load**   340
    Steven N. Singh and Pamela Karasik

48. **Mechanical heterogeneity and after
    contractions as trigger for
    Torsades de Pointes**   345
    Annerie M.E. Moers and Paul G.A. Volders

49. **Stretch-induced arrhythmias
    in ischaemia**   352
    Ruben Coronel, Natalia A. Trayanova,
    Xiao Jie and Michael J. Janse

CLINICAL RELEVANCE, SECTION VII
**Mechano-electric coupling
as a mechanism involved in
therapeutic interventions**

50. **Anti-arrhythmic effects of acute
    mechanical stimulation**   361
    Tommaso Pellis and Peter Kohl

51. **Termination of arrhythmias by
    haemodynamic unloading**   369
    Peter Taggart and Peter Sutton

52. **Mechanical modulation of defibrillation
    and resuscitation efficacy**   374
    Derek J. Dosdall, Harish Doppalapudi
    and Raymond E. Ideker

53. **Anti- and proarrhythmic effects of
    cardiac assist device implantation**   381
    Paul J. Joudrey, Roger J. Hajjar and Fadi G. Akar

54. **Anti- and proarrhythmic effects of
    cardiac resynchronisation therapy**   387
    Nico H.L. Kuijpers and Frits W. Prinzen

CLINICAL RELEVANCE, SECTION VIII
**Evidence for mechano-electric
coupling from clinical trials**

55. **Evidence for mechano-electric coupling
    from clinical trials on AF**   395
    Matthias Hammwöhner and Andreas Goette

56. **Evidence for mechano-electric coupling
    from clinical trials on heart failure**   402
    Paulus Kirchhof and Günter Breithardt

57. **Mechano-electric coupling and the
    pathogenesis of arrhythmogenic right
    ventricular cardiomyopathy**   407
    Hayden Huang, Angeliki Asimaki, Frank
    Marcus and Jeffrey E. Saffitz

58. **Evidence for mechano-electric coupling from clinical trials on cardiac resynchronisation therapy** 412
Nico R.L. Van de Veire and Jeroen J. Bax

59. **Mechano-electric coupling in patients treated with ventricular assist devices: insights from individual cases and clinical trials** 420
Cesare M. Terracciano, Michael Ibrahim, Manoraj Navaratnarajah and Magdi H. Yacoub

OUTLOOK, SECTION IX
Novel directions in cardiac mechano-electric coupling

60. **Measuring strain of structural proteins *in vivo* in real time** 431
Fanjie Meng and Frederick Sachs

61. **Roles of cardiac SAC beyond mechano-electric coupling: stretch-enhanced force generation and muscular dystrophy** 435
David G. Allen and Marie L. Ward

62. **Distributions of myocyte stress, strain and work in normal and infarcted ventricles** 442
Elliot J. Howard and Jeffrey H. Omens

63. **Evolving concepts in measuring ventricular strain in canine and human hearts: non-invasive imaging** 450
Elisa E. Konofagou and Jean Provost

64. **Evolving concepts in measuring ventricular strain in the human heart: impedance measurements** 456
Douglas A. Hettrick

65. **Mechano-sensitive channel blockers: a new class of antiarrhythmic drugs?** 462
Ed White

Index 469

Contributors

Takeshi Aiba, MD, PhD, Chief, Division of Arrhythmia and Electrophysiology, National Cerebral and Cardiovascular Center, Department of Cardiovascular Medicine, 5-7-1 Fujishirodai, Suita, Osaka, 565-8565, Japan
Chapter 46

Fadi G. Akar, PhD, Associate Professor of Medicine, Mount Sinai School of Medicine, Akar Laboratory, Atran Berg Laboratory Building Floor 5th, Floor Room 510, 1428 Madison Ave., New York, NY 10029, USA
Chapter 53

David G. Allen, MBBS, PhD, FAA, Professor of Physiology, University of Sydney, School of Medical Sciences F13, Fisher Road, Sydney, NSW 2006, Australia
Chapter 61

Evgeny P. Anyukhovsky, PhD, Research Scientist, Columbia University. Department of Pharmacology, 630 West 168 St., PH 7W-318, New York, NY 10032, USA
Chapter 42

Angeliki Asimaki, PhD, Research Associate/Harvard Medical School Instructor, Beth Israel Deaconess Medical Center, Department of Pathology, 330 Brookline Ave., Boston, MA 02215, USA
Chapter 57

Alexander Balakin, PhD, Researcher, Ural Branch of the Russian Academy of Sciences, Institute of Immunology and Physiology, Pervomayskaya Str., Bld. 106, Yekaterinburg, 6200049, Russia
Chapter 21

Jean-Luc Balligand, MD, PhD, FESC, FAHA, Chair of Medicine and Pharmacology, Université catholique de Louvain, Institut de Recherche Expérimentale et Clinique, FATH 5349, 52 Ave. E. Mounier, Brussels, 1200, Belgium
Chapter 11

Troy A. Baudino, PhD, Associate Professor, Texas A and M University, Department of Medicine, Division of Molecular Cardiology, Cardiovascular Research Institute, 1901 S. First St., Bldg. 205, Temple, TX 76504, USA
Chapter 19

Clive M. Baumgarten, PhD, FAHA, Professor of Physiology & Biophysics, Medical College of Virginia, Virginia Commonwealth University, Department of Physiology & Biophysics, 1101 E. Marshall, Richmond, VA 23298, USA
Chapter 4

Jeroen J. Bax, MD, PhD, FESC, Professor of Cardiology, Leiden University Medical Center, Department of Cardiology, Albinusdreef 2, PO Box 9600, Leiden, RC 2300, the Netherlands
Chapter 58

David Benoist, MSc, Emma and Leslie Reid endowed PhD student, University of Leeds, Institute of Membrane and Systems Biology, Garstang Building, Woodhouse Lane, Leeds, LS2 9JT, United Kingdom
Chapter 30

Omer Berenfeld, PhD, Assistant Professor of Internal Medicine, Center for Arrhythmia Research, Internal Medicine, 5025 Venture Drive, Ann Arbor, MI 48108, USA
Chapter 29

Olivier Bernus, PhD, Tenure Track Independent Research Fellow, University of Leeds Institute of Membrane and Systems Biology, Garstang Building, Woodhouse Lane, Leeds, LS2 9JT, United Kingdom
Chapter 30

Donald M. Bers, PhD, Professor and Chair, University of California, Department of Pharmacology, Genome Building, Room 3513, Davis, *CA* 95616, USA
Chapter 10

Yuri Blaauw, MD, PhD, Cardiologist, Maastricht University Medical Centre, Cardiovascular Research Institute Maastricht, Cardiology, PO Box 5800, Maastricht, AZ 6202, the Netherlands
Chapter 41

Frank Bode, MD, Head of Cardiac Electrophysiology, Universitätsklinikum Schleswig Holstein, Campus Lübeck, Medizinische Klinik II, Ratzeburger Allee 160, Lübeck, 23538, Germany
Chapters 23 and 31

Christian Bollensdorff, PhD, Senior Research Fellow, University of Oxford, Cardiac Mechano-Electric Feedback Lab, Sherrington Building, South Parks Road, Oxford, OX1 3QX, United Kingdom
Chapter 24

Thomas K. Borg, PhD, Professor, Medical University of South Carolina, Department of Regenerative Medicine and Cell Biology, 173 Ashley Ave., Suite 601, Charleston, SC 29425, USA
Chapter 19

Martin Borggrefe, MD, PhD, FESC, Head of Cardiology, Angiology, Pneumology, Intensive Care, Universitätsmedizin Mannheim, 1st Department of Medicine-Cardiology, Theodor-Kutzer-Ufer 1-3, Mannheim, 68167, Germany
Chapter 38

Penelope A. Boyden, PhD, Professor of Pharmacology, Columbia University, Centre for Molecular Therapeutics, 630 West 168th St., New York, NY 10032, USA
Chapter 16

Günter Breithardt, MD, FESC, FACC, FHRS, Professor (emer.) of Medicine and Cardiology, Hospital of the University of Münster, Department of Cardiology and Angiology, Von-Esmarch-Str. 117, Münster, 48149, Germany
Chapter 56

Sarah Calaghan, PhD, University Research Fellow, University of Leeds, Institute of Membrane and Systems Biology, Garstang Building, Woodhouse Lane, Leeds, LS2 9JT, United Kingdom
Chapter 7

Elizabeth M. Cherry, PhD, Assistant Professor, Rochester Institute of Technology, School of Mathematical Sciences, 85 Lomb Memorial Drive, Rochester, New York, NY 14623, USA
Chapter 35

Jason Constantino, BS, PhD Student, Johns Hopkins University, Department of Biomedical Engineering and Institute for Computational Medicine, 3400 N. Charles St., Hackerman Hall 218, Baltimore, MD 21218, USA
Chapter 36

Patricia J. Cooper, DPhil (Oxon), Post-doctoral Fellow, University of Auckland, Department of Physiology, 85 Parks Road, Grafton, Auckland, 1023, New Zealand
Chapter 13

Ruben Coronel, MD, PhD, Associate Professor, Academic Medical Centre, Laboratory of Experimental Cardiology, Meibergdreef 9, Amsterdam, AZ 1105, the Netherlands
Chapters 43 and 49

Harry J.G.M. Crijns, MD, PhD, Professor and Chairman of the Department of Cardiology, Maastricht University Medical Centre, Cardiovascular Research Institute Maastricht, Cardiology, PO Box 5800, Maastricht, AZ 6202, the Netherlands
Chapter 41

Nathan P. Deis, MSc, MD, Neurosurgery Resident, University of Alberta, Department of Surgery, 8440 - 112 St., Edmonton, Alberta, T6G 2B7, Canada
Chapter 16

Wu Deng, MD, PhD, Postdoctoral Fellow, Medical College of Virginia, Virginia Commonwealth University, Department of Physiology & Biophysics, 1101 E. Marshall, Richmond, VA 23298, USA
Chapter 4

Chantal Dessy, PhD, Associate Professor, Université catholique de Louvain, Institut de Recherche Expérimentale et Clinique, FATH 5349, 52 Ave. E. Mounier, Brussels, 1200, Belgium
Chapter 11

Ni Diao, MSc, Research Associate, Fudan University, Institute of Biomedical Sciences, 138 Yixueyuan Road, Shanghai, 200032, China
Chapter 16

Harish Doppalapudi, MD, Assistant Professor, University of Alabama, Department of Medicine, Division of Cardiovascular Disease, 2000 6th Ave. South, Birmingham, AL 35233, USA
Chapter 52

Derek J. Dosdall, PhD, FRHS, Assistant Professor, University of Utah, Department of Internal Medicine, Division of Cardiology, 675 Arapeen Drive, Salt Lake City, UT 84108, USA
Chapter 52

Yung E. Earm, MD, PhD, Professor Emeritus, Seoul National University Medical College, Department of Physiology, 28 Yeongeon-dong Jongno-gu, Seoul, 110-799, Republic of Korea
Chapter 15

Larissa Fabritz, MD, Principal Investigator, Hospital of the University of Münster, Department of Cardiology and Angiology, Von-Esmarch-Str. 117, Münster, 48149, Germany
Chapter 32

Michael R. Franz, MD, PhD, FHRS, Director, Cardiac Arrhythmias and Myocardial Research, Georgetown University and VA Medical Center, Division of Cardiology, Veteran Affairs Medical Center, 50 Irving St, NW, Washington, DC 20422, USA
Chapters 14, 23, and 31

Andreas Goette, MD, Senior Cardiologist, Otto-von-Guericke-University Hospital Magdeburg, Division of Cardiology, Leipziger Str. 44, Magdeburg, 39120, Germany
Chapter 55

Asger Granfeldt, MD, MD/PhD Trainee, Arhus University Hospital, Department of Anesthesiology, Nørrebrogade 44 Building 1C 1st. Floor, Aarhus, 8000, Denmark
Chapter 27

Henk Granzier, PhD, Professor of Molecular & Cellular Biology, University of Arizona, Molecular Cardiovascular Research Program, Medical Research Building, 1656 East Mabel St., Tucson, AZ 85719, USA
Chapter 9

Viatcheslav Gurev, PhD, Associate Research Scientist, Johns Hopkins University, Institute for Computational Medicine, 3400 N. Charles St., Hackerman Hall 218, Baltimore, MD 21218, USA
Chapter 36

Roger J. Hajjar, MD, Professor of Medicine, Mount Sinai School of Medicine, Wiener Family Cardiovascular Research Laboratories, Atran Berg Laboratory Building Floor 05, Room 08, 1428 Madison Ave., New York, NY 10029, USA
Chapter 53

Matthias Hammwöhner, MD, Staff Cardiologist, Otto-von-Guericke-University Hospital Magdeburg, Division of Cardiology, Leipziger Str. 44, Magdeburg, 39120, Germany
Chapter 55

Michiel Helmes, PhD, Visiting Industry Scientist, University of Oxford, Department of Physiology, Anatomy & Genetics, Sherrington Building, Parks Road, Oxford, OX1 3PT, United Kingdom
Chapter 9

Douglas A. Hettrick, PhD, Program Director, Medtronic, Inc., 710 Medtronic Pkwy, Minneapolis, MN 55432, USA
Chapter 64

Eric Honoré, PhD, Director of Research, CNRS, Institut de Pharmacologie Moléculaire et Cellulaire, 660, route des Lucioles, Sophia Antipolis, Valbonne, 06560, France
Chapter 3

Elliot J. Howard, MS, Graduate Student Researcher, University of California, San Diego, Department of Bioengineering, 9500 Gilman Drive, La Jolla, CA 92093, USA
Chapter 62

Yuxuan Hu, MS, PhD Student, Johns Hopkins University, Department of Biomedical Engineering and Institute for Computational Medicine, 3400 N. Charles St., Hackerman Hall 219, Baltimore, MD 21218, USA
Chapter 36

Hayden Huang, PhD, Assistant Professor of Biomedical Engineering, Columbia University, Department of Biomedical Engineering, 510 S.W. Mudd Building, 500 W. 120th St., New York, NY 10027, USA
Chapter 57

Peter J. Hunter, DPhil (Oxon), ME, FRSNZ, FRS, University Distinguished Professor, University of Auckland, Auckland Bioengineering Institute, Department of Physiology and Department of Anatomy with Radiology, 70 Symonds St., Auckland 1010, New Zealand
Chapter 34

Michael Ibrahim, MD, MB-PhD Track, Imperial College London, Heart Science Centre, Harefield, Middlesex, UB9 6JH, United Kingdom
Chapter 59

Raymond E. Ideker, MD, PHD, Professor, University of Alabama, Department of Medicine, Division of Cardiovascular Disease, 1530 3rd Ave. South, Birmingham, AL 35294, USA
Chapter 52

Gentaro Iribe, MD, PhD, FESC, Assistant Professor of Cardiovascular Physiology, Okayama University, Graduate School of Medicine, Dentistry and Pharmaceutical Sciences, 2-5-1, Shikata-cho, Kita-ku, Okayama, 700-8558, Japan
Chapter 5

Michiel J. Janse, MD, PhD, EFESC, FRCP, Emeritus Professor of Experimental Cardiology, Academic Medical Centre, Laboratory of Experimental Cardiology, Heart Failure Centre, Meibergdreef 9, Amsterdam, AZ 1105, the Netherlands
Chapters 43 and 49

Darwin Jeyaraj, MD, MRCP, Assistant Professor, Case Western Reserve University, The Heart and Vascular Research Center, and The Department of Biomedical Engineering, MetroHealth Campus, 10900 Euclid Ave., Cleveland, Ohio 44106, USA
Chapter 26

Rong Jiang, MD, PhD, Instructor, Emory University School of Medicine, Cardiothoracic Surgery (Research), Carlyle Fraser Heart Center, 550 Peachtree St. NE, Atlanta, GA 30308, USA
Chapter 27

Xiao Jie, PhD, Research Assistant, Oxford University, Computational Biology Group, Oxford University Computing Laboratory, Parks Road, Oxford, OX1 3QD, United Kingdom
Chapter 49

Paul J. Joudrey, MS, Research Associate, Mount Sinai School of Medicine, Cardiovascular Research Center, Division of Cardiology, 1 Gustave L. Levy Place, New York, NY 10029, USA
Chapter 53

Yutaka Kagaya, MD, PhD, Vice Director and Professor, Tohoku University, Graduate Medical Education Centre, 1-1 Seiryocho, Aoba-Ku, Sendai, 980-8574, Japan
Chapter 16

Jérôme Kalifa, MD, PhD, Assistant Professor, University of Michigan, Center for Arrhythmia Research, 5025 Venture Drive, Ann Arbor, MI 48108, USA
Chapter 44

Jonathan M. Kalman, MBBS, PhD, FACC, Director of Cardiac Electrophysiology, Royal Melbourne Hospital, Melbourne Heart Centre, Grattan St., Parkville, Melbourne, Victoria, VIC 3050, Australia
Chapter 40

Pamela Karasik, MD, Director, Washington DC Veterans Affairs Medical Center, Electrophysiology Lab, 50 Irving St. Northwest, Washington, DC 20010, USA
Chapter 47

Henk E.D.J. ter Keurs, MD, PhD, FRCPC, Professor, University of Calgary, Department of Cardiac Sciences, Faculty of Medicine, 3280 Hospital Drive, N.W. Calgary, Alberta, T2N 4Z6, Canada
Chapter 16

Won Tae Kim, BSc, University of Ulsan College of Medicine & Asan Medical Center, Department of Physiology, 388-1 Poongnap-Dong Songpa-Ku, Seoul, 138-736, Republic of Korea
Chapter 15

Paulus Kirchhof, Dr. med., Professor and Attending Physician, University Hospital Münster, Department of Cardiology and Angiology, Albert-Schweitzer-Str. 33, Münster, 48149, Germany
Chapters 32, 56

André G. Kléber, MD, FAHA, Visiting Professor of Pathology, Harvard Medical School, Beth Israel Deaconess Medical Center, Department of Pathology, 330 Brookline Ave., Boston, MA 02215, USA
Chapter 18

Anna Kloda, BSc, MSc, PhD, Australian Research Fellow, University of Queensland, School of Biomedical Sciences, Upland Road, St Lucia, Brisbane, 4067, Australia
Chapter 1

Peter Kohl, MD, PhD, FHRS, Professor and Chair of Cardiac Biophysics and Systems Biology, Imperial College London, National Heart and Lung Institute, Heart Science Centre, Harefield, Middlesex, UB9 6JH, United Kingdom
Chapters 5, 22, and 50

Elisa E. Konofagou, PhD, Associate Professor of Biomedical Engineering and Radiology, Columbia University, Department of Biomedical Engineering, 510 S.W. Mudd Building, 500 W. 120th St., New York, NY 10027, USA
Chapter 63

Nico H.L. Kuijpers, PhD, Assistant Professor, University of Maastricht, Department of Biomedical Engineering, Universiteitssingel 50, 6229 ER Maastricht, the Netherlands
Chapter 54

Max J. Lab, MD, PhD, Professor Emeritus & Senior Research Investigator, Imperial College London, National Heart & Lung Institute, Dovehouse St., London, SW3 6LY, United Kingdom
Chapter 24

Kenneth R. Laurita, PhD, Associate Professor, Case Western Reserve University, Heart and Vascular Research Center, MetroHealth Medical Center, 2500 MetroHealth Drive, Cleveland, OH 44109, USA
Chapter 17

Geoffrey Lee, MBCHB, FRACP, Cardiologist, The Royal Melbourne Hospital, Melbourne Heart Centre, Grattan St., Parkville, Melbourne, Victoria, 3050, Australia
Chapter 40

Chae Hun Leem, MD, PhD, Professor, University of Ulsan College of Medicine & Asan Medical Center, Department of Physiology, 388-1 Poongnap-Dong Songpa-Ku, Seoul, 138-736, Republic of Korea
Chapter 15

Ian J. LeGrice, BE, MBChB, PhD, DipTP, Associate Professor, Auckland Bioengineering Institute, Department of Physiology and Department of Anatomy with Radiology, University of Auckland, 70 Symonds St., Auckland 1010, New Zealand
Chapter 34

Mark S. Link, MD, FACC, FHRS, Professor of Medicine, Tufts Medical Center, Cardiac Arrhythmia Center, 800 Washington St., Tufts Medical Center Box #197, Boston, MA 02111, USA
Chapter 45

Frank Marcus, MD, Distinguished Professor of Medicine; Director of Arrhythmia Services at University Medical Center, University of Arizona, Department of Medicine, 1501 N. Campbell Ave., Tucson, AZ 85724, USA
Chapter 57

Vladimír S. Markhasin, Dr. Sci., Corr. Member of RAS, Professor and Principal Researcher, Ural Branch of the Russian Academy of Sciences, Institute of Immunology and Physiology, Mathematical Physiology, Pervomayskaya Str., Bld. 106, Yekaterinburg, 6200049, Russia
Chapter 21

Boris Martinac, BSc, PhD, Australian Professorial Fellow, Head of Laboratory, Victor Chang Cardiac Research Institute, Mechanosensory Biophysics Laboratory/Molecular Cardiology and Biophysics Division, Lowy Packer Building, 405 Liverpool St, Darlinghurst, Sydney, NSW 2010, Australia
Chapter 1

Michela Masè, PhD, Post-doctoral Fellow, University of Trento, Department of Physics, Laboratory of Biophysics and Biosignals, Via Sommarive 14, Povo (Trento), 38123, Italy
Chapter 33

Andrew D. McCulloch, PhD, Professor of Bioengineering and Medicine, University of California, San Diego, Department of Bioengineering, Cardiac Biomedical Science and Engineering Center, 9500 Gilman Drive, La Jolla, CA 92093, USA
Chapter 25

Fanjie Meng, PhD, Research Associate, SUNY Buffalo, Center for Single Molecule Biophysics, Physiology and Biophysics, 301 Cary Hall, 3435 Main St., Buffalo, NY 14214, USA
Chapter 60

Robert W. Mills, PhD, Research Fellow, Harvard University, School of Medicine, Cardiovascular Research Center, Massachusetts General Hospital, 149 13th St, Charlestown, MA 02129, USA
Chapter 25

Masahito Miura, MD, Associate Professor, Tohoku University, Graduate Medical Education Centre, 1-1 Seiryocho, Aoba-Ku, Sendai, 980-8574, Japan
Chapter 16

Annerie M.E. Moers, MD, PhD student, Maastricht University, Cardiovascular Research Institute Maastricht, Cardiology, PO Box 616, Maastricht, MD 6200, the Netherlands
Chapter 48

Catherine E. Morris, PhD, Senior Scientist, Ottawa Hospital Research Institute, Neuroscience, 451 Smyth Rd, Ottawa, Onatrio, K0J 1G0, Canada
Chapter 6

Joseph B. Morton, MBBS, Honorary Senior Fellow, Faculty of Medicine, Dentistry and Health Sciences Research, Cardiology Unit, The University of Melbourne, Parkville, Melbourne, Victoria, 3050, Australia
Chapter 40

Sanjiv M. Narayan, MD, FHRS, FRCP, Associate Professor of Medicine in Residence, UCSD School of Medicine, VA Medical Center, Division of Cardiology, 3350 La Jolla Village Drive, San Diego, CA 92161, USA
Chapter 25

Martyn P. Nash, BE, PhD, Associate Professor, University of Auckland, Auckland Bioengineering Institute, Department of Physiology and Department of Anatomy with Radiology, 70 Symonds St., Auckland, 1010, New Zealand
Chapter 34

Manoraj Navaratnarajah, MBBCh, MRCS, BSc, Cardiothoracic Surgery, Harefield Hospital, Heart Science Centre, Harefield, Middlesex, UB9 6JH, United Kingdom
Chapter 59

Jeffrey H. Omens, PhD, Professor of Medicine, University of California, San Diego, Department of Medicine, 9500 Gilman Drive, La Jolla, CA 92093, USA
Chapter 62

Jurren M. van Opstal, MD, PhD, Cardiologist, Cardiovascular Research Institute Maastricht, Maastricht University Medical Centre, Cardiology, PO Box 5800, Maastricht, AZ 6202, the Netherlands
Chapter 41

Kevin Kit Parker, PhD, Associate Professor of Biomedical Engineering, Harvard University, School of Engineering and Applied Sciences, 29 Oxford St., Cambridge, MA 02138, USA
Chapter 12

Amanda Patel, PhD, Researcher, CNRS, Institut de Pharmacologie Moléculaire et Cellulaire, 660, route des Lucioles, Sophia Antipolis, Valbonne, 06560, France
Chapter 3

Tommaso Pellis, MD, Consultant in Anaesthesia, A.O. Santa Maria degli Angeli Hospital, Anaesthesia, Intensive Care and Emergency Medical Service, Via Montereale 24, Porednone, 33170, Italy
Chapter 50

Guy Price, MD, PhD, Research Associate, University of Calgary, Department of Cardiac Sciences, Faculty of Medicine, 3280 Hospital Drive, N.W. Calgary, Alberta, T2N 4Z6, Canada
Chapter 16

Frits W. Prinzen, PhD, Professor of Physiology, Maastricht University, Department of Physiology, Universiteitssingel 50, Maastricht, ER 6229, the Netherlands
Chapter 54

Yuri Protsenko, Dr. Sci., Principal Researcher, Ural Branch of the Russian Academy of Sciences, Institute of Immunology and Physiology, Biological Motility, Pervomayskaya Str., Bld. 106, Yekaterinburg, 6200049, Russia
Chapter 21

Jean Provost, MS, Research Scientist, Columbia University, Department of Biomedical Engineering, 1210 Amsterdam Ave., New York, NY 10027, USA
Chapter 63

T. Alexander Quinn, PhD, EPSRC Postdoctoral Research Fellow, Imperial College London, National Heart and Lung Institute, Heart Science Centre, Harefield, Middlesex, UB9 6JH, United Kingdom
Chapter 22

Frank J. Raucci, Jr., MS, MD/PhD Program Student, Virginia Commonwealth University, Medical College of Virginia, Department of Physiology & Biophysics, 1101 E. Marshall, Richmond, VA, 23298, USA
Chapter 4

Flavia Ravelli, PhD, Senior Research Scientist, University of Trento, Department of Physics, Laboratory of Biophysics and Biosignals, Via Sommarive 14, Povo (Trento), 38123, Italy
Chapter 33

Ursula Ravens, MD, Dr. h.c., FESC, FAHA, Professor and Chair of the Department of Pharmacology and Toxicology, Dresden University of Technology, Medical Faculty Carl-Gustav Carus, Fetscher Str. 74, Dresden, 01307, Germany
Chapter 13

John Jeremy Rice, PhD, Research Staff Member, IBM Research, T.J. Watson Research Centre, Functional Genomics and Systems Biology Group, 1101 Kitchawan Road, Route 134, Yorktown Heights, New York, NY 10598, USA
Chapter 10

Michael R. Rosen, MD, FAHA, FHRS, Gustavus A. Pfeiffer Professor of Pharmacology, Professor of Pediatrics, Director, Columbia University, Center for Molecular Therapeutics, 630 West 168 St., PH 7W-321, New York, NY 10032, USA
Chapter 42

David S. Rosenbaum, MD, Director, Case Western Reserve University, The Heart and Vascular Research Center, and The Department of Biomedical Engineering, MetroHealth Campus, 2500 MetroHealth Drive, Hamman 3, Cleveland, OH 44109, USA
Chapter 26

Frederick Sachs, PhD, SUNY Distinguished Professor of Physiology and Biophysics, SUNY Buffalo, Physiology and Biophysics, 301 Cary Hall, Buffalo, NY 14214, USA
Chapters 2, 8, and 60

Jeffrey E. Saffitz, MD, PhD, Mallinckrodt Professor of Pathology, Harvard Medical School, Chairman, Department of Pathology, Beth Israel Deaconess Medical Center, 330 Brookline Ave., Boston, MA 02215, USA
Chapters 18 and 57

Prashanthan Sanders, PhD, FRACP, FCSANZ, FESC, Knapman - NHF Chair of Cardiology Research, University of Adelaide, Cardiovascular Centre, 52 Sydenham Rd., Norwood, Adelaide, SA 5067, Australia
Chapter 40

Rainer Schimpf, MD, PhD, Chair of Arrhythmia Clinic, Universitätsmedizin Mannheim, 1st Department of Medicine-Cardiology, Theodor-Kutzer-Ufer 1-3, Mannheim, 68167, Germany
Chapter 38

Ulrich Schotten, MD, PhD, Chair of Cardiac Electrophysiology, Maastricht University, Department of Physiology, Universiteitssingel 50, PO Box 616, Maastricht, ER 6229, the Netherlands
Chapter 28

Chang Ahn Seol, MD, BSc, University of Ulsan College of Medicine & Asan Medical Center, Department of Physiology, 388-1 Poongnap-Dong Songpa-Ku, Seoul,138-736, Republic of Korea
Chapter 15

Weiwei Shi, MD, PhD, Postdoctoral Fellow, Emory University School of Medicine, Cardiothoracic Surgery (Research), Carlyle Fraser Heart Center, 550 Peachtree St. NE, Atlanta, GA 30308, USA
Chapter 27

Yoshinao Shinozaki, MD, Research Associate, University of Calgary, Department of Cardiac Sciences, Faculty of Medicine, 3280 Hospital Drive, N.W. Calgary, Alberta, T2N 4Z6, Canada
Chapter 16

Steven N. Singh, MD, Internal Medicine Physician, Georgetown University and VA Medical Center, Division of Cardiology, Veteran Affairs Medical Center, 50 Irving St., NW, Washington, DC 20422, USA
Chapter 47

Bruce H. Smaill, PhD, Deputy Director, University of Auckland, Auckland Bioengineering Institute, Department of Physiology and Department of Anatomy with Radiology, 70 Symonds St., Auckland, 1010, New Zealand
Chapter 34

Olga Solovyova, Dr. Sci., Professor and Head of Laboratory, Ural Branch of the Russian Academy of Sciences, Institute of Immunology and Physiology, Mathematical Physiology, Pervomayskaya Str., Bld. 106, Yekaterinburg, 6200049, Russia
Chapter 21

Eugene A. Sosunov, PhD, Research Scientist, Columbia University, Department of Pharmacology, 630 West 168 St., PH 7W-318, New York, NY 10032, USA
Chapter 42

Bruno D.M. Stuyvers, PhD, Associate Professor - Biomedical Sciences, Memorial University, Division of Biomedical Sciences, Faculty of Medicine, 300 Prince Phillip Dr, St. John's, Newfoundland and Labrador, A1B 3V6, Canada
Chapter 16

Thomas M. Suchyna, PhD, Assistant Research Professor, SUNY Buffalo, Physiology and Biophysics, 301 Cary Hall, Buffalo, NY 14214, USA
Chapter 8

Yoshinao Sugai, MD, PhD, Principal Investigator, Hiraka General Hospital, 1-30 Ekimae-cho, Yokote, Akita, 013-8610, Japan
Chapter 16

Peter Sutton, PhD, Senior Lecturer and Assistant Director, University College London Medical School, The Hatter Institute and Centre for Cardiology, Grafton Way, London, WC1E 6DB, United Kingdom
Chapters 37 and 51

Peter Taggart, MD, DSc, FRCP, Professor of Cardiac Electrophysiology, University College London, Department of Medicine, The Heart Hospital, 16-18 Westmoreland St., London, W1G 8PH, United Kingdom
Chapters 37 and 51

Cesare Terracciano, PhD, Head of the Laboratory of Cellular Electrophysiology, Imperial College London, Heart Science Centre, Harefield, Middlesex, UB9 6JH, United Kingdom
Chapter 59

Susan A. Thompson, BS, Graduate student, Johns Hopkins University, Biomedical Engineering, 703 Traylor Building, 720 Rutland Ave., Baltimore, MD 21122, USA
Chapter 20

Gordon F. Tomaselli, MD, FAHA, FACC, FHRS, Chief, Johns Hopkins University, Division of Cardiology, School of Medicine, 720 North Rutland Ave., Baltimore, MD 21205, USA
Chapter 46

Natalia A. Trayanova, PhD, FHRS, FAHA, Professor, Johns Hopkins University, Department of Biomedical Engineering and Institute for Computational Medicine, 3400 N. Charles St., Hackerman Hall 216, Baltimore, MD 21218, USA
Chapters 36 and 49

Leslie Tung, PhD, Professor of Biomedical Engineering, The Johns Hopkins University, Cardiac Bioelectric Systems Laboratory, 720 North Rutland Ave., Baltimore, MD 21205, USA
Chapter 20

John V. Tyberg, MD, PhD, FACC, Professor of Cardiac Sciences and Physiology/Pharmacology, University of Calgary, Libin Cardiovascular Institute of Alberta, GAA 18, Health Research Innovation Centre, 3280 Hospital Drive N.W., Calgary, T2N 4Z6, Canada
Chapter 39

Nico R.L. Van de Veire, MD, PhD, FESC, Cardiologist, Leiden University Medical Center, Department of Cardiology, Albinusdreef 2, PO Box 9600, Leiden, RC 2300, the Netherlands
Chapter 58

Jakob Vinten-Johansen, MS, PhD, FAHA, FAPS, Professor, Emory University School of Medicine, Division of Cardiothoracic Surgery, Carlyle Fraser Heart Center, 550 Peachtree St. NE, Atlanta, GA 30308, USA
Chapter 27

Paul G.A. Volders, MD, PhD, FESC, Associate Professor, Cardiovascular Research Institute Maastricht, Maastricht University Medical Centre, Cardiology, PO Box 5800, Maastricht, AZ 6202, the Netherlands
Chapter 48

Yuji Wakayama, MD, Associate Professor, Tohoku University Graduate School of Medicine, 1-1 Seiryocho, Aoba-Ku, Sendai 980-8574, Japan
Chapter 16

Vicky Y. Wang, BE (Hons), Doctoral Candidate, Auckland Bioengineering Institute, Department of Physiology and Department of Anatomy with Radiology, University of Auckland, 70 Symonds St., Auckland 1010, New Zealand
Chapter 34

Ed White, PhD, Professor of Cardiac Physiology, University of Leeds, Institute of Membrane and Systems Biology, Woodhouse Lane, Leeds, LS2 9JT, United Kingdom
Chapters 30 and 65

Marie L. Ward, PhD, Senior Lecturer, University of Auckland, Department of Physiology, Faculty of Medical and Health Sciences, Private Bag 92019, Auckland, New Zealand
Chapter 61

Adam T. Wright, PhD, Post-doctoral Researcher, University of California, Department of Bioengineering, San Diego, 9500 Gilman Drive, La Jolla, CA 92093, USA
Chapter 25

Magdi H. Yacoub, MD, FRS, Professor of Cardiothoracic Surgery, Imperial College London, Heart Science Centre, Harefield, Middlesex, UB9 6JH, United Kingdom
Chapter 59

Masatoshi Yamazaki, MD, PhD, Research Fellow, University of Michigan, Center for Arrhythmia Research, 5025 Venture Drive, Ann Arbor, MI 48108, USA
Chapter 44

Jae Boum Youm, MD, PhD, Associate Professor, Inje University College of Medicine, Department of Physiology, 633-165 Gaegeum-Dong Busanjin-Gu, Busan, 614-735, Republic of Korea
Chapter 15

Alistair A. Young, PhD, Associate Professor, Auckland Bioengineering Institute, Department of Physiology and Department of Anatomy with Radiology, University of Auckland, 70 Symonds St., Auckland, 1010, New Zealand
Chapter 34

Mei L. Zhang, MD, PhD, Research Associate, University of Calgary, Dept. of Biomedical Engineering, 3380 Hospital Drive, N.W. Calgary, Alberta, T2N 4Z6, Canada
Chapter 16

List of abbreviations

$[ATP]_I$	adenosine triphosphate concentration
$[Ca^{2+}]_i$	intracellular (free) Ca^{2+} concentration
$[Ca^{2+}]_{MX}$	mitochondrial Ca^{2+} concentration
$[Ca^{2+}]_o$	extracellular Ca^{2+} concentration
$[Ca^{2+}]_{SR}$	Ca^{2+} concentration in the sarcoplasmic reticulum
$[Ca^{2+}]_{SS}$	sub-sarcolemmal Ca^{2+} concentration
$[K^+]_o$	extracellular potassium concentration
$[Na^+]_i$	intracellular Na^+ concentration
$[Na^+]_{SS}$	sub-sarcolemmal Na^+ concentration
1D	one-dimensional
2-APB	2-aminoethanoxydiphenyl borate
2D	two-dimensional
3D	three-dimensional
3T3	3-day transfer, inoculum 3×10^5 cells
9AC	9-anthracenecarboxylic acid
AA	arachidonic acid
ACE	angiotensin-converting enzyme
ACS	adrenocholinergic stimulation
ADONIS	American–Australian–African trial with DronedarONe In atrial fibrillation/flutter patients for the maintenance of Sinus rhythm
ADVANCE	Action in Diabetes and Vascular disease: preterAx and diamicroN-MR Controlled Evaluation
AERP	atrial effective refractory period
AF	atrial fibrillation
AFFIRM	Atrial Fibrillation Follow-up Investigation of Rhythm Management
AFL	atrial flutter
AFSS	average fractional shortening in the short-axis plane
AgTx	agkistrodon halys toxin
AHA	American Heart Association
AKAP	A-kinase anchoring protein
Akt	member of the serine/threonine-specific protein kinase family
ALS	advanced life support
ANDROMEDA	ANtiarrhythmic trial with DROnedarone in Moderate to severe heart failure Evaluating morbidity DecreAse
ANP	atrial natriuretic peptide
AoP	aortic pressure
AP	action potential
APD	action potential duration
$APD_{[number]}$	action potential duration at [number]% repolarization (e.g. APD_{90} = APD at 90% repolarization)
ARB	angiotensin receptor blocker
ARDA	atrial repolarization-delaying agents
ARI	activation recovery interval
ARP	absolute refractory period
ARVC	arrhythmogenic right ventricular cardiomyopathy
ASD	atrial septal defect
ASIC	acid sensing ion channel
ATHENA	a placebo-controlled, double-blind, parallel arm Trial to assess the efficacy of dronedarone 400 mg bid for the prevention of cardiovascular Hospitalization or death from any cause in patieNts with AF/atrial flutter
AT_1	angiotensin II receptor type 1
AT_2	angiotensin II receptor type 2
ATP	adenosine triphosphate
AV	atrio-ventricular
AWT	average wall thickening
BAEC	bovine aortic endothelial cell
BAPTA	1,2-bis(o-aminophenoxy)ethane-N,N,N',N'-tetraacetic acid
BAPTA-AM	1,2-bis(0-aminophenoxy)ethane-N,N,N',N'-tetraacetic acid (acetoxymethyl ester)
BBB	bundle branch block
BDM	2,3-butanedione monoxime
bFGF	basic fibroblast growth factor
BMI	body mass index
bpm	beats per minute
BR	beating rate

BZ	border zone	DDR2	discodin domain receptor 2
CABG	coronary artery bypass grafting	DENSE	displacement encoding with stimulated echoes
CaM	calmodulin	dF/dt_{max}	maximum rate of force change
CaMK	calmodulin kinase	DF	dominant frequency
CaMKII	Ca^{2+}/calmodulin-dependent protein kinase II	DF_{Max}	maximum dominant frequency
CaMKIV	Ca^{2+}/calmodulin-dependent kinase IV	DFT	defibrillation threshold
cAMP	cyclic adenosine monophosphate	DGC	dystrophin-associated glycoprotein complex
CAR	*Coxsackie*-adenovirus receptor	DHF	diastolic heart failure
Care-HF	Cardiac Resynchronization in Heart Failure	DIDS	4,4 -diisothiocyanatostilbene-2,2 -disulfonic acid
CaT	calcium transient	DMA	5-(N,N-dimethyl)amiloride
Ca-to-Vm	calcium to trans-membrane potential	DMD	Duchenne muscular dystrophy
cav	caveolin	dP/dt_{max}	maximum rate of pressure change
Cav	voltage-gated Ca^{2+} channel	DR	dispersion of repolarization
CC	*Commotio cordis*	DS	dynamic stiffness
CCS	cortical cytoskeleton	DT-MRI	diffusion tensor magnetic resonance imaging
CF	caffeine		
CF	carbon fibre	E_A	effective arterial elastance
CFTR	cystic fibrosis trans-membrane conductance regulator	EAD	early after-depolarization
		EC	excitation–contraction
cGMP	cyclic guanosine monophosphate	ECG	electrocardiogram
CHARM	Candesartan in Heart Failure – Assessment of Reduction in Mortality and Morbidity	ECM	extracellular matrix
		ED50	50% effective dose
CHD	congenital heart disease	EDPV	end-diastolic pressure–volume relationship
CHO	Chinese hamster ovary	EDP	end-diastolic Pressure
CHORD	cysteine and histidine-rich domain	EDV	end-diastolic volume
CICR	Ca^{2+}-induced Ca^{2+} release	EF	ejection fraction
CIZ	central ischaemic zone	EGF	epidermal growth factor
CK	creatine kinase	EGFR	epidermal growth factor receptor
CM	cardiac memory	EGTA	ethylene glycol tetraacetic acid
COMPANION	comparison of medical, pacing and defibrillation therapies in heart failure	EM	electron microscopy
		EMS	emergency medical service
C_p	patch capacitance	EMT	epithelial–mesenchymal transformation
CPA	cyclopiazonic acid	ENA/VASP	enabled vasodilator-stimulated phosphoprotein
CREATIVE-AF	Impact of Irbesartan on Oxidative Stress and C-Reactive Protein Levels in Patients with Persistent Atrial Fibrillation	ENaC	epithelial Na^{2+} channel
		ENDO	endocardium
		eNOS	endothelial type nitric oxide synthase
CREB	cAMP response element binding protein	EPDC	epicardial-derived cells
CREM	cAMP responsive element modulator	EPI	epicardium
CRT	cardiac resynchronization therapy	ER	endoplasmic reticulum
CRT-D	cardiac resynchronization therapy with implantable cardioverter-defibrillator	ERK	extracellular signal-regulated kinase
		ERM	Ezrin, Radixin and Moesin
CRT-P	cardiac resynchronization therapy without implantable cardioverter-defibrillator	ERP	effective refractory period
		ESC	embryonic stem cell
CSD	caveolin-scaffolding domain	ESPVR	end-systolic pressure–volume relationship
CSK	cell cytoskeleton	ESP	end-systolic pressure
CTAF	Canadian Trial of Atrial Fibrillation	ESV	end-systolic volume
CTGF	connective tissue growth factor	ET-1	endothelin-1
CV	conduction velocity	EURIDIS	EURopean trial In atrial fibrillation or flutter patients receiving Dronedarone for the maIntenance of Sinus rhythm
C_W	initial $[Ca^{2+}]_i$ rise		
Cx	connexin		
DAD	delayed after-depolarization	EWI	electro-mechanical wave imaging
DAG	diacylglycerol	F	force
DAVID	Dual Chamber and VVI Implantable Defibrillator	FACS	fluorescence-activated cell sorting
		FAK	focal adhesion kinase
DCM	dilated cardiomyopathy	F–Ca	force–Ca^{2+} relationship
DDD pacing	on demand and atrially triggered ventricular pacing with sensing and stimulating electrodes in the right atrium and ventricle	FCCP	carbonyl cyanide p-(trifluoromethoxy) phenylhydrazone
		FCT	fetal cardiac titin

FE	finite element
FGF	fibroblast growth factor
FHL	four-and-a-half LIM protein
FI	fibrillatory interval
FKBP	focal kinase binding protein
FN	fibronectin
FRNK	focal adhesion kinase-related non-kinase
FSLR	force–sarcomere length relationship
FSVR	force–sarcomere velocity relationship
$FSVR_{XB}$	force–sarcomere velocity relationship of the average cross-bridge
GABA	γ-aminobutyric acid
GAG	glycosaminoglycan
GFP	green fluorescence protein
GHK	Goldman–Hodgkin–Katz
GISSI-AF	Gruppo Italiano per lo Studio della Sopravvivenza nell'Infarto Miocardico
GPCR	G-protein coupled receptor
GsMTx-4	*Grammostola spatulata* mechano-toxin 4
GTP	guanosine-5'-triphosphatase
$G\alpha_I$	inhibitory G protein
HARP	harmonic phase imaging
HB-EGF	heparin-binding epidermal growth factor
HCM	hypertrophic cardiomyopathy
HCN	hyperpolarization-activated cyclic nucleotide gated (pacemaker) channel
HEK	human embryonic kidney cell line
HEPES	4-(2-hydroxyethyl)-1-piperazineethanesulfonic acid
HF	heart failure
hF	high frequency
IABCP	intra-aortic balloon counter pulsation
IAP	intra-atrial pressure
$I_{b,Ca}$	Ca^{2+} background current
$I_{b,Na}$	Na^+ background current
$I_{Ca,Cl}$	Ca^{2+}-activated Cl^- current
$I_{Ca,L}$	long-lasting Ca^{2+} current = L-type Ca^{2+} current
$I_{Ca,T}$	transient Ca^{2+} current = T-type Ca^{2+} current
ICD	implantable cardioverter-defibrillator
$I_{Cir,Swell}$	inwardly rectifying volume-activated cation channel
ICK	internal cysteine knot
$I_{Cl,swell}$	swelling-activated Cl^- current
I_f	hyperpolarization-activated inward current
IFR	immediate force response
Ig	immunoglobulin
I_K	delayed rectifier K^+ current
I_{K1}	inward rectifier K^+ current
$I_{K,ACh}$	acetylcholine-activated K^+ current
$I_{K,ATP}$	adenosine triphosphate-dependent K + current
I_{KH}	hyperpolarization-activated K^+ current
I_{Kr}	rapid component of the delayed rectifier K^+ current
I_{Ks}	slow component of the delayed rectifier K^+ current
I_{Kur}	ultra-rapid-component of the delayed K^+ rectifier current
ILCOR	International Liaison Committee on Resuscitation
ILK	integrin-linked kinase
I_{Na}	fast Na^+ current
$I_{Na,L}$	late Na^+ current
I_{NCX}	Na^+/Ca^{2+} exchange current
iNOS	inductible nitric oxide synthase
$I_{NS,(Ca)}$	calcium-activated non-selective current
$I_{NS,swell}$	non-selective swelling-activated cation current
IP_3R	inositol triphosphate receptor
I_{pCa}	sarcolemmal Ca^{2+} pump current
I_{pNaK}	Na^+/K^+ exchanger pump current
I-precon	ischaemic preconditioning
iPSC	induced pluripotent stem cell
IS	infarct size
$I_{SAC,Cl}$	stretch-activated Cl^- current
$I_{SAC,NS}$	stretch-activated non-selective cation current
I_{sus}	sustained rectifier K^+ current
I_{ti}	transient inward K^+ current
I_{to}	transient outward K^+ current
I_{to2}	Ca^{2+}-sensitive transient outward Cl^- current
I–V	current–voltage relationship
IVC	inferior *Vena cava*
JAK/STAT	janus kinase/signal transducer and activator of transcription
JNK	c-Jun-activated N-terminal kinase
JPV	pulmonary vein junction
JTc	heart rate-corrected JT interval
K_{2P}	two-pore domain K^+ channel
KAA	arachidonic acid-activated K^+ channel
K_{ACh}	acetylcholine-activated K^+ channel
K_{ATP}	adenosine triphosphate-sensitive K^+ channel
$K_{ATP,mito}$	mitochondrial K_{ATP} channel
$K_{ATP,sarc}$	sarcolemmal K_{ATP} channel
KChAP	K^+channel accessory protein channel
KChIP	voltage-gated K^+ channel interacting proteins
KO	knockout
Kv	voltage-gated K^+ channel
Kvβ	voltage-activated K^+channel beta subunit
LA	left atrium
LAD	left-anterior descending
LAFW	left atrial free wall
LAV	left atrial volume
LBBB	left bundle branch block
LDA	length-dependent activation
LDH	lactate dehydrogenase
lF	low frequency
LIFE	Losartan Intervention for Endpoint Reduction in Hypertension
L-NAME	N^G-nitro-L-arginine methyl ester
LPA	lysophosphatidic acid
LPC	lysophosphatidyl choline
LQT1	long QT 1 syndrome
LQT3	long QT 3 syndrome
LQTS	long QT syndrome
LSPV	left superior pulmonary vein
LV	left ventricle

LVAD	left ventricular assist device	NHE	Na^+/H^+ exchanger
LVEDD	left ventricular end-diastolic dimension	NHE1	cardiac Na^+/H^+ exchanger
LVEDP	left ventricular end-diastolic pressure	NIH	National Institutes of Health
LVEDV	left ventricular end-diastolic volume	NMDA	N-methyl-D-aspartic acid
LVESD	left ventricular end-systolic dimension	nNOS	neuronal type nitric oxide synthase
LVH	left ventricular hypertrophy	NO	nitric oxide
LVP	left ventricular pressure	NOX	nicotinamide-adenine dinucleotide phosphate oxidase
M	mid-myocardial		
MADIT-II trial	Multicenter Automatic Defibrillator Implantation Trial II	NPPB	5-nitro-2-(3-phenylpropylamino)benzoic acid
		N-RAP	nebulin-related anchoring protein
MAP	monophasic action potential	NRVM	neonatal rat ventricular myocyte
MAPD	monophasic action potential duration	NSR	normal sinus rhythm
$MAPD_{[number]}$	monophasic action potential duration at [number]% repolarization (e.g. $MAPD_{50}$ – MAPD at 50 % repolarization)	NSVT	non-sustained ventricular tachycardia
		NYHA	New York Heart Association
		ODQ	$1H$-[1,2,4]oxadiazolo[4,3,-a]quinoxalin-1-one
MAPK	mitogen-activated protein kinase	PAH	pulmonary artery hypertension
MARP	muscle ankyrin repeat proteins	PCI	percutaneous coronary intervention
MCG	magnetocardiography	PCWP	pulmonary capillary wedge pressure
MCT	monocrotaline	PEDF	pigment epithelium-derived factor
MDP	maximum diastolic potential	PEVK	titin segment rich in proline (P), glutamate (E), valine (V) and lysine (K)
mdx	muscular dystrophy mouse		
MEA	microelectrode array	PF	pressurized flow
MEC	mechano-electric coupling	pH_i	intracellular pH
MERLIN-TIMI	Metabolic Efficiency with Ranolazine for Less Ischaemia in Non-ST-elevation acute coronary syndrome Thrombolysis In Myocardial Infarction	PIP_3K	phosphatidylinositol-3,4,5-trisphosphate kinase
		PIP_2	phosphatidylinositol-4,5-bisphosphate
		PIP_3	phosphatidylinositol-3,4,5-trisphosphate
		PIP_4KI	phosphatidylinositol-4-phosphate kinase type I
MI	myocardial infarction	PI3K	Phosphoinositide 3-kinase
miR	micro ribonucleic acid	PKA	protein kinase A
MIRACLE	Myocardial Ischaemia Reduction with Acute Cholesterol LowEring	PKC	protein kinase C
		PKG	protein kinase G
MLC2	myosin light chain 2	PLB	phospholamban
MLCK	myosin light chain kinase	PLC	phospholipase C
MLP	muscle-specific LIM protein	P_o	open probability
MMP	matrix metalloproteinase	postcon	postconditioning
mPTP	mitochondrial permeability transition pore	PP	protein phosphatase
MR	magnetic resonance	PP1	protein phosphatase 1
mR	mitral regurgitation	PP2	protein phosphatase 2
mRNA	messenger ribonucleic acid	PP2A	protein phosphatase 2A
MS	mitral stenosis	PP2B	protein phosphatase 2B (calcineurin)
MSC	mechano-sensitive channel	P-postcon	pacing-induced postconditioning
MSC1	mechano-sensitive channel 1	P-precon	pacing-induced preconditioning
MSC_K	mechano-sensitive channel selective, for K^+	PROSPECT	Predictors of Response to Cardiac Resynchronization Therapy
MscL	mechano-sensitive channel of large conductance		
		PRSW	preload recruitable stroke work
MSC_{NS}	mechano-sensitive channel, cation non-selective	PS	phase singularity
		PT	precordial thump
MscS	mechano-sensitive channel of small conductance	PTK	protein tyrosine kinase
		PTP	protein tyrosine phosphatase
MSP	maximum systolic potential	PUFA	polyunsaturated fatty acids
MVT	monomorphic ventricular tachycardia	PV	pulmonary vein
MyBP-C	myosin binding protein C	PVC	premature ventricular contraction
NADPH	nicotinamide-adenine dinucleotide phosphate	PVT/VF	polymorphic ventricular tachycardia/ ventricular fibrillation
Nav	voltage-gated Na^+ channel		
NCX	Na^+/Ca^{2+} exchanger	Pyr3	ethyl-1-(4-(2,3,3-trichloroacrylamide)phenyl)-5-trifluoro-methyl)-1H-pyrazole-4-carboxylate
NCX_{mito}	mitochondrial Na^+/Ca^{2+} exchanger		
NFAT	calcineurin/nuclear factor of activated T-cells	Q–aU interval	time interval of Q wave until apex of U wave

QTc	corrected QT interval	sub-EPI	sub-epicardium
RA	right atrium	sub-ENDO	sub-endocardium
RALES	Randomized Aldactone Evaluation Study	SV	stroke volume
RCC	rapid cooling-induced contracture	SVC	superior *Vena cava*
REVERSE	Resynchronization Reverses Remodelling in Systolic Left Ventricular Dysfunction	SVT	supraventricular tachycardia
		TALK	two pore domain alkaline activated K$^+$ channel
RF	radiofrequency	TASK	TWIK-related acid-sensitive K$^+$ channel
RGD	arginine–glycine–aspartate	Tcap	titin-cap telethonin
RGS	regulators of G protein signalling	TDI	tissue Doppler imaging
RhoA	a member of the Ras homology family of small GTPases	TEM	transmission electron microscopy
		TGF-β	transforming growth factor-β
RIF	reduced injury factor	THIK	two pore domain halothane-inhibited K$^+$ channel
RMP	resting membrane potential		
RNAi	ribonucleic acid interference	T$_{LV,min}$	time required for reaching the lowest left ventricular diastolic pressure
RNS	reactive nitrogen species		
ROS	reactive oxygen species	TM	trans-membrane
RSA	respiratory sinus arrhythmia	TMEM43	trans-membrane protein 43
RT PCR	reverse transcription polymerase chain reaction	TnC	troponin C
		TOK1	outwardly rectifying K$^+$ channel
RT	restoring tension	TPC	triggered propagated contraction
Rt	tissue resistivity	TRAAK	TWIK-related arachidonic acid-activated K$^+$ channel
Ru360	ruthenium 360		
RV	right ventricle	TREK	TWIK-related K$^+$ channel
RVEDP	right ventricular end-diastolic pressure	TRESK	TWIK-related spinal cord K$^+$ channel
RVOT	right ventricular outflow tract	TRP	transient receptor potential
RyR	ryanodine receptor	TRPA	ankyrin transient receptor potential
RyR2	cardiac-specific ryanodine receptor	TRPC	transient receptor potential channel = canonical TRP
SAC	stretch-activated channel		
SAC$_K$	K$^+$-selective stretch-activated channel	TRPC6	transient receptor potential cation channel, member 6
SAC$_{NS}$	cation non-selective stretch-activated channel		
SAF	stretch acceleration factor	TRPCY1	Y1 sub-type of transient receptor potential channel group
SAFE-T	Sotalol Amiodarone Atrial Fibrillation Efficacy Trial		
		TRPM	melastatin transient receptor potential
SAN	sino-atrial node	TRPML	mucolipin transient receptor potential
sANK-1	small ankyrin-1	TRPP	polycystin transient receptor potential
SCD	sudden cardiac death	TRPV	vanilloid transient receptor potential
SENC	strain encoding	TSG	transseptal gradient
SERCA	sarcoplasmic/endoplasmatic reticulum calcium adenosine triphosphatase	TSH	thyroid stimulating hormone
		TSI	tissue synchronization imaging
SFR	slow force response	TTX	tetrodotoxin
SHR	spontaneously hypertensive rat	TWA	T-wave alternans
SKF96363	1-[2-(4-methoxyphenyl)-2-[3-(4-methoxyphenyl)propoxy]ethyl-1H-imidazole hydrochloride	TWIK	weak inwardly rectifying two pore domain K$^+$ channel
		VA	ventricular arrhythmia
SL	sarcomere length	VAC	volume-activated channel
sma	smooth muscle actin	VAC$_{CAT}$	weakly cation selective volume-activated channel
SAN	sinoatrial node		
SND	sinus node dysfunction	VAD	ventricular assist device
SOLVD	Studies of Left Ventricular Dysfunction	Val-HeFT	Valsartan Heart Failure Trial
SPWMD	septal-to-posterior wall motion delay	VDAC	voltage-dependent anion channel
SQTS	short QT syndrome	VEGF	vascular endothelial growth factor
SQUID	superconducting quantum interference device	VEP	virtual electrode polarization
SR	sarcoplasmic reticulum	VER	ventricular electrical remodelling
SRAF	stretch-related atrial fibrillation	VF	ventricular fibrillation
Src	sarcoma	VGC	voltage-gated channel
STOP H2	Swedish Trial in Old Patients with Hypertension	V$_m$	trans-membrane potential
		VMB	ventricular myocardial band
STP	spatio-temporal periodicity		

V_{prop}	propagation velocity	XB	cross-bridge
VT	ventricular tachycardia	β-AR	β-adrenergic receptor
VVI pacing	on-demand pacing with a single sensing and stimulating electrode in the right ventricle	λ_{cc}	circumferential stretch ratio
		λ_{ff}	fibre stretch ratio
WKY	Wistar Kyoto rat	λ_{ll}	longitudinal stretch ratio
WPW	Wolff–Parkinson–White syndrome	λ_{rr}	fibre radial stretch ratio
WT	wild-type	σ_{ff}	fibre stress ratio

SECTION 1

Sub-cellular mechanisms of cardiac mechano-electric coupling

1. **Evolutionary origins of stretch-activated ion channels** *3*
   Boris Martinac and Anna Kloda

2. **Stretch-activated channels in the heart** *11*
   Frederick Sachs

3. **The mechano-gated K_{2p} channel TREK-1 in the cardiovascular system** *19*
   Eric Honoré and Amanda Patel

4. **Cell volume-sensitive ion channels and transporters in cardiac myocytes** *27*
   Clive M. Baumgarten, Wu Deng and Frank J. Raucci, Jr

5. **Non-sarcolemmal stretch-activated channels** *35*
   Gentaro Iribe and Peter Kohl

6. **Pacemaker, potassium, calcium, sodium: stretch modulation of the voltage-gated channels** *42*
   Catherine E. Morris

7. **Role of caveolae in stretch-sensing: implications for mechano-electric coupling** *50*
   Sarah Calaghan

8. **The membrane/cytoskeleton interface and stretch-activated channels** *57*
   Thomas M. Suchyna and Frederick Sachs

9. **Cardiomyocyte stretch-sensing** *66*
   Michiel Helmes and Henk Granzier

10. **The response of cardiac muscle to stretch: calcium and force** *74*
    John Jeremy Rice and Donald M. Bers

11. **Stretch effects on second messengers** *81*
    Jean-Luc Balligand and Chantal Dessy

12. **Functional implications of myocyte architecture** *87*
    Kevin Kit Parker

Evolutionary origins of stretch-activated ion channels

Boris Martinac and Anna Kloda

Background

Stretch-activated channels (SAC) present the major type of mechano-sensitive channels (MSC) found in living cells. They convert mechanical stimuli acting upon membranes of biological cells into electrical or chemical signals in mechano-sensory transduction processes ranging from turgor control in bacteria and plant cells to hearing, touch, renal tubular function and blood pressure regulation in mammals[1]. In the evolution of different life forms on Earth these ion channels probably represent the oldest sensory transduction molecules that evolved as primary signalling elements in mechano-sensory physiology of living organisms. The concept of ion channels gated by mechanical stimuli arose originally from studies of specialized mechano-sensory neurons[1]. Their discovery in embryonic chick skeletal muscle[2] and in frog muscle[3] some 25 years ago confirmed this concept and, furthermore, it demonstrated their existence in many non-specialized cell types[4]. Instrumental for the discovery of SAC was the invention of the patch-clamp technique[5], which allowed the first direct measurements of single mechano-sensitive channel currents in a variety of non-specialized cells[1]. Although once considered an artefact of the patch-clamp recording[6], mechano-sensitive ion channels attracted revived interest after cloning and structural characterization of SAC in bacteria and *Archaea* and cloning of several SAC implicated in mechano-transduction processes in invertebrates and vertebrates[1]. Currently, mechano-sensitive channel proteins are at the focus of structural, spectroscopic, computational and functional studies aiming to understand the molecular basis of mechano-sensory transduction in living cells.

Mechano-transduction in microbial cells

Microbes have for many years been excellent experimental objects amenable to modern electrophysiological techniques[7]. Osmotic forces are omnipresent determinants of the everyday life of microbial cells. SAC are indispensable for microbial survival when an increase in cellular turgor caused by a sudden hypo-osmotic shift in osmolarity of external environment threatens to kill the microbe. Over the last 20 years the patch-clamp technique has been used to identify and characterize SAC activities in microorganisms from all three domains of life. Especially, SAC from the bacterium *Escherichia coli*[8], the yeast *Saccharomyces cerevisiae*[9,10] and the green algae *Chlamydomonas reinhardtii*[11] have been studied in more detail.

The ancient nature of mechano-sensory transduction

The Earth is 4.6 billion years old and for most of this time (~3.8 billion years) has been inhabited by innumerable life forms, with microbes of all provenances encompassing the largest group[12]. The diversity, number and adaptability of microorganisms to environments characterized by extreme temperatures, salinity or acidity have enabled them to inhabit all niches of life. From their early appearance they were exposed to changes in environmental osmolarity, which resulted in osmotic forces that could easily damage their cellular membranes. To prevent this from occurring microbial cells are usually protected by a cell wall and have a cell membrane equipped with different types of SAC, allowing the cells to adjust to a large range of osmotic forces acting upon them[7]. Importantly, a difference in osmotic forces of only a few milliosmols across a membrane of a cell is sufficient to fully activate most of the known SAC[13]. Consequently, from very early on SAC might have served as cellular osmoregulators that measured small changes in the concentration of solutes and water across microbial membranes[4,14]. Later during evolution of eukaryotic cells SAC could have been employed to function in the regulation of cell size and volume, and later with the appearance of multicellular organisms they may have further evolved into molecular sensors to function in more specialized forms of mechano-sensory transduction, such as gravitropism in plants or contractility of the heart.

Mechano-sensitive channels of prokaryotes

Initially, SAC from prokaryotes were first documented in the Gram-negative bacterium *E. coli*[8]. Later they were extensively studied in both Gram-negative and Gram-positive bacteria[7]. In *Archaea*, the third domain of the universal phylogenetic tree, they were identified in consecutive years[15] thanks to the cloning of the bacterial mechano-sensitive channel of large conductance (MscL) and mechano-sensitive channel of small conductance (MscS) channels[16,17] and a large number of bacterial and archaeal genome sequences available in the National Center for Biotechnology Information genomic database. What follows is a brief description of the structural and functional properties of the representative SAC from prokaryotic cells.

SAC of bacteria

Bacterial SAC were discovered in *E. coli* more than 20 years ago[8]. Since then they have been the subject of extensive multidisciplinary research, which has been greatly advanced by the cloning[17,18] and determination of the X-ray crystal structure[19,20] of MscL and MscS, the SAC of large and small conductance. The three-dimensional (3D) structures of MscL and MscS have provided the basis for further experimental and theoretical studies addressing the mechanism of membrane tension sensing defined by lipid–protein interactions, which direct the opening and closing of these structurally unrelated channels[21].

The X-ray crystal structure of Tb-MscL, the MscL homologue from *Mycobacterium tuberculosis*, revealed that the MscL channel is a homopentamer of monomers consisting of two trans-membrane helices TM1 and TM2, N- and C-terminal domains located at the cytoplasmic side and a flexible loop connecting the two helices at the periplasmic side of the bacterial cell membrane (Fig. 1.1A)[20,22]. The channel pore of MscL is lined by five TM1 helices. This structure is generally agreed to represent the oligomeric structure of MscL. Surprisingly, a recent study by Liu and colleagues[23], who also reported the 3D structure of Tb-MscL, showed that a truncated form of the MscL channel from *Staphylococcus aureus* (Δ26 SaMscL) is organized as a homotetramer rather than a homopentamer, suggesting an unusual plasticity in oligomerization of the MscL channel family.

The currently accepted oligomeric structure of MscS is that of a homoheptamer consisting of three trans-membrane helices, TM1, TM2 and TM3, and the N- and C-terminal domains located at the periplasmic and cytoplasmic end of the bacterial cell membrane, respectively (Fig. 1.1B). This structure is based on the X-ray crystal structure of an intermediate conformation of Eco-MscS, the MscS channel from *E. coli*[19,24]. According to this structure, the pore of MscS is formed by seven TM3 helices. Future structural studies may demonstrate whether the MscS family of SAC possesses similar plasticity of oligomerization to that of the MscL family.

MscL and MscS function as electromechanical switches with the capability to sense the membrane tension in the lipid bilayer. The bilayer deformations are transduced into open and closed conformations of the channel proteins. The conformational rearrangements generate large non-selective channel pores, allowing unhindered permeation of small solutes on a millisecond time scale, which serves as a defence mechanism in prokaryotic cells against sudden osmotic challenges[25]. Although the bilayer mechanism of gating MscL and MscS channels is generally undisputed, the specific lipid–protein interactions controlling the conformational changes in these channel proteins remain unresolved.

MscL and MscS families of SAC

The accessibility of a large number of genome sequences of bacteria and *Archaea* available in genomic databases has enabled the analysis of the phylogenetic distribution of SAC in these microbes. According to this analysis MscL and MscS form separate subfamilies of prokaryotic mechano-sensitive channels (Fig. 1.1A, B)[26], indicating that *mscL* and *mscS* genes followed separate evolutionary pathways[26]. A recent analysis of aligned sequences of 231 homologues of MscL and 309 homologues of MscS revealed that both types of channels can be found in all three domains of life, *Bacteria*, *Archaea* and *Eukarya*. MscS-like proteins, in particular,

are abundant in higher plants including *Arabidopsis* and *Oryza*, in the single-celled alga *Chlamydomonas* and in the fission yeast *Schizosaccaromyces pombe* (Fig. 1.1B)[27]. Neither MscL nor MscS homologues have been found in animal cells[26,27].

SAC of Archaea

SAC in *Archaea* were first documented in the halophilic archaeon *Haloferax volcanii* (formerly *Halobacterium volcanii*), followed by molecular cloning and characterization of SAC from methanogenic archaeon *Methanococcus jannashi*[7]. MscMJ and MscMJLR, the SAC from *M. jannashii*, share sequence homology with members of the MscS-like subfamily of mechano-sensitive channel proteins (Fig. 1.1B)[26].

Mechano-sensitive channels of microbial eukaryotes

In the past, classical electrophysiological measurements based on two-microelectrode voltage clamp technique in eukaryotic microbial cells could only be carried out in large protozoan cells (e.g. *Paramecium*) or giant algal cells (e.g *Chara*)[7]. The patch-clamp method[5] provided means to examine electrophysiologically for the first time cell membranes of very small cells including microbial eukaryotes, yeasts and algae, allowing study of the electrical properties of these cells by examining ion channels in their cellular membranes in situ[28]. Like bacteria, yeast and algal cells have to face rapid and large changes in osmolarity. Therefore it is not surprising that yeasts and green algae also harbour SAC.

Mechano-receptor currents in ciliates

A *Paramecium* cell has two types of mechano-receptor currents. One is a Ca^{2+}-dependent current elicited by a mechanical stimulus at the anterior end of the cell[29,30]. This mechano-receptor current is carried by Ca^{2+} ions depolarizing cell membrane and evoking a Ca^{2+}-dependent action potential, which causes ~6,000 cilia covering the body of a *Paramecium* cell to reverse their beating direction[31]. The ciliary reversal causes the cell to reverse its swimming direction, resulting in an 'avoiding reaction', which is a stereotypical behaviour observed in *Paramecium*[32]. The second type of mechano-receptor currents are elicited by a mechanical stimulus at the posterior end of the cell. It is a hyperpolarizing K^+-dependent current[33] propelling the cell rapidly forward due to an increase in the ciliary beating frequency in normal direction. This increase in the ciliary beat is an 'escape response', a second type of stereotypical behaviour[32]. Mechano-sensitive Ca^{2+} and K^+ channels, the conduits of the corresponding mechano-receptor currents, localized on the cell soma[34], are distributed over the somatic cell surface of a *Paramecium* cell in the manner of overlapping gradients[35]. Although both mechano-receptor currents have been well characterized by the voltage-clamp method the molecular identity of the corresponding mechano-sensitive ion channels is currently unknown.

Mechano-sensitive channels in yeast

There are two types of SAC found in yeast. The first type is located on the yeast plasma membrane and the second one is found in the vacuolar membrane[28]. A patch-clamp survey of the *S. cerevisiae* plasma membrane led to identification of an SAC of 36 pS[9]. A cation-selective SAC of 180-pS conductance was identified in *S. pombae*[36], whereas a highly cation-selective 600-pS SAC was

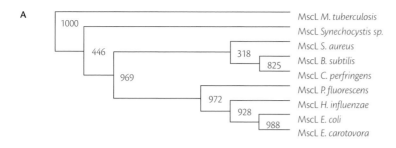

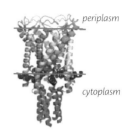

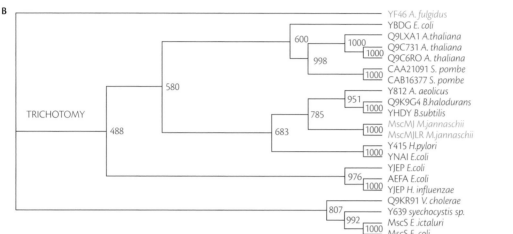

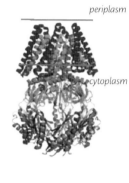

Fig. 1.1 Families of prokaryotic SAC. **A** A subfamily of MscL-like proteins found in bacteria. The structure of the MscL homopentamer from *Mycobacterium tuberculosis*[22,85] is shown on the right. The position of the lipid bilayer relative to the channel protein is indicated by red lines. The most divergent members of the MscL subfamily, the archaeal and fungal proteins, most closely resemble those of Gram-positive bacteria[26]. **B** A representative phylogenetic tree of MscS homologues found in three kingdoms of living organisms. The structure of the MscS heptamer from *E. coli*[24,85] is shown on the right. The position of the lipid bilayer relative to the channel protein is indicated by red lines. MscS-like proteins of bacteria are shown in black, those of *Archaea* are shown in red, whereas MscS homologues found in fungi and plants are shown in green. [Adapted, with permission from Elsevier, from Martinac B, Kloda A (2003) Evolutionary origins of mechanosensitive ion channels. *Prog Biophys Mol Biol* **82**:11–24.] (See color plate section.)

found in the growing germ tubes of *Uromyces appendiculatus*[37]. The physiological function of the SAC in *S. cerevisiae* and *S. pombe* is unknown to date. The SAC of *U. appendiculatus* is believed to be a component of the bean-leaf topography sensing mechanism serving as a transducer of the membrane tension induced by the leaf topography into a flux of Ca^{2+} ions, which is required for differentiation of the germ tubes into invading structures of this fungal parasite.

The second type of mechano-sensitive channel found in yeast is a 350-pS SAC that is activated by stretching the vacuolar membrane using a patch-clamp set-up[38]. At first named Yvc1, a yeast vacuolar channel, this SAC was renamed as a Y1 sub-type of transient receptor potential (TRP) channel group (TRPY1) because it was identified as a member of the superfamily of TRP-like channels (Fig. 1.2A) (see also section on TRP channels). Upon osmotic up-shock of the vacuole the channel releases calcium from the vacuole into the cytoplasm and thus plays a role in calcium homeostasis[39]. TRPY1 has direct homologues in over 30 species of fungi except *S. pombe* and the parasitic *Zygomycetes* (Fig. 1.2A). Upon heterologous expression in the vacuole of *S. cerevisiae* two ion channel genes from *Kluyveromyces lactis* and *Candida albicans* have been found to encode cation-selective SAC[40].

MscS-like channels of *Chlamydomonas*

Mechano-sensitive channel 1 (MSC1), an MscS-like SAC, has been identified in chloroplasts of the green alga *C. reinhardtii*[11]. Like any of the seven subunits of the MscS channel, MSC1 monomer consists of three putative trans-membrane domains. Its TM3 trans-membrane helix shows high structural homology to the TM3 helix of MscS. The MSC1 channel expressed in *E. coli* has a conductance of 400 pS. A striking feature of MSC1 is its stretch-dependent hysteresis behaviour, which depends on the way tension is applied to the membrane[11]. The origin of this behaviour remains unclear but probably reflects simply channel or membrane kinetics slower than the stimulus. MSC1 exhibits higher selectivity for anions over cations than MscS, which shows only a slight preference for anions over cations[8]. A physiological function of the MSC1 channels is unknown, although ribonucleic acid interference (RNAi) knockdown of MSC1 reduces chlorophyll autofluorescence in chloroplasts due to abnormal localization of chlorophyll, suggesting that MSC1 is an intracellular mechanosensitive channel responsible for the organization of chloroplasts in *Chlamydomonas*[11].

Mechano-sensory transduction in plants

Plants respond to a number of mechanical stimuli including touch, gravity and osmotic stress[41]. These stimuli cause rapid changes in proton and calcium concentration in plant cells. Mechano-sensitive ion channels that could mediate rapid responses to touch, gravity and changes in cell turgor have been reported in plants[42].

MscS-like channels in *Arabidopsis thaliana*

Phylogenetic analysis of the distribution of prokaryotic SAC proteins has revealed the presence of ten MscS-like genes phylogenetically divided into two groups in the experimental plant *Arabidopsis thaliana* (Fig. 1.2B)[26,42]. Two of them, MSL1 and MSL3, belong

to Class I *Arabidopsis* proteins and are localized to the inner membrane of the envelope of plastids, which are plant-specific endosymbiotic organelles responsible for photosynthesis, gravity perception and many metabolic reactions[42]. Upon expression in an *E. coli* strain lacking MS channel activity, both MSL1 and MSL3 can protect bacterial cells from hypo-osmotic shock similar to MscS[42]. Finding prokaryotic MscS-type SAC in plants may not be surprising given that, similar to mitochondria, plastids in green plants may have originated directly from a symbiont bacterium via primary endosymbiosis[43].

Diversity of mechano-sensitive channels in animal cells

Several different types of mammalian mechano-gated ion channels and receptors have been identified and cloned. They belong to several families with different structural characteristics. They include DEG/MEC/ENaC channels, 2P-type K+ SAC, TRP channels, and N-methyl-D-aspartic acid (NMDA) receptors (see Fig 1.3A–D) for further details).

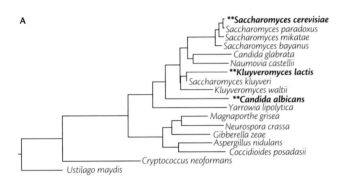

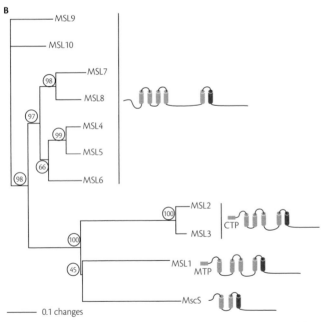

Fig. 1.2 Families of SAC from fungiand plants. **A** Dendrogram of members of the fungal TRP channel protein family showing the relatedness in amino acid sequence of the 18 TRPCY members. [Reproduced, with permission, from Zhou XL, Loukin SH, Coria R, Kung C, Saimi Y (2005) Heterologously expressed fungal transient receptor potential channels retain mechanosensitivity in vitro and osmotic response in vivo. *Eur Biophys J* **34**:413–422.] **B** Phylogenetic tree of the MscS-like MSL proteins from *Arabidopsis thaliana*. The predicted topologies of the MSL proteins are shown to the right of the tree. Cylinders indicate predicted trans-membrane domains. The cylinders marked in dark grey designate the pore-forming helix. MTP, mitochondrial permeability transition pore; CTP, chloroplast transit sequence. [Reproduced, with permission, from Haswell ES (2007) MscS-like proteins in plants. In: *Mechanosensitive Ion Channels, Part A* (ed OP Hamill). Academic Press, Amsterdam, pp 329–359.]

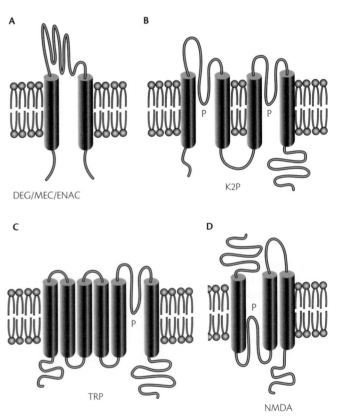

Fig. 1.3 Diversity in membrane topology of eukaryotic SAC. DEG/MEC/ENaC channels (**A**) assemble as tetramers, K2P channels (**B**) form dimers, whereas TRP channels (**C**) and NMDA receptors (**D**) assemble as heteromultimeric tetramers. Pore (P) domains are indicated for each channel. [Modified, with permission, from Folgering JH, Sharif-Naeini R, Dedman A, Patel A, Delmas P, Honore E (2008) Molecular basis of the mammalian pressure-sensitive ion channels: focus on vascular mechanotransduction. *Prog Biophys Mol Biol* **97**:180–195.]

DEG/MEC/ENaC channels

DEG/MEC and ENaC proteins belong to a family of eukaryotic ion channels which share an MscL-like structural motif of two trans-membrane domains connected by an extracellular loop and cytosolic C- and N-termini (Fig. 1.3A). Several members of this group are believed to be involved in mechano-sensory transduction. The DEG/MEC family of ion channels mediates responses to gentle touch in *Caenorhabditis elegans*[44]. The touch-sensitive channel is presumably formed by association of MEC4 and MEC10 pro-teins which are attached to a number of intracellular and extracellular MEC/DEG counterparts, forming a touch-sensitive complex[45].

The epithelial sodium channel (ENaC) is a structural homologue of the DEG/MEC family. The ENaC channel is expressed on the apical surfaces of a variety of epithelial cells including the kidney, lung and colon, where it is involved in maintenance of body salt and water homeostasis by absorption of sodium ions[46]. The ENaC channel is believed to be heteromultimer, formed of three subunits: alpha, beta and gamma[47]. Several studies have reported activation of ENaC channels by mechanical forces such as tension and shear stress. There is evidence that ENaC proteins are essential in mediating myogenic vasoconstriction in animal brain and renal arteries. Inhibition of ENaC subunits abolishes pressure-induced (but not agonist-induced) vasoconstriction[48], indicating that these proteins are required for mechano-sensation.

2P-type-K⁺ channels

A diverse family of potassium channels includes a structurally and functionally unique two-pore domain (2P-type K^+) subfamily also named K2P. These types of channels are widely distributed in excitable and non-excitable cells where they produce leak potassium conductance important for the establishment of membrane resting potential, cell excitability and transport of water and solutes. The membrane topology of the K2P subfamily is unique compared to other known potassium channels and is characterized by four trans-membrane domains (TM1–TM4) and two pore-forming domains (P1 and P2) (Fig. 1.3B). Both pore domains – P1 (located between M1 and M2) and P2 (located between M3 and M4) – contribute to a selectivity filter which forms a conduction pathway for K^+. The functional channel assembles as a dimer of subunits. The stretch-activated TWIK (**t**andem of P domains in a **w**eak **i**nwardly rectifying **K**⁺ channel) -**r**elated subgroup (TREK) subgroup comprises three members: TREK1, TREK2 and TRAAK[49].

The TREK1 channel is highly expressed in the brain as well as peripheral tissues including the hippocampus, prefrontal cortex, hypothalamus, serotoninergic neurons of the dorsal raphe nucleus, sensory neurons of the dorsal root ganglia, gastrointestinal tract, odontoblasts, myocytes and endothelial cells of some blood vessels[50]. The activity of the TREK1 channel is inhibited at negative resting membrane potentials by an external Mg^{2+} block and a voltage-dependent gating mechanism which is controlled by the C-terminal domain[51]. The TREK1 channel is regulated by a variety of physical and chemical stimuli including membrane stretch, intracellular acidosis, temperature, amphipathic molecules, antidepressants, volatile general anaesthetics, arachidonic acid and intracellular phospholipids[49].

The TREK2 channel displays 63% sequence identity with the TREK1 channel and its expression overlaps with the TREK1 channel in many brain regions and peripheral tissues including the kidney, pancreas, gastrointestinal tract, myometrium, heart and arteries[52]. The TREK2 channel shares all the functional properties of the TREK1 channel and, similar to TREK1, is modulated by membrane stretch, temperature, cytosolic pH, polyunsaturated fatty acids and phosphorylation[49,53].

TRAAK shares approximately 40% sequence identity with TREK1 and TREK2. Its expression has been detected mostly in the brain but also in several peripheral organs including the heart, liver, kidney, pancreas and placenta. Unlike TREK1 and TREK2 channels, TRAAK channels can be distinguished from other TREK isoforms by weak inward rectification and activation by increased cytosolic alkalinity[54]. TRAAK activity can be modulated by membrane tension or curvature in the lipid bilayer induced by stretch or amphipaths. Similar to TREK1, the mechano-sensitivity of TRAAK is potentiated by membrane depolarization[54]. Arachidonic acid, lysophospholipids and lysophosphatidic acid all stimulated TRAAK channel activity[54].

Transient receptor potential channels

TRP channels are members of a superfamily of cellular receptors responding to a large variety of extra- and intracellular signals, including temperature, membrane potential, osmolarity, membrane stretch and ligands. TRP channels were originally discovered in the *trp* mutant strain of a fruit fly, *Drosophila* which is characterized by transient photoreceptor activity in response to light[55]. In recent years, TRP channels from different subfamilies have been shown to function as Ca^{2+}-permeable mechano- and/or osmosensitive ion channels, which play a crucial role in the response to mechanical and osmotic perturbations in a wide range of cell types[56]. TRP channels play an important role in cellular calcium signalling and homeostasis. The secondary structure of TRP channels is comprised of six membrane-spanning helices with intracellular N- and C-termini (Fig. 1.3C). In mammals, the TRPC family is a product of at least 33 genes divided into the following families: TRPC (canonical TRP channel), TRPV (vanilloid), TRPA (ankyrin), TRPM (melastatin), TRPP (polycystin) and TRPML (mucolipin).

Within the TRPC family, TRPC1 and TRPC6 have been reported to be involved in the process of mechano-sensory transduction. TRPC1 protein is expressed in the brain, heart, testes, ovaries, smooth muscles, endothelium, salivary glands and liver[57]. They can be activated directly by membrane stretch[58]. TRPC1 and TRPP2 can assemble to form a heteromeric channel which may underlie mechano-transduction of cilium-based Ca^{2+} signalling in response to fluid flow shear stress[59]. The TRPC6 subfamily is expressed in the stomach, colon, oesophagus, myometrium and human brain[60]. TRPC6 may be activated by mechanically or osmotically induced membrane stretch. The activity of TRPC6 in the smooth muscle of resistance arteries was found to be modulated by blood pressure[61].

Heat-sensitive members of the TRPV family, TRPV1, TRPV2 and TRPV4, can function as mechano-sensors. Acid-sensitive TRPV1 channels are found in both the central and peripheral nervous systems. In the peripheral nervous system the TRPV1 is involved in modulation of responses during inflammatory thermal hyperalgesia[62]. In the central nervous system, TRPV1 appears to affect long-term depression and memory formation[63]. A recent report suggested that the *Trpv1* gene is also required for osmosensory transduction and osmoregulation in osmoreceptor neurons that control water balance[64].

TRPV2 receptor acts as a noxious heat thermosensor[65]. The TRPV2 homologues are expressed in sensory neurons, vascular smooth muscle and myocytes. These channels can be activated by stretch and osmotic changes[66]. The TRPV4 channel is expressed in a variety of neurosensory cells, inner-ear hair cells, Merkel cells, kidney, liver and heart cells[67]. Several polymodal stimuli including warm temperature, metabolites of arachidonic acid and hypotonicity activate the TRPV4 channel[68].

TRPM3, TRPM4 and TRPM7 have also been reported to be involved in mechano-transduction. The TRPM3 proteins are expressed in kidney, brain and pancreatic cells[69]. The activity of the TRPM3 splice variant was reported to be enhanced by cell swelling as well as sphingolipids[70]. The TRPM4 receptor is expressed in vascular endothelium and arterial smooth muscle cells[71]. TRPM4 channels can be activated directly by mechanical stimulation[72]. TRPM7 is expressed in vascular smooth muscle and endothelium and it is both an ion channel and a self-phosphorylating kinase[73]. The channel activity is enhanced by shear stress and osmotic swelling as well as direct stretching of the membrane[74].

The mechano-sensitive polycystin complex composed of TRPP1 and TRPP2 proteins is involved in autosomal dominant polycystic kidney disease. The TRPP1 protein is an integral membrane glycoprotein with 11 trans-membrane domains, whereas the membrane topology of the TRPP2 protein is similar to other TRPC. The TRPP1/TRPP2 complex is expressed in the cilia of renal epithelial cells and may act as a mechano-sensor which detects sheer stress from flow of fluid[75].

TRPA1 is the sole member of the TRP family characterized by a large number of ankyrin repeats. It has been proposed to function as a mechanical stress sensor. TRPA1 is expressed in nociceptive neurons as well as the mechano-sensory epithelia of the inner ear. TRPA1 has been proposed to function as the auditory transducer channel[76,77].

NMDA receptors

The NMDA receptor is an oligomeric cation channel which mediates long-term potentiation, synaptic plasticity and neurodegeneration via conditional Ca^{2+} signalling[78]. The channel requires co-activation by two ligands, glutamate and glycine. Although not canonical stretch-activated ion channels, NMDA receptors exhibit mechano-sensitive properties and can be activated by mechanical stimuli upon reconstitution into artificial liposomes[79,80].

Mechano-sensitivity in blood pressure regulation and heart function

Ion channels and transporters play an important role in myocyte response to mechanical stimulation caused by pressure or sheer stress. The expression of ENaC channels at the site of mechanoreceptors and arterial baroreceptors[81] has linked ENaC channels to the mechano-transduction processes associated with touch detection, blood pressure regulation and hypertension. Gain of function mutants of ENaC cause severe hypertension due to retention of salt and water leading to Liddle's syndrome, whereas loss of function mutations provoke hypotension (or pseudohypoaldosteronism type I) associated with salt wasting[82]. TREK1 channels expressed in myocytes and endothelial cells play an important role

in endothelium-dependent vasodilation and endothelial dysfunction. Deletion of TREK1 abolishes alpha-linolenic acid-induced vasodilation and alters cutaneous blood flow in response to local pressure application[83]. The activity of TRPC6 is regulated by the blood flow pressure. Decreased expression of TRPC6 reduces arterial smooth muscle depolarization and constriction of blood vessels in response to pressure[61]. In contrast, TRPC6 knockout mice show enhanced responsiveness of the smooth muscle to constrictor agonists in the thoracic aorta[84], which indicates the unique dual role of TRPC6 in the control of the vascular smooth muscle tone. The TRPV2 homologue expressed in murine aortic myocytes forms an osmotically sensitive cation channel, which can be activated by cell swelling in response to hypotonic solutions[66]. Attenuated expression of TRPM4 by antisense oligonucleotides reduces pressure-induced depolarization of myocytes and myogenic contraction. Furthermore, activation of TRPM4 channels by membrane stretch is believed to contribute to the depolarization, followed by vasoconstriction of cerebral arteries following mechanical stimulation[72].

Conclusions and outlook

In this brief overview we have summarized over 20 years of research into mechano-sensitive ion channels, which has developed from their serendipitous discovery in chick and frog muscle and gradually led to molecular identification and structural determination of a large number of SAC from organisms of diverse phylogenetic provenance. Cloning and structural determination of bacterial MscL and MscS channels, cloning and genetic analysis of the *mec* genes in *Cenorhabditis elegans*, genetic and functional studies of the TRP-type SAC as well as functional and genetic studies of the TREK and TRAAK 2P-type K^+ SAC continue promoting our understanding of the role that mechano-sensitive ion channels play in the physiology of mechano-sensory transduction in living organisms. In recent years the scientific and medical community has become more aware of the importance of aberrant mechano-sensitive channels contributing to pathophysiology of various diseases including heart failure and dysfunction, a topic highly relevant for the specialized research described in the consecutive chapters of this book. We may expect that further substantial developments of the research on SAC will continue so that we can look forward to solving additional molecular mysteries of these fascinating molecules, not only in order to satisfy our intellectual curiosity and enrich our knowledge, but also for the betterment of human health.

Acknowledgements

We thank Dr Ching Kung and Dr Elizabeth Haswell for sharing the material used in Fig. 1.2. This work was supported by grants from the Australian Research Council.

References

1. Hamill OP, Martinac B. Molecular basis of mechanotransduction in living cells. *Physiol Rev* 2001;**81**:685–740.
2. Guharay F, Sachs F. Stretch-activated single ion channel currents in tissue-cultured embryonic chick skeletal muscle. *J Physiol* 1984;**352**:685–701.
3. Brehm P, Kullberg R, Moody-Corbett F. Properties of non-junctional acetylcholine receptor channels on innervated muscle of *Xenopus laevis. J Physiol* 1984;**350**:631–648.

4. Sachs F. Mechanical transduction in biological systems. *Crit Rev Biomed Eng* 1988;**16**:141–169.

5. Hamill OP, Marty A, Neher E, Sakmann B, Sigworth FJ. Improved patch-clamp techniques for high-resolution current recording from cells and cell-free membrane patches. *Pflugers Arch* 1981;**391**:85–100.

6. Morris CE, Horn R. Failure to elicit neuronal macroscopic mechanosensitive currents anticipated by single-channel studies. *Science* 1991;**251**:1246–1249.

7. Martinac B, Saimi Y, Kung C. Ion channels in microbes. *Physiol Rev* 2008;**88**:1449–1490.

8. Martinac B, Buechner M, Delcour AH, Adler J, Kung C. Pressure-sensitive ion channel in *Escherichia coli*. *Proc Natl Acad Sci USA* 1987;**84**:2297–2301.

9. Gustin MC, Zhou XL, Martinac B, Kung C. A mechanosensitive ion channel in the yeast plasma membrane. *Science* 1988;**242**:762–765.

10. Zhou XL, Batiza AF, Loukin SH, Palmer CP, Kung C, Saimi Y. The transient receptor potential channel on the yeast vacuole is mechanosensitive. *Proc Natl Acad Sci USA* 2003;**100**:7105–7110.

11. Nakayama Y, Fujiu K, Sokabe M, Yoshimura K. Molecular and electrophysiological characterization of a mechanosensitive channel expressed in the chloroplasts of Chlamydomonas. *Proc Natl Acad Sci USA* 2007;**104**:5883–5888.

12. Woese CR. There must be a prokaryote somewhere: microbiology's search for itself. *Microbiol Rev* 1994;**58**:1–9.

13. Sachs F, Morris CE. Mechanosensitive ion channels in nonspecialized cells. In: *Reviews of Physiology Biochemistry and Pharmacology*. Springer, Berlin, 1998; Vol 33, pp. 1–77.

14. Kung C, Saimi Y, Martinac B. (1990) Mechanosensitive ion channels in microbes and the early evolutionary origin of solvent sensing. In: *Current Topics in Membranes and Transport*, (ed T Claudio). Academic Press, New York, pp. 9451–9455.

15. Kloda A, Martinac B. Structural and functional differences between two homologous mechanosensitive channels of *Methanococcus jannaschii*. *EMBO J* 2001;**20**:1888–1896.

16. Sukharev SI, Blount P, Martinac B, Blattner FR, Kung C. A large-conductance mechanosensitive channel in *E. coli* encoded by MscL alone. *Nature* 1994;**368**:265–268.

17. Levina N, Totemeyer S, Stokes NR, Louis P, Jones MA, Booth IR. Protection of *Escherichia coli* cells against extreme turgor by activation of MscS and MscL mechanosensitive channels: identification of genes required for MscS activity. *EMBO J* 1999;**18**:1730–1737.

18. Sukharev SI, Blount P, Martinac B, Kung C. Functional reconstitution as an assay for biochemical isolation of channel proteins: application to the molecular identification of a bacterial mechanosensitive channel. *Meth Companion Meth Enzymol* 1994;**6**:51–59.

19. Bass RB, Strop P, Barclay M, Rees D. Crystal structure of *Escherichia coli* MscS, a voltage-modulated and mechanosensitive channel. *Science* 2002;**298**:1582–1587.

20. Chang G, Spencer RH, Lee AT, Barclay MT, Rees DC. Structure of the MscL homolog from *Mycobacterium tuberculosis*: a gated mechanosensitive ion channel. *Science* 1998;**282**:2220–2226.

21. Corry B, Martinac M. Bacterial mechanosensitive channels: experiment and theory. *Biochim Biophys Acta-Biomembr* 2008;**1778**:1859–1870.

22. Steinbacher S, Bass R, Strop P, Rees DC. (2007) *Mechanosensitive Channel of Large Conductance (MscL)*. Protein Data Bank (PDB), DOI: 10.2210/pdb2oar/pdb.

23. Liu Z, Gandhi CS, Rees DC. Structure of a tetrameric MscL in an expanded intermediate state. *Nature* 2009;**461**:120–124.

24. Steinbacher S, Bass R, Strop P, Rees DC. (2007) *Mechanosensitive Channel of Small Conductance (MscS)*. Protein Data Bank (PDB), DOI: 10.2210/pdb2oau/pdb.

25. Booth IR, Edwards MD, Murray E, Miller S. (2005) The role of bacterial channels in cell physiology. In: *Bacterial Ion Channels and Their Eukaryotic Homologs* (eds A Kubalski, B Martinac). ASM Press, Washington, DC, pp. 291–312.

26. Pivetti D, Yen MR, Miller S, *et al*. Two families of mechanosensitive channel proteins. *Microbiol Mol Biol Rev* 2003;**67**:66–85, table of contents.

27. Balleza D, Gomez-Lagunas F. Conserved motifs in mechanosensitive channels MscL and MscS. *Eur Biophys J Biophys Lett* 2009;**38**: 1013–1027.

28. Martinac B, Saimi Y, Kung C. Ion channels in microbes. *Physiol Rev* 2008;**88**:1449–1490.

29. Eckert R. Bioelectric control of ciliary activity. *Science* 1972;**176**: 473–481.

30. Naitoh Y, Eckert R. Ionic mechanisms controlling behavioral responses of paramecium to mechanical stimulation. *Science* 1969;**164**:963–965.

31. Martinac B, Hildebrand E. Electrically induced Ca^{2+} transport across the membrane of *Paramecium caudatum* measured by means of flow-through technique. *Biochim Biophys Acta* 1981;**649**:244–252.

32. Jennings HS. (1906) *Behavior of Lower Organisms*. Indiana University Press, Bloomington.

33. Naitoh Y, Eckert R. Sensory mechanisms in paramecium. II. Ionic basis of the hyperpolarizing mechanoreceptor potential. *J Exp Biol* 1973;**59**:53–65.

34. Machemer H, Ogura A. Ionic conductances of membranes in ciliated and deciliated *Paramecium*. *J Physiol* 1979;**296**:49–60.

35. Ogura A, Machemer H. Distribution of mechanoreceptor channels in the *Paramecium* surface membrane. *J Comp Physiol A* 1980;**135**:233–242.

36. Zhou XL, Kung C. A mechanosensitive ion channel in *Schizosaccharomyces pombe*. *EMBO J* 1992;**11**:2869–2875.

37. Zhou XL, Stumpf MA, Hoch HC, Kung C. A mechanosensitive channel in whole cells and in membrane patches of the fungus *Uromyces*. *Science* 1991;**253**:1415–1417.

38. Saimi Y, Zhou XL, Loukin SH, Haynes WJ, Kung C. (2007) Microbial TRP channels and their mechanosensitivity. In: *Mechanosensitive Ion Channels*, Part A (ed OP Hamill). Academic Press, Amsterdam, pp. 311–327.

39. Denis V, Cyert MS. Internal Ca^{2+} release in yeast is triggered by hypertonic shock and mediated by a TRP channel homologue. *J Cell Biol* 2002;**156**:29–34.

40. Zhou XL, Loukin SH, Coria R, Kung C, Saimi Y. Heterologously expressed fungal transient receptor potential channels retain mechanosensitivity in vitro and osmotic response in vivo. *Eur Biophys J* 2005;**34**:413–422.

41. Pickard BG. (2007) Delivering force and amplifying signals in plant mechanosensing. In: *Mechanosensitive Ion Channels*, Part A (ed O P Hamill). Academic Press, Amsterdam, pp. 361–392.

42. Haswell ES. (2007) MscS-like proteins in plants. In: *Mechanosensitive Ion Channels*, Part A (ed OP Hamill). Academic Press, Amsterdam, pp. 329–359.

43. Nozaki H. A new scenario of plastid evolution: plastid primary endosymbiosis before the divergence of the "Plantae," emended. *J Plant Res* 2005;**118**:247–255.

44. Chalfie M, Au M. Genetic control of differentiation of the *Caenorhabditis elegans* touch receptor neurons. *Science* 1989;**243**: 1027–1033.

45. Goodman MB, Schwarz EM. Transducing touch in *Caenorhabditis elegans*. *Annu Rev Physiol* 2003;**65**:429–452.

46. Kellenberger S, Schild L. Epithelial sodium channel/degenerin family of ion channels: a variety of functions for a shared structure. *Physiol Rev* 2002;**82**:735–767.

47. Canessa CM, Schild L, Buell G, *et al*. Amiloride-sensitive epithelial Na^+ channel is made of three homologous subunits. *Nature* 1994;**367**: 463–467.

48. Jernigan NL, Drummond HA. Myogenic vasoconstriction in mouse renal interlobar arteries: role of endogenous beta and gammaENaC. *Am J Physiol* 2006;**291**:F1184–F1191.

49. Lesage F, Lazdunski M. Molecular and functional properties of two-pore-domain potassium channels. *Am J Physiol* 2000;**279**: F793–F801.

50. Blondeau N, Petrault O, Manta S, *et al.* Polyunsaturated fatty acids are cerebral vasodilators via the TREK-1 potassium channel. *Circ Res* 2007;**101**:176–184.

51. Maingret F, Honore E, Lazdunski M, Patel AJ. Molecular basis of the voltage-dependent gating of TREK-1, a mechano-sensitive K$^+$ channel. *Biochem Biophys Res Commun* 2002;**292**:339–346.

52. Medhurst AD, Rennie G, Chapman CG, *et al.* Distribution analysis of human two pore domain potassium channels in tissues of the central nervous system and periphery. *Brain Res Mol Brain Res* 2001;**86**: 101–114.

53. Kim Y, Gnatenco C, Bang H, Kim D. Localization of TREK-2 K$^+$ channel domains that regulate channel kinetics and sensitivity to pressure, fatty acids and pHi. *Pflugers Arch* 2001;**442**:952–960.

54. Kim Y, Bang H, Gnatenco C, Kim D. Synergistic interaction and the role of C-terminus in the activation of TRAAK K$^+$ channels by pressure, free fatty acids and alkali. *Pflugers Arch* 2001;**442**:64–72.

55. Cosens DJ, Manning A. Abnormal electroretinogram from a *Drosophila* mutant. *Nature* 1969;**224**:285–287.

56. Pedersen SF, Nilius B. Transient receptor potential channels in mechanosensing and cell volume regulation. *Meth Enzymol* 2007;**428**:183–207.

57. Beech DJ. TRPC1: store-operated channel and more. *Pflugers Arch* 2005;**451**:53–60.

58. Maroto R, Raso A, Wood TG, Kurosky A, Martinac B, Hamill OP. TRPC1 forms the stretch-activated cation channel in vertebrate cells. *Nat Cell Biol* 2005;**7**:179–185.

59. Chachisvilis M, Zhang YL, Frangos JA. G protein-coupled receptors sense fluid shear stress in endothelial cells. *Proc Natl Acad Sci USA* 2006;**103**:15463–15468.

60. Hofmann T, Schaefer M, Schultz G, Gudermann T. Cloning, expression and subcellular localization of two novel splice variants of mouse transient receptor potential channel 2. *Biochem J* 2000;**351**: 115–122.

61. Welsh DG, Morielli AD, Nelson MT, Brayden JE. Transient receptor potential channels regulate myogenic tone of resistance arteries. *Circ Res* 2002;**90**:248–250.

62. Davis JB, Gray J, Gunthorpe MJ, *et al.* Vanilloid receptor-1 is essential for inflammatory thermal hyperalgesia. *Nature* 2000;**405**:183–187.

63. Gibson HE, Edwards JG, Page RS, Van Hook MJ, Kauer JA. TRPV1 channels mediate long-term depression at synapses on hippocampal interneurons. *Neuron* 2008;**57**:746–759.

64. Sharif-Naeini R, Ciura S, Zhang Z, Bourque CW. Contribution of TRPV channels to osmosensory transduction, thirst, vasopressin release. *Kidney Int* 2008;**73**:811–815.

65. Caterina M, Rosen TA, Tominaga M, Brake AJ, Julius D. A capsaicin-receptor homologue with a high threshold for noxious heat. *Nature* 1999;**398**:436–441.

66. Muraki K, Iwata Y, Katanosaka Y, *et al.* TRPV2 is a component of osmotically sensitive cation channels in murine aortic myocytes. *Circ Res* 2003;**93**:829–838.

67. Strotmann R, Harteneck C, Nunnenmacher K, Schultz G, Plant TD. OTRPC4, a nonselective cation channel that confers sensitivity to extracellular osmolarity. *Nat Cell Biol* 2000;**2**:695–702.

68. Cohen DM. TRPV4 and the mammalian kidney. *Pflugers Arch* 2005;**451**:168–175.

69. Harteneck C, Reiter B. TRP channels activated by extracellular hypo-osmoticity in epithelia. *Biochem Soc Trans* 2007;**35**:91–95.

70. Grimm C, Kraft R, Schultz G, Harteneck C. Activation of the melastatin-related cation channel TRPM3 by D-erythro-sphingosine [corrected]. *Mol Pharmacol* 2005;**67**:798–805.

71. Earley S, Waldron BJ, Brayden JE. Critical role for transient receptor potential channel TRPM4 in myogenic constriction of cerebral arteries. *Circ Res* 2004;**95**:922–929.

72. Morita H, Honda A, Inoue R, *et al.* Membrane stretch-induced activation of a TRPM4-like nonselective cation channel in cerebral artery myocytes. *J Pharmacol Sci* 2007;**103**:417–426.

73. Runnels LW, Yue L, Clapham DE. TRP-PLIK, a bifunctional protein with kinase and ion channel activities. *Science* 2001;**291**:1043–1047.

74. Numata, T, Shimizu T, Okada Y. Direct mechano-stress sensitivity of TRPM7 channel. *Cell Physiol Biochem* 2007;**19**:1–8.

75. Nauli SM, Alenghat FJ, Luo Y, *et al.* Polycystins 1 and 2 mediate mechanosensation in the primary cilium of kidney cells. *Nat Genet* 2003;**33**:129–137.

76. Garcia-Anoveros, J, Nagata K. TRPA1. *Handb Exp Pharmacol* 2007;**179**:347–362.

77. Corey DP, Garcia-Anoveros J, Holt JR, *et al.* TRPA1 is a candidate for the mechanosensitive transduction channel of vertebrate hair cells. *Nature* 2004;**432**:723–730.

78. Cull-Candy S, Brickley S, Farrant M. NMDA receptor subunits: diversity, development and disease. *Curr Opin Neurobiol* 2001;**11**:327–335.

79. Casado M, Ascher P. Opposite modulation of NMDA receptors by lysophospholipids and arachidonic acid: common features with mechanosensitivity. *J Physiol* 1998;**513**(Pt 2):317–330.

80. Kloda A, Lua L, Hall R, Adams DJ, Martinac B. Liposome reconstitution and modulation of recombinant N-methyl-D-aspartate receptor channels by membrane stretch. *Proc Natl Acad Sci USA* 2007;**104**:1540–1545.

81. Drummond HA, Abboud FM, Welsh MJ. Localization of beta and gamma subunits of ENaC in sensory nerve endings in the rat foot pad. *Brain Res* 2000;**884**:1–12.

82. Oh YS, Warnock DG. Disorders of the epithelial Na$^+$ channel in Liddle's syndrome and autosomal recessive pseudohypoaldosteronism type 1. *Exp Nephrol* 2000;**8**:320-325.

83. Garry A, Fromy B, Blondeau N, *et al.* Altered acetylcholine, bradykinin and cutaneous pressure-induced vasodilation in mice lacking the TREK1 potassium channel: the endothelial link. *EMBO Rep* 2007;**8**:354–359.

84. Dietrich A, Mederos YSM, Gollasch M, *et al.* Increased vascular smooth muscle contractility in TRPC6–/– mice. *Mol Cell Biol* 2005;**25**:6980–6989.

85. Steinbacher S, Bass R, Strop P, Rees DC. (2007) Structures of the prokaryotic mechanosensitive channels MscL and MscS. In: *Mechanosensitive Ion Channels*, Part A. Elsevier/Academic Press, San Diego, pp. 1–24.

86. Martinac B, Kloda A. Evolutionary origins of mechanosensitive ion channels. *Prog Biophys Mol Biol* 2003;**82**:11–24.

87. Folgering JH, Sharif-Naeini R, Dedman A, Patel A, Delmas P, Honore E. Molecular basis of the mammalian pressure-sensitive ion channels: focus on vascular mechanotransduction. *Prog Biophys Mol Biol* 2008;**97**:180–195.

Stretch-activated channels in the heart

Frederick Sachs

Background

Mechano-sensitive channels (MSC) or stretch-activated channels (SAC) have gating rates sensitive to mechanical stress in their environment. That environment may include the lipid bilayer, the cytoskeleton and the extracellular matrix. Bacterial SAC are the only SAC that have been reconstituted in artificial lipid membranes so that their relevant stimulus can only be tension in the lipid bilayer[1,2]. Eukaryotic SAC seem to occur in two classes: those associated with specialized receptors, such as the cochlea, muscle spindles and Pacinian corpuscles, and those in all other cells. SAC have been reported in all cells tested, ranging from red blood cells[3] to epithelium, nerve and muscle[4–6]. This chapter focuses on cationic stretch-activated channels (SAC_{NS}) seen in cells not specialized for sensory transduction, notably the heart[7].

At the molecular level, all structures change with mechanical stress and whether that produces a physiological effect depends on the magnitude of the stress and the compliance of the physical structure. This sensitivity is the core of molecular dynamic simulations in which the conformation of molecules is calculated as they are deformed by forces arising from gradients in mechanical, chemical, electrical and thermal energy. This sensitivity can show up as modulation of the gating rates of channels that have been classified as voltage dependent (see Chapter 6) or ligand-gated channel or volume-activated channels (VAC) (see Chapter 4). I will focus on those SAC that can be driven over their full dynamic range by physiological levels of mechanical stress. A 'typical' SAC_{NS} record is shown in Fig. 2.1 taken from a cell-attached patch on a chick heart cell. The patch was stretched with a pulse of pipette suction. The figure illustrates several common features for cation non-selective SAC: (1) there are not many of them active in a patch; typical densities appear in the order of $1/\mu m^2$ and the area of inside-out and cell-attached patches tends to be in the order of $10–20~\mu m^{2(8,9)}$; (2) the gating rates may be voltage dependent; and (3) the channels can inactivate. In what follows I will be interspersing data on heart with data from other systems since there is a shortage of cardiac SAC data.

A critical factor that distinguishes the study of SAC from other channels is that the local stimulus, the one that the channel is actually exposed to, is not tightly controlled[10]. When one applies suction to a patch, stress is transferred to the bilayer, the cytoskeleton,

the glass of the pipette and probably the extracellular matrix since the patch is not a lipid bilayer. If stress in any one of those components changes over time, so does the stimulus. For example, we can ask whether the inactivation shown in Fig. 2.1 represents a property of the channels or transfer of stress from one component of the patch to another. At the present time there are no data to suggest that stress in the fibrous proteins of the cytoskeleton directly applies stress to the channels [but see[11]], so for simplicity we will assume that the gating stress is transmitted through the bilayer as occurs in bacterial MSC. However, the reader must remember that this is an assumption.

Even if the stress that a channel is exposed to arrives from the bilayer, that stress can be manipulated by the cytoskeleton and by phase separations of lipid/lipid or protein/lipid [cf[12–14]]. For example, the cartoon of Fig. 2.2 illustrates one way in which membrane-bound cytoskeletal corrals[15] can affect lipid tension. Bear in mind that any drugs that affect the cytoskeleton are also likely to affect lipid tension and channels embedded within.

Amphipaths can affect SAC gating in a number of ways[16]: they dissolve in the lipid and change the local stress on the channel[17], they can change the thickness of the bilayer relative to the channel favouring closed or open states[18], they can expand the membrane

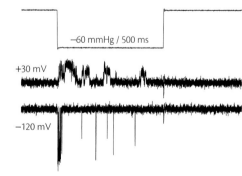

Fig. 2.1 Currents from a cationic SAC_{NS} from a cell-attached patch of a chick heart cell. The channels were stimulated by suction in the pipette, as shown in the top trace. The activity is shown at two membrane potentials and the data illustrate that the channels inactivate with time and voltage.

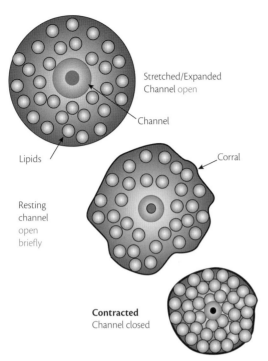

Fig. 2.2 Cartoon showing how a cytoskeletal corral containing a channel can compress and close the channel or expand and open it. Opening can be caused by external tension or only by expansion or contraction of the corral, say by a drug.

against a corral causing it to close, or they could expand the corral favouring the open state. The ability of amphipathic drugs to alter SAC kinetics was emphasized by work from Andersen's laboratory in which they showed that genistein, a commonly used kinase inhibitor, affects gramicidin channel gating in a planar bilayer even though there were no kinases or kinase substrates[19]. SAC are notoriously sensitive to multiple inputs[20] (see Chapter 3).

In addition to channels that are directly sensitive to mechanical stress, there are VAC activated by increased cell volume (see Chapter 4). It is not known whether these channels are mechanically sensitive themselves or may be activated by one of the many secondary processes that accompany swelling such as elevated Ca^{2+} and the drop in ionic strength (see Chapter 4).

Many channels with previously characterized non-mechanical gating properties have been shown to be mechano-sensitive. These channels include *Shaker*, voltage-dependent calcium and sodium channels (see Chapter 6), cyclic adenosine monophosphate (cAMP)[21], N-methyl-D-aspartic acid (NMDA) channels[22] and the antibiotic alamethicin[23]. Some channels, such as the nicotinic acetylcholine receptor, are not very mechano-sensitive.

There are no direct data on the stretch sensitivity of channels in organelles, but indirect data[24,25] suggest that these may exist, and that Ca^{2+} release channels are particularly significant candidates. Transporters may be stretch sensitive. Recent papers have suggested that stretch activates the Na/H exchanger elevating cell Na and thus Ca^{2+} via the Na/Ca^{2+} exchanger[26–28] (see Chapter 5 for details).

Structure

There is no generic molecular structure associated with SAC. The only eukaryotic SAC that have been cloned and reconstituted are

those of the K+ selective TREK-1 family (see Chapter 3) and a Ca^{2+} activated K+ channel from chick heart[29]. The channels that produce the commonly observed SAC_{NS} currents have not yet been cloned so we do not know if they are homomers or heteromers. The lack of homology between SAC has been most accurately demonstrated in *Escherichia coli* (see section 'Mechano-sensitive channels of prokaryotes' in Chapter 1), where the two most common SAC have no significant sequence homology and one channel is a pentamer while the other is a heptamer[30,31]. Site-directed spin labelling and crosslinking studies have shown that the larger conductance MSC in *E. coli* (MscL) tends to open like an iris; the alpha helices of the trans-membrane segments tilt and flatten, making the channel larger in diameter and thinner[32,33], as expected from the Poisson ratio for solid mechanics.

Evolution

SAC developed early in living cells[34] (see Chapter 1). They are found in bacteria, *Archaea*, fungi, higher plants and animals[35,36]. This primitive evolutionary origin in cells with cell walls probably reflects the need to solve a universal problem: osmotic regulation.

We have found that cationic SAC (VAC) generally do not open with osmotic swelling and thus are not universal volume sensors. Cell volume is determined by the cytoskeleton in nucleated animal cells and not the membrane (see Chapter 60). This is rather clear from the fact that cells challenged with a hypotonic stress are not spherical; the stress is contained primarily in the cytoskeleton. The evolutionary divergence of animal cells from plant cells was successful when the animal cell utilized the cytoskeleton to bear the osmotic strain rather than utilizing a rigid cell wall.

What makes channels mechanically sensitive?

Mechanical sensitivity of a channel arises from a significant change in channel dimensions between the closed and open states. Open SAC are bigger (in the plane of the membrane) than closed SAC. This 'size' does not refer to the diameter of the pore but to the outer physical dimensions where the protein meets the lipid that bears the tension. At tension T, the energy difference between the open and closed states is $\Delta G = T * \Delta A$, where ΔA is the difference in planar area between the closed and open states. There may also be secondary energy terms arising from thinning of the channel as it enlarges in circumference[32]. In addition to bilayer tension, there may also be local effects of curvature that can be modified by amphipaths[32].

The most extensive study on SAC kinetics was done with TREK-1[6] (see also Chapter 3). In that study, adhesion of the membrane to the glass of the pipette, the bond required to form the 'gigaseal', applies a resting tension to all patches on the order of the lytic strength of the membrane[8]. One must always consider the role of resting stress in studies of SAC. The presence of resting stress in a patch prevents a comparison with channel activity in a resting cell. The study with TREK also showed that wrinkling of the patch did not open the channels, so that micron-scale bending adds negligible energy to the opening process[16].

The dimensional changes required to produce SAC activation are minute. Quantitative analysis of the kinetics indicated that if the channel were a cylinder 5 nm in diameter, the entire stretch sensitivity could be accounted for if the closed and open diameters differed by only 2 Å (Angstroms).

What is membrane tension and how is tension generated?

Although tension sounds like a simple concept, the cell cortex is not mechanically homogeneous and the definition of 'membrane' tension becomes obscure. A homogeneous lipid bilayer is the simplest membrane and at equilibrium it has no gradients of tension. However, the lipid bilayer is not homogeneous (lipid phases, rafts, etc.). The cytoskeleton supports the bilayer by adding a binding energy to the lipids. It also supports static and time-dependent shear stresses in three dimensions (see Chapter 8).

The extracellular matrix is another component of the cell cortex that is likely to have an effect on membrane mechanics, but we do not yet know the magnitude of its contribution. However, the connective tissue outside cells clearly has a strong influence on the stress in the cortex where the channels are located. While the cytoskeleton is probably not explicitly required for mechanical sensitivity, it cannot be dismissed in animal cells. In what follows, I will use the term 'membrane tension' in its most crude form: some kind of average tension in the cell cortex. The recent development of stress-sensitive probes for the cytoskeleton will now begin to let us dissect the stress in individual proteins[37] (see Chapter 60).

In most quantitative experiments, tension is changed in a patch pipette by applying hydrostatic pressure (suction) to the inside of the pipette[10]. This causes the membrane to bulge and the tension to increase. However, SAC are not sensitive to the applied pressure[38] *per se*, they are sensitive to the tension. According to Laplace's law, the tension T in a patch of uniform curvature (a spherical cap) is proportional to $Pr/2$, where p is the *trans-membrane* pressure and r is the radius of curvature. With patch pipettes, SAC tend to be open significantly at pipette pressures in the range of −25 to −50 mmHg or −3,000 to −6,000 Pa [note that for elastic membranes, the tension is non-linearly related to the pressure[36]]. The formulation of membrane tension using Laplace's law ignores the effects of the membrane bending stiffness and the presence of the cytoskeleton.

Table 2.1 provides an illustration of the interrelation between several commonly used pressure and tension units. A useful reference value is that the lytic tension of a lipid bilayer, or a red blood cell, is in the region of 10 dyne/cm or 10 mN/m.

Limitations of patch measurements of SAC

Membrane patches cannot be formed within a pipette without a massive reorganization of the cell cortex [8,10,39,40], and there is a substantial resting tension due to adhesion of the membrane to

the glass[8,23]. These factors beg the question of whether patch currents can be used to judge the SAC' contribution to the resting conductance of a cell *in situ*. That question can be answered using whole cell recordings with specific pharmacologic SAC blockers such as *Grammostola spatulata* mechano-toxin 4 (GsMTx4)[41].

The absolute calibration of tension in a patch is difficult and rarely performed. Calculating the tension requires knowledge of patch geometry and the stress-strain properties of the membrane. Furthermore, the applied pressure is usually not accurately calibrated or recorded. A requisite initialization is to compensate for the negative pressure produced by the meniscus of the solution–capillary interface at the upper end of a patch pipette. The best calibration is to offset that negative pressure with a slight positive pressure that will eliminate fluid flow into the open pipette tip (including movement of debris present in the dish). (Note: planar bilayers cannot be used for stressing SAC. There is excess lipid at the partition, and capillary forces holding the bilayer to the partition will maintain a constant tension regardless of the trans-membrane pressure.)

Channel density

Most patch recordings show the activity of only a few SAC, suggesting a density of $\sim 1/\mu m^2$. There are no known tissues with a much higher density, including the cochlear hair cells. In any case, patch clamp is not a reliable tool to measure channel density since the area that is sampled is small and not representative of the whole cell[8]. For example, in adult striated muscle (including cardiac muscle), SAC may be located in the t-tubules, where they are not accessible to a pipette[42], 'hidden' in caveolae (see Chapter 7), or even located in intracellular membrane compartments[43] (see Chapter 5). Furthermore, channel proteins may preferentially attach to the glass walls of the pipette and then not appear in the membrane cap that spans the pipette[8,39].

Stimuli

Attention to stimulus detail is important when attempting to compare experiments on SAC. As opposed to voltage- or ligand-gated channels, mechanical channels have no trustworthy whole-cell current counterparts since uniform stress cannot be applied to a cell. Osmotic stress is commonly labeled a 'mechanical' stimulus, and perhaps in some cases it is, but the effects are very different from the effects of direct stress[44]. Hu and Sachs showed that in chick heart cells, direct mechanical stress activated a cation conductance, while osmotic stress activated an anion conductance[45]. Similarly, Kohl's group reported that stretching sinus node cells of the rabbit increases the spontaneous pacemaking rate, but swelling decreases it[46,47] (see Chapter 13).

Voltage clamp is the most accurate method to study channel currents, but it is difficult to voltage clamp and stretch cells. Pulling on isolated heart cells is particularly tedious because the force probes tend either to not stick or to damage the cells. In addition, the process of isolating cells with proteolytic enzymes removes the extracellular connections that normally transmit forces to cells. Recent work using graphite micro rods as levers attached to the surface of isolated cells to apply and measure force[43] has been reasonably successful in stretching isolated cells, but it avoids the question as to whether those forces are applied to physiologically relevant sites.

Table 2.1 Common units for pressure, and the tension (T) in a patch with a 1 μm radius of curvature.

Atm	mmHg	Pa	cm H$_2$O	T (mN/m)
1.00	760	101,325	1,033	200
0.06	50	6,666	68	13

Properties of cation non-selective SAC in the heart

As mentioned previously, there is no simple sequence homology between different SAC. There can be multiple types of mechanical channels in single cells, much as there are many types of voltage-gated channels in a cell. In early embryonic chick heart cells, for example, there are at least five different SAC, and their relative proportion changes during development[48]. In young embryos (7 days old), there are multiple SAC_{NS}, as well as K^+ selective SAC (SAC_K). One SAC_K appears to be a maxiK channel[49]. As the embryos get older (~17 days), cells express only two channel types: the high conductance (90 pS) SAC_K and a lower conductance (20 pS) SAC_{NS}[45]. Developmental changes in SAC distribution are undoubtedly present in the mammalian heart as well.

There is at least one successful experiment demonstrating SAC in fetal ventricular cells[50]. However, there are no published experiments showing single channel recordings of SAC in adult ventricular cardiomyocytes. This dearth of data on adult heart muscle cells fits the hypothesis that adult SAC are preferentially located in t-tubules[42]. In neonatal cells or cells in culture, the t-tubules are not fully developed, and hence the channels are accessible to a patch-clamp pipette.

A deliberate search for SAC in rat atria found only K^+ selective channels (probably of the 2P domain family) (see Chapter 3). This finding is also compatible with the t-tubule hypothesis since atrial cells have few, if any, t-tubules.

Permeation properties

As expected from other K^+ channels, SAC_K are highly selective for K^+ over other cations and their conductances are relatively large. For example, the conductance of TREK-1 is ~50 pS in symmetric K^+ salines. The channel displays a strong mean outward rectification that results from external Mg^{2+} block and from an intrinsic voltage-dependent gating. In chick heart, SAC_{NS} conductances are ~ 25 and 50 pS, while those of SAC_K are ~100 and 200 pS[48]. These numbers obviously depend upon the permeant ion species and are provided only as rough guidelines.

Time-dependent behaviour of SAC

In general, SAC responses inactivate with time, although they have mostly been studied with constant stimuli. In the extreme case of steady state stimulation, there may be no response because the channels are fully deactivated.

In the heart, the only dynamic properties of single channels came from atrial SAC_K channels[52]. There are dynamic whole-cell recordings of mechano-sensitive currents from rat and chick heart. In the study by Zeng et al. on rat ventricular cells[42], the stretch-sensitive currents did not show much inactivation. However, in studies by Bett and Sachs[51] and Hu and Sachs[45] on chick cells, inactivation was common. In the adult rat heart cells, studied by Bett and Sachs[51], mechanical stimuli evoked two different responses (Fig. 2.3).

Initially, the cells were insensitive to mechanical stimulation. Deformation produced no current. However, if the cell was repeatedly stimulated, responsiveness suddenly appeared as though a mechano-protective support had broken (Fig. 2.3). This endogenous protection of SAC in the resting cell is important when comparing studies of different cells or tissues, or even comparing results

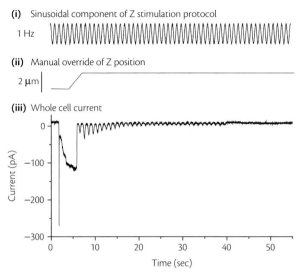

Fig. 2.3 Prolonged stimulation exposes mechano-sensitivity in rat ventricular cells. An isolated cell was squeezed sinusoidally against a coverslip using the side of a patch pipette (2 μm, 2 Hz) while recording the whole cell current. After 1–2 min of continuous stimulation, ending about 2 s into the above record, a spike of inward current appeared, followed by a sustained inward current (apparently the saturated value of the mechano-sensitive current). The mean position of the stimulation pipette was then lifted 2 μm, and the cell began to respond in phase with the stimulus and then inactivated. [Reproduced, with permission, from Bett GCL and Sachs F (2000) Whole-cell mechanosensitive currents in rat ventricular myocytes activated by direct stimulation. *J Membr Biol* **173**: 255–263.]

of a single preparation at different times. The observed mechanical sensitivity can depend upon the history of stimulation, and probably on the metabolic history as well. Single cell data suggest that chronic stretching should be more effective in exposing large electrophysiological effects than short-term stimulation. Stretch may cause the fusion of vesicles with the plasmalemma, changing the local stress, and perhaps delivering new channels to the surface (cf Chapter 7).

Resting activity

Possibly the most precise measurements to date of specificity and background current used whole cell currents with a permeabilized patch clamp of isolated rabbit atrial cells (Fig. 2.4). The peptide SAC-blocker grammostola spatulata mechano-toxin 4 (GsMTx-4)[41] had no effect on the action potential (AP), suggesting that under mechanically unloaded auxotonic conditions, there is little resting SAC activity and that other ion channels are unaffected by the blocker[53]. Consistent with this result, in the intact heart monophasic action potential (MAP) recordings showed that GsMTx-4 had little effect on the AP when the heart was mechanically unloaded[54], but in resting dystrophic muscle GsMTx4 decreased Ca^{2+} sparks[55] and sensitivity to extracellular Ca^{2+}[56].

Pharmacology of SAC

Given the wide variety of SAC, it is not surprising that there is no universal 'blocker'. However, the most general pharmacologic effectors are non-specific lanthanides, notably Gd^{3+} and La^{3+}[57]. Gd^{3+} sensitivity, while often used as a signature of SAC channels, is

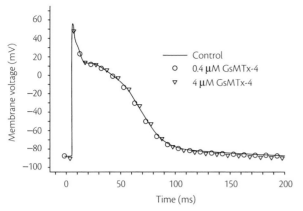

Fig. 2.4 Action potentials recorded from isolated rabbit atrial cells are unaffected by concentrations of GsMTx-4 that are ~10× the *in vitro* dissociation constant, K_d.

not reliable since it has significant reactivity with other channels. In addition, Gd^{3+} will readily precipitate many physiological anions including PO_4, HCO_3 and proteins[58], so it cannot be used in physiological conditions. The active form of Gd^{3+} is not known (e.g. a hydrate, an anionic salt) and Gd^{3+} has valences of $^+2$ or $^+3$. While there have been reports of Gd^{3+} effects when it was administered in bicarbonate buffered solutions or blood[59], the origin of these effects is not clear. (Note: in Gd^{3+} based MRI contrast agents, the Gd^{+3} is chelated, not free.)

Amiloride[57] and cationic antibiotics such as streptomycin have been used to block SAC_{NS}[60], but again, these agents are not specific for SAC. SAC may also be sensitive to 'specific' ion channel reagents such as tetrodotoxin (TTX) and diltiazem[48].

Amphiphilic compounds such as aracidonic acid, chlorpromazine and general anaesthetics can affect SAC[32] (see Chapter 3). They appear to act by changing local membrane curvature allowing SAC to be activated (or inactivated) in the absence of global changes in membrane tension. However, the sensitivity of SAC to amphipaths makes them vulnerable to modulation by amphiphilic members of the signal transduction pathways, such as inositol phosphates and lysolipids.

The discovery of GsMTx-4, a specific inhibitory peptide, isolated from tarantula venom[41,61–63] and now commercially available, has provided an important new tool to study SAC effects in cellular and multicellular preparations. This peptide blocks SAC in a number of cells including chick heart, rat heart and astrocytes and rabbit, sheep and dog ventricular cells. It is capable of blocking the mechanical augmentation of burst-pacing induced atrial fibrillation in rabbit heart at less than 200 nM[54]. GsMTx-4 seems remarkably specific, with no significant effects found thus far with other channels. For example, Fig. 2.4 shows action potentials from an isolated rabbit atrial cell exposed to GsMTx-4 at doses up to eight times that required to block SAC in rat astrocytes. The action potential is unaffected. Apparently GsMTx-4 affects none of the channels or transporters that generate the action potential. Recent results (Sachs *et al.*, unpublished) with implanted pumps in *mdx* mice with up to 5 mM GsMTx-4 solution administered over

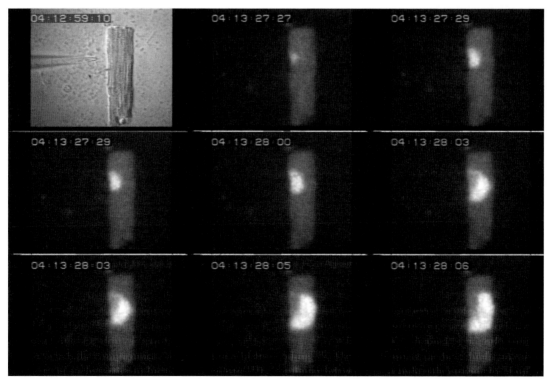

Fig. 2.5 Ca^{2+} waves induced in adult rat ventricular cells by gentle pressing with a fire-polished pipette. The cells were loaded with Fluo-3AM (the first frame is brightfield). The initiation of Ca^{2+} waves was blocked by the removal of extracellular Ca^{2+} or addition of Gd^{3+} to block SAC. The time code is h:min:s:frame.

42 days showed no toxic side effects even at the site of injection, although there was dose-dependent improvement in motor activity.

In a surprising observation, Clemo and Baumgarten found that **spontaneous depolarizations**[7,64], first reported by Nuss et al.[65], were blocked by GsMTx-4. Spontaneous depolarizations commonly occur in failing hearts and are distinguished from **delayed after-depolarizations** (DAD) by the effect of increased extracellular Ca^{2+}: DAD are potentiated and spontaneous depolarizations inhibited. Spontaneous depolarizations are not affected by the drugs that are commonly used to affect voltage-dependent channels. The origin of spontaneous depolarizations is not established, but their *de facto* sensitivity to GsMTx-4 suggests that they may be produced by SAC. We clearly have much to learn about the role of SAC in the heart and their potential roles as therapeutic targets (see Chapter 65).

Intracellular Ca^{2+} effects of SAC activation

Heart cells, like other cells[25], change their Ca^{2+} handling in response to mechanical stimulation. This effect is large enough to induce Ca^{2+} waves (Fig. 2.5),[7,66]. Iribe et al.[43] demonstrated an increase in Ca^{2+} spark rate from ryanodine receptors with mechanical stress, even in the presence of SAC blockers and in the absence of extracellular Na^+ and Ca^{2+}, so that there may be multiple mechano-sensitive sites for Ca^{2+} coupling.

As a final caveat to those new to mechano-electric coupling (MEC), there is another coupling pathway that probably does not involve SAC: auto- and paracrine activation of purinergic receptors. All cells release ATP upon mechanical stimulation, so that P2X and P2Y receptors may indirectly serve as mechanical transducers[67].

Conclusions and outlook

MEC translates variations in stress and strain, such as occurs during scarring and heterogeneity of relaxation, into changes of electrical activity. Electrical and mechanical heterogeneity is maximal during phase 3 when the chambers are still under systolic pressure. The pressure and larger radius create a high wall tension, making relaxed areas stretch and thereby activate SAC – a likely prelude to tachyarrhythmias[68].

The most likely rapidly responding transducers for MEC are SAC [although mechanical effects on Ca^{2+} binding are also rapid (cf Chapter 21)]. The mechano-sensitivity of cells seems not to be regulated by SAC expression density but by mechano-protection by the cytoskeleton and the extracellular matrix and by amphipaths such arachidonic acid[10]. Chronic remodelling of the heart must involve changes in mechano-sensitivity through cytoskeletal modifications and changes in gene transcription (cf Chapter 12).

The development of specific pharmacologic agents for SAC, such as GsMTx-4, should allow us to begin dissecting the contribution of SAC to cardiac function. They also represent a new class of antiarrhythmic drugs [cf Chapter 65 and[69]]. Interesting times are ahead.

References

1. Martinac B. Open channel structure of MscL: a patch-clamp and spectroscopic study. *Appl Magnet Reson* 2009;**36**:171–179.

2. Battle AR, Petrov E, Pal P, Martinac B. Rapid and improved reconstitution of bacterial mechanosensitive ion channel proteins MscS and MscL into liposomes using a modified sucrose method. *FEBS Letters* 2009;**583**:407–412.

3. Vandorpe DH, Xu C, Shmukler BE, Otterbein L, Trudel M, Sachs F, et al. Hypoxia activates a Ca^{2+}-permeable cation conductance sensitive to carbon monoxide and to GsMTx-4 in human and mouse sickle erythrocytes. *PLoS Biol* 2010;**5**:e8732.

4. Guharay F, Sachs F. Mechanotransducer ion channels in chick skeletal muscle: the effects of extracellular pH. *J Physiol* 1985;**353**:119–134.

5. Guharay F, Sachs F. Stretch-activated single ion channel currents in tissue-cultured embryonic chick skeletal muscle. *J Physiol* 1984;**352**:685–701.

6. Honore E, Patel AJ, Chemin J, Suchyna T, Sachs F. Desensitization of mechano-gated K-2P channels. *Proc Natl Acad Sci USA* 2006;**103**:6859–6864.

7. Sachs F, Jalife J, Zipes D. Heart mechanoelectric transduction. In: *Cardiac Electrophysiology: From Cell to Bedside*. Saunders (Elsevier), Philadelphia 2004; pp. 96–102.

8. Suchyna TM, Markin VS, Sachs F. Biophysics and structure of the patch and the gigaseal. *Biophys J* 2009;**97**:738–747.

9. Suchyna T, Sachs F. Dynamic regulation of mechanosensitive channels; capacitance used to monitor patch tension in real time. *Phys Biol* 2004;**1**:1–18.

10. Sachs F. Stretch activated ion channels; what are they? *Physiology* 2010;**25**:6.

11. Matthews BD, Thodeti CK, Ingber DE. Activation of mechanosensitive ion channels by forces transmitted through integrins and the cytoskeleton. In: *Mechanosensitive Ion Channels*, Part A Volume 58 (eds OP Hamill, SA Simon, DJ Benos). Elsevier/Academic Press, San Diego, 2007; pp. 59–85.

12. Apajalahti T, Niemela P, Govindan PN, et al. Concerted diffusion of lipids in raft-like membranes. *Faraday Discussions* 2010;**144**:411–430.

13. Raguz M, Widomska J, Dillon J, Gaillard ER, Subczynski WK. Physical properties of the lipid bilayer membrane made of cortical and nuclear bovine lens lipids: EPR spin-labeling studies. *Biochim Biophys Acta-Biomembr* 2009;**1788**:2380–2388.

14. Rawicz W, Smith BA, McIntosh TJ, Simon SA, Evans E. Elasticity, strength, and water permeability of bilayers that contain raft microdomain-forming lipids. *Biophys J* 2008;**94**:4725–4736.

15. Morone N, Nakada C, Umemura Y, Usukura J, Kusumi A. Three-dimensional molecular architecture of the plasma-membrane-associated cytoskeleton as reconstructed by freeze-etch electron tomography. In: *Introduction to Electron Microscopy for Biologists* (ed TD Allen). Elsevier/Academic Press, San Diego, 2008; pp. 207–236.

16. Markin VS, Sachs F. Thermodynamics of mechanosensitivity. *Phys Biol* 2004;**1**:110–124.

17. Andersen OS, Nielsen C, Maer AM, Lundbaek JA, Goulian M, Koeppe RE. Ion channels as tools to monitor lipid bilayer–membrane protein interactions: gramicidin channels as molecular force transducers. *Meth Enzymol* 1999;**294**:208–224.

18. Martinac B, Adler J, Kung C. Mechanosensitive ion channels of E. coli activated by amphipaths. *Nature* 1990;**348**:261–263.

19. Hwang TC, Koeppe RE, Andersen OS. Genistein can modulate channel function by a phosphorylation-independent mechanism: importance of hydrophobic mismatch and bilayer mechanics. *Biochemistry* 2003;**42**:13646–13658.

20. Chemin J, Patel AJ, Duprat F, Sachs F, Lazdunski M, Honore E. Up- and down-regulation of the mechano-gated K-2P channel TREK-1 by PIP2 and other membrane phospholipids. *Pflugers Arch* 2007;**455**:97–103.

21. Vandorpe DH, Morris CE. Stretch activation of the Aplysia S-channel. *J Membr Biol* 1992;**127**:205–214.

22. Paoletti P, Ascher P. Mechanosensitivity of NMDA receptors in cultured mouse central neurons. *Neuron* 1994;**13**:645–655.

23. Opsahl LR, Webb WW. Lipid–glass adhesion in giga-sealed patch-clamped membranes. *Biophys J* 1994;**66**:75–79.

24. Kondratev D, Gallitelli MF. Increments in the concentrations of sodium and calcium in cell compartments of stretched mouse ventricular myocytes. *Cell Calcium* 2003;**34**:193–203.

25. Niggel J, Sigurdson W, Sachs F. Mechanically induced calcium movements in astrocytes, bovine aortic endothelial cells and C6 glioma cells. *J Membr Biol* 2000;**174**:121–134.

26. Baartscheer A, Schumacher CA, van Borren MMGJ, Belterman CN, Coronel R, Fiolet JWT. Increased Na$^+$/H$^+$-exchange activity is the cause of increased [Na$^+$]$_{(i)}$ and underlies disturbed calcium handling in the rabbit pressure and volume overload heart failure model. *Cardiovasc Res* 2003;**57**:1015–1024.

27. Cingolani HE, Perez MG, Pieske B, von Lewinski D, de Hurtado MCC. Stretch-elicited Na$^+$/H$^+$ exchanger activation: the autocrine/paracrine loop and its mechanical counterpart. *Cardiovasc Res* 2003;**57**:953–960.

28. von Lewinski D, Stumme B, Maier LS, Luers C, Bers DM, Pieske B. Stretch-dependent slow force response in isolated rabbit myocardium is Na$^+$ dependent. *Cardiovasc Res* 2003;**57**:1052–1061.

29. Tang QY, Qi Z, Naruse K, Sokabe M. Characterization of a functionally expressed stretch-activated BKca channel cloned from chick ventricular myocytes. *J Membr Biol* 2003;**196**:185–200.

30. Bass RB, Strop P, Barclay M, Rees DC. Crystal structure of *Escherichia coli* MscS, a voltage-modulated and mechanosensitive channel. *Science* 2002;**298**:1582–1587.

31. Chang G, Spencer RH, Lee AT, Barclay MT, Rees DC. Structure of the MscL homolog from *Mycobacterium tuberculosis*: a gated mechanosensitive ion channel. *Science* 1998;**282**:2220–2226.

32. Perozo E, Kloda A, Cortes DM, Martinac B. Physical principles underlying the transduction of bilayer deformation forces during mechanosensitive channel gating. *Nature Struct Biol* 2002;**9**:696–703.

33. Betanzos M, Chiang CS, Guy HR, Sukharev S. A large iris-like expansion of a mechanosensitive channel protein induced by membrane tension. *Nature Struct Biol* 2002;**9**:704–710.

34. Martinac B, Kloda A. Evolutionary origins of mechanosensitive ion channels. *Prog Biophys Mol Biol* 2003;**82**:11–24.

35. Hamill OP, Martinac B. Molecular basis of mechanotransduction in living cells. *Physiol Rev* 2001;**81**:685–740.

36. Sachs F, Morris CE. Mechanosensitive ion channels in nonspecialized cells. *Rev Physiol Biochem Pharmacol* 1998;**132**:1–77.

37. Meng F, Suchyna TM, Sachs F. A fluorescence energy transfer-based mechanical stress sensor for specific proteins in situ. *FEBS J* 2008;**275**:3072–3087.

38. Moe P, Blount P. Assessment of potential stimuli for mechano-dependent gating of MscL: effects of pressure, tension, and lipid headgroups. *Biochemistry* 2005;**44**:12239–12244.

39. Ruknudin A, Song MJ, Sachs F. The ultrastructure of patch-clamped membranes: a study using high voltage electron microscopy. *J Cell Biol* 1991;**112**:125–134.

40. Wan X, Juranka P, Morris CE. Activation of mechanosensitive currents in traumatized membrane. *Am J Physiol* 1999;**276**:C318–C327.

41. Bowman CL, Gottlieb PA, Suchyna TM, Murphy YK, Sachs F. Mechanosensitive ion channels and the peptide inhibitor GsMTx-4: history, properties, mechanisms and pharmacology. *Toxicon* 2007;**49**:249–270.

42. Zeng T, Bett GCL, Sachs F. Stretch-activated whole-cell currents in adult rat cardiac myocytes. *Am J Physiol* 2000;**278**:H548–H557.

43. Iribe G, Ward CW, Camelliti P, *et al.* Axial stretch of rat single ventricular cardiomyocytes causes an acute and transient increase in Ca^{2+} spark rate. *Circ Res* 2009;**104**:787–795.

44. Spagnoli C, Beyder A, Besch S, Sachs F. Atomic force microscopy analysis of cell volume regulation. *Phys Rev E Stat Nonlin Soft Matter Phys* 2008;**78**:031916.

45. Hu H, Sachs F. Single-channel and whole-cell studies of mechanosensitive currents in chick heart. *Biophys J* 1996;**70**:A347.

46. Cooper PJ, Lei M, Cheng LX, Kohl P. Selected contribution: axial stretch increases spontaneous pacemaker activity in rabbit isolated sinoatrial node cells. *J Appl Physiol* 2000;**89**:2099–2104.

47. Lei M, Kohl P. Swelling-induced decrease in spontaneous pacemaker activity of rabbit isolated sino-atrial node cells. *Acta Physiol Scand* 1998;**164**:1–12.

48. Ruknudin A, Sachs F, Bustamante JO. Stretch-activated ion channels in tissue-cultured chick heart. *Am J Physiol* 1993;**264**:H960–H972.

49. Naruse K, Tang Q, Zhi Q, Sokabe M. Cloning and functional expression of a stretch-activated BK channel (SAKCa) from chick embryonic cardiomyocyte. *Biophys J* 2003;**84**:234A.

50. Craelius W, Chen V, El-Sherif N. Stretch activated ion channels in ventricular myocytes. *Biosci Rep* 1988;**8**:407–414.

51. Bet, GCL, Sachs F. Whole-cell mechanosensitive currents in rat ventricular myocytes activated by direct stimulation. *J Membr Biol* 2000;**173**:255–263.

52. Niu W, Sachs F. Dynamic properties of stretch-activated K$^+$ channels in adult rat atrial myocytes. *Prog Biophys Mol Biol* 2003;**82**:121–135.

53. Jacques-Fricke BT, Seow YQ, Gottlieb PA, Sachs F, Gomez TM. Ca^{2+} influx through mechanosensitive channels inhibits neurite outgrowth in opposition to other influx pathways and release from intracellular stores. *J Neurosci* 2006;**26**:5656–5664.

54. Bode F, Sachs F, Franz MR. Tarantula peptide inhibits atrial fibrillation. *Nature* 2001;**409**:35–36.

55. Suchyna T, Sachs F. Mechanical and electrical properties of membranes from dystrophic and normal mouse muscle. *J Physiol* 2007;**581**:369–387.

56. Yeung EW, Whitehead NP, Suchyna TM, Gottlieb PA, Sachs F, Allen DG. Effects of stretch-activated channel blockers on [Ca^{2+}]$_i$ and muscle damage in the mdx mouse. *J Physiol* 2005;**562**:367–380.

57. Hamill OP, McBride DW. The pharmacology of mechanogated membrane ion channels. *Pharmacol Rev* 1996;**48**:231–252.

58. Caldwell RA, Clemo HF, Baumgarten CM. Using gadolinium to identify stretch-activated channels: technical considerations. *Am J Physiol* 1998;**275**:C619–C621.

59. Vaz R, Sarmento A, Borges N, Cruz C, Azevedo I. Effect of mechanogated membrane ion channel blockers on experimental traumatic brain oedema. *Acta Neurochir* 1998;**140**:371–375.

60. Belus A, White E. Streptomycin and intracellular calcium modulate the response of single guinea-pig ventricular myocytes to axial stretch. *J Physiol* 2003;**546**:501–509.

61. Oswald RE, Suchyna TM, McFeeters R, Gottlieb P, Sachs F. Solution structure of peptide toxins that block mechanosensitive ion channels. *J Biol Chem* 2002;**277**:34443–34450.

62. Suchyna TM, Johnson JH, Hamer K, Leykam JF, Gage DA, Clemo HF, *et al.* Identification of a peptide toxin from *Grammostola spatulata* spider venom that blocks cation-selective stretch-activated channels. *J Gen Physiol* 2001;**115**:583–598.

63. Sachs F. Stretch activated channels in the heart. In: *Cardiac Mechano-Electric Feedback and Arrhythmias: From Pipette to Patient* (eds P Kohl, F Sachs, MR Franz). Saunders (Elsevier), Philadelphia, 2004;2–10.

64. Clemo HF, Hackenbracht JM, Patel DG, Baumgarten CM. Swelling-activated cation current causes spontaneous depolarizations in failing ventricular myocytes. *Biophys J* 2002;**82**:270A–271A.

65. Nuss HB, Kaab S, Kass DA, Tomaselli GF, Marban E. Cellular basis of ventricular arrhythmias and abnormal automaticity in heart failure. *Am J Physiol* 1999;**277**:H80–H91.

66. Sigurdson W, Ruknudin A, Sachs F. Calcium imaging of mechanically induced fluxes in tissue-cultured chick heart: role of stretch-activated ion channels. *Am J Physiol* 1992;**262**:H1110–H1115.

67. Near JT, Kang Y, Willoughby KA, Ellis EF. Activation of extracellular signal-regulated kinase by stretch-induced injury in astrocytes involves extracellular ATP and P2 purinergic receptors. *J Neurosci* 2003;**23**:2348–2356.

68. Franz MR, Bode F Mechano-electrical feedback underlying arrhythmias: the atrial fibrillation case. *Prog Biophys Mol Biol* 2003;**82**:163–174.

69. White E. Mechanosensitive channels: therapeutic targets in the myocardium? *Curr Pharm Des* 2006;**12**:3645–3663.

3

The mechano-gated K_{2P} channel TREK-1 in the cardiovascular system

Eric Honoré and Amanda Patel

Background

The versatility of cellular electrical activity is highly conditioned by the expression of different structural and functional classes of hyperpolarizing K^+ channels. More than 80 genes encoding the main K^+ channel alpha subunits have been identified in the human genome. Two-pore domain K^+ channel subunits (K_{2P}) are made up of four trans-membrane segments and two pore-forming domains, which are arranged in tandem and function as either homo- or heterodimeric channels. This structural arrangement is associated with unusual gating and pharmacological properties including stretch sensitivity and activation by polyunsaturated fatty acids. The K_{2P} channel TREK-1 is present in cardiac and arterial myocytes, as well as in the endothelium.

In this chapter, we focus on the physiological role of the mechano-gated K_{2P} channel TREK-1 in the cardiovascular system and we discuss the polymodal regulation of this 'unconventional' K^+ channel by various physical and chemical stimuli.

Introduction

Mammalian K^+ channel subunits can contain two, four or six/seven trans-membrane segments. Members of the two and six/seven trans-membrane segment classes (inward rectifiers, voltage-gated and calcium-dependent K^+ channels, see below) are characterized by the presence of a single pore-forming domain, whereas the more recently discovered class of four trans-membrane segment subunits contain two pore-forming domains in tandem[1–5]. In K_{1P} channels, four matching pore-forming loops are assembled in a homo- or heterotetramer (all subunits have a similar pore-forming domain sequence GYG), whereas in the dimeric K_{2P} channels the P1 and P2 domains are different[6,7]. Many K_{2P} channels have a phenylalanine in the GXG motif (where X represents any amino acid) of the selectivity filter in the second pore domain, instead of a tyrosine as in K_{1P} channels[2,3,7]. This means that in K_{2P} channels the pore is predicted to have a twofold symmetry, rather than the classical fourfold arrangement of other K^+ channels. Although the selectivity of K_{2P} channels for K^+ over Na^+ is

high [permeability ratio (P_{Na}/P_K) < 0.03], these structural differences suggest more varied permeation and gating properties compared to K_{1P} channels[1,7]. Alternative splicing, heteromultimeric assembly, post-translational modification and interaction with auxiliary regulatory subunits further increase the molecular and functional diversity of K^+ channels.

The *Saccharomyces cerevisiae* outwardly rectifying K^+ channel TOK-1 channel (composed of eight trans-membrane segments) was the first K^+ channel discovered to contain two pore-forming domains in tandem[8–12]. Subsequently, K_{2P} subunits have been cloned in plants, *Drosophila melanogaster*, *Caenorhabditis elegans* and mammals[8,13–15]. The class of mammalian K_{2P} channel subunits now includes 15 members. Although these subunits display the same structural arrangement, with four trans-membrane segments, two pore-forming domains and an extended M1P1 extracellular loop with intracellular N and C termini, they share rather low sequence identity outside the pore-forming regions[1,16]. The K_{2P} channel subunits are subdivided into six main structural and functional classes: **t**andem of pore-forming domains in a **w**eak **i**nwardly rectifying **K**$^+$ (TWIK)-1, TWIK-2 and KCNK7 channels (functional expression of KCNK7 has not yet been reported); mechano-gated and arachidonic acid-activated **TWIK-re**lated **K**$^+$ (TREK)-1, TREK-2 and **TWIK-re**lated **a**rachidonic **a**cid-activated K^+ channel (TRAAK) channels; **TWIK**-related **a**cid-**s**ensitive **K**$^+$ (TASK)-1, TASK-3 and TASK-5 channels (functional expression of TASK-5 has not yet been reported); **t**andem pore domain **h**alothane-**i**nhibited **K**$^+$ (THIK)-1 and THIK-2 channels (functional expression of THIK-2 has not yet been reported); **TWIK**-related **al**kaline-pH-activated **K**$^+$ (TALK-1), TALK-2 and TASK-2 channels; and the **TWIK-re**lated **s**pinal cord **K**$^+$ (TRESK) channel, which is regulated by intracellular calcium.

In this chapter, we review the functional properties of the mechano-gated K_{2P} channel TREK-1. The complex gating properties of TREK-1 and its modulation by cellular lipids, membrane-receptor-coupled second messengers and pharmacological agents are described. Finally, we discuss the possible pathophysiological role of TREK-1 in the cardiovascular system.

The native stretch-activated K⁺ channels in the heart

The patch-clamp technique was used to identify and characterize the stretch-activated K⁺ channels (SAC_K) in molluscan, chick and rat cardiac myocytes[17–26]. SAC_K are opened at the whole cell level by applying a stretch on single myocytes[27]. The cardiac SAC_K are K⁺-selective outward rectifiers with a large single channel conductance (in the range of 100 pS in a symmetrical K⁺ gradient). The density of these channels is about 0.2/μm² [25]. The pressure to induce half-maximal activation is –12 mm Hg at +40 mV in a cell-attached patch[17]. The latency for activation is 50–100 ms, with a time to peak of about 400 ms[25]. Stretch activation is not maintained and a time-dependent decrease in current amplitude occurs within 1 s[25]. A time-dependent adaptation is also observed at the whole cell level when isometric displacement is applied to chick heart cells[28]. This adaptation is thought to be due to channel inactivation[29]. SAC_K activity is independent of intracellular Ca^{2+} and the probability of opening is mildly voltage-dependent, with greater channel activity at depolarized potentials[17]. Mechano-activation persists upon patch excision, demonstrating that cell integrity is not required for stretch activation[17]. Tetraethylammonium (10 mM), 4-aminopyridine (5 mM), apamine (10 nM), nifedipine (10 μM), quinidine (100 μM), tetrodotoxin (10 μM), ouabain (100 μM), vanadate (1 mM), glibenclamide (10 μM), tolbutamide (10 μM) and 4,4′-di-isothiocyanatostilbene-2,2′-disulfonic acid (DIDS) (100 μM) fail to affect the rat cardiac SAC_K channels. However, these channels are inhibited by gadolinium in chick heart cells[26]. Cellular lipids including polyunsaturated fatty acids as well as phospholipids (phosphatidylcholine) are potent openers of SAC_K in cardiac cells[19]. Nevertheless, it is important to note that pressure activation of SAC_K occurs in the presence of lipid-free albumin, a fatty acid binding protein, demonstrating that pressure and arachidonic acid activate the same K⁺ channel via separate pathways[17]. Interestingly, both the SAC_K and the arachidonic acid (AA)-activated K⁺ channel (K_{AA}) are opened by intracellular acidosis, further suggesting that they correspond to the same channel[17,20]. The SAC_K/K_{AA} is more sensitive to pressure at acidic pH, analogous to the effect of pH on AA-activated K⁺ channel activity. The SAC_K/K_{AA} in rat atrium is additionally opened by clinical doses of volatile general anaesthetics including chloroform, halothane and isoflurane[22]. The cardiac SAC_K/K_{AA} is also apparently directly activated by intracellular adenosine triphosphate (ATP) in the millimolar range[21]. The response to intracellular ATP is rapid and occurs in isolated patches, which appears to preclude the action of a kinase. In rat ventricular cardiomyocytes, the SAC_K/K_{AA} is additionally activated by extracellular ATP via the phospholipase A_2 pathway[30]. The purinergic-dependent activation of $cPLA_2$ requires the simultaneous activation of both p38 mitogen-activated protein kinase (MAPK) and p42/44 MAPK by a cyclic adenosine monophosphate (cAMP)-dependent protein kinase and a tyrosine kinase-dependent pathway, respectively[17]. The SAC_K/K_{AA} in rat atrial myocytes is inhibited by protein kinase A activation with cAMP or by addition of the β1 adrenergic receptor agonist isoproterenol[22].

In single-channel recordings with symmetrical high K⁺ solution, two TREK-like channels with 'flickery-burst' kinetics were found in cardiomyocytes: a 'large conductance' K⁺ channel (132 +/–5 pS at positive potentials) and a 'low-conductance' channel (41 +/–5 pS at positive potentials)[27]. The low-conductance channel could be activated by negative pressure in inside-out patches, positive pressure in outside-out patches, intracellular acidification and application of arachidonic acid. Its open probability was strongly increased by depolarization, due to decreased duration of gaps between bursts. The biophysical properties of the two cardiac TREK-like channels were similar to those of TREK-1 channels expressed in human embryonic kidney cell-line (HEK293) cells, which both displayed low- and high-conductance modes[27]. It was proposed that the current flowing through SAC_K may serve to counterbalance the inward current flowing through depolarizing stretch-activated nonselective cation channels during the filling phase of the cardiac cycle and thus prevent the occurrence of ventricular extrasystoles[27].

SAC_K were similarly recorded from cardiac blebs which are lacking F actin[31]. Thus, the mechano-sensitivity of native SAC_K is likely to be the result of interaction with membrane lipids (the bilayer model) and not of direct involvement of the cytoskeleton with the channel (the tethered model). Native SAC_K in blebs also showed a time-dependent decrease in current amplitude corresponding to adaptation or inactivation[31]. Finally, SAC_K were also recently shown to have an essential role in determining membrane potential in embryonic atrial myocytes, where inward rectifier K⁺ current (I_{K1}) is absent[32]. SAC_K are encoded by the TREK/TRAAK K_{2P} channels[1,33].

Functional properties of cloned mammalian K_{2P} channels

Mammalian K_{2P} channels[1–5] show a weak inward rectification [as is the case for TWIK-1 channel[12]], an open rectification [as for TASK-1 channel[34]] or an outward rectification [as for TREK-1[35,36]]. Some channels, such as TASK-1 and TASK-3, are constitutively open at rest[34,37–40], whereas other channels, including TREK-1, require physical or chemical stimulation to open[36,41–44]. The key feature of the K_{2P} channels is that they open over the whole voltage range and therefore qualify as leak or background K⁺ channels[1,3,5,45].

Mammalian K_{2P} channels can pass large inward K⁺ currents in elevated concentrations of extracellular K⁺ at negative membrane potentials[8,12,34,46–48]. The rectification of a constitutively open K⁺-selective pore (leak channel) is a direct function of the difference in concentration of K⁺ across the membrane, as expected from the Goldman–Hodgkin–Katz (GHK) constant field theory[49]. The GHK equation predicts an increase in conductance when ions flow from the more concentrated side[49]. The equation also assumes that permeant ions are not interacting. However, K_{2P} channels, as previously demonstrated for the classical K_{1P} channels, fail to respect this rule of ionic independence, which indicates that the pore can simultaneously accommodate multiple ions, with their movement influenced by each other[50]. The GHK equation also anticipates that leak channels lack voltage and time dependency — that is, K⁺ flow should remain stable over time[49]. However, several mammalian K_{2P} channels, including TREK-1, show both striking voltage- and time-dependent gating[35,51–53] (see below).

Pattern of TREK-1 expression

Human TREK-1 is highly expressed in the brain, where it is particularly abundant in γ-aminobutyric acid (GABA)ergic interneurons of the caudate nucleus and putamen[54]. Moreover, TREK-1 is also found in peripheral tissues such as the gastrointestinal tract as well as in blood vessels[55–58].

Immunohistochemical labelling on mesenteric artery sections has shown that TREK-1 expression is distributed throughout the mesenteric wall in both myocytes and endothelial cell layers[58]. TREK-1 is also expressed in mouse cutaneous arteries[58]. A particularly strong staining, confirmed by electron microscopy analysis, is observed in the endothelium of the blood vessel network surrounding and interconnecting hair follicles[58]. Additionally, reverse transcription polymerase chain reaction (RT PCR) experiments have detected TREK-1 mRNA expression in rat and mouse basilar arteries, but this subunit is apparently absent from both carotid and femoral arteries[59]. Expression of TREK-1 in the myocytes and endothelial cells of the basilar artery was confirmed by *in-situ* hybridization, Western blot analysis and immunostaining[59].

TREK-1 is expressed in the murine heart, with a stronger expression in endocardial cells[60,61]. Increased expression of TREK-1 has been reported in hypertrophic hearts as well as in acutely pressurized rat hearts[62,63]. Immunohistochemistry with antibodies against TREK-1 showed localization of the channel in longitudinal stripes at the external surface membrane of rat ventricular cardiomyocytes[27]. TREK-1 is more abundant in rat atria as compared to ventricle (4.17-fold) and has been proposed to act as a regulator of atrial natriuretic peptide (ANP) secretion[64]. Strong expression of an amino terminal splice variant of TREK-1 was found in the rat heart[27]. Finally, TREK-1 expression has not been reported in healthy human heart[56]. However, the expression of TREK channels in specialized cardiac cells, such as the pacemaker cells or conductive tissue, needs to be carefully evaluated in the human heart.

TREK-1 voltage dependency

Deletional and chimeric analyses have shown that the C-terminal domain of TREK-1 conditions the voltage-dependent gating of the channel[35]. Phosphorylation by protein kinase A of serine 333 in the distal C-terminal domain has been proposed to be responsible for the interconversion between the voltage-dependent and the leak phenotype of rat TREK-1[52,65] (see below). However, there must be additional mechanisms controlling TREK-1 voltage-dependent gating because, in a significant number of recordings, the TREK-1 S333A mutant reveals an intermediate phenotype between leak and voltage dependency[52]. Furthermore, the activation kinetics and the voltage dependency of the mouse TREK-1 S333A mutant do not differ from those of the wild-type channel[35].

TREK-1 therefore combines a leak channel (an instantaneous component) with a voltage-dependent outward rectifier (a delayed component)[35,44,52,66] (Fig. 3.1). As K$_{2P}$ channels diverge from the constant-field GHK current formulation and are characterized by complex and sophisticated permeation and gating mechanisms, they should not be considered as genuine leak K$^+$ channels[52,67].

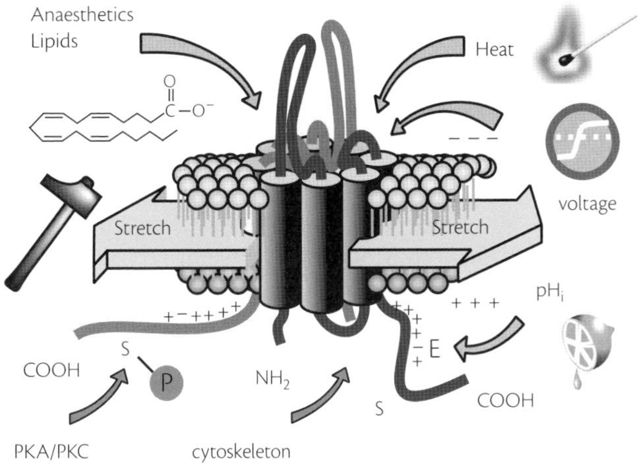

Mechano-activation of TREK-1

Membrane stretch reversibly induces TREK-1 channel opening in both cell-attached and excised inside-out configurations[36,43] (Figs 3.1 and 3.2). Mechano-activation of TREK-1 occurs independently of intracellular Ca^{2+} and ATP levels[36]. The relationship between channel activity and pressure is sigmoidal with half-maximal

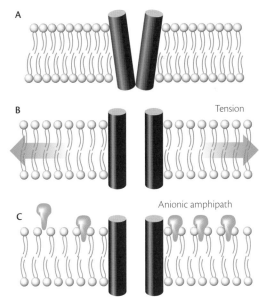

Fig. 3.1 Polymodal activation of TREK-1 by physical and chemical stimuli. TREK-1 is opened by stretch, heat, intracellular acidosis, depolarization, lipids and volatile general anaesthetics, but closed by protein kinase A (PKA) and protein kinase C (PKC) phosphorylation pathways. TREK-1 is tonically inhibited by the actin cytoskeleton. The cytosolic carboxy terminal domain plays a key role in the regulation of TREK-1 activity. Phosphorylation of S333 by PKA and phosphorylation of both S333 and S300 by PKC in this region inhibit TREK-1 opening. PIP$_2$ as well as AKAP interact with a cluster of positive charges (overlapping with E306) in the carboxy terminal domain. Protonation of E306 induces channel opening. (See color plate section.)

Fig. 3.2 The influence of tension and anionic amphipaths on TREK-1 channel activity. **A** The membrane at rest. **B** The effect of applied pressure. The tension in the membrane according to the law of Laplace is a function of pressure and of the radius of membrane curvature (T=Pr/2). **C** Insertion of an anionic amphipath (AA) or trinitrophenol (TNP) in the outer layer induces a coupled expansion of the inner layer which promotes TREK-1 opening.

activation at about –40 mm Hg[51]. At the whole cell level, when the osmolarity of the external solution is increased, the basal TREK-1 current amplitude is strongly reduced, which suggests that cellular volume (presumably by influencing tension on the cell membrane) also regulates channel activity[36,41].

The number of active TREK-1 channels is enhanced after treatment of cell-attached patches with agents that disrupt the actin cytoskeleton or after patch excision[36,51,68]. Mechanical force is likely to be transmitted to the channel through the bilayer, with the cytoskeleton acting as a tonic repressor, limiting channel activation by membrane tension[16,36,68]. Conversely, the expression of TREK-1 markedly alters the cytoskeletal network and induces the formation of membrane protrusions that are rich in actin and ezrin (a protein that links the cytoskeleton to the membrane)[68]. Thus, there is a dynamic interaction between TREK-1 and the actin cytoskeleton[68].

TREK-1 shows pronounced desensitization within 100 ms of membrane stretch[51]. This phenomenon is independent of the cytoskeleton and remains after patch excision. Mechano-sensitive currents can be assigned to a four-state cyclic kinetic model, without the need to introduce adaptation of the stimulus, which therefore implies the presence of an inactivation mechanism that is intrinsic to the channel[51]. Progressive deletion of the C-terminal domain of TREK-1 gradually renders the channels more resistant to stretch, with a faster inactivation demonstrating that this domain is central to channel mechano-gating[36,43,51].

Modulation of TREK-1 by internal pH

Lowering the internal pH shifts the pressure-activation relationship of TREK-1 toward positive pressure values (the opposite occurs following C-terminal deletion) and ultimately leads to channel opening at atmospheric pressure[43,69] (Fig. 3.1). Moreover, TREK-1 inactivation is gradually inhibited by intracellular acidosis[51]. Acidosis essentially converts a TREK-1 mechano-gated channel into a constitutively active, leak K^+ channel[43,69]. Residue E306 in the proximal C-terminal domain acts as a proton sensor and is therefore important in the internal pH modulation of TREK-1[69]. Removing this negative charge, by protonation or amino acid substitution, locks TREK-1 in the open conformation[69].

Temperature sensitivity of TREK-1

A progressive rise in temperature induces a gradual and reversible stimulation of TREK-1 activity[41] (Fig. 3.1). The maximal temperature sensitivity of TREK-1 is observed between 32°C and 37°C[41]. Patch excision results in the loss of the response of TREK-1 to heat, whereas stretch still maximally opens channels[41]. Therefore, thermal activation of TREK-1 critically requires cell integrity and implies that an indirect mechanism is acting on the channel.

Modulation of TREK-1 by membrane phospholipids

The cationic molecules poly-lysine or spermine have a high affinity for anionic phospholipids and inhibit TREK-1 currents when administered intracellularly on excised inside-out patches[70,71]. However, channel activity can be restored and even stimulated by applying phosphatidylinositol-4,5-bisphosphate (PIP_2) on the intracellular side of the channel[70,71]. Other inner leaflet phospholipids such as phosphatidylinositol, phosphatidylethanolamine and phosphatidylserine also increase the activity of TREK-1[70]. The presence of a large polar head is not an absolute requirement,

as phosphatidic acid [as well as lysophosphatidic acid (LPA)] also stimulates TREK-1 channel activity[44,70,72], but diacylglycerol cannot increase this activity, which indicates that the negative phosphate group at position 3 of the glycerol is critical[70,71].

A cluster of five positive charges in the proximal C-terminal domain of TREK-1, which encompass the proton sensor E306, is central to the effect of phospholipids[70] (Fig. 3.1). This cationic region is required for the interaction between the C-terminal domain of TREK-1 and the inner leaflet of the plasma membrane[70]. The positively charged nature of this region is increased at acidic pH_i (or by the E306A mutation), which probably favours a stronger electrostatic interaction with the inner leaflet phospholipids[70] (Fig. 3.1). This region is also involved in the interaction with A-kinase-anchoring protein (AKAP)] and comprises a serine residue that can be phosphorylated by protein kinase C (see below)[73,74].

Agonist-induced PIP_2 hydrolysis inhibits TREK-1 activity by shifting its voltage dependency of activation towards more depolarized voltages[71]. Conversely, stimulation of channel activity as a result of a left shift in the voltage dependency of TREK-1 currents occurs in response to addition of PIP_2[70,71]. The fine regulation of TREK-1 voltage dependency by PIP_2 might be involved in the downregulation of TREK-1 by G_q-coupled membrane receptors (see below)[71].

Polyunsaturated fatty acids modulation of TREK-1

The TREK-1 channel is reversibly opened by anionic amphipaths including polyunsaturated fatty acids, such as arachidonic acid[36] (Figs 3.1 and 3.2). The activation is observed in excised patch configurations and in the presence of cyclooxygenase and lipoxygenase inhibitors, which indicates that the effect is direct[16]. Chain length (docosahexaenoic acid C22:6 being the most potent polyunsaturated acid tested), the extent of unsaturation (at least one double bond) and a negative charge are critically required for channel stimulation[36].

The bilayer–couple hypothesis assumes that the effects of amphipaths derive entirely from interactions within the bilayer[75,76]. Anionic amphipaths, including arachidonic acid, preferentially insert into the outer leaflet, presumably because of the natural asymmetric distribution of negatively charged phosphatidylserines in the inner leaflet[75,76] (Fig. 3.2). This differential insertion produces a convex, positive curvature of the membrane. By contrast, positively charged amphipaths are expected to preferentially insert into the inner leaflet of the bilayer and thereby generate a concave negative curvature[75,76]. Assuming that TREK-1 is preferentially opened by tension (which causes convex or negative curvature of the membrane) rather than compression, it is indeed expected from the bilayer–couple hypothesis that anionic amphipaths such as trinitrophenol will open the channel[16,36]. The other possible explanation is that expansion of the outer layer by insertion of anionic amphipaths would stretch the inner layer (coupled expansion) which would promote the opening of TREK-1 [the bilayer is viewed as two monolayers with a fixed number of lipid molecules that could have different tension (Fig. 3.2)]. Deletional analysis demonstrates that the C-terminal domain of TREK-1 is critical for the response to arachidonic acid, as previously demonstrated for membrane stretch[36]. These results strongly suggest that activation of TREK-1 by polyunsaturated fatty acids and stretch are related. However, the possible existence of a specific binding site for polyunsaturated fatty acids on the channel protein itself cannot be entirely ruled out [5,16,36].

Lysophospholipid modulation of TREK-1

Extracellular lysophospholipids (including lysophosphatidylcholine), but not phospholipids, open TREK-1[42]. At low doses, arachidonic acid and lysophosphatidylcholine induce additive activation. The effect of lysophospholipids is critically dependent on the length of the carbonyl chain and the presence of a large polar head but is independent of the global charge of the molecule[42]. The conical shape of lysophospholipids is the key parameter conditioning TREK-1 stimulation. By contrast, intracellular lysophospholipids inhibit TREK-1 activation, further suggesting that expansion of the inner leaflet may promote channel opening, while compression would induce channel closing[16] (Fig. 3.2).

TREK-1 is also strongly activated by LPA, but only when applied on the intracellular side of the channel following patch excision in the inside-out patch configuration[44]. LPA reversibly converts the voltage-, internal pH- and stretch-sensitive K$^+$ channel TREK-1 into a leak conductance channel[44].

Membrane receptors and second messengers modulation of TREK-1

When co-expressed with the G$_s$-coupled 5HT$_4$ receptor, serotonin inhibits TREK-1[36,55]. This effect is mimicked by a membrane-permeant derivative of cAMP and is mediated by protein kinase A-mediated phosphorylation of S333 in the C-terminal domain of TREK-1[36]. Binding of AKAP150 to a key regulatory charged domain in the proximal C-terminal domain of TREK-1 [the same region that is involved in modulation by PIP$_2$ and internal pH (see above and Fig. 3.1)] dramatically stimulates TREK-1 activity[66,69,73]. Furthermore, in the presence of AKAP150, inhibition of TREK-1 by G$_s$-coupled receptors is enhanced, which suggests that AKAP150 might cluster TREK-1 with protein kinase A to facilitate protein kinase A-mediated phosphorylation of TREK-1[73].

Stimulation of G$_q$-coupled receptors, including metabotropic glutamate receptors 1 or 5, inhibits TREK-1[71,74,77]. Several pathways are involved: (1) phospholipase C hydrolyzes PIP$_2$[71]; (2) TREK-1 may be directly inhibited by diacylglycerol and/or phosphatidic acid[77]; and (3) protein kinase C sequentially phosphorylates S333 and S300 (which is also located in the AKAP150 binding site)[74]. As AKAP150 reverses the downregulation of TREK-1 by G$_q$-coupled receptor stimulation (or stimulation with the phorbol ester phorbol-12-myristate-13-acetate), this suggests that it might prevent the access of protein kinase C to the S300 phosphorylation site[73].

Finally, nitric oxide donors, as well as 8-bromo-cyclic guanosine monophosphate (cGMP), increase TREK-1 currents by protein kinase G-mediated phosphorylation of S351[78]. This effect is apparently very labile as it can only be detected using the perforated whole cell patch-clamp configuration[78].

Pharmacology of TREK-1

TREK-1 is unusual in terms of its pharmacology, as it is resistant to all the classical blockers of K$_{1P}$ channels, including tetraethylammonium and 4-aminopyridine[36,55]. However, it is inhibited by a variety of other pharmacological agents, including the antidepressant selective serotonin reuptake inhibitors such as fluoxetine[79,80]. This is apparently a direct effect, as channels are inhibited in the outside-out patch configuration[80]. TREK-1 is opened by the neuroprotective agent riluzole (100 μM)[81].

TREK-1 is opened by another important class of pharmacological agents, the volatile general anaesthetics[36,67,82–84]. Clinical doses of chloroform, diethyl ether, halothane and isoflurane open TREK-1[82]. Nitrous oxide, xenon and cyclopropane, which are gaseous anaesthetics known for their potent analgesic action in addition to their euphoric and neuroprotective effects, similarly stimulate TREK-1 at clinical doses[85], as does chloral hydrate[86]. Stimulation of TREK-1 activity by these anaesthetics occurs in excised patches, which again suggests a direct effect. The C-terminal domain of TREK-1 also has a major role in its modulation by anaesthetics[82,85,86].

TREK-1 and vascular physiology

Alpha-linolenic acid injections increase cerebral blood flow and induce vasodilation of the basilar artery, but not the carotid artery where TREK-1 is apparently absent[59]. The saturated fatty acid palmitic acid, which does not open TREK-1, fails to produce vasodilation. Vasodilation induced by polyunsaturated fatty acids (PUFA) in basilar artery and the resultant increase in blood flow are abolished in TREK-1 –/– mice[59]. Furthermore, deletion of TREK-1 leads to an important alteration in vasodilation of mesenteric arteries induced by acetylcholine and bradykinin[59]. Similarly, TREK-1 plays a major role in cutaneous endothelium-dependent vasodilation[58]. Additionally, the vasodilator response to local pressure application is markedly decreased in TREK-1 –/– mice, mimicking the decreased response to pressure observed in diabetes[58]. Therefore, deletion of TREK-1 is associated with a marked alteration in the efficacy of the G-protein-coupled receptor-associated cascade producing nitric oxide (NO) which leads to major endothelial dysfunction and impairment of vasodilation[58,59].

TREK-1 and cardiac function

K$^+$ channels that open at supra-threshold depolarized potentials will not affect threshold but will tend to facilitate recovery and repetitive re-firing[41,52]. TREK-1, similarly to cardiac SAC$_K$, preferentially opens at depolarized potentials with complex outward rectification[35]. Opening of TREK-1 will thus tend to increase repetitive activity and may contribute to the facilitation of heart rate observed during atria distension.

Stretch is the main stimulus of ANP secretion which is initiated by an increase in intracellular Ca^{2+}. Opening of TREK-1 by stretch may act as a negative feedback of ANP secretion by shortening action potential and thus decreasing intracellular Ca^{2+}. β adrenergic stimulation, by inhibiting TREK channels, would, on the contrary, stimulate ANP release from atrial myocytes[22].

In pathological conditions such as ischaemia, TREK-1 channel opening may become critical. Ischaemic insult induces phospholipase A2 activation, PUFA and lysophospholipid release, cell swelling and intracellular acidosis[1,33,83]. All these alterations will contribute to open TREK-1 and will tend to repolarize the membrane potential, reduce intracellular Ca^{2+} and thus protect ischaemic cardiomyocytes. It is interesting to note that chemical ischaemia induced by the uncoupling agent carbonyl cyanide p-(trifluoromethoxy) phenylhydrazone (FCCP) strongly opens TREK-1[69].

Conclusions and outlook

TREK-1 encodes the mechano-gated lipid-sensitive SAC_K/K_{AA}. TREK-1 is expressed at high levels in the cardiovascular system. Opening of TREK-1 by membrane stretch is relevant to both cardiac mechano-electric coupling (MEC) and the regulation of arterial tone. Because of the unusual polymodal behaviour of the TREK channels, including stretch sensitivity, it is anticipated that these 'unconventional' channels may have important implications in various cardiovascular disease states. In the future it will be important also to address the role of the mechano-gated K_{2P} channels in electrical remodelling of the heart and acquired arrhythmias.

Acknowledgements

We are grateful to the ANR 2008 du Gène à la Physiopathologie, to the Association for Information and Research on Genetic Kidney Disease France, to the Fondation del Duca, to the Fondation de la Recherche Médicale, to the Fondation de Recherche sur l'Hypertension Artérielle, to the Fondation de la Recherche sur le Cerveau, to Société Générale AM, to the Université de Nice-Sophia Antipolis and to the Centre National de la Recherche Scientifique for financial support.

References

1. Patel AJ, Honoré E. Properties and modulation of mammalian 2P domain K+ channels. *Trends Neurosci* 2001;**24**:339–346.

2. Lesage F, Lazdunski, M. Molecular and functional properties of two-pore-domain potassium channels. *Am J Physiol* 2000;**279**: F793–F801.

3. Goldstein SAN, Bockenhauer D, O'Kelly I, Zilberg N. Potassium leak channels and the KCNK family of two-P-domain subunits. *Nature Rev Neurosci* 2001;**2**:175–184.

4. Talley EM, Sirois JE, Lei Q, Bayliss DA. Two-pore-domain (KCNK) potassium channels: dynamic roles in neuronal function. *Neuroscientist* 2003;**9**:46–56.

5. Kim D. Fatty acid-sensitive two-pore domain K+ channels. *Trends Pharmacol Sci* 2003;**24**:648–654.

6. Doyle DA, Morais Cabral J, Pfuetzner RA, *et al.* The structure of the potassium channel: molecular basis of K+ conduction and selectivity. *Science* 1998;**280**:69–77.

7. O'Connell AD, Morton MJ, Hunter M. Two-pore domain K+ channels-molecular sensors. *Biochim Biophys Acta* 2002;**1566**: 152–161.

8. Goldstein SA, Price LA, Rosenthal DN, Pausch MH. ORK1, a potassium-selective leak channel with two pore domains cloned from *Drosophila melanogaster* by expression in *Saccharomyces cerevisiae*. *Proc Natl Acad Sci USA* 1996;**93**:13256–13261.

9. Ketchum KA, Joiner WJ, Sellers AJ, Kaczmarek LK, Goldstein SAN. A new family of outwardly rectifying potassium channel proteins with two pore domains in tandem. *Nature* 1995;**376**:690–695.

10. Reid JD, Lukas W, Shafaatian R, *et al.* The *S. cerevisiae* outwardly-rectifying potassium channel (DUK1) identifies a new family of channels with duplicated pore domains. *Receptors Channels* 1996;**4**: 51–62.

11. Zhou XL, Vaillant B, Loukin SH, Kung C, Saimi Y. YKC1 encodes the depolarization-activated K+ channel in the plasma membrane of yeast. *FEBS Lett* 1995;**373**:170–176.

12. Lesage F, Guillemare E, Fink M, *et al.* TWIK-1, a ubiquitous human weakly inward rectifying K+ channel with a novel structure. *EMBO J* 1996;**15**:1004–1011.

13. Lesage F, Guillemare E, Fink M, *et al.* A pH-sensitive yeast outward rectifier K+ channel with two pore domains and novel gating properties. *J Biol Chem* 1996;**271**:4183–4187.

14. Wei A, Jegla T, Salkoff L. Eight potassium channel families revealed by the *C. elegans* genome project. *Neuropharmacology* 1996;**35**: 805–829.

15. Czempinski K, Zimmermann S, Ehrhardt T, Muller-Rober B. New structure and function in plant K+ channels: KCO1, an outward rectifier with a steep Ca^{2+} dependency. *EMBO J* 1997;**16**:2565–2575.

16. Patel AJ, Lazdunski M, Honoré E. Lipid and mechano-gated 2P domain K+ channels. *Curr Opin Cell Biol* 2001;**13**:422–428.

17. Kim D. A mechanosensitive K+ channel in heart cells. Activation by arachidonic acid. *J Gen Physiol* 1992;**100**:1021–1040.

18. Kim D, Duff RA. Regulation of K+ channels in cardiac myocytes by free fatty acids. *Circ Res* 1990;**67**:1040–1046.

19. Kim D, Clapham DE. Potassium channels in cardiac cells activated by arachidonic acid and phospholipids. *Science* 1989;**244**:1174–1176.

20. Wallert MA, Ackerman MJ, Kim D, Clapham DE. Two novel cardiac atrial K+ channels, IK.AA and IK.PC. *J Gen Physiol* 1991;**98**:921–939.

21. Tan JH, Liu W, Saint DA. TREK-like potassium channels in rat cardiac ventricular myocytes are activated by intracellular ATP. *J Membr Biol* 2001;**185**:201–207.

22. Terrenoire C, Lauritzen I, Lesage F, Romey G, Lazdunski M. A TREK-1-like potassium channel in atrial cells inhibited by β-adrenergic stimulation and activated by volatile anesthetics. *Circ Res* 2001;**89**: 336–342.

23. Sigurdson W, Morris CE, Brezden BL, Gardner DR. Stretch activation of a K+ channel in molluscan heart cells. *J Exp Biol* 1987;**127**: 191–209.

24. Hu H, Sachs F. Mechanically activated currents in chick heart cells. *J Membr Biol* 1996;**154**:205–216.

25. Niu W, Sachs F. Dynamic properties of stretch-activated K+ channels in adult rat atrial myocytes. *Prog Biophys Mol Biol* 2003;**82**:121–135.

26. Ruknudin A, Sachs F, Bustamante JO. Stretch-activated ion channels in tissue-cultured chick heart. *Am J Physiol* 1993;**264**:H960–H972.

27. Li XT, Dyachenko V, Zuzarte M, *et al.* The stretch-activated potassium channel TREK-1 in rat cardiac ventricular muscle. *Cardiovasc Res* 2006;**69**:86–97.

28. Bett GC, Sachs F. Whole-cell mechanosensitive currents in rat ventricular myocytes activated by direct stimulation. *J Membr Biol* 2000;**173**:255–263.

29. Suchyna TM, Besch SR, Sachs F. Dynamic regulation of mechano-sensitive channels: capacitance used to monitor patch tension in real time. *Phys Biol* 2004;**1**:1–18.

30. Aimond F, Rauzier JM, Bony C, Vassort G. Simultaneous activation of p38 MAPK and p42/44 MAPK by ATP stimulates the K+ current ITREK in cardiomyocytes. *J Biol Chem* 2000;**15**:39110–39116.

31. Liu X, Huang H, Wang W, Wang J, Sachs F, Niu W. Stretch-activated potassium channels in hypotonically induced blebs of atrial myocytes. *J Membr Biol* 2008;**226**:17–25.

32. Zhang H, Shepherd N, Creazzo TL. Temperature-sensitive TREK currents contribute to setting the resting membrane potential in embryonic atrial myocytes. *J Physiol* 2008;**86**:3645–3656.

33. Honoré E. The neuronal background K_{2P} channels: focus on TREK-1. *Nature Rev Neurosci* 2007;**8**:251–261.

34. Duprat F, Lesage F, Fink M, Reyes R, Heurteaux C, Lazdunski M. TASK, a human background K+ channel to sense external pH variations near physiological pH. *EMBO J* 1997;**16**:5464–5471.

35. Maingret F, Honoré E, Lazdunski M, Patel AJ. Molecular basis of the voltage-dependent gating of TREK-1, a mechano-sensitive K+ channel. *Biochem Biophys Res Commun* 2002;**292**:339–346.

36. Patel AJ, Honoré E, Maingret F, *et al.* A mammalian two pore domain mechano-gated S-like K$^+$ channel. *EMBO J* 1998;**17**: 4283–4290.

37. Bayliss DA, Talley EM, Sirois JE, Lei Q. TASK-1 is a highly modulated pH-sensitive 'leak' K$^+$ channel expressed in brainstem respiratory neurons. *Respir Physiol* 2001;**129**:159–174.

38. Talley EM, Lei Q, Sirois JE, Bayliss DA. TASK-1, a two-pore domain K$^+$ channel, is modulated by multiple neurotransmitters in motoneurons. *Neuron* 2000;**25**:399–410.

39. Talley EM, Bayliss DA. Modulation of TASK-1 (Kcnk3) and TASK-3 (Kcnk9) potassium channels: volatile anesthetics and neurotransmitters share a molecular site of action. *J Biol Chem* 2002;**277**:17733–17742.

40. Kim D, Fujita A, Horio Y, Kurachi Y. Cloning and functional expression of a novel cardiac two-pore background K$^+$ channel (cTBAK-1). *Circ Res* 1998;**82**:513–518.

41. Maingret F, Lauritzen I, Patel A, *et al.* TREK-1 is a heat-activated background K$^+$ channel. *EMBO J* 2000;**19**:2483–2491.

42. Maingret F, Patel AJ, Lesage F, Lazdunski M, Honoré E. Lysophospholipids open the two P domain mechano-gated K$^+$ channels TREK-1 and TRAAK. *J Biol Chem* 2000;**275**:10128–10133.

43. Maingret F, Patel AJ, Lesage F, Lazdunski M, Honoré E. Mechano- or acid stimulation, two interactive modes of activation of the TREK-1 potassium channel. *J Biol Chem* 1999;**274**:26691–26696.

44. Chemin J, Patel A, Duprat F, Zanzouri M, Lazdunski M, Honoré E. Lysophosphatidic acid-operated K$^+$ channels. *J Biol Chem* 2005;**280**: 4415–4421.

45. Lesage F. Pharmacology of neuronal background potassium channels. *Neuropharmacology* 2003;**44**:1–7.

46. Fink M, Lesage F, Duprat F, *et al.* A neuronal two P domain K$^+$ channel activated by arachidonic acid and polyunsaturated fatty acid. *EMBO J* 1998;**17**:3297–3308.

47. Reyes R, Duprat F, Lesage F, Fink M, Farman N, Lazdunski M. Cloning and expression of a novel pH-sensitive two pore domain potassium channel from human kidney. *J Biol Chem* 1998;**273**:30863–30869.

48. Lesage F, Terrenoire C, Romey G, Lazdunski M. Human TREK2, a 2P domain mechano-sensitive K$^+$ channel with multiple regulations by polyunsaturated fatty acids, lysophospholipids, and Gs, Gi, and Gq protein-coupled receptors. *J Biol Chem* 2000;**275**:28398–28405.

49. Hille B (1992) *Ion Channels of Excitable Membranes*, 3rd edn. Sinauer Associates, Sunderland, Massachusetts.

50. Ilan N, Goldstein SA. Kcnko: single, cloned potassium leak channels are multi-ion pores. *Biophys J* 2001;**80**:241–253.

51. Honoré E, Patel AJ, Chemin J, Suchyna T, Sachs F. Desensitization of mechano-gated K$_{2P}$ channels. *Proc Natl Acad Sci USA* 2006;**103**: 6859–6864.

52. Bockenhauer D, Zilberberg N, Goldstein SA. KCNK2: reversible conversion of a hippocampal potassium leak into a voltage-dependent channel. *Nature Neurosci* 2001;**4**:486–491.

53. Lopes CM, Gallagher PG, Buck ME, Butler MH, Goldstein SA. Proton block and voltage gating are potassium-dependent in the cardiac leak channel Kcnk3. *J Biol Chem* 2000;**275**:16969–16978.

54. Hervieu GJ, Cluderay JE, Gray CW, *et al.* Distribution and expression of TREK-1, a two-pore-domain potassium channel, in the adult rat CNS. *Neuroscience* 2001;**103**:899–919.

55. Fink M, Duprat F, Lesage F, *et al.* Cloning, functional expression and brain localization of a novel unconventional outward rectifier K$^+$ channel. *EMBO J* 1996;**15**:6854–6862.

56. Medhurst AD, Rennie G, Chapman CG, *et al.* Distribution analysis of human two pore domain potassium channels in tissues of the central nervous system and periphery. *Mol Brain Res* 2001;**86**:101–114.

57. Talley EM, Solorzano G, Lei Q, Kim D, Bayliss DA. CNS distribution of members of the two-pore-domain (KCNK) potassium channel family. *J Neurosci* 2001;**21**:7491–7505.

58. Garry A, Fromy B, Blondeau N, *et al.* Altered acetylcholine, bradykinin and cutaneous pressure-induced vasodilation in mice lacking the TREK1 potassium channel: the endothelial link. *EMBO J* 2007;**8**: 354–359.

59. Blondeau N, Petrault O, Manta S, *et al.* Polyunsaturated fatty acids are cerebral vasodilators via the TREK-1 potassium channel. *Circ Res* 2007;**101**:176–184.

60. Kelly D, Mackenzie L, Hunter P, Smaill B, Saint DA. Gene expression of stretch-activated channels and mechanoelectric feedback in the heart. *Clin Exp Pharmacol Physiol* 2006;**33**:642–648.

61. Liu W, Saint DA. Heterogeneous expression of tandem-pore K$^+$ channel genes in adult and embryonic rat heart quantified by real-time polymerase chain reaction. *Clin Exp Pharmacol Physiol* 2004;**31**: 174–178.

62. Cheng L, Su F, Ripen N, *et al.* Changes of expression of stretch-activated potassium channel TREK-1 mRNA and protein in hypertrophic myocardium. *J Huazhong Univ Sci Technol Med Sci* 2006;**26**:31–33.

63. Zhao F, Dong L, Cheng L, Zeng Q, Su F. Effects of acute mechanical stretch on the expression of mechanosensitive potassium channel TREK-1 in rat left ventricle. *J Huazhong Univ Sci Technol Med Sci* 2007;**27**:385–387.

64. McGrath MF, de Bold AJ. Transcriptional analysis of the mammalian heart with special reference to its endocrine function. *BMC Genom* 2009;**10**:254.

65. Maylie J, Adelman JP. Beam me up, Scottie! TREK channels swing both ways. *Nature Neurosci* 2001;**4**:457–458.

66. Chemin J, Patel AJ, Duprat F, Lauritzen I, Lazdunski M, Honoré E. A phospholipid sensor controls mechanogating of the K$^+$ channel TREK-1. *EMBO J* 2005;**24**:44–53.

67. Patel AJ, Honoré E. Anesthetic-sensitive 2P domain K$^+$ channels. *Anesthesiology* 2001;**95**:1013–1025.

68. Lauritzen I, Chemin J, Honoré E, *et al.* Cross-talk between the mechano-gated K2P channel TREK-1 and the actin cytoskeleton. *EMBO J* 2005;**6**:642–648.

69. Honoré E, Maingret F, Lazdunski M, Patel AJ. An intracellular proton sensor commands lipid- and mechano-gating of the K$^+$ channel TREK-1. *EMBO J* 2002;**21**:2968–2976.

70. Chemin J, Patel A, Delmas P, Sachs F, Lazdunski M, Honoré E. Regulation of the mechano-gated K2P channel TREK-1 by membrane phospholipids. *Curr Topics Membr* 2007;**59**:155–170.

71. Lopes CM, Rohacs T, Czirjak G, Balla T, Enyedi P, Logothetis DE. PiP2-hydrolysis underlies agonist-induced inhibition and regulates voltage-gating of 2-P domain K$^+$ channels. *J Physiol* 2005;**564**: 117–129.

72. Chemin J, Patel A, Sachs F, Lazdunski M, Honoré E. Up- and down-regulation of the mechano-gated K2P channel TREK-1 by PIP2 and other membrane phospholipids. *Pflugers Archiv* 2007;**455**: 97–103.

73. Sandoz G, Thummler S, Duprat F, *et al.* AKAP150, a switch to convert mechano-, pH- and arachidonic acid-sensitive TREK K$^+$ channels into open leak channels. *EMBO J* 2006;**25**:5864–5872.

74. Murbartian J, Lei Q, Sando JJ, Bayliss DA. Sequential phosphorylation mediates receptor- and kinase-induced inhibition of TREK-1 background potassium channels. *J Biol Chem* 2005;**280**:30175–30184.

75. Sheetz MP, Singer SJ. Biological membranes as bilayer couples. A molecular mechanism of drug–erythrocyte interactions. *Proc Natl Acad Sci USA* 1974;**71**:4457–4461.

76. Martinac B, Adler J, Kung C. Mechanosensitive ion channels of *E. coli* activated by amphipaths. *Nature* 1990;**348**:261–263.

77. Chemin J, Girard C, Duprat F, Lesage F, Romey G, Lazdunski M. Mechanisms underlying excitatory effects of group I metabotropic glutamate receptors via inhibition of 2P domain K$^+$ channels. *EMBO J* 2003;**22**:5403–5411.

78. Koh SD, Monaghan KM, Sergeant GP, *et al.* TREK-1 regulation by nitric oxide and cGMP-dependent protein kinase. *J Biol Chem* 2001;**47**:44338–44346.

79. Heurteaux C, Lucas G, Guy N, *et al.* Deletion of the background potassium channel TREK-1 results in a depression-resistant phenotype. *Nature Neurosci* 2006;**9**:1134–1141.

80. Kennard LE, Chumbley JR, Ranatunga KM, Armstrong SJ, Veale EL, Mathie A. Inhibition of the human two-pore domain potassium channel, TREK-1, by fluoxetine and its metabolite norfluoxetine. *Br J Pharmacol* 2005;**144**:821–829.

81. Duprat F, Lesage F, Patel AJ, Fink M, Romey G, Lazdunski M. The neuroprotective agent riluzole activates the two P domain K⁺ channels TREK-1 and TRAAK. *Mol Pharmacol* 2000;**57**:906–912.

82. Patel AJ, Honoré E, Lesage F, Fink M, Romey G, Lazdunski M. Inhalational anaesthetics activate two-pore-domain background K⁺ channels. *Nature Neurosci* 1999;**2**:422–426.

83. Franks NP, Honoré E. The TREK K2P channels and their role in general anaesthesia and neuroprotection. *Trends Pharmacol Sci* 2004;**25**:601–608.

84. Franks NP, Lieb WR. Background K⁺ channels: an important target for volatile anesthetics? *Nature Neurosci* 1999;**2**:395–396.

85. Gruss M, Bushell TJ, Bright DP, Lieb WR, Mathie A, Franks NP. Two-pore-domain K⁺ channels are a novel target for the anesthetic gases xenon, nitrous oxide, and cyclopropane. *Mol Pharmacol* 2004;**65**:443–452.

86. Harinath S, Sikdar SK. Trichloroethanol enhances the activity of recombinant human TREK-1 and TRAAK channels. *Neuropharmacology* 2004;**46**:750–760.

Cell volume-sensitive ion channels and transporters in cardiac myocytes

Clive M. Baumgarten, Wu Deng and Frank J. Raucci, Jr

Background

In addition to stretch-activated channels (SAC) that respond to purely mechanical stimuli (e.g. Chapter 2), the heart possesses voltage- and ligand-gated channels and ion transporters that are modulated by cell volume. Volume-activated channels (VAC) and SAC are distinguished empirically by the nature of the stimulus. Both stimuli alter membrane tension and cytoskeletal stress and trigger overlapping signalling cascades; consequently the distinction between VAC and SAC is not absolute.

Insights into the role of VAC in the heart are still emerging. Myocyte volume increases acutely with ischaemia/reperfusion, chronically with hypertrophy and remodelling and is affected by disease-induced alterations of serum osmolarity. Atrial natriuretic peptide, autonomic stimulation and cardiovascular agents, including nitrates and diuretics, also regulate cell volume. Therefore, volume-sensitive channels and transporters contribute in multiple settings.

Transducing cell volume

How are alterations in cell volume converted into biologic responses? Parts of the process are known for several cases, but the initial step(s) remains elusive. The complexity of the transduction cascade and its tissue specificity have proven to be experimental and conceptual challenges[1,2].

An obvious effect of osmotic swelling and shrinkage is dilution or concentration of cytoplasmic ions and regulatory molecules and the resulting change in ionic strength. Such perturbations affect ionic fluxes, electrochemical gradients, surface potential and binding affinities of macromolecules. Isosmotic cell inflation by transient application of hydrostatic pressure is, however, an equally effective stimulus for VAC, although alterations of ion concentrations and ionic strength are minimized.

The consequences of osmotic stress depend, at least in part, on whether a cell is intact or dialyzed with whole-cell or perforated-patch methods. Initially, water flux during an osmotic challenge exceeds the ability of diffusion from the pipette to maintain cytoplasmic ion content[3]. As volume reaches a new steady state, water flux decreases and intracellular ionic concentrations again approach those in the pipette in whole-cell recordings. Transport numbers for anion and cation fluxes between the pipette and cell can effect steady-state volume, however[4].

Cell swelling also modifies membrane tension by stretch and altering membrane curvature. The resulting forces may directly regulate channels and membrane-bound signalling molecules. Specializations, such as caveolae, are proposed to serve as tension detectors that activate macromolecular signalosomes (see also Chapter 7). Effects of cell volume on membrane tension are, however, difficult to quantify because of sarcolemmal folding and the contributions of the viscoelastic cytoskeleton. Atomic force microscopy reveals that osmotic swelling softens the cell membrane rather than stiffens it, as would be expected from the elastic modulus[5,6].

Deformation and reorganization of the cytoskeleton in response to volume perturbations is important. Channels, transporters and signalling molecules are anchored to cytoskeletal components, and their activity is influenced by the cytoskeleton. Signalling cascades respond to volume perturbations and also may serve as volume sensors. Transduction may involve their altered binding to docking and adapter proteins that trigger phosphorylation or dephosphorylation. Binding affinities can be influenced by physical distortion of proteins, ionic strength, concentration of competing ions, or through macromolecular crowding, which reflects non-deal behaviour of proteins in solutions. Macromolecules that are neither substrate nor product exclude other molecules from a fraction of the cytoplasm. Consequently, diluting or concentrating inert macromolecules will significantly affect the reaction rate of signalling molecules and, thereby, the functions of target proteins.

Volume-activated channels

$I_{Cl,swell}$

The most extensively studied cardiac VAC is the cell volume-sensitive Cl^- channel, $I_{Cl,swell}$[7-9], shown in Fig. 4.1. $I_{Cl,swell}$ is elicited by

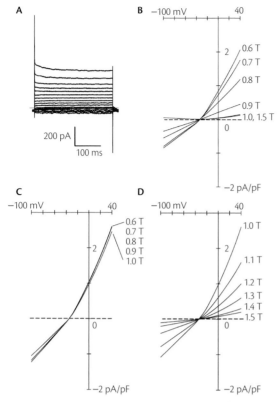

Fig. 4.1 Families of $I_{Cl,swell}$ and I-V relationships in control (**A, B**) and heart failure (**C, D**). **A** $I_{Cl,swell}$ measured as difference current (0.6–1T) in rabbit ventricle by perforated patch. Steps to −100 to +60 mV from −80 mV. [Modified, with permission, from Baumgarten CM, Clemo HF (2003) Swelling-activated chloride channels in cardiac physiology and pathophysiology. *Prog Biophys Mol Biol* **82**: 25–42.] **B** Activation of $I_{Cl,swell}$ is graded. 9-AC-sensitive currents during ramp clamps in 0.6T–1T and in 1.5T in dog ventricle. **C** Persistent activation of $I_{Cl,swell}$ in 1T in pacing-induced heart failure in the dog. Swelling in 0.9T–0.6T does not elicit additional current. **D** Osmotic shrinkage (1.1T–1.5T) inhibits $I_{Cl,swell}$ in heart failure. [Modified, with permission, from Clemo HF, Stambler BS, Baumgarten CM (1999) Swelling-activated chloride current is persistently activated in ventricular myocytes from dogs with tachycardia-induced congestive heart failure. *Circ Res* **84**:157–165.]

anisosmotic swelling in hyposmotic bath or hyperosmotic pipette solutions, isosmotic uptake of urea, or cell inflation by positive pipette pressure[10–13]. $I_{Cl,swell}$ is outwardly rectifying with both physiologic and symmetric Cl⁻ gradients, time-independent over most of the physiologic voltage range, but partially inactivates at positive potentials[14,15]. Although Cl⁻ is the primary charge carrier, organic anions are permeant, and the permeability sequence is: I⁻ > NO₃⁻ > Br⁻ > Cl⁻ > Asp⁻[12,13]. Activation of $I_{Cl,swell}$ shortens action potential duration, depolarizes the resting membrane potential and influences arrhythmogenesis; it also regulates cardiac cell volume, apoptosis and perhaps preconditioning[7–9].

DCPIB (4-[(2-butyl-6,7-dichloro-2-cyclopentyl-2,3-dihydro-1-oxo-1*H*-inden-5-yl)oxy]butanoic acid) is the most selective $I_{Cl,swell}$ inhibitor available and does not suppress native currents including I_{Ks}, I_{Kr}, I_{K1}, I_{Na}, I_{Ca}, $I_{Cl,CFTR}$, $I_{Cl,Ca}$ or expressed ClC, CFTR, Kv1.5, Kv4.3, hERG or MinK currents[16]. Tamoxifen and DIDS (4,4′-diisothiocyanatostilbene-2,2′-disulfonic acid) also

distinguish between $I_{Cl,swell}$ and cystic fibrosis trans-membrane conductance regulator (CFTR) and in some tissues $I_{Cl,Ca}$, but these agents affect several cation channels. With less selective anion channel blockers [e.g. 9AC (9-anthracenecarboxylic acid), NPPB (5-nitro-2-(3-phenylpropylamino)benzoic acid)][7,8,17], volume perturbations are needed to verify involvement of $I_{Cl,swell}$.

Background Cl⁻ current is due, in part, to $I_{Cl,swell}$[7], and its spontaneous activation may occur without an overt osmotic gradient[11]. A Donnan system exists between the cytoplasm, which contains charged proteins, and mobile ions in the pipette; the resulting distribution of mobile ions and water tends to cause cell swelling. Swelling also can arise from differences in permeability of pipette and bath ions – that is, the distinction between tonicity and osmolarity.

$I_{Cl,swell}$ is both a VAC and SAC because it is sensitive to mechanical stretch as well as volume. One way to modify membrane tension and shape is with amphipaths. Anionic amphipaths preferentially insert into the outer membrane leaflet causing convex curvature (crenation) that mimics swelling, whereas cationic amphipaths insert into the inner leaflet causing concave curvature (cupping) that mimics shrinkage. In the ventricle, $I_{Cl,swell}$ is activated by crenators and inhibited by cupping agents[10]. Modulation of mechano-gated two pore-domain K⁺ channels such as TREK (TWIK-related K⁺ channels) and TRAAK (TWIK-related arachidonic acid-activated K⁺ channel; note: TWIK stands for tandem of P domains in a weak inwardly rectifying K⁺ channel), by amphipaths also is attributed to altered membrane tension. Although these data are consistent with effects on membrane tension or shape, amphipaths have multiple additional actions.

The classic method for identifying SAC is to apply pressure to an attached or excised membrane patch. Whereas most find only cation SAC by this method, a linear Cl⁻ SAC (8.6 pS) is found in human atrial myocytes[18]. Open probability increased with positive pipette pressure in the outside-out and with negative pressure in the inside-out configurations. Swelling-induced $I_{Cl,swell}$ unitary currents are, however, larger (38–76 pS at positive potentials) and outwardly rectify[19–21]. Stretching β₁D integrins with monoclonal antibody-coated magnetic beads activates current resembling $I_{Cl,swell}$[22–24] via the same signalling cascade as osmotic swelling[25,26].

Clemo *et al.*[8,27,28] found that $I_{Cl,swell}$ is persistently activated in ventricular myocytes in models of dilated cardiomyopathy, ischaemia and atrial myocytes from patients with right atrial enlargement. An outwardly rectifying, tamoxifen- and 9AC-sensitive Cl⁻ current with I⁻ > Cl⁻ permeability is present under isosmotic conditions in heart failure and infarction myocytes, but not sham or control cells. $I_{Cl,swell}$ in diseased myocytes is turned off by osmotic shrinkage, whereas osmotic swelling does not activate more current[28]. Ventricular $I_{Cl,swell}$ also is upregulated in lipopolysaccharide-induced endotoxic shock[29] and by doxorubicin[30].

The molecular identity of $I_{Cl,swell}$ remains uncertain. Hume and co-workers[7] provided substantial evidence that ClC-3 underlies $I_{Cl,swell}$, but $I_{Cl,swell}$ is present in cardiac[20,31,32] and non-cardiac[33] cells from *Clcn3*⁻/⁻ mice. It remains possible that ClC-3 modulates $I_{Cl,swell}$; aspects of its regulation are distinct in native and *Clcn3*⁻/⁻ cells[31]. Recently, the calcium-dependent chloride channel TMEM16A (ANO1) was proposed as $I_{Cl,swell}$ in epithelial cells[34], but several of its features seem inconsistent with cardiac $I_{Cl,swell}$.

$I_{Cl,swell}$ signalling cascade

Activation of $I_{Cl,swell}$ lags behind a swelling or stretch by > 1 min, suggesting that signalling is required for stimulus transduction. An early response to swelling and stretch is protein tyrosine kinase (PTK) activation, which occurs in less than 5 s[35]. Sorota[36] found blocking PTK with genistein or herbimycin A, which are non-selective, suppresses stimulation of $I_{Cl,swell}$ in atrial myocytes. In contrast, differential effects of two PTK families, Src and EGFR kinase, were identified in atrial[37] and ventricular[25] myocytes. Genistein and the selective Src inhibitor PP2 substantially augment $I_{Cl,swell}$ after osmotic swelling but not under isosmotic conditions. In contrast, selective inhibitors of EGFR kinase reduce $I_{Cl,swell}$. The protein tyrosine phosphatase (PTP) inhibitor orthovanadate antagonized both stimulation and inhibition of $I_{Cl,swell}$ by PTK inhibitors and partially blocked $I_{Cl,swell}$ in their absence. Suppressing Src and focal adhesion kinase (FAK) by overexpressing FAK-related-non-kinase (FRNK), an endogenous FAK inhibitor, also augments $I_{Cl,swell}$, mimicking the action of PP2[38]. Thus, multiple PTK and PTP modulate $I_{Cl,swell}$ but fail to elicit current in isotonic media.

The role of protein kinase A (PKA) is controversial. Initial studies showed that neither organic nor specific peptide blockers of PKA inhibit $I_{Cl,swell}$[10,12]. A PKA-dependent slow inhibition was reported later[39], but it was argued that PKA might phosphorylate a protein kinase C (PKC) consensus site on ClC-3[7].

Duan, Hume and co-workers suggested that $I_{Cl,swell}$ is activated by dephosphorylation of ClC-3 by ser/thr protein phosphatases (PP) and is inhibited by phosphorylation by PKC[7,9] or via α-adrenergic stimulation[14]. They proposed that ClC-3 ser-51, a consensus PKC site, was responsible[40]. PKC-dependent regulation was compared in normal and failing hearts[8]. In normal myocytes, PP2a is responsible for current activation and $I_{Cl,swell}$ is independent of $[Ca^{2+}]$. In heart failure myocytes, however, calcineurin (PP2B), a Ca^{2+}-dependent PP, also regulates $I_{Cl,swell}$, and activation of $I_{Cl,swell}$ is inhibited by PP2B blockers, cyclosporin A, Fujimycin FK506 and the cell-permeable Ca^{2+} chelator BAPTA-AM [1,2-Bis (2-aminophenoxy)ethane-N,N,N',N'-tetraacetic acid (acetoxymethyl ester)]. In contrast, stimulation of $I_{Cl,swell}$ rather than inhibition was reported by others[32,41]. This discrepancy may reflect the complex role of various PKC isoforms.

Reactive oxygen species (ROS) are required for $I_{Cl,swell}$ activation by β_{1D} integrin stretch[22–24] and osmotic swelling[26,42]. Stretch and swelling evoke an autocrine/paracrine cascade that triggers in sequence: (1) angiotensin II type 1 receptors; (2) endothelin ET_A receptors; (3) EGFR kinase; (4) PI-3K; (5) production of $O_2^{-\bullet}$ by NADPH (nicotinamide-adenine dinucleotide phosphate) oxidase; and (6) dismutation of $O_2^{-\bullet}$ to H_2O_2. Block of $I_{Cl,swell}$ by AT_1, ET_A, EGFR kinase and PI-3K inhibitors is overcome by H_2O_2, indicating H_2O_2 is a downstream effector[26,42], and H_2O_2 scavengers, catalase and ebselen, suppress the current. Under isosmotic conditions, exogenous angiotensin II, endothelin, epidermal growth factor (EGF) and H_2O_2 (EC_{50} ~18 μM) also elicit $I_{Cl,swell}$.

Although NADPH oxidase is a required source of ROS in heart and other tissues, it is not a sufficient source. ET-1-induced $I_{Cl,swell}$ is fully suppressed by blocking either NADPH oxidase or mitochondrial ROS production in atrial myocytes[42]. Moreover, $I_{Cl,swell}$ is elicited by stimulating mitochondrial complex III ROS production with antimycin A or diazoxide, and antimycin- and diazoxide-induced $I_{Cl,swell}$ is unaffected by inhibiting NADPH oxidase. ROS (primarily H_2O_2) measurements by flow cytometry confirmed that ET-1-induced ROS production is fully suppressed by blocking NADPH oxidase or mitochondrial electron transport, whereas antimycin- and diazoxide-induced ROS production is unaffected on blocking NADPH oxidase. These data argue that mitochondrial ROS production – triggered by NADPH oxidase ROS – is ultimately responsible for activating $I_{Cl,swell}$ upon osmotic swelling. In contrast, certain HIV protease inhibitors[43] and sphingolipids elicit $I_{Cl,swell}$ via mitochondrial ROS without NADPH oxidase activity (see note added in print).

One difference in transduction of stretch and swelling was noted. Blocking Src with PP2 abrogates $I_{Cl,swell}$ activation by stretch[22], whereas swelling-induced $I_{Cl,swell}$ is augmented[25,37,38]. This suggests that swelling and stretch differently affect one or more Src family members that regulate $I_{Cl,swell}$.

ClC-2

In addition to $I_{Cl,swell}$, an inwardly rectifying Cl^- VAC, termed $I_{Cl,IR}$, is found in atrial and ventricular myocytes and attributed to ClC-2[44]. This channel slowly activates at negative potentials, exhibits $Cl^- > I^- > Asp^-$ permeability and is blocked by 9AC but neither tamoxifen nor DIDS. Osmotic swelling increases its amplitude and speeds activation; shrinkage causes inhibition. Current density of $I_{Cl,IR}$ is less than that of $I_{Cl,swell}$, however.

Non-selective cation volume-activated channels

Although most studies of VAC focus on $I_{Cl,swell}$, several weakly selective cation channels (VAC_{CAT}) are activated by osmotic swelling, as shown in Fig. 4.2. VAC_{CAT} in atrial myocytes exhibits nearly equal permeabilities for Na^+, K^+ and Cs^+ and a P_{Ca}/P_K ratio of 0.13[45]. Its time course of activation closely follows that of the volume change. Swollen myocytes in symmetrical K^+ produced 36 pS unitary currents, and open probability increases on depolarization. Curiously, applying negative pressure to the patch pipette increases VAC_{CAT} open probability in some patches but decreased it in others. This channel has different biophysical characteristics than cationic SAC activated through stretch of a patch by negative pipette pressure (see Chapter 1), and it is insensitive to Gd^{3+}. However, osmotic swelling of ventricular myocytes activates a Gd^{3+}-sensitive VAC_{CAT} with a nearly linear current–voltage (I–V) relationship[46].

An inwardly rectifying cation VAC, termed $I_{Cir,swell}$, with a P_K/P_{Na} ratio of 6 to 8 also is seen on swelling ventricular myocytes (Fig. 4.3)[4,7]. $I_{Cir,swell}$ is blocked by SAC blockers Gd^{3+} and GsMTx-4[4,27,47], but it is insensitive to Ba^{2+}, an inward-rectifier K^+ channel blocker. Importantly, $I_{Cir,swell}$, together with $I_{Cir,swell}$, are persistently activated in ventricular myocytes from dilated cardiomyopathies and are suppressed in diseased cells by osmotic shrinkage[27,28]. $I_{Cir,swell}$ activation in cardiomyopathies is responsible, at least in part, for spontaneous depolarizations that arise late in phase 4 and cause runs of tachycardia; the spontaneous depolarizations and spontaneous activity are blocked by GsMTx-4, Gd^{3+}, or osmotic shrinkage[8]. Moreover, this current contributes to volume regulation in normal and cardiomyopathy myocytes[4,27] and thereby may influence other volume-sensitive processes.

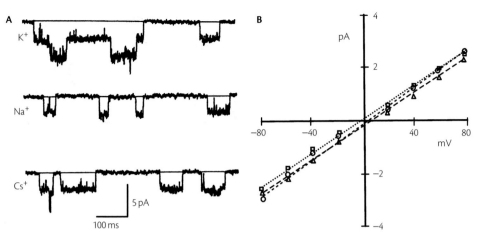

Fig. 4.2 Cation volume-activated channels in rat atrial myocytes do not distinguish among Na^+, K^+ and Cs^+. **A** Unitary currents recorded at -60 mV from cell-attached patches on osmotically swollen cell (0.73T) with 140 mM KCl, NaCl, or CsCl in the pipette. **B** I-V relations from inside-out patch with either 140 mM KCl, NaCl, or CsCl in the bath and 140 mM KCl in the pipette were linear and reversed at 0 mV. Unitary current amplitude, reversal potential and conductance were not significantly affected by choice of cation. [Modified, with permission, from Kim D, Fu C (1993) Activation of a nonselective cation channel by swelling in atrial cells. *J Membr Biol* **135**:27–37.]

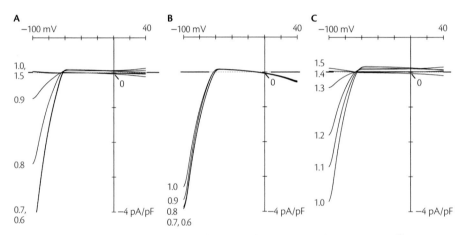

Fig. 4.3 Inwardly rectifying volume-activated cation current, $I_{Cir,swell}$, in control and heart failure dog ventricle measured as Gd^{3+}-sensitive current. **A** Activation is graded on osmotic swelling (0.9T–0.6T). **B** Persistent activation of $I_{Cir,swell}$ in pacing-induced heart. Swelling in 0.9T–0.6T elicits only a slight increase in current. **C** Osmotic shrinkage (1.1T–1.5T) inhibits $I_{Cir,swell}$ in heart failure. $I_{Cir,swell}$ is blocked by the SAC antagonist GsMT-4 but not by Ba^{2+}. Voltage ramp with perforated patch. [Modified, with permission, from Clemo HF, Stambler BS, Baumgarten CM (1998) Persistent activation of a swelling-activated cation current in ventricular myocytes from dogs with tachycardia-induced congestive heart failure. *Circ Res* **83**:147–157.]

Swelling effects on voltage-gated ion channels

I_{Ks}

Sasaki *et al.*[48] examined the effects of cell volume on cardiac delayed rectifier K^+ current, I_K. They found osmotic swelling increases I_K (not separated into rapid and slow components; I_{Kr} and I_{Ks} respectively), whereas osmotic shrinkage inhibits it[49–51]. Selective blockers and analysis of tail currents indicate that I_{Ks} is responsible for augmenting I_K on swelling[46,52–54], and isosmotic cell inflation gives a similar enhancement of I_{Ks}[55]. Whereas swelling selectively augments I_{Ks}, shrinkage inhibits both I_{Kr} and I_{Ks}[51].

Swelling stimulates I_{Ks} by activating PTK[36]. Genistein, but not its inactive analogue daidzein, blocks stimulation of I_{Ks} on cell swelling[54,56]. Moreover, genistein reduces I_{Ks} under isosmotic conditions, suggesting basal PTK activity supports I_{Ks}[54,56].

Caution is warranted, however, because genistein displays non-specific actions. PTK-independent inhibition of I_{Ks} is seen with daidzein[54], and other PTK blockers, lavendustin A and tyrphostin A51, fail to suppress I_{Ks} activation[56].

Cardiac I_{Ks} arises from KCNQ1 (Kv7.1) and an accessory subunit KCNE1 (MinK). KCNQ1 expressed either alone or with KCNE1 in COS-7 cells gives a twofold augmentation of current on swelling, recapitulating activation of I_{Ks}[57]. This suggests KCNQ1 is the osmotically responsive component. Moreover, swelling-induced expressed currents are insensitive to genistein, orthovanadate and AMP-PNP. These data argue that swelling-induced I_{Ks} is independent of PTK, although the native signalling cascade may not be present in COS-7 cells.

Blockers of PKC, PKA and other ser/thr kinases do not prevent enhancement of I_{Ks}[53–55]. Disrupting the actin cytoskeleton with cytochalasin B and D and microtubules with vinblastine and colchicines also is ineffective[55], and the signalling process is insensitive to $[Ca^{2+}]_i$ [49,52,54,55].

I_{Kr}

The responses of I_{Kr} and I_{Ks} to swelling are distinct. Swelling of ventricular myocytes decreases I_{Kr} by 25%[52] (but see[53]). I_{Kr} also is suppressed by swelling sinoatrial node myocytes, which contributes to slowing of automaticity[58].

Osmotic swelling reduces the sensitivity of I_{Kr} to several pharmacologic agents. Normally I_{Kr} is fully blocked by 0.2 μmol/L dofetilide, but after swelling less than 50% inhibition is observed[52]. Swelling also reduces action potential prolongation by E-4031, but this is attributed to multiple plateau currents rather than a specific effect on I_{Kr} [53]. Volume-dependent alterations in drug potency and efficacy may be important issues during ischaemia/reperfusion and in other settings where cell volume changes. This may result from effects on drug binding or, secondarily, because volume alters action potential trajectory and, thus, other conductances.

I_{Ca-L}

Osmotic swelling is reported to stimulate[59,60], inhibit[60,61], or have no effect[48,53,54,62] on L-type Ca^{2+} channels, I_{Ca-L}. At least in rabbit ventricle, however, the effect of swelling on I_{Ca-L} is biphasic. There is an initial increase followed by a decrease under perforated patch conditions[60]. Thus, timing and other experimental details may contribute to these discrepancies.

A detailed study by Matsuda et al.[59] compared responses to hyposmotic bath solution, hyperosmotic pipette solution and hydrostatic cell inflation. In each case, I_{Ca-L} increased by ~35%, without altering its voltage-dependence or inactivation kinetics. Noise analysis indicates that swelling increases open probability by 33%, but unitary current amplitude and the number of active channels are unchanged. Inhibiting PKA or maximizing Ca^{2+} channel phosphorylation with cAMP and forskolin fails to suppress swelling-induced I_{Ca-L} activation. Moreover, strong Ca^{2+} buffering fails to interrupt enhancement of I_{Ca-L} upon hydrostatic inflation.

Hyperosmotic shrinkage also modulates I_{Ca-L}. Shrinkage under ruptured or perforated patch conditions reduces I_{Ca-L} amplitude (~30% in 1.5T) and slows inactivation[50].

I_{Ca-T}

Effects of osmotic stress on T-type Ca^{2+} channels (I_{CaT}) have not been extensively studied. Pascarel et al.[62] showed that osmotic swelling of ventricle stimulates I_{Ca-T} sixfold at a time when I_{Ca-L} is unaffected. Disruption of the actin cytoskeleton with cytochalasin D or microtubules with colchicines prevents swelling-induced I_{Ca-T} activation, but taxol, a microtubule stabilizer, has no effect.

Other cation channels

Osmotic swelling dilutes cytoplasmic K^+ as water flows into the cell, and appropriate shifts of the K^+ equilibrium potential, E_K, are detected under some situations. I_{K1} is, however, unaltered by osmotic swelling[48,52–54,59] or cell inflation[3,55]. I_{to} also is insensitive to volume changes; only a 10% inhibition of I_{to} is seen acutely on swelling of canine ventricle[54], where Kv4.3 is responsible for I_{to}. However, chronic angiotensin II exposure and mechanical stretch destabilize Kv4.3 mRNA via NADPH oxidase-dependent $O_2^{-\bullet}$ production[63], and presumably chronic swelling would have

similar effects. In contrast, these interventions did not affect Kv4.2 expression or that of Kv1.5[63], which is responsible for atrial I_{Kur}. Furthermore, inflation of sino-atrial node myocytes does not significantly alter I_f [59].

Ligand-gated ion channels

I_{K-ATP}

The adenosine triphosphate (ATP)-sensitive K^+ channel, I_{K-ATP}, activates with delay upon hyposmotic swelling, and stretch of cell-attached and inside-out patches by pipette suction provokes single-channel openings[64]. The I-V relationship for VAC I_{K-ATP} is similar to that for pinacidil-activated I_{K-ATP}, and both are blocked by glibenclamide (also see[65,66]). Swelling-induced I_{K-ATP} activation and shortening of action potential duration are enhanced under ischaemic conditions and when $[ATP]_i$ is reduced, suggesting heightened importance during ischaemia and reperfusion. Disruption of the actin cytoskeleton by swelling and ischaemia may trigger these effects because I_{K-ATP} is regulated by f-actin.

I_{K-ACh}

Cardiac muscarinic K^+ channel activity is mechano-sensitive. Stretching patches with pipette suction increases open probability without altering cholinergic agonist affinity[67]. This stimulation is independent of G_i because stretch still augments I_{K-ACh} after its maximal activation with GTPγS. The response to cell swelling is different, however. Inflation myocytes rapidly inhibit carbachol-induced current by 15%[68]. To identify the mechanism, Ji et al.[68] expressed Kir3.1 and Kir3.4 with an excess of Gβγ and osmotically swelled the oocytes. Swelling reduces Kir3.1/3.4 current by 18%, whereas Kir2.1 currents responsible for I_{K1} are unaffected. Furthermore, both Kir3.1[69] and Kir3.4[68] homomeric channels are inhibited by osmotic swelling. The target of swelling may be phosphatidylinositol-4,5-bisphosphate (PIP$_2$). The volume sensitivity of Kir3.4 and native myocytes is abolished by inhibiting PKC[69], and PKC regulates I_{K-ACh} through PIP$_2$ production.

To test the role of PIP$_2$, PIP$_2$ binding to Kir3.4 was enhanced by replacing the binding domain of Kir3.4 with that of Kir2.1, which strengthens the interaction with PIP$_2$[69]. Both volume sensitivity and regulation by PKC is eliminated in these chimeric or mutant Kir3.4. In contrast, mutants of Kir2.1 that weaken association with PIP$_2$ induce volume sensitivity in Kir2.1 not present in wild-type channels.

Pumps and exchangers

Na^+-K^+ pump

Osmotic swelling of ventricular myocytes rapidly stimulates the Na^+-K^+ pump, whereas osmotic shrinkage causes inhibition[49,70]. These responses reflect altered affinity for intracellular free Na^+ concentration ($[Na^+]_i$), whereas the maximum pump current, I_p, and the Hill coefficient for Na^+ are unchanged[70]. Voltage- and $[Na^+]_i$-dependence of swelling-induced I_p may vary in different preparations, however[49,70]. Na^+ affinity is increased by PP1-dependent dephosphorylation on swelling and reduced by PKC-dependent phosphorylation on shrinkage, and it is independent of $[Na^+]_i$ and $[Ca^{2+}]_i$ [71]. PP1 is downstream of PTK, which is rapidly activated on swelling, and PTK and PI-3K inhibitors block Na^+-K^+ pump stimulation.

It is important to remember that I_p with $[Na^+]_i$ fixed by pipette dialysis does not fully reflect I_p in intact myocyte. Swelling causes a persistent decrease of $[Na^+]_i$, whereas shrinkage causes an increase. $[Na^+]_i$ is regulated as a pump-leak system that strives to exactly balance Na^+ influx and efflux. If Na^+ influx is constant, alterations in pump Na^+ affinity during an osmotic challenge necessarily will cause $[Na^+]_i$ to change just enough to restore the pump rate to its original value. Thus, effects of swelling and shrinkage on Na^+ influx ultimately control the Na^+-K^+ pump. Nevertheless, changes in $[Na^+]_i$ required to adjust Na^+ efflux to match the leak will have consequences for other transport processes.

Na^+-Ca^{2+} exchange

The Na^+-Ca^{2+} exchanger (NCX) also is modulated by cardiac cell volume. Hyposmotic swelling decreases I_{NCX}, whereas hyperosmotic shrinkage stimulates the current[72]. Volume-sensitivity is blocked by Ca^{2+}-free bathing solution containing EGTA and by intracellular dialysis with the NCX inhibitory peptide to the XIP region of the exchanger The mechanism by which cardiac NCX is modulated by anisosmotic solutions is unclear but may, in part, reflect altered $[Na^+]_i$.[51]

Na^+-H^+ exchange

Rasmussen's laboratory[73] found that hyperosmotic shrinkage causes intracellular alkalinization due to Na^+-H^+ exchanger (NHE) stimulation. Reducing the gradient driving H^+ extrusion by decreasing extracellular Na^+ ($[Na^+]_o$) or blocking NHE with dimethylamiloride converts alkalinization on shrinkage to acidification, and there is a DMA (5-(N,N-dimethyl)amiloride)-sensitive increase in $[Na^+]_i$ on exposure to hyperosmotic solutions after blocking the Na^+-K^+ pump. As judged by the rate of recovery of intracellular pH (pH_i) from an NH_4Cl pulse, NHE is progressively stimulated over the entire range of hyperosmotic solutions examined. Nevertheless, strong osmotic shrinkage causes acidification rather than alkalinization. This is attributed to Ca^{2+} release from the sarcoplasmic reticulum and the competition between Ca^{2+} and H^+ for binding sites.

Effects of hyposmotic swelling on NHE also were studied[73]. Although pH_i is unchanged, the rate of recovery of pH_i from an NH_4Cl pulse is significantly slowed despite the decrease in cytoplasmic buffer capacity. Thus, swelling causes inhibition of NHE.

Alkalinization in hyperosmotic media and stimulation of H^+ efflux was confirmed by membrane-permeable pH indicator BCECF-AM fluorescence[74]. In these neonatal myocytes, NHE stimulation is Ca^{2+}-dependent and involves calmodulin, CaMKII and myosin light-chain kinase. The effect of swelling and shrinkage on pH_i in intact heart was confirmed by ^{31}P nuclear magnetic resonance[75]. This study concluded, however, that NHE does not control pH_i during a volume change, but rather Cl^--HCO_3^- exchange alters intracellular bicarbonate.

Interestingly, mechanical stretch activates cardiac NHE by autocrine–paracrine signalling involving AT_1 and ET_A receptors and PKC and is thought to cause the slow phase of stretch-induced force development, at least in some species[76]. Cingolani and co-workers[77,78] recently implicated ROS production in this signalling cascade. Therefore, stretch and osmotic swelling activate NHE and $I_{Cl,swell}$[23,24,26,42] by the same pathway. Is there a physiologic benefit from this parallel regulation? NHE-induced alkalinization

in response to stretch[76] and swelling[75] are countered by Cl^--HCO_3^- exchange, which drives Cl^- uptake. One might thus speculate that parallel activation of $I_{Cl,swell}$ permits Cl^- efflux and helps maintain pH_i in these settings.

Conclusions and outlook

Substantial evidence indicates that cell volume modulates a variety of anion and cation channels and transporters in the heart. A critical future goal is to understand the initial steps in transduction and the signalling cascades. Channels and transporters that respond to cell volume (and stretch) are likely to multitask. Nominally 'volume-sensitive' processes can be elicited without altering cell volume, and it will be important to understand how this influences cardiac function. On the other hand, disease processes clearly alter cell volume and VAC, but we are uncertain how this is accomplished and how it influences cardiac electrical activity. Thus, volume sensitivity represents an additional dimension for mechano-electrical coupling.

Acknowledgements

Original studies were supported by grants from the National Institutes of Health (HL-46764 and HL-65435) and American Heart Association (0855044E and 10GRNT3740003).

References

1. Baumgarten CM, Feher JJ (2001) Osmosis and the regulation of cell volume. In: *Cell Physiology Source Book: A Molecular Approach* (ed N Sperelakis). Academic Press, New York, pp. 319–355.

2. Baumgarten CM (2007) Origin of mechanotransduction: stretch-activated ionic channels. In: *Mechanotransduction* (eds M Weckstrom, P Tavi). Landes Bioscience, Georgetown, Texas, pp. 8–27.

3. Du XY, Sorota S. Cardiac swelling-induced chloride current depolarizes canine atrial myocytes. *Am J Physiol* 1997;**272**: H1904–H1916.

4. Clemo HF, Baumgarten CM. Swelling-activated Gd^{3+}-sensitive cation current and cell volume regulation in rabbit ventricular myocytes. *J Gen Physiol* 1997;**110**:297–312.

5. Steltenkamp S, Rommel C, Wegener J, Janshoff A. Membrane stiffness of animal cells challenged by osmotic stress. *Small* 2006;**2**:1016–1020.

6. Spagnoli C, Beyder A, Besch S, Sachs F. Atomic force microscopy analysis of cell volume regulation. *Phys Rev E Stat Nonlin Soft Matter Phys* 2008;**78**:031916.

7. Hume JR, Duan D, Collier ML, Yamazaki J, Horowitz B. Anion transport in heart. *Physiol Rev* 2000;**80**:31–81.

8. Baumgarten CM, Clemo HF. Swelling-activated chloride channels in cardiac physiology and pathophysiology. *Prog Biophys Mol Biol* 2003; **82**:25–42.

9. Duan D. Phenomics of cardiac chloride channels: the systematic study of chloride channel function in the heart. *J Physiol* 2009;**587**:2163–2177.

10. Tseng GN. Cell swelling increases membrane conductance of canine cardiac cells: evidence for a volume-sensitive Cl channel. *Am J Physiol* 1992;**262**:C1056–C1068.

11. Sorota S. Swelling-induced chloride-sensitive current in canine atrial cells revealed by whole-cell patch-clamp method. *Circ Res* 1992;**70**: 679–687.

12. Hagiwara N, Masuda H, Shoda M, Irisawa H. Stretch-activated anion currents of rabbit cardiac myocytes. *J Physiol* 1992;**456**:285–302.

13. Vandenberg JI, Yoshida A, Kirk K, Powell T. Swelling-activated and isoprenaline-activated chloride currents in guinea pig cardiac myocytes have distinct electrophysiology and pharmacology. *J Gen Physiol* 1994; **104**:997–1017.

14. Duan D, Fermini B, Nattel S. α-Adrenergic control of volume-regulated Cl⁻ currents in rabbit atrial myocytes: characterization of a novel ionic regulatory mechanism. *Circ Res* 1995;**77**:379–393.

15. Shuba LM, Ogura T, McDonald TF. Kinetic evidence distinguishing volume-sensitive chloride current from other types in guinea-pig ventricular myocytes. *J Physiol* 1996;**491**:69–80.

16. Decher N, Lang HJ, Nilius B, Bruggemann A, Busch AE, Steinmeyer K. DCPIB is a novel selective blocker of $I_{Cl,swell}$ and prevents swelling-induced shortening of guinea-pig action potential duration. *Br J Pharmacol* 2001;**134**:1467–1479.

17. Sorota S. Pharmacologic properties of the swelling-induced chloride current of dog atrial myocytes. *J Cardiovasc Electrophysiol* 1994;**5**: 1006–1016.

18. Sato R, Koumi S. Characterization of the stretch-activated chloride channel in isolated human atrial myocytes. *J Membr Biol* 1998;**163**: 67–76.

19. Duan D, Nattel S. Properties of single outwardly rectifying Cl⁻ channels in heart. *Circ Res* 1994;**75**:789–795.

20. Wang J, Xu H, Morishima S, *et al.* Single-channel properties of volume-sensitive Cl⁻ channel in ClC-3-deficient cardiomyocytes. *Jpn J Physiol* 2005;**55**:379–383.

21. Demion M, Guinamard R, El CA, Rahmati M, Bois P. An outwardly rectifying chloride channel in human atrial cardiomyocytes. *J Cardiovasc Electrophysiol* 2006;**17**:60–68.

22. Browe DM, Baumgarten CM. Stretch of β1 integrin activates an outwardly rectifying chloride current via FAK and Src in rabbit ventricular myocytes. *J Gen Physiol* 2003;**122**:689–702.

23. Browe DM, Baumgarten CM. Angiotensin II (AT1) receptors and NADPH oxidase regulate Cl⁻ current elicited by β1 integrin stretch in rabbit ventricular myocytes. *J Gen Physiol* 2004;**124**:273–287.

24. Browe DM, Baumgarten CM. EGFR kinase regulates volume-sensitive chloride current elicited by integrin stretch via PI-3K and NADPH oxidase in ventricular myocytes. *J Gen Physiol* 2006;**127**: 237–251.

25. Ren Z, Baumgarten CM. Antagonistic regulation of swelling-activated chloride current in rabbit ventricle by Src and EGFR protein tyrosine kinases. *Am J Physiol* 2005;**288**:H2628–H2636.

26. Ren Z, Raucci FJ Jr, Browe DM, Baumgarten CM. Regulation of swelling-activated Cl current by angiotensin II signalling and NADPH oxidase in rabbit ventricle. *Cardiovasc Res* 2008;**77**:73–80.

27. Clemo HF, Stambler BS, Baumgarten CM. Persistent activation of a swelling-activated cation current in ventricular myocytes from dogs with tachycardia-induced congestive heart failure. *Circ Res* 1998;**83**: 147–157.

28. Clemo HF, Stambler BS, Baumgarten CM. Swelling-activated chloride current is persistently activated in ventricular myocytes from dogs with tachycardia-induced congestive heart failure. *Circ Res* 1999;**84**: 157–165.

29. Chiang CE, Luk HN, Wang TM. Swelling-activated chloride current is activated in guinea pig cardiomyocytes from endotoxic shock. *Cardiovasc Res* 2004;**62**:96–104.

30. d'Anglemont de Tassigny A, Souktani R, Henry P, Ghaleh B, Berdeaux A. Volume-sensitive chloride channels $I_{Cl,vol}$ mediated doxorubicin-induced apoptosis through apoptotic volume decrease in cardiac myocytes. *Fundam Clin Pharmacol* 2004;**18**:531–538.

31. Yamamoto-Mizuma S, Wang GX, Liu LL, *et al.* Altered properties of volume-sensitive osmolyte and anion channels (VSOACs) and membrane protein expression in cardiac and smooth muscle myocytes from Clcn3⁻/⁻ mice. *J Physiol* 2004;**557**:439–456.

32. Gong W, Xu H, Shimizu T, *et al.* ClC-3-independent, PKC-dependent activity of volume-sensitive Cl channel in mouse ventricular cardiomyocytes. *Cell Physiol Biochem* 2004;**14**:213–224.

33. Jentsch TJ, Stein V, Weinreich F, Zdebik AA. Molecular structure and physiological function of chloride channels. *Physiol Rev* 2002;**82**: 503–568.

34. Almaca J, Tian Y, Aldehni F, *et al.* TMEM16 proteins produce volume-regulated chloride currents that are reduced in mice lacking TMEM16A. *J Biol Chem* 2009;**284**:28571–28578.

35. Sadoshima J, Qiu ZH, Morgan JP, Izumo S. Tyrosine kinase activation is an immediate and essential step in hypotonic cell swelling-induced ERK activation and c-*fos* gene expression in cardiac myocytes. *EMBO J* 1996;**15**:5535–5546.

36. Sorota S. Tyrosine protein kinase inhibitors prevent activation of cardiac swelling-induced chloride current. *Pflug Arch* 1995;**431**: 178–185.

37. Du XL, Gao Z, Lau CP, *et al.* Differential effects of tyrosine kinase inhibitors on volume-sensitive chloride current in human atrial myocytes: evidence for dual regulation by Src and EGFR kinases. *J Gen Physiol* 2004;**123**:427–439.

38. Walsh KB, Zhang J. Regulation of cardiac volume-sensitive chloride channel by focal adhesion kinase and Src kinase. *Am J Physiol* 2005; **289**:H2566–H2574.

39. Du XY, Sorota S Modulation of dog atrial swelling-induced chloride current by cAMP: protein kinase A-dependent and -independent pathways. *J Physiol* 1997;**500**:111–122.

40. Duan D, Cowley S, Horowitz B, Hume JR. A serine residue in ClC-3 links phosphorylation–dephosphorylation to chloride channel regulation by cell volume. *J Gen Physiol* 1999;**113**:57–70.

41. Du XY, Sorota S. Protein kinase C stimulates swelling-induced chloride current in canine atrial cells. *Pflug Arch* 1999;**437**:227–234.

42. Deng W, Baki L, Baumgarten CM. Endothelin signalling regulates volume-sensitive Cl⁻ current via NADPH oxidase and mitochondrial reactive oxygen species. *Cardiovasc Res* 2010;**88**:93–100.

43. Deng W, Baki L, Yin J, Zhou H, Baumgarten CM. HIV protease inhibitors elicit volume-sensitive Cl⁻ current in ventricular myocytes via mitochondrial ROS. *J Mol Cell Cardiol* 2010;**49**: 746–752.

44. Duan D, Ye L, Britton F, Horowitz B, Hume JR. A novel anionic inward rectifier in native cardiac myocytes. *Circ Res* 2000;**86**: E63–E71.

45. Kim D, Fu C. Activation of a nonselective cation channel by swelling in atrial cells. *J Membr Biol* 1993;**135**:27–37.

46. Kocic I, Hirano Y, Hiraoka M. Ionic basis for membrane potential changes induced by hypoosmotic stress in guinea-pig ventricular myocytes. *Cardiovasc Res* 2001;**51**:59–70.

47. Suchyna TM, Johnson JH, Hamer K, *et al.* Identification of a peptide toxin from *Grammostola spatulata* spider venom that blocks cation-selective stretch-activated channels. *J Gen Physiol* 2000;**115**:583–598.

48. Sasaki N, Mitsuiye T, Noma A. Effects of mechanical stretch on membrane currents of single ventricular myocytes of guinea-pig heart. *Jpn J Physiol* 1992;**42**:957–970.

49. Sasaki N, Mitsuiye T, Wang Z, Noma A. Increase of the delayed rectifier K⁺ and Na⁺-K⁺ pump currents by hypotonic solutions in guinea pig cardiac myocytes. *Circ Res* 1994;**75**:887–895.

50. Ogura T, You Y, McDonald TF. Membrane currents underlying the modified electrical activity of guinea-pig ventricular myocytes exposed to hyperosmotic solution. *J Physiol* 1997;**504**:135–151.

51. Ogura T, Matsuda H, Shibamoto T, Imanishi S. Osmosensitive properties of rapid and slow delayed rectifier K⁺ currents in guinea-pig heart cells. *Clin Exp Pharmacol Physiol* 2003;**30**:616–622.

52. Rees SA, Vandenberg JI, Wright AR, Yoshida A, Powell T. Cell swelling has differential effects on the rapid and slow components of delayed rectifier potassium current in guinea pig cardiac myocytes. *J Gen Physiol* 1995;**106**:1151–1170.

53. Groh WJ, Gibson KJ, Maylie JG. Hypotonic-induced stretch counteracts the efficacy of the class III antiarrhythmic agent E-4031 in guinea pig myocytes. *Cardiovasc Res* 1996;**31**:237–245.

54. Zhou YY, Yao JA, Tseng GN. Role of tyrosine kinase activity in cardiac slow delayed rectifier channel modulation by cell swelling. *Pflug Arch* 1997;**433**:750–757.

55. Wang ZR, Mitsuiye T, Noma A. Cell distension-induced increase of the delayed rectifier K$^+$ current in guinea pig ventricular myocytes. *Circ Res* 1996;**78**:466–474.

56. Washizuka T, Horie M, Obayashi K, Sasayama S. Does tyrosine kinase modulate delayed-rectifier K channels in guinea pig ventricular cells?. *Heart Vessels* 1997;**12**(Suppl):173–174.

57. Kubota T, Horie M, Takano M, Yoshida H, Otani H, Sasayama S. Role of KCNQ1 in the cell swelling-induced enhancement of the slowly activating delayed rectifier K$^+$ current. *Jpn J Physiol* 2002;**52**:31–39.

58. Lei M, Kohl P. Swelling-induced decrease in spontaneous pacemaker activity of rabbit isolated sino-atrial node cells. *Acta Physiol Scand* 1998;**164**:1–12.

59. Matsuda N, Hagiwara N, Shoda M, Kasanuki H, Hosoda S. Enhancement of the L-type Ca^{2+} current by mechanical stimulation in single rabbit cardiac myocytes. *Circ Res* 1996;**78**:650–659.

60. Li GR, Zhang M, Satin LS, Baumgarten CM. Biphasic effects of cell volume on excitation–contraction coupling in rabbit ventricular myocytes. *Am J Physiol* 2002;**282**:H1270–H1277.

61. Brette F, Calaghan SC, Lappin S, White E, Colyer J, Le Guennec J. Biphasic effects of hyposmotic challenge on excitation-contraction coupling in rat ventricular myocytes. *Am J Physiol* 2000;**279**: H1963–H1971.

62. Pascarel C, Brette F, Le Guennec JY. Enhancement of the T-type calcium current by hyposmotic shock in isolated guinea-pig ventricular myocytes. *J Mol Cell Cardiol* 2001;**33**:1363–1369.

63. Zhou C, Ziegler C, Birder LA, Stewart AF, Levitan ES. Angiotensin II and stretch activate NADPH oxidase to destabilize cardiac Kv4.3 channel mRNA. *Circ Res* 2006;**98**:1040–1047.

64. Van Wagoner DR. Mechanosensitive gating of atrial ATP-sensitive potassium channels. *Circ Res* 1993;**72**:973–983.

65. Priebe L, Beuckelmann DJ. Cell swelling causes the action potential duration to shorten in guinea-pig ventricular myocytes by activating I$_{K,ATP}$. *Pflug Arch* 1998;**436**:894–898.

66. Baron A, van Bever L, Monnier D, Roatti A, Baertschi AJ. A novel K$_{ATP}$ current in cultured neonatal rat atrial appendage cardiomyocytes. *Circ Res* 1999;**85**:707–715.

67. Pleumsamran A, Kim D. Membrane stretch augments the cardiac muscarinic K$^+$ channel activity. *J Membr Biol* 1995;**148**:287–297.

68. Ji S, John SA, Lu Y, Weiss JN. Mechanosensitivity of the cardiac muscarinic potassium channel. A novel property conferred by Kir3.4 subunit. *J Biol Chem* 1998;**273**:1324–1328.

69. Zhang L, Lee JK, John SA, Uozumi N, Kodama I. Mechanosensitivity of GIRK channels is mediated by protein kinase C-dependent channel-phosphatidylinositol 4,5-bisphosphate interaction. *J Biol Chem* 2004; **279**:7037–7047.

70. Whalley DW, Hool LC, Ten Eick RE, Rasmussen HH. Effect of osmotic swelling and shrinkage on Na$^+$-K$^+$ pump activity in mammalian cardiac myocytes. *Am J Physiol* 1993;**265**:C1201–C1210.

71. Bewick NL, Fernandes C, Pitt AD, Rasmussen HH, Whalley DW. Mechanisms of Na$^+$-K$^+$ pump regulation in cardiac myocytes during hyposmolar swelling. *Am J Physiol* 1999;**276**:C1091–C1099.

72. Wright AR, Rees SA, Vandenberg JI, Twist VW, Powell T. Extracellular osmotic pressure modulates sodium-calcium exchange in isolated guinea-pig ventricular myocytes. *J Physiol* 1995;**488**:293–301.

73. Whalley DW, Hemsworth PD, Rasmussen HH. Regulation of intracellular pH in cardiac muscle during cell shrinkage and swelling in anisosmolar solutions. *Am J Physiol* 1994;**266**:H658–H669.

74. Moor AN, Murtazina R, Fliegel L. Calcium and osmotic regulation of the Na$^+$/H$^+$ exchanger in neonatal ventricular myocytes. *J Mol Cell Cardiol* 2000;**32**:925–936.

75. Befroy DE, Powell T, Radda GK, Clarke K. Osmotic shock: modulation of contractile function, pH$_i$, an ischemic damage in perfused guinea pig heart. *Am J Physiol* 1999;**276**:H1236–H1244.

76. Cingolani HE, Ennis IL. Sodium-hydrogen exchanger, cardiac overload, and myocardial hypertrophy. *Circulation* 2007;**115**:1090–1100.

77. Caldiz CI, Garciarena CD, Dulce RA, Novaretto LP, Yeves AM, Ennis IL, *et al.* Mitochondrial reactive oxygen species activate the slow force response to stretch in feline myocardium. *J Physiol* 2007; **584**:895–905.

78. De Giusti V, Correa MV, Villa-Abrille MC, Beltrano C, Yeves AM, de Cingolani GE, *et al.* The positive inotropic effect of endothelin-1 is mediated by mitochondrial reactive oxygen species. *Life Sci* 2008; **83**:264–271.

Note added in Print

The observation that sphingolipids elicit I$_{Cl, swell}$ via mitochondrial ROS without NADPH oxidase activity has been recently been communicated in by Raucci FJ, Jr, and Baumgarten CM: Ceramide activates I$_{Cl, swell}$ in rabbit ventricular myocytes via mitochondrial ROS production. *Biophys J* 2009;**96**:258a (abstract).

5

Non-sarcolemmal stretch-activated channels

Gentaro Iribe and Peter Kohl

Background

Stretch-activated ion channels (SAC) in the mammalian heart were initially identified as structures in the sarcolemma of cardiomyocytes[1]. It would be wrong, though, to assume that this is the only location where SAC can be found. Mechanical stimuli, applied to cardiac myocytes, affect the whole cell. Therefore, ion channels in any intracellular membrane structure may be subject of mechanical modulation. In this chapter we briefly review the myocytes as an integrated mechanical substrate and then discuss the currently available evidence on non-sarcolemmal SAC.

Force transmission between 'outside' and 'inside' of cells

Mechanical integration of the contractile machinery

The contractile machinery of the cardiomyocyte consists of overlapping arrangements of (thin) actin and (thick) myosin filaments that are aligned in parallel with the long axis of the myocyte. Filaments are integrated into sarcomeres where, at the z-line, a multilayered structure anchors the thin filaments of adjacent sarcomeres, as well as the N-termini of opposite titin strands. Mechanical coupling between cells occurs at the intercalated discs (essentially a merger between z-disks of neighbouring cells). At the cell sides, the extracellular matrix (ECM) connects to the contractile apparatus via protein complexes involving integrin and dystrophin that link through to the z-disks via costameric structures[2,3]. These cell–cell and cell–ECM–cell connections help to transmit the forces generated by contractile proteins between 'in' and 'out' sides of the cell (see Fig. 9.1).

Cytoskeleton

Cellular shape stability is a consequence of force balance between opposing structural components, involving pre-stressed and tensile components ('struts' and 'springs'; see tensegrity model reviews[4,5] and Chapter 12). In the cell, force balance is governed by cytoskeleton and the extracellular matrix. In the tensegrity model[4,5] the prestressed struts are microtubules (for example, anchored between integrin sites that mechanically connect the 'inside' to the 'outside' of the cell), while tensile spring components

include non-sarcomeric actin filaments and titin. Mechanical signals can propagate rapidly and efficiently through the cell (essentially at the speed of sound)[5,6].

Membranes

The cell membrane delineates the inside from the outside of cells. In the case of acute mechanical deformation, cells are presumed to retain their volume. Thus, shape changes should affect the surface-to-volume ratio. However, the lipid bilayer—while fluid—is relatively resistant to area expansion, so it will not behave like an elastic sheet (an increase in lipid bilayer membrane area of more than 3% will cause membrane rupture)[7]. This apparent contradiction is explained by the fact that cell membranes contain folds; in cardiomyocytes these may include invaginations at the z-lines (whether or not continous with t-tubules that penetrate the cell interior), microfolds and caveolae. When cells are stretched, the membrane is partially unfolded (a bit like a concertina), giving rise to an *apparent* increase in surface area[8]. In this context, sub-sarcolemmal caveolae may be integrated into the surface membrane in response to stretch, thereby potentially increasing actual membrane area[8] (see also Chapter 7).

Cytosolic viscosity

Cells are viscoelastic bodies[9]. Elasticity and viscosity interact. For example, neighbouring microtubules in cardiomyocytes 'buckle' in a spatially and temporally coordinated way[10]. Thus, cytosolic viscosity contributes to structural coupling (as a function of spatial proximity and relative velocity of deformation), in addition to tensile and elastic coupling, and provides high-speed and steady-state constraints to deformation[6].

The cell as an integrated mechanical substrate

Cardiomyocytes are continuously exposed to a dynamically changing mechanical environment as they cycle through contraction, relaxation and passive distension. Mechano-sensitive responses range from adaptation to chronic challenges (e.g. via cell signalling cascades that adjust the 'trophic state' of cardiac cells to elevated mechanical demands, such as in pregnancy-induced hypertrophy), to acute responses such as the classic Frank–Starling and Bainbridge responses (for details see Chapters 10 and 13).

Responses to stretch of non-sarcolemmal ion channels

Sarcoplasmic reticulum

Cardiomyocyte Ca^{2+} handling is modified by the mechanical environment at various levels (see Chapters 10, 16 and 21).

For instance, stretching cardiac muscle will, over several minutes, lead to an increase in peak intracellular free Ca^{2+} concentration ($[Ca^{2+}]_i$) during the Ca^{2+} transient and correspondingly raise twitch force[11]. This is caused by an increase in Ca^{2+} concentration in the sarcoplasmic reticulum (SR) ($[Ca^{2+}]_{SR}$). This increase is generally attributed to factors external to the SR itself. One explanation is based on a stretch-induced increase in Na^+ influx (via cation non-selective stretch-activated channels, SAC_{NS}, or through altered activity of the Na^+/H^+ exchanger, NHE). An increase in intracellular free Na^+ concentration ($[Na^+]_i$) would affect the ability of the Na^+/Ca^{2+} exchanger (NCX) to extrude Ca^{2+}, causing partial preservation of $[Ca^{2+}]_i$ and, hence, accumulation of $[Ca^{2+}]_{SR}$[12,13]. $[Ca^{2+}]_{SR}$ is, therefore, both a slave and a master of the cyclically changing $[Ca^{2+}]_i$. Both are affected by a number of time-, voltage- and ligand-dependent processes, including finely balanced trans-sarcolemmal Ca^{2+} influx and extrusion, as well as SR uptake and release (in steady state, the opposite fluxes between spatial domains must be pair-wise equivalent over time)[14].

Given this complexity, experimental insight can be gained from studies under quiescent conditions, i.e. when key ion fluxes associated with excitation–contraction coupling are excluded. Even in the quiescent state, $[Ca^{2+}]_{SR}$ is determined by the balance of Ca^{2+} release (leak) and (re)uptake via SR and sarcolemmal membranes[15]. In the rat, this leads to an increase of $[Ca^{2+}]_{SR}$ with rest time. This 'post-rest potentiation' in $[Ca^{2+}]_{SR}$ is illustrated in Fig. 5.1; rapid cooling-induced contracture (RCC) of rat papillary

muscle increases with the duration of quiescence after termination of the conditioning pacing run. However, if exposed to diastolic stretch, the relative gain of $[Ca^{2+}]_{SR}$ is reduced (after 1 min of rest; Fig. 5.1)[16]. Thus, in rat myocardium, diastolic stretch counters SR Ca^{2+} accumulation.

In contrast to rat, guinea pig cardiomyocytes show a 'post-rest decay' in $[Ca^{2+}]_{SR}$. The magnitude of $[Ca^{2+}]_{SR}$ reduction in guinea pig single cardiomyocytes (after 1 min rest) is greater in axially stretched cells[17] (Fig. 5.2A). Thus, in guinea pig, diastolic stretch enhances SR Ca^{2+} loss.

These stretch effects on SR Ca^{2+} handling (both in rat and guinea pig) could be explained either by an increase in Ca^{2+} leak from the SR or by a decrease in SR Ca^{2+} uptake. However, considering the effects of stretch on the trans-sarcolemmal Ca^{2+} flux balance (see above), a decrease in SR Ca^{2+} uptake seems unlikely. Indeed, if one starts off with an emptied SR (depleted by caffeine exposure), a stretch-induced increase in the rate of SR Ca^{2+} recovery can be observed (Fig. 5.2B)[17]. Therefore, it would seem that stretch induces an increase in both SR Ca^{2+} leak and uptake, whose balance – which is affected by the initial $[Ca^{2+}]_{SR}$ and by species differences – determines SR content.

Ca^{2+} leak from the SR can be observed in the form of individual Ca^{2+} sparks[18] – spontaneous and local Ca^{2+} release events from SR Ca^{2+} release channels (aka ryanodine receptors, RyR). During application of axial stretch, Ca^{2+} spark rate increases (Fig. 5.3A)[19]. In intact rat myocytes 8% strain, applied using the carbon fibre technique, gives rise to an immediate and transient increase in Ca^{2+} spark rate by ~30%, without changes in individual spark dynamics. Large stretch-induced SR Ca^{2+} release can sum up sparks to trigger full-blown Ca^{2+} waves (Fig. 5.3B; see also Chapter 2). This suggests that the open probability of RyR is increased acutely by stretch. The stretch-induced increase in Ca^{2+} spark rate is transient and recovers to the original level after 1 min, probably because the gradually reduced $[Ca^{2+}]_{SR}$ (a main driver of SR spark release) moves the system back towards a lower spark rate equilibrium.

The acute increase in Ca^{2+} sparks is different from that observed after prolonged periods of sustained stretch (over 10 min), where a nitric oxide (NO)-mediated pathway has been identified[20]. Of note, the acute stretch-induced increase in Ca^{2+} spark rate is not affected by incubation with L-NAME (N^G-nitro-L-arginine methyl ester) to inhibit NO synthase.[19]

How is the open probability of RyR affected by externally applied cell stretch? Membrane potential changes would not explain the local nature of the stretch-induced increase in Ca^{2+} spark frequency, as observed during mechanical distension of only half the cell (Fig. 5.3A). Possible contributions from stretch-induced trans-sarcolemmal Ca^{2+} influx, followed by Ca^{2+}-induced Ca^{2+} release (CICR) from the SR were excluded by conducting the same experiments in the absence of external Ca^{2+} and Na^+[19]. A possible source of trigger-Ca^{2+} for CICR could be mitochondria, as mitochondrial Ca^{2+} concentration ($[Ca^{2+}]_{MX}$) is reduced during fluid shear-induced slow Ca^{2+} transients, observed in rat cardiomyocytes with chemically permeabilized sarcolemma (see next section)[21,22].

Alternatively, RyR may be SAC in their own right. While currently unconfirmed in direct recordings, this hypothesis is supported by cytostructural analysis. Disruption of cytoskeletal integrity (by prolonged incubation with colchicine) abolishes the acute stretch-induced increase in Ca^{2+} spark rate. It is not clear how the cytoskeleton modifies the behaviour of RyR, but electron

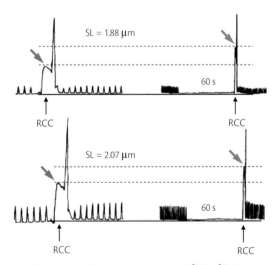

Fig. 5.1 Stretch-induced reduction in post-rest SR Ca^{2+} ($[Ca^{2+}]_{SR}$) increase, assessed by rapid cooling contracture (RCC) in rat papillary muscle. The ratio of post-rest RCC (red arrows) to steady state RCC (grey arrows) is smaller at increased diastolic sarcomere length (SL). Top: slack length; bottom: during stretch. [Reproduced, with permission, from Gamble J, Taylor PB, Kenno KA (1992) Myocardial stretch alters twitch characteristics and Ca^{2+} loading of sarcoplasmic reticulum in rat ventricular muscle. *Cardiovasc Res* **26**:865–870.]

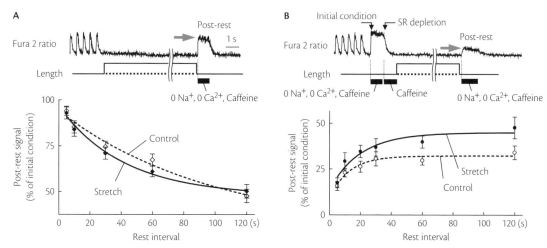

Fig. 5.2 Stretch-induced enhancement of SR Ca^{2+} leak (**A**) and reuptake after initial emptying of the SR by caffeine prepulse (**B**) in guinea pig myocyte. Post-rest [Ca^{2+}]$_{SR}$ (red arrow) is assessed by the amplitude of the Fura 2 ratio, measured from a caffeine-induced [Ca^{2+}]$_i$ transient in Na$^+$/Ca^{2+} free solution (top panels: Fura 2 ratio and stretch marker). Summary data are plotted as a function of the rest interval duration (bottom panels). [Reproduced, with permission, from Iribe G, Kohl P (2008) Axial stretch enhances sarcoplasmic reticulum Ca^{2+} leak and cellular Ca^{2+} reuptake in guinea pig ventricular myocytes: experiments and models. *Prog Biophys Mol Biol* **97**:298–311.]

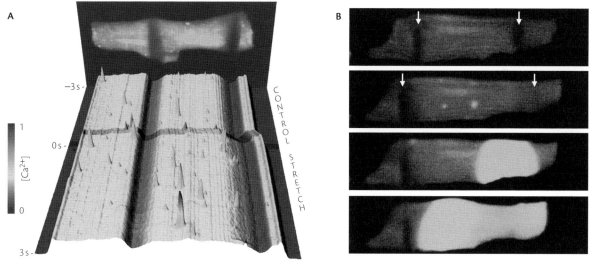

Fig. 5.3 A Acute stretch-induced increase in Ca^{2+} spark rate. Stretch (8%) was applied, at time 0 s, to the right half of the cell only, using carbon fibres attached to centre of the cell (anchor) and the right cell-end (low signal intensity regions on cell image panel at rear and 'canyons' in space–time plot at front). Spark rate increased after stretch only at the stretched part of the cell. **B** Acute application of large whole-cell axial stretch (> 20%, compare first and second row) increases spark rate (see bright spots in second row) and gives rise to a mechanically induced full Ca^{2+} wave (third and fourth rows). (See color plate section.)

microscopic tomography confirmed that microtubules approach the SR–t-tubular membrane complex to within 10 nm (Fig. 5.4), suggesting that the cytoskeleton may transmit physical deformation from the cell exterior to the SR, potentially modifying RyR gating.

Mitochondria

Mitochondria occupy ~35% of cardiomyocyte cell volume and are important not only for adenosine triphosphate (ATP) production,

but also for regulation of Ca^{2+} signalling, for instance in apoptosis[23]. Cytosolic ions can permeate the mitochondrial outer membrane through voltage-dependent anion channel (VDAC)[24]. As a consequence, Ca^{2+} concentration in the mitochondrial intermembrane space follows [Ca^{2+}]$_i$. In contrast, the mitochondrial inner membrane has a number of selective ion channels and exchangers that generate a steep ion concentration gradient[25], which also determines [Ca^{2+}]$_{MX}$.

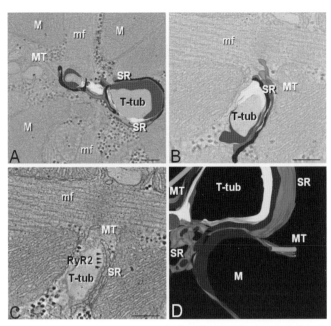

Fig. 5.4 Electron microscopic tomography (EMT) images of an SR–t-tubular membrane complex with associated microtubules from a rat ventricular cardiomyocyte. **A** and **B** Three-dimensional (3D) reconstructions, superimposed on single EMT sections. **C** Single EMT X–Y plane with outline of relevant structures. **D** Detail of 3D reconstruction showing close approximation of SR–t-tubular membrane complex, mitochondria and microtubules. Microtubules approach ryanodine receptor locations to within ~10 nm. T-tub, t-tubular membrane; SR, sarcoplasmic reticulum; MT, microtubule; M, mitochondria; mf, myofilaments; RyR2, ryanodine receptor. Scale bars: 200 nm. (See color plate section.)

As mentioned above, application of fluid shear stress by local pressurized flow (PF) induces a slow Ca^{2+} transient in rat cardiomyocytes[21,22,26,27], which has been associated with a reduction in $[Ca^{2+}]_{MX}$ in permabilized cells (Fig. 5.5). Possible sources for the slow Ca^{2+} transient include CICR from the SR, Ca^{2+} release via inositol triphosphate receptors (IP_3R) from the endoplasmic reticulum (ER) and mitochondria. Neither Na^+/Ca^{2+} free extracellular perfusion (to prevent Ca^{2+} influx required for CICR) nor block of IP_3R prevented PF-induced slow Ca^{2+} transients. In contrast, carbonyl cyanide-p-trifluoromethoxyphenylhydrazone (FCCP: a proton ionophore that is commonly used to uncouple ATP synthesis) and ruthenium 360 (Ru360: a mitochondrial Ca^{2+} uniporter blocker), applied to suppress Ca^{2+} uptake by mitochondria, blocked PF-induced slow Ca^{2+} transients. Therefore, mitochondria could be a source for PF-induced Ca^{2+} release (direct mechanically induced release of Ca^{2+} from the SR, described above, was not assessed in these studies).

Direct fluorometric measurement of $[Ca^{2+}]_{MX}$ (using Rhod-2 in permeabilized cardiomyocytes) confirmed that PF reduces mitochondrial Ca^{2+} in rat cardiac myocytes (Fig. 5.5). In atrial myocytes, the PF-induced increase in Ca^{2+} sparks can give rise to whole cell Ca^{2+} waves[27]. As mitochondria are located in close proximity to the dyadic space (200 nm or less; see Fig. 5.4)[28,29], it is possible that release from mitochondria may increase Ca^{2+} concentration in the dyadic space, inducing CICR.

Current questions in this context include: What is the identity of the mitochondrial Ca^{2+} transporter involved in PF-induced release? What is the means of mechanical impulse transmission from the cell surface to mitochondria? What is the interrelation of stretch with RyR open probability? PF-induced Ca^{2+} transients are suppressed by blocking mitochondrial NCX (mNCX), either by applying CGP-37157 (7-chloro-5-(2-chlorophenyl)1,5-dihydro-4, 1-benzothiazepin-2(3H)-one) or by exposure to a Na^+ free mitochondrial environment, which makes mNCX a possible substrate of the response to PF. Mechano-sensitivity of mNCX has also been confirmed in electrophysiological recordings. The transmission of mechanical deformation from externally applied PF to mitochondria may involve viscous coupling that links the velocity of sarcolemmal indentation to deformation of underlying mitochondria. That said, in atrial cardiomyocytes, even centrally located mitochondria respond to the mechanical stimulus. A possible link between them may be the z-disk, or microtubules that can be traced in close proximity to mitochondrial outer membranes (see Fig. 5.4D). Insight into the effects of partial disruption of cytoskeletal structures on PF-induced slow Ca^{2+} transients, and the associated Ca^{2+} sources, is still missing.

Nucleus

Nuclei are mechanically linked to integrins via the cytoskeleton[30]. Nuclear shape changes, for example caused by cell spreading on a solid substrate, are accompanied by an increase in perinuclear Ca^{2+} concentration. This Ca^{2+} is taken up into the nucleus via cation channels in the nuclear envelope, where it induces intra-nuclear signal transduction[6], for example leading to hypertrophic changes in cardiac myocytes[31]. Stretch sensitivity of nuclear cation channel has been confirmed directly in patch-clamp experiments, where an decrease in pipette pressure (suction) raised channel open probability (Fig. 5.6)[32].

Cytoskeleton-dependent nuclear signal transduction does not require acute mechanical stimulation. For instance, pharmacological modulation of actin filament structural integrity may alter nuclear envelope channel activity, in the absence of additional external mechanical stimulation[33]. That said, cytoskeletal properties (chemical equilibria, molecular polymerization) are modulated by the mesoscopic mechanical environment[34,35], while contributing to microscopic mechanical conditions (see also Chapters 8 and 12).

Connexin channels

The cytosols of neighbouring cardiomyocytes (and other cells, including cardiac fibroblasts)[36] are connected via gap junctions. Gap junctions consist of two interconnected hemichannels, each located in the sarcolemma of one of the adjacent cells (see Chapter 18). Hemichannels are formed from six connexins. If not connected to another hemichannel, they can act as trans-sarcolemmal pathways for ion fluxes.

Connexin 43 (Cx43) is the main connexin in ventricular myocardium. Cx43 hemichannels are closed at physiological extracellular Ca^{2+} concentrations. This helps to explain why cells can survive enzymatic isolation. Nonetheless, hemichannel opening is believed to be a contributor to ischaemic injury in the heart[37].

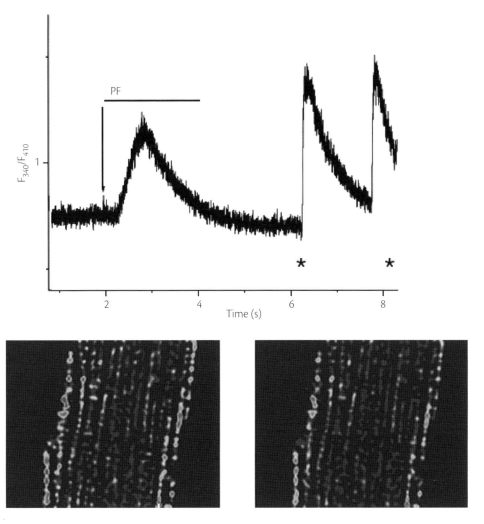

Fig. 5.5 Pressure flow (PF)-induced slow [Ca^{2+}]$_i$ transient (top: ratiometric measurement using Fura 2) and mitochondrial Ca signal (rhod-2) before applying PF (bottom left) and 6 s after applying PF in permeabilized ventricular myocytes (bottom right). PF-induced Ca^{2+} transients are accompanied by a reduction in mitochondrial [Ca^{2+}]. [Reproduced, with permission, from Belmonte S, Morad M (2008) 'Pressure-flow'-triggered intracellular Ca^{2+} transients in rat cardiac myocytes: possible mechanisms and role of mitochondria. *J Physiol* **586**:1379–1397.] (See color plate section.)

In addition, mechanical stimulation upregulates Cx43 expression in cultured cardiomyocytes[38].

In contrast to this slow (trophic) response, some connexin hemichannels [such as connexin 46 (Cx46), expressed in lens tissue] respond to mechanical stimulation by an acute increase in their open probability[39]. Whether coupled hemichannels (gap junctional channels) retain the ability to alter gating in response to their mechanical environment is unknown. Equally, the question whether cardiac connexin hemichannels display mechano-sensitivity needs further research.

Conclusions and outlook

Cardiomyocytes are integrated mechanical systems, in which stresses and/or strains can affect all organelles in the cell, potentially activating non-sarcolemmal SAC. Evidence for the presence of internal SAC has been reported for SR, mitochondria and the nuclear envelope. Direct electrophysiological investigation of these putative SAC is more difficult than for their sarcolemmal counterparts (even though many of the latter tend to 'hide' in adult ventricular cells inside surface membrane invaginations). Experimental access and application of

mechanical stimulation to non-sarcolemmal SAC is limited to local interventions, such as patching isolated organelles or liposomes, but these techniques are difficult to implement, and they do not preserve the normal intracellular mechanical environment.

The (patho-)physiological relevance of non-sarcolemmal SAC is largely speculative at this time. It has been proposed, for example, that mechano-sensitivity of RyR gating may not only form a contribution to the Frank–Starling response, but also be involved in terminating Ca^{2+} release from the SR as heart muscle cells shorten[40]. If present in pacemaker cells, a stretch-induced increase in Ca^{2+} release from intracellular stores could contribute to the Bainbridge effect, via actions on the 'Ca^{2+} clock'[41,42]. SAC in the nuclear envelope might contribute to mechano-sensitive signalling, for example in the context of switching 'on' hypertrophic signalling cascades in cardiac myocytes. The role of mitochondrial SAC is, perhaps, less intuitively obvious, as there is significant beat-by-beat deformation of mitochondria, sandwiched between contractile filament bundles. Clearly further research is required to elucidate the physiological relevance of non-sarcolemmal SAC. Equally, the pathophysiological potential of non-sarcolemmal SAC requires further elucidation. In the case of ischaemic uncoupling, connexin

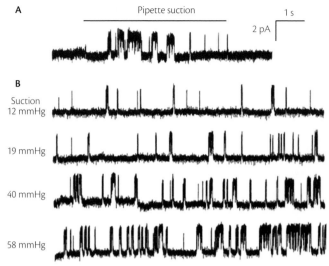

Fig. 5.6 *Mechano-sensitive single channel currents from the nuclear membrane.* **A** Typical recording from a nucleus-attached patch-clamp recording, showing increased channel opening probability during pipette suction (40 mmHg, holding potential +40 mV). **B** Pipette pressure dependence of channel open probability (holding potential +40 mV). [Reproduced, with permission, from Itano N, Okamoto S, Zhang D, Lipton SA, Ruoslahti E (2003) Cell spreading controls endoplasmic and nuclear calcium: a physical gene regulation pathway from the cell surface to the nucleus. *Proc Natl Acad Sci USA* **100**:5181–5186.]

hemichannel mechano-sensing may become a relevant contributor to pathogenesis. Equally, stretch-induced release of Ca^{2+} from internal stores (whether SR or mitochondria) may trip the balance in Ca^{2+} overloaded states towards induction of Ca^{2+} waves via CICR and/or arrhythmogenic NCX-mediated depolarizations.

References

1. Craelius W, Chen V, el-Sherif N. Stretch activated ion channels in ventricular myocytes. *Biosci Rep* 1988;**8**:407–414.

2. Ervasti JM. Costameres: the Achilles' heel of Herculean muscle. *J Biol Chem* 2003;**278**:13591–13594.

3. Samarel AM. Costameres, focal adhesions, and cardiomyocyte mechanotransduction. *Am J Physiol* 2005;**289**:H2291–H2301.

4. Ingber DE. Tensegrity I. Cell structure and hierarchical systems biology. *J Cell Sci* 2003;**116**:1157–1173.

5. Ingber DE. Tensegrity II. How structural networks influence cellular information processing networks. *J Cell Sci* 2003;**116**:1397–1408.

6. Wang N, Tytell JD, Ingber DE. Mechanotransduction at a distance: mechanically coupling the extracellular matrix with the nucleus. *Nature Rev* 2009;**10**:75–82.

7. Hamill OP, Martinac B. Molecular basis of mechanotransduction in living cells. *Physiol Rev* 2001;**81**:685–740.

8. Kohl P, Cooper PJ, Holloway H. Effects of acute ventricular volume manipulation on in situ cardiomyocyte cell membrane configuration. *Prog Biophys Mol Biol* 2003;**82**:221–227.

9. Heidemann SR, Kaech S, Buxbaum RE, Matus A. Direct observations of the mechanical behaviors of the cytoskeleton in living fibroblasts. *J Cell Biol* 1999;**145**:109–122.

10. Brangwynne CP, MacKintosh FC, Kumar S, *et al.* Microtubules can bear enhanced compressive loads in living cells because of lateral reinforcement. *J Cell Biol* 2006;**173**:733–741.

11. Allen DG, Kurihara S. The effects of muscle length on intracellular calcium transients in mammalian cardiac muscle. *J Physiol* 1982;**327**:79–94.

12. Calaghan SC, White E. Contribution of angiotensin II, endothelin 1 and the endothelium to the slow inotropic response to stretch in ferret papillary muscle. *Pflugers Arch* 2001;**441**:514–520.

13. Le Guennec JY, White E, Gannier F, Argibay JA, Garnier D. Stretch-induced increase of resting intracellular calcium concentration in single guinea-pig ventricular myocytes. *Exp Physiol* 1991;**76**: 975–978.

14. Dibb KM, Graham HK, Venetucci LA, Eisner DA, Trafford AW. Analysis of cellular calcium fluxes in cardiac muscle to understand calcium homeostasis in the heart. *Cell Calcium* 2007;**42**:503–512.

15. Diaz ME, Graham HK, O'Neill SC, Trafford AW, Eisner DA. The control of sarcoplasmic reticulum Ca content in cardiac muscle. *Cell Calcium* 2005;**38**:391–396.

16. Gamble J, Taylor PB, Kenno KA. Myocardial stretch alters twitch characteristics and Ca^{2+} loading of sarcoplasmic reticulum in rat ventricular muscle. *Cardiovasc Res* 1992;**26**:865–870.

17. Iribe G, Kohl P. Axial stretch enhances sarcoplasmic reticulum Ca^{2+} leak and cellular Ca^{2+} reuptake in guinea pig ventricular myocytes: experiments and models. *Prog Biophys Mol Biol* 2008;**97**:298–311.

18. Cheng H, Lederer WJ, Cannell MB. Calcium sparks: elementary events underlying excitation–contraction coupling in heart muscle. *Science (N Y)* 1993;**262**:740–744.

19. Iribe G, Ward CW, Camelliti P, Bollensdorff C, Mason F, Burton RA, *et al.* Axial stretch of rat single ventricular cardiomyocytes causes an acute and transient increase in Ca^{2+} spark rate. *Circ Res* 2009;**104**: 787–795.

20. Petroff MG, Kim SH, Pepe S, *et al.* Endogenous nitric oxide mechanisms mediate the stretch dependence of Ca^{2+} release in cardiomyocytes. *Nature Cell Biol* 2001;**3**:867–873.

21. Belmonte S, Morad M. Shear fluid-induced Ca^{2+} release and the role of mitochondria in rat cardiac myocytes. *Annals N Y Acad Sci* 2008;**1123**:58–63.

22. Belmonte S, Morad M. 'Pressure-flow'-triggered intracellular Ca^{2+} transients in rat cardiac myocytes: possible mechanisms and role of mitochondria. *J Physiol* 2008;**586**:1379–1397.

23. Zhu LP, Yu XD, Ling S, Brown RA, Kuo TH. Mitochondrial Ca^{2+} homeostasis in the regulation of apoptotic and necrotic cell deaths. *Cell Calcium* 2000;**28**:107–117.

24. Colombini M. VDAC: the channel at the interface between mitochondria and the cytosol. *Molec Cell Biochem* 2004;**256–257**:107–115.

25. Bernardi P. Mitochondrial transport of cations: channels, exchangers, and permeability transition. *Physiol Rev* 1999;**79**:1127–1155.

26. Morad M, Javaheri A, Risius T, Belmonte S. Multimodality of Ca^{2+} signaling in rat atrial myocytes. *Annals N Y Acad Sci* 2005;**1047**:112–121.

27. Woo SH, Risius T, Morad M. Modulation of local Ca^{2+} release sites by rapid fluid puffing in rat atrial myocytes. *Cell Calcium* 2007;**41**: 397–403.

28. Sanchez JA, Garcia MC, Sharma VK, Young KC, Matlib MA, Sheu SS. Mitochondria regulate inactivation of L-type Ca^{2+} channels in rat heart. *J Physiol* 2001;**536**:387–396.

29. Ramesh V, Sharma VK, Sheu SS, Franzini-Armstrong C. Structural proximity of mitochondria to calcium release units in rat ventricular myocardium may suggest a role in Ca^{2+} sequestration. *Annals N Y Acad Sci* 1998;**853**:341–344.

30. Maniotis AJ, Chen CS, Ingber DE. Demonstration of mechanical connections between integrins, cytoskeletal filaments, and nucleoplasm that stabilize nuclear structure. *Proc Natl Acad Sci USA* 1997;**94**: 849–854.

31. Passier R, Zeng H, Frey N, *et al.* CaM kinase signaling induces cardiac hypertrophy and activates the MEF2 transcription factor in vivo. *J Clin Invest* 2000;**105**:1395–1406.

32. Itano N, Okamoto S, Zhang D, Lipton SA, Ruoslahti E. Cell spreading controls endoplasmic and nuclear calcium: a physical gene regulation pathway from the cell surface to the nucleus. *Proc Natl Acad Sci USA* 2003;**100**:5181–5186.

33. Prat AG, Cantiello HF. Nuclear ion channel activity is regulated by actin filaments. *Am J Physiol* 1996;**270**:C1532–C1543.

34. Buxbaum RE, Heidemann SR. A thermodynamic model for force integration and microtubule assembly during axonal elongation. *J Theoret Biol* 1988;**134**:379–390.

35. Putnam AJ, Schultz K, Mooney DJ. Control of microtubule assembly by extracellular matrix and externally applied strain. *Am J Physiol* 2001;**280**:C556–C564.

36. Camelliti P, Borg TK, Kohl P. Structural and functional characterisation of cardiac fibroblasts. *Cardiovasc Res* 2005;**65**:40–51.

37. Shintani-Ishida K, Uemura K, Yoshida K. Hemichannels in cardiomyocytes open transiently during ischemia and contribute to reperfusion injury following brief ischemia. *Am J Physiol* 2007;**293**:H1714–H1720.

38. Zhuang J, Yamada KA, Saffitz JE, Kleber AG. Pulsatile stretch remodels cell-to-cell communication in cultured myocytes. *Circ Res* 2000;**87**:316–322.

39. Bao L, Sachs F, Dahl G. Connexins are mechanosensitive. *Am J Physiol* 2004;**287**:C1389–C1395.

40. Cannell MB. Pulling on the heart strings: a new mechanism within Starling's law of the heart? *Circ Res* 2009;**104**:715–716.

41. Bogdanov KY, Vinogradova TM, Lakatta EG. Sinoatrial nodal cell ryanodine receptor and Na^+–Ca^{2+} exchanger: molecular partners in pacemaker regulation. *Circ Res* 2001;**88**:1254–1258.

42. Huser J, Blatter LA, Lipsius SL. Intracellular Ca^{2+} release contributes to automaticity in cat atrial pacemaker cells. *J Physiol* 2000;**524**:415–422.

6

Pacemaker, potassium, calcium, sodium: stretch modulation of the voltage-gated channels

Catherine E. Morris

Background

Cardiomyocyte voltage-gated channels (VGC) are abundant, ubiquitous and continuously at work. They are also inherently susceptible to bilayer stretch[1–5]. When dysfunctional, VGC can cause life-threatening arrhythmias and their contributions to mechano-transduction in stretch-induced cardiac arrhythmias are beginning to receive attention[6–10]. Wherever bilayer deformations occur, beat-to-beat cardiac electrical activity should reflect stretch-modulated feedback.

This chapter first briefly explains what underlies the susceptibility of VGC to stretch, at the same time pointing out why this is difficult to study *in situ*. Next it explores how and why pharmacologically modified and disease-mutated VGC might be used to explore the roles of VGC in cardiac mechano-electric coupling (MEC). The last section briefly covers selected features of stretch-modulated gating kinetics in different families of VGC: pacemaker (HCN), potassium (Kv), calcium Cav and sodium (Nav) channels.

VGC and the lipid bilayer

The susceptibility of VGC to mechanical stimuli is now broadly understood[11–14]. VGC are exquisitely structured membrane proteins that adopt various conformations (closed, open, inactivated, etc.) (Fig. 6.1A). Importantly, the diverse bilayers in which VGC are embedded are also structured – bilayers are not merely 2D solvents[15]. Physical events (stretch, bending, shear, hyperbaric pressure, cold) and chemical variation in the bilayer's make-up (e.g. cholesterol, lysophospholipid, sphingomyelin, ethanol) perturb the structure and hence energetics (summarized by profiles of **lateral pressure** of the bilayer as exemplified in Fig. 6.1B). Each VGC has four laterally located voltage sensors that respond to voltage. With voltage sensor motions occurring at the lateral interface, Δ[bilayer mechanics] = Δ[voltage sensor motions] = Δ[VGC activity] during any voltage excursion. If a bilayer thickens, if its

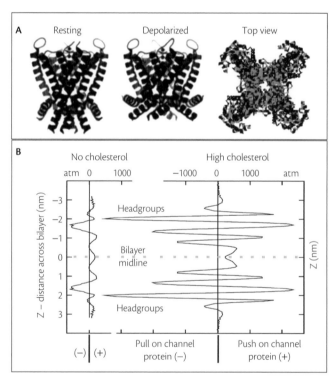

Fig. 6.1 Bilayer mechanics and voltage-gated channels. **A** VGC shape (modified from homotetrameric Kv channel structures[12], shown resting (left) and in an open-like conformation plus a top view (plane of bilayer), emphasizing the extensive periphery for lateral protein–lipid interactions. **B** Lateral pressure profiles (from simulated symmetrical bilayers without/with cholesterol) illustrate the link between bilayer structure/mechanics. Over < 1 nm, lateral pressures change dramatically (+/– thousands of atm). Embedded proteins experience localized push/pull forces (at equilibrium, balancing to zero across the bilayer) whose patterns would vary with lipid composition, stretch, hyperbaric pressure, temperature, etc. (modified from [15] which should be consulted for further explanation; see also [14,17]). Native bilayers, unlike what is depicted here, have non-identical leaflets.

molecular packing gets denser, more orderly (as with hyperbaric pressure or cholesterol-enrichment or cold), voltage sensor movements are impeded and VGC activation becomes sluggish. If, by contrast, a bilayer thins, becomes less orderly, less densely packed (as with membrane stretch, high temperature, elevated fatty acid content), voltage sensor movements speed up, causing VGC to operate more quickly and, typically, at 'lower' voltage thresholds.

Summarizing, *VGC behaviour is inextricably linked to bilayer mechanics because lateral interactions between the structured bilayer and the structured protein must adjust when either bilayer structure or protein structure changes.*

Stretch-modulated VGC activity and myocardial physiology

What do these biophysical basics signify for complex cardiac electrical events? Statements 1 and 2 provide a rapid overview of where things stand regarding this question.

◆ **Statement 1**: *Channel 'X' of cardio-membrane 'Y' contributes to rhythmic cardiac excitation phenomenon 'Z' and implicates channel 'X' in abnormailty 'D' causing cardiac dys-rhythmia 'Q'.*

As suggested by many recent reviews, many of the variables of Statement 1 can be filled in – the challenge is to be able to do likewise for Statement 2.

◆ **Statement 2**: *Stretch-modulated VGC 'X' (altered, perhaps, by 'D') of cardio-membrane 'Y' experiences mechanical deformation 'S' under mechanical condition 'W', thereby contributing to normo-rhythmic cardiac excitation phenomenon 'Z' and to dys-rhythmic phenomenon 'Q'.*

Choose (for either statement) from:

X = Nav (1.5, 1.6), Cav (L-type and T-type, etc.), Kv (1, 2, 3…11; including HERG, KvCa), HCN[1–4].

Y = sarcoplasmic membrane, intercalated disc, transverse tubule, sarcoplasmic reticulum (SR), caveolae, raft. Any of the above in multiple myocardial cell subtypes (sinoatrial node and Purkinje fibre cells, ventricular and atrial myocytes). Membranes of cardiovascular cells and intrinsic cardiac neurons (nerve endings ramify in the myocardial wall).

Z = action potentials (or refractoriness) for: pacemaking, conduction, calcium influx, excitation–contraction (EC) coupling

D = mutation, drug effect, developmental/physiological/pathological change, etc.

S = bilayer deformation

W = every beat, each respiratory cycle, increased blood volume (Δ atrial/ventricular distension), modified blood flow (Δ wall shear), externally imposed organ deformation (e.g. chest thump, compressions), altered ambient pressure, altered core temperature, etc.

Q = tacchycardia, bradycardia, atrial flutter, etc.

For Statement 2, the only strong area at present is '**X**'. This is based on recombinant channel electrophysiology, plus native channel work in several cardiomyocytes and other primary cell preparations. Taken together (see[4,5,9,16,17]) that body of work suggests that all VGC are susceptible to stretch. The weakest area, that most

in need of fresh approaches, continues to be *in situ* cytomechanics, i.e. the interplay of '**Y/S/W**'. The fundamental problem regarding **Y/S/W** is: *for the working myocardium, it is not known when or where or if bilayers deform enough to modulate VGC activity.* This is problematic not only for VGC but also for all stretch-susceptible membrane proteins. Where channels link to the cytoskeleton, stresses normal to the membrane may also play a role, but I will focus on the membrane.

Tools to study VGC mechano-sensitivity

A stretch-sensitive voltage sensor toxin?

Resolving the Y/S/W problem might become easier if there were drugs that inhibited only the 'stretch-modulated' component of VGC currents. However, the action potential (AP) generating machinery (i.e. voltage sensor-bearing channels) are inherently stretch-sensitive, making the prospects for finding such drugs difficult. On the other hand, VGC toxins that showed selectively higher (or lower) affinity to their VGC targets *during bilayer stretch* could be useful.

The molecular actions of some voltage sensor toxins are quite well understood[18]. However, might any of them bind differently during stretch? GsMTx4, from tarantula venom, would appear to be an excellent candidate for further investigation. Grammostola spatulata mechano-toxin 4 (GsMTx4) is an internal cysteine knot (ICK) peptide structurally similar to several other voltage sensor toxins of the same venom. A decade ago an exciting report revealed that in perfused rabbit heart, without affecting resting cardiac behaviour or AP shape, submicromolar GsMTx4 strongly inhibits stretch-induced atrial fibrillation[19]. The mechanism is still not understood.

Like voltage sensor toxins, GsMTx4 is amphiphilic and accumulates in the bilayer's outer leaflet[18,20]. In planar bilayers doped with gramicidin, GsMTx4 (concentrates ~300-fold in the bilayer leaflet) alters gramicidin gating by bilayer deformation[20], but the gramicidin assay was not applied to the venom's other ICK peptides, so whether GsMTx4 is unusual in this regard is unknown. Also unknown is the molecular identity of the GsMTx4 target in the atrial fibrillation experiments, but it appears to be stretch-sensitive cation (K^+, Na^+, Ca^{2+}) conductance[21,22]. In addition to strongly inhibiting stretch-fibrillation at 170 nM[19], 400 nM GsMTx4 in ventricular myocytes almost completely abolishes a swelling-enhanced inwardly rectifying macroscopic cation conductance[21]. This GsMTx4-sensitive myocardial conductance shows hallmark traits of an HCN-based cation-selective channel. In oocytes, HCN2 channels pass inwardly rectifying stretch-sensitive (Fig. 6.2A) and swell-sensitive macroscopic current[5,23]. Both atrial and ventricular myocytes (mammalian) express HCN channel isoforms[24]. HCN channel unitary conductance is too small for single channel activity to be evident and, consistent with this, ventricular myocytes exhibit no unitary stretch-activated cation channel events[10,25] and yet do exhibit small HCN currents whose role, except in the atrial-ventricular conducting system, is unknown[24]. In non-myocardial cells, partial (~75%) inhibition of the stretch-activated cation current can require 5 [μ]M GsMTx-4[20,21], unlike its inhibitory actions in rabbit heart (at ~170 nM). Binding of voltage sensor toxins to their targets is exceptionally sensitive to perturbations of bilayer lipids[13,18]. Thus, it seems plausible that, during

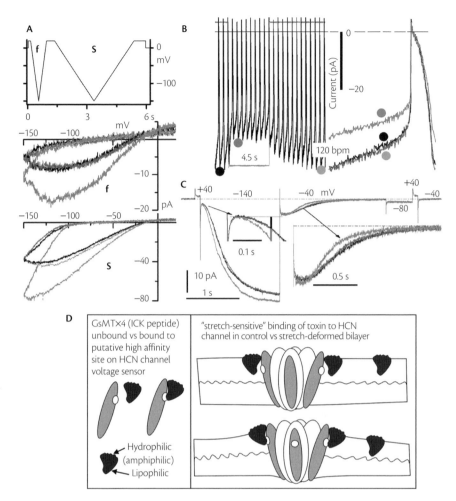

Fig. 6.2 Pacemaker currents (HCN2, oocyte patches) before/during/after stretch. **A** Fast (f), slow (s) sawtooth ramp clamp (voltages, top, currents, below; before/after = black/light grey, during stretch = red). Net effect: stretch-augmented current. **B** Purkinje fibre AP clamp, with 4.5 s stretch step; selected traces expanded, overlapped, right. Net effect: stretch-inhibited pacemaker current during diastole. **C** Both effects are seen in a step regime (see expanded insets): stretch augments current turn-on (hyperpolarize, −140 mV) and accelerates turn-off (depolarize, −40 mV). HCN2 turn-off (equivalent to Kv1 turn-on) depends on stretch-acceleratable outward voltage sensor movements. Hyperpolarization-induced HCN2 turn-on is limited by a voltage-independent transition[47] which could be favoured by stretch if it expands the channel. **D** GsMTx4 as a putative stretch- (and/or swell- and/or lipid-) sensitive voltage sensor toxin that targets HCN-based channels (four inhibitory sites per channel). [Modified, with permission, from Lin W, Laitko U, Juranka PF, Morris CE (2007) Dual stretch responses of mHCN2 pacemaker channels: accelerated activation, accelerated deactivation. *Biophys J* **92**:1559–1572.]

stretch perturbations of bilayer structure (caveolar deformations?) but not in unstressed membrane, GsMTx4 may bind with high affinity to HCN-based myocardial channels (see Fig. 6.2B) whose activity would otherwise contribute to hyperexcitation during stretch. Interestingly, peripheral nerve ending HCN channels contribute, as we pointed out[5], to a form of mechanically induced neuronal 'hyperexcitation', i.e. mechanical allodynia. Might submicromolar GsMTx4 also be inhibitory in that context? Preliminary behavioural data show GsMTx4 inhibition of mechanically induced pain in rats[26].

In summary, *pacemaker-type channels in stretched/deformed cardiac membranes represent a possible target for the voltage-sensor-toxin-like ICK peptide GsMTx4.*

Impaired stretch responses in arrhythmia-inducing mutants of VGC

Arrhythmia-inducing VGC mutants linked to distinctive mechano-physiological phenotypes could also be leverage tools for the Y/S/W (*in situ* cytomechanics) problem. Relevant phenotypes could include hypersensitivity to volume-induced atrial distension, susceptibility to exercise- or load-induced arrhythmias, hypersensitivity to chest compression and arrhythmias linked to cardio-respiratory abnormalities. The strong connection between sudden

cardiac events and respiratory disturbances[27,28], such as that demonstrated in recent observations on the so-called sudden unexpected nocturnal death syndrome SCN5A(Nav1.5 gene)-linked patients[53] seems particularly worth exploiting given the potentially rich veins of physiology-level information of malfunctioning coupled oscillator systems.

This approach recently provided fascinating new evidence in humans, implicating respiratory and ventricular motions as elements in an MEC loop[29]. That experimental paradigm involved having patients with atrial flutter undertake metronomic breathing at various rates. Changes in the electrocardiogram (ECG) flutter pattern were compared with expectations from a mathematical model in which atrial flutter variability is related to the phase of re-entrant activity in ventricular and respiratory cycles. Mechanosensors are required in the feedback loop, with stretch-sensitive myocardial currents considered likely candidates. WT vs mutant VGC with key roles in pacemaking and conduction would be particularly interesting candidates. Arrhythmias linked to known VGC abnormalities and to respiratory behaviour might be fruitfully exploited (with appropriate adjustments of experiment and feedback theory) using non-invasive (or minimally invasive) tests of cardio-respiratory mechano-electric coupling (MEC) on animal models of the VGC arrhythmia (with/without corrective drugs). As an example, long QT 3 syndrome (LQT3) is caused by Nav1.5

channel mutations that prolong inactivation and that can be mimicked by 'site-3' toxins (that bind Nav1.5 at the domain-4 voltage sensor)[30,31]. The sudden cardiac events of LQT3 syndrome in humans are typically sleep-related (i.e. low heart rate related [see[32]]) and associated with respiratory abnormalities (e.g. in sudden infant death syndrome).

Nav1.5 channels, like HCN and Kv1 (in fact, like all VGC), make multiple time-and-voltage-dependent (plus voltage-independent) transitions. Not surprisingly, some of this complexity is mirrored in the effects of mutations and in the wild-type (WT) and mutant channels' stretch responses.

Adult rat ventricular myocyte Nav1.5 channels [Fig. 6.3A; see **stretch difference currents** (SDC)] respond like recombinant Nav1.5 channels in oocyte patches[4]. From a family of WT Nav1.5 SDC (Fig. 6.3B) it can be inferred that during an AP, stretch would initially be excitatory, but quickly, as depolarization proceeded, it

would become inhibitory. Stretch accelerates both activation and inactivation processes that in Nav1.5 are kinetically coupled, meaning that an X-fold change in current onset speed is accompanied by an X-fold change in current decay speed. This co-acceleration persists during stretch – the 'stretch acceleration factor' (SAF) gives the 'X' (e.g. see double rescaled stretch/no stretch currents in Fig. 6.3D from which the SAF is determined, and for a stretch-intensity 'dose-response' for a LQT3 mutant of Nav1.5 see Fig. 6.3C).

Do LQT3-Nav1.5 stretch responses differ from WT-Nav1.5 responses in ways that could exacerbate the already pro-arrhythmic nature of LQT3 mutations? We are pursuing this at a biophysical level[10] via disease mutants R1623Q[33] and R1626P[34]. In WT Nav1.5, inactivation picks up speed with increasing depolarization; in the LQT3 mutants that we examined, the effect is weak (R1623Q) or absent [R1626P; see flat Tau-inactivation (V) (Fig. 6.3D)], though *kinetic* coupling persists in both[10]. At voltages near threshold,

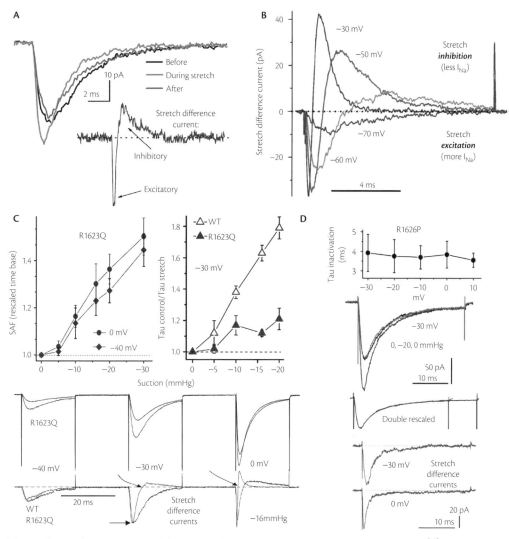

Fig. 6.3 Stretch-modulation of WT and LQT3 Nav1.5. **A** Adult rat ventricular myocyte I_{Na} and stretch difference current (SDC)[10]. **B** SDC for recombinant hNav1.5, depolarizing steps. I_{Na} SDC represent stretch inhibition/excitation when +ve/−ve, respectively[4]. **C** Stretch dose-responses for hNav1.5-R1623Q, two well-separated voltages; increasing stretch intensity (from pipette suction) accelerates currents. Right, inactivation speed is *more* stretch-sensitive in WT than in the LQT3-mutant. Bottom, R1623Q I_{Na} (voltages indicated) without (black)/with (light grey) stretch and below, the associated SDC normalized (arrow) and compared to a WT SDC (same step protocol). Curved arrows: WT SDC is inhibitory far sooner than for the LQT3 mutant[10]. **D** Top, inactivation speed is voltage independent in hNav1.5-R1626P. Bottom, R1626P I_{Na}, as labelled and described in the text.

stretch can more than double the peak I_{Na} in WT and LQT3 channels (e.g. see Fig. 6.3C); clearly, stretch excitation is not impaired. Nevertheless, in both mutants, the SAF is substantially smaller than in WT. Correspondingly, Tau-inactivation stretch-dose responses [blinded comparison, WT vs R1623Q (Fig. 6.3C, top right)] show stretch has a significantly weaker effect on the LQT3 mutant. An overlay comparison of normalized stretch difference currents for R1623Q vs WT shows the consequence: stretch excitation persists far longer in the mutant than in WT (Fig. 6.3C, bottom). R1626P is even more problematic: stretch inhibition never develops, there is only stretch excitation (Fig. 6.3D, bottom).

KCNQ (Kv7) channels are slow delayed rectifier channels. Native and recombinant WT Kv7 currents are sensitive to cell volume but are also dubbed 'stretch sensitive' (but see[35]). Among a familial cohort with a high incidence of hypertension-linked late onset (atrial dilation induced) atrial fibrillation, affected individuals expressed Kv7-R14C[9]. Possible links to atrial stretch were sought by examining responses to cell swelling (stretch responses *per se* were not tested). Baseline behaviour and adenylate cyclase modulation were normal, but cell swelling elicited larger currents with left-shifted kinetics that, in an AP model, yielded atrial fibrillation. Animal model work would help establish whether the defective VGC kinetics and hence defective stretch responses cause defective MEC.

Impaired MEC and toxin-induced long QT syndrome?

To test for the direct involvement of VGC in MEC, intact heart investigations are needed (e.g. akin to those of Zabel and colleagues[36] who applied volume pulses at various points during AP). Transgenic and knock-out mouse models of VGC function and VGC-linked cardiac pathophysiologies might be used, but whole animal and perfused heart physiology procedures for studying MEC are challenging with rodents and might not be feasible with mice. The idea that VGC reagents (HMR1556, antagonist of slow delayed rectifier, plus isoproteronol stimulation) can unmask long QT 1 syndrome (LQT1-related aspects of MEC in whole heart preparations has been discussed by Fabritz[8]. For LQT3, sea anemone and scorpion toxins whose specific target is the domain-4 voltage sensor of Nav1.5[29,30] could be used. For example, WT Nav1.5 exposed to agkistrodon halys toxin (AgTx) yields a key biophysical trait of the LQT3 mutant Nav1.5-R1626P, i.e. an inactivation rate insensitive to voltage. Stretch-modulation of AgTx-bound Nav1.5 channels should therefore be strictly excitatory (i.e. no inhibitory stretch difference current; this needs to be confirmed *in vitro*). AP behaviour in both AgTx-treated WT cardiomyocytes[30] and an R1626P patient[34] can be largely normalized by the anti-arrhythmic agent mexiletine. One can therefore envisage driving ventricular volume changes while monitoring APs, as per Zabel *et al.*[35]. MEC testing would be done before then during AgTx-induced LQT3-like prolongation of APs and again during AP recovery (due, for example, to mexiletine). To finesse more information about possible MEF, it should be helpful to drive volume changes smoothly using frequencies and electrical/pressure synchronies resembling slow, normal and fast respiration. The goal would be to echo, *in vitro*, the *in vivo* approach of Masé *et al.*[29] with MEC in atrial flutter patients. Toxins highly specific to other VGC subclasses implicated in cardiac arrhythmias would be similarly useful (e.g. Kv channel toxins[37] and LQT1).

Additional details on stretch responses of individual VGC

Kv channels and stretch

Multiple Kv channel subtypes with radically different kinetic properties contribute to cardiac APs and studies on recombinant Kv1 and Kv3 show that responses to stretch reflect that diversity.

Kv1: see Fig. 6.4A–E. In Kv1-WT Shaker, stretch accelerates the current onset (A), yielding a hyperpolarizing shift of activation [i.e. g(V)] (D). An explanation (supported by preliminary gating current data; A. Correa and C.E. Morris, unpublished) is that the rate-limiting voltage sensor movement in the activation path (C) accelerates with stretch. By contrast, in Kv1-ILT (mutant in which the high entropy concerted movement of all four voltage sensors just prior to opening limits the rate of opening), stretch slows ionic current onset (B), yielding a depolarizing g(V) shift [in both WT and another mutant, 5AA, the independent voltage sensor motions limit opening (C)][38]. In Kv1, slow inactivation also accelerates with stretch, an effect *not* kinetically coupled to the effect of stretch on activation, in spite of the fact that both processes accelerate to the same extent (E); the molecular mechanism for this phenomenon is not known[39].

Kv3: these channels respond like L- and N-type Cav channels, insofar as stretch increases Kv3 (and Cav) current amplitude without changing onset kinetics[39]. The fraction of Kv3 channels occupying a state between fully resting and open must therefore increase with stretch. The rate-limiting transition in the activation path does not, evidently, appreciably perturb the lateral interface with the bilayer (since, vice versa, the onset kinetics are unresponsive to stretch). This bilayer mechanical trait might be relevant for Kv3 (as opposed, say, to Kv1) gating behaviour in different lipid domains and/or for Kv3 responses to drugs that perturb bilayer structure[15].

Kv7: these 'cell volume sensitive' channels have been termed 'stretch-sensitive', albeit based on responses to cell swelling[9]. Recently, explicit tests for stretch sensitivity were done, in which a Kv7 and a KvCa were tested under the same recording conditions (large oocyte patches): KvCa channel activity responded to stretch but the Kv7 channel did not[35]. Given the involvement of 'LQT1' mutant Kv7 channels in atrial distension-linked fibrillation[9], it will be important to pursue this discrepancy.

KvCa: patch stretch (oocytes) can increase recombinant 'BK' (KvCa) patch current amplitude several-fold[35].

Nav1.5 vs Nav1.6 channels and stretch – reversible vs irreversible effects

Nav1.5 is the major cardiac Nav isoform and, as already described (Fig. 6.3), Nav1.5 current onset and decay co-accelerate reversibly during membrane stretch such that the net effect of stretch would normally be a pro-rhythmic *net decrease of sodium current*.

In addition, the 'neuronal' isoform, Nav1.6, is crucial for sinoatrial node cells pacing. With other 'neuronal' Nav isoforms it is also the major type of ventricular myocyte t-tubule Nav channel[40]. Nav1.6 channels respond reversibly to stretch (like Nav1.5), but if the stretch stimulus causes the membrane's bilayer to bleb away from the underlying membrane skeleton, this is discernible only after the dramatic *irreversible bleb-induced* left-shift of

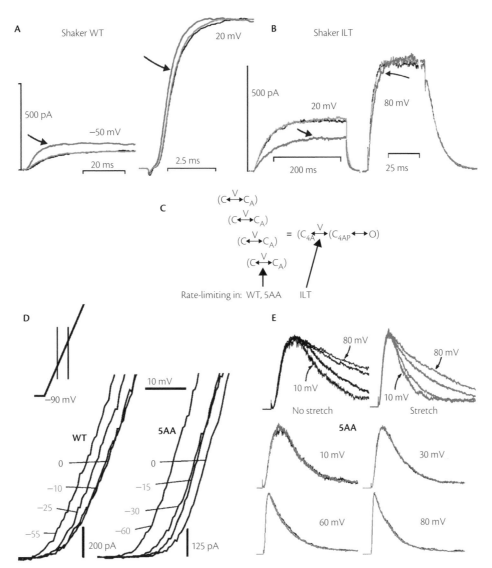

Fig. 6.4 Kv1 (Shaker) channels have three distinct stretch-sensitive transitions. **A** *Transition 1: independent motion of each subunit's voltage sensor:* for WT Shaker Kv1 and, not shown, for 5AA Shaker (mutant with simplified voltage sensor paddle[12] and especially 'clean' kinetics[40]), stretch accelerates I_K turn-on, increases steady-state I_K and left-shifts g(V); see WT I_K before, during (arrows) and after stretch. **B** *Transition 2: concerted pre-opening step:* for ILT Shaker stretch decelerates I_K turn-on, decreases steady-state I_K and right-shifts g(V). **C** Shaker activation (A) path from closed (C) to open (O), with independent and concerted voltage (V) dependent transitions labelled. Opening of the activated pore (4AP) is voltage *in*dependent. **D** Ramp I_K for WT and 5AA Shaker left-shift with stretch (suction, mmHg, labelled; patches ruptured after largest suctions; only I_K near foot of g(V) is shown; see verticals on ramp schematic). **E** *Transition 3: slow inactivation* (voltage *in*dependent transition, not depicted in C): at voltages where slow inactivation is demonstrably not limited by activation[39] Shaker Kv1-5AA reveals that slow inactivation (= 'collapse' of selectivity filter) is stretch sensitive. Top, overlapping amplitude normalized I_K without/with stretch, time bases adjusted so activation (current turn-on) overlaps perfectly at all voltages. Performing this double normalization causes the entirety of the without/with stretch time course at any given voltage to overlap. Restated: the extent of stretch acceleration is the same for voltage dependent activation and voltage *in*dependent inactivation (as if the rate limiting steps for these very different transitions feel the same perturbation during stretch). The explanation for this stretch co-acceleration must differ from that for Nav1.5 channel stretch co-acceleration; the Kv1 channels have no inactivation particle. [**A–C**: Modified, with permission, from Laitko U, Juranka PF, Morris CE (2006) Membrane stretch slows the concerted step prior to opening in a Kv channel. *J Gen Physiol* **127**:687–701. **D**: Modified, with permission, from Tabarean IV, Morris CE (2002) Membrane stretch accelerates activation and slow inactivation in Shaker channels with S3–S4 linker deletions. *Biophys J* **82**:2982–2994. **E**: Modified, with permission, from Laitko U, Morris CE (2004) Membrane tension accelerates rate-limiting voltage-dependent activation and slow inactivation steps in a Shaker channel. *J Gen Physiol* **123**:135–154.]

Nav1.6 operation is complete. At that point, availability and g(V) are both left-shifted by ~20 mV[17]. One consequence is an elevated Nav1.6 channel leak due to shifted window and persistent currents[17]. Thus, if metabolic compromise causes t-tubular blebbing (or dilation; e.g. in tachycardia-induced heart failure[41]), 'leaky' Nav1.6 channels might be an exacerbating factor and thus a target for Nav channel drugs like riluzole and ranolazine[42,43].

In healthy ventricular myocytes, t-tubules have a precise microarchitecture and are a putative mechano-transduction site for MEC (e.g[44].). While Nav1.5 channels evidently suffice for EC coupling[40], Nav1.6 channels in these high-curvature deformable tubular bilayers might indirectly provide local information about the (bilayer) mechanical status of this multi-branched conduction pathway.

Pacemaker channels and stretch

HCN channels open with hyperpolarization. Their slow beat-to-beat 'mode switching' (possibly due to voltage sensor shape changes) contributes strongly to rhythmic stability[45,46]. Stretch has at least two discrete effects on HCN2 current (Fig. 6.2); whether stretch augments or inhibits HCN2 current at any given moment depends on the voltage regime (i.e. pattern of voltage excursions and their speed)[5].

During the diastolic period of sinoatrial node cell AP clamp at low and high frequencies, HCN2 stretch-difference currents were positive (less current) or negative (more current) respectively[5]. In current-clamped guinea pig (low intrinsic rate) and mouse (high intrinsic rate) sinoatrial node cells subjected to stretch or swelling, the AP rate in guinea pig cells increased and that in mouse cells slowed[47]. Insofar as stretch modulation of VGC underlies these changes, combined changes in the many VGC species present are presumably responsible (see also Chapter 13).

Pacemaker channel swelling-sensitivity[23] and stretch-sensitivity[5] may be different phenomena, since swelling increases HCN2 current amplitude without changing the channel's kinetics.

Cav channels and stretch

Cardiac Cav channel mechano-sensitivity has been discussed previously (such as in[16]) and that material is not repeated here. Whole cell inflation studies of N-type Cav channels showed that a 'threshold' mechanical disruption, possibly bleb formation, was needed for responses to membrane stretch[48]. With whole cell inflation, reversibility is difficult to confirm. Irreversible stretch-induced changes bespeak trauma[17,49]. Nevertheless, our procedures taken together [intracellular 1,2-bis(o-aminophenoxy) ethane-N,N,N',N'-tetraacetic acid (BAPTA) controls, monitoring of cell volume and comparison of whole-cell inflation data to cell-attached patch single-channel data] established that N-type channel open probability increases reversibly with membrane stretch.

Timothy syndrome is caused by mutant L-type Cav channels; the phenotype includes long QT and severe cardiac arrhythmias due to overly slow activation and overly slow open state inactivation[50]. In N-type Cav channels, stretch reversibly accelerates open state inactivation[48]. If stretch-accelerated inactivation is impaired in, for example, Cav1.2-G406R[50], this might provide a useful tool for Cav channels and MEC, as envisaged for the Nav channels and MEC with LQT3 mutants (recall that Nav1.5-R1623Q has slowed activation and slowed inactivation and poor stretch acceleration of both processes[10]).

Conclusions and outlook

Cardiac VGC are abundant and inherently sensitive to bilayer deformation, making them serious contenders for roles in MEC. I argue that case here from a largely cellular/biophysical standpoint. Simultaneously I suggest feasible new ways to explore VGC involvement in MEC at whole tissue levels. I now end by pointing to an under-studied phenomenon likely to be crucial for VGC and MEC: caveolar deformation. Many myocardial VGC channels, including Cav, Nav, HERG and HCN channels, plus other membrane proteins (e.g. Na^+/Ca^{2+} exchanger) traffic to elaborate caveolin-based lipid microdomains[51]. Various mechanical events must reversibly and/or irreversibly flex the caveolar environment (as an analogy, depending on how force was applied, a metal hoop

could experience elastic flex or plastic strain). Deformations of these membrane microdomains[52] during developmental, physiological and/or pathological (ischaemic, inflammatory, traumatic) membrane remodelling might be mimicked by some experimental stretch regimes[17,48,49]. When classifying responses to such stimuli, therefore, multiple categories should be considered. Relying solely on 'artifact-versus-real' would be an oversimplification likely to obscure the point that VGC behave differently whenever their bilayer mechanical environments change[13]. I predict that this attribute of VGC will prove to be exceptionally relevant to the developmental, physiological and pathological aspects of cardiac MEC.

References

1. Langton PD. Calcium channel currents recorded from isolated myocytes of rat basilar artery are stretch sensitive. *J Physiol* 1993;**471**: 1–11.
2. Gu CX, Juranka PF, Morris CE. Stretch-activation and stretch-inactivation of Shaker-IR, a voltage-gated K^+ channel. 2001;**80**: 2678–2693.
3. Tabarean IV, Morris CE. Membrane stretch accelerates activation and slow inactivation in Shaker channels with S3–S4 linker deletions. *Biophys J* 2002;**82**:2982–2994.
4. Morris CE, Juranka PF. Nav channel mechanosensitivity: activation and inactivation accelerate reversibly with stretch. *Biophys J* 2007;**93**:822–833.
5. Lin W, Laitko U, Juranka PF, Morris CE. Dual stretch responses of mHCN2 pacemaker channels: accelerated activation, accelerated deactivation. *Biophys J* 2007;**92**:1559–1572.
6. Eijsbouts SC, Houben RP, Blaauw Y, Schotten U, Allessie MA. Synergistic action of atrial dilation and sodium channel blockade on conduction in rabbit atria. *J Cardiovasc Electrophysiol* 2004;**15**: 1453–1461.
7. Kalifa J, Bernard M, Gout B, *et al.* Anti-arrhythmic effects of I_{Na}, I_{Kr}, and combined I_{Kr}-I_{CaL} blockade in an experimental model of acute stretch-related atrial fibrillation. *Cardiovasc Drugs Ther* 2007;**21**: 47–53.
8. Fabritz L. Drug-induced torsades de pointes – a form of mechano-electric feedback? *Cardiovasc Res* 2007;**76**:202–203.
9. Otway R, Vandenberg JI, Guo G, *et al.* Stretch-sensitive KCNQ1 mutation A link between genetic and environmental factors in the pathogenesis of atrial fibrillation? *J Am Coll Cardiol* 2007;**49**:578–586.
10. Banderali U, Juranka PF, Clark RB, Giles W, Morris CE. Impaired stretch modulation in potentially lethal cardiac sodium channel mutants. *Channels* 2010;**4**:12–21.
11. Morris CE, Juranka PF. Lipid stress at play: mechanosensitivity of voltage-gated channels. In: *Mechanosensitive Ion Channels*, Part B (eds O Hamill, S Simon, D Benos). *Curr Topics Membr* 2007;**59**:297–337.
12. Long SB, Tao X, Campbell EB, MacKinnon R. Atomic structure of a voltage-dependent K^+ channel in a lipid membrane-like environment. *Nature* 2007;**450**:376–382.
13. Schmidt D, MacKinnon R. Voltage-dependent K^+ channel gating and voltage sensor toxin sensitivity depend on the mechanical state of the lipid membrane. *Proc Natl Acad Sci USA* 2008;**105**:19276–19281.
14. Phillips R, Ursell T, Wiggins P, Sens P. Emerging roles for lipids in shaping membrane–protein function. *Nature* 2009;**459**:379–385.
15. Finol-Urdaneta RK, Juranka PF, French RJ, Morris CE. Modulation of KvAP unitary conductance and gating by 1-alkanols and other surface active agents. *Biophys J* 2010;**98**:762–772.
16. Morris CE, Laitko U. (2005) The mechanosensitivity of voltage-gated channels may contribute to cardiac mechano-electric feedback. In: *Cardiac Mechano-Electric Feedback and Arrhythmias: from Pipette to Patient* (eds P Kohl F Sachs MR Franz). Elsevier Saunders, Philadelphia, pp. 33–41.

17. Wang JA, Lin W, Morris T, Banderali U, Juranka PF, Morris CE. Membrane trauma and Na$^+$-leak from Nav1.6 channels. *Am J Physiol* 2009;**297**:C823–C834.

18. Milescu M, Vobecky J, Roh SH, et al. Tarantula toxins interact with voltage sensors within lipid membranes. *J Gen Physiol* 2007;**130**:497–511.

19. Bode F, Sachs F, Franz MR. Tarantula peptide inhibits atrial fibrillation. *Nature* 2001;**409**:35–36.

20. Suchyna TM, Tape SE, Koeppe RE 2nd, Andersen OS, Sachs F, Gottlieb PA. Bilayer-dependent inhibition of mechanosensitive channels by neuroactive peptide enantiomers. *Nature* 2004;**430**:235–240.

21. Suchyna TM, Johnson JH, Hamer K, et al. Identification of a peptide toxin from *Grammostola spatulata* spider venom that blocks cation-selective stretch-activated channels. *J Gen Physiol* 2000;**115**:583–598.

22. Gottlieb P, Folgering J, Maroto R, et al. Revisiting TRPC1 and TRPC6 mechanosensitivity. *Pflugers Arch* 2008;**455**:1097–1103.

23. Calloe K, Elmedyb P, Olesen SP, Jorgensen NK, Grunnet M. Hypoosmotic cell swelling as a novel mechanism for modulation of cloned HCN2 channels. *Biophys J* 2005;**89**:2159–2169.

24. Baruscotti M, Barbuti A, Bucchi A. The cardiac pacemaker current. *J Mol Cell Cardiol* 2010;**48**:55–64.

25. Zeng T, Bett GC, Sachs F. Stretch-activated whole cell currents in adult rat cardiac myocytes. *Am J Physiol* 2000;**278**:H548–H557.

26. Park SP, Kim BM, Koo JY, et al. A tarantula spider toxin, GsMTx4, reduces mechanical and neuropathic pain. *Pain* 2008;**137**:208–217.

27. Orban M, Bruce CJ, Pressman GS, et al. Dynamic changes of left ventricular performance and left atrial volume induced by the Mueller maneuver in healthy young adults and implications for obstructive sleep apnea, atrial fibrillation, and heart failure. *Am J Cardiol* 2008;**102**:1557–1561.

28. Sredniawa B, Lenarczyk R, Kowalski O, et al. Sleep apnoea as a predictor of mid- and long-term outcome in patients undergoing cardiac resynchronization therapy. *Europace* 2009;**11**:106–114.

29. Masé M, Glass L, Ravelli F. A model for mechano-electrical feedback effects on atrial flutter interval variability. *Bull Math Biol* 2008;**70**:1326–1347.

30. Priori SG, Napolitano C, Cantù F, Brown AM, Schwartz PJ. Differential response to Na$^+$ channel blockade, beta-adrenergic stimulation, and rapid pacing in a cellular model mimicking the SCN5A and HERG defects present in the long-QT syndrome. *Circ Res* 1996;**78**:1009–1015.

31. Hanck DA, Sheets MF. Site-3 toxins and cardiac sodium channels. *Toxicon* 2007;**49**:181–193.

32. Horner SM, Dick DJ, Murphy CF, Lab MJ. Cycle length dependence of the electrophysiological effects of increased load on the myocardium. *Circulation* 1996;**94**:1131–1136.

33. Kambouris NG, Nuss HB, Johns DC, Marban E, Tomaselli GF, Balser JR. A revised view of cardiac sodium channel "blockade" in the long-QT syndrome. *J Clin Invest* 2000;**105**:1133–1140.

34. Ruan Y, Liu N, Bloise R, Napolitano C, Priori SG. Gating properties of SCN5A mutations and the response to mexiletine in long-QT syndrome type 3 patients. *Circulation* 2007;**116**:1137–1144.

35. Hammami S, Willumsen NJ, Olsen HL, Morera FJ, Latorre R, Klaerke DA. Cell volume and membrane stretch independently control K$^+$ channel activity. *J Physiol* 2009;**587**:2225–2231.

36. Zabel M, Koller BS, Sachs F, Franz MR. Stretch-induced voltage changes in the isolated beating heart: importance of the timing of stretch and implications for stretch-activated ion channels. *Cardiovasc Res* 1996;**32**:120–130.

37. Diochot S, Lazdunski M. Sea anemone toxins affecting potassium channels. *Prog Mol Subcell Biol* 2009;**46**:99–122.

38. Laitko U, Juranka PF, Morris CE. Membrane stretch slows the concerted step prior to opening in a Kv channel. *J Gen Physiol* 2006;**127**:687–701.

39. Laitko U, Morris CE. Membrane tension accelerates rate-limiting voltage-dependent activation and slow inactivation steps in a Shaker channel. *J Gen Physiol* 2004;**123**:135–154.

40. Brette F, Orchard CH. Density and sub-cellular distribution of cardiac and neuronal sodium channel isoforms in rat ventricular myocytes. *Biochem Biophys Res Commun* 2006;**348**:1163–1166.

41. Cannell MB, Crossman DJ, Soeller C. Effect of changes in action potential spike configuration, junctional sarcoplasmic reticulum micro-architecture and altered t-tubule structure in human heart failure. *J Muscle Res Cell Motil* 2006;**27**:297–306.

42. Mestre M, Djellas Y, Carriot T, Cavero I. Frequency-independent blockade of cardiac Na$^+$ channels by riluzole: comparison with established anticonvulsants and class I anti-arrhythmics. *Fundam Clin Pharmacol* 2000;**14**:107–117.

43. Dhalla AK, Wang WQ, Dow J, Shryock JC, Belardinelli L, Bhandari A, et al. Ranolazine, an antianginal agent, markedly reduces ventricular arrhythmias induced by ischemia and ischemia-reperfusion. *Am J Physiol* 2009;**297**:H1923–H1929.

44. Dyachenko V, Christ A, Gubanov R, Isenberg G. Bending of z-lines by mechanical stimuli: an input signal for integrin dependent modulation of ion channels? *Prog Biophys Mol Biol* 2008;**97**:196–216.

45. Elinder F, Männikkö R, Pandey S, Larsson HP. Mode shifts in the voltage gating of the mouse and human HCN2 and HCN4 channels. *J Physiol* 2006;**575**:417–431.

46. Chen S, Wang J, Zhou L, George MS, Siegelbaum SA. Voltage sensor movement and cAMP binding allosterically regulate an inherently voltage-independent closed-open transition in HCN channels. *J Gen Physiol* 2007;**129**:175–188.

47. Cooper PJ, Kohl P. Species- and preparation-dependence of stretch effects on sino-atrial node pacemaking. *Ann N Y Acad Sci* 2005;**1047**:324–335.

48. Calabrese B, Tabarean IV, Juranka P, Morris CE. Mechanosensitivity of N-type calcium channel currents. *Biophys J* 2002;**83**:2560–2574.

49. Wan X, Juranka P, Morris CE. Activation of mechanosensitive currents in traumatized membrane. *Am J Physiol* 1999;**276**:C318–C327.

50. Yarotskyy V, Gao G, Peterson BZ, Elmslie KS. The Timothy syndrome mutation of cardiac CaV1.2 (L-type) channels: multiple altered gating mechanisms and pharmacological restoration of inactivation. *J Physiol* 2009;**587**:551–565.

51. Balijepalli RC, Kamp TJ. Caveolae, ion channels and cardiac arrhythmias. *Prog Biophys Mol Biol* 2008;**98**:149–160.

52. Sens P, Turner MS. Budded membrane microdomains as tension regulators. *Phys Rev E Stat Nonlin Soft Matter Phys* 2006;**73**:031918.

53. Cheng J, Makielski JC, Yuan P, Shi N, Zhou F, Ye B, et al. Sudden unexplained nocturnal death syndrome in southern China: an epidemiological survey and SCN5A gene screening. *Am J Forensic Med Pathol* 2010; doi:10.1097/PAF.0b013e3181d03d02.

Role of caveolae in stretch-sensing: implications for mechano-electric coupling

Sarah Calaghan

Background

Introduction to caveolae

Caveolae are small flask-like invaginations of the cell membrane, first identified in the 1950s by electron microscopy (EM). They represent a specialized form of lipid raft (an area of the cell membrane enriched in cholesterol and sphingolipids) characterized by the presence of a small protein, caveolin (cav) (see Fig. 7.1). A proportion of caveolae exist as closed submembrane vesicles (Fig. 7.1C)[1,2].

The lipid environment, caveolin content and morphology of caveolae are central to their diverse functional roles which include co-ordination of signal transduction, cholesterol homeostasis and endocytosis. One of caveolae's best characterized roles is as a signalosome – a compartment that brings together components of signal transduction cascades (receptors, G proteins, kinases), thereby increasing the efficiency and fidelity of signalling [see[3] for review]. Within caveolae, caveolin provides an additional level of regulatory control via its 20-residue caveolin-scaffolding domain (CSD) (Fig. 7.1B) which interacts with a complementary caveolin binding domain in select proteins, generally stabilizing these in an inactive conformation[3]. This enables oligomeric caveolin to act as a regulatory scaffold for macromolecular signalling complex formation[4].

Caveolae as mechano-sensors and mechano-transducers

Some three decades ago it was proposed that caveolae serve as miniature stretch-receptors within the cell[5]. Since then it has become clear that mechanical stimuli can alter the morphology, lipid environment and caveolin content of caveolae. These characteristics regulate the activity of proteins in caveolae, thereby supporting the view of caveolae as a component of the cellular machinery that senses and transduces mechanical stimuli. Here, the role of caveolae in stretch-sensing and mechano-electric coupling (MEC) in the heart will be considered. The focus will be the cardiac myocyte, as this is a major site of MEC in the heart.

Stretch-sensing and mechano-electric coupling

Overview

Mechanical stimuli regulate cardiac function physiologically and pathologically [see[6]]. Specifically in terms of MEC, this can occur directly through mechano-sensitive ion channels [including transient receptor potential cation channels (TRPC), volume-regulated anion channels such as the swelling activated Cl$^-$ channel ($I_{Cl,swell}$), and K$^+$ channels]. However, a direct effect on mechano-sensitive channels is not the only mechanism for MEC. Intracellular Ca^{2+} ($[Ca^{2+}]_i$) is exquisitely dependent on mechanical stimulation and alters electrical activity through the Ca^{2+}-dependence of certain membrane currents ($I_{Ca,L}$, I_{Ks}, I_{NCX})[6]. In response to stretch, $[Ca^{2+}]_i$ may increase by Ca^{2+} entry through TRPC, or on the Na$^+$/Ca^{2+} exchanger (NCX) secondary to increased $[Na^+]_i$ through TRPC or Na$^+$/H$^+$ exchange (NHE) (7–9). Furthermore, the activity of ion channels and Ca^{2+}-regulatory proteins is altered by post-translational modification (phosphorylation, s-nitrosylation) which is, in turn, under the control of mechano-gated receptors [e.g. angiotensin II type 1 receptor (AT-1)] and signal components [e.g. the endothelial nitric oxide synthase (eNOS)][10,11]. Caveolae are linked with mechano-sensitive ion channel function[12,13], with regulation of $[Ca^{2+}]_i$[14] and with numerous mechano-sensitive signal cascades[3], strongly supporting an important role in MEC.

Properties of caveolae important for stretch-sensing

There are several properties of caveolae that may promote – or protect against – the sensing and/or transducing of mechanical stimuli.

Morphology

The distinct morphology of caveolae is due to their lipid and protein content. Line tension between immiscible raft and non-raft phases is minimized by membrane budding and caveolin promotes membrane curvature because of its asymmetric membrane

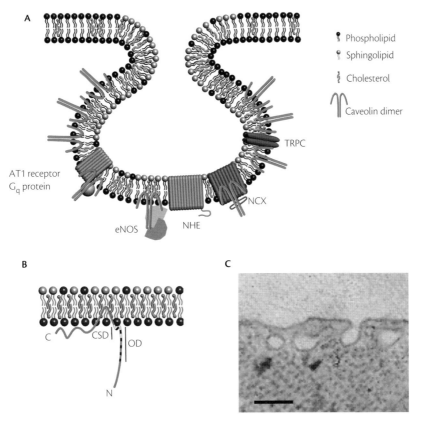

Fig. 7.1 Caveolae and caveolin. **A** Caveolae are invaginated lipid rafts, enriched in cholesterol and sphingolipids and lined with the protein caveolin (shown as a dimer, although it usually exists as oligomers of 14–16 caveolins). Within the caveola, key proteins that may be relevant for cardiac MEC are shown (see text for details). **B** Caveolin inserts assymetrically into the inner leaflet of the membrane. It oligomerizes via its oligomerization domain (OD) and interacts with binding partners via its scaffolding domain (CSD). Caveolin exists in three isoforms: cav1 and cav2 (ubiquitously expressed) and cav3 (the predominant isoform in muscle). (Figures courtesy of Tim Lee, Faculty of Biological Sciences, University of Leeds.) **C** Caveolae visualized using EM in the adult rat ventricular myocyte. Both open and closed vesicles of a size consistent with caveolae are seen. Scale bar represents 200 nm.

insertion and tendency to cluster[15]. Proteins in the caveolar membrane will be protected, to some extent, from mechanical stimuli because the more curved a membrane is, the less tension will be experienced for a given trans-membrane pressure, according to Laplace [see[16,17]]. However, any increase in tension could selectively regulate caveolar proteins that interact with caveolin because this can cause a structural change in the membrane which disperses caveolin, relieving constitutive inhibition[18].

As a membrane reserve

The lipid bilayer can only increase in area by around 3% before rupture, so membrane reserves are essential to allow changes in cell surface area to occur during stretching or swelling without irreversible cell damage[17]. In the cardiac myocyte, Z-line folds and caveolae (both as open invaginations and closed subsarcolemmal vesicles) act as membrane reserves[1,2,19]. We have recently estimated that open and closed caveolae contribute around 12% to available membrane area in the adult cardiac myocyte[2]. As cells are stretched or swollen, membrane tension increases, mechanically accessible membrane (including that from open and closed caveolae) is inserted and membrane tension is reduced[16]. Thus the presence of caveolae may effectively buffer increases in membrane tension which are required to gate mechano-sensitive channels. This potentially protective mechanism is likely to take place over a longer timescale than mechano-sensitive mechanisms which rely on dispersion of caveolin or changes in the lipid environment of caveolae.

Lipid environment

Protein function is affected by the lipid composition of the bilayer[20]. Caveolae have a particular profile of membrane lipids (sterols, sphingolipids and phospholipids) which has the capacity to regulate channel/exchanger function. For example, cholesterol is a well-established modulator of ion channel activity; it suppresses activation of the volume-regulated anion channel in endothelial cells, either through stiffening of the bilayer (which increases membrane deformation energy) or by specific sterol–protein interactions[21]. In the cardiac cell, lipid rafts (caveolar and non-caveolar) are enriched in pools of phosphatidylinositol 4,5, bisphosphate (PIP_2)[22] which show stimuli-specific depletion[23]. Phospholipase C (PLC), which hydrolyzes PIP_2 to diacylglycerol (DAG), is activated by mechanical stimulation[24] and this will have consequences for the activity of PIP_2-sensitive ion channels (e.g. TRPC) and transporters (NCX)[25] and for DAG-activated TRPC [see[26]]. Thus caveolae-specific phospholipid pools that are mechanically regulated provide a mechanism by which caveolae can contribute to MEC.

As a compartment

Caveolae are essentially a compartment that brings together elements of signal transduction cascades and their targets. This may be relevant to their role in mechano-sensation as well as in the co-ordination of downstream mechano-transductive signalling [see[27]].

Proteins in caveolae

The conformation and activity of proteins embedded in the membrane is dependent on properties of the membrane including physical parameters (tension/curvature/stiffness), lipid content and protein (e.g. caveolin) content. Caveolae represent a distinct membrane microenvironment, and this environment is subject to mechanically induced changes (see section on 'Properties of caveolae important for stretch-sensing'). Therefore in order to define a role for caveolae in MEC, the way in which relevant proteins are distributed within or outside of caveolae, and their interactions with caveolin, must be considered.

Ion channels

Here the focus will be on two types of ion channel which are linked with mechano-transduction in the heart: TRPC and volume-regulated anion channels (see Chapters 2 and 4).

TRPC

TRPC have been reported to respond to a range of stimuli including stretch, depletion of intracellular Ca^{2+} stores and DAG[26]. TRPC1 and 6 have attracted particular attention with regard to MEC in the heart[26]. A clear link exists between caveolae and TRPC in non-cardiac cells (including endothelial, vascular smooth muscle and skeletal muscle cells). For example, TRPC 1, 3 and 4 are found in caveolar membrane fractions[28], TRPC1 interacts with cav1 and cav3 (probably through a CSD binding sequence in its C terminus)[12,29] and disruption of the TRPC1–cav1 interaction regulates store-operated Ca^{2+} entry[12,30]. Recent findings have suggested that TRPC are not directly mechanically gated but rather respond to mechano-sensitive Gq-coupled receptors in a PLC-dependent manner[31]. In human embryonic kidney (HEK) cells, DAG activation of TRPC6 is dependent on intact rafts[32]; data specifically for caveolae are not available. In the adult cardiac myocyte Ang II activation of PLC triggers Na^+ entry through TRPC3 and consequent Ca^{2+} entry via NCX[9]. Thus the presence of particular TRPC isoforms in caveolae may define their functional role in MEC by providing the opportunity to interact with particular up/downstream signal molecules (see section on 'G_q protein-coupled receptors').

$I_{Cl,swell}$

In the heart, $I_{Cl,swell}$ is the main volume-regulating ion channel activated by swelling [see[33]]. This channel is considered to be acting as a mechano-sensor responding to changes in membrane tension, rather than decreased intracellular osmolarity, because it can be activated by other mechanical stimuli[34]. A clear link between caveolae and $I_{Cl,swell}$ was made by Trouet et al.[13] who showed that cav1 expression (in a caveolin-free cell line) was required for swelling-induced current characteristic of $I_{Cl,swell}$. Furthermore, in endothelial cells, displacement of cav1 from caveolae attenuated $I_{Cl,swell}$ activation during swelling[35]. These authors proposed that caveolae's role in $I_{Cl,swell}$ is as a compartment that brings the channel together with regulatory tyrosine kinases (although, because the molecular identity of the $I_{Cl,swell}$ channel is unknown, this could not be shown directly; see section on 'Morphology and sarcolemmal incorporation').

Other

The subcellular localization of ion channels is vital for rapid and efficient integration of signalling, and therefore the enrichment of many channels in caveolae comes as no surprise [see[36] for a review]. However, not all channels are found in caveolae; e.g. the mechano-sensitive TREK1 channel is found almost exclusively outside caveolar fractions in the adult heart (Fig. 7.2; see also Chapter 3).

Ca^{2+}-regulating proteins

Ca^{2+} is a key regulator of electrical activity and caveolae have been linked with control of $[Ca^{2+}]_i$ in many different cell types over the years since Popescu[37] first proposed caveolae as the site of Ca^{2+} entry in smooth muscle. In the adult cardiac myocyte, although caveolae are not a major site of Ca^{2+} entry on $I_{Ca,L}$, they do enhance sarcoplasmic reticulum Ca^{2+} release, perhaps through an effect of nitric oxide (NO) on ryanodine receptor (RyR) activity (see section on 'Other signal components')[14]. Other Ca^{2+}-regulatory proteins have been linked with caveolae. For example, in the bovine heart NCX is enriched in caveolae and positively regulated by interaction with cav3[38]. NCX is important for stretch- and AT-1 receptor-induced elevations in $[Ca^{2+}]_i$ secondary to increased $[Na^+]_i$ via NHE and TRPC3[7,9]. NHE is found exclusively in caveolae fractions in the adult myocardium (Fig. 7.2). Thus caveolae may act as an MEC microdomain which allows efficient coupling of stretch-induced Na^+ entry with Ca^{2+} entry on NCX.

G_q protein-coupled receptors

A role for G protein-coupled receptors in mechano-sensation has attracted particular interest since the discovery that mechanical stress leads directly to a conformational change and activation of the AT-1 receptor without requirement for a ligand[11,39]. The concept of the 'mechano-sensitive receptor' has recently been expanded to include the idea that Gq-coupled receptors are ultimately responsible for activation of some TRPC in response to stretch (in a PLC-dependent manner) (see section on 'Ion channels'). Therefore two important questions are: Where are the Gq-coupled

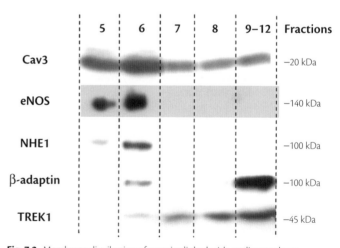

Fig. 7.2 Membrane distribution of proteins linked with cardiac mechano-transduction in the adult rat myocardium. Fractions 5 and 6 represent buoyant caveolae-containing sucrose gradient fractions (containing the majority of cav3, the marker protein for caveolae). Fractions 9–12 represent heavy fractions (non-cholesterol enriched membranes and cytosolic proteins); the marker protein for these fractions is β-adaptin.

receptors within the membrane? Do caveolae provide a compartment to promote signalling downstream of these receptors? Direct evidence in the cardiac cell is lacking. AT-1 receptors do interact with caveolin, but whether this is within caveolae is a point of debate. In cultured cell lines cav1 acts as a molecular chaperone for the receptor through the exocytotic pathway, rather than as a plasma membrane scaffold[40]. However, agonist stimulation has been shown to promote AT-1 receptor translocation to caveolae in vascular smooth muscle[41]. The idea of caveolae as a microdomain of mechano-sensitive Gq-coupled receptor signalling is an attractive one, given evidence (from endothelial and epithelial cells) that caveolin acts as a scaffold to trap and stabilize the Gq protein within caveolae[42].

Other signal components

Any discussion of mechano-sensation and caveolae would be incomplete without mention of NO (although this subject is dealt with in more depth in Chapter 11). In endothelial cells and cardiac myocytes, NO production is mechano-sensitive[10,43]. The major constitutively expressed NOS isoform in the cardiovascular system, eNOS, is exquisitely dependent on caveolae; dual palmitoylation of eNOS directs it to caveolae (Fig. 7.2) where interaction with cav clamps the enzyme in an inactive conformation [see[44]]. Activation of eNOS occurs predominantly through Ca^{2+}-calmodulin disruption of the inhibitory cav interaction and/or Akt-dependent phosphorylation at Ser^{1177} [45]. There are multiple interrelated mechanisms by which mechanical stimuli can activate caveolar eNOS: translocation of cav/eNOS from caveolae (see section on 'Calveolar protein distribution'); elevated $[Ca^{2+}]_i$[10,43]; and PI3 kinase/Akt phosphorylation of eNOS[46]. These regulatory mechanisms rely on caveolae as a compartment bringing together eNOS with inhibitory cav, acting as a site of entry of Ca^{2+} (e.g. through TRPC) and allowing access from Akt[47]. Indeed, a recent study suggests that, at the cellular level, multiple eNOS-activating mechanisms operate in response to a given form of mechanical stimulus; cyclically stretched endothelial cells show early eNOS activation via Ca^{2+} entry on stretch-activated channels and subsequent eNOS activation via PI3 kinase/Akt-dependent phosphorylation[48]. NO effects on the heart are complex and outside the scope of this chapter. Essentially, caveolae-dependent NO production in response to mechanical stimulation is likely to affect electrical activity either by direct regulation of ion channel function (e.g. $I_{Ca,L}$ through phosphorylation, s-nitrosylation) or by indirect effects on $[Ca^{2+}]_i$ (e.g. s-nitrosylation of RyR)[27]. In the intact heart, NO effects on the cardiac myocyte may be autocrine or paracrine (from endothelial cells).

How do caveolae change with mechanical stimuli?

A fundamental question to consider with regard to a role for caveolae in MEC is how the properties of caveolae change with mechanical stimulation.

Morphology and sarcolemmal incorporation

In the cardiac muscle cell, does membrane tension increase sufficiently with physiological degrees of stretch to promote flattening and/or sarcolemmal incorporation of closed caveolae? Early studies using freeze-fracture EM showed that the number of caveolae necks does not vary as a function of sarcomere length in the physiological range[19]. This is in contrast to more recent work using transmission EM (TEM) which shows caveolae in cross section. A preliminary study by Kohl et al.[1] reported that stretch to sarcomere length of 2.1 μm smoothes Z-line folds and causes surface membrane incorporation of subsarcolemmal caveolae (Fig. 7.3). Osmotic swelling also affects caveolar morphology in the cardiac myocyte.

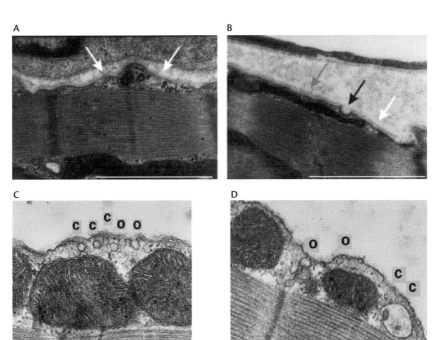

Fig. 7.3 Effect of stretch and swelling on caveolae morphology. TEM of adult rabbit myocardium fixed during contraction (**A**) or after balloon inflation of the ventricle to yield a diastolic pressure of 30 mm Hg (**B**), showing stretch-induced incorporation of closed caveolae (white arrows) into open (black arrow) or flattened (grey arrow) caveolae. Scale bar is 1 μm. [Reprinted, with permission from Elsevier, from Kohl P, Cooper PJ, Holloway H (2003) Effects of acute ventricular volume manipulation on in situ cardiomyocyte cell membrane configuration. *Prog Biophys Mol Biol* **82**:221–227.] **C** Rat ventricular myocytes under normosmotic conditions and following 15 min exposure to 0.64T hyposmotic solution (**D**). Caveolae density was reduced following hyposmotic swelling due to a reduction in the closed (C) rather than the open (O) population of caveolae [see [2]]. Scale bar is 200 nm.

A complete absence of subsarcolemmal caveolae in myocytes from hearts swollen with 0.75T solution for 30 min has been reported[1]. We have shown that exposure of cells to 0.64T solution for 15 min reduces the number of caveolae by 50%, due entirely to a reduction in the population of closed caveolae (for which no connecting neck was visible by TEM; see Fig. 7.3)[2]. We propose that this is due to flattening of open caveolae balanced by sarcolemmal incorporation of closed caveolae (changes that would not be detected by freeze-fracture EM). How do these morphological effects of swelling on caveolae relate to activation of $I_{Cl,swell}$? In the cardiac myocyte, our data show that pharmacological inhibition of $I_{Cl,swell}$ and disruption of caveolae (with the cholesterol-depleting agent methyl-β-cyclodextrin) increase the rate of hyposmotic cell swelling in an identical, non-additive manner[2], which is consistent with the view that caveolae are required for $I_{Cl,swell}$ activation as proposed by Trouet et al.[13] (see section on 'Ion channels'). However, we have also shown that disrupting caveolae enhances the negative inotropic response to cell swelling [a consequence of $I_{Cl,swell}$ activation (2, 49)]. Given the morphological changes in caveolae during swelling, we propose an alternative role for caveolae in $I_{Cl,swell}$ activation in the cardiac myocyte – not as a compartment that promotes kinase activation of the channel, but as a membrane reserve which normally acts to limit $I_{Cl,swell}$ activation. In a hyposmotic environment, $I_{Cl,swell}$ protects cells, regulating cell volume by promoting loss of osmotically obliged water. Our data suggest, in the cardiac cell at least, that the presence of caveolae as a membrane reserve may reduce the requirement for $I_{Cl,swell}$ activation.

Morphological changes in caveolae with mechanical stimuli may also be relevant to MEC by disrupting caveolin's regulatory interactions (see next section) and by increasing membrane capacitance, if this allows access to previously electrically inaccessible membrane [e.g. see[50]].

Caveolar protein distribution

Caveolin

Curvature of the caveolar membrane is dependent on the presence of caveolin; therefore flattening of the membrane in response to swelling or stretch could cause dissociation of caveolin from caveolae, with consequences for signal cascades regulated by caveolin[15] (see section on 'Properties of caveolae important for stretch-sensing'). Indeed, in vascular smooth muscle, translocation of cav1 and 3 from caveolar membrane fractions is seen in response to 30-min cyclic stretch[51]. Likewise, in adult myocardium we have reported a time-dependent translocation of cav3 from caveolae-containing membranes with 30 min of left ventricular pressure inflation[52]. However, cav translocation is not a universal finding with mechanical stimulation; in neonatal cardiac myocytes 15 min biaxial stretch has no effect on cav3 distribution[53]. We see no effect of osmotic swelling on cav3 distribution in the adult cardiac myocyte, despite changes in caveolae morphology[2]. These data suggest that translocation of caveolin may be dependent on the type of mechanical stimulus and the cells to which it is applied.

eNOS

Caveolar eNOS has also been shown to be affected by mechanical stimuli. For example, increased vascular flow and pressure in situ dissociates eNOS from its inhibitory interaction with cav in the endothelium[45]. We have reported a trend for translocation of eNOS from caveolae in the pressure-inflated left ventricle[52].

Conclusions and outlook

Various levels of information are available regarding the caveolar dependence of mechano-sensation. These include demonstration of the presence of mechano-sensitive proteins in membrane fractions that contain caveolae, interaction of such proteins with caveolin, stretch-induced changes in morphology/lipid/protein and functional consequences of disrupting rafts/caveolae for mechano-sensitive processes. Whilst comprehensive data confirm a role for caveolae in, for example, eNOS activation during shear stress in endothelial cells, data for MEC in the cardiac myocyte are still fragmentary. Direct extrapolation of caveolae's role in endothelial cells to the cardiac myocyte is not possible because of differences in, for example, caveolin isoform expression and the form of mechanical stimuli experienced by these cells.

Caveolae are implicated in cardiac diseases which show dysregulation of electrical activity; e.g. cav3 mutations promote long QT syndrome via effects on $Na_v1.5$[54]. Furthermore, caveolin expression increases in conditions in which abnormal mechanical stress is applied to cells, such as Duchenne muscular dystrophy[55], chronic shear[56]. Whilst a direct link between cardiac myocyte caveolae and MEC which causes disease has yet to be shown, evidence suggests that this connection exists.

It is difficult to argue against a role for caveolae in sensing and transducing mechanical stimuli, given that these 'little caves' are sensitive to varied mechanical stimuli, and that one of their key roles is to assemble signal complexes and co-ordinate specific molecular interactions. However, we must not lose sight of the fact that several properties of caveolae (membrane curvature, cholesterol content, membrane reserve) are actually mechano-protective and may limit activation of mechano-sensitive proteins. There is a paucity of cardiac-specific research in the caveolae field and more work is required to fully understand the potentially complex role of caveolae in MEC in the heart.

Acknowledgements

Sarah Calaghan's work is supported by the British Heart Foundation and the Medical Research Council.

References

1. Kohl P, Cooper PJ, Holloway H. Effects of acute ventricular volume manipulation on in situ cardiomyocyte cell membrane configuration. *Prog Biophys Mol Biol* 2003;**82**:221–227.

2. Kozera L, White E, Calaghan S. Caveolae act as membrane reserves which limit mechanosensitive $I_{Cl,swell}$ channel activation during swelling in the rat ventricular myocyte. *PLoS One* 2009; **4**:e8312.

3. Razani B, Woodman SE, Lisanti MP. Caveolae: from cell biology to animal physiology. *Pharmacol Rev* 2002;**54**:431–467.

4. Sargiacomo M, Scherer PE, Tang Z, et al. Oligomeric structure of caveolin: implications for caveolae membrane organization. *Proc Natl Acad Sci USA* 1995;**92**:9407–9411.

5. Prescott L, Brightman MW. The sarcolemma of Aplysia smooth muscle in freeze-fracture preparations. *Tissue Cell* 1976;**8**: 248–258.

6. Calaghan SC, Belus A, White E. Do stretch-induced changes in intracellular calcium modify the electrical activity of cardiac muscle? *Prog Biophys Mol Biol* 2003;**82**:81–95.

7. Perez NG, de Hurtado MC, Cingolani HE. Reverse mode of the Na+-Ca2+ exchange after myocardial stretch: underlying mechanism of the slow force response. *Circ Res* 2001;**88**:376–382.

8. Calaghan S, White E. Activation of Na$^+$-H$^+$ exchange and stretch-activated channels underlies the slow inotropic response to stretch in myocytes and muscle from the rat heart. *J Physiol* 2004; **559**:205–214.

9. Eder P, Probst D, Rosker C, *et al*. Phospholipase C-dependent control of cardiac calcium homeostasis involves a TRPC3–NCX1 signaling complex. *Cardiovasc Res* **73**:111–119.

10. Vila Petroff MG, Kim SH, Pepe S, *et al*. Endogenous nitric oxide mechanisms mediate the stretch dependence of Ca^{2+} release in cardiomyocytes. *Nat Cell Biol* 2001;**3**:867–873.

11. Zou Y, Akazawa H, Qin Y, *et al*. Mechanical stress activates angiotensin II type 1 receptor without the involvement of angiotensin II. *Nat Cell Biol* 2004;**6**:499–506.

12. Sundivakkam PC, Kwiatek AM, Sharma TT, Minshall RD, Malik AB, Tiruppathi C. Caveolin-1 scaffold domain interacts with TRPC1 and IP3R3 to regulate Ca^{2+} store release-induced Ca^{2+} entry in endothelial cells. *Am J Physiol* 2009;**296**:C403–C413.

13. Trouet D, Nilius B, Jacobs A, Remacle C, Droogmans G, Eggermont J. Caveolin-1 modulates the activity of the volume-regulated chloride channel. *J Physiol* 1999;**520**:113–119.

14. Calaghan S, White E. Caveolae modulate excitation–contraction coupling and beta2-adrenergic signalling in adult rat ventricular myocytes. *Cardiovasc Res* 2006;**69**:816–824.

15. Sens P, Turner MS (2007) The forces that shape caveolae. In: *Lipid Rafts and Caveolae* (ed CJ Fielding).Wiley, Weinheim, pp. 25–44.

16. Morris CE, Homann U. Cell surface area regulation and membrane tension. *J Membr Biol* 2001;**179**:79–102.

17. Hamill OP, Martinac B. Molecular basis of mechanotransduction in living cells. *Physiol Rev* 2001;**81**:685–740.

18. Kosawada T, Inoue K, Schmid-Schonbein GW. Mechanics of curved plasma membrane vesicles: resting shapes, membrane curvature, and in-plane shear elasticity. *J Biomech Eng* 2005;**127**:229–236.

19. Levin KR, Page E. Quantitative studies on plasmalemmal folds and caveolae of rabbit ventricular myocardial cells. *Circ Res* 1980;**46**:244–255.

20. Loukin SH, Kung C, Saimi Y. Lipid perturbations sensitize osmotic down-shock activated Ca^{2+} influx, a yeast "deletome" analysis. *FASEB J* 2007;**21**:1813–1820.

21. Levitan I, Christian AE, Tulenko TN, Rothblat GH. Membrane cholesterol content modulates activation of volume-regulated anion current in bovine endothelial cells. *J Gen Physiol* 2000;**115**:405–416.

22. Morris JB, Huynh H, Vasilevski O, Woodcock EA. Alpha1-adrenergic receptor signaling is localized to caveolae in neonatal rat cardiomyocytes. *J Mol Cell Cardiol* 2006;**41**:17–25.

23. Fujita A, Cheng J, Tauchi-Sato K, Takenawa T, Fujimoto T. A distinct pool of phosphatidylinositol 4,5-bisphosphate in caveolae revealed by a nanoscale labeling technique. *Proc Natl Acad Sci USA* 2009;**106**:9256–9261.

24. Ruwhof C, van Wamel JT, Noordzij LA, Aydin S, Harper JC, van der LA. Mechanical stress stimulates phospholipase C activity and intracellular calcium ion levels in neonatal rat cardiomyocytes. *Cell Calcium* 2001;**29**:73–83.

25. Suh BC, Hille B. PIP2 is a necessary cofactor for ion channel function: how and why? *Annu Rev Biophys* 2008;**37**:175–195.

26. Sharif-Naeini R, Folgering JH, Bichet D, *et al*. Sensing pressure in the cardiovascular system: Gq-coupled mechanoreceptors and TRP channels. *J Mol Cell Cardiol* 2009;**48**:83–89.

27. Calaghan S. (2008) Caveolae: co-ordinating centres for mechanotransduction in the heart? In: *Mechanosensitive Ion Channels* (eds A Kamkin, I Kiseleva). Springer, Berlin, pp. 267–289.

28. Yao X, Garland CJ. Recent developments in vascular endothelial cell transient receptor potential channels. *Circ Res* 2005;**97**:853–863.

29. Gervasio OL, Whitehead NP, Yeung EW, Phillips WD, Allen DG. TRPC1 binds to caveolin-3 and is regulated by Src kinase – role in Duchenne muscular dystrophy. *J Cell Sci* 2008;**121**:2246–2255.

30. Bergdahl A, Gomez MF, Dreja K, *et al*. Cholesterol depletion impairs vascular reactivity to endothelin-1 by reducing store-operated Ca^{2+} entry dependent on TRPC1. *Circ Res* 2003;**93**:839–847.

31. Schnitzler M, Storch U, Meibers S, *et al*. Gq-coupled receptors as mechanosensors mediating myogenic vasoconstriction. *EMBO J* 2008;**27**:3092–3103.

32. Aires V, Hichami A, Boulay G, Khan NA. Activation of TRPC6 calcium channels by diacylglycerol (DAG)-containing arachidonic acid: a comparative study with DAG-containing docosahexaenoic acid. *Biochimie* 2007;**89**:926–937.

33. Baumgarten CM, Clemo HF. Swelling-activated chloride channels in cardiac physiology and pathophysiology. *Prog Biophys Mol Biol* 2003;**82**:25–42.

34. Browe DM, Baumgarten CM. Stretch of beta 1 integrin activates an outwardly rectifying chloride current via FAK and Src in rabbit ventricular myocytes. *J Gen Physiol* 2003;**122**:689–702.

35. Trouet D, Hermans D, Droogmans G, Nilius B, Eggermont J. Inhibition of volume-regulated anion channels by dominant-negative caveolin-1. *Biochem Biophys Res Commun* 2001;**284**: 461–465.

36. Martens JR, Sakamoto N, Sullivan SA, Grobaski TD, Tamkun MM. Isoform-specific localization of voltage-gated K$^+$ channels to distinct lipid raft populations. Targeting of Kv1.5 to caveolae. *J Biol Chem* 2001;**276**:8409–8414.

37. Popescu LM, Diculescu I, Zelck U, Ionescu N. Ultrastructural distribution of calcium in smooth muscle cells of guinea-pig taenia coli. A correlated electron microscopic and quantitative study. *Cell Tissue Res* 1974;**154**:357–378.

38. Bossuyt J, Taylor BE, James-Kracke M, Hale CC. The cardiac sodium–calcium exchanger associates with caveolin-3. *Ann N Y Acad Sci* 2002;**976**:197–204.

39. Yasuda N, Miura S, Akazawa H, *et al*. Conformational switch of angiotensin II type 1 receptor underlying mechanical stress-induced activation. *EMBO Rep* 2008;**9**:179–186.

40. Wyse BD, Prior IA, Qian H, *et al*. Caveolin interacts with the angiotensin II type 1 receptor during exocytic transport but not at the plasma membrane. *J Biol Chem* 2003;**278**:23738–23746.

41. Ishizaka N, Griendling KK, Lassegue B, Alexander RW. Angiotensin II type 1 receptor: relationship with caveolae and caveolin after initial agonist stimulation. *Hypertension* 1998;**32**:459–466.

42. Oh P, Schnitzer JE. Segregation of heterotrimeric G proteins in cell surface microdomains. *Mol Biol Cell* 2001;**12**:685–698.

43. Dimmeler S, Fleming I, Fisslthaler B, Hermann C, Busse R, Zeiher AM. Activation of nitric oxide synthase in endothelial cells by Akt-dependent phosphorylation. *Nature* 1999;**399**:601–605.

44. Balligand JL, Feron O, Dessy C. eNOS activation by physical forces: from short-term regulation of contraction to chronic remodeling of cardiovascular tissues. *Physiol Rev* 2009;**89**:481–534.

45. Rizzo V, McIntosh DP, Oh P, Schnitzer JE. In situ flow activates endothelial nitric oxide synthase in luminal caveolae of endothelium with rapid caveolin dissociation and calmodulin association. *J Biol Chem* 1998;**273**:34724–34729.

46. Sedding DG, Hermsen J, Seay U, *et al*. Caveolin-1 facilitates mechanosensitive protein kinase B (Akt) signaling in vitro and in vivo. *Circ Res* 2005;**96**:635–642.

47. Takeda H, Komori K, Nishikimi N, Nimura Y, Sokabe M, Naruse K. Bi-phasic activation of eNOS in response to uni-axial cyclic stretch is mediated by differential mechanisms in BAECs. *Life Sci* 2006;**79**: 233–239.

48. Rastaldo R, Pagliaro P, Cappello S, *et al*. Nitric oxide and cardiac function. *Life Sci* 2007;**81**:779–793.

49. Brette F, Calaghan SC, Lappin S, White E, Colyer J, Le Guennec JY. Biphasic effects of hyposmotic challenge on excitation–contraction coupling in rat ventricular myocytes. *Am J Physiol* 2000;**279**: H1963–H1971.

50. Suchyna TM, Sachs F. Mechanosensitive channel properties and membrane mechanics in mouse dystrophic myotubes. *J Physiol* 2007;**581**:369–387.

51. Kawabe J, Okumura S, Lee MC, Sadoshima J, Ishikawa Y. Translocation of caveolin regulates stretch-induced ERK activity in vascular smooth muscle cells. *Am J Physiol* 2004;**286**:H1845–H1852.

52. Calaghan S, White E. Location and stretch-induced translocation of mechanotransductive proteins to and from caveolae in the adult heart. *Proc Physiol Soc* 2008;**10**:C16.

53. Kawamura S, Miyamoto S, Brown JH. Initiation and transduction of stretch-induced RhoA and Rac1 activation through caveolae: cytoskeletal regulation of ERK translocation. *J Biol Chem* 2003;**278**:31111–31117.

54. Vatta M, Ackerman MJ, Ye B, *et al.* Mutant caveolin-3 induces persistent late sodium current and is associated with long-QT syndrome. *Circulation* **114**:2104–2112.

55. Repetto S, Bado M, Broda P, *et al.* Increased number of caveolae and caveolin-3 overexpression in Duchenne muscular dystrophy. *Biochem Biophys Res Commun* 1999;**261**:547–550.

56. Rizzo V, Morton C, DePaola N, Schnitzer JE, Davies PF. Recruitment of endothelial caveolae into mechanotransduction pathways by flow conditioning in vitro. *Am J Physiol* 2003;**285**:H1720–H1729.

The membrane/cytoskeleton interface and stretch-activated channels

Thomas M. Suchyna and Frederick Sachs

Background

Stretch-activated channels (SAC) have been implicated in cardiac arrhythmias and other vascular pathologies[1–3]. SAC gating is controlled by intrinsic channel kinetics and the mechanical properties of the membrane in which it is embedded. Unlike voltage and ligand gated channels, SAC gating is highly dependent on the local 'mechano-physical' environment. The mechanical properties of the membrane are governed not only by the lipid composition, but also by membrane interactions with the cytoskeleton and extracellular matrix (ECM). Cytoskeleton–membrane–ECM interactions are tightly regulated by multiple stress sensors that activate a variety of secondary messenger pathways to control membrane tension.

Due to the complexity of mechanical studies *in vivo*, much of our understanding of the functional role of vertebrate SAC comes from experiments on cultured cells where the cytoskeletal architecture is distorted by adherence to a rigid two-dimensional (2D) coverslip[4]. Furthermore, SAC gating properties are measured in membrane patches that are under non-physiological levels of stress due to the adherence of the membrane to the glass walls of the pipette[5]. Even so, much has been learned about the potential chemical identity of SAC subunits [e.g. two-P domain (TREK), acid sensing ion channel (ASIC) and transient receptor potential channel (TRPC) families of channel subunits][3] and their regulation by the cytoskeleton[1]. This chapter focuses on the regulation of SAC by the cytoskeleton. Before delving into the structure of the plasma membrane–cytoskeleton interface, it is helpful to review the basic physical properties of lipid membranes.

Mechanical properties of a homogeneous membrane

There are two categories of SAC: those that may be activated by tension transmitted through an associated protein tether and those that appear to be activated by the tension in the bilayer[3]. Here we focus on the latter mechanism.

The cell membrane is a 2D fluid containing peptides that form channels, transporters and various receptors. A channel sensitive to bilayer tension is intimately linked to the dynamic mechanical properties of the membrane. There are four primary modes of deformation in a naked bilayer (Fig. 8.1). A fifth mode of deformation is hydrostatic membrane compression. However, like most liquids, the membrane is relatively incompressible [10^9–10^{10} N/m^2,[6]] and so this mode will not be considered in detail.

Stretching will increase membrane surface area and apply tension to the channel perimeter. However, membranes will resist stretching because of the high surface tension of the polar interface (~70 mN/m) which keeps head groups tightly packed (Fig. 8.1, part 1). The maximum area strain ($\Delta A/A$) that a lipid membrane can withstand at steady state without lysis is < 4%[7]. For small deformations (as in a Hookean spring) a linear relationship exists between the membrane tension (T) and the area strain:

$$T = K_A \cdot \Delta A / A$$

where K_A is the area expansion modulus [10^2–10^3 mN/m for biological membranes[8]], ΔA is the change in area and A is the initial area. Membrane expansion can occur, for example, during hypotonic cell swelling (although unfolding of membrane invaginations is likely to confound this process in cardiac cells[30]), or during pressure changes applied to membranes in a patch pipette. In a subsequent section, we will describe a method for measuring changes in membrane area via capacitance when a patch is stretched. For a constant volume membrane, the change in capacitance with stretch is twice the change in area (as thickness decreases since the membrane volume is fixed).

The stiffness with respect to membrane bending (Fig. 8.1, part 2) arises because curvature causes stretching of one monolayer and compression of the other. However, the energy to bend a bilayer is quite small (~10^{-19} N•m), so that large unsupported bilayers (but also red blood cells) undergo measurable thermal fluctuations in curvature[9]. Membranes may also have a natural curvature due to differences in the area occupied by the head groups and the acyl chains (see section on 'Membrane modifiers: amphipaths, polyvalent cations and peptides'). The bending stiffness depends on the degree of coupling or shear between the bilayers (Fig. 8.1, part 4, intermonolayer slip). Viscous drag may be negligible for slow

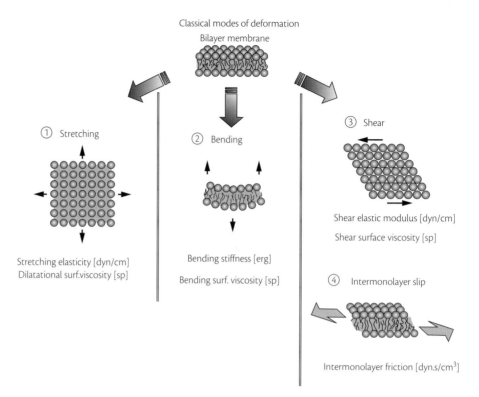

Classical modes of deformation
Bilayer membrane

① Stretching

② Bending

③ Shear

Shear elastic modulus [dyn/cm]

Shear surface viscosity [sp]

④ Intermonolayer slip

Stretching elasticity [dyn/cm]
Dilatational surf.viscosity [sp]

Bending stiffness [erg]

Bending surf. viscosity [sp]

Intermonolayer friction [dyn.s/cm³]

Fig. 8.1 Cartoon showing four physiologically relevant modes of lipid bilayer deformation that may affect SAC gating. [Courtesy of Rumiana Dimova, *Lipids and Membrane Mechanics*, Max Planck Institute of Colloids and Interfaces, Golm. http://www.mpikg-golm.mpg.de/th/people/dimova/courses/handouts/l3handouts.pdf.]

deformations, but it can significantly affect the dynamics of tension relaxation for rapidly applied stresses[10].

All of the deformations in Fig. 8.1 are sensitive to the concentration of cholesterol, the degree of saturation and the length of acyl chains[8–9], and the physical characteristics of the head groups. Shear, bending and area elasticity (K_A) increase with the cholesterol concentration, lipid saturation and chain length. Components such as saturated sphingolipids may aggregate into a new phase forming ordered domains called 'rafts'[11]. Proteins adjacent to or within rafts will experience different mechanical stresses from those in the more fluid portions of the membrane outside the raft[8]. Raft membranes are major components of caveolae, curved structures at equilibrium that form flask-like membrane invaginations and appear intimately involved in mechano-sensing[12] (see also Chapter 7).

In order for a channel to respond robustly to membrane stress, it must undergo a significant change in dimensions between the closed and open state [see Chapter 2 and ref.[13]]. Figure 8.2 shows the forces in a 2D bilayer that can cause conformational changes in a channel. The far-field membrane tension (i.e. stretching) favours states that are larger in area and the energy change is proportional to the area of the channel (the square of a linear dimension) (Fig. 8.2a). There is also an interfacial line tension between the channel and the surrounding boundary lipids that is proportional to the perimeter of the channel. The line tension is produced by the difference in area expansion modulus between the protein and the surrounding lipids. Line-tension is affected by all of the physico-chemical properties of the bilayer–channel interface such

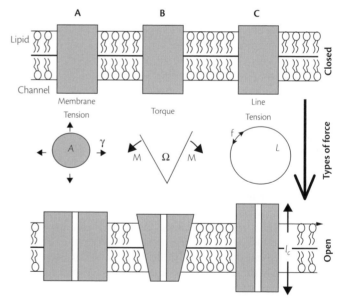

Fig. 8.2 Cartoon of three basic types of SAC deformation during transition between closed and open states. (**A**) Change of area A occupied by the channel in the plane of the membrane also changes the length L of the border between the channel complex and surrounding lipid where the line tension f resides. (**B**) Change of shape of the SAC expressed as a body angle Ω produced by torque during membrane bending. (**C**) Change of length l_c of the MS complex normal to the membrane; it can lead to changes in line tension f at the border with lipid. γ, membrane tension; M, torque. [Adapted, with permission, from Markin VS, Sachs F (2004) Thermodynamics of mechanosensitivity. *Phys Biol* **1**:110–124.]

as thickness, bending rigidity and hydrophobic mismatch with the channel. The corresponding decrease in membrane thickness that occurs during membrane stretching can create a hydrophobic mismatch between the trans-membrane domains of a protein and the boundary lipids, which could induce a conformational change (Fig. 8.2c). In addition to the area and linear strains, membrane curvature (spontaneous or pressure induced) can produce torque on the channel (Fig. 8.2b).

It is important to recall that, in general, biological membranes are fluid, so there can be no tension gradients at equilibrium. However, there are two common methods to generate gradients. First, the addition of membrane-soluble amphipaths exerts stress on the membrane-bound components such as channels. Second, for rapidly changing stimuli, the viscosity of the system can create stress gradients both parallel and perpendicular to the plane of the membrane.

Mechanics of heterogeneous membranes: cortical cytoskeleton support

The bilayer and cortical cytoskeleton (CCS) should be considered a composite mechanical structure. The physical modes of deformation described above are either intensified or buffered, depending on the strength and arrangement of membrane interactions with the CCS. Thus, it is not surprising that SAC gating properties (activation and inactivation) are intimately connected to the state of the CCS[14–16].

The CCS is a specialized region of the cytoskeleton forming a thin [< 200 nm[17]] protein lattice that provides bilayer support, localizes membrane proteins and governs the interaction of the membrane with the deeper cytoskeleton. Even without deeper cytoskeletal connections, the CCS–membrane association creates a mechanical composite material with a greater bending modulus and shear rigidity than a naked bilayer[7]. For example, red blood cells possess CCS without a deeper cytoskeleton, which increases the elastic shear modulus of the membrane to 10^{-2} mN/m. Thus, unlike naked lipid bilayers, red blood cells recover rapidly from large extensions[18] and are able to withstand the shear forces of the circulatory system.

The CCS is composed of a multitude of linking elements that connect the ECM and the deeper cytoskeleton to the bilayer [reviewed in[19]]. Intra-membrane proteins (e.g. integrins, dystroglycan, cadherins) connect the cytoskeleton and the ECM. Many small hetero-bifunctional adapter elements crosslink membrane proteins or form connections between the membrane and other proteins [e.g. ERM (Ezrin, Radixin and Moesin) proteins, vinculin, caveolin, syntrophin, homer], creating complexes of signalling molecules near membrane stress points. There are also numerous fibrous elements (e.g. spectrin, dystrophin, talin, spectraplakins) linked between focal stress complexes and the deeper cytoskeleton.

The CCS crosslinking proteins are especially important in the regulation of SAC gating. They localize ion channels and transporters to stress sensing regions and the fibrous rod-like proteins contain flexible domains that allow them to absorb mechanical stress [20–21]. These fibres are critical components for the formation and stabilization of mechanically sensitive structures such as caveolae, microvilli, t-tubules and costameres (see below).

The strength of the CCS interaction with the membrane is governed by regulatory proteins (e.g. small guanosine-5'-triphosphatases (GTPases), kinases, calpains, SAC). These effectors are induced by multiple signalling agents like phosphatidylinositol-4,5-bisphosphate (PIP_2), diacyl glycerol, aracidonic acid and Ca^{2+} [reviewed in[22,23]]. PIP_2 appears central to controlling membrane–cytoskeletal interactions such as membrane ruffling and filopodial extensions and the formation of more permanent structures such as microvilli and focal adhesions. Most cytoskeletal proteins that associate with the membrane have cationic binding sites that favourably interact with the negatively charged PIP_2 lipids. Elevated levels of PIP_2 increase membrane/cytoskeleton adhesion energy and strengthen the CCS by recruiting proteins for actin crosslinking, bundling, nucleating and capping.

Bilayer adhesion strength to the CCS has been investigated by measuring the amount of force necessary to pull a bilayer tether away from a cell. The calculated adhesion energy density for a variety of different cells ranges from 1 to 10×10^{-16} J/μm^2 [24], corresponding to hundreds of linkage sites per micrometre squared of membrane[25]. Thus, bilayer deformations are controlled primarily by a multitude of weak protein–lipid surface interactions, with different domains experiencing different amounts of stress depending on the degree of cytoskeletal adhesion and the rate of stress change[15].

The dystrophin-associated glycoprotein complex (DGC; Fig. 8.3A) is the main cortical anchoring system of muscle cells. β-dystroglycan is a trans-membrane protein linked to actin by the fibrous protein dystrophin. Dystrophin is critical for adhesion between actin and the sarcolemma[26]. In dystrophic muscle, the membrane–costamere adhesion is weaker and the shear elasticity of the membrane is lower[27], leading to hyperactive SAC[14]. In heart muscle, mutations that disrupt dystrophin lead to weakening of the ventricular wall and dilated cardiomyopathy[28].

Specialized cardiomyocyte membranes: role in mechano-sensitivity

Costameres, caveolae and the transverse (T)-tubular system, present in both skeletal and cardiac muscle cells, are regions of cytoskeletal–membrane interaction that illustrate many of the concepts described above. Costameres are located at the Z-lines, which are like circumferential focal adhesion plaques rich in CSS components such as DGC and integrins (Fig. 8.3B). They adhere to the sarcolemma, the deeper cytoskeleton and to adjacent cardiomyocyte costameres, helping to distribute force laterally between cardiomyocytes[29]. In the intercostameric region, the sarcolemma is weakly associated with deeper cytoskeleton and festoons outward during contraction[30]. There are also membrane folds at the costameres that can unfold when the cardiomyocyte is stretched.

T-tubules (200–300 nm diameter) and caveolae (50–100 nm diameter) are highly curved membranes that are tightly associated with the CSS[12,31]. Respectively, they make up > 50% and > 15% of the total sarcolemma surface area. On the cell surface, t-tubule pores are located along the costameres, while caveolae are fairly evenly distributed over the sarcolemma. Both membrane systems are cholesterol-rich and contain many signalling proteins.

Costamere membrane folds and caveolae have been shown to undergo radical shape changes under osmotic and axial stress[30,32].

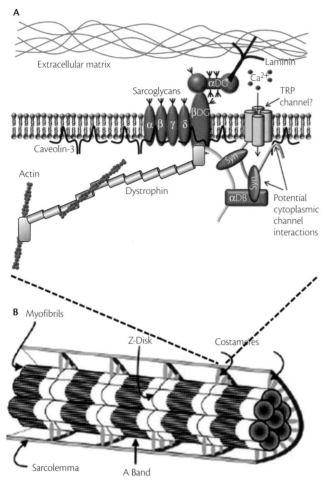

Fig. 8.3 A Cartoon of the molecular structure of the dystroglycan complex and its potential associations with MSC. It is a primary component of the costameres (**B**) that forms tightly coupled cytoskeletal–membrane regions around the Z-disks. The DGC forms links with the deeper cytoskeleton primarily through dystrophin (red). Beta-dystroglycan (βDG) forms a trans-membrane connection to the extracellular matrix so that the whole complex is designed to regulate membrane tension. Syn, α-syntrophin; αDB, α-dystrobrevin; αDG, α-dystroglycan; α, β, γ and δ, sarcoglycans. [Adapted, with permission, from Ervasti JM (2003) Costameres: the Achilles' heel of Herculean muscle. *J Biol Chem* **278**:13591–13594.]

where mechano-sensitive whole-cell currents can be elicited[36], while single channel currents in patch-clamp studies remained elusive. This can be explained if SAC are 'hidden' in membrane invaginations, such as t-tubules. This reverse behaviour appears to be the result of mechano-protection, or shielding, of SAC from mechanical strain by the cytoskeleton.

Voltage- and ligand-gated channels can be responsive to mechanical stress [see reference[37] and Chapter 6]. In fact most cardiomyocyte channels involved in excitation–contraction coupling are associated with the specialized membrane structures described above[31,38] and are thus exposed to relatively high resting membrane curvatures. The sarcomeric and t-tubular membranes contain most of the Ca^{2+} transporters (L-type Ca^{2+} channels, Na^+/Ca^{2+} and Na^+/H^+ exchangers) and many other voltage-gated channels (see Chapter 6).

Channels such as TRPC have been implicated in cardiac physiology usually related to Ca^{2+} influx induced by mechanical stimuli[1]. Their activity has been linked to cytoskeletal remodelling and strengthening of CCS adhesion under normal conditions[3,39]. Elevated TRPC activity, such as occurs in dystrophies, has been linked to excess protease activity leading to CCS degradation. In skeletal myocytes, TRPC1 and 4 activation is controlled by scaffolding proteins like α-syntrophin, Homer and Caveolin-3 that crosslink the channels to the DGC (Fig. 8.3A)[40]. Immunofluorescence staining in cardiac tissue shows that TRPC1 and 6 localize along the t-tubules in myofibres but not the surface sarcolemma[41,42]. Thus, TRPC are strategically localized in membrane regions associated with significant mechanical deformation and/or with molecular structures that control membrane stress.

However, channel localization in specific membrane regions is not the only factor that confers mechano-sensitivity. TRPC6, for example, was reported to be mechano-sensitive and activated by second messengers[42,43]. However, the channels proved to be mechanically insensitive in patch studies, even when the channels were present in the patch dome[5]. Recent evidence shows that TRPC6[44], like other TRPC[45], becomes mechanically sensitive only after receptor-mediated production of secondary messengers, suggesting that other factors are required to induce mechano-sensitivity. In addition, there is no *a prioi* reason to suspect that SAC are homomers of any channel subunit and may only express this sensitivity as heteromers.

SAC – activated by membrane tension but regulated by cytoskeleton

Cation non-selective SAC (SAC_{NS}) are found in all tissues of the body and are considered stimulatory due to their permeability for Na^+ and Ca^{2+}. In the heart, stretching can activate these channels to increase background and transient cytoplasmic Ca^{2+} levels and increase force production[41]. Chronic mechanical stress[1,3] or pathological inability to control SAC_{NS} activation[46] may lead to cardiomyopathies.

In patches, SAC activation is intimately connected to the state of the cytoskeleton[5,16,47]. This is best observed when the cytoskeleton of the patch membrane is disrupted during excision to form the inside-out conformation. Images of inside-out patches have an optical density tenfold lower than cell-attached patches [see reference[5] and Fig. 8.4A]. In patches with mechanically or chemically disrupted cytoskeleton, the likelihood of SAC activation is

Caveolae will actually splay up to the sarcolemmal surface, becoming almost planar with the surrounding membrane. Whether the internal portion of t-tubules experiences significant stress remains unknown. However, in contrast to skeletal myofibres that only have surface expression of dystrophin and caveolae, cardiomyocytes have internal dystrophin associated with the t-tubules[33] and caveolae that bud off the t-tubule surface[32]. This may suggest differing mechanical stress-bearing abilities of the two cell types.

The question of how the ultrastructure of the membrane affects SAC gating has been a focus of investigation since Morris and Horn[34] raised the question of why it was difficult to observe mechano-sensitive whole-cell current in nerve cells. In oocytes, where SAC are easily observed in patches, a variety of mechanical deformations did not produce significant whole-cell currents either[35]. The discrepancy is reversed in cardiac ventricular cells,

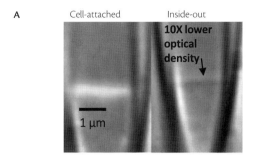

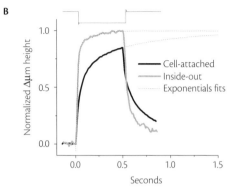

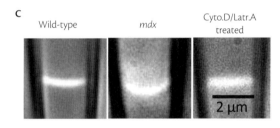

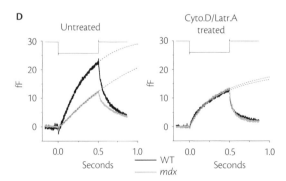

increased (astrocytes – Table 8.1, myotubes –[47], TREK transfected cells – unpublished observations). Effects of the disruption of cytoskeletal support can also be shown by the difference in mechanical relaxation rates between the two types of patches (Fig. 8.4B).

Dystrophin has a central role in regulating overall cytoskeletal association with the sarcolemma. In patches formed from muscular dystrophy mouse (*mdx*) myotubes, the dome membrane is more compliant than the wild-type. As actin pulls normal to the membrane, a cell-attached *mdx* patch bends toward the cell [Fig. 8.4C and ref.[47]].

Patch capacitance (C$_p$, measured using a phase lock amplifier) can be tracked while measuring channel current[16]. Membrane capacitance will change as the membrane area changes. Since tension will produce an area change, monitoring C$_p$ provides a convenient indication of the dynamic tension change in the patch dome. In response to step pressure changes, patches lacking dystrophin are four times less elastic than patches from normal myotubes and have slower relaxation times and extended SAC activation periods [Fig. 8.4D and ref.[47]]. These properties are related to the interaction of dystrophin with the underlying actin network, since by depolymerizing actin the patches become flat and their relaxation kinetics become equivalent (Fig. 8.4C, D).

Another form of SAC regulation is a rapid, voltage-sensitive, inactivation phase [Fig. 8.5 and refs[16,48,49]]. Inactivation is a common process that minimizes charge transfer and provides a higher 'differential' sensitivity to changing stimuli. It is important to examine these dynamic properties of SAC since the magnitude and timing of the responses may profoundly alter the resulting steady state effects. The SAC inactivation mechanism seems to be sensitive to cytoskeletal integrity, since mechanical or chemical disruption eliminates inactivation in astrocytes (Table 8.1). In myocytes this function appears connected to the presence of dystrophin, since patches without dystrophin lose inactivation[47]. The loss of inactivation and slower relaxation times are likely to contribute to the elevated activity of SAC in dystrophic skeletal and cardiac myofibres.

In mammalian cells, the decline in channel activity over time is best termed inactivation, not adaptation[16] since there is no evidence of a decrease in the local stimulus, as has been suggested for amphibian and bacterial SAC[48,50]. This conclusion is based on two lines of evidence: (1) since inactivation can be eliminated with cytoskeletal disruption, the more robust activation response can be studied in isolation. In this condition, non-inactivating channels

Fig. 8.4 Cortical cytoskeleton plays a crucial role in membrane mechanics as observed in the patch. **A** Side-by-side comparison of the optical density difference between cell-attached and excised inside-out patches. **B** Average inside-out patch motion shows a much faster relaxation time in response to pressure steps than the cell attached patch. **C** Patches from *mdx* myotubes that are missing dystrophin are more compliant than wild-type. At rest (0 mmHg applied pressure) and *mdx* patches bend toward the inside of the cell due to the pull of actin. Actin inhibitors make the patch flat. **D** Capacitance measurements show that *mdx* patches relax slower than patches from wild-type fibres, suggesting a loss of stiffness. This difference is due to the interaction of dystrophin with actin since this difference is eliminated by actin disruption.

Table 8.1 SAC inactivation is lost when the cytoskeleton is disrupted in adult rat astrocytes

	Number of patches	Number with active MSC	Number showing inactivation
Cell-attached patches, untreated	123	41 (33%)	17 (14%)
Outside-out patches, mechanical disruption	42	21 (50%)	1 (2%)
Cell-attached + cytoskeleton inhibitors, chemical disruption	36	17 (47%)	0 (0%)

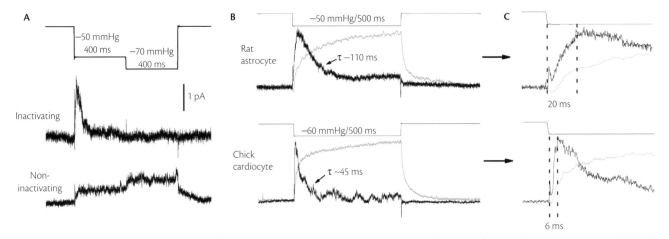

Fig. 8.5 SAC activation and inactivation analyzed with high speed pressure stimuli and patch capacitance. **A** The current from the inactivating rat astrocyte SAC$_{NS}$ does not respond to increased pressure, but channels in which the inactivation process is disrupted do respond. **B** Average inactivating currents (black, normalized) are shown for rat astrocytes and chick heart cells with the corresponding ΔCp records (light grey). The patch potential is −90 mV in both cases. The kinetics of chick heart SAC activation and inactivation phases (panel **C**, expanded views) are approximately three times faster than that observed for the astrocyte SAC. In both cases the activation rate appears to roughly follow the rate of capacitance change, which again is more rapid in chick heart cell patches.

respond to increased stimulus strength with increased open probability, while inactivating channels that have reached a steady state show no response to an increasing stimulus (Fig. 8.5A); (2) for inactivating channels, the average patch current starts its decay phase while patch area is still increasing (Fig. 8.5B). This shows that tension relaxation (adaptation) is not the cause of the current decay.

The kinetics of SAC can be sensitive to voltage and to the membrane environment. Figure 8.5B, C compares the phasic response of two cell types containing distinctly different cytoskeletal properties. The channels are both cation selective, show a voltage sensitive response, are sensitive to the same range of pressures and have nearly identical unitary conductance and inward rectification (rat astrocyte, 1.25 pA at +50 mV/1.75 pA at −50 mV; chick heart cells, 1.1 pA at +50 mV/1.75 pA at −50 mV). Thus, although these channels are from different species, they appear to be the same 'ubiquitous' SAC$_{NS}$ that occurs in many vertebrate cell types. The one significant difference between these two channels is their phasic responses to pressure steps. Channels from the chick heart inactivate (Fig. 8.4B) and activate (Fig. 8.4C) nearly three times faster than that in rat astrocytes (21°C). Interestingly, the mechanically induced changes in patch dimensions of chick heart membranes are also three times faster than in astrocytes, suggesting that the difference is due to the membrane/cytoskeletal relaxation time, rather than differences in channel structure.

Membrane modifiers: amphipaths, polyvalent cations and peptides

SAC are sensitive to agents that modify the physical properties of the bilayer, such as amphiphiles – chemicals with polar and apolar regions. The physico-chemical characteristics of an amphiphile dictate how it inserts into the bilayer. This determines effects on membrane curvature, thickness and stiffness[51]. Exogenous amphiphiles may produce complex phase separations in association with, or separate from, the endogenous phases. In addition to

modifying membrane mechanical properties, exogenous amphiphiles may show distinct interactions with membrane proteins.

Amphipath activity is determined by the shape (conical or cylindrical), head group charge, saturation and dimensions of the hydrophobic region. If the amphipath has a hydrophobic:hydrophilic area ratio ≠ 1, it will tend to behave as conical, and its insertion into a bilayer will create an area difference between the interior and exterior. This causes changes in curvature and imposes torque on embedded proteins[51]. Some common natural amphipaths are products of phospholipases, e.g. lysophospholipids, diacylglycerol (DAG) and arachidonic acid (AA) and its metabolites[52]. Phospholipases cleave acyl chains from the phosphate head group, resulting in single acyl chains or diglycerides that differ in area ratio and charge.

For small amphiphiles like AA that can traverse the bilayer[53], headgroup charge will affect preferential insertion into one of the two leaflets of the bilayer. Biological membranes are normally more negative on the inside, so anionic amphiphiles will tend to partition into the outer leaflet (Fig. 8.6, crenator, e.g. AA, trinitrophenol, salicylate). Cationic amphiphiles will tend to partition into the inner leaflet (Fig. 8.5, cup-former, e.g. chlorpromazine, tetracaine).

Cytoplasmic and extracellular phospholipase A2 can produce lysophophatidyl choline (LPC) and AA on either leaflet. These amphiphiles activate K$^+$ selective SAC such as TREK and TRAAK[55] (see Chapter 3). However, LPC only activates these two channels from the outer leaflet where it acts as a crenator (Fig. 8.5). AA also acts as a crenator, but it can be produced at either leaflet since it can flip between them. Thus, activation of these channels appears to require crenators with an outward bending torque.

Obviously the action of amphiphiles (especially AA) is more complicated than their ability to affect membrane curvature. They can affect regulatory proteins such as G-proteins and kinases that may have secondary effects. However, some TRPC forms appear to be activated by internal cup-forming agents[44,52,56], but not by

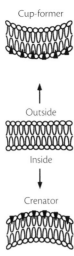

Cup-former

↑

Outside

Inside

↓

Crenator

Fig. 8.6 Differential effects of anionic and cationic amphiphiles. [Reproduced, with permission, from Patel AJ, Honoré E, Maingret F, *et al.* (1998) A mammalian two pore domain mechano-gated S-like K+ channel. *EMBO J* **17**:4283–4290.]

external crenators[52]. Thus, the gating of SAC$_{NS}$ TRPC that depolarize resting membranes may occur by significantly different mechanisms than those activating 2P domain K+ channels that hyperpolarize the cell. This raises the intriguing possibility that one and the same regulatory pathway may induce an excitatory effect by simultaneously activating TRPC and inhibiting 2P channels.

Among polyvalent cations, Gd^{3+} is a potent blocker of SAC[57]. In contrast to amphiphiles, polyvalent cations appear to exert their effect primarily by interaction with the lipid head groups. These effects include compression of the membrane and changes in the membrane dipole potential[58]. Exposure of the outer surface of negative-charged lipid vesicles to Gd^{3+} causes cup formation. Lipid bonding may also increase the line tension surrounding the channels, causing inhibition[13]. In addition, polyvalent cations shift the internal electric field of the membrane and this will affect voltage sensitive channels. This may explain the variable effects of Gd^{3+} on different channels.

GsMTx-4 is a small amphiphilic peptide that inhibits SAC$_{NS}$but not K+ selective SAC). It acts as a gating modifier, rather than a pore blocker[59]. Despite being specific for SAC$_{NS}$, there is no stereospecific binding as demonstrated when the D and L enantiomers were found to behave equivalently[59]. This is surprising since GsMTx-4 is ~10 times more potent than Gd^{3+}, with a K$_D$ of 200–500 nM. GsMTx-4 appears to interact closely with the channel since, during extracellular inhibition, inward currents are reduced while outward currents are unaffected. This suggests that a charged portion of the peptide is within a Debye (~10Å) of the pore. However, unlike Gd^{3+} which is somewhat promiscuous, GsMTx-4 is remarkably selective for SAC$_{NS}$[59] and has no known effect on other channels at micromolar concentrations[49,60,61], including K+ selective SAC such as TREK and TRAAK. Specificity may arise from the channels themselves, since the gating inhibition is due to a change in stress on the channel, while most channels with interior gates are not sensitive to stress in the outer monolayer. Because cardiovascular disease is often related to mechanical dysfunction or excess mechanical stimulation, substances affecting the heart like

GsMTx-4 may prove to be a useful therapeutic [see references [1,41] and Chapter 65]. Since the D-peptide is effective, it could represent an interesting drug development paradigm with reduced immunogenicity and susceptibility to degradation.

Conclusions and outlook

SAC exist in a complex mechanical environment where the properties of individual components are not easily tractable. We cannot predict the effect of an intervention on SAC activity unless we know the effect on the local environment. Recent work has shown that cytoskeletal stiffness and adhesion strength are two of the main factors regulating SAC activity. However, for structures as complex and elaborate as the cell cortex, the material properties are known well enough to enable useful analytic models, and it is important to remain wary of generalized interpretations. For example, if an agent produces a drop in SAC current, the inhibition could arise from a range of effects, including block of the pore, change in the channel gating properties, change in properties of the local lipids or changes in cytoskeleton. SAC may have originally evolved as amphipath receptors, and the mechano-sensitivity is simply a by-product.

The sensitivity of SAC to a wide range of inputs creates an effective integrator of information, but we cannot directly transfer patch data to *in vivo* behaviour since adhesion to the glass of the pipette creates stresses much larger than in resting cells. However, there is evidence for SAC activity *in vivo* from GsMTx-4 inhibition of spontaneous Ca^{2+} entry in dystrophic muscle cells in culture. Development of drugs active on SACs may have potential in a wide range of pathologies.

References

1. Stiber JA, Seth M, Rosenberg PB. Mechanosensitive channels in striated muscle and the cardiovascular system: not quite a stretch anymore. *J Cardiovasc Pharmacol* 2009;**54**:116–122.

2. Watanabe H, Murakami M, Ohba T, Ono K, Ito H. The pathological role of transient receptor potential channels in heart disease. *Circ J* 2009;**73**:419–427.

3. Inoue R, Jian Z, Kawarabayashi Y. Mechanosensitive TRP channels in cardiovascular pathophysiology. *Pharmacol Ther* 2009;**123**: 371–385.

4. Larsen M, Artym VV, Green JA, Yamada KM. The matrix reorganized: extracellular matrix remodeling and integrin signaling. *Curr Opin Cell Biol* 2006;**18**:463–471.

5. Suchyna TM, Markin VS, Sachs F. Biophysics and structure of the patch and the gigaseal. *Biophys J* 2009;**97**:738–747.

6. Andersen OS, Koeppe RE. 2nd Bilayer thickness and membrane protein function: an energetic perspective. *Annu Rev Biophys Biomol Struct* 2007;**36**:107–130.

7. Hamill OP,Martinac B. Molecular basis of mechanotransduction in living cells. *Physiol Rev* 2001;**81**:685–740.

8. Rawicz W, Smith BA, McIntosh TJ, Simon SA, Evans E. Elasticity, strength, and water permeability of bilayers that contain raft microdomain-forming lipids. *Biophys J* 2008;**94**:4725–4736.

9. Rawicz W, Olbrich KC, McIntosh T, Needham D, Evans E. Effect of chain length and unsaturation on elasticity of lipid bilayers. *Biophys J* 2000;**79**:328–339.

10. Evans E, Yeung A. Hidden dynamics in rapid changes of bilayer shape. *Chem Phys Lipids* 1994;**73**:39–56.

11. Alonso MA, Millan J. The role of lipid rafts in signalling and membrane trafficking in T lymphocytes. *J Cell Sci* 2001;**114**:3957–3965.

12. Parton RG, Simons K. The multiple faces of caveolae. *Nat Rev Mol Cell Bio* 2007;**8**:185–194.

13. Markin VS, Sachs F. Thermodynamics of mechanosensitivity. *Phys Biol* 2004;**1**:110–124.

14. Franco-Obregon A, Lansman JB. Changes in mechanosensitive channel gating following mechanical stimulation in skeletal muscle myotubes from the mdx mouse. *J Physiol* 2002;**539**:391–407.

15. Morris CE. Mechanoprotection of the plasma membrane in neurons and other non-erythroid cells by the spectrin-based membrane skeleton. *Cell Mol Biol Lett* 2001;**6**:703–720.

16. Suchyna TM, Besch SR, Sachs F. Dynamic regulation of mechanosensitive channels: capacitance used to monitor patch tension in real time. *Phys Biol* 2004;**1**:1–18.

17. Masuda T, Fujimaki N, Ozawa E, Ishikawa H. Confocal laser microscopy of dystrophin localization in guinea pig skeletal muscle fibers. *J Cell Biol* 1992;**119**:543–548.

18. Discher DE, Mohandes N, Evans EA. Molecular maps of red cell deformation: hidden elasticity and in situ connectivity. *Science* 1994;**266**:1032–1036.

19. Doherty GJ, McMahon HT. Mediation, modulation, and consequences of membrane–cytoskeleton interactions. *Ann Rev Biophys* 2008;**37**:65–95.

20. Roper K, Gregory SL, Brown NH. The 'spectraplakins': cytoskeletal giants with characteristics of both spectrin and plakin families. *J Cell Sci* 2002;**115**:4215–4225.

21. Bretscher A, Edwards K, Fehon RG. ERM proteins and merlin: integrators at the cell cortex. *Nat Rev Mol Cell Biol* 2002;**3**:586–599.

22. Sheetz MP, Sable JE, Dobereiner HG. Continuous membrane–cytoskeleton adhesion requires continuous accommodation to lipid and cytoskeleton dynamics. *Annu Rev Biophys Biomol Struct* 2006;**35**:417–434.

23. Janmey PA, McCulloch CA. Cell mechanics: integrating cell responses to mechanical stimuli. *Annu Rev Biomed Eng* 2007;**9**:1–34.

24. Ermilov SA, Murdock DR, Qian F, Brownell WE, Anvari B. Studies of plasma membrane mechanics and plasma membrane–cytoskeleton interactions using optical tweezers and fluorescence imaging. *J Biomech* 2007;**40**:476–480.

25. Raucher D, Stauffer T, Chen W, et al. Phosphatidylinositol 4,5-bisphosphate functions as a second messenger that regulates cytoskeleton–plasma membrane adhesion. *Cell* 2000;**100**:221–228.

26. Rybakova IN, Patel JR, Ervasti JM. The dystrophin complex forms a mechanically strong link between the sarcolemma and costameric actin. *J Cell Biol* 2000;**150**:1209–1214.

27. Pasternak C, Wong S, Elson EL. Mechanical function of dystrophin in muscle cells. *J Cell Biol* 1995;**128**:355–361.

28. Muntoni F, Torelli S, Ferlini A. Dystrophin and mutations: one gene, several proteins, multiple phenotypes. *Lancet Neurol* 2003;**2**:731–740.

29. Ervasti JM. Costameres: the Achilles' heel of Herculean muscle. *J Biol Chem* 2003;**278**:13591–13594.

30. Kohl P, Cooper PJ, Holloway H. Effects of acute ventricular volume manipulation on in situ cardiomyocyte cell membrane configuration. *Prog Biophys Mol Biol* 2003;**82**:221–227.

31. Brette F, Orchard C. T-tubule function in mammalian cardiac myocytes. *Circ Res* 2003;**92**:1182–1192.

32. Levin KR, Page E. Quantitative studies on plasmalemmal folds and caveolae of rabbit ventricular myocardial cells. *Circ Res* 1980;**46**:244–255.

33. Kaprielian RR, Stevenson S, Rothery SM, Cullen MJ, Severs NJ. Distinct patterns of dystrophin organization in myocyte sarcolemma and transverse tubules of normal and diseased human myocardium. *Circulation* 2000;**101**:2586–2594.

34. Morris CE, Horn R. Failure to elicit neuronal macroscopic mechanosensitive currents anticipated by single-channel studies. *Science* 1991;**251**:1246–1249.

35. Zhang Y, Hamill OP. On the discrepancy between whole-cell and membrane patch mechanosensitivity in *Xenopus* oocytes. *J Physiol* 2000;**523**:101–115.

36. Zeng T, Bett GCL, Sachs F. Stretch-activated whole-cell currents in adult rat cardiac myoctes. *Am J Physiol* 2000;**278**:H548–H557.

37. Gu CX, Juranka PF, Morris CE. Stretch-activation and stretch-inactivation of Shaker-IR, a voltage- gated K+ channel. *Biophys J* 2001;**80**:2678–2693.

38. Balijepalli RC, Kamp TJ. Caveolae, ion channels and cardiac arrhythmias. *Prog Biophys Mol Biol* 2008;**98**:149–160.

39. Clark K, Middelbeek J, van Leeuwen FN. Interplay between TRP channels and the cytoskeleton in health and disease. *Eur J Cell Biol* 2008;**87**:631–640.

40. Sabourin J, Lamiche C, Vandebrouck A, et al. Regulation of TRPC1 and TRPC4 cation channels requires an alpha1-syntrophin-dependent complex in skeletal mouse myotubes. *J Biol Chem* 2009;**284**:36248–36261.

41. Ward ML, Williams IA, Chu Y, et al. Stretch-activated channels in the heart: contributions to length-dependence and to cardiomyopathy. *Prog Biophys Mol Biol* 2008;**97**:232–249.

42. Dyachenko V, Husse B, Rueckschloss U, Isenberg G. Mechanical deformation of ventricular myocytes modulates both TRPC6 and Kir 2.3 channels. *Cell Calcium* 2009;**45**:38–54.

43. Spassova MA, Hewavitharana T, Xu W, Soboloff J, Gill DL. A common mechanism underlies stretch activation and receptor activation of TRPC6 channels. *Proc Natl Acad Sci USA* 2006;**103**:16586–16591.

44. Inoue R, Jensen LJ, Jian Z, et al. Synergistic activation of vascular TRPC6 channel by receptor and mechanical stimulation via phospholipase C/diacylglycerol and phospholipase A2/omega-hydroxylase/20-HETE pathways. *Circ Res* 2009;**104**:1399–1409.

45. Watanabe H, Vriens J, Prenen J, et al. Anandamide and arachidonic acid use epoxyeicosatrienoic acids to activate TRPV4 channels. *Nature* 2003;**424**:434–438.

46. Fanchaouy M, Polakova E, Jung C, et al. Pathways of abnormal stress-induced Ca2+ influx into dystrophic mdx cardiomyocytes. *Cell Calcium* 2009;**46**:114–121.

47. Suchyna TM Sachs F. Mechanosensitive channel properties and membrane mechanics in mouse dystrophic myotubes. *J Physiol* 2007;**581**:369–387.

48. McBride DW Jr, Hamill OP. Pressure-clamp: a method for rapid step perturbation of mechanosensitive channels. *Pflugers Arch* 1992;**421**:606–612.

49. Suchyna TM, Johnson JH, Kamer K, et al. Identification of a peptide toxin from *Grammostola spatulata* spider venom that blocks stretch activated channels. *J Gen Physiol* 2000;**115**:583–598.

50. Koprowski P, Kubalski A. Voltage-independent adaptation of mechanosensitive channels in *Escherichia coli* protoplasts. *J Membr Biol* 1998;**164**:253–262.

51. Perozo E, Kloda A, Cortes DM, Martinac B. Physical principles underlying the transduction of bilayer deformation forces during mechanosensitive channel gating. *Nat Struct Biol* 2002;**9**:696–703.

52. Beech DJ, Bahnasi YM, Dedman AM, Al-Shawaf E. TRPC channel lipid specificity and mechanisms of lipid regulation. *Cell Calcium* 2009;**45**:583–588.

53. Kamp F, Zakim D, Zhang F, Noy N, Hamilton JA. Fatty acid flip-flop in phospholipid bilayers is extremely fast. *Biochemistry* 1995;**34**:11928–11937.

54. Patel AJ, Honoré E, Maingret F, Lesage F, Fink M, Duprat F, et al. A mammalian two pore domain mechano-gated S-like K+ channel. *EMBO J* 1998;**17**:4283–4290.

55. Maingret F, Patel AJ, Lesage F, Lazdunski M, Honore E. Lysophospholipids open the two-pore domain mechano-gated K+ channels TREK-1 and TRAAK. *J Biol Chem* 2000;**275**:10128–10133.

56. Andersson DA, Nash M, Bevan S. Modulation of the cold-activated channel TRPM8 by lysophospholipids and polyunsaturated fatty acids. *J Neurosci* 2007;**27**:3347–3355.

57. Caldwell RA, Clemo HF, Baumgarten CM. Using gadolinium to identify stretch-activated channels: technical considerations. *Am J Physiol* 1998;**275**:C619–C621.

58. Ermakov YA, Averbakh AZ, Yusipovich AI, Sukharev S. Dipole potentials indicate restructuring of the membrane interface induced by gadolinium and beryllium ions. *Biophys J* 2001;**80**:1851–1862.

59. Suchyna TM, Tape SE, Koeppe RE, Andersen OS, Sachs F, Gottlieb PA, *et al.* Bilayer-dependent inhibition of mechanosensitive channels by neuroactive peptide enantiomers. *Nature* 2004;**430**: 235–240.

60. Bode F, Sachs F, Franz MR. Tarantula peptide inhibits atrial fibrillation – a peptide from spider venom can prevent the heartbeat from losing its rhythm. *Nature* 2001;**409**:35–36.

61. Ruta V, MacKinnon R. Localization of the voltage-sensor toxin receptor on KvAP. *Biochemistry* 2004;**43**:10071–10079.

9

Cardiomyocyte stretch-sensing

Michiel Helmes and Henk Granzier

Background

The heart is an organ of amazing adjustability and resilience. Both acute and chronic responses take place with precision and effectiveness. A prime example of the former is the onset of exercise which increases cardiac output more than fivefold, and of the latter the nearly twofold increase in cardiac muscle mass with sustained training, as well as the return to the original size after training stops. An intimate role in this remarkable adaptability is played by the cytoskeleton which consists of an intricate network of filaments and accessory proteins (Fig. 9.1). These filaments allow the cells to withstand the large mechanical stresses that are experienced during each heart beat and, furthermore, they sense when biomechanical stresses and strains exceed physiological levels and, in response, trigger cardiac adaptations. The cytoskeleton is comprised of microtubules, intermediate filaments and microfilaments with membrane-associated proteins linking the cytoskeleton to the extracellular matrix. In addition, the intrasarcomeric skeleton contains the giant protein titin and a multitude of titin-binding proteins. In this chapter we first discuss the microtubules, intermediate filaments and microfilaments and dedicate much of the discussion to the recent progress in understanding the role of titin system.

Cytoskeletal filaments

The cytoskeletal filaments support the fragile cell membranes, position organelles, provide for intracellular transport, organize myofilaments and provide mechanical strength and structural integrity to the cardiac myocyte. Recent work, especially involving titin, has revealed important functions in mechano-sensing and feedback control. In cardiac myocytes from normal hearts, microtubules form a fine network that is most prominent in the perinuclear region. One of the hallmarks of human heart failure is the increase in microtubular networks[1]. The role that microtubules play in hypertrophy and cardiac failure has been investigated in animal models and revealed increases in density as well as in the total amount of tubulin[2]. It is likely that this increase reflects cellular growth (hypertrophy) and increased protein turnover, processes' that require enhanced microtubular-based transport systems. The increased microtubular networks result in contractile abnormalitie s of cardiac myocytes (reduction in extent of unloaded shortening) that can be normalized by colchicine (a drug

that depolymerizes microtubules)[2]. Thus the microtubular network constitutes an internal viscous load that might contribute to contractile dysfunction when these networks are upregulated (see also Chapter 12).

The main intermediate filament type in cardiac myocytes is desmin, where it constitutes ~2% of the total protein[3]. Desmin monomers polymerize into long rope-like filaments (diameter of ~12 nm) that provide mechanical integrity and strength to the cardiac myocyte. Desmin filaments surround myofibrils and laterally connect adjacent Z-disks (inter-sarcomeric disk; 'Z' from zwischen – German for in-between) and M-lines (sarcomeric mid-line; also referred to as M-band), ensuring that during contraction sarcomeres of adjacent myofibrils remain in register. In addition to connecting Z-disks of adjacent myofibrils, desmin filaments connect successive Z-disks longitudinally[4]. These longitudinally oriented desmin filaments bear force in myocytes stretched beyond their physiological sarcomere length[5] and desmin filaments might provide thereby a safety mechanism against over-distension of sarcomeres. Desmin filaments also form physical links between myofibrils, mitochondria, nuclei and the sarcolemma. This cytoplasmic network maintains the spatial relationship between the contractile apparatus and other organelles of the myocyte. Desmin is especially abundant at the intercalated disks[3] and contributes to the strong links that connect adjacent cells. Changes in the expression and distribution of desmin have been reported in many cardiac diseases, such as human idiopathic hypertrophy and failure, where desmin protein expression is upregulated and desmin filaments are disorganized. In transgenic mouse lines in which wild-type desmin is overexpressed, specifically in the heart[6], desmin is increased at the Z-disk and intercalated disk but no other structural abnormalities were present. Isolated myocyte mechanics, isolated heart mechanics and in vivo haemodynamics and echocardiography were all normal[6]. It is possible that upregulation of desmin expression in hypertrophy reflects a need to counteract elevated wall stress but is not in itself detrimental to the heart.

Actin filaments (also known as F-actin) consist of actin monomers that polymerize head-to-tail to form slender filaments. In the sarcomere, F-actin filaments are associated with regulatory proteins to form thin filaments and are crosslinked by α-actinin in the Z-disk. During contraction, actin interacts with myosin and the

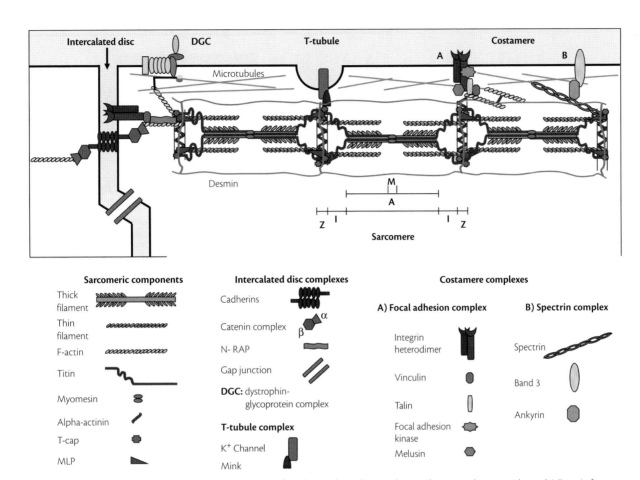

Fig. 9.1 Cytoskeletal elements of the cardiac myocyte. Microtubules are found throughout the cytoplasm and are most dense near the nuclei. Desmin forms intermediate filaments that connect myofibrils laterally at the level of the Z-disk and M-line and that connect successive Z-disks longitudinally. They also link myofibrils to nuclei and cell membranes. F-actin filaments are part of the sarcomeric thin filaments and constitute various linking systems that connect Z-disks to the plasma membrane and intercalated disk. They are linked to the cadherins of the intercalated disks by interacting with catenins and to the dystrophin–glycoprotein complex (DGC) via binding to dystrophin. Titin spans half-sarcomeres, with its terminal ends overlapping in the Z-disk and at the M-line. Titin is associated with the other parts of the cytoskeleton at various locations. T-cap interacts with the Z-disk end of titin and with MLP, forming part of an MLP-dependent stretch sensing complex. MLP interacts with N-RAP, a protein that may be involved in mediating interactions between myofibrils and the cell membrane at adherens junctions through its possible interactions with cadherin-based protein complexes and/or integrin-associated vinculin. T-cap also interacts with the potassium channel subunit minK at T-tubules, forming a complex that may be involved in the stretch-dependent regulation of potassium flux. (See color plate section.)

resulting force is transmitted via the thin filament to the Z-disk. Actin filaments also link the terminal half-sarcomere of the cell to the intercalated disk, by binding to catenins that in turn bind to the cytoplasmic domain of cadherins which mediate cell–cell attachment[7]. Thus, actin filaments transmit force between adjacent sarcomeres and neighbouring myocytes. Actin filaments also link to the sarcolemma in structural complexes known as costameres (present at the level of the Z-disk) by binding to the amino terminus of dystrophin. Dystrophin is part of a complex that consists of peripheral and integral proteins, known as the dystrophin-associated–glycoprotein complex (DGC)[8]. This complex forms a structural linkage between the cytoskeleton and the extracellular matrix and provides mechanical support to the plasma membrane during contraction. Multiple mutations in the genes encoding DGC proteins have been shown to underlie dilated cardiomyopathy[8,9]. That linking of the DGC to the actin-based cytoskeleton is important is also shown by actin mutations that reduce actin's ability to bind dystrophin and that give rise to dilated

cardiomyopathy (DCM)[10]. These DCM-causing mutations in actin are thought to result in disease by causing force transmission abnormalities. Thus actin performs critically important roles in force transmission, with mutations that cause defects in force transmission giving rise to DCM.

The giant protein titin

Among the multiple intracellular mechanisms involved in the heart's adaptability, the giant protein titin (Mw 3–4 MDa) is considered to be a key player in the organization and development of the sarcomere, in protein turnover and in sensing mechanical stresses and mediating these both acutely and chronically by initiating hypertrophy.

A single titin polypeptide spans from the Z-disk to the M-band region of the sarcomere (Fig. 9.2). The ~140 kDa N terminus is located in the Z-disk and overlaps with titin molecules from the adjacent sarcomere. The I-band region of the titin molecule is

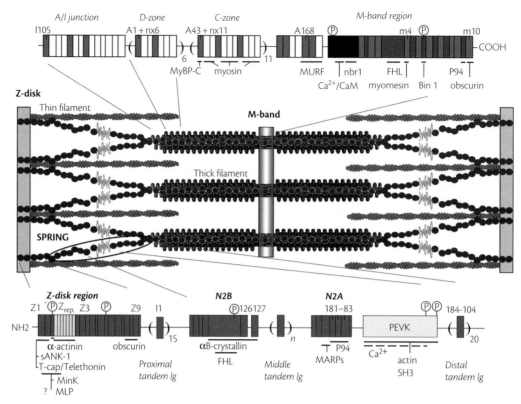

Fig. 9.2 Schematic of titin in sarcomere. The sarcomere contains thin, thick and titin filaments. Titin filaments span the half sarcomere from the Z-disk to the M-band. The domain composition of the various regions of the titin molecule is shown. The various known titin-binding proteins and their bindings sites are also shown. P, phosphorylation sites. See text for details. (See color plate section.)

extensible and consists of tandem immunoglobulin (Ig)-like domains that make up proximal (near Z-disk) and distal (near A–I junction) segments, interspersed by the N2B and N2A elements (titin segments) and the PEVK sequence (titin segment rich in proline (P), glutamate (E), valine (V) and lysine (K))[11]. Each functions as a distinct spring element. The C-terminal ~2 MDa of titin is located in the A-band and is inextensible, due to its interaction with thick filament-based proteins. Titin's ~250-kDa C-terminal region is an integral part of the M-band and contains a kinase domain. As in the Z-disk, where titin filaments from opposite sarcomeres overlap, titin filaments from opposite half-sarcomeres overlap within the M-band, where they are interconnected by M-band proteins. Thus, titin filaments with opposite polarity overlap in both Z-disk and M-band, forming a contiguous filament along the myofibril.

Titin produces passive tension in response to stretch

The best understood property of titin is its role in producing passive tension in response to stretch. Passive tension results from its extensible I-band region, which elongates in a complex fashion as sarcomere length (SL) increases. Tandem Ig segments are extended first, followed by the PEVK segment, with the N2B segment elongating last. The spring elements behave according to the worm-like chain entropic model, applicable to flexible polymers, with the three spring regions of cardiac titin (tandem Ig segments, PEVK and N2B) having different bending rigidities. In the unstressed state the spring segments have an end-to-end length close to zero. External force increases the end-to-end length in association with reduced bending movements. The latter results in decreased entropy, manifested as increased passive force generation. This model is consistent with the non-linear relation between SL and cardiomyocyte passive tension (Fig. 9.3) and explains elongation of the various segments of I-band titin as external force is applied[12].

Titin is encoded by a single gene[13]. Multiple splice pathways in the I-band encoding region give rise to isoforms with different spring composition[13]. The relatively small ~3.0-MDa isoform is known as N2B titin (it contains the N2B element)[13]. A second class also contains the N2A element and is termed N2BA titin. N2BA titins have a longer PEVK segment and a variable number of additional Ig domains resulting in a 3.3–3.5 MDa size[13]. The third class includes isoforms that predominate in fetal–neonatal life which contain additional spring elements in both tandem Ig and PEVK regions, resulting in a 3.6–3.8 MDa size protein[14]. These isoforms gradually disappear during postnatal development. The titin isoform N2BA has a longer extensible I-band region and is more compliant than N2B titin[15]. Both isoforms are co-expressed within the sarcomere; their ratio determines passive stiffness of the myocytes[16]. In adult rodents, N2B titin predominates in the left

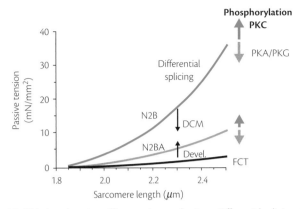

Fig. 9.3 Titin-based passive stiffness tuning mechanisms. Differential splicing gives rise to isoforms of varying stiffness. During postnatal development (Devel) passive stiffness increases due to switching of fetal cardiac titin (FCT) to adult N2B and N2BA isoforms; dilated cardiomyopathy (DCM) alters splicing in the opposite direction. PKA and PKG phosphorylation reduce and PKC phosphorylation increases passive stiffness.

ventricle (LV) and passive stiffness is therefore high[17]. In larger mammals, the proportion of N2BA titin increases, roughly paralleling body size. In human LV, the N2B/N2BA ratio is ~0.6. The atria contain largely N2BA titin. Reflecting their isoform composition, rodent LV cardiomyocytes are stiffer than cardiomyocytes from larger mammals[17]. Figure 9.3 depicts the force–extension relation of the three main classes of cardiac titin isoforms.

Titin is the main element responsible for passive tension of the cardiac myocyte. *Myocardial* passive tension includes contributions from cardiomyocytes (i.e. titin-dependent force) and collagen[18]. Titin's contribution is larger than collagen's at shorter SL. At longer SL, collagen fibrils straighten and their stiffness increases. However, even at long SL, titin-dependent tension remains a substantial portion of total tension. Both titin- and collagen-dependent passive tension are higher in rodents than in larger mammals[18]. In consequence, passive *myocardial* stiffness and diastolic LV *chamber* stiffness are also greater in rodents. Recently, two mouse knockout(KO) models were generated in which N2B or PEVK elements were excised[19,20]. The remaining spring elements (the tandem Ig and PEVK segments in the N2B KO; the tandem Ig and N2B segments in the PEVK KO) extend to a greater degree, explaining the increased titin-based passive tension of KO myocytes. Furthermore, *in vivo* pressure–volume loops revealed increased chamber stiffness[19], further establishing the importance of titin for diastolic function.

Titin isoform shifts have been reported in several diseases. Modest shifts can have significant effects because of the marked stiffness difference between N2B and N2BA titin. A disease-related shift in a large mammal was first reported using the pacing tachycardia canine model[21,22]. Here, the N2BA/N2B ratio was decreased in association with increased titin-dependent myocardial stiffness. Subsequently, opposite results have been found in explanted hearts from patients with end-stage DCM, i.e. increased N2BA/N2B ratio and decreased titin-dependent tension[23–25].

Titin produces restoring tension in response to shortening

Cardiomyocytes recoil after contracting because they develop a restoring tension (RT) at systolic SL below their slack value. It has been estimated that titin accounts for the majority of RT[26]. The mechanism of titin-based RT is thought to be reverse extension at short SL during contraction, i.e. movement of the thick filament during shortening extends the spring segments of titin in the opposite direction from where they are passively lengthened. With relaxation, the stretched springs recoil. The magnitude of RT and the velocity of recoil are proportional to the stiffness of titin. Titin RT may contribute to diastolic suction[21], an important mechanism of early ventricular filling. Another physiologically important feature of titin-based restoring tension is that it might terminate contraction by exerting so-called length-dependent deactivation[27] (see also below). Since rapid termination of myocardial activation is a key to fast ventricular filling *in vivo*, length-dependent deactivation might be an important physiological mechanism of the cardiac sarcomere.

Post-translational modification of titin's passive tension response to stretch

Although it was originally thought that titin is a static molecular spring, this view has been disproved in recent years by work that showed that titin-dependent passive tension can be modulated by post-translational modification, primarily phosphorylation. Yamasaki *et al.*[28] discovered that β-adrenergic stimulation of intact rat cardiac myocytes results in protein kinase A (PKA) phosphorylation of the cardio-specific N2B sequence, which reduces passive stiffness. This occurs in many species, including canines and humans, and is more pronounced in N2B than N2BA titin[28–30]. Kruger *et al.*[31] showed that cyclic guanosine monophosphate (cGMP)-dependent protein kinase G (PKG) phosphorylates titin in canines and human. cGMP is a second messenger of nitric oxide (NO) and natriuretic peptides. The cGMP/PKG signalling cascade phosphorylates many sarcomeric and cytosolic proteins, with effects that include improvement in diastolic function (reviewed in[32]). Like PKA, PKG phosphorylates the N2B element; in human titin, this takes place on serine (S) 469[31]. Interestingly, sequence analysis indicates that S469 is not conserved in other species. Similar to PKA, PKG phosphorylation reduces passive stiffness[30]. Thus, the N2B element is a cardiac-specific sequence that can be phosphorylated by both PKA and PKG, resulting in decreased stiffness.

Hidalgo *et al.*[33] recently demonstrated that titin is also phosphorylated by protein kinase C (PKC). PKC regulates cardiac contractility by phosphorylating multiple thin- and thick-filament proteins. Titin phosphorylation was observed in skinned myocardium following incubation with PKCα. *In vitro* phosphorylation of recombinant protein representing titin's spring elements showed that PKCα targets the PEVK element at two highly conserved serine residues (S11,878 and S12,022). Mechanical experiments in both mouse and pig myocardium revealed that PKCα *increases* titin-based passive tension. Thus, PKCα phosphorylation of titin links myocardial signalling and stiffness[33]. It is noteworthy that PKCα phosphorylation increases passive tension, whereas

PKA/PKG produce the opposite effect. This is analogous to kinase effects on thin filament regulatory proteins where, for example, phosphorylation of TnI by PKA lowers and phosphorylation by PKC increases calcium sensitivity. The role of this novel PKC pathway for altering passive stiffness under physiological and pathological conditions remains to be established.

Recent studies indicate that alterations in titin phosphorylation occur in various disease states. Borbely and colleagues have shown[34,35] that in skinned cardiomyocytes from patients with diastolic heart failure (DHF), passive tension is markedly increased. This was reversed by PKA treatment. These results suggest that PKA phosphorylation of titin is reduced in DHF, which would raise resting tension. Clearly, it will be important to study the phosphorylation state of titin's PEVK segment in various disease states including heart failure, where PKC protein levels and PKC activity are increased. Inhibiting PKCα has been proposed as a therapeutic strategy for treating heart failure; improving diastolic function via lowering titin phosphorylation could be one of its benefits.

Differential splicing is highly effective in altering titin-based passive stiffness but is a slow process. Changes in passive tension resulting from PKA, PKG and PKC phosphorylation allow for rapid modulation of passive stiffness. PKA effects on passive stiffness are most prominent at shorter SL[28], whereas PKC effects are more prominent at longer SL[33].

Titin and length-dependent activation

Increases in SL within the physiologic range result in increased myofilament calcium sensitivity, i.e. length-dependent activation (LDA). LDA is an important mechanism of the Frank–Starling relation of the heart and involves length-dependent thin filament activation[36]. Titin is often regarded as a passive spring, unrelated to active force generation. However, contrary to this view, recent evidence indicates that titin is involved in increasing active force generation at submaximal calcium levels. Cazorla et al.[37,38] measured force–pCa^{2+} relations in skinned rat cardiomyocytes at differing levels of passive force, modulated by stretch history, and found that the magnitude of the SL-dependent increase in Ca^{2+} sensitivity depends on passive force. Similar findings were obtained in studies with bovine cardiac muscle that took advantage of the differing expression profiles of titin in the heart[39]. As discussed above, in the adult heart two classes of titin isoform co-exist: N2B and N2BA. Their expression profiles are species- and location-dependent[17]. In the cow, N2B and N2BA isoforms are similarly expressed in the ventricle while N2BA titin is predominantly expressed in the atrium, and this differential expression profile of titin results in different levels of passive force[18]. It was found that length-dependent activation is markedly more pronounced in the ventricle than in the atrium in the cow, consistent with its higher level of passive tension.

The mechanisms by which titin increases active tension at submaximal calcium levels need to be further established. One possible mechanism is through an effect of titin on myofilament lattice spacing. Titin is an integral component of the thick filament and near the Z-disk titin binds to the thin filament . As a result, titin does not run parallel to the thin and thick filaments, but it is oblique, so that titin produces a radial force which reduces myofilament lattice spacing during stretch. Several X-ray diffraction studies have also found a reciprocal relationship between titin-dependent passive tension and inter-filament lattice spacing[38]. Another possibility is that longitudinal strain, exerted by titin on the thick filament, increases actin-myosin interaction[38,40].

Titin and long-term adaptations to stretch

A variety of titin-binding proteins have been discovered (Fig. 9.1) that play structural roles and roles in the adaptations of the heart to chronic pressure and volume overload. Titin's two N-terminal domains (Z1 and Z2) bind to small ankyrin-1 (sANK-1), a 17-kDa sarcoplasmic reticulum (SR) trans-membrane protein[41]. This interaction is thought to play a role in organizing the SR around the contractile apparatus at the Z-disk. Furthermore, Z1 and Z2 interact with Tcap (the titin-cap telethonin), which assembles titin filaments into a tightly packed anti-parallel sandwich structure that is resistant to stretch[42]. Additional Z-disk strength is provided by titin's Z-repeats, 45-amino-acid repeats that bind α-actinin[43,44]. Tcap also interacts with the potassium-channel subunit MinK found in T-tubules[45], which may modulate stretch-sensitive ion channel function. Furthermore, it has been suggested that Tcap is part of a mechano-sensor by virtue of its interaction with muscle-specific LIM protein (MLP), with MLP regulating gene expression[46]. Thus, the Z-disk region of the sarcomere is a hotspot for biomechanical sensing and titin plays an intimate role in this.

The central sarcomeric isotropic (I)-band region of titin is a second hotspot for protein interactions. The N2B element has two established binding partners. One is αB-crystallin, a member of the small heatshock protein family that functions as a molecular chaperone[47]. Upregulation of αB-crystallin occurs in several cardiac disorders. Overexpression protects the cardiomyocyte from ischaemia-reperfusion injury (for review see[48]). Titin's N2B element also interacts with members of the four-and-a-half LIM (FHL) protein family, a newly identified group of LIM proteins characterized by four complete LIM domains and an N-terminal half LIM domain. FHL-1 is found in cardiac and skeletal muscle and FHL-2 mainly in myocardium. FHL-1 and -2 bind to the extensible region of the N2B element[19,49]. FHL proteins have varied biological functions[50]. Lange et al.[51] showed that FHL-2 couples metabolic enzymes. Sheikh et al.[49] showed that FHL-1 deficiency protects from pathological hypertrophy. Interestingly, we recently found that in PEVK KO, where N2B element strain is enhanced (see above), FHL-1 and FHL-2 are upregulated and hypertrophy occurs[19]. Furthermore, the N2B KO, in which the N2B element is absent, has cardiac *atrophy* and *decreased* FHL levels[20]. Additionally, FHL-1 interacts with members of the mitogen-activated protein kinases (MAPK) signalling pathways (Raf1, MEK1/2 and ERK2) that co-localize with N2B in the sarcomere[49]. Together, these findings suggest that N2B facilitates assembly of a signalling complex that triggers hypertrophy in response to non-physiological N2B strain (as in volume overload[49] or the PEVK KO[19]). The blunted hypertrophy obtained when Gq overexpressing mice are crossed with FHL1 KO mice, a finding reported by Sheik et al.[49], suggests that the N2B-FHL-based signalosome receives input from G-protein receptors. It has been proposed that the FHL-based signalosome is a strain sensor that triggers hypertrophy in response to excessive titin strain.

Additionally, the N2A element binds to three homologous muscle ankyrin repeat proteins (MARP): CARP, ankrd2 and DARP[52]. MARP participate in stress-activated pathways and are

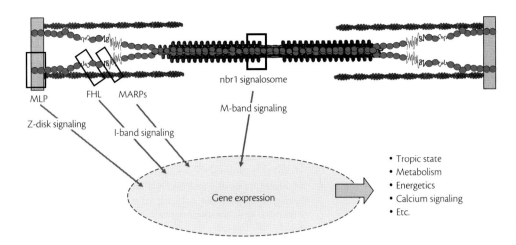

Fig. 9.4 Titin-based signalling pathways. See text for details.

upregulated after mechanical or metabolic challenge. Cyclic stretching of cultured cardiomyocytes induces expression of MARP in the nucleus and the sarcomeric I-bands[52]. Analogous to the regulatory mechanism for MLP, dual localization of MARP (titin's I-band region and the nucleus) may link stretch to gene expression. The N2A element also interacts with the Ca^{2+}-dependent muscle protease calpain3/P94; this interaction may modulate P94 function in protein degradation[53].

In the sarcomeric anisotropic (A)-band, the first Ig domain of each 11-domain super-repeat interacts with myosin binding protein C (MyBP-C), whereas the titin segment FN3domains bind to myosin[54]. Because A-band titin provides regularly spaced binding sites for myosin and MyBP-C, it may function as a molecular ruler which controls assembly and length of the thick filament. The M-line region of titin contains a serine/threonine kinase domain[55], but little is known about its function or substrates. *In vitro* studies with a mutant kinase domain indicate that T-cap is a substrate in embryonic muscle[56]. Furthermore, titin kinase may play a role in embryonic sarcomere development, specifically, integration of titin in the A-band[57] and sarcomere structure maintenance[58]. Recent studies from our laboratory suggest that titin kinase affects cardiac contractility due to decreased SR calcium uptake[59]. Lange *et al.*[60] provided evidence that the titin kinase assembles an nbr1 scaffold protein -based signalosome that communicates with the nucleus and modulates, in a stretch-dependent manner, protein expression and turnover.

Known titin-based signalling pathways are depicted in Fig. 9.4. The FHL and MARP pathways are located in the extensible I-band region and are well positioned to respond to changes in sarcomere strain during diastole. It is important to note that MARP-based signalling requires the presence of the N2A element, which is only found in the N2BA titin isoform. Thus, as titin isoform composition changes during various cardiac diseases, the prevalence of MARP signalling is likely to vary as well. Indeed MARP signalling has been found to be increased in end-stage DCM where N2BA titin is upregulated[24]. The Z-disk and the M-band signalling pathways, on the other hand, experience only limited changes in strain during diastole and it is likely that these sites are more responsive to the large actomyosin-based stresses produced during systole, which are transmitted via the Z-disks and M-bands. It is probable, therefore, that the various titin-based signalling pathways are specialized for sensing a variety of signals with graded responses.

Conclusions and outlook

Cardiac myocytes contain an intricate network of cytoskeletal filaments that are essential for providing strength and mechanical integrity to the cell as well as for sensing stress and strain and triggering changes in cardiac function. The most recently discovered filament, titin, develops passive force that determines diastolic filling and tunes the Frank–Starling mechanism, allowing the heart to respond to acute changes in demand. Length-dependent activation can be modulated in an intermediate-acute response by titin phosphorylation, and long-term by changes in the ratio of stiffer (N2B) to more compliant (N2BA) isoforms. Titin senses stress during systole primarily via the Z-disk and M-band signalling pathways, and strain during diastole via the N2B and N2A pathways. When stress and/or strain exceed physiological boundaries adaptive signalling pathways are triggered. Titin's role extends beyond a direct effect on myofilament function and is likely to include modulation of stretch-sensitive ion channel function. It is also worthwhile noting that several titin mutations have been identified in recent years that are linked to various cardiac diseases, with many more likely to be discovered. It is of interest to note that the titin gene locus is near the arrhythmogenic right ventricular cardiomyopathy (ARVC) locus that has been identified, and it will be exciting to sequence titin in ARVC patients and study titin's role in mechano-electric coupling. Although many functions of titin have been discovered in recent years, undoubtedly many more remain to be discovered. Future challenges also include the elucidation of the detailed mechanisms by which altered mechanical environments are sensed and the detailed signalling response pathways. It is likely that the cytoskeleton-based sensing and signalling pathways are central to adapting cardiac function and that they will be instrumental in devising successful therapeutic strategies in combating cardiac dysfunction and disease.

Acknowledgements

We thank the National Institute for Health (grant NIH HL062881) for financial support.

References

1. Zile MR, Green GR, Schuyler GT, Aurigemma GP, Miller DC, Cooper G. Cardiocyte cytoskeleton in patients with left ventricular pressure overload hypertrophy. *J Am Coll Cardiol* 2001;**37**:1080–1084.

2. Cooper Gt. Cytoskeletal networks and the regulation of cardiac contractility: microtubules, hypertrophy, and cardiac dysfunction. *Am J Physiol* 2006;**291**:H1003–H1014.

3. Price MG. Molecular analysis of intermediate filament cytoskeleton – a putative load-bearing structure. *Am J Physiol* 1984;**246**:H566–H572.

4. Wang K, Ramirez-Mitchell R. A network of transverse and longitudinal intermediate filaments is associated with sarcomeres of adult vertebrate skeletal muscle. *J Cell Biol* 1983;**96**:562–570.

5. Granzier HL, Irving TC. Passive tension in cardiac muscle: contribution of collagen, titin, microtubules, and intermediate filaments. *Biophys J* 1995;**68**:1027–1044.

6. Wang X, Osinska H, Dorn GW 2nd, et al. Mouse model of desmin-related cardiomyopathy. *Circulation* 2001;**103**:2402–2407.

7. Alberts B (2007) *Molecular Biology of the Cell*, 5th edn. Garland, Oxford.

8. Durbeej M, Campbell KP. Muscular dystrophies involving the dystrophin–glycoprotein complex: an overview of current mouse models. *Curr Opin Genet Dev* 2002;**12**:349–361.

9. Towbin JA, Bowles NE. The failing heart. *Nature* 2002;**415**:227–233.

10. Olson TM, Michels VV, Thibodeau SN, Tai YS, Keating MT. Actin mutations in dilated cardiomyopathy, a heritable form of heart failure. *Science* 1998;**280**:750–752.

11. Labeit S, Kolmerer B. Titins: giant proteins in charge of muscle ultrastructure and elasticity. *Science* 1995;**270**:293–296.

12. Watanabe K, Nair P, Labeit D, et al. Molecular mechanics of cardiac titin's PEVK and N2B spring elements. *J Biol Chem* 2002;**277**: 11549–11558.

13. Bang ML, Centner T, Fornoff F, et al. The complete gene sequence of titin, expression of an unusual approximately 700-kDa titin isoform, and its interaction with obscurin identify a novel Z-line to I-band linking system. *Circ Res* 2001;**89**:1065–1072.

14. Lahmers S, Wu Y, Call DR, Labeit S, Granzier H. Developmental control of titin isoform expression and passive stiffness in fetal and neonatal myocardium. *Circ Res* 2004;**94**:505–513.

15. Trombitas K, Redkar A, Centner T, Wu Y, Labeit S, Granzier H. Extensibility of isoforms of cardiac titin: variation in contour length of molecular subsegments provides a basis for cellular passive stiffness diversity. *Biophys J* 2000;**79**:3226–3234.

16. Trombitas K, Wu Y, Labeit D, Labeit S, Granzier H. Cardiac titin isoforms are coexpressed in the half-sarcomere and extend independently. *Am J Physiol* 2001;**281**:H1793–H1799.

17. Cazorla O, Freiburg A, Helmes M, Centner T, McNabb M, Wu Y, Trombitas K. Differential expression of cardiac titin isoforms and modulation of cellular stiffness. *Circ Res* 2000;**86**:59–67.

18. Wu Y, Cazorla O, Labeit D, Labeit S, Granzier H. Changes in titin and collagen underlie diastolic stiffness diversity of cardiac muscle. *J Mol Cell Cardiol* 2000;**32**:2151–2162.

19. Granzier HL, Radke MH, Peng J, et al. Truncation of titin's elastic PEVK region leads to cardiomyopathy with diastolic dysfunction. *Circ Res* 2009;**105**:557–564.

20. Radke MH, Peng J, Wu Y, et al. Targeted deletion of titin N2B region leads to diastolic dysfunction and cardiac atrophy. *Proc Natl Acad Sci USA* 2007;**104**:3444–3449.

21. Bell SP, Nyland L, Tischler MD, McNabb M, Granzier H, LeWinter MM. Alterations in the determinants of diastolic suction during pacing tachycardia. *Circ Res* 2000;**87**:235–240.

22. Wu Y, Bell SP, Trombitas K, et al. Changes in titin isoform expression in pacing-induced cardiac failure give rise to increased passive muscle stiffness. *Circulation* 2002;**106**:1384–1389.

23. Neagoe C, Kulke M, del Monte F, et al. Titin isoform switch in ischemic human heart disease. *Circulation* 2002;**106**:1333–1341.

24. Nagueh SF, Shah G, Wu Y, et al. Altered titin expression, myocardial stiffness, and left ventricular function in patients with dilated cardiomyopathy. *Circulation* 2004;**110**:155–162.

25. Makarenko I, Opitz CA, Leake MC, et al. Passive stiffness changes caused by upregulation of compliant titin isoforms in human dilated cardiomyopathy hearts. *Circ Res* 2004;**95**:708–716.

26. Helmes M, Trombitas K, Granzier H. Titin develops restoring force in rat cardiac myocytes. *Circ Res* 1996;**79**:619–626.

27. Helmes M, Lim CC, Liao R, Bharti A, Cui L, Sawyer DB. Titin determines the Frank–Starling relation in early diastole. *J Gen Physiol* 2003;**121**:97–110.

28. Yamasaki R, Wu Y, McNabb M, Greaser M, Labeit S, Granzier H. Protein kinase A phosphorylates titin's cardiac-specific N2B domain and reduces passive tension in rat cardiac myocytes. *Circ Res* 2002;**90**:1181–1188.

29. Fukuda N, Wu Y, Nair P, Granzier HL. Phosphorylation of titin modulates passive stiffness of cardiac muscle in a titin isoform-dependent manner. *J Gen Physiol* 2005;**125**:257–271.

30. Kruger M, Linke WA. Protein kinase-A phosphorylates titin in human heart muscle and reduces myofibrillar passive tension. *J Muscle Res Cell Motil* 2006;**27**:435–444.

31. Kruger M, Kotter S, Grutzner A, et al. Protein kinase G modulates human myocardial passive stiffness by phosphorylation of the titin springs. *Circ Res* 2009;**104**:87–94.

32. Burley DS, Ferdinandy P, Baxter GF. Cyclic GMP and protein kinase-G in myocardial ischaemia-reperfusion: opportunities and obstacles for survival signaling. *Br J Pharmacol* 2007;**152**:855–869.

33. Hidalgo C, Hudson B, Bogomolovas J, et al. PKC phosphorylation of titin's PEVK element: a novel and conserved pathway for modulating myocardial stiffness. *Circ Res* 2009;**105**:631–638.

34. Borbely A, Falcao-Pires I, van Heerebeek L, et al. Hypophosphorylation of the Stiff N2B titin isoform raises cardiomyocyte resting tension in failing human myocardium. *Circ Res* 2009;**104**:780–786.

35. Borbely A, van der Velden J, Papp Z, et al. Cardiomyocyte stiffness in diastolic heart failure. *Circulation* 2005;**111**:774–781.

36. Tachampa K, Wang H, Farman GP, de Tombe PP. Cardiac troponin I threonine 144: role in myofilament length dependent activation. *Circ Res* 2007;**101**:1081–1083.

37. Cazorla O, Vassort G, Garnier D, Le Guennec JY. Length modulation of active force in rat cardiac myocytes: is titin the sensor? *J Mol Cell Cardiol* 1999;**31**:1215–1227.

38. Cazorla O, Wu Y, Irving TC, Granzier H. Titin-based modulation of calcium sensitivity of active tension in mouse skinned cardiac myocytes. *Circ Res* 2001;**88**:1028–1035.

39. Fukuda N, Wu Y, Farman G, Irving TC, Granzier H. Titin isoform variance and length dependence of activation in skinned bovine cardiac muscle. *J Physiol* 2003;**553**:147–154.

40. Fukuda N, Sasaki D, Ishiwata S, Kurihara S. Length dependence of tension generation in rat skinned cardiac muscle: role of titin in the Frank–Starling mechanism of the heart. *Circulation* 2001;**104**:1639–1645.

41. Kontrogianni-Konstantopoulos A, Bloch RJ. The hydrophilic domain of small ankyrin-1 interacts with the two N-terminal immunoglobulin domains of titin. *J Biol Chem* 2003;**278**:3985–3991.

42. Zou P, Pinotsis N, Lange S, et al. Palindromic assembly of the giant muscle protein titin in the sarcomeric Z-disk. *Nature* 2006;**439**:229–233.

43. Sorimachi H, Freiburg A, Kolmerer B, et al. Tissue-specific expression and alpha-actinin binding properties of the Z-disc titin: implications for the nature of vertebrate Z-discs. *J Mol Biol* 1997;**270**:688–695.

44. Gautel M, Goulding D, Bullard B, Weber K, Furst DO. The central Z-disk region of titin is assembled from a novel repeat in variable copy numbers. *J Cell Sci* 1996;**109**:2747–2754.

45. Furukawa T, Ono Y, Tsuchiya H, *et al.* Specific interaction of the potassium channel beta-subunit minK with the sarcomeric protein T-cap suggests a t-tubule-myofibril linking system. *J Mol Biol* 2001;**313**:775–784.

46. Knoll R, Hoshijima M, Hoffman HM, *et al.* The cardiac mechanical stretch sensor machinery involves a Z disc complex that is defective in a subset of human dilated cardiomyopathy. *Cell* 2002;**111**:943–955.

47. Bullard B, Ferguson C, Minajeva A, *et al.* Association of the chaperone alphaB-crystallin with titin in heart muscle. *J Biol Chem* 2004;**279**: 7917–7924.

48. Wang X, Osinska H, Gerdes AM, Robbins J. Desmin filaments and cardiac disease: establishing causality. *J Card Fail* 2002;**8**:S287–S292.

49. Sheikh F, Raskin A, Chu PH, *et al.* An FHL1-containing complex within the cardiomyocyte sarcomere mediates hypertrophic biomechanical stress responses in mice. *J Clin Invest* 2008;**118**: 3870–3880.

50. Chu PH, Ruiz-Lozano P, Zhou Q, Cai C, Chen J. Expression patterns of FHL/SLIM family members suggest important functional roles in skeletal muscle and cardiovascular system. *Mech Dev* 2000;**95**:259–265.

51. Lange S, Auerbach D, McLoughlin P, *et al.* Subcellular targeting of metabolic enzymes to titin in heart muscle may be mediated by DRAL/FHL-2. *J Cell Sci* 2002;**115**:4925–4936.

52. Miller MK, Bang ML, Witt CC, *et al.* The muscle ankyrin repeat proteins: CARP, ankrd2/Arpp and DARP as a family of titin filament-based stress response molecules. *J Mol Biol* 2003;**333**:951–964.

53. Ono Y, Torii F, Ojima K, *et al.* Suppressed disassembly of autolyzing p94/CAPN3 by N2A connectin/titin in a genetic reporter system. *J Biol Chem* 2006;**281**:18519–18531.

54. Muhle-Goll C, Habeck M, Cazorla O, Nilges M, Labeit S, Granzier H. Structural and functional studies of titin's fn3 modules reveal conserved surface patterns and binding to myosin S1 – a possible role in the Frank–Starling mechanism of the heart. *J Mol Biol* 2001;**313**:431–447.

55. Labeit S, Gautel M, Lakey A, Trinick J. Towards a molecular understanding of titin. *EMBO J* 1992;**11**:1711–1716.

56. Mayans O, van der Ven PF, Wilm M, *et al.* Structural basis for activation of the titin kinase domain during myofibrillogenesis. *Nature* 1998;**395**:863–869.

57. Weinert S, Bergmann N, Luo X, Erdmann B, Gotthardt M. M line-deficient titin causes cardiac lethality through impaired maturation of the sarcomere. *J Cell Biol* 2006;**173**:559–570.

58. Gotthardt M, Hammer RE, Hubner N, *et al.* Conditional expression of mutant M-line titins results in cardiomyopathy with altered sarcomere structure. *J Biol Chem* 2003;**278**:6059–6065.

59. Peng J, Raddatz K, Molkentin JD, *et al.* Cardiac hypertrophy and reduced contractility in hearts deficient in the titin kinase region. *Circulation* 2007;**115**:743–751.

60. Lange S, Xiang F, Yakovenko A, *et al.* The kinase domain of titin controls muscle gene expression and protein turnover. *Science* 2005;**308**:1599–1603.

61. Miller MK, Granzier H, Ehler E, Gregorio CC. The sensitive giant: the role of titin-based stretch sensing complexes in the heart. *Trends Cell Biol* 2004;**14**:119–126.

The response of cardiac muscle to stretch: calcium and force

John Jeremy Rice and Donald M. Bers

Background

Mammalian muscle is characterized by a biphasic force response to stretch. In isolated myocardium, stretch induces an immediate increase in twitch force [immediate force response (IFR)], followed by a slowly developing second phase [slow force response (SFR)] as first described by Parmley and Chuck[1]. The IFR is the result of a length-dependent increase in myofilament Ca^{2+} sensitivity of cardiac muscle. Whereas the acute increase in Ca^{2+} sensitivity is well characterized and generally accepted as the cellular basis of the Frank–Starling mechanism, the underlying mechanisms of the length dependence remain controversial. After the immediate increase in force, SFR is characterized by a gradual increase in force that saturates over a time course of minutes. This increase is probably involved in the classic Anrep effect (afterload-induced increase in myocardial contractility, described first by Russian Physiologist Gleb Anrep in *J Physiol* in 1912), because it is assumed to correspond to the secondary increase in developed pressure found in whole heart. The increase in force is paralleled by an increase in the Ca^{2+} transient amplitude[2], but the source of the increase is still under debate. Several mechanisms have been suggested to contribute to the SFR, including changes in direct or indirect trans-membrane Ca^{2+} influx via stretch-activated channels (SAC) or second messenger systems. These mechanisms are reviewed in this chapter.

Immediate force response

Length-dependent changes in Ca^{2+} sensitivity

Changing cardiac muscle length has an immediate effect on myofilament force production that is quantified by the force–Ca^{2+} (F–Ca) relation that shows developed force as a function of steady-state activator Ca^{2+} concentration (see Fig. 10.1). The F–Ca relations show a steep dependence on activator $[Ca^{2+}]$ at each length, although the exact mechanisms remain highly controversial. Specifically, the single regulatory binding site on troponin predicts a Hill coefficient of 1, whereas Hill coefficients up to the range of 7–8 have been reported [such as those in Fig. 10.1 from[3]]. The length-dependent changes in the F–Ca relations can be separated into two main categories: changes in plateau or maximal force and changes in the Ca^{2+} sensitivity.

The changes in plateau force at high Ca^{2+} are likely the result of recruitment based on filament overlap, as detailed in classical work

from Gordon and colleagues[4]. In skeletal muscle, the ascending limb of the force—sarcomere length (SL) relation extends to 2.0 µm, after which there is a plateau to 2.2 µm followed by the descending limb. Extending this scheme to cardiac muscle requires an extended ascending limb of the Force-SL relation in cardiac versus skeletal muscle, based on different thin filament lengths[5].

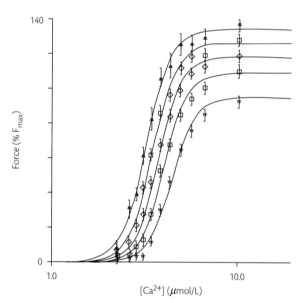

Fig. 10.1 Average force-Ca^{2+} (F–Ca) relationships from pooled data in skinned rat cardiac trabeculae ($n=10$) at five sarcomere lengths (SL = 1.85, 1.95, 2.05, 2.15 and 2.25 µm). Force measurements were made with SL controlled at each SL to the values shown during steady-state activation at varying Ca^{2+} concentrations. Force is normalized to maximum force measured at SL = 1.9 µm (trace not shown). Data are fit to a modified single Hill relationship:

$$F = F_{max}\left[Ca^{2+}\right]^{n_H} / \left(EC_{50}^{n_H} + \left[Ca^{2+}\right]^{n_H}\right)$$

Increases in SL induced a significant increase in maximum Ca^{2+}-saturated force (F_{max}, mean values = 49.1, 56.8. 60.6, 65.3 and 72.9 mN/mm^2) and Ca^{2+} sensitivity (EC_{50}, mean values = 4.43, 4.03, 3.74, 3.51 and 3.21 µM); however, the level of cooperativity as assessed by the Hill coefficient (n_H, mean values = 7.4, 7.2, 7.3, 7.0 and 6.9) was not affected by SL. Force measurements were made with SL controlled during steady-state activation [see[3] for details]. [Reproduced, with permission, from Dobesh DP, Konhilas JP, de Tombe PP (2002) Cooperative activation in cardiac muscle: impact of sarcomere length. *Am J Physiol* **282**:H1055–H1062]

Anatomical data show the mean length of rat and mouse cardiac thin filament to be roughly 0.1 μm longer than in frog skeletal muscle[6]. However, this length difference is too small to account for the functionally longer ascending limb, and the physiological data are compelling. In cardiac muscle at a fixed activation level, the developed force and adenosine triphosphatase (ATPase) rate is an increasing linear function of the change in SL in the range 2.0–2.2 μm[7]. In trabeculae preparations, further increases in SL are prevented by the high passive force. However, skinned cells can be stretched to reveal a peak in force at 2.2–2.4 μm followed by a descending limb[8]. In both datasets mentioned, the changes in force or ATPase rates are linear with SL, suggesting a simple recruitment phenomenon based on filament overlap.

The second primary length-dependent change is an increase in Ca^{2+} sensitivity that is shown by the decreasing EC50 values in Fig. 10.1. The SL-dependent Ca^{2+} sensitivity plays a much larger role in shaping responses because cardiac muscle is typically operating under sub-maximal activation (i.e. the plateau force is not achieved in typical contractions). The source of this length sensitivity is still under debate. One hypothesis suggests that length changes the lattice spacing of the thick and thin filaments as a result of the iso-volumetric properties (at least over the short term) of heart cells[9]. As SL increases, the thick and thin filaments become closer and thus increase the local concentration cross-bridge sites with subsequent effects on attachment rates to increase the developed force. For example, Fuchs and Wang[10] showed that SL sensitivity disappears when muscle diameter is held constant via application of dextran. Another study by Smith and Fuchs suggests that weak- rather than strong-binding cross-bridge states convey the SL-dependence on Ca and force generation. In addition, the fraction of weakly bound cross-bridges is found to be dependent on lattice spacing as assessed by X-ray diffraction and stiffness[11]. Hence, the effects of SL could be transduced before the actual strong-binding cross-bridges that generate force. Note the lattice spacing hypothesis could also potentially explain the changes in plateau force at high Ca^{2+} instead of the simple recruitment based on longitudinal filament overlap as proposed above.

While the lattice spacing hypothesis is attractive, not all data agree with this mechanism. Estimates of myofilament lattice spacing by synchrotron X-ray diffraction suggest that the changes in lattice spacing occurring over the physiologic range cannot fully account for length-dependent changes in Ca^{2+} sensitivity in cardiac muscle[12,13]. Some authors suggest that titin may play a role[14–16]; this protein is situated between the thick filament and the Z-disk, and hence its length will be modulated by the SL. Another possibility is that the SL-dependent Ca^{2+} sensitivity may result from the interplay of recruitable cross-bridges and the cooperative mechanisms that generate the high Hill coefficients found in cardiac muscle[17]. The Ca^{2+} binding affinity of regulatory proteins appears to be modulated by the number of attached or force-generating cross-bridges, instead of length itself[18]. Moreover, end-to-end interactions between troponin and tropomyosin may allow the effects of attached cross-bridges to propagate along the thin filament[17].

Effects on the Ca^{2+} transient

While the underlying cooperative mechanisms that bring about steep F–Ca relations are under debate, the exact mechanisms may not be important to understand the effects of length-dependent changes of Ca^{2+} transients. The Ca^{2+} affinity of troponin should change in accordance with the number of attached cross-bridges (XB) that can be modulated by cooperative thin filament activation, sarcomere length or the interaction of the two. This change in Ca^{2+} buffering strength can produce secondary effects on the intracellular Ca^{2+} transient, as shown in Fig. 10.2 and reported in other studies[2,19–21]. However, the effects on the Ca^{2+} transient tend to be rather small, and sometimes no change is reported[22,23]. These observations suggest that the changes in force, secondary to length modulation, are unlikely to produce large perturbations in intracellular Ca^{2+} concentration that could be pro-arrhythmic by activating Ca^{2+}-dependent inward currents. For example, one would not expect the amount of Ca^{2+} released by the myofilaments to trigger delayed after-depolarizations as seen in some pathological conditions such as heart failure[24]. This can also be appreciated by considering that the local sub-sarcolemmal calcium concentration $[Ca^{2+}]_{SS}$ sensed by Ca^{2+}-activated currents is elevated more dramatically by SR Ca^{2+} release or L-type Ca^{2+} current influx than would be expected by $[Ca^{2+}]_{SS}$ changes in the myofilament matrix[25].

Slow force response

As first described by Parmley and Chuck[1], after the immediate increase in force, there is an SFR in a staircase-like fashion that eventually reaches a plateau. The increase is variable but generally 20–30% over the IFR[26]. This increase is thought to correspond to the Anrep effect, the secondary increase in developed pressure found in whole heart[27]. The increase in force is closely mirrored by an increase in the Ca^{2+} transient amplitude[2], as shown in Fig. 10.2 from[20]. Note that the relative change in Ca^{2+} is smaller than force because of the steep Ca^{2+} sensitivity of cardiac muscle. Results presented in[20] are similar to the data in Fig. 10.1 which reveal a high Hill coefficient and length-dependent increases in Ca^{2+} sensitivity. Importantly, results from[20] also demonstrate that there are no slow time-dependent changes in Ca^{2+} sensitivity at the level of the myofilaments, and hence this does not account for the SFR. In other studies[19,28], length changes during the diastolic period alone are sufficient to generate the SFR, again suggesting mechanisms other than the myofilaments themselves. However, a role for the myofilaments may not be completely discounted. Stretch is reported to increase phosphorylation of myosin light chain 2 (MLC2), and inhibition of myosin light chain kinase (MLCK) attenuated the SFR in atrium and ventricle[29]. Here, the proposed SFR mechanism is that phosphorylation of MLC2 increases myofilament Ca^{2+} sensitivity. While some exceptions exist, the general assumption has been that the IFR results from intrinsic properties of the myofilaments whereas membrane events produce the SFR[26]. Below we discuss the origin of the SFR in terms of mechanisms that mostly increase the amplitude of the Ca^{2+} transient, although alternative mechanisms are possible.

The role of Na^+/Ca^{2+} exchanger and increased $[Na^+]_i$

The Na^+/Ca^{2+} exchanger (NCX) is the primary Ca^{2+} extrusion pathway from the cell, and rising intracellular Na^+ concentration ($[Na^+]_i$) will thermodynamically limit Ca^{2+} efflux and can even favour Ca^{2+} entry via NCX in its reverse mode[30]. The 3:1 stoichiometry generally assumed for this transporter will generate a cubic dependence on intra- and extracellular $[Na^+]$, and, thus, a small

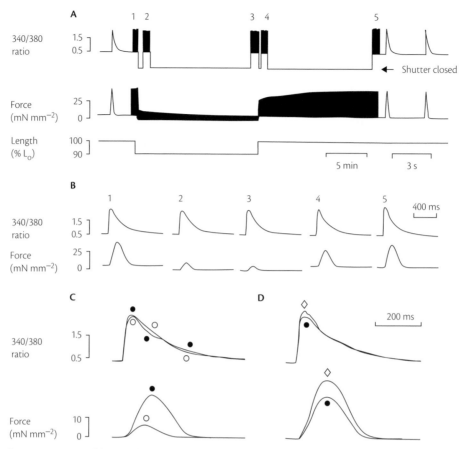

Fig. 10.2 Changes in fura2 fluorescence ratio and force produced by shortening a rat trabecula by 10% for 15 min. **A** Chart records of 340 nm/380 nm fluorescence ratio and force, with a representation of the length change from the initial length (L_0). A shutter in the excitation light pathway was opened only for discrete 48 s recording periods (labelled 1–5) in order to avoid photobleaching of fura2. The shutter was closed also during the adjustment of muscle length using a micromanipulator. Traces were scanned digitally from the original records (filtered at 15 Hz). Note the slow changes in twitch force after the changes in muscle length. **B** Mean records (from 16 twitches) of fluorescence ratio and force measured during periods 1–5 in **A**. **C** Unfiltered records with overlaid traces of the fluorescence ratio and force averaged during periods 3 (solid circles) and 4 (open circles) to illustrate the rapid effects of the length increase. Resting forces have been subtracted from these traces. **D** Similar overlaid traces averaged during periods 4 (O) and 5 (◊) to illustrate the delayed effects of the length increase. 24°C, 1 mM external Ca^{2+}, 0.33 Hz stimulation rate. [Reproduced, with permission, from Kentish JC, Wrzosek A (1998) Changes in force and cytosolic Ca^{2+} concentration after length changes in isolated rat ventricular trabeculae. *J Physiol* **506**:431–144.]

increase in $[Na^+]_i$ can bias the exchanger to lessen the forward mode and increase the reverse mode that brings in Ca^{2+}. The slow increase in the amplitude of the Ca^{2+} transient in SFR is often attributed to elevated $[Na^+]_i$ that decreases Ca^{2+} efflux in the forward mode of the NCX and increases Ca^{2+} influx in the reverse mode[31]. Experimental studies have shown the SFR to be closely mirrored by increases in $[Na^+]_i$[25]. Also, the role of elevated $[Na^+]_i$ is strongly suggested by theoretical studies[33,34].

While there is some consensus as to the important role of elevated $[Na^+]_i$, the source of the Na^+ is still quite controversial. Two leading hypotheses are sarcolemma influx via SAC (see Chapters 1–6) and activation of the Na^+/H^+ exchanger (NHE) by cellular signalling mechanisms. The story is further complicated as there have been recent reports that cellular signalling mechanisms may activate SAC rather than direct activation by mechanical stimuli (see section on 'SFR resulting from second messenger systems' below). Hence the SFR may involve an interplay of several

mechanisms rather than a single pathway (even if increased $[Na^+]_i$ and NCX effects are a final common pathway).

Stretch-induced changes in sarcolemmal ionic influx

The primary source of Ca^{2+} influx in cardiac cells is the L-type channel, but these have not shown sensitivity to stretch in numerous species [guinea pig[35]; rat:[36]; rabbit[37]] and have even been shown to decrease in response to membrane stretch[38]. Ca^{2+} influx via L-type channels occurs throughout the whole action potential, so prolonged action potential duration (APD) is another possible mechanism to increase Ca^{2+} influx, sarcoplasmic reticulum (SR) load and the Ca^{2+} transient[39]. While a complete treatment of stretch-induced changes in APD is beyond the scope of this work, APD changes do not appear to be a prerequisite for the SFR in all species and/or tissues. For example, the SFR is observed with little change in APD in isolated rabbit trabeculae[40], isolated sheep Purkinje fibres[41] and Langendorff-perfused canine hearts[42].

The role of stretch-activated channels

While some early reports indicated Ca^{2+} influx via SAC[43,44], most other reports have shown cation-non-selective SAC (SAC_{NS}) in which inward current is mostly carried by Na^{+}[38,43,45,46]. SAC_{NS} permeable to Na^{+} will increase in $[Na^{+}]_i$ or perhaps the local sub-sarcolemmal $[Na^{+}]$ ($[Na^{+}]_{SS}$). For example, studies with fluorescent imaging and electron probe analysis show stretch-induced hotspots with $[Na^{+}]_{SS} > 24$ mM that appeared close to the surface membrane and t-tubules[38]. The important role of SAC_{NS} is also suggested by a modelling study[33] that concluded that this mechanism is more likely to produce SFR than other mechanisms such as stretch-activation of NHE or nitric oxide (NO) production. However, the role of SAC_{NS} in SFR in failing human ventricle has been questioned because SFR is unaffected after blocking SAC_{NS} using a number of agents [70 μM streptomycin and 10 μM gadolinium[47] and 500 nM and 1000 GsMtx-4[29]].

Stretch-induced changes in SR release and uptake

If SFR is the result of an increased Ca^{2+} transient, then a change in SR release is expected as SR is the source of most of the Ca^{2+} in the transient[48]. One plausible mechanism is that SR Ca^{2+} load increases during SFR. Such a result has been reported for rabbit ventricle[40,49]. An alternative is that Ca^{2+} loading of SR does not change, but a greater fraction of SR is released. However, the limited data do not point to this mechanism. In rat ventricle, the fraction of release is 32–35% and independent of length, and, interestingly, the loading capacity of the SR is greater when the muscle operates at a shorter diastolic length[50]. These features are counter to the SFR where greater release is found for long, not short, diastolic length.

While a functional SR is required to generate the intracellular Ca^{2+} transient, the role of SR in stretch effects appears to be as an accomplice (managing the rise in Na^{+} and Ca^{2+}) rather than the primary culprit in inducing SFR. Inhibition of SR release by ryanodine[49] or caffeine[51] has no effect on the relative magnitude of SFR. Another possibility to load SR is to increase uptake via the sarco/endoplasmic reticulum Ca^{2+}-ATPase (SERCA) pump. However, disruption of the Ca^{2+}-induced Ca^{2+} release (CICR) system by blocking both release by ryanodine and uptake by cyclopiazonic acid (CPA), a blocker of the SERCA pump, still had little effect on SFR[20,49]. These results should not be overinterpreted to say that SR has no role. That is, while SR Ca^{2+} is not required to see a SFR, the effective removal of SR does change the time course of SFR[20] and could amplify any change in diastolic $[Ca^{2+}]_i$ or Ca^{2+} influx. To be sure, without the SR Ca^{2+} transients will be relatively smaller, because both systolic level will decrease and diastolic level between transient will increase.

SFR resulting from second messenger systems

Until very recently, SFR was assumed to result from one of several proposed mechanisms that were considered distinct and unconnected. For example, the modelling study of Niederer and Smith[33] considered the separate stretch-activated contributions of SAC_{NS}, NHE and NO production as separate pathways. However, the emerging picture shows second messenger systems that are complex, redundant and with the potential for substantial crosstalk. Figure 10.3 summarizes several proposed mechanisms to transduce

stretch into the increase in Ca^{2+} influx that is generally assumed to underlie the SFR. The mechanisms are described in more detail below.

Angiotensin II and endothelin-1 leading to ROS activation of NHE

One proposed mechanism of SFR involves stretch-induced autocrine/paracrine release of angiotensin II (AT-II) and endothelin-1 (ET-1) which can activate Na^{+} influx via a pathway that produces increased Ca^{2+} via the NCX[31,52,53]. Recent studies[54] have suggested a complex pathway so that stretch-induced release of Ang-II stimulates myocardial reactive oxidative species (ROS) production from nicotinamide-adenine dinucleotide phosphate (NADPH) oxidases (NOX). Stretch causes integrins to produce exocytosis of AT-II and activation of the receptor AT_1. Then a secondary release of ET-1 and activation of its receptor ET_A causes downstream activations of NOX leading to O_2^{-} production, opening of mitochondrial K^{+} ATP channels and increased mitochondrial O_2^{-} production. The mitochondria appeared to amplify NOX-dependent ROS by a mechanism of ROS-induced ROS release[55]. The mitochondrial O_2^{-} or H_2O_2 (via dismutation) may activate a cascade including extracellular signal-regulated kinases 1 and 2 (ERK1 and 2) and p90 ribosomal S6 kinase (p90RSK), leading to phosphorylation and activation of the NHE[54].

Angiotensin II and endothelin-1 leading to protein kinase activation of NHE

Stretch-induced autocrine/paracrine release of AT-II and ET-1 has also been proposed to activate NHE via the pathway involving phospholipase C (PLC) and protein kinase C (PKC). PKC inhibition blocks the ionotropic effects of ET-1 in ventricular myocytes of guinea pig[56] and cat[57]. The latter study suggests that PKC has a secondary activation of the NCX although the primary effect was activation of NHE[57]. An alternative target of ET-1 activation is PKC which subsequently increases L-type Ca channel current[58]. A role for PKA is demonstrated by studies showing cyclic adenosine monophosphate (cAMP) increases in response to stretch in rat[59] and dog[60] ventricles. ET-1 activation of ET_A is shown to produce positive increases in cAMP in rat myocytes[61] and mixed positive and negative effects, depending on concentration, in rat atria[62].

Stretch-activation of AT_1 leads to superoxide-based activation of SAC current

A recent study[63] suggests that stretch produces AT-II which ultimately opens SAC via superoxide pathways, as shown in Fig. 10.3. Stretch causes integrins to produce exocytosis of AT-II and activation of AT_1. The AT_1 then activates phosphatidylinositol 3-kinase (PI_3K) which in turn activates NOX and nitric oxide synthases 3 (eNOS) localized to the caveolae of the sarcolemma and the t-tubules. NOX and eNOS produce O_2^{-} and NO, respectively, and these species can combine into peroxynitrite ($ONOO^{-}$) which is thought to activate phospholipases. NO and peroxynitrite are reactive nitrogen species (RNS) that can modulate a diverse set of Ca^{2+}-handling proteins (see below). Two targets of peroxynitrite are phospholipases PLC and PLA_2 which can generate amphipaths (diacyl glycerol and arachidonic acid, respectively) which may change membrane curvature to activate transient receptor potential cation channel, member 6 (TRPC6), a cation non-specific SAC[64]. Stretch-activation of TRPC6 channels may increase Ca^{2+}

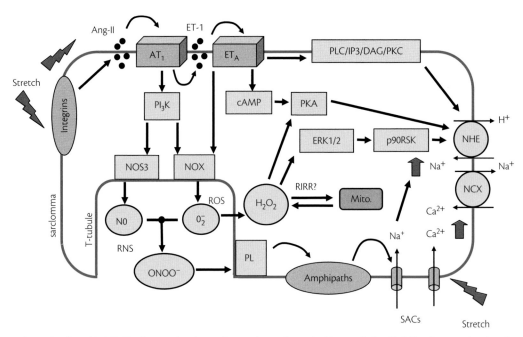

Fig. 10.3 Signalling pathways implicated in SFR. The illustrated pathways show an input of stretch either applied to SAC directly or causing the release of Ang-II triggered by integrins. The output is an increased $[Ca^{2+}]$ from either direct influx through SAC or the action of the NCX which raises $[Ca^{2+}]_i$ in response to elevated $[Na^+]_i$. The $[Na^+]$ is elevated by influx through SAC or activation of the NHE. The intermediate signalling is described in the text. NOX, NADPH oxidases; AT_1, Ang-II receptor; ET-1, endothelin-1; ET_A, ET-1 receptor; PLC/IP3/DAG/PKC, pathway with phospholipase C, inositol trisphosphate, diacylglycerol and protein kinase C; ROS, reactive oxidative species including O_2- and H_2O_2; RIRR, ROS-induced ROS release; Mito., mitochondria; ERK1/2, extracellular signal-regulated kinases 1 and 2; p90RSK, p90 ribosomal S6 kinase; PI_3K, phosphatidylinositol 3-kinases; NOS3, nitric oxide synthases 3; RNS, reactive nitrogen species including NO and $ONOO^-$; PL, phospholipases including PLC and PLA_2; vcAMP, cyclic adenosine monophosphate, PKA, protein kinase A.

influx directly and indirectly by membrane depolarization (activating voltage-gated Ca^{2+} channels) and by elevated $[Na^+]_i$ via NCX.

Additional potential mechanisms of SFR involving second messengers

The signalling pathways in Fig. 10.3 are a compilation from a specific set to hypotheses that SFR results from increased $[Ca^{2+}]_i$ via SAC or augmented activation of the NHE. However, many other possibilities exist because the signalling cascades described above affect an extremely wide range of Ca^{2+}-handling mechanisms. A detailed enumeration of all possible mechanisms is not possible here; however, we present a brief description of some modulatory effects on Ca^{2+}-handling mechanisms that could be in involved in the SFR.

IP$_3$-induced effects

While ryanodine receptors (RyR) are the primary method of Ca^{2+} release in cardiac cells, IP_3 receptors (IP_3R) are expressed in cardiac cells and some evidence suggests a modulatory role in excitation–contraction (EC) coupling [for review see[65]]. For example, IP_3R activation via ET-1 is found to enhance systolic and diastolic Ca^{2+} levels and increase spontaneous release[66,67]. Moreover, the activation of $InsP_3$ production can also increase influx through L-type channels[56,58].

Redox regulation of Ca^{2+}-handling proteins

Redox modification of the sulph-hydryl groups of neighbouring cysteine residues leads to formation or breaking of disulphide

bonds that can affect the function of ion channels, pumps and exchangers [for review see[68]]. ROS and RNS are the two main biologically active molecules that can have diverse and often complementary regulatory effects on RYR, L-type Ca channels, SERCA pump, sarcolemmal Ca^{2+}-ATPase and NCX [see Table 1 in[68]].

A full description of these effects is beyond the scope of this chapter, but a few brief points related to SFR will be discussed. There is evidence of downstream regulation by S-nitrosylation of the RYR which increases RYR open probability[69,70]. One end effect of this signalling cascade is increased Ca^{2+} sparks and electrically stimulated Ca^{2+} transients. However, changing RYR properties alone may have little effect on sustained changes in the Ca^{2+} transient such as those in SRF. Specifically, changing RYR release properties alone produces only transient changes in the Ca^{2+} transient in experimental[71] and modelling[33] studies. Note that modulation of SR-based Ca^{2+}-handling mechanisms alone is unlikely to be sufficient to completely account for SFR because SFR still occurs after disruption of SR function, although the time course is altered.

Conclusions and outlook

Mammalian muscle is characterized by a biphasic force response to stretch. In the first phase, stretch induces an immediate increase in twitch force which is the result of a length-dependent increase in Ca^{2+} sensitivity of cardiac muscle that is generally accepted as the cellular basis of the Frank-Starling mechanism. Considerable controversy exists over what is the sensor of muscle length that brings about the increased Ca^{2+} sensitivity. After the immediate increase in force, the second phase is characterized by a slow increase in force that saturates over a time course of minutes. The increase in force is most often reported to include Ca^{2+} influx via SAC or Na^+ influx via SAC that leads to a secondary increase in $[Ca^{2+}]_i$ via the NCX. Another proposed mechanism is Na^+ influx via the NHE that is activated by a signalling mechanism involving stretch-induced autocrine/paracrine release of angiotensin II and endothelin-1. Downstream activation of the NOX and NOS can potentially modulate a diverse set of targets including the L-type channels, SAC, RYR and SERCA pumps directly to increase Ca^{2+} cycling. Recent work has revealed a complicated picture in which the second messenger systems are complex, redundant and with the potential for substantial crosstalk. Further work will be required to elucidate the exact contribution of these, or perhaps other mechanisms, to the SFR. Specifically, considerable differences are reported across tissues and species which suggest more than one mechanism could be responsible for the SFR. Moreover, the possibility exists that some stretch-induced changes in Ca^{2+} are not related to SFR *per se* but instead are epiphenomena of other roles in inducing gene expression or other cellular signalling.

References

1. Parmley WW, Chuck L. Length-dependent changes in myocardial contractile state. *Am J Physiol* 1973;**224**:1195–1199.

2. Allen DG, Kurihara S. The effects of muscle length on intracellular calcium transients in mammalian cardiac muscle. *J Physiol* 1982;**327**:79–94.

3. Dobesh DP, Konhilas JP, de Tombe PP. Cooperative activation in cardiac muscle: impact of sarcomere length. *Am J Physiol.* 2002;**282**:H1055–H1062.

4. Gordon AM, Huxley AF, Julian FJ. The variation in isometric tension with sarcomere length in vertebrate muscle fibres. *J Physiol* 1966;**184**:170–192.

5. Rice JJ, Wang F, Bers DM, de Tombe PP. Approximate model of cooperative activation and crossbridge cycling in cardiac muscle using ordinary differential equations. *Biophys J* 2008;**95**:2368–2390.

6. Burgoyne T, Muhamad F, Luther PK. Visualization of cardiac muscle thin filaments and measurement of their lengths by electron tomography. *Cardiovasc Res* 2008;**77**:707–712.

7. Wannenburg T, Heijne GH, Geerdink JH, Van Den Dool HW, Janssen PM, De Tombe PP. Cross-bridge kinetics in rat myocardium: effect of sarcomere length and calcium activation. *Am J Physiol* 2000;**279**:H779–H790.

8. Weiwad WK, Linke WA, Wussling MH. Sarcomere length–tension relationship of rat cardiac myocytes at lengths greater than optimum. *J Mol Cell Cardiol* 2000;**32**:247–259.

9. McDonald KS, Moss RL. Osmotic compression of single cardiac myocytes eliminates the reduction in Ca^{2+} sensitivity of tension at short sarcomere length. *Circ Res* 1995;**77**:199–205.

10. Fuchs F, Wang YP. Sarcomere length versus interfilament spacing as determinants of cardiac myofilament Ca^{2+} sensitivity and Ca^{2+} binding. *J Mol Cell Cardiol* 1996;**28**:1375–1383.

11. Martyn DA, Adhikari BB, Regnier M, Gu J, Xu S, Yu LC. Response of equatorial x-ray reflections and stiffness to altered sarcomere length and myofilament lattice spacing in relaxed skinned cardiac muscle. *Biophys J* 2004;**86**:1002–1011.

12. Konhilas JP, Irving TC, de Tombe PP. Length-dependent activation in three striated muscle types of the rat. *J Physiol* 2002;**544**:225–236.

13. Farman GP, Allen EJ, Gore D, Irving TC, de Tombe PP. Interfilament spacing is preserved during sarcomere length isometric contractions in rat cardiac trabeculae. *Biophys J* 2007;**92**:L73–L75.

14. Le Guennec JY, White E, Gannier F, Argibay JA, Garnier D. Stretch-induced increase of resting intracellular calcium concentration in single guinea-pig ventricular myocytes. *Exp Physiol* 1991;**76**:975–978.

15. Fukuda N, Sasaki D, Ishiwata S, Kurihara S. Length dependence of tension generation in rat skinned cardiac muscle: role of titin in the Frank–Starling mechanism of the heart. *Circulation* 2001;**104**:1639–1645.

16. Cazorla O, Vassort G, Garnier D, Le Guennec JY. Length modulation of active force in rat cardiac myocytes: is titin the sensor? *J Mol Cell Cardiol* 1999;**31**:1215–1227.

17. Rice JJ, De Tombe PP. Approaches to modeling crossbridges and calcium-dependent activation in cardiac muscle. *Prog Biophys Mol Biol* 2004;**85**:179–195.

18. Guth K, Potter JD. Effect of rigor and cycling cross-bridges on the structure of troponin C and on the Ca^{2+} affinity of the Ca^{2+}-specific regulatory sites in skinned rabbit psoas fibers. *J Biol Chem* 1987;**262**:13627–13635.

19. Allen DG, Nichols CG, Smith GL. The effects of changes in muscle length during diastole on the calcium transient in ferret ventricular muscle. *J Physiol* 1988;**406**:359–370.

20. Kentish JC, Wrzosek A. Changes in force and cytosolic Ca^{2+} concentration after length changes in isolated rat ventricular trabeculae. *J Physiol* 1998;**506**:431–444.

21. Tavi P, Han C, Weckstrom M. Mechanisms of stretch-induced changes in $[Ca^{2+}]_i$ in rat atrial myocytes: role of increased troponin C affinity and stretch-activated ion channels. *Circ Res* 1998;**83**:1165–1177.

22. Saeki Y, Kurihara S, Hongo K, Tanaka E. Tension and intrac-ellular calcium transients of activated ferret ventricular muscle in response to step length changes. *Adv Exp Med Biol* 1993;**332**:639–647.

23. Steele DS, Smith GL. Effects of 2,3-butanedione monoxime on sarcoplasmic reticulum of saponin-treated rat cardiac muscle. *Am J Physiol* 1993;**265**:H1493–H1500.

24. Pogwizd SM, Bers DM. Cellular basis of triggered arrhythmias in heart failure. *Trends Cardiovasc Med* 2004;**14**:61–66.

25. Weber CR, Piacentino V 3rd, Ginsburg KS, Houser SR, Bers DM. Na^+–Ca^{2+} exchange current and submembrane $[Ca^{2+}]$ during the cardiac action potential. *Circ Res* 2002;**90**:182–189.

26. Fuchs F, Smith SH. Calcium, cross-bridges, and the Frank–Starling relationship. *News Physiol Sci* 2001;**16**:5–10.

27. Sarnoff SJ, Mitchell JH, Gilmore JP, Remensynder JP. Homeometric autoregulation in the heart. *Circ Res* 1960;**8**:1077–1091.

28. Nichols CG. The influence of 'diastolic' length on the contractility of isolated cat papillary muscle. *J Physiol* 1985;**361**:269–279.

29. Kockskamper J, von Lewinski D, Khafaga M, *et al*. The slow force response to stretch in atrial and ventricular myocardium from human heart: functional relevance and subcellular mechanisms. *Prog Biophys Mol Biol* 2008;**97**:250–267.

30. Blaustein MP, Lederer WJ. Sodium/calcium exchange: its physiological implications. *Physiol Rev* 1999;**79**:763–854.

31. Alvarez BV, Perez NG, Ennis IL, Camilion de Hurtado MC, Cingolani HE. Mechanisms underlying the increase in force and Ca^{2+} transient that follow stretch of cardiac muscle: a possible explanation of the Anrep effect. *Circ Res* 1999;**85**:716–722.

32. Luers C, Fialka F, Elgner A, *et al*. Stretch-dependent modulation of $[Na^+]_i$, $[Ca^{2+}]_i$, and pH_i in rabbit myocardium – a mechanism for the slow force response. *Cardiovasc Res* 2005;**68**:454–463.

33. Niederer SA, Smith NP. A mathematical model of the slow force response to stretch in rat ventricular myocytes. *Biophys J* 2007;**92**:4030–4044.

34. Bluhm WF, Lew WY, Garfinkel A, McCulloch AD. Mechanisms of length history-dependent tension in an ionic model of the cardiac myocyte. *Am J Physiol* 1998;**274**:H1032–H1040.

35. Sasaki N, Mitsuiye T, Noma A. Effects of mechanical stretch on membrane currents of single ventricular myocytes of guinea-pig heart. *Jpn J Physiol* 1992;**42**:957–970.

36. Hongo K, White E, Le Guennec JY, Orchard CH. Changes in $[Ca^{2+}]_i$, $[Na^+]_i$ and Ca^{2+} current in isolated rat ventricular myocytes following an increase in cell length. *J Physiol* 1996;**491**:609–619.

37. Kentish JC, Davey R, Largen P. Isoprenaline reverses the slow force responses to a length change in isolated rabbit papillary muscle. *Pflugers Arch* 1992;**421**:519–521.

38. Isenberg G, Kazanski V, Kondratev D, Gallitelli MF, Kiseleva I, Kamkin A. Differential effects of stretch and compression on membrane currents and $[Na^+]_c$ in ventricular myocytes. *Prog Biophys Mol Biol* 2003;**82**: 43–56.

39. Bouchard RA, Clark RB, Giles WR. Effects of action potential duration on excitation–contraction coupling in rat ventricular myocytes. Action potential voltage-clamp measurements. *Circ Res* 1995;**76**: 790–801.

40. von Lewinski D, Stumme B, Maier LS, Luers C, Bers DM, Pieske B. Stretch-dependent slow force response in isolated rabbit myocardium is Na^+ dependent. *Cardiovasc Res* 2003;**57**:1052–1061.

41. Dominguez G, Fozzard HA. Effect of stretch on conduction velocity and cable properties of cardiac Purkinje fibers. *Am J Physiol* 1979; **237**:C119–C124.

42. Calkins H, Maughan WL, Kass DA, Sagawa K, Levine JH. Electrophysiological effect of volume load in isolated canine hearts. *Am J Physiol* 1989;**256**:H1697–H1706.

43. Naruse K, Sokabe M. Involvement of stretch-activated ion channels in Ca^{2+} mobilization to mechanical stretch in endothelial cells. *Am J Physiol* 1993;**264**:C1037–C1044.

44. Sigurdson W, Ruknudin A, Sachs F. Calcium imaging of mechanically induced fluxes in tissue-cultured chick heart: role of stretch-activated ion channels. *Am J Physiol* 1992;**262**:H1110–H1115.

45. Zhang YH, Youm JB, Sung HK, *et al*. Stretch-activated and background non-selective cation channels in rat atrial myocytes *J Physiol* 2000; **523**:607–619.

46. Kamkin A, Kiseleva I, Isenberg G. Ion selectivity of stretch-activated cation currents in mouse ventricular myocytes. *Pflugers Arch* 2003; **446**:220–231.

47. von Lewinski D, Stumme B, Fialka F, Luers C, Pieske B. Functional relevance of the stretch-dependent slow force response in failing human myocardium. *Circ Res* 2004;**94**:1392–1398.

48. Bers DM. (2001) *Excitation–Contraction Coupling and Cardiac Contractile Force*, 2nd edn. Kluwer Academic Publishers, Boston.

49. Bluhm WF, Lew WY. Sarcoplasmic reticulum in cardiac length-dependent activation in rabbits. *Am J Physiol* 1995;**269**: H965–H972.

50. Gamble J, Taylor PB, Kenno KA. Myocardial stretch alters twitch characteristics and Ca^{2+} loading of sarcoplasmic reticulum in rat ventricular muscle. *Cardiovasc Res* 1992;**26**:865–870.

51. Chuck LH, Parmley WW. Caffeine reversal of length-dependent changes in myocardial contractile state in the cat. *Circ Res* 1980; **47**:592–598.

52. Cingolani HE, Alvarez BV, Ennis IL, Camilion de Hurtado MC. Stretch-induced alkalinization of feline papillary muscle: an autocrine-paracrine system. *Circ Res* 1998;**83**:775–780.

53. Aiello EA, Villa-Abrille MC, Cingolani HE. Autocrine stimulation of cardiac Na^+–Ca^{2+} exchanger currents by endogenous endothelin released by angiotensin II. *Circ Res* 2002;**90**:374–376.

54. Caldiz CI, Garciarena CD, Dulce RA, *et al*. Mitochondrial reactive oxygen species activate the slow force response to stretch in feline myocardium *J Physiol* 2007;**584**:895–905.

55. Garciarena CD, Caldiz CI, Correa MV, *et al*. Na^+/H^+ exchanger-1 inhibitors decrease myocardial superoxide production via direct mitochondrial action. *J Appl Physiol* 2008;**105**:1706–1713.

56. Woo SH, Lee CO. Effects of endothelin-1 on Ca^{2+} signaling in guinea-pig ventricular myocytes: role of protein kinase C. *J Mol Cell Cardiol* 1999;**31**:631–643.

57. Aiello EA, Villa-Abrille MC, Dulce RA, Cingolani HE, Perez NG. Endothelin-1 stimulates the Na^+/Ca^{2+} exchanger reverse mode through intracellular Na^+: Na^+_i-dependent and Na^+_i-independent pathways. *Hypertension* 2005;**45**:288–293.

58. He JQ, Pi Y, Walker JW, Kamp TJ. Endothelin-1 and photo released diacylglycerol increase L-type Ca^{2+} current by activation of protein kinase C in rat ventricular myocytes. *J Physiol* 2000;**524**:807–820.

59. Watson PA, Haneda T, Morgan HE. Effect of higher aortic pressure on ribosome formation and cAMP content in rat heart. *Am J Physiol* 1989;**256**:C1257–C1261.

60. Todaka K, Ogino K, Gu A, Burkhoff D. Effect of ventricular stretch on contractile strength, calcium transient, and cAMP in intact canine hearts. *Am J Physiol* 1998;**274**:H990–H1000.

61. Rebsamen MC, Church DJ, Morabito D, Vallotton MB, Lang U. Role of cAMP and calcium influx in endothelin-1-induced ANP release in rat cardiomyocytes. *Am J Physiol* 1997;**273**:E922–E931.

62. Sokolovsky M, Shraga-Levine Z, Galron R. Ligand-specific stimulation/ inhibition of cAMP formation by a novel endothelin receptor subtype. *Biochemistry* 1994;**33**:11417–11419.

63. Dyachenko V, Rueckschloss U, Isenberg G. Modulation of cardiac mechanosensitive ion channels involves superoxide, nitric oxide and peroxynitrite. *Cell Calcium* 2009;**45**:55–64.

64. Dyachenko V, Husse B, Rueckschloss U, Isenberg G. Mechanical deformation of ventricular myocytes modulates both TRPC6 and Kir2.3 channels. *Cell Calcium* 2009;**45**:38–54.

65. Kockskamper J, Zima AV, Roderick HL, Pieske B, Blatter LA, Bootman MD. Emerging roles of inositol 1,4,5-trisphosphate signaling in cardiac myocytes. *J Mol Cell Cardiol* 2008;**45**:128–147.

66. Mackenzie L, Bootman MD, Laine M, *et al*. The role of inositol 1,4,5-trisphosphate receptors in Ca^{2+} signalling and the generation of arrhythmias in rat atrial myocytes. *J Physiol* 2002;**541**:395–409.

67. Li X, Zima AV, Sheikh F, Blatter LA, Chen J. Endothelin-1-induced arrhythmogenic Ca^{2+} signaling is abolished in atrial myocytes of inositol-1,4,5-trisphosphate(IP3)-receptor type 2-deficient mice. *Circ Res* 2005;**96**:1274–1281.

68. Zima AV, Blatter LA. Redox regulation of cardiac calcium channels and transporters. *Cardiovasc Res* 2006;**71**:310–321.

69. Xu L, Eu JP, Meissner G, Stamler JS. Activation of the cardiac calcium release channel (ryanodine receptor) by poly-S-nitrosylation. *Science* 1998;**279**:234–237.

70. Stoyanovsky D, Murphy T, Anno PR, Kim YM, Salama G. Nitric oxide activates skeletal and cardiac ryanodine receptors. *Cell Calcium* 1997; **21**:19–29.

71. Trafford AW, Diaz ME, Sibbring GC, Eisner DA. Modulation of CICR has no maintained effect on systolic Ca^{2+}: simultaneous measurements of sarcoplasmic reticulum and sarcolemmal Ca^{2+} fluxes in rat ventricular myocytes. *J Physiol* 2000;**522**:259–270.

Stretch effects on second messengers

Jean-Luc Balligand and Chantal Dessy

Background

Despite years of research, our understanding of the intracellular signalling pathway(s) that modulate cardiac contractility and remodelling in response to stretch remains limited. Although the length-dependent increase in contraction force underlying the rapid Frank–Starling law of the heart[1] and the more slowly occurring Anrep effect[2] could be assigned to specific changes in excitation–contraction (EC) coupling, in crossbridge formation or myofilaments Ca^{2+} sensitivity (see also Chapter 10), the signalling pathway(s) mediating these changes largely remain elusive. The fact that (at least some of) the same pathways may be implicated in the trophic effects following chronic application of physical forces adds yet another level of complexity. The final responses are probably dictated by time-dependent recruitment of specific receptors and effectors reversibly assembled in 'signalosomes' at discrete locales at or near the cell surface where signalling from neurohormones and physical forces may intersect. In this chapter, we review some of these elements including membrane-associated proteins, channels, kinases and small molecular messengers such as nitric oxide (NO).

Integrins

Integrins have long been recognized as critical for the transmission of outside-in signalling from extracellular matrix proteins and have been implicated in the formation of multiprotein complexes responding to mechanical forces in a variety of cell types, including endothelial cells and myocytes. Baumgarten et al. used antibodies against ß1-integrins coupled to magnetic beads to demonstrate the activation of tamoxifen-sensitive Cl^- currents upon cardiomyocyte stretch with a magnetic field[3]. Others used arginine–glycine–aspartate (RGD) peptides that disrupt integrin binding to the extracellular matrix to establish connections to stretch-activated currents and stretch-mediated responses. The connection of integrins (through a variety of adaptor proteins) to the actin cytoskeleton both relays the mechanical stimulus to distant intracellular targets [including the nucleus, with potential long-term transcriptional regulation[4]] and focuses the stimulus to specific transduction sites. In the 'tensegrity' model of a cell, pre-tensed cytoskeletal elements play a critical role in transmission of mechanical forces throughout the cell[5–7] (see also Chapter 12).

Downstream effectors of integrin-mediated stretch signalling in cardiac myocytes

At costameres, integrins (containing the ß1D isoform in adult cardiac myocytes, mostly as the laminin-binding α7/ß1 heterodimer) are connected to the sarcomere through dynamically regulated multiprotein complexes linking their cytoplasmic domains to actin filaments (Fig. 11.1). These complexes include integrin-like kinase/paxillin/parvin and vinculin/talin/α-actinin, as well as filamin/migfilin. Upon stretch, other protein partners are added to these complexes and control downstream signalling through the activation of specific kinases.

A paradigmatic example is the enhanced recruitment of talin/vinculin together with integrins at sites of increased mechanical stress to increase integrin anchoring to the actin filaments (thereby providing adaptation to altered physical forces in the 'tensegrity' model). This is initiated by activation of focal adhesion kinase (FAK) and sarcoma (Src)-kinase upon integrin stimulation, which phosphorylates phosphatidylinositol-4,5-phosphate (PIP) kinase I-gamma. The latter then binds the head domain of talin[8], which induces a transition to its extended/active conformation, more prone to integrin binding, resulting in more talin recruitment on the integrin complex. Reciprocally, talin binding increases phosphatidylinositol-4-phosphate kinase type I (PIP_4KI)-gamma catalytic activity, with sustained production of phosphatidylinositol-4,5-bisphosphate (PIP_2) at the membrane. The latter favours the binding of vinculin to both talin and actin, thereby promoting anchoring of integrins to actin[9,10]. Similarly, integrin-linked kinase (ILK) binding to paxillin and parvin, itself bound to actin, provides another physical link between integrin and actin[11]. In addition to this structural role, ILK controls the phosphorylation of Akt/PKB and GSK-3ß[12], both implicated in cell survival and cardiomyocyte hypertrophy[13]. Likewise, FAK, cooperatively with Src and the binding of p85 subunit of phosphatidylinositol-3,4,5-trisphosphate (PIP_3) kinases (PIP_3K), initiates the local production of PIP_3 to mediate critical signals for cell survival and proliferation, as well as cardiomyocyte hypertrophy, possibly through activation of ERK1/2 and Akt/PKB[14]. Notably, this signalling machinery seems specifically sensitive to stretch and pro-hypertrophic autacoids [e.g. catecholamines and endothelin[15,16]], but not to increased contractile activity[17]. Whether these two modes of activation will result in a similar biological response remains to be

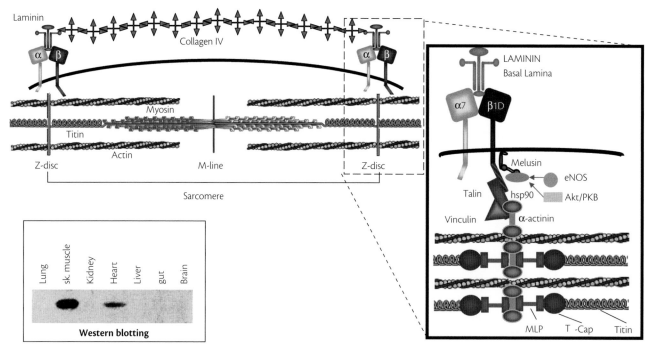

Fig. 11.1 Representation of the sarcomeric structure and its junction with the plasma membrane. The contractile unit lies between two Z-discs. The boxed area is magnified to illustrate the junctional complex connecting the Z-disc structure to integrins at the plasma membrane[60]. Melusin acts as a co-chaperone with Hsp90. Stretch-dependent signalosome assembly results in Akt activation and subsequent eNOS phosphorylation. Insert: muscle-specific expression of melusin in newborn mouse tissue[61]. [Reproduced, with permission, from Tarone G, Lembo G (2003) Molecular interplay between mechanical and humoral signalling in cardiac hypertrophy. *Trends Mol Med* **9**:376–382.] (See color plate section.)

determined. Indeed, integrins may transmit mechanical signals cooperatively with other membrane-associated proteins in cardiac myocytes, most notably receptor tyrosine kinases, such as the epidermal growth factor (EGF) receptor (EGFR), and G-protein coupled receptors (GPCR), such as the angiotensin II type 1 (AT-I) receptor.

Membrane receptor-mediated stretch effects

Not only do cardiac myocytes release angiotensin II upon stretching[18], providing an autocrine/paracrine signal to AT-I, but also the receptor itself was shown to be stretch-sensitive and to participate in integrin clustering[19]. Accordingly, losartan (an AT-I blocker) blocks stretch-activated Cl⁻ currents[20], including after osmotic swelling[21]. Likewise, EGFR transactivation participates in the stretch-evoked chloride current [which could also be activated by exogenous EGF, or endogenous heparin-binding EGF-like growth factor (HB-EGF) upon release from the extracellular matrix after the activation of matrix metalloproteinases (MMP)] but not the non-selective cation current. This involves PIP_3K and reactive oxidative species (ROS) production, e.g. by nicotinamide-adenine dinucleotide phosphate (NADPH) oxidase, as Cl⁻ currents were blocked by the NADPH oxidase inhibitor peptide, gp91ds-tat[22].

Angiotensin II and endothelin-1 act in series to promote strain-dependent activation of cardiac-specific gene expression [as demonstrated in cultured neonatal rat ventricular myocytes[23] and in wall-stretch-stimulated ventricles[24]]. As proposed by Alvarez[25], stretch causes the release of angiotensin II, which triggers the release of endothelin-1, consequently stimulating Na⁺/H⁺ exchanger (NHE) through ET-A and ET-B receptors[26] and protein kinase C (PKC). The increased $[Na^+]_i$ transient results in activation of the Na⁺/Ca²⁺ exchanger (NCX) in the reverse mode and the development of slow force response[25]. Whether cardiomyocytes are the target and the source of angiotensin II and endothelin-1 is still a matter of controversy. Arguments for an autocrine regulation arise notably from the observations that slow force develops in response to stretch in isolated cardiomyocytes[27]. However, the removal of endocardial endothelium abrogates the slow increase in the contraction force of papillary muscles, suggesting a paracrine regulation[26]. The possibility remains that signalling pathway(s) that operate in single cardiomyocytes may be different from those mediating the slow increase in contraction force in intact muscle, where another cell population – cardiac fibroblasts – is omnipresent and sensitive to angiotensin and other stimuli, including stretch (see Chapter 19).

Nitric oxide

As in endothelial cells, some GPCR in cardiomyocytes are coupled to an NO synthase with the subsequent release of NO. We and others have provided evidence that NO modulates EC coupling in response to acute stretch, as well as cardiac muscle remodelling in response to a chronic haemodynamic challenge, such as pressure overload. Given the short half-life of this highly reactive radical (especially in contracting cells with constitutive production of superoxide anions), time and spatial control of its production is mandatory for efficient signalling to specific targets. In this section, we briefly review 'endothelial type' nitric oxide synthase (eNOS) expression and compartmentation in the heart and describe the effects of stretch-activated NO production on cardiac contraction.

Expression and compartmentation of the NOS in the heart and cardiac myocytes

Three NOS isoforms are profusely expressed in myocardial tissues, albeit with major differences in terms of cell type, myocardial location and specific subcellular compartment. The importance of such compartmentation was highlighted by evidence accumulated over the last few years[28–32] that the effect of NO on cardiac physiology depends both on the specific stimulus acting on a specific NOS isoform and on the spatial confinement of the NOS isoform. 'Neuronal type' nitric oxide synthase (nNOS) regulates Ca^{2+}-handling proteins, so that changes in expression or activity of myocardial nNOS are believed to participate in the myocardial response to stretch. Direct evidence for this, however, is still lacking. Implication of inductible nitric oxide synthase (iNOS) is also very unlikely. Although iNOS is expressed in cardiac tissues between embryonic days 9–14, iNOS is present in neither the healthy nor the hypertrophic adult heart[33]. By contrast, the eNOS isoform has been implicated in both rapid and slow components of the cardiac response to stretch[34,35].

eNOS (encoded by *NOS3*) is abundantly expressed in normal heart, as demonstrated in the ferret. It clearly predominates over and follows a gradient opposite to nNOS[36]. It is highly expressed in the left ventricular apical and midventricular epicardium, is intermediate in the right ventricular free wall and is virtually absent in the left ventricular endocardium and left ventricular side of the septum. eNOS is also prominently expressed in the right atrium and sino-atrial node[36]. This reflects eNOS expression in human left ventricular tissue, although a predominant epicardial expression has been observed[36].

In canine cardiac vasculature, coronary microvessels contain 15-fold more eNOS messenger ribonucleic acid (mRNA) than larger arteries. The circumflex coronary artery shows the highest eNOS mRNA content, followed by the right coronary artery, left anterior descending coronary artery and the aorta, respectively[37]. Cardiomyocyte expression represents only 20% of total cardiac eNOS[38] which does not rule out physiologically important roles in the cardiomyocytes themselves.

Myocyte subcellular localization of NOS

In adult cardiomyocytes, eNOS is predominantly located in caveolae[39] in the external envelope and t-tubular sarcolemma[40,41]. eNOS expression at the sarcoplasmic reticulum (SR) itself remains controversial. In rat hearts, mitochondrial NOS activity accounts for as much as 55% of the cytosolic NO[42]. However, it seems to contribute little to basal NO production, as demonstrated in the porcine heart. Mitochondrial NOS activity was first attributed to both iNOS and eNOS[43,44] or nNOS and eNOS[45] isoforms. Purification of the mitochondrial isoform in the rat liver identified a variant of nNOS-α to support this activity[46]. Notably, eNOS-derived NO, via a cyclic guanosine monophosphate (cGMP)-dependent mechanism, modulates cardiac mitochondrial biogenesis[47]. In endothelial cells, translocation of eNOS to the cytoskeleton mediates shear-stress signalling, but evidence for a similar subcellular translocation in cardiomyocytes is lacking[48].

Activation of cardiac eNOS by stretch: molecular mechanisms

Petroff et al.[34] studied the involvement of NO as a mediator for the slow increase in calcium and contractile force following stretch (resulting in an 8–10% increase in sarcomere length) in isolated rat and mouse ventricular myocytes. Using confocal microscopic analysis of fluo4-loaded cardiomyocytes, they observed that stretch increased the calcium spark rate (but produced no change in spark characteristics, such as distributions of spontaneous spark amplitudes). These increases were fully abrogated upon pre-incubation of single cardiomyocytes with the NOS inhibitor N^G-nitro-L-arginine methyl ester (L-NAME). As this effect was totally absent in single cells from eNOS deficient mice, it was assigned specifically to activation of eNOS within the cardiomyocytes. The activation of the NOS by stretch was also demonstrated using the NO-sensitive fluorescent dye, DAF2, in single, isolated cardiomyocytes[34]. These effects were seen upon application of stretch for about 10 min, a notable difference from the experimental conditions used in another study[49] which observed a more acutely occurring (and transient) increase in Ca spark rate after 5 s, which appeared to be independent of NOS but related to direct mechano-sensitivity of ryanodine receptors (RyR). This does not contradict the activation of eNOS by stretch, as independently observed by others in single cardiomyocytes (also in comparison with eNOS$^{-/-}$ cardiomyocytes)[50], but points to different signalling downstream stretch for the acute versus slow effects on EC coupling.

In the Petrof study[34], the mechanism underlying the increased calcium sparks rate (reflecting SR calcium release) was not due to an increased SR calcium load (which was unchanged by stretch), nor to an indirect effect secondary to stretch-activated non-specific cationic currents, since it was unaffected by treatment with the GsMTx-4 peptide from *Grammostola spatulata* (or gadolinium; Gd^{3+}). Since the L-type calcium current (the trigger for SR calcium-induced calcium release) was reported to be unchanged by stretch, these observations led to the conclusion that intracellular NO production acted as a gain amplifier for EC coupling. Note, the increase in calcium sparks rate was unaffected by treatment with the guanylyl cyclase-inhibitor, ODQ [(1*H*-[1,2,4]oxadiazolo[4,3,-a] quinoxalin-1-one)], suggesting that this effect of NO was independent from cyclic guanosine monophosphate (cGMP), its classical downstream second messenger. Conversely, the effect of stretch on Ca^{2+} sparks rate could be reproduced with S-nitroso-acetyl-penicillamine or S-nitrosocysteine, which both release the S-nitrosylating species NO^+, while the reducing agent, dithiothreitol, prevented it[34]. Together with previous evidence that the cardiac-specific ryanodine receptor (RyR2) can be regulated by S-nitrosylation of critical cysteine residues, these results suggested a cGMP-independent effect of autocrine NO through S-nitrosylation of RyR2, although this was not directly demonstrated. Such post-translational modification would be favoured by the close proximity of eNOS in t-tubular caveolae with the SR RyR2 in the dyads.

eNOS activation by stretch was mediated by PI3K, since pre-treatment with LY294002 (a PI3K inhibitor) inhibited both the increase in Ca^{2+} sparks rate and phosphorylation of Akt/protein kinase B, as well as eNOS on Ser1177 (reflective of its activation) (Fig. 11.2). Possibly, oxidant radicals from NADPH oxidase may be involved in PI3K activation (e.g. following AT-I stimulation by

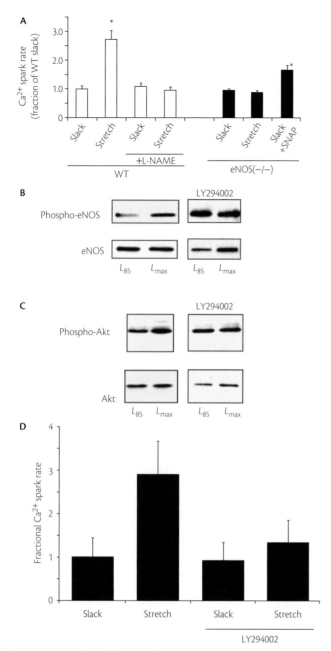

Fig. 11.2 Nitric oxide mediates stretch-sensitive Ca release in cardiomyocytes. **a** The stretch-induced increase in Ca^{2+} spark rate is observed in fluo-4-loaded cardiac myocytes from wild type (WT) but is absent in myocytes from eNOS-deficient mice ($n = 38$). The increase in Ca^{2+} spark rate in wild-type myocytes following stretch is abolished by pre-treatment with L-NAME. Superfusion of eNOS-deficient myocytes with S-nitroso-N-acetyl-penicillamine (SNAP) produces a significant increase in Ca^{2+}-spark frequency. **b–d** Stretch increases Akt and eNOS phosphorylation and Ca^{2+} spark frequency in a PI3K-dependent fashion. **b, c** Stretch increases Akt and eNOS phosphorylation in cardiac trabeculae; both phosphorylation events are inhibited by the PI3K inhibitor LY294002. **d** The stretch-induced increase of Ca^{2+} spark frequency is mediated by a PI3K-dependent signalling pathway. [Reproduced, with permission, from Petroff MG, Kim SH, Pepe S, et al. (2001) Endogenous nitric oxide mechanisms mediate the stretch dependence of Ca^{2+} release in cardiomyocytes. *Nat Cell Biol* **3**:867–873.]

autocrine/paracrine production of angiotensin II in response to stretch), a mechanism previously proposed for other stretch-activated channels (see above). Alternatively, transduction of mechanical stretch may implicate another muscle-specific protein, melusin (see Fig. 11.1). Melusin was identified as a muscle-specific cytoplasmic, CHORD (cysteine and histidine-rich domain) protein interacting with surface integrins in costameres near the Z-disk. Genetic deletion of melusin completely abrogates the phosphorylation of Akt/protein kinase B in response to acute pressure overload in left ventricular muscle[51]. Conversely, basal as well as stretch-induced phosphorylation of Akt is increased in left ventricular muscle from mice with cardiac-specific transgenic overexpression of melusin[52]. Although melusin is probably only one among several mediators of stretch-induced signalling to specific kinases, it may be critical for the recruitment of multiprotein complexes (including Akt) in the vicinity of Z-disk proteins implicated in both acute and chronic regulation of cardiac mechanics and remodelling in response to stretch. Indeed, recent work has shown that melusin directly interacts with the chaperone, hsp90, not as a client protein, but rather as a co-chaperone[53]; since both eNOS and Akt/PKB were clearly identified as client proteins for hsp90, at least in endothelial cells, it is likely (but not yet formally proven) that melusin participates in the stretch-dependent assembly of a 'signalosome', leading to Akt-dependent phosphorylation and activation of eNOS in cardiac muscle.

Additional proteins that participate in the anchoring of integrins to actin may be sensitive to NO and modify the adaptive response of the myocardium to increased mechanical forces. One of these is ENA/VASP (enabled vasodilator-stimulated phosphoprotein), a well-known target for cGMP-activated PKG, itself a mediator downstream of NO). ENA/VASP, in turn, binds to Zyxin and this interaction controls its localization at cell adhesion points for the modulation of actin assembly and organization. Although genetic deletion of both Zyxin and VASP does not interfere with proper cardiac development and basal function[54], transgenic mice with a dominant negative VASP develop dilated cardiomyopathy with early mortality[55]. This suggests a role for VASP in the dynamic regulation of sarcomere–plasmalemma anchoring. Whether this function is modulated by NO (and cGMP/PKG) in response to stretch, however, remains unclear. Still, these observations point to *NOS3* as a potential 'modifier gene' affecting the biological response of the myocardium to mechanical stress.

eNOS-dependent regulation of cardiac EC coupling in response to stretch

The eNOS-mediated increase in Ca^{2+} sparks rate resulted in a slow (i.e. over 10 min) increase in whole-cell Ca^{2+} transient and cell shortening in electrically stimulated cardiac myocytes[34]. This was proposed to contribute to the Anrep effect, i.e. the slowly evolving increase in cardiac contractility beyond that immediately achieved as the result of ordinary length-dependent mechanisms. Therefore, NO produced by eNOS in the cardiomyocytes may add its effects to those of NO produced by paracrine effects from surrounding capillary endothelial cells, to cooperatively orchestrate the length-dependent changes in contractility in response to increased preload. Indeed, coronary endothelial NO, produced in response to shear (mostly during diastole, when coronary flow is maximal), would promote myocyte relaxation through cGMP-dependent desensitization of cardiac myofilaments[31,56]. The ensuing myocyte elongation, in turn, would recruit the length-dependent cardiac reserve through the slow stretch- and NO-dependent adaptive increase in contractility.

Conclusions and outlook

Among molecular elements transducing external physical forces into intracellular signals, integrins and membrane GPCR play a key role not only in cell anchoring to the extracellular matrix (for the former), but also as stretch-sensitive receptors within signal 'interactomes' where they activate intracellular effectors in specific subcellular locales such as caveolae. Among the effectors, the 'endothelial type' of nitric oxide synthase, or eNOS, expressed in cardiomyocytes is the only stretch-sensitive isoform identified so far with profound effects on EC coupling. Stretch-dependent activation of eNOS is accompanied by its Akt-dependent phosphorylation. Akt activation by haemodynamic overload in left ventricular muscle is controlled by the recently identified muscle-specific cytoplasmic CHORD protein, melusin, interacting both with surface integrins and the chaperone, hsp90, for which eNOS is a well-characterized client protein. This would support the formation of stretch-sensitive multiprotein complexes in costameres near the Z-disk, with a potential NO-mediated regulation of multiple proteins involved both in EC coupling (such as the ryanodine receptor) and hypertrophic remodelling (such as ENA/VASP and Zyxin).

Future work needs to directly verify the post-translational regulation of these target proteins by NO (and/or downstream PKG) in response to acute or chronic stretch in cardiomyocytes. Important consideration should be given to modifications of such post-translational regulation in circumstances of excessive stretch or cardiomyopathies. In skeletal muscle from dystrophic mice, for example, recent work has identified hypernitrosylation of RyR1 causing loss of focal kinase binding protein FKBP12.6 (calstabin) association and calcium 'leaks' from the SR. This is thought to participate in skeletal muscle degeneration through activation of calcium-sensitive proteases[57]. Similar hypernitrosylation of RyR2 may cause calcium leaks in cardiac SR, leading to arrhythmia. NO-mediated signalling can also be profoundly modified by concurrent oxidant stress, as commonly produced in pathophysiologic conditions such as ischaemia-reperfusion or heart failure. Oxidant radicals produced (e.g. from NADPH oxidases) are known to produce 'uncoupling' of the NOS, with a shift towards more superoxide anions production by the enzymes[58]. This in turn will produce peroxinitrite and subsequent oxidation-dependent signalling driving maladaptive remodelling. This was exemplified in single cardiac myocytes by peroxinitrite-dependent activation of mechano-sensitive depolarizing currents potentially leading to arrhythmia[50]. *In vivo*, excessive haemodynamic overload was shown to produce eNOS uncoupling which, in turn, aggravates oxidant stress and maladaptive remodelling[59]. Therefore, a better understanding of the mechanisms controlling NOS 'coupled' enzymatic activity in subcellular compartments close to the EC machinery should yield promising therapeutic approaches to prevent arrhythmias as well as progression to heart failure in response to haemodynamic overload.

References

1. Kentish JC, Wrzosek A. Changes in force and cytosolic Ca^{2+} concentration after length changes in isolated rat ventricular trabeculae. *J Physiol* 2005;**506**:431–444.

2. Cingolani HE, Pérez NG, Aiello EA, de Hurtado MC. Intracellular signaling following myocardial stretch: an autocrine/paracrine loop. *Regul Pept* 2005;**128**:211–220.

3. Browe DM, Baumgarten CM. Stretch of beta 1 integrin activates an outwardly rectifying chloride current via FAK and Src in rabbit ventricular myocytes. *J Gen Physiol* 2005;**122**:689–702.

4. Meyer CJ, Alenghat FJ, Rim P, Fong JH, Fabry B, Ingber DE. Mechanical control of cyclic AMP signalling and gene transcription through integrins. *Nat Cell Biol* 2000;**2**:666–668.

5. Ingber DE. Cellular mechanotransduction: putting all the pieces together again. *FASEB J* 2000;**20**:811–827.

6. Matthews BD, Overby DR, Mannix R, Ingber DE. Cellular adaptation to mechanical stress: role of integrins, Rho, cytoskeletal tension and mechanosensitive ion channels. *J Cell Sci* 2006;**119**:508–518.

7. Lele TP, Pendse J, Kumar S, Salanga M, Karavitis J, Ingber DE. Mechanical forces alter zyxin unbinding kinetics within focal adhesions of living cells. *J Cell Physiol* 2006;**207**:187–194.

8. Di Paolo G, Pellegrini L, Letinic K, *et al.* Recruitment and regulation of phosphatidylinositol phosphate kinase type 1 gamma by the FERM domain of talin. *Nature* 2002;**420**:85–89.

9. Critchley DR. Focal adhesions – the cytoskeletal connection. *Curr Opin Cell Biol* 2000;**12**:133–139.

10. Brancaccio M, Hirsch E, Notte A, Selvetella G, Lembo G, Tarone G. Integrin signalling: the tug-of-war in heart hypertrophy. *Cardiovasc Res* 2006;**70**:422–433.

11. Brakebusch C, Fassler R. The integrin-actin connection, an eternal love affair. *EMBO J* 2003;**22**:2324–2333.

12. Wu C, Dedhar S. Integrin-linked kinase (ILK) and its interactors: a new paradigm for the coupling of extracellular matrix to actin cytoskeleton and signaling complexes. *J Cell Biol* 2001;**155**:505–510.

13. Chen H, Huang XN, Yan W, *et al.* Role of the integrin-linked kinase/PINCH1/alpha-parvin complex in cardiac myocyte hypertrophy. *Lab Invest* 2005;**85**:1342–1356.

14. Franchini KG, Torsoni AS, Soares PH, *et al.* Early activation of the multicomponent signaling complex associated with focal adhesion kinase induced by pressure overload in the rat heart. *Circ Res* 2000;**87**:558–565.

15. Pham CG, Harpf AE, Keller RS, *et al.* Striated muscle-specific beta(1D)-integrin and FAK are involved in cardiac myocyte hypertrophic response pathway. *Am J Physiol* 2000;**279**:H2916-H2926.

16. Taylor JM, Rovin JD, Parsons JT. A role for focal adhesion kinase in phenylephrine-induced hypertrophy of rat ventricular cardiomyocytes. *J Biol Chem* 2000;**275**:19250–19257.

17. Domingos PP, Fonseca PM, Nadruz W, Jr. *et al.* Load-induced focal adhesion kinase activation in the myocardium: role of stretch and contractile activity. *Am J Physiol* 2002;**282**:H556-H564.

18. Sadoshima J, Xu Y, Slayter HS, *et al.* Autocrine release of angiotensin II mediates stretch-induced hypertrophy of cardiac myocytes in vitro. *Cell* 1993;**75**:977–984.

19. Zou Y, Akazawa H, Qin Y, *et al.* Mechanical stress activates angiotensin II type 1 receptor without the involvement of angiotensin II. *Nat Cell Biol* 2004;**6**:499–506.

20. Browe DM, Baumgarten CM. Angiotensin II (AT1) receptors and NADPH oxidase regulate Cl⁻ current elicited by beta1 integrin stretch in rabbit ventricular myocytes. *J Gen Physiol* 2004;**124**:273–287.

21. Ren Z, Baumgarten CM. Antagonistic regulation of swelling-activated Cl⁻ current in rabbit ventricle by Src and EGFR protein tyrosine kinases. *Am J Physiol* 2005;**288**:H2628-H2636.

22. Browe DM, Baumgarten CM. EGFR kinase regulates volume-sensitive chloride current elicited by integrin stretch via PI-3K and NADPH oxidase in ventricular myocytes. *J Gen Physiol* 2006;**127**:237–251.

23. Liang F, Gardner DG. Autocrine/paracrine determinants of strain-activated brain natriuretic peptide gene expression in cultured cardiac myocytes. *J Biol Chem* 1998;**273**:14612–14619.

24. Hautala N, Tenhunen O, Szokodi I, *et al.* Direct left ventricular wall stretch activates GATA4 binding in perfused rat heart: involvement of autocrine/paracrine pathways. *Pflugers Arch* 2002;**443**:362–369.

25. Alvarez BV, Perez NG, Ennis IL, *et al.* Mechanisms underlying the increase in force and Ca^{2+} transient that follow stretch of cardiac muscle: a possible explanation of the Anrep effect. *Circ Res* 1999;**85**: 716–722.

26. Calaghan SC, White E. Contribution of angiotensin II, endothelin 1 and the endothelium to the slow inotropic response to stretch in ferret papillary muscle. *Pflugers Arch* 2001;**441**:514–520.

27. Perez NG, de Hurtado MC, Cingolani HE. Reverse mode of the Na^+-Ca^{2+} exchange after myocardial stretch: underlying mechanism of the slow force response. *Circ Res* 2001;**88**:376–382.

28. Barouch LA, Harrison RW, Skaf MW, *et al.* Nitric oxide regulates the heart by spatial confinement of nitric oxide synthase isoforms. *Nature* 2002;**416**:337–339.

29. Hare JM, Stamler JS. NOS: modulator, not mediator of cardiac performance. *Nat Med* 1999;**5**:273–274.

30. Ziolo MT, Bers DM. The real estate of NOS signaling: location, location, location. *Circ Res* 2003;**92**:1279–1281.

31. Massion PB, Feron O, Dessy C, *et al.* Nitric oxide and cardiac function: ten years after, and continuing. *Circ Res* 2003;**93**:388–398.

32. Hare JM. Spatial confinement of isoforms of cardiac nitric-oxide synthase: unravelling the complexities of nitric oxide's cardiobiology. *Lancet* 2004;**363**:1338–1339.

33. Bloch W, Fleischmann BK, Lorke DE, *et al.* Nitric oxide synthase expression and role during cardiomyogenesis. *Cardiovasc Res* 1999;**43**:675–684.

34. Petroff MG, Kim SH, Pepe S, *et al.* Endogenous nitric oxide mechanisms mediate the stretch dependence of Ca^{2+} release in cardiomyocytes. *Nat Cell Biol* 2001;**3**:867–873.

35. Prendergast BD, Sagach VF, Shah AM. Basal release of nitric oxide augments the Frank–Starling response in the isolated heart. *Circulation* 1997;**96**:1320–1329.

36. Brahmajothi MV, Campbell DL. Heterogeneous basal expression of nitric oxide synthase and superoxide dismutase isoforms in mammalian heart: implications for mechanisms governing indirect and direct nitric oxide-related effects. *Circ Res* 1999;**85**:575–587.

37. Fulton D, Papapetropoulos A, Zhang X, *et al.* Quantification of eNOS mRNA in the canine cardiac vasculature by competitive PCR. *Am J Physiol* 2000;**278**:H658-H665.

38. Godecke A, Heinicke T, Kamkin A, *et al.* Inotropic response to beta-adrenergic receptor stimulation and anti-adrenergic effect of ACh in endothelial NO synthase-deficient mouse hearts. *J Physiol* 2001; **532**:195–204.

39. Feron O, Belhassen L, Kobzik L, *et al.* Endothelial nitric oxide synthase targeting to caveolae. Specific interactions with caveolin isoforms in cardiac myocytes and endothelial cells. *J Biol Chem* 1996;**271**: 22810–22814.

40. Levin KR, Page E. Quantitative studies on plasmalemmal folds and caveolae of rabbit ventricular myocardial cells. *Circ Res* 1980;**46**: 244–255.

41. Parton RG, Way M, Zorzi N, *et al.* Caveolin-3 associates with developing t-tubules during muscle differentiation. *J Cell Biol* 1997;**136**:137–154.

42. Zaobornyj T, Valdez LB, La Padula P, *et al.* Effect of sustained hypobaric hypoxia during maturation and aging on rat myocardium. II. mtNOS activity. *J Appl Physiol* 2005;**98**:2370–2375.

43. Gonzales GF, Chung FA, Miranda S, *et al.* Heart mitochondrial nitric oxide synthase is upregulated in male rats exposed to high altitude (4,340 m). *Am J Physiol* 2005;**288**:H2568-H2573.

44. Zanella B, Giordano E, Muscari C, *et al.* Nitric oxide synthase activity in rat cardiac mitochondria. *Basic Res Cardiol* 2004;**99**: 159–164.

45. Hare JM. Nitric oxide and excitation-contraction coupling. *J Mol Cell Cardiol* 2003;**35**:719–729.

46. Kanai AJ, Pearce LL, Clemens PR, *et al.* Identification of a neuronal nitric oxide synthase in isolated cardiac mitochondria using electrochemical detection. *Proc Natl Acad Sci USA* 2001;**98**: 14126–14131.

47. Nisoli E, Tonello C, Cardile A, *et al.* Calorie restriction promotes mitochondrial biogenesis by inducing the expression of eNOS. *Science* 2005;**310**:314–317.

48. Su Y, Kondrikov D, Block ER. Cytoskeletal regulation of nitric oxide synthase. *Cell Biochem Biophys* 2005;**43**:439–449.

49. Iribe G, Ward CW, Camelliti P, *et al.* Axial stretch of rat single ventricular cardiomyocytes causes an acute and transient increase in Ca^{2+} spark rate. *Circ Res* 2009;**104**:787–795

50. Dyachenko V, Rueckschloss U, Isenberg G. Modulation of cardiac mechanosensitive ion channels involves superoxide, nitric oxide and peroxynitrite. *Cell Calcium* 2009;**45**:55–64.

51. Brancaccio M, Fratta L, Notte A, *et al.* Melusin, a muscle-specific integrin beta1-interacting protein, is required to prevent cardiac failure in response to chronic pressure overload. *Nat Med* 2003; **9**:68–75.

52. De Acetis M, Notte A, Accornero F, *et al.* Cardiac overexpression of melusin protects from dilated cardiomyopathy due to long-standing pressure overload. *Circ Res* 2005;**96**:1087–1094.

53. Sbroggio M, Ferretti R, Percivalle E, *et al.* The mammalian CHORD-containing protein melusin is a stress response protein interacting with Hsp90 and Sgt1. *FEBS Lett* 2008;**582**:1788–1794.

54. Hauser W, Knobeloch KP, Eigenthaler M, *et al.* Megakaryocyte hyperplasia and enhanced agonist-induced platelet activation in vasodilator-stimulated phosphoprotein knockout mice. *Proc Natl Acad Sci USA* 1999;**96**:8120–8125.

55. Eigenthaler M, Engelhardt S, Schinke B, *et al.* Disruption of cardiac Ena-VASP protein localization in intercalated disks causes dilated cardiomyopathy. *Am J Physiol* 2003;**285**:H2471-H2481.

56. Kaye DM, Wiviott SD, Kelly RA. Activation of nitric oxide synthase (NOS3) by mechanical activity alters contractile activity in a Ca^{2+}-independent manner in cardiac myocytes: role of troponin I phosphorylation. *Biochem Biophys Res Commun* 1999;**256**: 398–403.

57. Bellinger AM, Reiken S, Carlson C, *et al.* Hypernitrosylated ryanodine receptor calcium release channels are leaky in dystrophic muscle. *Nat Med* 2009;**15**:325–330.

58. Balligand JL, Feron O, Dessy C. eNOS activation by physical forces: from short-term regulation of contraction to chronic remodeling of cardiovascular tissues. *Physiol Rev* 2009;**89**:481–534

59. Takimoto E, Champion HC, Li M, *et al.* Oxidant stress from nitric oxide synthase-3 uncoupling stimulates cardiac pathologic remodeling from chronic pressure load. *J Clin Invest* 2005;**115**:1221–31

60. Tarone G, Lembo G. Molecular interplay between mechanical and humoral signalling in cardiac hypertrophy. *Trends Mol Med* 2003;**9**: 376–382.

61. Brancaccio M, Guazzone S, Menini N, *et al* Melusin is a new muscle-specific interactor for beta(1) integrin cytoplasmic domain. *J Biol Chem* 1999;**274**:29282–29288.

Functional implications of myocyte architecture

Kevin Kit Parker

Background

Cardiac muscle growth underlies the morphogenetic and, often, the pathogenic processes that begin and end the lives of complex organisms. Excitation–contraction (EC) coupling and the role of soluble hormones and growth factor signalling represent areas where our understanding of cardiac muscle development and control is well developed. However, a growing number of reports indicate that the paradigm of reception of these factors at the cell surface, and subsequent intracellular cascades of signalling events, are insufficient to elucidate the switches that differentiate spatially and temporally distinct populations of mesodermal progenitors into cardiac muscle, or potentiate the transition from the stable, characteristic genetic programme of a healthy adult cardiac myocyte to the unstable expression of fetal gene patterns such as seen in heart failure. In other cell types, studies suggest that cells can be switched from one genetic programme to another by alterations of the extracellular matrix (ECM) environment, or by mechanical perturbations that produce changes in cell shape independent of growth factor reception or integrin binding[1]. These studies suggest that ECM and cell cytoskeleton (CSK) should be considered as an integrated structure, maintaining the structural integrity of a cell, and facilitating mechano-transduction events in the cell. In the case of the latter, the architecture of the ECM and CSK networks endow the cell with a massively parallel polymer network for processing signals, encoded as mechanical forces, to potentiate its function.

This chapter explores the dynamic nature of myocyte architecture and its role in electrical excitability. It is impossible to review the myocyte's architecture without considering the ECM and the CSK, as they are continuous networks of discrete structural elements that maintain the structural integrity of the myocyte and also serve as a bi-directional signalling substrate as mechanical stresses are transmitted into, and out of, the myocyte. We discuss how the principal components of the myocyte remodel, and how this can be associated with cardiac pathogenesis. Finally, we summarize the discussion with take-home messages for researchers and clinicians to consider when pondering mechano-electrical signalling in cardiac myocytes.

Myocyte strategies for mechano-electrical coupling

Recent work suggests that ionic currents, with specific attention to calcium metabolism, are affected by microenviromental cues that guide myocyte shape. In work by Walsh and Parks[2], the expression and regulatory properties of voltage-gated calcium channels were modified during changes in neonatal rat myocyte shape *in vitro*. The expression of the calcium channel alpha(1C) subunit was increased in myocytes grown on substrata to encourage aligned growth as compared to myocytes cultured on substrates that promoted only pleomorphic growth. Data from Entcheva's laboratory[3] in myocyte tissues cultured on microgrooved substrata showed slow diastolic rise and increased systolic intracellular Ca^{2+} over a broad range of pacing frequencies. The results ask why elongated myocytes, more closely resembling the morphologies observed *in vivo*, have different electrophysiological properties.

One hypothesis is that altered myocyte shape is coupled to unique cytoskeletal architectures, resulting in unique regulatory mechanisms for ion channel kinetics. Pharmacological agents targeting cytoskeletal proteins have been shown to have a variety of effects on ion channels. For example, colchicine, which depolymerizes microtubules, and taxol, which stabilizes tubulin in the polymer form, have been show to influence the kinetics for the L-type Ca^{2+} channel. In patch-clamp experiments, Galli and DeFelice[4] showed that hyperpolymerization of tubulin increased the mean open time of the channel and their open probability, whereas their depolymerization with colchicines increased the probability for the channels being found in the closed state. In cardiac myocytes and neurons, different effects of tubulin binding agents on the L-type current have been debated, including: (1) restriction of Ca^{2+}-dependent conformation change in the cytoskeleton[5], (2) effects on the concentration of inactivating ions near the mouths of the channels[4], and (3) increased direct interaction between microtubules and the Ca^{2+} channels[4]. In isolated rabbit hearts, an extension of the Galli and DeFelice experiments demonstrated that taxol-induced microtubule stabilization increased the probability of stretch-induced arrhythmias during transient diastolic stretch of the left ventricle[6]. These results are important because they suggest a possible link between the proliferation of polymerized tubulin in pressure-overloaded hearts and their increased propensity for arrhythmias.

Similar observations regarding the role of actin in modulating ion channel kinetics have been reported in the adenosine triphosphate (ATP)-sensitive K^+ channel (K_{ATP}). This channel, inhibited by ATP, was found to have its ATP sensitivity suppressed by actin filament disruptors, suggesting this channel is a unique coupler of the electrical, mechanical and metabolic conditions of the myocyte[7]. These results suggest that myocyte shape and the cytoskeleton are regulatory mechanisms for ion channel expression and activity in the cardiac myocyte.

It is helpful to consider the extracellular matrix, integrins and cytoskeleton as a single mechanical network when considering how mechanical forces may modulate ion channel kinetics. For example, in many cell types, integrins are hypothesized to modulate ion channel kinetics via mechanical linkage through the cytoskeleton and by integrin-linked tyrosine kinases[8]. In atrial myocytes, laminin has been shown to attenuate the L-type Ca^{2+} current[9]. In neuronal cells, the binding of integrins by ligands has been shown to alter pacemaker properties, intracellular free Ca^{2+} concentration ($[Ca^{2+}]_i$) and voltage-gated Ca^{2+} currents[10]. Recently, cytoskeletal-mediated interaction of integrins with L-type Ca^{2+} channels has been demonstrated in vascular smooth muscle[11]. Taken together, these results suggest an integrated network of discrete proteins that not only maintain the structural integrity of the myocyte, but also facilitate its contractility and modulate its excitability by effects on ion channels. How myocyte shape acts as a biological signal is poorly understood.

Myocyte shape

At the cellular level, form is a signal. The question as to whether a muscle's form follows its function, or vice versa, is difficult to solve because the processes of muscle growth and contraction have many nested feedback loops that make linear correlations difficult[12,13]. A cell's shape is a function of its external boundary conditions, such as the ECM, adjacent cells and sinuses, and its internal architecture, the CSK and nucleus. Through the integrins that maintain the mechanical continuity between the extra- and intracellular space, mechanical forces potentiate the activation of chemical signalling pathways[14,15], the opening of ion channels[5], contractile behaviour[16] and the potentiation of unique gene expression profiles[17]. Morphogenetic processes, such as angiogenesis and the formation of lung buds, have been attributed to intercellular variations in architecture and mechanical signal processing that potentiate localized, cellular responses that are unique with respect to neighbouring cells.

In the heart, alterations in myocyte shape during disease have been extensively documented[18]. The changes in myocyte shape during heart disease vary according to the etiology of the disease. Modest changes in myocyte length from about 93 μm to 109 μm have been reported, while heart mass more than doubled in humans[19], suggesting an increase in either cell numbers or cell diameters. Others found more pronounced increases of length per nucleus in multinucleated myocytes, up to 51%, while diameter increased by only 16% and cross-sectional area by 34% in cells from the dilated left ventricle of ischaemic hearts[20]. In contrast, larger changes in cell diameter have been observed, such as by 39% in studies of intact tissue from hearts with dilated cardiomyopathy[21] and 45–50% in myocytes from failing human left ventricle[22]. Most of these studies agree that the length-to-width ratio (aspect ratio) of myocytes changes, decreasing substantially in hypertrophied hearts with increased wall thickness. In failing human hearts due to ischaemic cardiomyopathy, the aspect ratio approaches 11, compared to a normal value of 7.5[23]. These changes, consistent in both rodent and humans, suggest that strategies for compensatory remodelling of the ventricular muscle are genetically conserved across species and represent a fundamental mechanism for myocyte growth and remodelling. As suggested by Gerdes, the unique correlation of myocyte shapes with specific myopathic aetiologies suggests that there may be a direct correlation between a myocyte's shape and its contractile strength[23].

To put cell shape in a different context, the work of Ingber and colleagues[17] demonstrated with micro-contact printing that by controlling the shape of capillary endothelial cells *in vitro* one can drive cells to divide, enter apoptosis or differentiate. This is a notable result in considering angiogenesis, and this has been replicated in other cell types. However, this particular phenomenon has yet to be studied in cardiac myocytes.

Extracellular matrix and the cardiac myocyte

A potential contributor to the changes in myocyte shape is fibrosis, commonly defined as an increased collagen concentration[24]; additionally, enhanced fibronectin (FN) expression is activated initially and is then followed rapidly by collagen messenger ribonucleic acid (mRNA) synthesis[25,26]. This is important because FN anchors cells to other ECM proteins via multiple ligand domains, which connect collagen scaffolding and basement membrane to the integrin proteins that traverse the plasma membrane of the cell[27]. When these trans-membrane receptors interact with FN, they maintain mechanical continuity between the ECM and CSK. Thus, FN is a major component of the mechano-transductive pathways that regulate cell phenotype, and it has been demonstrated to do so by modulating cell shape in non-muscle cells[28]. Fibrotic alterations of the extracellular environment can also occur quickly, for example after myocardial infarction[29,30], or more slowly, such as during aging.

Changes in extracellular matrix and cytoskeletal remodelling in the myocyte

Fibrosis in the extracellular space is concurrent with changes in the myocyte CSK. In normal hearts, only 30% of total tubulin is present in the polymerized form, whereas the remainder occurs as non-polymerized protein[31]. This ratio is reversed in heart failure, during fibrosis in the extracellular space. Extensive work has detailed the role of microtubules in contractile dysfunction during hypertrophy[32,33] and arrhythmogenesis[6]. However, the biophysical mechanisms by which they contribute to contractile dysfunction in the ventricle proved elusive. Recently, mechanisms by which microtubules may contribute to contractile dysfunction in pressure-overload hypertrophy were reported by Brangwynne *et al.*[34]. In isolated neonatal rat ventricular myocytes transfected with green fluorescent tubulin, systolic microtubule buckling was measured during high-speed fluorescent video microscopy. These data suggested that microtubules bear compressive loads during cell shortening. Isolated microtubules in solution buckle with a single long-wavelength arc, whereas microtubules in beating ventricular myocytes have a buckling wavelength of ~3 μm. The latter suggests that, intracellularly, microtubules are mechanically coupled to other elements of the cytoskeletal network (Fig. 12.1) which structurally reinforce their ability to bear compressive forces during myocyte shortening. In pressure overload hypertrophy, where microtubules are hyperpolymerized, the increased number of microtubules increases the intracellular resistance to systolic shortening, contributing to reduced cardiac output.

Desmin, an intermediate filament which maintains Z-line registration in the transverse direction, is irregularly distributed and overexpressed in failing human myocardium. This accompanies the appearance of perturbations in Z-line registration and the lack of contractile filaments[35–38]. Enhanced expression and disorderly arrangement of desmin, as well as disorganization of α-actinin, suggests that myofibril structure is perturbed due to extracellular stimuli. Increased expression of titin during experimental decompensated cardiac hypertrophy in the guinea pig heart and in the failing human heart suggests sarcomeric remodelling[39]. Focal adhesion proteins, such as vinculin, dystrophin, talin and spectrin, were observed in increased amounts in failing human hearts[37,40] and in dilated cardiomyopathy[41]. These reports indicate tight coupling of ECM and CSK remodelling, a process that includes intermediate filaments, focal adhesions and sarcomeres.

Fibrosis and alterations in CSK architecture may be due to stretch-induced hypertrophy, or aberrant strain distributions, in regions of the myocardium that surround an infarct or fibrotic scar[42,43]. Cell-scale variations in the strain patterns of tissue *in vivo* have been hypothesized to regulate cellular growth differentials on the micron scale, thus potentiating directed growth in microenvironments where saturating concentrations of growth factors do not provide the chemotactic cues required for directed cell migration and tissue morphogenesis[1]. In the tissue microenvironment of the

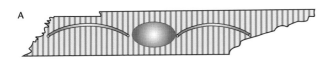
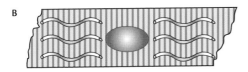

Fig. 12.1 Schematic illustrating how microtubule buckling resists myocyte shortening during systole. **A** In healthy myocardium, most tubulin is unpolymerized; however, because the microtubules are mechanically reinforced by their attachment to other components of the cytoskeletal network, they buckle with a shorter wavelength. **B** During pressure-overload hypertrophy, the balance of tubulin shifts towards polymerization. In this case, the systolic buckling wavelength is still short, but the greater number of microtubules increases the resistance to myocyte shortening. In the schematic, sarcomeric Z-lines are represented in red, the microtubules are the wavy grey tubes and nuclear DNA is indicated by the central ellipsoid.

failing heart, this might explain the appearance of vacuoles, myelin figures and lipid droplets, all of which are morphological signs of myocyte degeneration, in myocytes whose neighbouring myocytes have a normal appearance[37]. These heterogeneities may be a consequence of altered boundary conditions that potentiate myocyte remodelling; however, they are usually studied in the context of being an obstacle to action potential wavefront propagation and the substrate of cardiac arrhythmias.

Cardiac myofibrillogenesis

Cardiac myocyte growth is marked by the serial alignment and parallel bundling of sarcomeres, referred to as myofibrillogenesis. This process is required for the temporal and spatial synchronization required for uniform contraction of a muscle cell[44]. Several models of myofibrillogenesis have been proposed[45–48]. The Sanger model[46,47] proposes that premyofibril-containing banded Z-bodies, consisting of α-actinin and non-muscle myosin IIB, form at the edges of spreading cardiac myocytes. The non-muscle myosin IIB filaments are exchanged for muscle myosin II filaments, and the Z-bands are formed from the fusion of Z-bodies. As the myofibrils increase in width, they align laterally and are characterized by continuous bands of α-actinin (Fig. 12.1).

Holtzer's model describes Sanger's premyofibrils as stress-fibre-like structures that form at the periphery of spreading cardiac myocytes and serve as the scaffold for myofibril assembly[45]. The fibres contain discrete complexes that form along their length, containing sarcomeric α-actinin, Z-bodies, α-actin and muscle tropomyosin. The lateral aggregation of these structures forms the nascent myofibrils of the Sanger model. Finally, myofibrils are completed by the incorporation of titin and the replacement of non-muscle myosin by muscle myosin. The maturity of myofibrils is marked by the disappearance of nebulin-related anchoring protein (N-RAP), hypothesized to be an organizing centre in the initial phase of myofibril assembly. N-RAP binds actin and links it to vinculin. Supporting this hypothesis is the observation that N-RAP binds directly to talin *in vitro*. This, potentially, plays a role in positioning Z-line components with respect to the actin filaments[49].

Sarcomeregenesis and myofibrillogenesis are important because remodelling of the hypertrophying, mature myocyte is marked by changes in cytoskeletal architecture. They may also contribute to improved, or diminished, myocyte contraction. Changes in myofibrillar structure and myocyte shape are concurrent with changes in contractility in failing hearts[22]. This is important because the myofibrils are mechanically coupled to the nucleus and may propagate mechanical signals to the nucleus in a manner that may affect gene expression[36]. The coupling of the ECM to the myofibrillar structures[50] also suggests that changes in the matrix structure of the extracellular space are a direct gene regulatory pathway. While there are circumstantial data suggesting mechano-regulation of gene expression, the kinetics of the signalling pathway represented by the ECM, integrins, the CSK and the nuclear matrix is unknown.

Closing the loop: extracellular matrix, myocyte shape and myofibrillogenesis

Our group has spent considerable time trying to understand the cardiac myocyte's capacity to rebuild itself with respect to boundary conditions imposed by geometric templating of the ECM [51–53].

Using soft lithography techniques to pattern ECM on coverslips, in several studies we cultured freshly harvested neonatal rat ventricular myocytes on protein islands of varying size and shape to quantify how the myocytes changed their shape and how these shape changes affected myofibrillogenesis (Fig. 12.2). Given sufficient time in culture, those ventricular myocytes will assume the shape of the protein islands they are cultured on and rebuild their myofibrils in distinct, repeatable patterns. These data suggest that the translation of sarcomeric proteins is necessary but not sufficient to define the cardiac myocyte as striated muscle. Rather, a distinct process of self-assembly and self-organization must follow translation, along the lines of the theories of myofibrillogenesis offered by Holtzer and Sanger. What our work suggests is that extracellular cues, in the form of a matrix boundary, can catalyze and spatially organize these processes. This is important because changes in the ECM in the various cardiomyopathies are concurrent with muscle cell shape and reorganization of the contractile apparatus. The functional implications of this reorganization are yet to be explored but promise to help validate or refute the Gerdes hypothesis.

The points in this chapter can be summarized as follows:

◆ Remodelling of ECM, myocyte shape and myocyte CSK are hallmarks of cardiac morpho- and pathogenesis, and they are coupled events.

◆ Form is a biological signal, and changes to the boundary conditions and myocyte senses, including changes in ECM composition and remodelling of adjacent cells, will alter the myocyte's shape and the topology of the intracellular cytoskeletal networks.

◆ These changes can be adaptive or maladaptive, depending on the nature of the stimulus.

◆ Changes in CSK network architecture may change the myocyte's contractility and its response to external stimuli.

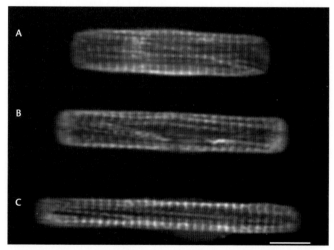

Fig. 12.2 Neonatal rat ventricular myocytes cultured on microcontact printed fibronectin islands with aspect rations of 5:1 (**A**), 7:1 (**B**) and 10:1 (**C**) and stained for DNA [using 4′,6-diamidino-2-phenylindole (DAPI), staining nucleus blue], F-actin (phalloidin, staining inter-Z-disc space of sarcomeres green) and sarcomeric α-actinin (red, thin striations that appear red, or yellow in co-stained areas; see full-colour insert). Scale bar is 10 μm.

Conclusions and outlook

What guidance for future work can be drawn from the reports discussed in this chapter in understanding arrhythmogenic mechano-electrical coupling and heart failure?

First, fundamental cardiac cell biology must be aggressively pursued. The role of the cardiac tissue microenvironment is poorly understood and progress in elucidating its dynamic role in health and disease lags behind other fields, such as oncology, where attention to the tumor microenvironment decades ago spurred new therapeutic directions in anti-angiogenesis therapy and drug delivery. In the case of the heart, these studies will be multidisciplinary, taking into account the micromechanics and metabolic and electrophysiological behaviour of cardiac muscle cells as a function of their surroundings.

Second, if modelling studies are to be relevant to our understanding of cardiac physiology, they must take into account the cardiac tissue microenvironment. These studies could benefit from two advances: (1) new imaging technologies that allow unprecedented spatial and molecular resolution and may accelerate coarse-grain modelling of the cardiac syncitium, and (2) cell and tissue engineering techniques that can be used to understand the scaling laws of the heart, the testing of theoretical predictions and fine-grain analysis of mechano-transduction events over spatial scales ranging from focal adhesion to three-dimensional anisotropic cardiac tissue.

Acknowledgements

I would like to thank all past and present members of the Disease Biophysics Group for their careful tutelage over the last 7 years at Harvard and the help of Sean Sheehy and Nicholas Geisse with figure preparation. We acknowledge financial support from the Defence Advanced Research Projects Agency (DARPA) Biomolecular Motors Program, the Air Force Office of Sponsored Research, the Harvard Materials Research Science and Engineering Center (MRSEC), the Harvard Nanoscale Science and Engineering Center and NIH/NHLBI 5 R01 HL079126-02.

References

1. Huang S, Ingber DE. The structural and mechanical complexity of cell-growth control. *Nat Cell Biol* 1999;**1**:E131–E138.

2. Walsh KB, Parks GE. Changes in cardiac myocyte morphology alter the properties of voltage-gated ion channels. *Cardiovasc Res* 2002;**55**:64–75.

3. Yin L, Bien H, Entcheva E. Scaffold topography alters intracellular calcium dynamics in cultured cardiomyocyte networks. *Am J Physiol* 2004;**287**:H1276–H1285.

4. Galli A, DeFelice LJ. Inactivation of L-type Ca channels in embryonic chick ventricle cells: dependence on the cytoskeletal agents colchicines and taxol. *Biophys J* 1994;**67**:2296–2304.

5. Johnson BD, Byerly L. Acytoskeletal mechanism for Ca²⁺ channel metabolic dependence and inactivation by intracellular Ca²⁺. *Neuron* 1993;**10**:797–804.

6. Parker KK, Taylor LK, Atkinson JB, *et al.* The effects of tubulin-binding agents on stretch-induced ventricular arrhythmias. *Eur J Pharmacol* 2001;**417**:131–40.

7. Van Wagoner DR. Mechanosensitive gating of atrial ATP-sensitive potassium channels. *Circ Res* 1993;**72**:973–83.

8. Davis MJ, Wu X, Nurkiewicz TR, Kawasaki J, Gui P, Hill MA, Wilson E. Regulation of ion channels by integrins. *Cell Biochem Biophys* 2002;**36**:41–66.

9. Wang YG, Samarel AM, Lipsius SL. Laminin acts via beta 1 integrin signalling to alter cholinergic regulation of L-type Ca^{2+} current in cat atrial myocytes. *J Physiol* 2000;**526**:57–68.

10. Wildering WC, Hermann PM, Bulloch AG. Rapid neuromodulatory actions of integrin ligands. *J Neurosci* 2002;**22**:2419–2426.

11. Wu X, Davis GE, Meininger GA, Wilson E, Davis MJ. Regulation of the L-type calcium channel by alpha 5beta 1 integrin requires signaling between focal adhesion proteins. *J Biol Chem* 2001;**276**:30285–30292.

12. Onodera T, Tamura T, Said S, *et al*. Maladaptive remodeling of cardiac myocyte shape begins long before failure in hypertension. *Hypertension* 1998;**32**:753–757.

13. Russell, B, Motlagh, D, Ashley WW, *et al*. Form follows function: how muscle shape is regulated by work. *J Appl Physiol* 2000;**88**:1127–1132.

14. Meyer CJ, Alenghat FJ, Rim P, *et al*. Mechanical control of cyclic AMP signalling and gene transcription through integrins. *Nat Cell Biol* 2000;**2**:666–668.

15. Parker KK, Brock AL, Brangwynne, C, *et al*. Directional control of lamellipodia extension by constraining cell shape and orienting cell tractional forces. *FASEB J* 2002;**16**:1195–1204.

16. Shiels HA, White E. The Frank–Starling mechanism in vertebrate cardiac myocytes. *J Exp Biol* 2008;**211**:2005–2013.

17. Chen CS, Mrksich M, Huang S, Whitesides GM, Ingber DE. Geometric control of cell life and death. *Science* 2007; **276**:1425–1428.

18. Gerdes AM, Capasso JM. Structural remodeling and mechanical dysfunction of cardiac myocytes in heart failure. *J Mol Cell Cardiol* 1995;**27**:849–856.

19. Shozawa T, Okada E, Kawamura K, *et al*. Development of binucleated myocytes in normal and hypertrophied human hearts. *Am J Cardiovasc Pathol* 1990;**3**:27–36.

20. Beltrami CA, Finato N, Roeco M, *et al*. Structural basis of end-stage failure in ischemic cardiomyopathy in humans. *Circulation* 1994;**89**:151–163.

21. Scholz D, Diener W, Schaper J, *et al*. Altered nucleus/cytoplasm relationship and degenerative structural changes in human dilated cardiomyopathy. *Cardioscience* 1994;**5**:127–138.

22. Del Monte F, O'Gara P, Poole-Wilson PA, *et al*. Cell geometry and contractile abnormalities of myocytes from failing human left ventricle. *Cardiovasc Res* 1995;**30**:281–290.

23. Gerdes AM. Remodeling of ventricular myocytes during cardiac hypertrophy and heart failure. *J Fla Med Assoc* 1992;**79**:253–255.

24. Assayag P, Carré F, Chevalier B, *et al*. Compensated cardiac hypertrophy: arrhythmogenicity and the new myocardial phenotype. I. Fibrosis. *Cardiovasc Res* 1997;**34**:439–444.

25. Armstrong PB, Armstrong MT. Regulation of tissue patterning in the developing heart by fibronectin. *Prog Clin Biol Res* 1986;**217B**:177–185.

26. Swynghedauw B. Molecular mechanisms of myocardial remodeling. *Physiol Rev* 1999;**79**:215–262.

27. Ross RS, Borg TK. Integrins and the myocardium. *Circ Res* 2001;**88**:1112–1119.

28. Ingber DE. Fibronectin controls capillary endothelial cell growth by modulating cell shape. *Proc Natl Acad Sci USA* 1990;**87**:3579–3583.

29. Knowlton AA, Connelly CM, Romo GM, *et al*. Rapid expression of fibronectin in the rabbit heart after myocardial infarction with and without reperfusion. *J Clin Invest* 1992;**89**:1060–1068.

30. Casscells W, Kimura H, Sanchez JA, *et al*. Immunohistochemical study of fibronectin in experimental myocardial infarction. *Am J Pathol* 1990;**137**:801–810.

31. Tagawa H, Wang N, Narishige T, *et al*. Cytoskeletal mechanics in pressure-overload cardiac hypertrophy. *Circ Res* 1997;**80**:281–289.

32. Tsutsui H, Ishihara K, Cooper G, 4th, *et al*. Cytoskeletal role in the contractile dysfunction of hypertrophied myocardium. *Science* 1993;**260**:682–687.

33. Tsutsui H, Tagawa H, Kent RL, *et al*. Role of microtubules in contractile dysfunction of hypertrophied cardiocytes. *Circulation* 1994;**90**:533–555.

34. Brangwynne CP, Mackintosh FC, Kumar S, *et al*. Microtubules can bear enhanced compressive loads in living cells due to lateral reinforcement. *Jour Cell Bio* 2006;**173**:733–741.

35. Hatt PY, Berjal G, Moravec D, *et al*. Heart failure: an electron microscopic study of the left ventricular papillary muscle in aortic insufficiency in the rabbit. *J Mol Cell Cardiol* 1970;**1**:235–247.

36. Ferrans VJ, Roberts WC. Intermyofibrillar and nuclear-myofibrillar connections in human and canine myocardium. An ultrastructural study. *J Mol Cell Cardiol* 1973;**5**:247–257.

37. Schaper J, Hein S, Scholz D, *et al*. Multifaceted morphological alterations are present in the failing human heart. *J Mol Cell Cardiol* 1995;**27**:857–861.

38. Hein S, Kostin S, Heling A, *et al*. The role of the cytoskeleton in heart failure. *Cardiovasc Res* 2000;**45**:273–278.

39. Collins JF, Pawloski-Dahm C, Davis MG, *et al*. The role of the cytoskeleton in left ventricular pressure overload hypertrophy and failure. *J Mol Cell Cardiol* 1996;**28**:1435–1443.

40. Kostin S, Scholz D, Shimada T, *et al*. The internal and external protein scaffold of the t-tubular system in cardiomyocytes. *Cell Tissue Res* 1998;**294**:449–460.

41. Schwartz K, Carrier L, Guicheney P, *et al*. Molecular basis of familial cardiomyopathies. *Circulation* 1995;**91**:532–540.

42. Gopalan SM, Flaim C, Bhatia SN, *et al*. Anisotropic stretch-induced hypertrophy in neonatal ventricular myocytes micropatterned on deformable elastomers. *Biotechnol Bioeng* 2003;**81**:578–587.

43. Latimer DC, Roth BJ, Parker KK, *et al*. Analytical model for predicting mechanotransduction effects in engineered cardiac tissue. *Tissue Eng* 2003;**9**:283–289.

44. Gregorio CC, Antin PB. To the heart of myofibril assembly. *Trends Cell Biol* 2000;**10**:355–362.

45. Dlugosz AA, Antin PB, Nachmias VT, *et al*. The relationship between stress fiber-like structures and nascent myofibrils in cultured cardiac myocytes. *J Cell Biol* 1984;**99**:2268–2278.

46. Rhee D, Sanger JM, Sanger JW, *et al*. The premyofibril: evidence for its role in myofibrillogenesis. *Cell Motil Cytoskeleton* 1994;**28**:1–24.

47. Dabiri GA, Turnacioglu KK, Kenan K, *et al*. Myofibrillogenesis visualized in living embryonic cardiomyocytes. *Proc Natl Acad Sci USA* 1997;**94**:9493–9498.

48. Ehler E, Rothen BM, Hammerle SP, *et al*. Myofibrillogenesis in the developing chicken heart: assembly of Z-disk, M-line and the thick filaments. *J Cell Sci* 1999;**112**:1529–1539.

49. Carroll SL, Horowits R. Myofibrillogenesis and formation of cell contacts mediate the localization of NRAP in cultured chick cardiomyocytes. *Cell Motil Cytoskeleton* 2000;**47**:63–76.

50. Hilenski LL, Terracio L, Sawyer R, Borg TK. Effects of extracellular matrix on cytoskeletal and myofibrillar organization in vitro. *Scanning Microsc* 1989; **3**:535–548.

51. Bray MA, Sheehy SP, Parker KK. Sarcomere alignment is regulated by myocyte shape. *Cell Motil Cytoskeleton* 2008;**65**:641–651.

52. Parker KK, Tan J, Chen CS, Tung L. Myofibrillar architecture in engineered cardiac myocytes. *Circ Res* 2008;**103**:340–342.

53. Geisse NA, Sheehy SP, Parker KK. Control of myocyte remodeling in vitro with engineered substrates. *In Vitro Cell Dev Biol Anim* 2009; **45**:343–350.

SECTION 2

Cellular manifestations of cardiac mechano-electric coupling

13. **Mechanical modulation of pacemaker electrophysiology** 95
Patricia J. Cooper and Ursula Ravens

14. **Mechano-electric coupling in working cardiomyocytes: diastolic and systolic effects** 103
Michael R. Franz

15. **Mechano-sensitivity of pulmonary vein cells: implications for atrial arrhythmogenesis** 110
Chang Ahn Seol, Won Tae Kim, Jae Boum Youm, Yung E. Earm and Chae Hun Leem

16. **Heterogeneity of sarcomere length and function as a cause of arrhythmogenic calcium waves** 117
Henk E.D.J. ter Keurs, Ni Diao, Nathan P. Deis, Mei L. Zhang, Yoshinao Sugai, Guy Price, Yuji Wakayama, Yutaka Kagaya, Yoshinao Shinozaki, Penelope A. Boyden, Masahito Miura and Bruno D.M. Stuyvers

17. **Cellular mechanisms of arrhythmogenic cardiac alternans** 125
Kenneth R. Laurita

18. **Remodelling of gap junctions in ventricular myocardium, effects of cell-to-cell adhesion, mediators of hypertrophy and mechanical forces** 132
André G. Kléber and Jeffrey E. Saffitz

19. **The origin of fibroblasts, extracellular matrix and potential contributions to cardiac mechano-electric coupling** 138
Troy A. Baudino and Thomas K. Borg

20. **Advantages and pitfalls of cell cultures as model systems to study cardiac mechano-electric coupling** 143
Leslie Tung and Susan A. Thompson

13

Mechanical modulation of pacemaker electrophysiology

Patricia J. Cooper and Ursula Ravens

(With special thanks to Peter Kohl for contributions to this chapter in the first edition)

Background

'*It is well known that when [...] venous inflow to the heart increases, the venous pressure rises and the output of the heart becomes larger. At the same time the heart beats more frequently and the increase in the rate of the pulse may be very considerable.*'[1]

This observation by Francis A. Bainbridge of the positive chronotropic response of the heart to stretch has given rise to numerous studies into the mechanisms and relevance of venous return induced changes in heart rate. This chapter reviews these studies and presents evidence beyond the original nervous reflex theory towards intrinsic cardiac mechanisms and mechano-electric coupling (MEC).

The Bainbridge Reflex

The studies by Bainbridge[1] used volume loading via injection of fluids into the jugular vein of anaesthetized dogs to elevate venous return. Arterial and venous pressures, respiration and pulse rate were monitored. These studies showed that an increase in venous pressure could raise cardiac beating rate (BR) in the absence of changes in arterial pressure. This was attributed to a vagal reflex-based response, subsequently referred to as the Bainbridge Reflex.

Several investigators have repeated Bainbridge's experiments, and the majority indeed observed tachycardia with increased venous return, although some found little change, or the opposite response, as reviewed in detail elsewhere[2].

The relevance of the Bainbridge Reflex for human physiology is a subject of contention. Its principal applicability, however, has been confirmed in a study where passive elevation of the legs of human volunteers in supine position raised BR. This is caused by an increase in venous return (so-called auto-transfusion of blood), as witnessed by an increase in central venous pressure in the absence of changes in arterial pressure [an important difference to standard tilt-table studies where both venous return and arterial pressure are changed, resulting in the opposite effect when both pressures are raised[3]].

In contrast to the original reflex-based explanation, a stretch-induced increase in BR was subsequently observed in isolated hearts[4] and isolated sino-atrial node (SAN) tissue[5], suggesting that the Bainbridge effect may be, in part at least, determined at the level of the SAN pacemaker.

Physiological stimuli

The majority of atrial filling is, as in the ventricles, caused by a shift in atrio-ventricular border position. In contrast to ventricular filling, this is an active process, caused by ventricular contraction. This pulls the atrio-ventricular border towards the cardiac apex, thereby distending the atria, which fill with blood from the *Venae cavae* (i.e. the heart is a combined pressure and suction pump). The extent of atrial filling depends crucially on the available venous blood volume, determined by venous return. Increased venous return will increase right atrial filling, thereby distending the atrial wall, including the SAN.

Mechanisms that affect venous return include activities that cause undulation in venous pressure which – in the presence of competent semi-lunar valves in the venous vasculature – direct blood flow towards the heart. Such pressure changes are caused by arterial pulse wave effects on neighbouring veins, skeletal muscle activity and respiratory fluctuations in the thoraco-abdominal pressure gradient.

The latter may underlie the non-neuronal component of respiratory sinus arrhythmia (RSA)[6]. During inspiration, the thoraco-abdominal pressure gradient favours venous return to the heart, while the opposite prevails during expiration. These respiratory-induced fluctuations in venous return may promote matching changes in SAN stretch and BR: an increase during inspiration and a decrease during expiration. While this non-neuronal component of RSA plays little, if any, role in normal subjects at rest (< 1%), it may account for up to a third of RSA during heavy exercise, and explain the presence of RSA in heart transplant recipients.

Thus, mechanical stimuli affect SAN pacemaking. In order to discuss potential mechanisms of this form of cardiac MEC, we will briefly review basic SAN cell electrophysiology.

The sino-atrial node

SAN pacemaker electrophysiology

Pacemaker cells are characterized by the absence of a stable resting membrane potential (see Figs 13.1–13.4). Instead, they display spontaneous diastolic depolarization, from their maximum diastolic potential (MDP) towards threshold for action potential (AP) generation. *In situ*, cells in the SAN centre show the least negative

MDP, fastest rate of diastolic depolarization and – despite having the slowest rate of AP upstroke – they set BR[7]. The SAN is located at the junction of the superior *Vena cava* with the right atrium, extending roughly in parallel with the *Crista terminalis* towards the inferior *Vena cava*. The precise location of the SAN differs from species to species.

The SAN is the site of initiation of primary pacemaker activity in the mammalian heart[8]. Other regions of the heart that may spontaneously generate rhythmic AP, such as the atrio-ventricular node and Purkinje fibres, do so at lower intrinsic rates. These pacemakers will not, therefore, determine normal cardiac BR. However, when subjected to stretch, Purkinje fibres – like SAN may depolarize and accelerate the rate of spontaneous activity[5,9,10]. Therefore during acute dilation of the ventricles, Purkinje fibre firing rate could override SAN rate leading to stretch-induced arrhythmia. Incidentally, even ventricular trabeculae can produce pacemaker-like automaticity when exposed to stretch[10].

The cycle of spontaneous electrical activity in SAN cells is brought about by the finely balanced interaction of a number of interdependent processes including surface membrane ion channels and intracellular Ca^{2+} handling mechanisms. Figure 13.1

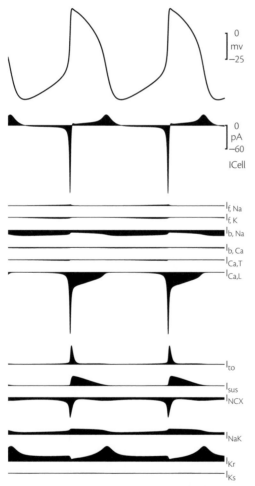

begins with repolarization from a preceding AP, generated with a mathematical model of SAN pacemaking that includes these mechanisms[11,12].

Outward (i.e. hyperpolarizing) K^+ currents (including, in varying amounts in different species, rapidly, I_{Kr}, and slowly, I_{Ks}, activating components of the delayed rectifier potassium current) drive the membrane potential towards the MDP. As the SAN cell membrane becomes more negative, these channels progressively inactivate, while the hyperpolarization-activated inward (i.e. depolarizing) current, I_f, is activated. Also, with the increasingly negative membrane potential, the inward Na^+ and Ca^{2+} background currents ($I_{b,Na}$ and $I_{b,Ca}$) reach their maximum (determined by the difference in actual membrane potential and reversal potential of these currents). Together, these currents force a change in net membrane current from outward to inward (see I_{Cell} in Fig. 13.1), thereby turning the direction of membrane potential dynamics from hyperpolarizing to depolarizing.

Progressive diastolic depolarization causes activation of the inward transient Ca^{2+} current ($I_{Ca,T}$)[13]. In addition, recent studies suggest an additional and independent contribution of local Ca^{2+} release from the sarcoplasmic reticulum (SR)[14]. Both then may contribute to an increase in sub-sarcolemmal $[Ca^{2+}]$, activating additional inward current via the Na^+/Ca^{2+} exchanger, I_{NaCa}[14,15].

The above inward currents drive the SAN membrane potential toward threshold for activation of the long-lasting Ca^{2+} current ($I_{Ca,L}$), triggering action potential upstroke and global release of Ca^{2+} from the SR[13,14]. In most species, the rapid depolarization to the maximum systolic potential (MSP) is carried chiefly by $I_{Ca,L}$ in primary SAN pacemaker cells [the fast Na^+ current (I_{Na}) contributes to SAN activity mainly in the periphery of the SAN, but in species with very high BR, such as mice, also in the centre of the node[16]].

Depolarization to MSP causes inactivation of potential-sensitive inward currents, reduces the driving force for depolarizing background currents and re-activates I_{Kr} and I_{Ks}, as well as the transient, I_{to}, and sustained, I_{sus}, outward currents, where present. The inward current generated by I_{NCX} diminishes as intracellular Ca^{2+} is taken back up into the SR, and/or extruded from the cell. Collectively, this activity causes membrane repolarization, until the subsequent SAN cycle begins.

The relative contribution of individual currents and Ca^{2+}-dependent processes varies with location of cells in the SAN[14,17] and between species. SAN beating frequency is modulated by the autonomic nervous system, circulating hormones [for reviews see[14,17,18]], electrotonic interaction with surrounding atrial muscle and stretch.

Pacemaker architecture and conduction pathways

SAN pacemaker excitation drives global atrial and ventricular activity via electrotonic interaction.

Central SAN cells synchronize their activity via gap junctions, formed predominantly by Connexin 45[19], that allow exchange of electrical and chemical information between neighbouring cells. The extent of direct coupling between adjacent cells, and effects from surrounding tissue, dictate how stable the pacemaking site is, and how fast and securely the electrical signal is propagated[7,17].

The electrotonic interaction between the atrium and nodal cells has an essential influence on SAN pacemaking. Peripheral SAN cells have, after isolation, a higher intrinsic BR than central SAN cells. Their activity is suppressed, *in situ*, by the electrotonic effects

Fig. 13.1 Mathematical model of SAN action potential (AP) and contributing ionic currents. Upper trace: SAN AP, based on a rabbit central SAN cell model[12]. Lower traces: contributing ionic currents, computed using Cellular Open Resource (COR; http://cor.physiol.ox.ac.uk/)[11]. Each current is scaled to the same extent, illustrating the large magnitude of $I_{Ca,L}$ and I_{Kr} in this model.

from surrounding atrial tissue whose stable resting potential counteracts depolarization in peripheral SAN[20]. This can be illustrated by cutting the SAN free from atrial tissue, which causes a shift of the leading pacemaker site from SAN centre to its periphery, and an overall increase in BR[21].

The central SAN is protected from atrial electrotonic inactivation by distance and low levels of intercellular coupling. An indication of the limited electrical coupling is the low conduction velocity in central SAN (2–8 cm/s)[7]. As the wavefront moves toward the SAN periphery, it speeds up (20–80 cm/s)[7] due to increased connectivity between adjacent cells. Excitation finally invades atrial muscle, predominantly via the *Crista terminalis* where cellular coupling is about one order of magnitude higher than in the node[22].

Gap junctions in the SAN are not restricted to a single cell type; pacemaker cells can be electrically connected to the extensive network of SAN fibroblasts (via Connexin 45)[19]. The functional significance of this heterogeneous cell coupling in native SAN is currently unknown, but it is interesting, in the context of MEC, to note that cardiac fibroblasts are mechano-sensitive cells [[23,24]; see also Chapter 19].

SAN mechanical stimulation

As highlighted above, the heart is able to respond to an increase in venous return with earlier initiation of the subsequent contraction. Investigations into underlying mechanisms have used a range of experimental models, from human volunteers to isolated SAN cells, each with its own advantages and limitations.

The heart *in vivo*

In vivo investigations offer the most relevant but least reproducible model system[25]. The experimental evidence resulting from this type of research has been highlighted in the 'Background' section of this chapter. Historically, it gave rise to the concept of a reflex-mediated stretch-induced rise in cardiac BR.

For the study of underlying mechanisms, *in vivo* models need to be combined with lower order experimental tools that offer more control and less variability.

Isolated heart or atrium

Isolated organ preparations allow near-physiological application of stretch, e.g. via intra-atrial volume control, potentially in the presence of preserved vagal innervation[26]. A rise in right atrial pressure by up to 20 mmHg has been found to increase BR in this type of preparation and has established the concept of an intra-cardiac BR response to stretch[4].

Isolated SAN tissue

SAN tissue preparations allow stable simultaneous recordings of electrophysiological and mechanical parameters (either of these parameters allow identification of BR)[5,27]. Stretch is usually applied uni-axially, often in parallel to the *Crista terminalis* (via attachment of mechanical probes to the *Venae cavae*).

In his pioneering study, Deck used a photographic iris to apply concentric stretch to isolated SAN preparations, which may be more representative of *in vitro* mechanics[5]. Using microelectrode recordings he observed that the stretch-induced increase in BR is accompanied by a decrease in MSP and MDP (see Fig. 13.2).

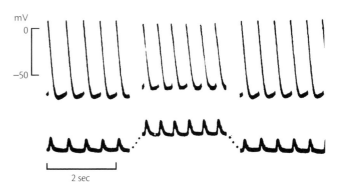

Fig. 13.2 Effect of stretch on cat isolated SAN pacemaking. Upper trace: AP recording illustrating a stretch-induced reduction in MDP, decreased AP amplitude and increased BR. Lower trace: mechanical activity with contractions pointing upwards; the shift in passive tension indicates stretch timing. [Reproduced, with permission, from Deck KA (1964) Dehnungseffekte am spontanschlagenden, isolierten Sinusknoten. *Pflügers Arch* **280**:120–130.]

The potential contribution of intra-cardiac neuronal pathways ('intramural reflexes') to this response was ruled out in a study by Wilson and Bolter[26]. In this study, atropine, propranolol or tetrodotoxin (TTX) were used to exclude the involvement of intra-cardiac neuronal activity in acutely denervated right atrial preparations subjected to increased atrial pressure. Still, native tissue preparations have one major drawback: due to the visco-elastic properties of cardiac tissue, there is always a difference in both the timing and the extent of the external 'command' mechanical intervention and its *in situ* equivalent at the cellular level. It is therefore difficult to grade, maintain and repeat mechanical stimulation of SAN cells in native tissue. This can be overcome using isolated cells.

Isolated SAN pacemaker cells

Cell swelling

Isolation of spontaneously beating, Ca^{2+}-tolerant SAN cells and maintenance of stable electrophysiological AP recordings is no minor task. Additional mechanical stimulation has therefore initially been attempted by osmotic challenges and cell inflation, which require no additional probe attachment and do not cause significant lateral translocation of the cell membrane relative to the recording electrode.

Hagiwara *et al.* identified a swelling-activated Cl^- current ($I_{Cl,swell}$) in rabbit SAN cells, whose electrophysiological properties, together with a cell-volume-related increase in $I_{Ca,L}$ open probability, could underlie the stretch-induced increase in cardiac BR[28].

Subsequent research by Lei and Kohl, however, showed that hyposmotic swelling actually reduces BR of spontaneously active SAN cells (Fig. 13.3A)[29]. Pharmacological block of $I_{Cl,swell}$ reduced BR further (in swollen cells only), reconfirming that this channel has indeed a positive chronotropic effect. This does not, however, dominate the pacemaker response to swelling. Cell swelling is, therefore, not a suitable model for the study of mechanisms involved in the positive chronotropic response of the SAN to stretch.

In fact, cell swelling and stretch cause very different micromechanical changes (swelling increases SAN cell diameter but not

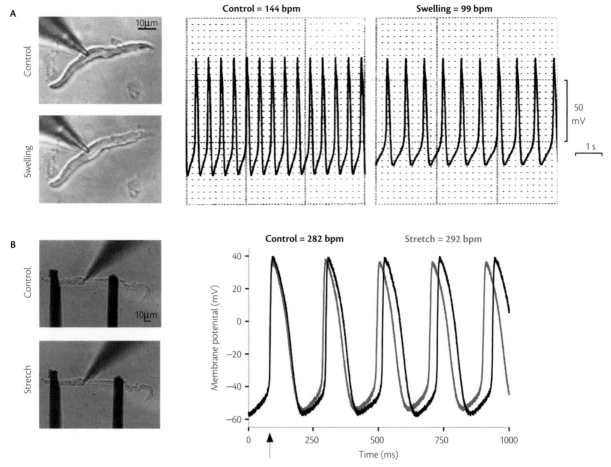

Fig. 13.3 Comparison of swelling- and axial stretch-induced changes in spontaneous BR of rabbit SAN cells. **A** Swelling, induced by perfusion with 75% hyposmotic solution, causes a 32% increase in cell area (see inset) and slowing of SAN cell BR[27]. **B** Axial stretch by 7% of cell length (see inset) increases spontaneous BR in SAN cells (grey trace: control; black trace: stretch)[29]. [Reproduced, with permission, from Lei M, Kohl P (1998) Swelling-induced decrease in spontaneous pacemaker activity of rabbit isolated sino-atrial node cells. *Acta Physiol Scand* **164**:1–12; and Cooper PJ, Lei M, Cheng L-X, Kohl P. (2000). Axial stretch increases spontaneous pacemaker activity in rabbit isolated sinoatrial node cells. *J Appl Physiol* **89**: 2099–2104.]

length, whereas stretch increases length and – since cell volume is understood to remain constant – reduces cell diameter). Additionally, cell-volume-controlled ion channels usually activate with a marked lag-time (one or more minutes compared to cell volume dynamics), suggesting the presence of intermediary reaction steps in their response to a mechanical event (for detail see Chapter 4).

Cell stretch

A number of experimental approaches have been deployed to stretch individual cardiac myocytes, including suction pipettes attached to opposite cell ends, glass probes or cantilevers for local deformation and magnetic beads (although the latter do not, at present, allow application of axial stretch, but rather cause 'centrifugal' membrane deformation that is, perhaps, more akin to cell swelling). Attachment of probes can be by negative pressure, various glues or electrostatic surface interactions. The carbon fibre technique, in particular, allows application of reasonably homogeneous cell distension, judging by the consistency of sarcomere lengthening established in ventricular myocytes[30].

Using this technique, Cooper *et al.* applied axial stretch to single, spontaneously beating SAN cells[31]. AP were recorded before,

during and after application of stretch (increasing cell length by 5–10% of control; see Fig. 13.3B). Stretch results in an instantaneous and reversible increase in BR (by about +5% in this study), combined with a reduction in MDP and MSP, as observed by Deck in the intact SAN[5]. This, along with the isolated heart and SAN tissue experiments described above, confirms that at least part of the Bainbridge effect is intrinsic to the heart and encoded at the level of individual SAN pacemaker cells.

Magnitude of the SAN stretch response

The stretch-induced increase in BR of single rabbit SAN cells (+5%)[31] is significantly smaller than that observed in multicellular preparations (often +15% to +40%)[4,5]. While the observed increase in whole animal experiments is variable, it tends to exceed +10% of control BR.

This difference in the magnitude of SAN responses to stretch may have several reasons. Isolation of single pacemaker cells from SAN tissue involves digestion of the extracellular matrix and may, therefore, remove or uncouple essential elements of the mechano-electrical transduction mechanism (it is also conceivable that some of the removed components may normally protect a mechano-sensitive pathway from activation, thereby potentially yielding false-positive findings in isolated cells). Also, intercellular interaction of SAN cells *in situ* may reinforce the dynamic response to a stimulus. In this context, the nature of SAN histoarchitecture may confer additional mechano-sensitivity via stretch-activated fibroblasts[23], electrically coupled to pacemaker cells[19].

There are major discrepancies in the amount of stretch that can be reversibly applied to single SAN cells (5–8% increase in cell length) and SAN/right atrial tissue preparations. Tissue preparations have been successfully stretched by an order of magnitude more than isolated cells[27]. The extent of actual SAN pacemaker cell stretch *in situ* remains unknown, even though Kamiyama notes that the peripheral SAN region is more distensible than the central SAN, presumably due to a lower connective tissue content[32].

In situ, stretch caused three-dimensional changes in each cell which, given that SAN tissue behaves largely like an incompressible body, must involve both positive *and* negative strain. This is further affected by the anatomical constraints placed on the heart *in situ*, e.g. by the pericardium, which affects the interrelation of venous return, atrial filling and transmural pressure (see Chapter 39). For example, it has been known since 1915 that the rise in BR produced by venous return is more pronounced when the pericardium is intact[33], suggesting a possible contribution of lateral tissue compression to the BR increase.

Stretch modality is another important determinant of the SAN response. Concentric stretch of isolated SAN tissue has a greater effect on BR (+16%) than uni-axial stretch (+9%)[5]. Also, fast stretch is more efficient in increasing BR than slow distension, and stretch timed to occur during the electrical diastole has a greater effect than during systole[27,34,35].

Molecular mechanisms of the SAN response to stretch

Current evidence

The observation that axial stretch of isolated SAN cells leads to an instantaneous and reversible increase in BR was followed up by the identification of a stretch-induced whole cell current with a reversal potential near –11 mV and a conductivity of 6 nS/pF[31]. The amplitude and current-voltage characteristics of this current are compatible with activation of cation non-selective stretch-activated channels (SAC$_{NS}$). Implementation of a matching ion current, I$_{SAC,NS}$, in quantitative mathematical models of SAN pacemaker activity confirmed that this electrophysiological mechanism would be sufficient to cause the changes in BR observed in isolated cells[31].

To what extent can this activation of I$_{SAC,NS}$ be reconciled with pre-existing observations? Ju and Allen review the identification of transient receptor potential (TRP) channels as potential candidates for I$_{SAC,NS}$ and provide immunohistological evidence that these proteins exist in SAN pacemaker cells[36]. The contribution of I$_{SAC,NS}$ to pacemaking depends not only on its mechano-sensitive open probability, expressed via the effective whole-cell conductance G$_{SAC,Cat}$, but also on the effective driving force for ions to pass the channel. This is largely determined by the voltage difference between the channel's reversal potential, E$_{SAC,Cat}$, and the actual membrane potential, E$_M$, according to the following equation:

$$I_{SAC,NS} = G_{SAC,NS} \left(E_{SAC,NS} - E_M \right).$$

This voltage dependence of the current helps to explain why stretch during spontaneous diastolic depolarization is more efficient in increasing BR than during systole or maintained distension[27]. SAC$_{NS}$ activation at an E$_M$ negative to E$_{SAC,NS}$ will promote depolarization. If this coincides with the spontaneous diastolic depolarization of SAN cells, the threshold for subsequent AP activation will be reached faster, thereby increasing BR.

This model is also in keeping with the general observation that the positive chronotropic response of the SAN to stretch is enhanced by reduction in background BR of the preparation[24,37]. This was reflected even in the 1882 study of Sewall and Donaldson, who found that the effect of stretch on SAN BR is greatly enhanced by vagal stimulation[38]. The rationale is that a reduction in BR predominantly prolongs the diastolic interval – the phase during which SAC$_{NS}$ activation will have its most pronounced positive chronotropic effect.

More precisely, SAC$_{NS}$ activation at membrane potentials that are different from but *moving towards* E$_{SAC,NS}$ will have a positive chronotropic effect by enhancing the prevailing change in voltage (↑ΔV, e.g. during spontaneous diastolic depolarization; see Fig. 13.4), while SAC$_{NS}$ activation during all other times will have the opposite effect (↓ΔV).

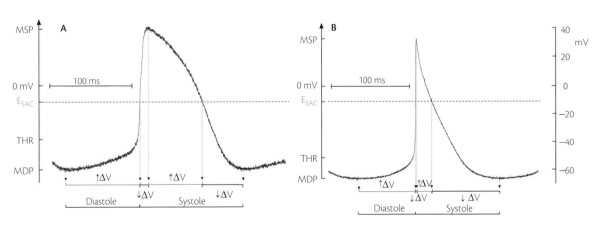

Fig. 13.4 Species differences in potential SAC$_{NS}$ effects on SAN cell AP. Membrane potential recordings illustrate the interrelation of cell electrophysiological parameters [MSP; MDP; THR (threshold for activation of AP)] and E$_{SAC}$. Electrical diastole, systole and time periods during which SAC$_{NS}$ activation would cause either positive (↑ΔV) or negative (↓ΔV) chronotropic effects are labelled. **A** Rabbit SAN cell; **B** mouse SAN cell.

This suggests that the actual shape of the SAN AP will have a major effect on stretch-induced changes in BR. Figure 13.4 compares how the SAN AP, recorded from rabbit (Fig. 13.4A) and mouse (Fig. 13.4B), relates to $E_{SAC,NS}$ (at −11 mV).

As indicated above, stretch during electrical diastole is characterized by $\uparrow\Delta V$ effects. During systole, both $\uparrow\Delta V$ and $\downarrow\Delta V$ effects can be observed, although with species-dependent differences in their relative duration. In rabbit, systolic $\uparrow\Delta V$ and $\downarrow\Delta V$ effects are of roughly equal duration, while in mouse, SAN systole is dominated by $\downarrow\Delta V$ effects.

The actual net charge transfer by SAC_{NS} activation can be approximated by taking into account the potential difference between E_M and $E_{SAC,NS}$ (driving force for $I_{SAC,NS}$) during $\uparrow\Delta V$ and $\downarrow\Delta V$ phases. This is illustrated in Table 13.1, where both the relative duration of these phases and the product of time and driving force (area between E_M and $E_{SAC,NS}$ in Fig. 13.4) are listed.

The data suggest that murine SAN is a model where stretch – depending on the actual $\uparrow\Delta V$:$\downarrow\Delta V$ ratio of the leading pacemaker – may have little effect on BR, or even cause a negative chronotropic response (if, as in the given example, the ratio is < 0.5). These responses have indeed been observed in isolated murine SAN tissue, where uni-axial stretch (parallel to the *Crista terminalis*) by 40–80% of resting tissue length most frequently (84% of cases) caused a reduction in spontaneous beating rate, while an increase or lack of change was observed more rarely (8% each, $n = 25$; changes were fully reversible, authors' observation; see Fig. 13.5 B).

Although it is intriguing that a majority of stretch-induced changes in SAN activity can be mathematically reproduced solely on the basis of SAC_{NS} activation, this does not mean that they are the only contributors to observed responses. Additional direct and indirect effects of stretch include changes in other ion-transporting systems and second messenger activity. An influx of Na^+ via $I_{SAC,NS}$, for example, may lead to a local (sub-membrane) increase in Na^+ concentration, thereby reducing the ability of the Na^+-Ca^{2+} exchanger to extrude Ca^{2+} (or, potentially, activating reverse mode Na^+-Ca^{2+} exchange). This would raise intracellular Ca^{2+} levels[39] and affect pacemaking[14]. Stretch effects on ion channels that are not customarily considered to be SAC are discussed in more detail in Chapter 6.

Stretch furthermore may cause nitric oxide (NO)-mediated[40] enhancement of SR Ca^{2+} release[41], probably via s-nitrosylation of the ryanodine-sensitive SR Ca^{2+} release channel. There is constitutive NO synthase in SAN cells[42]. Since block of SR Ca^{2+} release by ryanodine reduces the heart's positive chronotropic response to stretch[27], it is possible that NO-mediated effects on ryanodine-sensitive SR Ca^{2+} release contribute to the SAN response to stretch. Additionally, a recent study by Iribe *et al.*[43] in ventricular myocytes has shown that stretch may have a direct mechanical effect on

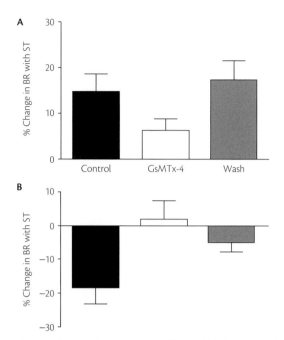

Fig. 13.5 Stretch effects on SAN BR in absence (Control, black; Wash, grey) and presence of SAC-specific blocker (GsMTx-4, 10 μM, white). **A** Guinea pig, $p = 0.013$, $n = 6$. **B** Mouse, $p = 0.038$, $n = 5$. (From Cooper and Kohl, unpublished observations.)

SR ryanodine receptors, increasing the rate of spontaneous Ca^{2+} release events. In SAN cells, this may result in increased diastolic depolarization rate, thereby increasing BR.

Ongoing investigations

In order to re-integrate findings at the (sub-)cellular level with tissue and organ function, selective pharmacological tools are ideally required to modulate the transduction of a mechanical event into an electrophysiologically relevant signal *in situ*. While gadolinium ions (Gd^{3+}) are a potent blocker of $I_{SAC,NS}$, their use is limited by non-selectivity[44,45] and precipitation in physiological buffers[46]. In experiments on rabbit SAN strips, Gd^{3+} had no effect on the stretch-induced increase in BR[27]. The aminoglycoside antibiotic streptomycin has been shown to efficiently block SAC_{NS} in isolated cardiomyocytes at concentrations below 50 μM[39,47] [at higher concentrations, streptomycin also affects $I_{Ca,L}$[48]]. However, streptomycin is ineffective in blocking SAC_{NS} if applied to SAN tissue preparations[49], as has occasionally been seen also in isolated whole heart preparations[50], suggesting that its utility for acute block of SAC_{NS} *in situ* may be limited (potential for false-negative conclusions).

More recently, GsMTx-4, a peptide isolated from the venom of the Chilean tarantula *Grammostola spatulata*, has been identified as a potent SAC_{NS} blocker[51]. It is highly specific (100 nM range), and has been shown to inhibit atrial arrhythmogenesis in isolated hearts during pressure overload[52]. GsMTx-4 has a +5 charge and a hydrophobic face, and therefore it can act as an amphipath. Cationic amphipaths insert into the inner leaflet of the lipid bilayer, and in doing so they may alter the mechanical integration of SAC. Application of GsMTx-4 (10 μM) blocked the stretch-induced change in BR in both guinea pig (Fig. 13.5A) and mouse (Fig. 13.5B)

Table 13.1 Species dependence of SAC_{NS} effects on SAN electrophysiology. Relation of duration (T) and net charge transport capacity (ΔQ) of positive ($\uparrow\Delta V$) and negative ($\downarrow\Delta V$) chronotropic effects.

Species	$T_{\uparrow\Delta V}$	$T_{\downarrow\Delta V}$	$Q_{\uparrow\Delta V}$	$Q_{\downarrow\Delta V}$
Rabbit SAN	70.8	29.2	72.7	27.3
Mouse SAN	46.4	53.6	47.5	52.5

SAN tissue. The effect was reversible, albeit only partially in the mouse. Additionally, the peptide did not affect the background BR or force, nor did it blunt the typically enhanced force development during stretch of the SAN/atrial tissue preparation used for either species. This is additional evidence that GsMTx-4 is specific for SAC and suitable for use in native tissue preparations (Cooper and Kohl, unpublished observations).

Conclusions and outlook

The stretch-induced increase in SAN BR has been observed in many different cardiac preparations from whole organism to single cell, in the presence and absence of sympathetic and parasympathetic control pathways, and using a multitude of methods to apply the mechanical stimulus. Studies, dating back to the 1880s, show that this response is observed both in amphibians and mammals, including man. The magnitude of the SAN response to stretch depends on a large variety of parameters, including background BR, modalities of mechanical stimulation and pacemaker AP shape. While the exact cellular mechanisms of this expression of cardiac MEF require further investigation, SAC_{NS} would appear to play an important role. Stretch of Purkinje fibres during ventricular loading may lead to faster depolarization of these cells, potentially overriding the SAN BR and thereby contributing to stretch-induced arrhythmia. More studies using Purkinje fibres are required to elucidate this potential role and mechanism.

Effects of NO on the SAN stretch response have not yet been addressed directly. The mechanism that links stretch and NO release is unknown. In cardiac myocytes *in situ*, stretch promotes the integration of caveolae [the location of endothelial NO synthase[53]] into the sarcolemma[54]. The relevance of this effect and its presence in SAN are unknown (see Chapter 7). Another possible mechanism of the positive chronotropic response to stretch – direct electrotonic interaction of SAN pacemaker cells with mechano-sensitive[23,24] cardiac fibroblasts[19] – has been assessed in mathematical models[55] but not yet in direct experiments.

References

1. Bainbridge FA. The influence of venous filling upon the rate of the heart. *J Physiol* 1915;**50**:65–84.
2. Hakumäki MO. Seventy years of the Bainbridge reflex. *Acta Physiol Scand* 1987;**130**:177–185.
3. Donald DE, Shepherd JT. Reflexes from the heart and lungs: physiological curiosities or important regulatory mechanisms. *Cardiovasc Res* 1978;**12**:449–469.
4. Blinks JR. Positive chronotropic effect of increasing right atrial pressure in the isolated mammalian heart. *Am J Physiol* 1956;**186**:299–303.
5. Deck KA. Dehnungseffekte am spontanschlagenden, isolierten Sinusknoten. *Pflügers Arch* 1964;**280**:120–130.
6. Kohl P, Hunter P, Noble D. Stretch-induced changes in heart rate and rhythm: clinical observations, experiments and mathematical models. *Prog Biophys Mol Biol* 1999;**71**:91–138.
7. Bleeker WK, Mackaay AJC, Masson-Pévet M, Bouman LN, Becker AE. Functional and morphological organization of the rabbit sinus node. *Circ Res* 1980;**46**:11–22.
8. Keith A, Flack MW. The form and nature of the muscular connections between the primary divisions of the vertebrate heart. *J Anat Physiol* 1907;**41**:172–189.
9. Deck KA, Änderungen des Ruhepotentials und der Kabeleigenschaften von Purkinje-Fäden bei der Dehnung. *Pflügers Arch* 1964;**280**:131–140.
10. Kaufmann R, Theophile U, Automatie fördernde Dehnungseffekte an Purkinjefäden, Papillarmuskeln und Vorhoftrabekeln von Rhesus-Affen. *Pflügers Arch* 1967;**297**:174–189.
11. Garny A, Kohl P, Noble D. Cellular Open Resource (COR): a public CellML based environment for modelling biological function. *Int J Bifur Chaos* 2003;**13**:3579–3590.
12. Maltsev VA, Lakatta EG. Synergism of coupled subsarcolemmal Ca^{2+} clocks and sarcolemmal voltage clocks confers robust and flexible pacemaker function in a novel pacemaker cell model. *Am J Physiol* 2009;**286**:H594-H615.
13. Hüser J, Blatter LA, Lipsius SL. Intracellular Ca^{2+} release contributes to automaticity in cat atrial pacemaker cells. *J Physiol* 2000;**524**: 415–422.
14. Vinogradova TM, Lakatta EG. Regulation of basal and reserve cardiac pacemaker function by interactions of cAMP-mediated PKA-dependent Ca^{2+} cycling with surface membrane channels. *J Mol Cell Cardiol* 2009;**47**:456–474.
15. Kimura J, Noma A, Iriswara H. Na-Ca exchange current in mammalian heart cells. *Nature* 1986;**319**:596–597.
16. Mangoni ME, Nargeot J. Properties of the hyperpolarization-activated current (If) in isolated mouse sino-atrial cells. *Cardiovasc Res* 2001;**52**: 51–64.
17. Boyett MR, Honjo H, Kodama I. The sinoatrial node, a heterogeneous pacemaker structure. *Cardiovasc Res* 2000;**47**:658–687.
18. Beaulieu P, Lambert C. Peptidic regulation of heart rate and interactions with the autonomic nervous system. *Cardiovasc Res* 1998;**37**:578–585.
19. Camelliti P, Green CR, LeGrice I, Kohl P. Fibroblast network in rabbit sinoatrial node: structural and functional identification of homogeneous and heterogeneous cell coupling. *Circ Res* 2004;**94**: 828–835.
20. Garny A, Noble D, Kohl P. Dimensionality in cardiac modelling. *Prog Biophys Mol Biol* 2005;**87**:47–66.
21. Kirchhof CJHJ, Bonke FIM, Allessie MA, Lammers WJEP. The influence of the atrial myocardium on impulse formation in the rabbit sinus node. *Pflügers Arch* 1987;**410**:198–203.
22. Verheule S, van Kempen MJA, Postma S, Rook MB, Jongsma HJ. Gap junctions in the rabbit sinoatrial node. *Am J Physiol* 2001;**280**: H2103-H2115.
23. Stockbridge LL, French AS. Stretch-activated cation channels in human fibroblasts. *Biophys J* 1988;**54**:187–190.
24. Kohl P, Kamkin AG, Kiseleva IS, Noble D. Mechanosensitive fibroblasts in the sino-atrial node region of rat heart: interaction with cardiomyocytes and possible role. *Exp Physiol* 1994;**79**:943–956.
25. Hearse DJ, Sutherland FJ. Experimental models for the study of cardiovascular function and disease. *Pharmacol Res* 2000;**41**: 597–603.
26. Wilson SJ, Bolter CP. Do cardiac neurons play a role in the intrinsic control of heart rate in the rat? *Exp Physiol* 2002;**87**:675–682.
27. Arai A, Kodama I, Toyama J. Roles of Cl⁻ channels and Ca^{2+} mobilization in stretch-induced increase of SA node pacemaker activity. *Am J Physiol* 1996;**270**:H1726-H1735.
28. Hagiwara N, Masuda H, Shoda M, Irisawa H. Stretch-activated anion currents of rabbit cardiac myocytes. *J Physiol* 1992;**456**:285–302.
29. Lei M, Kohl P. Swelling-induced decrease in spontaneous pacemaker activity of rabbit isolated sino-atrial node cells. *Acta Physiol Scand* 1998;**164**:1–12.
30. Le Guennec J-Y, Peinau N, Argibay JA, Mongo KG, Garnier D. A new method for attachment of isolated mammalian ventricular myocytes for tension recording: length dependence of passive and active tension. *J Mol Cell Cardiol* 1990;**22**:1083–1093.
31. Cooper PJ, Lei M, Cheng L-X, Kohl P. Axial stretch increases spontaneous pacemaker activity in rabbit isolated sinoatrial node cells. *J Appl Physiol* 2000;**89**:2099–2104.

32. Kamiyama A, Niimura I, Sugi H. Length-dependent changes of pacemaker frequency in the isolated rabbit sinoatrial node. *Jap J Physiol* 1984;**34**:153–165.

33. Kuno Y. The significance of the pericardium. *J Physiol* 1915;**50**:1–46.

34. Brooks CM, Lu H-H, Lange G, Mangi R, Shaw RB, Geoly K. Effects of localized stretch of the sinoatrial node region of the dog heart. *Am J Physiol* 1966;**211**:1197–1202.

35. Lange G, Lu H-H, Chang A, Brooks CM. Effect of stretch on the isolated cat sinoatrial node. *Am J Physiol* 1966;**211**:1192–1196.

36. Ju Y-K, Allen DG. Store-operated Ca^{2+} entry and TRPC expression; possible roles in cardiac pacemaker tissue. *Heart Lung Circ* 2007;**16**:349–355.

37. Barrett CJ, Bolter CP, Wilson SJ. The intrinsic rate response of the isolated right atrium of the rat, *Rattus norvegicus. Comp Biochem Physiol - A* 1998;**120**:391–397.

38. Sewall H, Donaldson F. On the influence of variations of intracardiac pressure upon the inhibitory action of the vagus nerve. *J Physiol* 1882;**3**:358–368.

39. Gannier F, White E, Lacampagne A, Garnier D, Le Guennec J-Y. Streptomycin reverses a large stretch induced increase in $[Ca^{2+}]_i$ in isolated guinea pig ventricular myocytes. *Cardiovasc Res* 1994;**28**:1193–1198.

40. Pinksy DJ, Patton S, Mesaros S, *et al.* Mechanical transduction of nitric oxide synthesis in the beating heart. *Circ Res* 1997;**81**:372–379.

41. Vila-Petroff MG, Kim SH, Pepe S, *et al.* Endogenous nitric oxide mechanisms mediate the stretch dependence of Ca^{2+} release in cardiomyocytes. *Nat Cell Biol* 2001;**3**:867–873.

42. Han X, Kobzik L, Severson D, Shimoni Y. Characteristics of nitric oxide-mediated cholinergic modulation of calcium current in rabbit sino-atrial node. *J Physiol* 1998;**509**:741–754.

43. Iribe G, Ward CW, Camelliti P, *et al.* Axial stretch of rat single ventricular cardiomyocytes causes an acute and transient increase in Ca^{2+} spark rate. *Circ Res* 2009;**104**:787–795.

44. Lacampagne A, Gannier F, Argibay J, Garnier D, Le Guennec J-Y. The stretch-activated ion channel blocker gadolinium also blocks L-type calcium channels in isolated ventricular myocytes of the guinea-pig. *Biochim Biophys Acta* 1994;**1191**:205–208.

45. Pascarel C, Hongo K, Cazorla O, White E, Le Guennec JY. Different effects of gadolinium on I_{Kr}, I_{Ks} and I_{K1} in guinea-pig isolated ventricular myocytes. *Br J Pharmacol* 1998;**124**:356–360.

46. Caldwell RA, Clemo HF, Baumgarten CM. Using gadolinium to identify stretch-activated channels: technical considerations. *Am J Physiol* 1998;**275**:C619-C621.

47. Belus A, White E. Streptomycin and intracellular calcium modulate the response of single guinea-pig ventricular myocytes to axial stretch. *J Physiol* 2003;**546**:501–509.

48. Belus A, White E. Effects of streptomycin sulphate on ICaL, IKr and IKs in guinea-pig ventricular myocytes. *Eur J Pharmacol* 2002;**445**:171–178.

49. Cooper PJ, Kohl P. Species- and preparation-dependence of stretch effects on sino-atrial node pacemaking. *Ann N Y Acad Sci* 2005;**1047**:324–335.

50. Sung D, Schettler J, Omens JH, McCulloch AD. Ventricular filling slows epicardial conduction and increases action potential duration in an optical mapping study of the isolated rabbit heart. *J Cardiovasc Electrophysiol* 2003;**14**:739–749.

51. Suchyna TM, Johnson JH, Hamer K, *et al.* Identification of a peptide toxin from *Grammostola spatulata* spider venom that blocks cation-selective stretch-activated channels. *J Gen Physiol* 2000;**115**:583–98

52. Bode F, Sachs F, Franz MR. Tarantula peptide inhibits atrial fibrillation. *Nature* 2001;**409**:35–36.

53. Feron O, Belhasson L, Kobzik L, Smith TW, Kelly RA, Michel T. Endothelial nitric oxide synthase targetting to caveolae: specific interactions with caveolin isoforms in cardiac myocytes and endothelial cells. *J Biol Chem* 1996;**271**:22810–22814.

54. Kohl P, Cooper PJ, Holloway H. Effects of acute ventricular volume manipulation on *in situ* cardiomyocyte cell membrane configuration. *Prog Biophys Mol Biol* 2003;**82**:221–227.

55. Kohl P, Noble D. Mechanosensitive connective tissue: potential influence on heart rhythm. *Cardiovasc Res* 1996;**32**:62–68.

Mechano-electric coupling in working cardiomyocytes: diastolic and systolic effects

Michael R. Franz

Background

Cells responding to mechanical stimuli were among the first cells on earth. An amoeba does not have many senses, but when it encounters an obstacle in its path, it reacts. Mechano-sensitive cells exist in almost every part of the body, from cochlear hair cells to digestive tract cells to bone cells to cardiac cells. While some of these mechano-sensitive properties make sense at first sight (for instance bone cells adjusting to the force of gravity, or intestinal cells responding to filling of the gut, or blood vessels responding to volume and pressure), the mechano-sensitive role or purpose of other cells in the body is less obvious, especially its secondary, electrophysiological effects.

Diastole and systole of the heart

The haemodynamic cycle of the heart is commonly separated into diastole and systole, the former being the relaxation period when blood filling from the venous system to the ventricles occurs, the latter the period of contraction and blood ejection into the arterial systems. Loading the ventricle with 'new' blood volume during diastole is known as **preload**. The filling phase pre-stretches the ventricular myocardium and, as the Frank–Starling mechanism describes, enhances the subsequent systolic force. Systolic mechanical stress refers to the events experienced by the ventricular walls during contraction (with subsequent intraventricular pressure rise) and ejection of blood. Since the ejection of blood needs to occur against the aortic and pulmonary artery impedance, mechanical systole works against **afterload**. While preload is a volume (or length, in mainly one-dimensional preparations such as cells or trabeculae), afterload is a pressure (or tension). Thus, despite their name similarity, they are actually different physical entities.

The realistic situation in the heart, however, is not this simply divided into these two categories. The ventricles are not homogeneous in wall thickness, and contractile properties vary between regions and across the wall. Electrical activation and therefore mechanical activation, albeit swift in normal hearts, is not synchronous throughout the ventricles. In diseased hearts, especially in hearts with contractile failure and/or conduction disease [e.g. left

bundle branch block (LBBB)] the degree of dysynchronous electrical and mechanical activation can be severe. There, contraction in early-activated parts can raise intraventricular pressure while segments still in diastole experience additional preloading. This intraventricular mechanical interaction during early systole is also known as 'tethering'. Even in the healthy heart, endocardial mechanical activation pre-strains epicardial layers, during normal iso-volumetric contraction[1]. The clinical determination of this, haemodynamically potentially adverse, scenario and its remedies are discussed in Chapter 62.

Cardiac mechano-sensitivity

At the cellular level, patch-clamp studies identified stretch-activated ion channels (SAC) in myocytes from several species, including chick[2] and rabbit[3], and helped explain electrophysiological effects of myocardial stretch at the channel level. The first mammalian SAC was reported in rat by Craelius et al.[4].

In the intact heart, microelectrode recordings of transmembrane action potentials (AP) are difficult to perform and have been impossible in the in situ human heart. The surface electrocardiogram (ECG), on the other hand, is too insensitive to detect electrophysiological stretch effects, probably due to the fact that such electrical effects are either (1) too slow, (2) too small, (3) too global within the heart or (4) masked by other electrophysiological changes occurring during repolarization (the U wave in the ECG is a special case and is discussed in great detail in Chapter 38). Thus, a significant body of information regarding electrophysiological stretch effects has been acquired utilizing monophasic action potential (MAP) recordings[5–7]. Such recordings, if done with proper technique and controls, can detect local AP waveforms in the vigorously beating heart, including the clinical setting. More recently, optical mapping of transmembrane potentials has provided further information on mechano-electrical coupling (MEC) and its heterogeneity (see below).

Cardiac cells respond to mechanical stimuli almost as readily as they do to electrical stimuli. Franz et al. (3) showed in isolated perfused rabbit hearts with atrio-ventricular (AV) block, instrumented with an intraventricular fluid-filled balloon connected to a computer-driven piston, that volume pulses of lower amplitude cause membrane depolarizations during diastole (see Fig. 14.1). When volume pulses were gradually ramped up, a threshold was seen beyond which each volume pulse triggered a beat (mechanical pacing). This is surprisingly similar to electrical pacing.

Mechanical pacing has been shown to also work in the human heart. Zoll and other inventors[9] have devised mechanical transthoracic pacing by applying mechanical stimuli to the asystolic heart to revive beating in emergency situations. Chest thumps also have been shown to start up an asystolic human heart and sometimes, but rarely, even convert ventricular fibrillation to sinus rhythm (see Chapter 50). Clinical electrophysiologists know that even a casual but sudden contact with a catheter to the endocardium usually elicits an ectopic beat at the site of contact. So there is little doubt that heart tissue (including human myocardium) is electrically responsive to mechanical stimuli. This phenomenon, which includes changes in the shape of the AP and secondary cellular effects, is known as MEC.

Electrophysiological effects of acute stretch: *ex vivo* studies

Numerous studies have shown that the action potential duration (APD), particularly at its plateau level, *shortens* during interventions that produce either greater intraventricular pressure or greater myocardial contractility, either by inotropic agents or by indigenous catecholamines. This early APD shortening, including that caused by stretch, is often heterogeneous (see below).

The first intracellular studies found stretch to shorten APD[10,11]. In MAP recordings from the left ventricular epicardium of the isolated canine heart, acutely increased mechanical load resulted in a decrease of APD as well as of effective refractory period (ERP)[12–14]. Similar results were found in isolated rabbit hearts[8]. Other investigators, however, reported a *lengthening* of APD in response to direct myocardial stretch[15,16]. Stretch-induced electrophysiological changes appeared to differ depending on whether acute mechanical stretch was applied in the form of increased preload or increased afterload[12,16–18]. The repolarization level at which APD was measured, as well as the mode of ventricular contraction, may offer an explanation. Franz et al.[16] studied stretch-induced changes in the isovolumically beating canine ventricle and demonstrated that an increase in ventricular volume load with a simultaneous increase in ventricular pressure shortened the APD at early repolarization levels, while APD near complete repolarization was lengthened (Fig. 14.2). Similar findings were reported by Hansen[17] from isolated canine hearts. Both investigators noted that the

increase in overall APD under increased isovolumic load occurred in the shape of early after-depolarizations (EAD)[16,17]. These divergent results were later reconciled by the time- and voltage-dependent characteristics of SAC, in direct comparison between computer simulation and experimental data (see below)[19].

Diastolic depolarization and a decrease in peak systolic AP amplitude were reported under various conditions of isovolumic loading in both dog[16] and rabbit[3] studies. These findings were in line with data reported from intracellular recordings in sinus node, Purkinje and ventricular muscle fibres exhibiting both less negative resting potential levels and reduced AP amplitudes under stretch[20–22]. The studies by Franz et al.[16] and Hansen[17] also addressed the question whether preload (i.e. diastolic volume increase) or systolic outflow impedance (afterload) are more important for inducing stretch-induced electrophysiological changes. Both studies showed that only *preload* increases lead to the acute electrophysiological changes described above. Changing the ventricular contraction mode from isovolumic to ejecting, despite elevated preload, abolished EAD induction immediately[16] (Fig. 14.3).

In the *in situ* heart setting, a strict separation between preload and afterload is not practical. When in open-chest dogs the ascending aorta was transiently occluded with large rubber-coated haemostats, it was the outflow tract obstruction that led to the sudden increase in left ventricular pressure (LVP), resulting in EAD induction and premature beats, thereby obfuscating the separate roles of preload and afterload. In the example shown in Fig. 14.4, the first beat after the onset of the clamp [evidenced by loss of aortic pressure (AoP) pulses] is followed by a premature depolarization that generates relatively little pressure. The beat following the compensatory pause exhibits post-extrasystolic potentiation with a much higher LVP and an EAD that triggers another premature depolarization. This sequence repeats itself four times, until release of the aortic clamp. What does this mean? There are two compatible explanations. First, the added stretch from enhanced preload and afterload during aortic occlusion leads to electrophysiological effects that reach threshold for ectopic depolarization. Second, the potentiated post-pause beat involves increased sarcoplasmic reticulum calcium load, leading to greater, spontaneous EAD.

Electrophysiological effects of short transient stretch – importance of timing during systole or diastole

Short rapid stretch pulses seem very adept at causing premature ventricular depolarizations in myocardial tissue of various species[15,23–25]. The velocity with which acute stretch pulses are applied (i.e. the stretch ramp velocity) was found to be an independent contributor to the induction of premature beats[8].

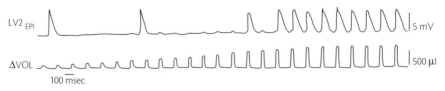

Fig. 14.1 Volume pulses of increasing amplitude applied to rabbit heart with intraventricular fluid-filled balloon. Note diastolic depolarizations during subthreshold pulses and ectopic beats during suprathreshold pulses. ΔVOL denotes balloon volume changes; LV2$_{EPI}$, one of two epicardial MAP recordings. [Reproduced, with permission, from Franz MR, Cima R, Wang D, Profitt D, Kurz R (1992) Electrophysiological effects of myocardial stretch and mechanical determinants of stretch-activated arrhythmias. *Circulation* **86**:968–978.]

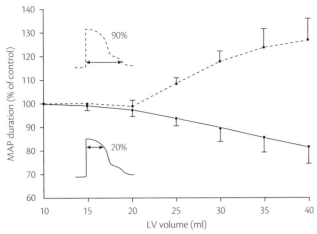

Fig. 14.2 MAP recordings were obtained from epicardium of isolated cross-perfused canine left ventricles (LV) instrumented with servo-controlled intracavity balloon. Data are average +/− SD from six ventricles beating isovolumically at constant cycle length of 500 msec during seven volume loading interventions. APD responded divergently depending on the level of repolarization. Plateau duration (APD at 20% repolarization) shortened with increasing volume, while APD at 90% repolarization lengthened due to the occurrence of after-depolarizations (see also Fig. 14.4). [Reproduced, with permission, from Franz MR, Burkhoff D, Yue DT, Sagawa K (1989) Mechanically induced action potential changes and arrhythmia in isolated and in situ canine hearts. *Cardiovasc Res* **23**:213–223.]

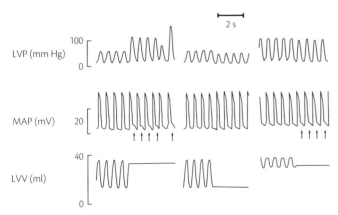

Fig. 14.3 MAP recordings from epicardium of isolated cross-perfused canine left ventricle (same preparation as in Fig. 14.1). LV volume (LVV, bottom) and outflow impedance were controlled by an intraventricular fluid-filled balloon coupled to a servo-controlled piston pump, while MAP (middle) and LV pressure (LVP, top) were recorded. Left column: normal MAP shapes were observed when the LV was allowed to eject freely, but with sudden clamping of LV volume at end-diastolic level, early after-depolarizations immediately occurred (arrows). Middle column: clamping LVV at end-systole did not cause after-depolarizations in the MAP recording. Right column: small after-depolarizations were recorded when ventricular contractions started at high diastolic volume and also had to eject against increased afterload. These after-depolarizations increased when the volume was clamped at end-systole. LV pressure (LVP) was measured with a catheter-tip transducer inserted within the balloon. [Reproduced, with permission, from Franz MR, Burkhoff D, Yue DT, Sagawa K (1989) Mechanically induced action potential changes and arrhythmia in isolated and in situ canine hearts. *Cardiovasc Res* **23**:213–223.]

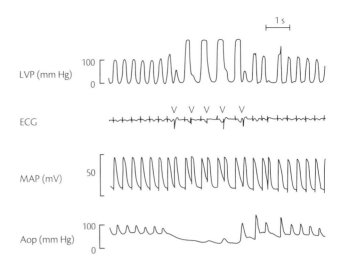

Fig. 14.4 After-depolarizations and ventricular arrhythmia with bigeminal pattern during transient aortic occlusion. See text for details. [Reproduced, with permission, from Franz MR, Burkhoff D, Yue DT, Sagawa K (1989) Mechanically induced action potential changes and arrhythmia in isolated and in situ canine hearts. *Cardiovasc Res* **23**:213–223.]

Zabel *et al.*[19] investigated the effects of short volume pulses administered at different times during systole and diastole, in comparison to longer, static stretch of the same amplitude. In this study, both repolarizing and depolarizing responses were observed with a remarkable dependence on the timing of the stretch pulse with respect to the MAP phase. A short transient stretch pulse elicited either transient *de*polarizations when applied during late systole or diastole, or transient *re*polarizations when applied during the plateau of the MAP. A stretch pulse placed towards the end of the MAP caused depolarizations that mimicked EAD or, if timed to occur after completion of the MAP, mimicked a delayed after-depolarization (DAD). With sufficient amplitude of the stretch-induced diastolic depolarizations, premature ventricular contractions were caused, confirming earlier results (see Fig. 14.1).

Stacy *et al.*[25] also confirmed these results but postulated an accelerated phase 4 depolarization of Purkinje fibres as the mechanism for premature beats. In contrast to 'classical' early or delayed after-depolarizations, stretch-activated depolarizations did not depend on the trigger of a preceding AP. The studies by Zabel *et al.*[19] and Stacy *et al.*[25] could together demonstrate that the amplitude of a stretch-activated depolarization is linearly correlated with the amplitude of the underlying stretch-pulse. In addition to that, Zabel *et al.*[19] found that the amplitude of a stretch-related repolarization 'dip' during the plateau phase of the MAP exhibited a similar linear relationship to the stretch pulse amplitude as did the diastolic depolarization 'hump' (Fig. 14.5). Stretch pulses during the early phase 3 of the AP (downward from the plateau) caused smaller repolarizing deflections than during the plateau of the AP. Similarly, stretch-activated depolarizations became smaller when the pulse was moved from full repolarization levels towards a less complete repolarization level. Halfway between these opposite responses, at the midway between peak electrical systole and full membrane repolarization, a neutral response to stretch was found: no discernable changes in the shape of the AP were noted (Fig. 14.5d). It is noteworthy that this MEC 'immunity'

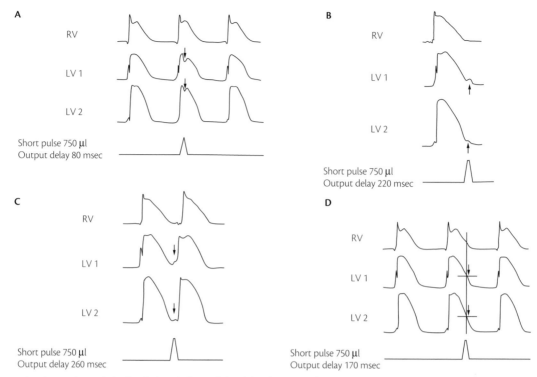

Fig. 14.5 Short stretch pulses evoke repolarization during AP plateau **(A)** and depolarization when applied during late phase 3 **(B)** or diastole **(C)**. Minimal effects are seen when stretch pulse is given at mid of phase 3 (**(D)**, arrows and bars). RV, right ventricular MAP recording; LV1 and LV2, MAP recordings from two left ventricular sites (all epicardial). [Reproduced, with permission, from Zabel M, Koller BS, Sachs F, Franz MR (1996) Stretch-induced voltage changes in the isolated beating heart: importance of the timing of stretch and implications for stretch-activated ion channels. *Cardiovasc Res* **32**:120–130.]

usually coincides with the peak ventricular pressure in most mammalian species, with the kangaroo heart being a notable exception[26].

Electrophysiological effects of sustained acute stretch – dispersion of repolarization

Slowly applied and sustained stretch interventions do not trigger ventricular arrhythmias[3,19]. Sodium channel activation is required to occur before voltage-dependent inactivation renders further depolarization futile. Zabel *et al.*[27] therefore explored the electrophysiological effects of sustained stretch, and showed that a static load of the isolated rabbit ventricle influences several electrophysiological parameters, including repolarization and activation. APD at 90% repolarization (APD_{90}) was shortened in the volume-loaded LV. At the same time, the refractory period was shortened. While the common effect of mechanical loading was to shorten the APD and refractoriness, that study also observed lengthening of APD_{90} in some parts of the heart (compare with Fig. 14.2). The disparity of stretch effects between various locations in the ventricle, particularly between the loaded LV and the non-stretched RV, resulted in an increased dispersion of ventricular repolarization. The latter parameter is known to be arrhythmogenic in many experimental models[28–30]. The activation time – measured as the longest interval between the pacing stimulus and the earliest MAP upstroke – was prolonged, particularly during premature extra-stimulation. A prolongation of conduction time by stretch was also found by Dominguez and Fozzard[31] in Purkinje fibres and Calkins *et al.*[13] in the intact canine heart. Conduction time is a second

arrhythmogenic parameter influenced by stretch or load. Arrhythmogenicity of sustained stretch could be demonstrated in dog models[13,14,24], where the induction of sustained ventricular arrhythmias was facilitated by loading (for more detail see Chapter 25). Stretch also enhances the inducibility and sustenance of atrial fibrillation and is antagonized by application of GsMTx-4, a highly selective SAC blocker (see Chapters 2 and 65).

Ionic basis for stretch-induced effects in intact heart studies – SAC

The myocardium contains SAC that allow both inward and outward currents, depending on their ion selectivity and the actual membrane potential of affected cells[2,32,33]. Whole-cell patch-clamp recordings of non-selective cation SAC (SAC_{NS}) currents in the heart indicated a reversal potential in the range of −10 to −30 mV at 35°C[34]. Characteristics of SAC_{NS} channels from patch-clamp studies were added to a computer heart model in order to simulate the effects of short, pulsatile stretch on the MAP. A remarkable agreement was found between the simulation data derived from guinea-pig[19] and experimental results from intact rabbit heart studies[19] (Fig. 14.6).

The computer model predicted that SAC_{NS} activation during the diastolic resting potential should result in an inward current (i.e. depolarization) and, conversely, that activation during the AP plateau should result in an outward current (i.e. repolarization). This is in keeping with experimentally observed data (Fig. 14.7). Reversal potential and linearity of the current-voltage relation underscore

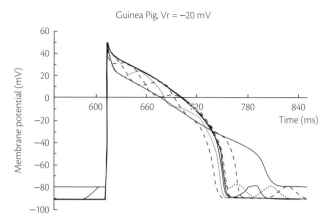

Guinea Pig, Vr = −20 mV

Fig. 14.6 Computer simulation of the effect of trapezoidal stretch pulses (20 ms rise and fall, 10 ms plateau) on the AP, using the program HEART (Oxsoft Ltd, Oxford, UK) with integrated SAC$_{NS}$. [Reproduced, with permission, from Zabel M, Koller BS, Sachs F, Franz MR (1996) Stretch-induced voltage changes in the isolated beating heart: importance of the timing of stretch and implications for stretch-activated ion channels. *Cardiovasc Res* **32**:120–130.]

the voltage-independence of SAC$_{NS}$. Deviations between the experimental data and the computer simulations occur mainly in late repolarization when the AP time course is most sensitive to voltage changes[5,35].

Additional experimental evidence for a role of SAC$_{NS}$ in mediating APD shortening was provided by Eckardt *et al.*[36] who in isolated perfused rabbit hearts showed that streptomycin (an SAC blocker) but not verapamil (a Ca-channel blocker) prevented APD shortening during acute ventricular dilatation.

Heterogeneity of ventricular stretch during loading

Ventricles, even in their normal physiological states, do not contract synchronously due to differences in their regional activation

times, wall thickness, intrinsic contractility differences, 'fibre' orientation and fibro-elastic compliance. Thus, a simple uniform stretch model cannot describe MEC in a clinically relevant manner, let alone the impact of LBBB in patients with heart failure.

The recent study by Seo *et al.*[37] elegantly demonstrates the heterogeneous effects of ventricular wall stretch (see Fig. 14.8). The investigators used optical voltage dye-mapping in isolated perfused rabbit hearts to study the electrophysiological effects of myocardial stretch across the right ventricle during diastole and early systole. Myocardial strain was tagged by markers while voltage mapping provided both AP displays and activation wave fronts, and thus also conduction velocities. The authors found that heterogeneity in wall thickness was a major predictor of stretch-induced electro-physiological events, with thinner wall segments being the most responsive. Also, most APs started at the point where the RV tissue was glued to the holding clamp, i.e. where the largest stress gradients and strain heterogeneity occurred. Mid-level stretch pulses were most likely to induce focal ectopic beats. Low-level activations fell below the threshold for electrical activation, while high-level stretch induced synchronous activation of the whole tissue. This is reminiscent of the upper level of vulnerability observed in implantable cardiac defibrillator studies and MEC research in isolated rabbit hearts (see Chapter 31 for details). Based on these careful mapping studies the authors concluded that high-level stretch pulses causing depolarization in all parts of the stretched preparation were less arrhythmogenic than mid-level stretch pulses which created a milieu of dispersed depolarization and only focal excitation. In fact, sustained re-entrant tachyarrhythmias were noted, some with spiral wave pattern.

Conclusions and outlook

There is ample experimental evidence to suggest that myocardial mechanical load alters myocardial electrophysiology in a way that is likely to facilitate the induction and/or sustenance of ventricular arrhythmias.

The electrophysiological effects of pulsatile stretch, stretch generated by increased preload and afterload, and acute static

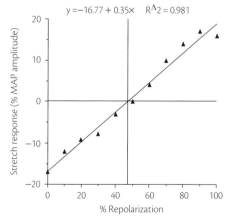

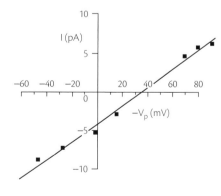

Fig. 14.7 Left, IV plot constructed from MAP data during stretch at various times of the depolarization and repolarization phase (see Fig. 14.5). Right, IV graph from the study by Craelius *et al.* [4] Note that data were plotted in reference to resting potential, rather than true zero mV, so the reversal potential is +36 mV 'depolarized from resting' potential (i.e. in the typical range of reversal potentials for SAC$_{NS}$), and that currents were measured in cell-attached mode. [Left graph reproduced, with permission, from Zabel M, Koller BS, Sachs F, Franz MR (1996) Stretch-induced voltage changes in the isolated beating heart: importance of the timing of stretch and implications for stretch-activated ion channels. *Cardiovasc Res* **32**:120–130. Right graph reproduced, with permission, from Craelius W, Chen V, El-Sherif N (1988) Stretch activated ion channels in ventricular myocytes. *Biosci Rep* **8**:407–414.]

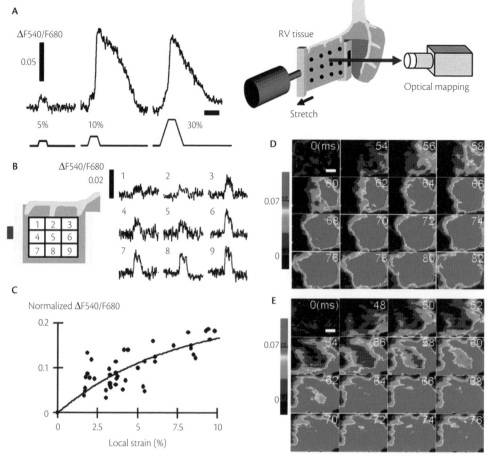

Fig. 14.8 Alterations in the electrical response in right-ventricular (RV) tissue from isolated perfused rabbit heart. **A** Ratiometric optical signals in response to 5%, 10% and 30% stretches (from left to right; scale bar: 100 ms). **B** Spatiotemporal pattern of the depolarizations in response to a 5% stretch. **C** Relationship between the changes in the normalized optical signals and the local strain under the excitation threshold ($n = 5$). **D** and **E** Representative action potentials and optical maps in response to 10% and 30% stretches. [Reproduced, with permission, from Seo K, Inagaki M, Nishimura S, *et al.* (2010) Structural heterogeneity in the ventricular wall plays a significant role in the initiation of stretch-induced arrhythmias in perfused rabbit right ventricular tissues and whole heart preparations. *Circ Res* **106**:176–184.] (See color plate section.)

mechanical stretch can be explained by the existence of SAC. As expected from the known characteristics of these channels, stretch generates a repolarizing response during systole, a neutral response in the middle of phase 3 near the reversal potential of SAC_{NS} and a depolarizing response during diastole. The latter response may mimic EAD that can induce propagated ventricular excitations. Sustained stretch increases dispersion of ventricular excitability and repolarization, refractoriness and opportunity for functional re-entry arrhythmias, further aided by disparate effects on conduction velocity.

The fact that the myocardium is protected from the highest stress occurring at peak systolic contraction and intraventricular pressure rise is not only explained by its highest myocardial stiffness at that time; the myocardial cells also enjoy the benefit of being at their most 'immune' state for stretch at this time, due to the equilibrium potential of SAC_{NS}.

In the near future, MEC effects may hopefully be open to faithful recording in the human heart, to provide new understanding of arrhythmias in the failing heart and to devise new therapies.

References

1. Ashikaga H, van der Spoel TI, Coppola BA, Omens JH. Transmural myocardial mechanics during isovolumic contraction. *JACC Cardiovasc Imag* 2009;**2**:202–211.
2. Ruknudin A, Sachs F, Bustamante JO. Stretch-activated ion channels in tissue-cultured chick heart. *Am J Physiol* 1993;**264**:H960–H972.
3. Hagiwara N, Masuda H, Shoda M, Irisawa H. Stretch-activated anion currents of rabbit cardiac myocytes. *J Physiol* 1992;**456**:285–302.
4. Craelius W, Chen V, El-Sherif N. Stretch activated ion channels in ventricular myocytes. *Biosci Rep* 1988;**8**:407–414.
5. Franz MR, Burkhoff D, Spurgeon H, Weisfeldt ML, Lakatta EG. In vitro validation of a new cardiac catheter technique for recording monophasic action potentials. *Eur Heart J* 1986;**7**: 34–41.
6. Franz MR. Method and theory of monophasic action potential recording. *Prog Cardiovasc Dis* 1991;**33**:347–368.
7. Franz MR, Chin MC, Sharkey HR, Griffin JC, Scheinman MM. A new single catheter technique for simultaneous measurement of action potential duration and refractory period in vivo. *J Am Coll Cardiol* 1990;**16**:878–886.

8. Franz MR, Cima R, Wang D, Profitt D, Kurz R. Electrophysiological effects of myocardial stretch and mechanical determinants of stretch-activated arrhythmias. *Circulation* 1992;**86**:968–978.

9. Zoll PM, Belgard AH, Weintraub MJ, Frank HA. External mechanical cardiac stimulation. *N Engl J Med* 1976;**294**:1274–1275.

10. Dudel J, Trautwein W. Das Aktionspotential und Mechanogramm des Herzmuskels unter dem Einfluss der Dehnung. *Cardiologie* 1954;**25**:344.

11. Kaufmann R, Lab MJ, Hennekes R, Krause H. Feedback interaction of mechanical and electrical events in the isolated ventricular myocardium (cat papillary muscle). *Pflugers Arch* 1971;**332**:96.

12. Lerman BB, Burkhoff D, Yue DT, Franz MR, Sagawa K. Mechanoelectrical feedback: independent role of preload and contractility in modulation of canine ventricular excitability. *J Clin Invest* 1985;**76**:1843–1850.

13. Calkins H, Maughan WL, Kass DA, Sagawa K, Levine JH. Electrophysiological effect of volume load in isolated canine hearts. *Am J Physiol* 1989;**256**:H1697–H1706.

14. Calkins H, Maughan WL, Weisman HF, Sugiura S, Sagawa K, Levine JH. Effect of acute volume load on refractoriness and arrhythmia development in isolated, chronically infarcted canine hearts. *Circulation* 1989;**79**:687–697.

15. Lab MJ. Mechanically dependent changes in action potentials recorded from the intact frog ventricle. *Circ Res* 1978;**42**:519–528.

16. Franz MR, Burkhoff D, Yue DT, Sagawa K. Mechanically induced action potential changes and arrhythmia in isolated and in situ canine hearts. *Cardiovasc Res* 1989;**23**:213–223.

17. Hansen DE. Mechanoelectrical feedback effects of altering preload, afterload, and ventricular shortening. *Am J Physiol* 1993;**264**: H423-H432.

18. Coulshed DS, Cowan JC. Contraction-excitation feedback in an ejecting whole heart model– dependence of action potential duration on left ventricular diastolic and systolic pressures. *Cardiovasc Res* 1991;**25**:343–352.

19. Zabel M, Koller BS, Sachs F, Franz MR. Stretch-induced voltage changes in the isolated beating heart: importance of the timing of stretch and implications for stretch- activated ion channels. *Cardiovasc Res* 1996;**32**:120–130.

20. Deck KA, Dehnungseffekte am spontanschlagenden, isolierten Sinusknoten. *Pflügers Arch* 1964;**280**:120–130.

21. Penefsky ZJ, Hoffman BF. Effects of stretch on mechanical and electrical properties of cardiac muscle. *Am J Physiol* 1963;**204**:433.

22. Boland J, Troquet J. Intracellular action potential changes induced in both ventricles of the rat by an acute right ventricular pressure overload. *Cardiovasc Res* 1980;**14**:735–740.

23. Dean JW, Lab MJ. Effect of changes in load on monophasic action potential and segment length of pig heart in situ. *Cardiovasc Res* 1989;**23**:887–896.

24. Hansen DE, Craig CS, Hondeghem LM. Stretch-induced arrhythmias in the isolated canine ventricle. Evidence for the importance of mechanoelectrical feedback. *Circulation* 1990;**81**:1094–1105.

25. Stacy GP, Jr., Jobe RL, Taylor LK, Hansen DE. Stretch-induced depolarizations as a trigger of arrhythmias in isolated canine left ventricles. *Am J Physiol* 1992;**263**:H613–621.

26. Surawicz B. U wave emerges from obscurity when the heart pumps like in a kangaroo. *Heart Rhythm* 2008;**5**:246–247.

27. Zabel M, Portnoy S, Franz MR. Electrocardiographic indexes of dispersion of ventricular repolarization: an isolated heart validation study. *J Am Coll Cardiol* 1995;**25**:746–752.

28. Han J, Moe GK. Nonuniform recovery of excitability in ventricular muscle. *Circ Res* 1964;**14**:44–60.

29. Kuo CS, Munakata K, Reddy CP, Surawicz B. Characteristics and possible mechanism of ventricular arrhythmia dependent on the dispersion of action potential durations. *Circulation* 1983;**67**: 1356–1367.

30. Opthof T, Misier AR, Coronel R, *et al.* Dispersion of refractoriness in canine ventricular myocardium. Effects of sympathetic stimulation. *Circ Res* 1991;**68**:1204–1215.

31. Dominguez G, Fozzard HA. Effect of stretch on conduction velocity and cable properties of cardiac Purkinje fibers. *Am J Physiol* 1979;**237**:C119-C124.

32. Bustamante JO, Ruknudin A, Sachs F. Stretch-activated channels in heart cells: relevance to cardiac hypertrophy. *J Cardiovasc Pharmacol* 1991;**17**:S110–S113.

33. Sigurdson W, Ruknudin A, Sachs F. Calcium imaging of mechanically induced fluxes in tissue-cultured chick heart: role of stretch-activated ion channels. *Am J Physiol* 1992;**262**:H1110–H1115.

34. Hu H, Sachs F. Mechanically activated currents in chick heart cells. *J Membr Biol* 1996;**154**:205–216.

35. Ino T, Karagueuzian HS, Hong K, Meesmann M, Mandel WJ, Peter T. Relation of monophasic action potential recorded with contact electrode to underlying transmembrane action potential properties in isolated cardiac tissues: a systematic microelectrode validation study. *Cardiovasc Res* 1988;**22**:255–264.

36. Eckardt L, Kirchhof P, Monnig G, Breithardt G, Borggrefe M, Haverkamp W. Modification of stretch-induced shortening of repolarization by streptomycin in the isolated rabbit heart. *J Cardiovasc Pharmacol* 2000;**36**:711–721.

37. Seo K, Inagaki M, Nishimura S, Hidaka I, Sugimachi M, Hisada T, Sugiura S. Structural heterogeneity in the ventricular wall plays a significant role in the initiation of stretch-induced arrhythmias in perfused rabbit right ventricular tissues and whole heart preparations. *Circ Res* 2010;**106**:176–184.

Mechano-sensitivity of pulmonary vein cells: implications for atrial arrhythmogenesis

Chang Ahn Seol, Won Tae Kim, Jae Boum Youm, Yung E. Earm and Chae Hun Leem

Background

After the discovery that the ectopic foci of paroxysmal atrial fibrillation (AF) were mainly located in the pulmonary vein[1], studies of the relationship between the pulmonary veins (PV) and AF rapidly increased. In this chapter we briefly review the anatomical and electrical characteristics of the PV and the possible linkage between the stretch of PV and the development of AF.

Anatomical structure at the junction between the pulmonary veins and the left atrium

Typically, four main PV (superior and inferior branch from each right and left lung) are connected to the left atrium (LA). At the junction between the LA and PV, sphincter-like formations of myocardium and myocardial sleeves are usually found[2]. Superior PV have thicker sphincter-like structures and longer myocardial sleeves than inferior PV[2]. The histology of PV shows that a longitudinal internal layer is composed of a myocardial sleeve and a circular external layer is composed of the sphincter-like structure[3,4].

A possible role of PV in the transition from paroxysmal AF to chronic AF

The causes of developing AF are still obscure. Two independent studies[5,6] showed that tachycardia-induced electrical remodelling in atria could occur and this phenomenon was referred as 'AF begets AF'[6]. Atrial tachycardias can induce changes in the activities of ion channels underlying the L-type Ca^{2+} current ($I_{Ca,L}$), transient outward K^+ current (I_{to})[7], the fast Na^+ current (I_{Na})[8] and Ca^{2+} handling[9]. Also, connexins governing cell-to-cell communication are changed in their expression level and compositions in an AF model of goat[10]. Ca^{2+} overload may be an important contributor as an early and common signalling mechanism[11,12],

even though those concepts still need to be proven. Recently, arrhythmia mechanisms related to ion-channel remodelling have been thoroughly reviewed by Nattel *et al.*[13]. Therefore, the mechanism of the transition from paroxysmal AF to chronic AF is likely explained by ion-channel remodelling induced by tachycardia. However, the causes of tachycardia are still in need of further explanation.

The most important report on the relationship between AF and PV came from Haissaguerre's group in 1998[1]. They demonstrated that over 90% of patients with paroxysmal AF had an ectopic focus in PV, and their AF could be successfully treated by disconnecting electrical connection between PV and the LA using radiofrequency ablation. They found the largest number of foci in the left superior PV and then the right superior, the left inferior and the right inferior PV in order of the foci number. The number of foci and the maximal distance of the myocardial sleeve in each PV showed a significant correlation[4]. After Haissaguerre's study, more than several thousand papers on the relationship between PV and AF were published, most of them suggesting that the ectopic activity in PV is one of the major causes of developing AF. From the clinical and experimental results it can be inferred that ectopic activities in PV cause the re-entrant activities in atria, which, in turn, develop into chronic AF by the mechanism of tachycardia-induced ion-channel remodelling[14,15].

Electrical characteristics of PV

The first electrophysiological studies of extrapulmonary veins were done in 1969[16]. This report showed that action potentials similar to that of the atrium could be recorded and that epinephrine or isoproterenol could evoke pacemaker activity in the extrapulmonary vein of guinea pig which could be propagated to the atrium retrogradely. Cheung[17,18] showed that the spontaneous action potentials (AP) could be generated in myocardial sleeves in PV and that PV could be ectopic foci in digitalis-induced arrhythmia.

The spontaneous AP with diastolic depolarization were observed in more than 75% of tested cardiac myocytes in PV of rabbit[19–21]. Studies of ionic currents in canine and rabbit PV cardiomyocytes have identified several types of currents, including acetylcholine-activated K^+ current ($I_{K,Ach}$), I_{Na}, $I_{Ca,L}$, Na^+/Ca^{2+} exchange current (I_{NCX}), T-type Ca^{2+} current ($I_{Ca,T}$), inward rectifier K^+ current (I_{K1}), slow and rapid component of the delayed rectifier K^+ currents (I_{Ks}, I_{Kr}), hyperpolarization-activated K^+ current (I_{KH}) and Ca^{2+}-activated Cl^- current ($I_{Ca,Cl}$)[19,21–25]. Also, recently, the first simulation of the spontaneous AP model was reported[19]. Automaticity in isolated cardiomyocytes in PV was shown in dog and rabbit [19–21,26], but was not observed in single isolated PV cardiomyocytes from dog[24] or in rabbit PV *in situ*[27]. Honjo *et al.*[27] showed that PV could elicit automaticity by pacing in the presence of low-concentration ryanodine, which suggested the possibility that Ca^{2+} dysregulation may generate automaticity in PV. However, the fundamental question of what causes such an ectopic activity in PV is not clearly answered yet.

AF vs the stretch of atrium and PV

The heart itself is physiologically a stretch-sensing organ that controls its own beating frequency and contractility and the whole body water balance by releasing an atrial natriuretic peptide. In pathological conditions, the stretch of myocardium may cause arrhythmia[28,29]. Several cardiac disorders may predispose subjects to AF, including coronary artery disease, pericarditis, mitral valve disease, congenital heart disease (CHD), thyrotoxic heart disease and hypertension[30,31]. Those cardiac disorders are thought to promote AF by increasing atrial pressure and/or by causing atrial dilatation[32–35]. It is still unclear whether the atrial dilatation is a consequence or a cause of AF[36]; however, it may be true that atrial dilatation and AF are mutually dependent and constitute a vicious circle[37].

Experimentally induced atrial dilatation could also induce AF in dog, feline and rabbit[38–41]. The mechanical stretch of the cardiac cell membrane can activate stretch-activated cation currents in ventricular or atrial cardiomyocytes[42–44] and also stretch-activated anion currents in rabbit ventricular myocyte[45]. AF inducibility by the burst-pacing was increased as intra-atrial pressure became larger and these effects were attenuated by stretch-activated channel (SAC) blockers such as gadolinium and GsMTx-4[46,47].

Atrial dilation, therefore, may activate SAC and contribute to AF induction.

Several reports showed the dilatation of PV in AF patients[48–52]. Those studies showed that superior PV had larger diameters in AF patients regardless of paroxysmal or chronic AF. They also showed the possibility that PV dilatation may be a crosslink between LA enlargement and AF[53]. Based on the relationships between PV and AF, it may be possible that stretch of PV increases the ectopic activity in PV. However, there is no direct evidence that PV stretch by dilatation induces AF. Direct distension of the PV–atrial junction by balloon in dogs may change heart rate, but all those effects were abolished by blocking vagal nerve activity[54,55]. Kalifa *et al.*[56] reported that an increase in intra-atrial pressure in sheep heart increases the rate of wave production emanating from superior PV[56]. There was also a report that the incidence and firing rates of spontaneous activity and the incidence of early after-depolarizations (EAD) and delayed after-depolarizations (DAD) were increased in PV after stretching a dissected tissue of the PV–atrial junction of rabbit and that stretch-activated channel blockers such as gadolinium and streptomycin reduced the stretch-induced spontaneous activities[57]. Unfortunately it was not clear where the spontaneous activities originated from, PV or atrium, which made it difficult to identify where the critical stretch effect occurred.

Characteristics of stretch-activated currents in single isolated cardiomyocytes in PV

Anatomically, the myocardial sleeve is much thinner than that of atrial myocardium and is probably more vulnerable to pathological conditions that stretch both PV and the atrium. Therefore, the existence of a stretch-sensing mechanism in PV would be important when PV stretch was expected. Seol *et al.*[58] reported that membrane stretch induced currents in single isolated cardiomyocytes in main PV of rabbit. They induced membrane stretch by two different ways, hypo-osmotic swelling and mechanical axial extension of the cardiomyocytes. The hypo-osmotic swelling could slowly activate the well-known swelling-activated Cl^- current ($I_{Cl,swell}$). They also found that hypo-osmotic swelling activates Gd^{3+}-sensitive and non-selective cation currents ($I_{NS,swell}$) (Fig. 15.1). The order of ion permeability for the $I_{NS,swell}$ was $K^+ > Cs^+ > Na^+ > Li^+$. The activation of $I_{NS,swell}$ was faster than that of

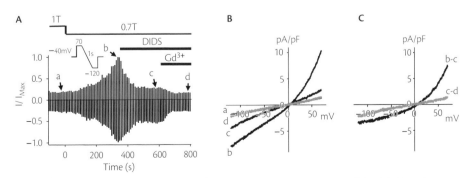

Fig. 15.1 The effect of DIDS and Gd^{3+} on swelling-induced stretch-activated cationic currents. **A** Time course analysis of the inward current amplitude at -100 mV and the outward current amplitude at $+60$ mV during swelling (see voltage clamp waveform insert). **B** I–V curves in 1 T (a), 0.7 T (b), 0.7 T + 100 μM DIDS (c) and 0.7 T + 100 μM Gd^{3+} (d). **C** I–V curves of the subtracted currents (for details see[19]). [Reproduced, with permission, from Seol CA, Kim J, Kim WT, *et al.* (2008) Simulation of spontaneous action potentials of cardiomyocytes in pulmonary veins of rabbits. *Prog Biophys Mol Biol* **96**:132–151.]

$I_{Cl,swell}$ and had a similar time course as the membrane area change. $I_{NS,swell}$ was easily blocked by 100 μM Gd^{3+}.

They also applied the mechanical stretch by axial lengthening of cardiomyocytes with two electrodes. The mechanical stretch instantaneously activated currents ($I_{SAC,NS}$) that were cation selective. K^+ had a higher permeability than Na^+. $I_{SAC,NS}$ was completely blocked with 100 μM Gd^{3+} or 100 μM streptomycin. The block by streptomycin seemed to be voltage-dependent. Interestingly, long-term application of mechanical stretch gradually activated a Cl^--dependent current ($I_{SAC,Cl}$) (Fig. 15.2). $I_{SAC,Cl}$ was blocked by 4,4'-di-isothiocyanatostilbene-2,2'-disulfonic acid (100 μM, DIDS). Blocking effects of streptomycin on $I_{SAC,NS}$ and $I_{NS,swell}$ were different. Streptomycin did not block $I_{NS,swell}$ but did block $I_{SAC,NS}$. Therefore $I_{NS,swell}$ may be a different entity from $I_{SAC,NS}$. Similar blocking action of DIDS, Cl^- sensitivity and slow activation of $I_{Cl,swell}$ and $I_{SAC,Cl}$ suggested that both channels may be the same, but this was not proven beyond doubt.

Possible arrhythmogenic role of stretch-activated currents in PV

Stretch-sensing ion currents may contribute to arrhythmogenesis in four different ways. One way is direct contribution to the ectopic activity by depolarizing membrane potential. Another way is the change of internal milieu, which, in turn, causes the change of the activity of the membrane currents and the generation of ectopic activity. The third way is a change of ion channel expression that causes overall changes in ion channel activity. The fourth way is a generation of the electrical heterogeneity in tissue, which may increase vulnerability of arrhythmogenesis. All four mechanisms are possible; however, there are very few studies on these aspects with PV. Supporting evidence for the first mechanism was reported by Chang et al.[57], as introduced in the previous section. They showed in tissue of the PV–atrial junction that stretch induced higher prevalence of EAD and DAD. This EAD or DAD activity could be attenuated by Gd^{3+} application. We also found the beating frequency of PV cardiomyocytes was slightly increased by the mechanical stretch or hypo-osmotic swelling. These results are compatible with the report by Cooper et al.[59] that the mechanical stretch increases the beating frequency, but not with the report by Lei and Kohl[60] that the hypo-osmotic swelling decreased the beating frequency in SA nodal cell. The discrepancies between PV cardiomyocytes and SA nodal cardiomyocytes cannot be explained clearly, but may be caused by different composition of ion channels or disparities in experimental conditions (such as the extent of cytosol dilution induced by hypo-osmotic cell swelling[60]).

One of the characteristics of PV compared to atrial myocytes is that cardiomyocytes in PV can generate spontaneous AP, even though not all reports support this. We have found that the increase of intracellular Na^+ or Ca^{2+} could increase the beating frequency in a concentration-dependent manner (Fig. 15.3). Stretch may induce an increase in intracellular Na^+ or Ca^{2+}[61]. In stretch simulations of atrial myocytes, the mechanical stimulus could gradually increase intracellular Ca^{2+}, secondary to an increase in intracellular Na^+[62]. Therefore, SACs activation may increase intracellular Na^+ and Ca^{2+}, which could increase the beating frequency of cardiomyocytes in PV and increase the chance of developing ectopic activity.

Another interesting feature of cardiomyocytes in PV is Ca^{2+}-dependent activation of the oscillatory current. When long positive step pulses (> 20 mV) were applied, oscillating currents were activated (Fig. 15.4A,B). Intracellular Na^+ increased the oscillating frequency and the current amplitude in a concentration-dependent manner. These oscillating currents were identified as Ca^{2+}-dependent Cl^- currents. Interestingly, when the voltage was returned to the holding potential, there were still residual oscillatory currents (see arrows in Fig. 15.4). The nature of Ca^{2+} loading dependency was tested by sequential application of positive step pulse (80 mV) for 1 s every 30 s. As the step pulses were applied, the residual oscillatory current became larger and lasted longer (Fig. 15.4C). When current traces at the 27th step pulse were checked, inward transient current could be observed at the starting point (see arrow in Fig. 15.4C) and was regularly activated. Since the pulses were applied every 30 s, the activation of the inward transient current persisted more than 30 s. The 80 mV step pulse can increase intracellular Ca^{2+} by the reverse mode of Na^+/Ca^{2+} exchanger (NCX) and the oscillating currents were abolished by the high concentration of the Ca^{2+} chelator ethylene glycol tetraacetic acid (EGTA). Therefore, the current activation of oscillating nature must be dependent on intracellular Ca^{2+} oscillation. Oscillating currents or residual oscillating currents were never observed in atrial myocytes isolated from atrial appendage. Therefore, these phenomena appear to be specific characteristics of PV cardiomyocytes.

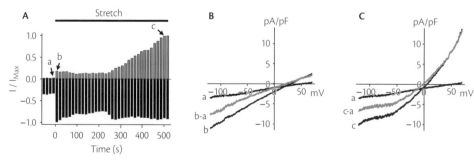

Fig. 15.2 Time course of the mechanical stretch-activated current. **A** Time course of the inward current amplitude at −100 mV and the outward current amplitude at +60 mV during stretching. **B** I–V curves immediately after stretching: control current (a), activated current (b) and subtracted current (b–a). **C** I–V curves 500 s after stretching: control current (a), activated current (c) and subtracted current (c–a) (for details see[19]). [Reproduced, with permission, from Seol CA, Kim J, Kim WT, *et al.* (2008) Simulation of spontaneous action potentials of cardiomyocytes in pulmonary veins of rabbits. *Prog Biophys Mol Biol* **96**:132–151.]

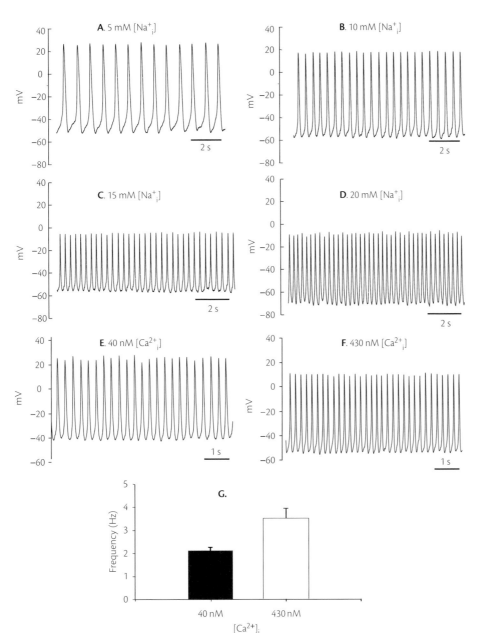

Fig. 15.3 Internal Na⁺ and Ca²⁺ concentration-dependent change of the beating frequency of cardiomyocytes in main PV. Intracellular K⁺ was substituted by Na⁺. **A** 5 mM Na⁺, **B** 10 mM Na⁺, **C** 15 mM Na⁺, **D** 20 mM Na⁺, **E** 40 nM Ca²⁺, **F** 430 nM Ca²⁺, **G** summary data on Ca²⁺ dependency of spontaneous beating rate.

These characteristics in relation to AF and PV stretch are quite suggestive. The activation of SACs by stretch can increase intracellular Na⁺ and Ca²⁺. The cardiomyocytes in PV have the potential to generate oscillating current which can become more persistent as Ca²⁺ overload increases. The persistent oscillating inward current probably facilitates the ectopic activity in PV. Honjo *et al.*[27] showed the interesting relationship between intracellular Ca²⁺ dysregulation and the persistent spontaneous AP in PV. In the presence of low concentration of ryanodine, rapid pacing could induce subsequently persistent activation of spontaneous AP. The low concentration of ryanodine may facilitate Ca²⁺ dysregulation and rapid pacing may facilitate intracellular Ca²⁺ increase. Depletion of sarcoplasmic Ca²⁺ and NCX block attenuated the pacing-induced activity while ß-adrenergic stimulation potentiated it. Recently, in

addition to an 'ion channel clock' for the initiation of spontaneous AP, a 'Ca²⁺ clock' for cardiac pacemaker function was suggested and reviewed[63]. In relation to Ca²⁺ clock for the initiation of spontaneous AP, the Ca²⁺-dependent oscillatory nature of PV cardiomyocytes may potentiate and facilitate the generation of spontaneous AP. However, it is still unclear whether the generation of Ca²⁺-dependent oscillating currents in PV cardiomyocytes is a physiological function or a pathological status.

Conclusions and outlook

It is too early to say whether stretch of PV is one of main causes of AF. The development of AF usually requires a long-term process and the causes of that are multifactorial. The stretch itself may not

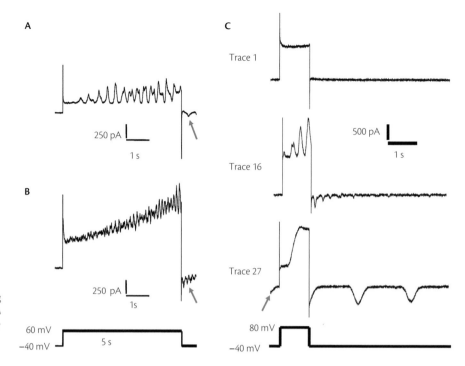

Fig. 15.4 Activation of the oscillating current in cardiomyocytes and residual inward currents at the holding potential in PV. **A** 5 mM Na⁺, **B** 15 mM Na⁺, **C** 5 mM Na⁺. Arrows indicate the residual inward oscillating currents at the holding potential.

be the direct initiation factor for the generation of AF. However, the characteristics of cardiomyocytes in PV, as shown above and in various reports in relation to stretch and AF, suggest that stretch of PV may be one of the factors for the generation of AF. The following hypothesis may be valid: atrial dilatation → PV dilatation and stretch → intracellular Ca^{2+} load and dysregulation → ectopic activities in PV → paroxysmal AF → ionic remodelling in atrium → chronic AF. SAC could be an important link between stretch and ectopic activity in PV in the course of establishment of AF. Experimental data on SACs were mainly obtained from rabbit, and there is a strong possibility that the electrical activity of PV cardiomyocytes in human is different from small animals. If ectopic beats in PV cause atrial arrhythmia, it is still unclear which mechanism is responsible for re-entrant activity or rapid focal discharges in PV. Stretch-induced changes must not be regarded as the sole contributor to atrial arrhythmogenesis, but should be thought of in conjunction with other humoral and neural changes. It is clear that many aspects still need to be clarified in order to understand the linkage between PV stretch and AF.

References

1. Haissaguerre M, Jais P, Shah DC, *et al.* Spontaneous initiation of atrial fibrillation by ectopic beats originating in the pulmonary veins. *N Engl J Med* 1998;**339**:659–666.
2. Nathan H, Eliakim M. The junction between the left atrium and the pulmonary veins. An anatomic study of human hearts. *Circulation* 1966;**34**:412–422.
3. Roux N, Havet E, Mertl P. The myocardial sleeves of the pulmonary veins: potential implications for atrial fibrillation. *Surg Radiol Anat* 2004;**26**:285–289.
4. Tagawa M, Higuchi K, Chinushi M, *et al.* Myocardium extending from the left atrium onto the pulmonary veins: a comparison between subjects with and without atrial fibrillation. *Pacing Clin Electrophysiol* 2001;**24**:1459–1463.
5. Morillo CA, Klein GJ, Jones DL, Guiraudon CM. Chronic rapid atrial pacing. Structural, functional, and electrophysiological characteristics of a new model of sustained atrial fibrillation. *Circulation* 1995;**91**:1588–1595.
6. Wijffels MC, Kirchhof CJ, Dorland R, Allessie MA. Atrial fibrillation begets atrial fibrillation. A study in awake chronically instrumented goats. *Circulation* 1995;**92**:1954–1968.
7. Yue L, Feng J, Gaspo R, Li GR, Wang Z, Nattel S. Ionic remodeling underlying action potential changes in a canine model of atrial fibrillation. *Circ Res* 1997;**81**:512–525.
8. Gaspo R, Bosch RF, Bou-Abboud E, Nattel S. Tachycardia-induced changes in Na⁺ current in a chronic dog model of atrial fibrillation. *Circ Res* 1997;**81**:1045–1052.
9. Sun H, Gaspo R, Leblanc N, Nattel S. Cellular mechanisms of atrial contractile dysfunction caused by sustained atrial tachycardia. *Circulation* 1998;**98**:719–727.
10. vander Velden HM, Ausma J, *et al.* Gap junctional remodeling in relation to stabilization of atrial fibrillation in the goat. *Cardiovasc Res* 2000;**46**:476–486.
11. Nattel S, Li D. Ionic remodeling in the heart: pathophysiological significance and new therapeutic opportunities for atrial fibrillation. *Circ Res* 2000;**87**:440–447.
12. Nattel S. Atrial electrophysiological remodeling caused by rapid atrial activation: underlying mechanisms and clinical relevance to atrial fibrillation. *Cardiovasc Res* 1999;**42**:298–308.
13. Nattel S, Maguy A, Le Bouter S, Yeh YH. Arrhythmogenic ion-channel remodeling in the heart: heart failure, myocardial infarction, and atrial fibrillation. *Physiol Rev* 2007;**87**:425–456.
14. Waldo AL. Mechanisms of atrial fibrillation. *J Cardiovasc Electrophysiol* 2003;**14**:S267–S274.
15. Nattel S. Basic electrophysiology of the pulmonary veins and their role in atrial fibrillation: precipitators, perpetuators, and perplexers. *J Cardiovasc Electrophysiol* 2003;**14**:1372–1375.
16. Tasaki H. Electrophysiological study of the striated muscle cells of the extrapulmonary vein of the guinea-pig. *Jpn Circ J* 1969;**33**:1087–1098.

17. Cheung DW. Pulmonary vein as an ectopic focus in digitalis-induced arrhythmia. *Nature* 1981;**294**:582–584.

18. Cheung DW. Electrical activity of the pulmonary vein and its interaction with the right atrium in the guinea-pig. *J Physiol* 1981;**314**:445–456.

19. Seol CA, Kim J, Kim WT, *et al.* Simulation of spontaneous action potentials of cardiomyocytes in pulmonary veins of rabbits. *Prog Biophys Mol Biol* 2008;**96**:132–151.

20. Nam GB, Choi KJ, Leem CH, Kim YH. The characteristics of spontaneous action potentials if myocytes in rabbit pulmonary vein : Implication ininitiation mechanism of focal atrial fibrillation. *PACE* 2000;**23**:206P.

21. Chen YJ, Chen SA, Chen YC, Yeh HI, Chang MS, Lin CI. Electrophysiology of single cardiomyocytes isolated from rabbit pulmonary veins: implication in initiation of focal atrial fibrillation. *Basic Res Cardiol* 2002;**97**:26–34.

22. Leem CH, Kim WT, Ha JM, *et al.* Simulation of Ca^{2+}-activated Cl$^-$ current of cardiomyocytes in rabbit pulmonary vein: implications of subsarcolemmal Ca^{2+} dynamics. *Phil Trans R Soc (Lond) A* 2006;**364**:1223–1243.

23. Ehrlich JR, Cha TJ, Zhang L, Chartier D, Villeneuve L, Hébert TE, Nattel S. Characterization of a hyperpolarization-activated time-dependent potassium current in canine cardiomyocytes from pulmonary vein myocardial sleeves and left atrium. *J Physiol* 2004;**557**:583–597.

24. Ehrlich JR, Cha TJ, Zhang L, Chartier D, Melnyk P, Hohnloser SH, Nattel S. Cellular electrophysiology of canine pulmonary vein cardiomyocytes: action potential and ionic current properties. *J Physiol* 2003;**551**:801–813.

25. Choi KJ, Kim WT, Nam GB. The characteristics of spontaneous action potential of cardiac myocytes in rabbit pulmonary veins. *Korean Circ J* 2001;**31**:94–105.

26. Chen YJ, Chen SA, Chen YC, Yeh HI, Chan P, Chang MS, Lin CI. Effects of rapid atrial pacing on the arrhythmogenic activity of single cardiomyocytes from pulmonary veins: implication in initiation of atrial fibrillation. *Circulation* 2001;**104**:2849–2854.

27. Honjo H, Boyett MR, Niwa R, *et al.* Pacing-induced spontaneous activity in myocardial sleeves of pulmonary veins after treatment with ryanodine. *Circulation* 2003;**107**:1937–1943.

28. Kohl P, Ravens U. Cardiac mechano-electric feedback: past, present, and prospect. *Prog Biophys Mol Biol* 2003;**82**:3–9.

29. Ravens U. Mechano-electric feedback and arrhythmias. *Prog Biophys Mol Biol* 2003;**82**:255–66.

30. Benjamin EJ, Levy D, Vaziri SM, D'Agostino RB, Belanger AJ, Wolf PA. Independent risk factors for atrial fibrillation in a population-based cohort. The Framingham Heart Study. *JAMA* 1994;**271**:840–844.

31. Nattel S. New ideas about atrial fibrillation 50 years on. *Nature* 2002;**415**:219–226.

32. Psaty BM, Manolio TA, Kuller LH, *et al.* Incidence of and risk factors for atrial fibrillation in older adults. *Circulation* 1997;**96**:2455–2461.

33. Vasan RS, Larson MG, Levy D, Evans JC, Benjamin EJ. Distribution and categorization of echocardiographic measurements in relation to reference limits: the Framingham Heart Study: formulation of a height- and sex-specific classification and its prospective validation. *Circulation* 1997;**96**:1863–1873.

34. Vaziri SM, Larson MG, Benjamin EJ, Levy D. Echocardiographic predictors of nonrheumatic atrial fibrillation. The Framingham Heart Study. *Circulation* 1994;**89**:724–730.

35. Tsang TS, Barnes ME, Bailey KR, *et al.* Left atrial volume: important risk marker of incident atrial fibrillation in 1655 older men and women. *Mayo Clin Proc* 2001;**76**:467–475.

36. Cheng TO. Atrial fibrillation and left atrial enlargement: the hen or the egg? *Int J Cardiol* 2007;**118**:107.

37. Liu T, Li GP, Li LJ. Atrial dilatation and atrial fibrillation: a vicious circle? *Med Hypotheses* 2005;**65**:410–411.

38. Boyden PA, Tilley LP, Albala A, Liu SK, Fenoglio JJ, Jr. and Wit AL. Mechanisms for atrial arrhythmias associated with cardiomyopathy: a study of feline hearts with primary myocardial disease. *Circulation* 1984;**69**:1036–1047.

39. Boyden PA, Tilley LP, Pham TD, Liu SK, Fenoglic JJ, Jr., Wit AL. Effects of left atrial enlargement on atrial transmembrane potentials and structure in dogs with mitral valve fibrosis. *Am J Cardiol* 1982;**49**:1896–1908.

40. Ravelli F, Allessie M. Effects of atrial dilatation on refractory period and vulnerability to atrial fibrillation in the isolated Langendorff-perfused rabbit heart. *Circulation* 1997;**96**:1686–1695.

41. Sideris DA, Toumanidis ST, Thodorakis M, *et al.* Some observations on the mechanism of pressure related atrial fibrillation. *Eur Heart J* 1994;**15**:1585–1589.

42. Bett GCL, Sachs F. Cardiac Mechanosensitivity and Stretch-Activated Ion Channels. *Trends Cardiovasc Med* 1997;**7**:4–8.

43. Cazorla O, Pascarel C, Brette F, Le Guennec JY. Modulation of ions channels and membrane receptors activities by mechanical interventions in cardiomyocytes: possible mechanisms for mechanosensitivity. *Prog Biophys Mol Biol* 1999;**71**:29–58.

44. Hu H, Sachs F. Stretch-activated ion channels in the heart. *J Mol Cell Cardiol* 1997;**29**:1511–1523.

45. Browe DM, Baumgarten CM. Stretch of beta1 integrin activates an outwardly rectifying chloride current via FAK and Src in rabbit ventricular myocytes. *J Gen Physiol* 2003;**122**:689–702.

46. Bode F, Katchman A, Woosley RL, Franz MR. Gadolinium decreases stretch-induced vulnerability to atrial fibrillation. *Circulation* 2000;**101**:2200–2205.

47. Bode F, Sachs F, Franz MR. Tarantula peptide inhibits atrial fibrillation. *Nature* 2001;**409**:35–36.

48. Lin WS, Prakash VS, Tai CT, *et al.* Pulmonary vein morphology in patients with paroxysmal atrial fibrillation initiated by ectopic beats originating from the pulmonary veins: implications for catheter ablation. *Circulation* 2000;**101**:1274–1281.

49. Tsao HM, Yu WC, Cheng HC, *et al.* Pulmonary vein dilation in patients with atrial fibrillation: detection by magnetic resonance imaging. *J Cardiovasc Electrophysiol* 2001;**12**:809–813.

50. Yamane T, Shah DC, Jais P, *et al.* Dilatation as a marker of pulmonary veins initiating atrial fibrillation. *J Interv Card Electrophysiol* 2002;**6**:245–249.

51. Takase B, Nagata M, Matsui T, *et al.* Pulmonary vein dimensions and variation of branching pattern in patients with paroxysmal atrial fibrillation using magnetic resonance angiography. *Jpn Heart J* 2004;**45**:81–92.

52. Herweg B, Sichrovsky T, Polosajian L, Rozenshtein A, Steinberg JS. Hypertension and hypertensive heart disease are associated with increased ostial pulmonary vein diameter. *J Cardiovasc Electrophysiol* 2005;**16**:2–5.

53. Liu T, Li G. Pulmonary vein dilatation: another possible crosslink between left atrial enlargement and atrial fibrillation? *Int J Cardiol* 2008;**123**:193–194.

54. Edis AJ, Donald DE, Shepher JT. Cardiovascular reflexes from stretch of pulmonary vein-atrial junctions in the dog. *Circ Res* 1970;**27**:1091–1100.

55. Moore-Gillon MJ, Fitzsimons JT. Pulmonary vein-atrial junction stretch receptors and the inhibition of drinking. *Am J Physiol* 1982;**242**:R452–R457.

56. Kalifa J, Jalife J, Zaitsev AV, *et al.* Intra-atrial pressure increases rate and organization of waves emanating from the superior pulmonary veins during atrial fibrillation. *Circulation* 2003;**108**:668–671.

57. Chang SL, Chen YC, Chen YJ, Wangcharoen W, Lee SH, Lin CI, Chen SA. Mechanoelectrical feedback regulates the arrhythmogenic activity of pulmonary veins. *Heart* 2007;**93**:82–88.

58. Seol CA, Kim WT, Ha JM, *et al.* Stretch-activated currents in cardiomyocytes isolated from rabbit pulmonary veins. *Prog Biophys Mol Biol* 2008;**97**:217–231.

59. Cooper PJ, Lei M, Cheng LX, Kohl P. Axial stretch increases spontaneous pacemaker activity in rabbit isolated sinoatrial node cells. *J Appl Physiol* 2000;**89**:2099–2104.

60. Lei M, Kohl P. Swelling-induced decrease in spontaneous pacemaker activity of rabbit isolated sino-atrial node cells. *Acta Physiol Scand* 1998;**164**:1–12.

61. Calaghan SC, Belus A, White E. Do stretch-induced changes in intracellular calcium modify the electrical activity of cardiac muscle?. *Prog Biophys Mol Biol* 2003;**82**:81–95.

62. Youm JB, Han J, Kim N, *et al.* Role of stretch-activated channels on the stretch-induced changes of rat atrial myocytes. *Prog Biophys Mol Biol* 2006;**90**:186–206.

63. Maltsev VA, Lakatta EG. Dynamic interactions of an intracellular Ca^{2+} clock and membrane ion channel clock underlie robust initiation and regulation of cardiac pacemaker function. *Cardiovasc Res* 2008;**77**: 274–284.

Heterogeneity of sarcomere length and function as a cause of arrhythmogenic calcium waves

Henk E.D.J. ter Keurs, Ni Diao, Nathan P. Deis, Mei L. Zhang, Yoshinao Sugai, Guy Price, Yuji Wakayama, Yutaka Kagaya, Yoshinao Shinozaki, Penelope A. Boyden, Masahito Miura and Bruno D.M. Stuyvers

Background

Electrical non-uniformity plays a major role in the re-entry mechanism of arrhythmia and has been well investigated[1]. Much less is known about arrhythmogenicity of non-uniform segmental wall motion, with areas of hypokinesis, akinesis and dyskinesis, which are well known signs of ischaemic heart disease[2,3]. Differences in the motion pattern around the left ventricle (LV) may result from different distributions of elastic structures compared to muscle elements. For example, systolic shortening in a region of the LV where myocardium has largely been replaced by a fibrotic scar is severely reduced. Alternatively changes in the intrinsic force-generating capacity of the myocytes in the fascicles may cause reduced systolic shortening or even lead to segment lengthening during contraction of surrounding healthy tissue. Thus, acute ischaemia causes acute loss of force-generating capacity of the cardiac cell by impairment of excitation–contraction (EC) coupling and may lead to non-uniform systolic strain distribution in the LV wall. Although non-uniform EC coupling has been linked to a variety of arrhythmogenic heart diseases[4], the role of non-uniform contraction in arrhythmogenesis has received far less attention.

Following the theme of this book we explore the contribution of the mechanics in non-uniform muscle to arrhythmias (see also Chapter 21). We explore in the first part of this chapter force development and strain distribution in cardiac trabeculae composed of 'acutely weak' and 'normal' muscle segments of equal lengths, in order to define the fundamental processes that dictate the force balance in non-uniform myocardium. The paradigm used to render part of the muscle weak mimics a scenario where a large part of the myocardium loses acutely 90% of its force-generating capacity. The results will show that a force balance can be maintained by muscle segments that operate in series owing to the combined effects of the force–sarcomere length relationship (FSLR) and force–sarcomere velocity relationship (FSVR). Both relationships behave in a way that can be predicted by modelling the response of the contractile apparatus to EC coupling and to load. Furthermore, these results show that a force balance is maintained in the presence of modest stretch of the weakened myocytes. These studies are an extension of the work on duplex muscle models[5] in which two muscles are mounted in series. The muscles used for our studies exhibited uniform properties under control conditions, which allowed conclusions to be drawn at the level of sarcomere length and velocity of sarcomere shortening.

In the second part of this chapter we explore the effects of non-uniform contraction on the generation of propagated Ca^{2+} waves. In particular we show the effects of shortening and stretch during the relaxation phase, which support the notion that it is the rapid force decline in the weaker segment of muscle that causes the Ca^{2+} surge that triggers the Ca^{2+} waves. The increased free $[Ca^{2+}]$ of these waves activates Na^+/Ca^{2+} exchange and Ca^{2+}-sensitive non-selective channels in the sarcolemma and therefore induces delayed after-depolarizations (DAD) that trigger action potentials[6]. This arrhythmogenic phenomenon in non-uniform myocardium has been coined reverse EC coupling[6–10]. Reverse EC coupling may be clinically relevant as it has been shown that when patients receive resynchronization pacing which can improve the mechanical uniformity, both the incidence of sudden death and the degree of heart failure is reduced[11].

Force maintenance and Ca²⁺ waves in non-uniform cardiac muscle

Force (F) measurement by a silicon strain gauge and sarcomere length (SL) detection by laser diffraction techniques together with intracellular [Ca²⁺] measurement by fluorescent dyes[12,13] allow the study of the effects of non-uniformity in several paradigms (Fig. 16.1). The reference scenario is uniform sarcomere behaviour in the muscle when superfused by one solution at a fixed extracellular Ca²⁺ concentration ($[Ca^{2+}]_o$; usually 1.2 mM). Arrhythmogenic effects of non-uniform contraction can be studied by exposing a restricted region of the muscle to a small 'jet' of solution[10] applied from a glass pipette ($\approx$ 100 μm tip) perpendicular to the trabecula (Fig. 16.1). The jet solution can be composed of standard 4-(2-hydroxyethyl)-1-piperazineethanesulfonic acid (HEPES)-buffered solution containing either caffeine to deplete Ca²⁺ content in the sarcoplasmic reticulum (SR)[14,15] or 2,3-butanedione monoxime (BDM) to suppress the activation of cross-bridges[16,17], or either low Ca²⁺ concentration in the fluid jet $[Ca^{2+}]_{jet}$ (LC) or high $[Ca^{2+}]_{jet}$ (HC). This approach caused sarcomere stretch in the jet-exposed region during the stimulated twitches[10] and led to the generation of arrhythmogenic Ca²⁺ waves starting in the exposed area. Alternatively, sarcomere dynamics in non-uniform muscle could be studied by mounting two inflow ports for solution in the bath: the main HEPES solution with 1.2 mM $[Ca^{2+}]_o$ ran (2.5 ml/min) longitudinally through the bath; the other inflow of HEPES saline entered from a side port in the bath (0.5 ml/min) and covered exactly half the muscle (Fig. 16.1 inset). Exposure of the muscle to HEPES solution with low $[Ca^{2+}]_o$ (0.4 mM) from the side port created non-uniform EC coupling consisting of a weak force-generating segment in low $[Ca^{2+}]_o$ and a strong segment in $[Ca^{2+}]_o$ 1.2 mM, thereby creating a variant duplex model (see also Chapter 21).

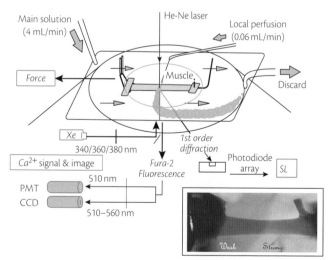

Fig. 16.1 The experimental paradigm to study non-uniform contraction in rat cardiac trabeculae. A fluid jet renders a segment weaker than the remainder of the muscle. The jet can cover either a small region of the muscle (main panel) or 50% of the muscle (inset). He-Ne, helium-neon; XE, xenon; PMT, photomultiplier tube; CCD, charge-coupled device camera [For detail see reference[10]].

Effects of FSLR and FSVR in uniform and non-uniform muscle

The FSLR of uniform muscles shows the expected shapes at homogeneous normal and low $[Ca^{2+}]_o$[13] (Fig. 16.2). Reducing $[Ca^{2+}]_o$ uniformly along the muscle to 0.4 mM caused a reduction of twitch force by 90%. In contrast, when only half of the length of the muscle was exposed to 0.4 mM $[Ca^{2+}]_o$, force decreases by only 60%, raising the question whether the force generation by the weak segment can fully be explained by the mechanics of contraction and specifically by the FSLR and FSVR of the sarcomeres. Indeed, Fig. 16.2 shows that stretching of the weak segment during contraction allowed it to support a fourfold higher force than it would when the whole muscle was uniformly exposed to 0.4 mM $[Ca^{2+}]_o$. The FSLR at lowered $[Ca^{2+}]_o$ shows that maintaining a longer SL in the weak segment is responsible for a 2.5-fold increase of force in the weak segment.

The remainder of the force enhancement may have been due to the act of stretching the weak segment during the contraction, as is shown by analysis of the effect of stretch on the FSVR measured by iso-velocity releases at the peak of contraction[18]. The FSVR and maximal shortening velocity shown in Fig. 16.2 match closely the well-known FSVR in cardiac muscle previously reported [18–20], but the data extend the FSVR to the force range where the muscle is stretched[18,19,21]. Figure 16.2 shows that the shortening velocity in the strong muscle segment matched the lengthening velocity in the weak segment as one would expect when overall muscle length is constant. Based on the FSVR (Fig. 16.2), F increased 1.6-fold due to the stretch of the weak segment.

Combining FSLR and FSVR, the increase in SL and the act of stretching both contribute to the force enhancement during non-uniform contraction. The product of the FSLR- and FSVR-based force increase explains that force in the non-uniform contraction is fourfold higher than the force when the whole muscle is exposed to 0.4 mM $[Ca^{2+}]_o$. Along the same line of reasoning, sarcomere shortening in the strong segments appears to be responsible for a force deficit of 30% by the FSVR (Fig. 16.2) and another 30% by the FSLR. These data show that the force-generating capacity in non-uniform muscle is completely explained by the FSLR and FSVR of the weak and strong segments of the muscle.

Proposed mechanism underlying the FSLR: feedback of force to Ca²⁺ binding by troponin C

Landesberg and Sideman proposed a positive feedback of force on Ca²⁺ binding to explain the cooperativity in the cardiac F–[Ca²⁺] relationship underlying the FSLR, as well as negative feedback between filament sliding velocity and number of cross-bridges underlying the FSVR[22]. We have recently proposed a simple mechanism based on the analysis of the FSLR at a wide range of [Ca²⁺] near the filaments[6,23]. The principal assumption, illustrated in Fig. 16.3, is that cross-bridge force on the actin filament decreases the rate of dissociation of Ca²⁺ that is bound to troponin C (TnC). Test of this assumption evidently requires measurement of the kinetics of Ca²⁺ bound to TnC, but computational modelling faithfully reproduces the observed intracellular Ca²⁺ concentration $[Ca^{2+}]_i$ transients[24–28], twitch time course (Fig. 16.3), FSLR and F–pCa relationship in intact and skinned cardiac muscle. Moreover, the model reproduces observations by Allen and Kurihara[27] that a rapid force decrease by a quick release of cardiac

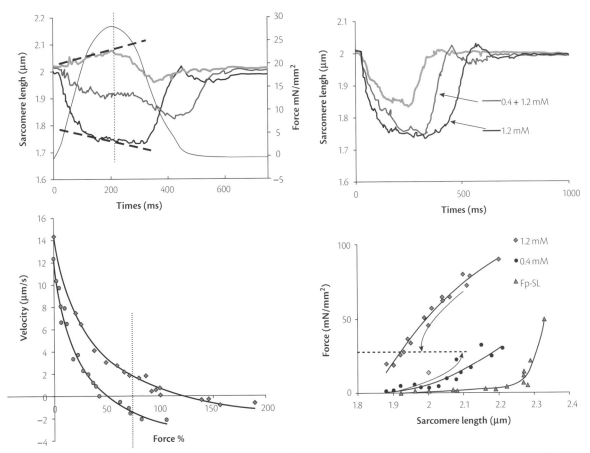

Fig. 16.2 Top left: SL versus time during a twitch force in a trabecula at normal [Ca^{2+}] during non-uniform contraction in the strong segment, as well as during uniform contraction of the same trabecula. Top right: simultaneous SL records in the strong and weak segment of a non-uniform muscle as well as SL in the border zone (see text). FSVR (bottom left) and FSLR (bottom right) of the same muscle as in the top panels. The passive and active FSLRs are shown for 0.4 mM [Ca^{2+}]$_o$ and 1.2 mM [Ca^{2+}]$_o$. Force in the weak segment is enhanced 2.5-fold by the fact that the sarcomeres of the weak segment are forced to operate at a higher SL (black arrow). The FSVR shows that the shortening velocity in the 'strong' segment is offset by the lengthening velocity from the 'weak' segment at peak force of the non-uniform muscle (dashed lines), thereby enhancing force another 1.5-fold. The dashed lines show a balance of V$_{SL}$ in the strong and weak segments (for further explanation see text).

muscles causes a substantial transient cytosolic Ca^{2+} increase (Fig. 16.3), which is important for the arrhythmogenic nature of non-uniform contraction (see below).

The FSVR and cross-bridge dynamics

The interpretation of the velocity of shortening in the FVR is unambiguous: velocity reflects twice the speed of actin propulsion by myosin cross-bridges. On the other hand, the force/load supported by the muscle at any velocity depends on the load per cross-bridge and the number of cross-bridges. We can use dynamic stiffness [(DS) or $\Delta F/\Delta SL$ during 1% SL perturbations at 200 Hz] of the muscles as an indicator of the number of strongly attached cross-bridges. DS appears proportional to the load on the muscle[20] up to loads 80% above isometric force (DS = 0.94 × F + 14; R^2 = 0.91), irrespective of the [Ca^{2+}] at which DS is measured.

Since force is determined by the number of attached cross-bridges and the unitary force produced by the single cross-bridge, the force–velocity curve of the average cross-bridge (FSVR$_{XB}$) can be calculated by dividing the force/load by DS at each force level. This correction converts Hill's hyperbola into a linear FSVR$_{XB}$ for the average single cross-bridge[20] (Fig. 16.4). The linear FSVR$_{XB}$ extends to stretch and appears independent of the level of activation,

i.e. independent of [Ca^{2+}]$_o$. The linear FSVR$_{XB}$ in Fig. 16.4 also shows that F$_{XB}$ is increased by only about 10% of isometric force during stretch, i.e. clearly less than the force increase in the whole muscle brought about by stretching, and supports the notion that the stretch-induced increase of force is dominated by an increased number of cross-bridges.

The number of attached cross-bridges is dictated by the transition rate (g) of the cross-bridge from the strong force-generating state to the weak state and has been postulated to be a linear function of the sarcomere shortening velocity[29]: g = g$_0$ + g$_1$V, where g$_0$ is the rate of cross-bridge detachment/weakening in the isometric regime and g$_1$ is the mechanical feedback coefficient that reflects the effect of the sliding velocity (V; being positive in a shortening sarcomere) on cross-bridge weakening[30]. It follows that in Hill's equation for the FSVR [(P–P$_0$) = (P+a)V][31] the parameter b approximates to b ≈ g$_0$/g$_1$ and g ≈ g$_1$ (V+b). As a result, g$_0$/g$_1$ = aV$_0$/ P$_0$.

Shortening at constant velocity results in a diminished force of contraction compared to an isometric twitch; this force deficit, normalized for the corresponding isometric twitch force at the same moment, increases progressively after an initial delay of a few milliseconds[29]. The slope of the progressively increasing force deficit is proportional to V and can be used to calculate g$_1$

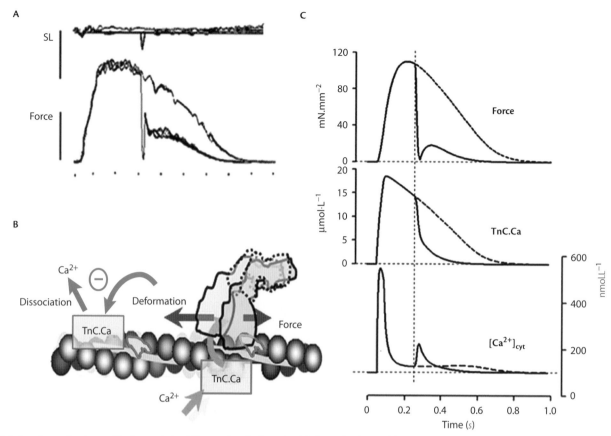

Fig. 16.3 Experimentally observed SL–force relation (**A**), reproduced using a simplified cross-bridge model where force exerted on the actin filament induces a deformation of the actin–troponin complex which reduces the dissociation rate of Ca^{2+} ions from TnC (**B**). Implementation of this feedback in a model of EC coupling generates both realistic cytosolic Ca^{2+} ($[Ca^{2+}]cyt$) and force transients (**C**), and the effect of a quick release on the force transient (compare panels **A** and **C**). (See color plate section.)

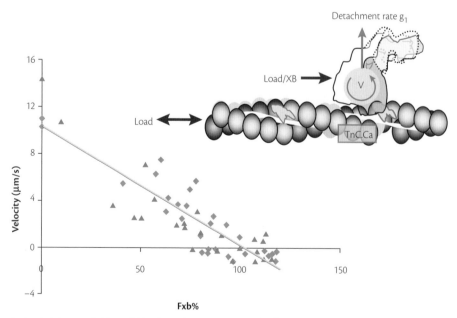

Fig. 16.4 Unique $FSVR_{XB}$ at the level of the cross-bridges, which is linear (V = 10.33–0.102 Fxb, R^2 = 0.81) and identical at 1.2 mM (red triangles) compared to 0.4 mM $[Ca^{2+}]_o$ (blue diamonds). Inset: assumed feedback between the velocity of cycling of the cross-bridge during sliding of the filaments and the weakening rate of the cross-bridges. (See color plate section.)

(see[29] for details). The calculated g_1 shows no variation for shortening ramps started at varied SL or at various times during the twitch, suggesting that the effect of shortening is independent of the level of activation of the muscle, which makes it unlikely that g_1 relates to Ca^{2+} kinetics[29]. We have shown that g_1 is about $6.15/\mu m^{[29]}$, while work on isolated myofibrils suggests that $g_0 = 13.7^{[32]}$, predicting a 45% increase in the number of cross-bridges and thus of force during stretch at a stretch 1 $\mu m/s$, which is very close to the above-mentioned results (Fig. 16.2).

In conclusion, cardiac sarcomere mechanics in uniform and non-uniform cardiac muscle can quantitatively be explained by two feedback mechanisms: (1) feedback of generated force to Ca^{2+} by TnC (Fig. 16.3) and (2) feedback of actin sliding to the detachment rate of the cross-bridges that propel actin (Fig. 16.4).

Arrhythmogenic Ca^{2+} waves in non-uniform muscle

Exposure of a small segment of muscle to a jet that contains (1) caffeine, (2) BDM or (3) low-$[Ca^{2+}]^{[10]}$ reduces electrically driven Ca^{2+} release from the SR and/or the contractile response to Ca^{2+} ions and weakens the jet-exposed segment. Consequently, twitch force decreases (by ~40–50%) and the sarcomeres in the segment exposed to the jet are stretched by shortening of the regions outside the jet (Fig. 16.5A). The behaviour of the weak and strong segments[10] is again consistent with a force balance owing to the FSLR and FSVR of the sarcomeres. During relaxation, the sarcomeres in the weak segment shorten rapidly; Fig. 16.5 shows that the maximal rate of shortening occurs at ~25% of peak force[10]. Furthermore, the phase of rapid force decline is followed by a Ca^{2+} surge which triggers propagated Ca^{2+} waves from the border of the jet-exposed segment (Fig. 16.5A).

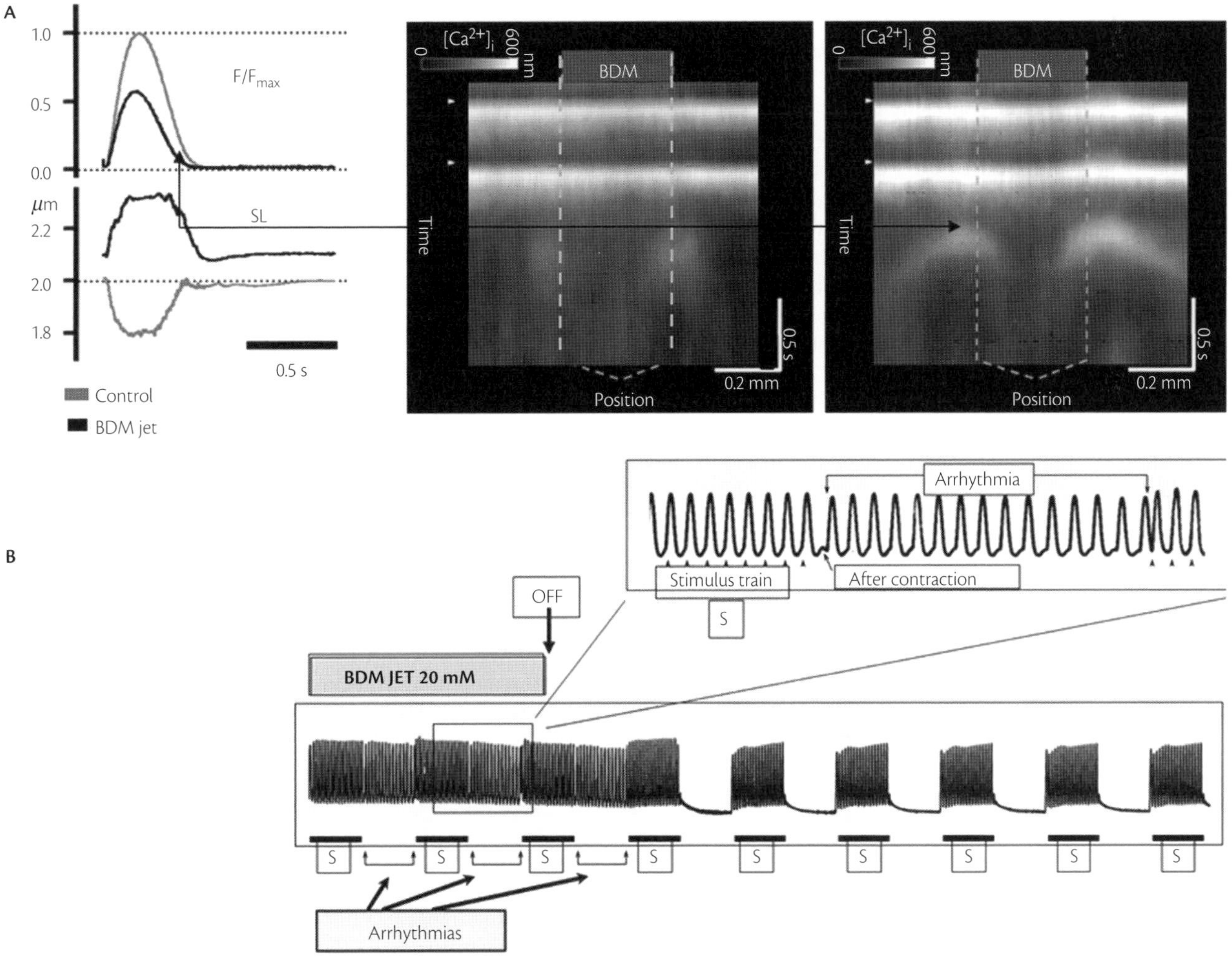

Fig. 16.5 **A** A jet containing BDM inhibits the contraction of local sarcomeres resulting in regional stretch (black trace), while SL behaviour is uniform and twitch force larger without the jet (grey trace). The spatio-temporal Ca^{2+} distribution shows that Ca^{2+} waves arise from the border between regions with and without the BDM jet at the time of relaxation of the last twitch. At low levels of activation this region generates only a localized Ca^{2+} surge during the late part of the relaxation phase (middle panel), but generates Ca^{2+} waves at higher $[Ca^{2+}]$ (right panel). **B** Non-uniform EC coupling caused by the jet containing BDM (20 mmol/L) is arrhythmogenic. Stimulus trains during local exposure to BDM (grey bars below the tracings) consistently induced arrhythmias. An expanded force tracing shows that spontaneous contractions were both preceded and followed by after-contractions induced by the stimulus train (arrowheads indicate electrical stimulation). OFF arrow indicates when the jet was turned off; this rapidly eliminated the contractile non-uniformity and its arrhythmogenic effects. S indicates stimulus trains repeated every 15 s. [Reproduced, with permission, from Wakayama Y, Miura M, Stuyvers BD, Boyden PA, ter Keurs HE (2005) Spatial nonuniformity of excitation–contraction coupling causes arrhythmogenic Ca^{2+} waves in rat cardiac muscle. *Circ Res* **96**:1266–1273.]

The jet-exposed segment can also be weakened by exposure of the muscle to high $[Ca^{2+}]_o$ (> 4 mM), which causes SR-Ca^{2+} over-load, witnessed by spontaneous diastolic contractile waves inside individual myocytes[33,34]. Exposure of the muscle segment to a high $[Ca^{2+}]_o$ jet consistently reduces twitch force and turns the normal monophasic twitch shortening into a pattern in which initial shortening was followed by stretch, or into frank stretch during the whole twitch despite the fact that the $[Ca^{2+}]_i$ transient during the electrically stimulated twitch is increased (by ~25%) and always leads to the generation of Ca^{2+} waves that start in the jet segment. It appears unlikely that SR-Ca^{2+} overload induces Ca^{2+} release in the segment exposed to the HC jet and accounts for the initiation of Ca^{2+} waves, because inhibition of cross-bridge activity by HC + BDM in the jet shifted the site of origin of the Ca^{2+} waves to the border zone of the jet[35].

Arrhythmias in non-uniform muscle

Short trains of rapid stimulation consistently caused a local Ca^{2+} transient in the border of the jet region as well as Ca^{2+}-waves starting in this area (Fig. 16.5A)[10]. These Ca^{2+}-waves start during force relaxation of the last stimulated twitch and propagate into segments both inside and outside of the jet. Exposure to high $[Ca^{2+}]_o$ cause local $[Ca^{2+}]_i$ transients which occur at the same moment during relaxation, as in muscle exposed to caffeine, BDM or low $[Ca^{2+}]_o$ jets and induced Ca^{2+} waves, but the waves now start in the centre of the jet with high $[Ca^{2+}]_o$. Arrhythmias in the form of non-driven rhythmic activity are triggered when the amplitude of the Ca^{2+} wave is increased, e.g. by raising $[Ca^{2+}]_o$. The arrhythmias disappear when the muscle uniformity is restored by turning the jet off (Fig. 16.5)[10]. The highest incidence of arrhythmias was found in muscles exposed to the jet of high $[Ca^{2+}]_o$. These observations suggest that arrhythmogenic Ca^{2+} waves arise in regions of the muscle with a Ca^{2+}-loaded SR, where the contractile apparatus exhibits active contraction owing to Ca^{2+}-dependent TnC activation of cross-bridges, albeit weaker than that of the adjacent regions.

Effects of stretch on Ca^{2+} waves

If the above-mentioned requirement for the initiation of arrhythmogenic Ca^{2+} waves is correct, one would expect that enhancing the amount of Ca^{2+} bound to TnC, e.g. by stretch of the sarcomeres, would increase the Ca^{2+} surge during the relaxation phase and would accelerate Ca^{2+} waves.

Sarcomere stretch indeed increased both the initial $[Ca^{2+}]_i$ rise (C_W) during initiation of Ca^{2+} waves and propagation velocity (V_{prop}) of Ca^{2+} waves as well as the amplitude of the $[Ca^{2+}]_i$ transients during the waves. Stretch increased V_{prop} twofold in caffeine and fourfold in BDM proportional to the increase of C_W. SL did not affect SR Ca^{2+} loading (reflected by the peak of the last stimulated Ca^{2+} transient)[36] in the region of the wave initiation (i.e. border zone) and in the region where the Ca^{2+} wave propagated outside the jet, suggesting that changes in C_W and V_{prop} were independent of SR Ca^{2+} load. In contrast, V_{prop} correlated strongly and linearly with C_W ($p < 0.001$), independent of the composition of the jet solution, suggesting that changes in V_{prop} induced by stretch depend on the magnitude of the initial $[Ca^{2+}]$ surge[35].

In summary, when non-uniform cardiac muscle operates at higher SL, TnC binds more Ca^{2+}; this causes more Ca^{2+} release during relaxation and leads to a larger Ca^{2+} surge which triggers larger, faster and more arrhythmogenic Ca^{2+} waves. In part this

may be due to stretch dependence of the ryanodine receptors (RyR), although this has not been proven yet.

Effect of force development and relaxation on Ca^{2+} waves

Cooperativity of force and Ca^{2+} binding by TnC[23,37] predicts that the initial Ca^{2+} surge is proportional to the amount of Ca^{2+} bound to TnC and to the rate of force decline during relaxation (Fig. 16.3A). Analysis of the factors for wave initiation suggest that the initial $[Ca^{2+}]$ rise is probably due to Ca^{2+} dissociation from myofilaments as a result of quick release of active sarcomeres[37,38]. The amount of Ca^{2+} binding and dissociation from myofilaments by length changes has been shown to correlate with force development[39]. Therefore, we compared the peak of force (F_T) and the maximum rate of force relaxation ($-dF/dt_{max}$) with subsequent initiation and propagation of Ca^{2+} waves. F_T and $-dF/dt_{max}$ increased in a similar manner with stretch during exposure to jets with both caffeine and BDM. Changes in C_W and V_{prop} of the Ca^{2+} waves correlated clearly with F_T and $-dF/dt_{max}$. These results strongly suggest that force development and relaxation of the twitch determine the initiation and subsequent propagation of Ca^{2+} waves.

Effect of dynamic stretch of the muscle during relaxation on Ca^{2+} waves

The rate of force decline is determined by the interplay between the strong and weak muscle segments. This interplay leads to rapid shortening of the weak, but still contracting, sarcomeres exposed to the jet. The effect of shortening of the weak segment during relaxation on Ca^{2+} wave generation can be tested in several ways. Wakayama et al. showed that quick release during relaxation indeed increases the amplitude of the initial Ca^{2+} transient and accelerates the Ca^{2+} waves[38]. The opposite test is to maintain SL in the weakened segment constant during relaxation. After correction for length dependence of active force development, i.e. the FSLR, the force of the triggered propagated contraction accompanying the Ca^{2+} wave following the dynamic stretch during the relaxation was substantially smaller and started later than the triggered propagated contraction at the same length without dynamic stretch[10].

Conclusions and outlook

Muscles made non-uniform so that a segment becomes weaker than the adjacent muscle segments show three patterns of response in or near the weakened segment: (1) a local Ca^{2+} surge late during relaxation; (2) the surge triggers propagated Ca^{2+} waves; (3) the Ca^{2+} wave may trigger arrhythmias[10,35]. SR loading facilitates the generation of Ca^{2+} waves. Figure 16.5 clearly shows that these arrhythmias are completely reversible and disappear when uniformity in the muscle is restored. The requirements for the initiation of arrhythmogenic Ca^{2+} waves are that the region from where the Ca^{2+} waves start has a Ca^{2+}-loaded SR and exhibits active contraction, albeit weaker than that of the adjacent muscle. These requirements are met in the border of the weak segment if the paradigm to weaken the segment lowers intracellular $[Ca^{2+}]$ or SR-Ca^{2+} load, or reduces cross-bridge activity. The same requirements are met inside the weak segment following exposure of the muscle to high $[Ca^{2+}]_o$ and this reduces contractile force in proportion to an increase in spontaneous Ca^{2+} release by the overloaded SR, as in normal cardiac muscle[33] and in failing heart[34]. The mechanism of propagation of the Ca^{2+} waves needs further study in order to fully explain the high propagation velocity of the waves and test the hypothesis of Ca^{2+} release coupled by Ca^{2+} diffusion, which permits a high propagation velocity as the Ca^{2+} ligands in the cells are still partially occupied[40].

The initial Ca^{2+} surge following rapid force relaxation can be explained by force feedback to Ca^{2+} binding by TnC, because the rapid force decline is expected to accelerate Ca^{2+} dissociation from TnC. Other feedback mechanisms, including feedback between TnC units and the number of cross-bridges, were not able to explain the Ca^{2+} surge[23]. We speculate that the molecular mechanism underlying force dependence of Ca^{2+} binding to TnC is probably that cross-bridge force exerted on the actin filament deforms the TnC molecule, thus retarding the dissociation of Ca^{2+} from TnC (Fig. 16.3)[35]. This mechanism is bound to be stretch-sensitive – thereby providing another means of mechano-electric feedback – since the number of myosin cross-bridges attaching to actin increases with SL over the range of operation, and removal of external load during the twitch causes a robust additional $[Ca^{2+}]_i$ transient[41]. Increased net Ca^{2+} binding by TnC with stretch accelerates the decline of the cytosolic $[Ca^{2+}]_i$ transient[36]. The Ca^{2+} surge and ensuing Ca^{2+} waves start during the rapid decline of twitch-force when the sarcomeres in the strong segments relax and lengthen while rapidly releasing the sarcomeres in the weak segment. It follows that Ca^{2+} release from TnC upon rapid unloading will increase at greater SL and, therefore, increase the Ca^{2+} surge in the non-uniform muscle and accelerate propagation of the Ca^{2+} waves, providing another pathway for mechano-electric feedback.

In summary, the mechanics of uniform and non-uniform cardiac muscle can largely be explained by the two feedback mechanisms illustrated in this chapter. Unloading of stretched weakened segments in non-uniform cardiac muscle during relaxation leads to mechano-electric feedback, i.e. an extra Ca^{2+} transient probably caused by the rapid force decrease during the relaxation phase[41], consistent with the hypothesis that force feeds back to the affinity of TnC for Ca^{2+} [23,42]. These rapid force changes in non-uniform muscle may cause arrhythmogenic Ca^{2+} waves to propagate by activation of neighbouring SR by diffusing Ca^{2+} ions[43,44].

Acknowledgements

This work was supported by grants HL-58860-O6A2 and HL-66140 from the National Heart and Lung Institute of the NIH, by the Canadian Institutes for Health Research, and the Heart and Stroke Foundation of Alberta, the North West Territories and Nunavut. H.E.D.J. ter Keurs is Senior Scientist of the Alberta Heritage Foundation for Medical Research.

References

1. Kleber AG, Rudy Y. Basic mechanisms of cardiac impulse propagation and associated arrhythmias. *Physiol Rev* 2004;**84**:431–488.

2. Young AA, Dokos S, Powell KA, *et al.* Regional heterogeneity of function in nonischemic dilated cardiomyopathy. *Cardivasc Res* 2001;**49**:308–318.

3. Siogas K, Pappas S, Graekas G, Goudevenos J, Liapi G, Sideris DA. Segmental wall motion abnormalities alter vulnerability to ventricular ectopic beats associated with acute increases in aortic pressure in patients with underlying coronary artery disease. *Heart* 1998;**79**: 268–273.

4. Janse MJ. Electrophysiological changes in heart failure and their relationship to arrhythmogenesis. *Cardiovasc Res* 2004;**61**:208–217.

5. Markhasin VS, Solovyova O, Katsnelson LB, Protsenko Y, Kohl P, Noble D. Mechano-electric interactions in heterogeneous myocardium: development of fundamental experimental and theoretical models. *Prog Biophys Mol Biol* 2003;**82**:207–220.

6. ter Keurs HEDJ, Shinozaki T, Zhang YM, *et al.* Sarcomere mechanics in uniform and nonuniform cardiac muscle – a link between pump function and arrhythmias. *Prog Biophys Mol Biol* 2008;**97**: 312–331.

7. ter Keurs HEDJ, Zhang YM, Miura M. Damage induced arrhythmias: reversal of excitation–contraction coupling. *Cardiovasc Res* 1998; **40**:444–455.

8. Wier WG, Hess P. Excitation-contraction coupling in cardiac purkinje fibers: Effects of cardiotonic steriods on the intracellular $[Ca^{2+}]$ transient, membrane potential, and contraction. *J Gen Physiol* 1984;**83**:395–415.

9. Miura M, Wakayama Y, Endoh H, *et al.* Spatial non-uniformity of excitation-contraction coupling can enhance arrhythmogenic-delayed afterdepolarizations in rat cardiac muscle. *Cardiovasc Res* 2008;**80**:55–61.

10. Wakayama Y, Miura M, Stuyvers BD, Boyden PA, ter Keurs HE. Spatial nonuniformity of excitation-contraction coupling causes arrhythmogenic Ca^{2+} waves in rat cardiac muscle. *Circ Res* 2005;**96**:1266–1273.

11. Cleland JGF, Daubert JC, Erdmann E, Freemantle N, Gras D, Kappenberger L, Tavazzi L. Longer-term effects of cardiac resynchronization therapy on mortality in heart failure [the CArdiac REsynchronization-Heart Failure (CARE-HF) trial extension phase]. *Europ Heart J* 2006;**27**:1928–1932.

12. Miura M, Boyden PA, ter Keurs HEDJ. Ca^{2+} waves during triggered propagated contractions in intact trabeculae. *Am J Physiol* 1998;**274**: H266-H276.

13. ter Keurs HEDJ, Rijnsburger WH, van Heuningen R, Nagelsmit MJ. Tension development and sarcomere length in rat cardiac trabeculae. Evidence of length-dependent activation. *Circ Res* 1980;**46**:703–714.

14. Konishi M, Kurihara S, Sakai T. The effects of caffeine on tension development and intracellular calcium transients in rat ventricular muscle. *J Physiol* 1984;**355**:605–618.

15. Sitsapesan R, Williams AJ. Mechanisms of caffeine activation of single calcium-release channels of sheep cardiac sarcoplasmic reticulum. *J Physiol* 1990;**423**:425–439.

16. Sellin LC, McArdle JJ. Multiple effects of 2,3-butanedione monoxime. *Pharmacol Toxicol* 1994;**74**:305–313.

17. Backx PHM, Gao WD, Azan-Backx MD, Marban E. Mechanism of force inhibition by 2,3-butanedione monoxime in rat cardiac muscle: roles of $[Ca^{2+}]_i$ and cross-bridge kinetics. *J Physiol* 1994;**476**:487–500.

18. Daniels MCG, Noble MIM, ter Keurs HEDJ, Wohlfart B. Velocity of sarcomere shortening in rat cardiac muscle: relationship to force, sarcomere length, calcium, and time. *J Physiol* 1984;**355**: 367–381.

19. Edman KAP, Mulieri LA, Scubon-Mulieri B. Non-hyperbolic force-velocity relationship in single muscle fibres. *Acta Physiol Scand* 1976; **98**:143–156.

20. de Tombe PP, ter Keurs HEDJ. An internal viscous element limits unloaded velocity of sarcomere shortening in rat myocardium. *J Physiol* 1992;**454**:619–642.

21. Hill AV. The heat of shortening and the dynamic constants of muscle. *Proc R Soc Lond* 1919;**126**:136–195.

22. Landesberg A, Sideman S. Mechanical regulation in the cardiac muscle by coupling calcium kinetics with crossbridge cycling; a dynamic model. *Am J Physiol* 1994;**267**:H779-H795.

23. ter Keurs HEDJ, Shinozaki T, Zhang YM, *et al.* Sarcomere mechanics in uniform and non-uniform cardiac muscle: A link between pump function and arrhythmias. *Prog Biophys Mol Biol* 2008;**97**: 312–331.

24. Backx PHM, ter Keurs HEDJ. Fluorescent properties of rat cardiac trabecule microinjected with fura-2 salt. *Am J Physiol* 1993;**264**: H1098-H1110.

25. Kurihara S, Komukai K. Tension-dependent changes of the intracellular Ca^{2+} transients in ferret ventricular muscles. *J Physiol* 1995;**489**:617–625.

26. Housmans PR, Lee NKM, Blinks JR. Active shortening retards the decline of the intracellular calcium transient in mammalian heart muscle. *Science* 1983;**221**:159–161.

27. Allen DG, Kurihara S. The effects of muscle length on intracellular calcium transients in mammalian cardiac-muscle. *J Physiol* 1982;**327**: 79–94.

28. Jiang Y, Patterson MF, Morgan DL, Julian FJ. Basis for late rise in fura 2 R signal reporting $[Ca^{2+}]_i$ during relaxation in intact rat ventricular trabeculae. *Am J Physiol* 1998;**274**:C1273-C1282.

29. Landesberg A, Livshitz L, ter Keurs HE. The effect of sarcomere shortening velocity on force generation, analysis, and verification of models for crossbridge dynamics. *Ann Biomed Eng* 2000;**28**: 968–978.

30. Landesberg A, Sideman S. Force-velocity relationship and biochemical-to-mechanical energy conversion by the sarcomere. *Am J Physiol* 2000;**278**:H1274-H1284.

31. Hill AV. The heat of shortening and the dynamic constants of muscle. *Proc R Soc Lond A* 1919;**126**:136–195.

32. Poggesi C, Tesi C, Stehle R. Sarcomeric determinants of striated muscle relaxation kinetics. *Pflug Arch* 2005;**449**:505–517.

33. Capogrossi MC, Stern MD, Spurgeon HA, Lakatta EG. Spontaneous calcium release from the sarcoplasmic reticulum limits calcium-dependent twitch potentiation in individual cardiac myocytes. *J Gen Physiol* 1988;**91**:133–155.

34. Obayashi M, Xiao B, Stuyvers BD, Davidoff AW, Mei J, Chen SR, ter Keurs HE. Spontaneous diastolic contractions and phosphorylation of the cardiac ryanodine receptor at serine-2808 in congestive heart failure in rat. *Cardiovasc Res* 2006; **69**:140–151.

35. ter Keurs HEDJ, Wakayama Y, Sugai Y, Stuyvers BD, Miura M, Kagaya Y. Role of sarcomere mechanics and Ca^{2+} overload in Ca^{2+} waves and arrhythmias in rat cardiac muscle. *Ann NY Acad Sci* 2006; **1080**:248–267.

36. Backx PH, ter Keurs HEDJ. Fluorescent properties of rat cardiac trabeculae microinjected with fura-2 salt. *Am J Physiol* 1993;**264**:H1098-H1110.

37. Hunter PJ, McCulloch AD, ter Keurs HEDJ. Modelling the mechanical properties of cardiac muscle. *Prog Biophys Mol Biol* 1998;**69**:289–331.

38. Wakayama Y, Sugai Y, Kagaya Y, Watanabe J, ter Keurs HEDJ. Stretch and quick release of cardiac trabeculae accelerates Ca^{2+} waves and triggered propagated contractions. *Am J Physiol* 2001;**281**: H2133–H2142.

39. Allen DG, Kentish JC. The cellular basis of the length-tension relation in cardiac muscle. *J Mol Cell Cardiol* 1985;**17**:821–840.

40. Backx PHM, de Tombe PP, van Deen JHK, Mulder BJM, ter Keurs HEDJ. A model of propagating calcium-induced calcium release mediated by calcium diffusion. *J Gen Physiol* 1989;**93**: 963–977.

41. Allen DG, Kurihara S. The effects of muscle length on intracellular calcium transients in mammalian cardiac muscle. *J Physiol* 1982;**327**:79–94.

42. Landesberg A, Sideman S. Coupling calcium binding to troponin-C and cross-bridge cycling in skinned cardiac cells. *Am J Physiol* 1994;**266**:H1260-H1271.

43. ter Keurs HEDJ, Boyden PA. Calcium and arrhythmogenesis. *Physiol Rev* 2007;**87**:457–506.

44. Boyden PA, Ter Keurs H. Would modulation of intracellular Ca^{2+} be antiarrhythmic? *Pharmacol Ther* 2005;**108**:149–179.

Cellular mechanisms of arrhythmogenic cardiac alternans

Kenneth R. Laurita

Background

Sudden cardiac death (SCD) resulting from ventricular arrhythmias is a major cause of mortality in Western societies. Despite its prevalence, the mechanisms of SCD remain unclear. Mechanical dysfunction is one of the best predictors of SCD; however, its relationship with electrical instability is not fully understood. For example, effects of electrical instability on mechanical dysfunction of the heart are well appreciated and relatively clear; however, the reverse effects of mechanical dysfunction on electrical instability, or mechano-electrical coupling (MEC), are not. Stretch activated channels are one way mechanical function can directly influence electrical activity at the cellular level (see Chapters 1–6). Intracellular free calcium concentration ($[Ca^{2+}]_i$), a key signalling mechanism of contraction, is also sensitive to the mechanical environment (see Chapter 10) and can also significantly influence electrical activity of the heart. The mechanisms by which $[Ca^{2+}]_i$ can provoke electrical instability and ventricular arrhythmias are the main focus of this chapter. In particular, this chapter focuses on how cardiac alternans, a mechanism of re-entrant excitation, is another significant way mechanical dysfunction and arrhythmogenesis are mechanistically linked.

Alternans-mediated arrhythmogenesis

Cardiac alternans can refer to either mechanical (contractile) or electrical (repolarization) oscillations that occur on an 'every other beat basis'. Cardiac alternans has been recognized for more than 100 years and is associated with a poor prognosis[1]. Until recently, however, the mechanistic relationship between cardiac alternans and mortality was unknown. It is generally accepted that T-wave alternans is caused by beat-to-beat changes in repolarization that increase in magnitude with increasing heart rate[2,3]. Alternans of the QRS complex of the electrocardiogram (ECG) can occur as well, but typically at faster heart rates, secondary to repolarization alternans[4]. In a nutshell, repolarization alternans significantly amplifies repolarization gradients such that unidirectional block may occur. Importantly, this is true even in the absence of large ion channel heterogeneities. Figure 17.1 shows the initiation of ventricular fibrillation (VF) by repolarization alternans[5]. Above a critical heart rate, repolarization alternans occurs with the same long–short phase across all regions of the heart (i.e. spatially concordant alternans). During spatially concordant alternans (not shown), the gradient of repolarization is relatively small and similar to that during baseline pacing. However, at faster heart rates, repolarization alternans between neighbouring regions occurs with opposite phase (i.e. spatially discordant alternans, not to be confused with electrical–mechanical discordance). As a result, steep gradients of repolarization form, as evidenced by marked crowding of repolarization isochrone lines with a range of repolarization times > 100 ms (Fig. 17.1 bottom, beats 1–3). Moreover, the orientation of repolarization gradients undergoes a nearly complete reversal in direction from beat-to-beat, as indicated by the arrows in Fig. 17.1. Although repolarization patterns are complex, they are highly reproducible on alternate beats (Fig. 17.1, compare repolarization maps of beat 1 and beat 3). The pattern of depolarization during spatially discordant repolarization alternans remains stable, without any significant evidence of conduction alternans (see depolarization maps). Finally, the introduction of a premature beat during discordant alternans results in conduction block (beat 4, depolarization map) into a region having delayed repolarization from the previous beat (beat 3, repolarization map). The impulse then propagates around both sides of the line of functional block (hatched area) and re-enters from outside the mapping field, forming the first spontaneous beat of re-entrant VF. These data demonstrate one way in which repolarization alternans can dynamically transform physiological gradients of repolarization into pathophysiological gradients that may give rise to VF. Importantly, spatially discordant alternans is a consistent precursor to re-entrant arrhythmogenesis because of its effect on repolarization gradients in the heart. Clearly, this cascade of events critically depends on the development of electrical alternans. Thus, what causes alternans in the first place?

Coupling between voltage and calcium

Electrical and mechanical alternans are often observed concurrently at the cellular and whole heart levels[2,6], suggesting that

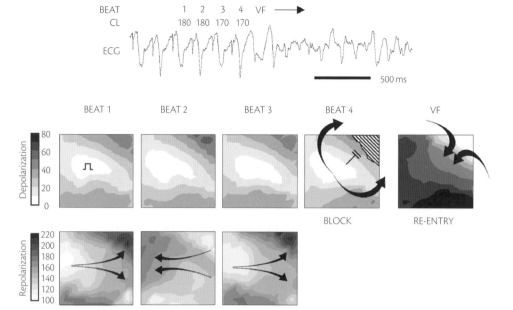

Fig. 17.1 Representative example demonstrating the mechanism linking repolarization alternans to the genesis of re-entrant VF. Contour maps indicate the pattern of depolarization (top) and repolarization (bottom) across the epicardial surface of guinea pig ventricle (times shown in milliseconds). The ECG across the top is shown for reference. CL, cycle length. [Reproduced, with permission, from Laurita KR, Rosenbaum DS (2008) Cellular mechanisms of arrhythmogenic cardiac alternans. *Prog Biophys Mol Biol* **97**: 332–347.]

$[Ca^{2+}]_i$ regulation plays a role. The numerous molecular processes involved in $[Ca^{2+}]_i$ homeostasis (see Chapter 10) highlight the complex nature of its regulation and, thus, the many pathways in which calcium dysregulation can occur. Consequently, how $[Ca^{2+}]_i$ regulation influences membrane potential and vice versa is key to understanding calcium-mediated repolarization alternans. During normal excitation–contraction coupling, trans-membrane voltage changes initiate the process of calcium-induced calcium release, raising $[Ca^{2+}]_i$. This, in turn, affects the trans-membrane potential. The complex interplay between trans-membrane potential and $[Ca^{2+}]_i$ has been referred to as 'bi-directional' coupling[7]. For example, the Na^+/Ca^{2+} exchanger (NCX) is electrogenic (importing three positive changes in exchange for extrusion of two), resulting in a net depolarizing current. Consequently, increased $[Ca^{2+}]_i$ would be expected to prolong action potential duration (APD). This type of coupling between calcium release and APD is referred to as positive calcium to trans-membrane potential (Ca-to-Vm) coupling[7]. Figure 17.2 shows an example of positive Ca-to-Vm coupling (also known as electrical–mechanical concordance) during cardiac alternans[2]. In the presence of significant ECG

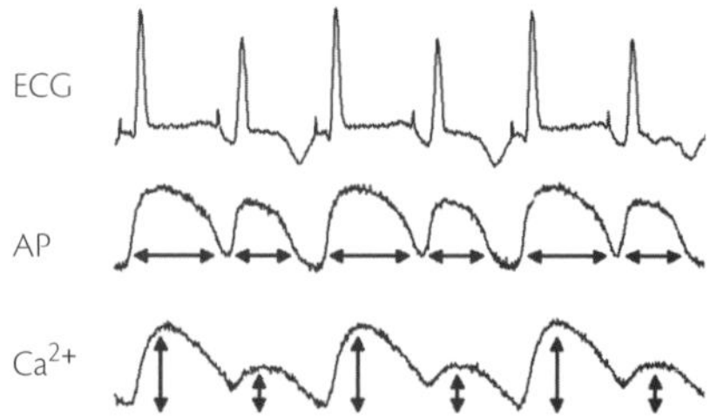

T-wave alternans, APD alternates as well. Significant calcium transient amplitude alternans also occurs, indicating alternating calcium release from the sarcoplasmic reticulum (SR). In this example of positive Ca-to-Vm coupling, a larger calcium release is associated with a longer APD, while smaller releases coincide with shorter APD.

Negative Ca-to-Vm coupling can also occur. For example, when calcium is released from the SR, it may inactivate L-type Ca^{2+} current ($I_{Ca,L}$), which would decrease net depolarizing current during the early action potential (AP) and shorten APD. In this case, a larger than normal calcium release would shorten APD, and vice versa. Additionally, the slow component of the delayed rectifier K^+ current (I_{Ks}) is enhanced by $[Ca^{2+}]_i$, which can contribute to calcium transient amplitude-dependent APD shortening. Finally, the calcium-activated transient outward chloride current (I_{to2}) and calcium-activated non-selective current $[I_{NS,(Ca)}]$ can also influence membrane potential, but their effect on APD is not as clear.

Overall, Ca-to-Vm coupling depends on the balance of calcium-sensitive currents, which may vary with species and disease conditions. This will determine the direction of APD changes for a given change in SR calcium release. For the most part, we see electrical–mechanical concordance, but discordance (short APD associated with large calcium transient) is possible, especially on a microscopic scale when electrotonic forces constrain local spatial discontinuities of voltage but not calcium[8,9]. There are also several reports of electrical–mechanical discordance in the whole heart[6,10].

In the case of Vm-to-Ca coupling, APD governs calcium release from the SR. For example, at constant heart rate, a sudden prolongation of APD will shorten the subsequent diastolic interval and thus provide less time for $I_{Ca,L}$ to fully recover. Consequently, $I_{Ca,L}$ will be reduced and so will calcium release from the SR. So, if APD alternates on a beat-to-beat basis, calcium release (or mechanical) alternans will follow. Rate dependence of repolarizing ion channels may be responsible for electrical alternans. This can be demonstrated by APD restitution, which describes how APD responds to

Fig. 17.2 ECG, AP and Ca^{2+} transients recorded simultaneously in a Langendorff-perfused guinea pig heart during alternans. Alternans was induced by pacing at a cycle length of 170 ms. The arrows below each AP and Ca^{2+} transient represent APD and Ca^{2+} transient amplitude, respectively. [Reproduced, with permission, from Laurita KR, Rosenbaum DS (2008) Cellular mechanisms of arrhythmogenic cardiac alternans. *Prog Biophys Mol Biol* **97**:332–347.]

heart rate. The basic premise of the 'restitution hypothesis' says that repolarization alternans will occur when the slope of the restitution curve is > 1, which has been taken as evidence that sarcolemmal ion channels, rather than SR calcium regulation, determine repolarization alternans[11,12]. However, restitution is a product of multiple ionic mechanisms, including $[Ca^{2+}]_i$ cycling. Therefore analysis of APD restitution can yield conflicting results[13]. Nonetheless, there are instances when membrane ionic current kinetics are a likely cause of alternans[14]. So, one should not rule out membrane ion channel kinetics as a mechanism of alternans. Nevertheless, in the setting of mechanical dysfunction, a more likely scenario is $[Ca^{2+}]_i$ dysfunction and its effects on electrical instability.

Cellular mechanisms of alternans

It has been hypothesized that repolarization alternans is caused by beat-to-beat alternans of SR calcium release[2,15]. In isolated cells, Chudin *et al.*[16]. demonstrated alternans of the calcium transient in the presence *and* absence of AP alternans (i.e. AP clamped). Similarly, measurements *in situ* (without voltage clamping)[9] found calcium transient alternans in intact myocardium using confocal imaging techniques. At fast heart rates, local calcium transient alternans could occur with opposite phase in adjoining cells. Membrane potential was not measured simultaneously, but assuming that electrotonic interaction would prevent significant discontinuities in membrane potential between adjoining cells, it is likely that APD alternated with similar phase. Thus, at the cellular and tissue level, calcium transient alternans may occur independent of voltage. Similar results have been reproduced in modelling studies[8]. These findings strongly support the notion that repolarization alternans may arise from calcium transient alternans.

We have used naturally occurring heterogeneities of repolarization alternans in the whole heart to understand the underlying cellular mechanisms. For example, in the guinea pig we consistently found that sites showing the first signs of alternans with increasing heart rate were at the base of the left ventricle (LV). These sites were defined as alternans-prone regions, in contrast to regions where alternans occurred at faster pacing rates (alternans-resistant regions). Figure 17.3A shows the alternans-prone region (hatched area) near the LV base, superimposed on baseline APD gradients in normal guinea pig heart. The alternans-prone region did not correlate with APD (panels A and B) or restitution kinetics (not shown), as would be expected if APD restitution was the underlying mechanism[2]. In a separate study we found that the alternans-prone region corresponded to tissue where calcium release is weakest (LV base)[17]. Figure 17.3C shows the spatial heterogeneity of calcium transient amplitudes in normal guinea pig heart, which is smallest near the LV base. This is consistent with the notion that a weaker calcium release may be a mechanism of repolarization alternans in the heart[18]. These findings provide further evidence that calcium transient alternans causes repolarization alternans.

Calcium transient alternans caused by heart rate and calcium cycling

If calcium transient alternans causes repolarization alternans, then what would be the molecular mechanisms of calcium transient alternans? Clinically[3], the appearance of cardiac alternans has

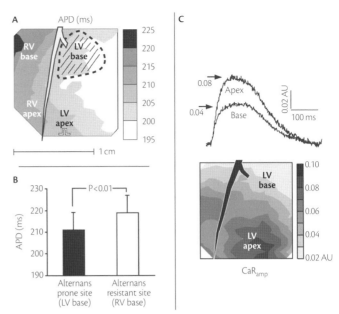

Fig. 17.3 Spatial heterogeneity of APD and alternans. APD gradient was oriented from the right ventricle (RV) base to the left ventricle (LV) free wall, orthogonal to the left anterior descending (LAD) artery (**A**). The onset of APD and Ca^{2+} transient alternans (hatched area) consistently occurred at the LV base (*n* = 7), independent of pacing site. Alternans onset did not occur where APD was longest (i.e. at the RV base), nor where APD was shortest (i.e. toward LV free wall). Similar results were observed in all experiments (**B**). **C** Heterogeneity of Ca^{2+} transient amplitudes (CaR_{amp}), measured using ratiometric optical mapping techniques. [Reproduced, with permission, from Laurita KR, Rosenbaum DS (2008) Cellular mechanisms of arrhythmogenic cardiac alternans. *Prog Biophys Mol Biol* **97**: 332–347.]

been linked to increased heart rate. Therefore, a simple explanation is that when heart rate is faster than the ability of a cell to release and reuptake (i.e. cycle) calcium, then alternans of calcium release will occur. For example, if an AP is initiated before SR calcium content returns to steady-state levels, then the amount released on the subsequent beat will be reduced. Given a smaller release, yet the same time to reclaim calcium, more calcium will end up in the SR on the subsequent beat, giving rise to calcium alternans. The calcium transients shown in Fig. 17.2 (bottom) illustrate this behaviour. Figure 17.4 shows another example of calcium alternans that depends on the rate of calcium cycling, in particular its uptake by the SR. Calcium transients were measured near the epicardium (EPI) and endocardium (ENDO) during an abrupt decrease in pacing cycle length (see arrow in Fig. 17.4). Calcium transient alternans is evident at ENDO and EPI locations. After approximately 4 s, steady-state calcium alternans is greater at ENDO compared to EPI. The decay phase of the calcium transient recorded just before the step change indicates that the rate of calcium decline to diastolic levels (Tau) is significantly slower near the ENDO compared to the EPI. Similar heterogeneities of alternans across the transmural wall have been reported by others and linked to SR calcium regulation[19].

Investigating protein expression in tissue samples taken from alternans-prone and alternans-resistant sites may provide clues to the underlying molecular mechanisms. We found reduced expression of SERCA2a[20,21], in ENDO compared to EPI, consistent with previous studies[22]. In contrast, NCX appeared the same across all

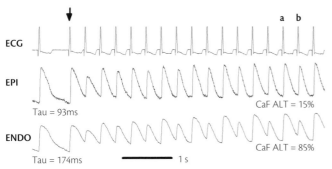

Fig. 17.4 ECG and Ca²⁺ transients near the EPI and ENDO recorded during an abrupt increase in pacing cycle length from 600 to 300 ms (arrow). Near ENDO and EPI, Ca²⁺ transient alternans (CaF ALT) was persistent following 4 s of rapid pacing. At ENDO, where the decay of the Ca²⁺ transient was slower (174 ms) compared to EPI (93 ms), the magnitude of Ca²⁺ transient alternans was greater. At ENDO, the Ca²⁺ transient amplitude for beat (a) was 68% larger than that for beat (b). In contrast, at EPI the degree of Ca²⁺ transient alternans was less obvious (9%). [Reproduced, with permission, from Laurita KR, Katra R, Wible B, Wan X, Koo MH (2003) Transmural heterogeneity of calcium handling in canine. *Circ Res* **92**:668–675.]

layers, a finding similar to that in humans[22], Zygmunt *et al.*[23]. suggests elevated NCX activity in midmyocardial canine LV, and Xiong *et al.*[24] found the highest NCX mRNA and protein expression from EPI in normal canine tissue. In guinea pig, we also found significantly less ryanodine receptors (RyR) at the ENDO compared to the EPI, suggesting a molecular basis of alternans due to SR release. Experiments performed in isolated myocytes subjected to pharmacological inhibition of either RyR or SERCA2a suggest that either of these calcium cycling proteins can cause calcium alternans[21,24]. Finally, we have also shown that *in vivo* gene transfer of a recombinant adenoviral vector with the transgene for SERCA2a suppressed repolarization alternans and, importantly, alternans-mediated ventricular arrhythmias[26]. Thus, the molecular mechanisms of calcium transient alternans appear to be related to not only the reuptake of calcium into the SR (SERCA2a), but also calcium release from the SR (RyR).

Calcium transient alternans caused by SR calcium release

Alternans of SR calcium release can also occur even if heart rate is much slower than the rate at which calcium is cycled. Diaz *et al.*[18] used a voltage-clamp pulse protocol that intentionally avoided $I_{Ca,L}$ activation, producing weak Ca²⁺-induced Ca²⁺ release (CICR). As a result, most RyR channels did not open by CICR, but rather by calcium released from neighbouring RyR, causing a spatially desynchronized calcium release. This gave rise to calcium waves only when SR calcium content was above a certain threshold. So, when an SR calcium release does occur, the SR will become depleted below this threshold, such that on the subsequent voltage clamp pulse no release will occur. The absence of a release will leave enough calcium in the SR so that the next voltage clamp pulse will trigger (a desynchronized) release, perpetuating alternans. Under these conditions, calcium transient alternans occurs at stimulation rates much slower than what is required when CICR is normal. Importantly, this protocol enhances the gain between SR calcium

content and SR calcium release so that small alternans of SR calcium content promote large alternans of SR calcium release. In a theoretical study, Shiferaw *et al.*[27] incorporated similar local dynamics of calcium release and found that alternans is dependent on a steep, non-linear relationship between calcium release and SR content. These findings suggest that the SR calcium store is an important contributor to alternans. However, Picht *et al.*[28] used direct measurements of intra-SR free calcium to show that pacing-induced calcium alternans does not require SR calcium content alternans but, rather, may depend more on RyR recovery.

In addition to voltage clamp protocols to weaken SR calcium release, ischaemia[29,30], and metabolic inhibition[25,31], have been associated with calcium transient alternans. The study of Qian *et al.*[4] showed the development of significant alternans during the acute phases of ischaemia. Interestingly, they found that during acute ischaemia arrhythmogenic alternans occurred at much slower heart rates than under normal conditions, and that repolarization alternans occurred in the absence of conduction alternans[4]. This finding suggests that during ischaemia the rate of calcium cycling (e.g. slow calcium reuptake) may not be the mechanism of alternans, but that RyR dysfunction may be a cause. Local inhibition of glycolysis impairs RyR function and is also associated with calcium transient alternans in the absence of beat-to-beat fluctuations in SR content[25,31]. Taken together, it is clear that RyR dysfunction is an important mechanism of alternans, independent of the rate of calcium cycling[32]. Finally, it is possible that other changes associated with abnormal RyR function can impact calcium transient alternans. For example, detubulation[33], disruption of the regular organization of transverse tubules[34] and a leaky RyR[35] may desynchronize calcium release in ventricular cells and promote the development of alternans.

Mechano-electrical coupling and alternans

As describe above, [Ca²⁺]ᵢ release from the SR, an indirect measure of contraction, plays an important role in repolarization alternans. It is also possible that contraction itself can directly affect repolarization alternans. For example, Murphy *et al.*[6,36], observed electrical alternans during simulated pulse alternans, which was achieved by clamping the aorta on every other beat. What is interesting is that SR calcium release alternans was probably not the primary cause. Enhanced T-wave alternans has also been associated with acute volume overload in structurally normal hearts[37]. These findings suggest that direct MEC may cause repolarization alternans. For example, mechano-sensitive ion channels are able to significantly change membrane potential on a beat-to-beat basis and may be playing a role[38]. Additionally, since these channels conduct sodium (and, in some cell types, calcium) they may affect cellular calcium balance. Furthermore, there is a growing body of evidence showing that stretch affects SR calcium regulation. Iribe and Kohl[39] demonstrated that when myocytes are stretched during diastole, calcium reuptake is enhanced. It is possible that when stretch is reduced (e.g. during mechanical dysfunction) calcium reuptake will be slower and, thus, promote alternans. It is also possible that alternating contraction strength is modulating the binding affinity of troponin C, resulting in alternans of [Ca²⁺]ᵢ[40]. As mentioned earlier, beat-to-beat changes in [Ca²⁺]ᵢ are likely to affect several calcium-sensitive ion channels and, thus, beat-to-beat APD. Despite these possibilities, the exact mechanisms by which mechanical alternans can directly affect electrical alternans are not well understood and are worthy of further investigation[2].

Alternans and heart failure

As mentioned at the beginning of this chapter, there is a very close but not well understood relationship between mechanical dysfunction and SCD (see also Chapter 43). Cardiac alternans is an important mechanistic link. Studies in isolated cells[41] and whole hearts[42] show diminished amplitudes and longer duration of calcium transients in heart failure (HF) compared to normal. Likewise, reduced expression of SERCA2a[43], phospholamban (PLB, a 52-amino-acid trans-membrane protein that reversibly inhibits Ca^{2+} transport by SERCA2a)[44] and 12.6-kDa FK506-binding protein (FKBP12.6)[45] have been reported in HF. Upregulation of

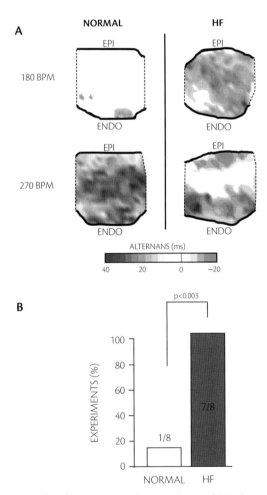

Fig. 17.5 Discordant alternans in HF. **A** Transmural maps of APD alternans magnitude (contour intensity) and phase (contour colour). At a lower heart rate (top) concordant alternans (i.e. one colour) is extensively distributed across the transmural surface in HF but not in normal hearts. At a faster heart rates (bottom), concordant alternans is transformed to discordant alternans in HF only, as myocytes near the EPI and ENDO surfaces begin alternating with opposite phase, depicted by the presence of both red and grey contours. **B** Development of discordant alternans was associated with a higher incidence of inducible VF in HF than in normal hearts. [Reproduced, with permission, from Wilson LD, Jeyaraj D, Wan X, et al. (2009) Heart failure enhances susceptibility to arrhythmogenic cardiac alternans. *Heart Rhythm* **6**:251–259.]

NCX is almost uniformly reported in human and animal models of HF[43,46] and may be a compensatory response[47]. The effect of increased NCX on alternans may be primarily through Ca-to-Vm coupling (positive coupling of Ca-to-Vm is expected to be greater in HF amplifying repolarization alternans). In addition, faster heart rates result in decreased SR calcium reuptake in HF, indicating a decreased ability of the failing heart to cycle calcium[48]. This, in addition to abnormalities of SR calcium release, may explain why alternans is increased in failing myocytes.

We have reported in experimental models that the magnitude of alternans is greater in HF compared to normal over a broad range of pacing cycle lengths across all transmural layers[49]. Importantly, the heart rate threshold for spatially discordant alternans is also greater in HF compared to normal canine wedge preparations. Figure 17.5A shows a representative example of APD alternans contour maps measured across the transmural wall of the canine wedge preparation. At a baseline heart rate (180 bpm), APD alternans is absent in normal but is widespread and spatially concordant in HF. At a faster heart rate (270 bpm) APD alternans is widespread and spatially concordant in the normal preparation; however, in the HF preparation APD alternans is spatially discordant, as indicated by the presence of +phase and –phase alternans. Consistent with this finding is the increased occurrence of arrhythmias in the HF preparation compared to normal (Fig. 17.5B). Wasserstrom et al.[50] also reported a lower heart rate threshold for calcium transient alternans at the subcellular level in spontaneously hypertensive rats compared to controls.

There are several possible reasons why calcium transient alternans is elevated in HF compared to normal, which could be related to SR release or reuptake. The decay phase of the calcium transient is significantly slower in canine ventricular wedge preparations isolated from HF hearts compared to normal[42,49]. Enhanced susceptibility to alternans in HF has also been associated with abnormal RyR function. Lehnart et al.[35] showed that FKBP12.6-deficient mice, which may be more likely to develop HF, are less prone to electrical alternans when pretreated with JTV519, a 1,4-benzothiazepine derivative that increases the binding affinity of FKBP12.6 for RyR and is thought to have cardio-protective actions. This may explain why mechanical and electrical dysfunction are linked; however, the role FKBP12.6 plays in HF and arrhythmogenesis is controversial[51].

Mechanical and $[Ca^{2+}]_i$ dysfunction is also associated with non-re-entrant arrhythmias caused by spontaneous (i.e. non-electrically driven) calcium release from the SR during diastole (see Chapter 16). In addition, we have recently reported spontaneous calcium release from large aggregates of cells in LV wedge preparations isolated from canines with HF[42]. These findings raise an interesting question. What is the mechanism of arrhythmias in the failing heart when calcium handling is abnormal; alternans-induced re-entrant excitation or non-re-entrant excitation caused by spontaneous calcium release? These two mechanisms are not mutually exclusive. Given that alternans and spontaneous calcium release occur at rapid rates, both mechanisms may be operative. Additional studies are required to determine the natural occurrence of arrhythmias in the failing heart.

Conclusions and outlook

To better understand the mechanisms of SCD, a more complete understanding of the complex feedback relationship between cardiac mechanical and electrophysiological dysfunction is essential. Cardiac alternans mediated by $[Ca^{2+}]_i$ may provide a critical link. It is very exciting to imagine the new therapeutic targets that calcium-mediated alternans suggests. For example, accelerating SR uptake of calcium could suppress alternans and reduce the risk of SCD in patients with HF[26], but this may come at the cost of SR calcium overload. Likewise, improving the efficiency of calcium release from the SR by restoring FKBP12.6 binding may also suppress alternans[35]. As an added advantage, targets that can enhance calcium cycling may also improve contractile function. This is in stark contrast to targets that reside on the cell membrane (such as the L-type calcium channels) which, when blocked, can suppress alternans but may also reduce contraction. Pharmacological blockade of membrane K^+ channels not only fails to ameliorate arrhythmias, but also often provokes them (i.e. the 'proarrhythmic effect'). Therefore, new therapeutic targets such as calcium cycling proteins need to be evaluated both for their anti-arrhythmic activity and proarrhythmic potential.

Cardiac alternans represents a unique link between electrical and mechanical dysfunction because it is a mechanism of abnormal impulse conduction (i.e. re-entrant excitation), unlike calcium-mediated arrhythmias caused by abnormalities of impulse formation. The relative importance of SR reuptake, SR release and SR calcium load for alternans is likely to depend on the disease and species. Therefore improved knowledge of calcium dysregulation at the cellular and molecular level is essential. However, relating such abnormalities to arrhythmias that occur in the intact heart remains a challenging task. In sum, it is not a coincidence that mechanical dysfunction remains as one of the best predictors of SCD. Therefore a better appreciation and understanding of MEC-mediated arrhythmogenesis could lead to the identification of novel targets and therapy for treating patients at risk of SCD.

References

1. Windle JD. The incidence and prognostic value of the pulsus alternans in myocardial and arterial disease. *Quart J Med* 1913;**6**:453–462.

2. Pruvot EJ, Katra RP, Rosenbaum DS, Laurita KR. Role of calcium cycling versus restitution in the mechanism of repolarization alternans. *Circ Res* 2004;**94**:1083–1090.

3. Rosenbaum DS, Jackson LE, Smith JM, Garan H, Ruskin JN, Cohen RJ. Electrical alternans and vulnerability to ventricular arrhythmias. *N Engl J Med* 1994;**330**:235–241.

4. Qian YW, Sung RJ, Lin SF, Province R, Clusin WT. Spatial heterogeneity of action potential alternans during global ischemia in the rabbit heart. *Am J Physiol* 2003;**285**:H2722–H2733.

5. Pastore JM, Girouard SD, Laurita KR, Akar FG, Rosenbaum DS. Mechanism linking T-wave alternans to the genesis of cardiac fibrillation. *Circulation* 1999;**99**:1385–1394.

6. Murphy CF, Lab MJ, Horner SM, Dick DJ, Harrison FG. Regional electromechanical alternans in anesthetized pig hearts: modulation by mechanoelectric feedback. *Am J Physiol* 1994;**267**:H1726–H1735.

7. Shiferaw Y, Sato D, Karma A. Coupled dynamics of voltage and calcium in paced cardiac cells. *Phys Rev E Stat Nonlin Soft Matter Phys* 2005;**71**:021903.

8. Sato D, Shiferaw Y, Garfinkel A, Weiss JN, Qu Z, Karma A. Spatially discordant alternans in cardiac tissue: role of calcium cycling. *Circ Res* 2006;**99**:520–527.

9. Aistrup GL, Kelly JE, Kapur S, *et al.* Pacing-induced heterogeneities in intracellular Ca^{2+} signaling, cardiac alternans, and ventricular arrhythmias in intact rat heart. *Circ Res* 2006;**99**:e65–e73.

10. Lee HC, Mohabir R, Smith N, Franz MR, Clusin WT. Effect of ischemia on calcium-dependent fluorescence transients in rabbit hearts containing Indo-1: correlation with monophasic action potentials and contraction. *Circulation* 1988;**78**:1047–1059.

11. Garfinkel A, Kim YH, Voroshilovsky O, *et al.* Preventing ventricular fibrillation by flattening cardiac restitution. *Proc Natl Acad Sci USA* 2000;**97**:6061–6066.

12. Riccio ML, Koller ML, Gilmour RF, Jr. Electrical restitution and spatiotemporal organization during ventricular fibrillation. *Circ Res* 1999;**84**:955–963.

13. Laurita KR. Role of action potential duration restitution in arrhythmogenesis. *J Cardiovasc Electrophysiol* 2004;**15**:464–465.

14. Hua F, Johns DC, Gilmour RF, Jr. Suppression of electrical alternans by overexpression of HERG in canine ventricular myocytes. *Am J Physiol* 2004;**286**:H2342–H2351.

15. Weiss JN, Karma A, Shiferaw Y, Chen PS, Garfinkel A, Qu Z. From pulsus to pulseless: the saga of cardiac alternans. *Circ Res* 2006;**98**:1244–1253.

16. Chudin E, Goldhaber J, Garfinkel A, Weiss J, Kogan B. Intracellular Ca^{2+} dynamics and the stability of ventricular tachycardia. *Biophys J* 1999;**77**:2930–2941.

17. Katra RP, Pruvot E, Laurita KR. Intracellular calcium handling heterogeneities in intact guinea pig hearts. *Am J Physiol* 2004;**286**:H648-H656.

18. Diaz ME, O'Neill SC, Eisner DA. Sarcoplasmic reticulum calcium content fluctuation is the key to cardiac alternans. *Circ Res* 2004;**94**:650–656.

19. Cordeiro JM, Malone JE, Di Diego JM, *et al.* Cellular and subcellular alternans in the canine left ventricle. *Am J Physiol* 2007;**293**:H3506–H3516.

20. Laurita KR, Katra R, Wible B, Wan X, Koo MH. Transmural heterogeneity of calcium handling in canine. *Circ Res* 2003;**92**:668–675.

21. Wan X, Laurita KR, Pruvot E, Rosenbaum DS. Molecular correlates of repolarization alternans in cardiac myocytes. *J Mol Cell Cardiol* 2005;**39**:419–428.

22. Prestle J, Dieterich S, Preuss M, Bieligk U, Hasenfuss G. Heterogeneous transmural gene expression of calcium-handling proteins and natriuretic peptides in the failing human heart. *Cardiovasc Res* 1999;**43**:323–331.

23. Zygmunt AC, Goodrow RJ, Antzelevitch C. I(NaCa) contributes to electrical heterogeneity within the canine ventricle. *Am J Physiol* 2000;**278**:H1671-H1678.

24. Xiong W, Tian Y, DiSilvestre D, Tomaselli GF. Transmural heterogeneity of Na^+-Ca^{2+} exchange: evidence for differential expression in normal and failing hearts. *Circ Res* 2005;**97**:207–209.

25. Hüser J, Wang YG, Sheehan KA, Cifuentes F, Lipsius SL, Blatter LA. Functional coupling between glycolysis and excitation–contraction coupling underlies alternans in cat heart cells. *J Physiol* 2000;**524**:795–806.

26. Cutler MJ, Wan X, Laurita KR, Hajjar RJ. *et al.* Targeted SERCA2a gene expression identifies molecular mechanism and therapeutic target for arrhythmogenic cardiac alternans. *Circ Arrhythm Electrophysiol* 2009;**2**:686–694.

27. Shiferaw Y, Watanabe MA, Garfinkel A, Weiss JN, Karma A. Model of intracellular calcium cycling in ventricular myocytes. *Biophys J* 2003;**85**:3666–3686.

28. Picht E, DeSantiago J, Blatter LA, Bers DM. Cardiac alternans do not rely on diastolic sarcoplasmic reticulum calcium content fluctuations. *Circ Res* 2006;**99**:740–748.

29. Mohabir R, Lee HC, Kurz RW, Clusin WT. Effects of ischemia and hypercarbic acidosis on myocyte calcium transients, contraction, and pHi in perfused rabbit hearts. *Circ Res* 1991;**69**:1525–1537.

30. Wilson LD, Wan X, Rosenbaum DS. Cellular alternans: a mechanism linking calcium cycling proteins to cardiac arrhythmogenesis. *Ann N Y Acad Sci* 2006;**1080**:216–234.

31. Kockskamper J, Blatter LA. Subcellular Ca^{2+} alternans represents a novel mechanism for the generation of arrhythmogenic Ca^{2+} waves in cat atrial myocytes. *J Physiol* 2002;**545**:65–79.

32. Pieske B, Kockskamper J. Alternans goes subcellular: a "disease" of the ryanodine receptor? *Circ Res* 2002;**91**:553–555.

33. Louch WE, Bito V, Heinzel FR, *et al.* Reduced synchrony of Ca^{2+} release with loss of t-tubules-a comparison to Ca^{2+} release in human failing cardiomyocytes. *Cardiovasc Res* 2004;**62**:63–73.

34. Song LS, Sobie EA, McCulle S, Lederer WJ, Balke CW, Cheng H. Orphaned ryanodine receptors in the failing heart. *Proc Natl Acad Sci USA* 2006;**103**:4305–4310.

35. Lehnart SE, Terrenoire C, Reiken S, *et al.* Stabilization of cardiac ryanodine receptor prevents intracellular calcium leak and arrhythmias. *Proc Natl Acad Sci USA* 2006;**103**:7906–7910.

36. Murphy CF, Horner SM, Dick DJ, Coen B, Lab MJ. Electrical alternans and the onset of rate-induced pulsus alternans during acute regional ischaemia in the anaesthetised pig heart. *Cardiovasc Res* 1996;**32**:138–147.

37. Narayan SM, Drinan DD, Lackey RP, Edman CF. Acute volume overload elevates T-wave alternans magnitude. *J Appl Physiol* 2007;**102**:1462–1468.

38. Kohl PSF. Mechanoelectric feedback in cardiac cells. *Phil Trans R Soc (Lond) A* 2001;**359**:1173–1185.

39. Iribe G, Kohl P. Axial stretch enhances sarcoplasmic reticulum Ca^{2+} leak and cellular Ca^{2+} reuptake in guinea pig ventricular myocytes: experiments and models. *Prog Biophys Mol Biol* 2008;**97**:298–311.

40. Housmans PR, Lee NK, Blinks JR. Active shortening retards the decline of the intracellular calcium transient in mammalian heart muscle. *Science* 1983;**221**:159–161.

41. O'Rourke B, Kass DA, Tomaselli GF, Kääb S, Tunin R, Marbán E. Mechanisms of altered excitation–contraction coupling in canine tachycardia-induced heart failure, I – Experimental studies. *Circ Res* 1999;**84**:562–570.

42. Hoeker GS, Katra RP, Wilson LD, Plummer BN, Laurita KR. Spontaneous calcium release in tissue from the failing canine heart. *Am J Physiol* 2009;**297**:H1235–H1242.

43. Tomaselli GF, Marbán E. Electrophysiological remodeling in hypertrophy and heart failure. *Cardiovasc Res* 1999;**42**:270–283.

44. Schwinger RHG, Böhm M, Schmidt U, *et al.* Unchanged protein levels of SERCA II and phospholamban but reduced Ca^{2+} uptake and Ca^{2+}-ATPase activity of cardiac sarcoplasmic reticulum from dilated cardiomyopathy patients compared with patients with nonfailing hearts. *Circulation* 1995;**92**:3220–3228.

45. Yano M, Ono K, Ohkusa T, *et al.* Altered stoichiometry of FKBP12.6 versus ryanodine receptor as a cause of abnormal Ca^{2+} leak through ryanodine receptor in heart failure. *Circulation* 2000;**102**:2131–2136.

46. Hasenfuss G. Alterations of calcium-regulatory proteins in heart failure. *Cardiovasc Res* 1998;**37**:279–289.

47. Hobai IA, O'Rourke B. Enhanced Ca^{2+}-activated Na$^+$-Ca^{2+} exchange activity in canine pacing-induced heart failure. *Circ Res* 2000;**87**:690–698.

48. Pieske B, Kretschmann B, Meyer M, *et al.* Alterations in intracellular calcium handling associated with the inverse force–frequency relation in human dilated cardiomyopathy. *Circulation* 1995;**92**:1169–1178.

49. Wilson LD, Jeyaraj D, Wan X, *et al.* Heart failure enhances susceptibility to arrhythmogenic cardiac alternans. *Heart Rhythm* 2009;**6**:251–259.

50. Wasserstrom JA, Sharma R, Kapur S, *et al.* Multiple defects in intracellular calcium cycling in whole failing rat heart. *Circ Heart Fail* 2009;**2**:223–232.

51. Xiao B, Sutherland C, Walsh MP, Chen SR. Protein kinase A phosphorylation at serine-2808 of the cardiac Ca^{2+}-release channel (ryanodine receptor) does not dissociate 12.6-kDa FK506-binding protein (FKBP12.6). *Circ Res* 2004;**94**:487–495.

52. Laurita KR, Rosenbaum DS. Cellular mechanisms of arrhythmogenic cardiac alternans. *Prog Biophys Mol Biol* 2008;**97**:332–347.

Remodelling of gap junctions in ventricular myocardium, effects of cell-to-cell adhesion, mediators of hypertrophy and mechanical forces

André G. Kléber and Jeffrey E. Saffitz

Background

Integration of individual cells into tissue involves binding of cells to the extracellular matrix, cell-to-cell adhesion and functional cell-to-cell communication. The functions of cell–matrix and cell-to-cell adhesion are not only to anchor cells and determine architecture and passive mechanical properties of tissue, cell–matrix interactions are also important for signalling processes in development and homeostasis in adult tissues.

The transition from normal heart function to cardiac hypertrophy and failure is associated with changes in the gene expression programme and resultant changes in phenotype. Besides intrinsic genetic diseases leading to cardiac failure, the upstream external stimuli leading to hypertrophy include chronically increased sympathetic tone and mechanical overload. The downstream changes in cellular function occur at all levels, including metabolism, electromechanical coupling, the contractile apparatus and electrical function. Changes in electrical function are accompanied by tachyarrhythmias, which are a major cause of sudden death in the setting of cardiac hypertrophy and failure. Remodelling of gap junctions is a major component of the molecular changes that determine altered electrical function in hypertrophied or failing hearts. The questions of whether or how adhesion and electrical junctions interact and how mechanical signalling may affect gap junction expression have been addressed only recently, although there is a relatively large body of literature on the role of cellular adhesion molecules as transmitters of signals from the extra- to the intracellular space. This chapter provides an overview of the work published in this field over the last 10 years. The role of mechanical and electrical coupling between myocytes and non-myocytes, especially fibroblasts, and the involvement of mechanical forces in this process is treated in Chapter 19.

Interaction between cell-to-cell adherens junctions and gap junctions

Molecular structure of cell junctions

Mechanical junctions between cells are composed of discrete clusters of adhesion molecules that connect the membranes of adjacent cells. In addition they form a continuum with the cytoskeleton of the intracellular space[1]. Extracellular binding is Ca^{2+}-dependent, and intracellular binding to components of the cytoskeleton is achieved via linker proteins that form a submembranous scaffold.

As shown schematically in Fig. 18.1, the two types of adhesion junctions in heart are **fascia adherens junctions** and **desmosomes**. The main adhesion molecules that span the cell membranes in the intercalated disks of cardiac myocytes are the **N-cadherins** (fascia adherens junctions) and the **desmogleins** and **desmocollins** (desmosomes). The major linker proteins include members of the catenin and plakin families. In fascia adherens junctions of cardiac myocytes, N-cadherins are linked to actin in sarcomeres by both β-catenin and γ-catenin (**plakoglobin**). In desmosomes, the desmosomal cadherins are associated with intracellular **desmoplakin** and plakoglobin, which in turn bind to desmin, the intermediate filament protein of the myocyte cytoskeleton[1].

Gap junction plaques exhibit a close spatial relationship with fascia adherens junctions as shown in ultrastructural analyses of intercalated disks in dog ventricular myocardium[2,3]. At the ends of ventricular myocytes, in the so-called terminal intercalated disks, large ribbon-like gap junctions oriented perpendicularly to the long cell axis alternate with interdigitated fascia adherens junctions. The fact that gap junctions are oriented in parallel to the long axis of the contractile apparatus[2] is generally interpreted as reflecting mechanical protection of the gap junction

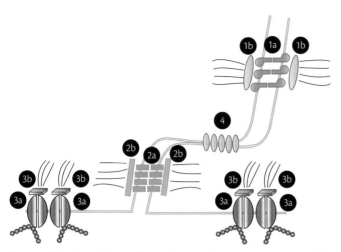

Fig. 18.1 The cell membranes of two adjacent cardiomyocytes are connected by fascia adherens junctions (1), desmosomes (2) and gap junctions (4). The surface membranes are connected to extracellular matrix proteins via cell adherens molecules(3). Fascia adherens junctions consist of the transmembrane spanning Ca^{2+}-dependent adherens proteins [N-cadherins (1a)] that are anchored in a submembranous scaffold (1b) consisting of several proteins (plakoglobin, catenins). The submembranous complex binds to the microfilaments of the cytoskeleton (actin). Desmosomes are formed by the transmembrane spanning proteins desmocollin and desmoglein (2a), anchored in a submembranous scaffold of plakoglobin and desmoplakin (2b). The latter proteins are bound to intermediate filaments (desmin). Gap junctions (4) consist of clustered gap junction channels each formed by two juxtaposed hemichannels (each formed by six connexin proteins). The extracellular matrix is connected to integrin (3a) via fibronectin. Intracellularly, integrins bind to cytoskeletal proteins via a number of intermediate proteins (3b) that cluster intergrin molecules and can induce intracellular signals when activated by extracellular mechanical stimuli. (See color plate section.)

plaque (consisting of channels clustered at high density) against contraction[3].

Interaction between mechanical junctions and gap junctions

A number of studies in cardiac and non-cardiac tissues suggest regulatory interaction between the number of channels clustered in the gap junction plaque and the function and integrity of adhesion junctions. For example, epidermal CA3/7 carcinoma cells have fewer gap junctions *and* adherens junctions than normal mouse epidermal cells of the same type (3PC)[4]. Tumour promoters such as phorbol esters and benzoyl peroxide diminish both connexin (Cx) and E-cadherin expression in 3PC and CA3/7 cells. This indicates that dysregulation of cell growth in tumours is associated with diminished cell-to-cell adhesion and communication[4].

In the heart, evidence for a close interaction between regulation of cell-to-cell adhesion and functional cell-to-cell coupling has been obtained from the neoformation of cell-to-cell junctions during experimental cell apposition, trafficking of connexins, experiments involving mechanical stretch of cardiac myocytes and rare human diseases caused by mutations in linker proteins at fascia adherens junctions and/or desmosomes.

Neoformation of adherens junctions and gap junctions has been studied in cell culture in which dissociated adult rat ventricular myocytes were observed during neoformation of cell-to-cell coupling[5–8].

Disaggregated myocytes start to lose their typical rod-like shape and remodel intracellular architecture within 24 h after seeding[9]. During this process of de-differentiation, the membrane regions corresponding to former intercalated disks become smooth and unstructured. Reformation of intercalated disks with increasing age in culture (culture days 3 to 4) is characterized by initial formation of intercellular fibrillar structures and subsequent appearance of subsarcolemmal plaques. These nascent adhesion junctions subsequently differentiate to intercalated disks. Immunohistochemical analysis at this early stage shows positive signals for N-cadherin, β-catenin and plakoglobin, but only very minor amounts of connexin. Gap junctions containing connexin 43 (Cx43) become evident only once complete adherens junctions have formed. The new gap junctions are located adjacent to the adherens junctions after 6–12 days in culture.

Several studies have suggested an important role for β-catenin in assembly and/or maintenance of adherence junctions and gap junctions and in regulating connexin expression. β-Catenin acts as a transcription factor in early embryonic development and is also a component of the submembranous scaffolding complex of adherens junctions, as described above (Fig. 18.1). Ai *et al.*[10] used immunohistochemical and biochemical approaches to show that Cx43 and β-catenin co-localize in cardiac myocytes and that Cx43/β-catenin complexes can be immunoprecipitated from Triton X100-soluble lysates, suggesting co-localization in the membranous compartment. Wu *et al.*[11] showed a consistent temporal sequence in the reappearance of α-catenin, β-catenin and Cx43 in the membrane. First, immunoreactive signals for α-catenin, β-catenin and Cx43 were redistributed to intracellular loci by culturing neonatal rat cardiac myocytes under low Ca^{2+} conditions. Then, addition of Ca^{2+} at physiologic concentration led to the appearance of α-catenin and β-catenin in the cell surface membrane at sites of cell–cell contacts within 10 min. Cx43 signal was observed at the cell surface only after these catenin proteins accumulated at apparent junctions.

A close association between proteins forming the scaffolds of fascia adherens junctions and Cx43 was also inferred from experiments assessing the introduction of Cx43 hemichannels to gap junctions along microtubular pathways[12]. This process depends on the integrity of protein–protein interactions between the microtubule plus-end-tracking protein EB1, the intermediate protein p150, β-catenin and N-cadherin.

The question of whether protein–protein interactions between elements of the mechanical junctions and the molecules forming gap junction channels are specific for a given connexin isoform was recently raised from the observation of the effects of *Coxsackie*-adenovirus receptor (CAR) protein on electrical coupling. CAR is located at intercalated disks and interacts with β-catenin, ZO-1[13] and N-cadherin[14]. ZO-1 by itself is a regulator of gap junction size[15]. Genetic deletion of CAR decreases the levels of ZO-1 at the intercalated disks and produces a specific deletion of connexin 45 (Cx45) in the sino-atrial and atrio-ventricular nodes accompanied by block of electrical propagation.

Desmosomal diseases affect expression of connexin 43

A fascinating new facet of interaction between expression of adhesion junctions and gap junctions has become evident from the analysis of cardiomyopathies caused by mutations in desmosomal proteins.

The first diseases to be described were two familial diseases (Naxos disease and Carvajal syndrome) characterized by mutations in the plakoglobin[16] and the desmoplakin genes[17], respectively. Among multiple symptoms, these patients suffer from arrhythmogenic right ventricular cardiomyopathy (ARVC; see Chapter 57 for detail). Subsequently, large cohorts of patients have been analyzed with several mutations affecting desmosomal proteins[18–20]. In the context of the topic of this chapter, it seems important to note that downregulation of Cx43, the main ventricular connexin, is a common endpoint in these mutations[21]. This change in functional, electrical cell-to-cell coupling in ARVC is likely to contribute to arrhythmogenesis.

Mediators of hypertrophy and mechanical stretch remodel gap junctions

Remodelling in hypertrophy and failure

The amount of connexin expression at gap junctions depends on the balance between connexin synthesis, channel assembly and connexin degradation. The turnover of connexins in the junctional plaques is very rapid, with half-lives of one to a few hours[22–25]. New connexons assembled in the endoplasmic reticulum (ER) and the Golgi apparatus travel in vesicles to the plasma membrane where they are added to the periphery of existing junctional plaques. Steady state is maintained by continuous movement of protein from the periphery to the centre where protein is removed[26] and subsequently degraded via both lysosomal and proteasomal pathways[24,25]. This continuous trafficking has been associated with phosphorylation of specific amino acids in the C-terminus of connexin proteins[27,28].

Connexin phosphorylation in its totality and integrity has not been fully elucidated. However, it has been shown that specific phosphorylation sites are responsive to typical molecules involved in signalling cascades[27,28]. Enzymes that phosphorylate connexins at serine residues include mitogen-activated protein kinase (MAPK) activity[29], protein kinase C (PKC)[30], protein kinase A[31] and casein kinase. Tyrosine phosphorylation occurs in cells that express activated tyrosine kinases and usually causes a decrease in junctional conductance[32–35]. Information about transcriptional regulation of connexin expression is scarce and relates to transcription factors that are also involved in cell fate determination during early development. Nkx2.5 is a homeodomain transcription factor involved in fate determination of embryonic cells to procardiomyocytes during early development[36]. It has been shown to regulate connexin 40 (Cx40) gene expression during this embryonic stage[37]. In adult cardiomyocytes, Nkx2.5 has been shown to reduce Cx43 expression[38], a change that may be responsible for atrio-ventricular node conduction disturbances and bradycardia[39]. Wnt1, another important factor involved in embryonic development, induces Cx43 expression, probably through pathways involving β-catenin as a transcription factor[10]. Further studies will be needed to define the exact role of transcriptional regulation of connexin expression in adult cardiomyocytes[40].

Cardiac hypertrophy and failure are associated with changes in electrical function caused by disturbances of impulse initiation and propagation, leading to an increased propensity to tachyarrhythmias. Electrical propagation velocity first increases in hypertrophied ventricles but then decreases as hypertrophy becomes more severe[41–43]. Decrements in conduction velocity and conduction block may be related to discontinuities in extracellular resistance caused by interstitial fibrosis[44–46] and an increase in intercellular resistance due to decreased connexin expression[47–49]. In patients with chronic ischaemic heart disease, Cx43 expression in the gap junctions of the ventricular myocardium is reduced[50]. These results and others suggest that reduced gap junction channel protein levels occur as a general rule in chronic myocardial disease states, such as healed myocardial infarction[47–49], chronic hibernation[50] and end-stage aortic stenosis[51]. In the setting of hypertrophy and failure the signalling mechanisms leading to connexin downregulation have not yet been fully defined. An important role may be played by c-Jun-activated N-terminal kinase (JNK). Indeed, a rapid and massive decrease of Cx43 expression (up to 90%) was consistently observed with activation of JNK in cultured cardiac myocytes or in vivo[52].

In contrast to the findings observed in advanced stages of heart failure, compensatory **myocardial hypertrophy** leads to increased connexin levels, increased number of gap junctions and enhanced intercellular coupling. With respect to mediators of myocardial hypertrophy, cyclic adenosine monophosphate (cAMP) and angiotensin II (AT-II) have been shown to upregulate gap junctions. Exposure of cultured neonatal rat ventricular myocytes to a membrane-permeable form of cAMP for 24 h increases the tissue content of Cx43 by approximately twofold and increases the number of gap junctions interconnecting cells[53]. These changes are associated with a significant increase in electrical propagation velocity[53]. Cultured neonatal rat ventricular myocytes exposed for 24 h to AT-II exhibit a twofold increase in Cx43 content and an increase in the number of gap junctions interconnecting cells[54].

Effect of acute stretch on connexin expression

Numerous studies have characterized changes in cardiac myocytes subjected to mechanical load in vitro. Early studies demonstrated that brief intervals of static stretch of neonatal rat myocytes induced features of the hypertrophic response including increases in protooncogene and contractile protein expression, and activation of signal transduction pathways including those mediated by MAPKs, tyrosine kinases, PKC and phospholipases C and D[55–58]. More recent experiments in which myocytes have been subjected to pulsatile stretch have demonstrated activation of numerous signal transduction pathways including all three members of the MAPK family, focal adhesion kinase (FAK) and the janus kinase/signal transducers and activators of transcription (JAK/STAT) pathway[59,60]. Mechanical stretch of cultured neonatal rat ventricles induces release of growth-promoting factors including AT-II, endothelin I, vascular endothelial growth factor (VEGF) and transforming growth factor-β (TGF-β)[55,61–64]. Shyu et al. reported a threefold increase in AT-II in the culture media of rat neonatal myocytes stretched for 1 h[61]. Seko et al. demonstrated that 5 min of pulsatile stretch is sufficient to induce rapid secretion of VEGF and increased expression of both VEGF and VEGF receptor mRNA in cultured cardiac myocytes[62].

Recent experiments carried out in our laboratories indicate that a number of the above-mentioned signalling pathways also exert an effect on connexin expression in gap junctions. Stretching monolayers of neonatal rat ventricular myocytes to 110% of resting cell length at a frequency of 3 Hz produced marked upregulation of Cx43 after only 1 h[65]. A further increase occurred after 6 h of stretch. The increase in gap junctional Cx43 was accompanied by a significant increase in electrical propagation velocity[65], suggesting that the change in conduction velocity was related mainly to enhanced electrical coupling[65].

VEGF and TGF-β are both known to be synthesized and secreted by cardiac myocytes in response to pulsatile stretch[62]. These same molecules, when added to the culture medium, also upregulate Cx43[66]. Thus, addition of either exogenous TGF-β (10 ng/ml) or VEGF (100 ng/ml) to unstretched neonatal rat ventricular myocytes for 1 h increases Cx43 expression by as much as ~1.8-fold, an amount comparable to that observed in cells subjected to pulsatile stretch for 1 h. A close association between stretch-induced Cx43 upregulation and VEGF or TGF-β is suggested by the observation that the stretch-induced effect is blocked by either anti-VEGF or anti-TGF-β antibodies[66]. Anti-VEGF antibodies also block the stretch-induced increase in electrical propagation velocity. Complementary results, confirming the involvement of VEGF or TGF-β, include the observation of stretch-induced VEGF release into the culture medium[66]. Upregulation of Cx43 expression stimulated by exogenous TGF-β was blocked by anti-VEGF antibody, but VEGF stimulation of Cx43 expression was not blocked by anti-TGF-β antibody, confirming that TGF-β was acting upstream of VEGF. In similar studies on AT-II, Shyu et al.[61] showed that upregulation of Cx43 following several hours of stretch could be blocked by addition of the AT_1-antagonist losartan. It is very likely that multiple chemical signals released from cells in response to stretch, in addition to those described above, may act on connexin regulation via complex interacting signalling pathways during different intervals of mechanical stimulation.

It needs to be emphasized that mechanical forces may affect cardiac propagation via modulation of factors other than cell-to-cell coupling, such as changes in the shape and passive electrical properties of the intra- and extracellular domains and changes in resting membrane potential. An extensive discussion of these factors is provided in Chapter 25 of this book.

Integrin signalling, focal adhesion kinases and their potential role in stretch-activated upregulation of Cx43

Interactions between integrins and extracellular matrix proteins are known to play a pivotal role in stretch-activated changes of cardiac myocyte structure and function. Overexpression of integrins, by itself, can induce a hypertrophic response in neonatal rat ventricular myocytes in vitro and enhance the effects of α_1 adrenergic stimulation[67]. Inhibition of β1 integrin function and signalling reduces the hypertrophic response. The effect of pulsatile longitudinal stretch to upregulate Cx43 in cultures of neonatal ventricular myocytes is mediated by interaction between the arginine–glycine–aspartate (RGD) motif in extracellular matrix proteins and β1-integrin[68]. This conclusion was made from the observation that exposure of RGD motifs in extracellular matrix (ECM) proteins (denaturation of collagen, fibronectin) increased while antibody-mediated inhibition of β1-integrin signalling decreased Cx43 expression[67].

FAK, a primary mediator of integrin signalling, may also play a role in the hypertrophic and adhesive responses of neonatal rat ventricular myocytes in culture[69–72]. FAK is also activated by VEGF[69] and translocates to costameres in cardiac myocytes subjected to stretch[73]. Whereas pulsatile stretch induces rapid common upregulation of Cx43 and mechanical junction proteins[74] via β1-integrin-mediated signalling and activation of FAK[68], regulation downstream of FAK seems more complex. In contrast to Cx43, upregulation of plakoglobin, desmoplakin and N-cadherin is mediated by a VEGF-independent mechanism[75]. Transfection of cells with a dominant-negative inhibitor of FAK blocked both stretched-induced upregulation of Cx43 and contractile proteins (plakoglobin, desmoplakin and N-cadherin). Application of VEGF to transfected cells upregulated Cx43. By contrast, application of an src kinase inhibitor blocked stretch-induced upregulation of mechanical junction proteins but not Cx43. This indicates that upregulation of Cx43 by acute stretch is mediated by FAK-dependent secretion of VEGF, whereas upregulation of mechanical junction proteins is induced by FAK-mediated activation of src kinase. The further pathways downstream of src kinase and the mechanisms by which VEGF upregulates Cx43 remain to be determined.

Conclusions and outlook

The discussion of the role of mechanical forces in mechanical and electrical cell-to-cell coupling makes it evident that research in this field is just at the beginning of a fascinating era. The interactions between mechanical junctions and gap junctions, which were originally described in experiments involving neoformation of cell junctions in cell cultures many years ago, have suddenly become important in the context of desmosomal diseases that show highly significant remodelling of electrical junctions. Yet, the exact molecular pathways linking genetic defects in multiple proteins of the mechanical junctions to decreased connexin expression have not been elucidated. Remodelling of electrical junctions in cardiac hypertrophy and failure is another field where our knowledge is largely incomplete. In particular, relatively little is known about the signalling pathways and molecular mechanisms that downregulate connexins in the chronic stage of heart failure. Moreover, research over the past years has shown that connexin may contribute to functions other than cell-to-cell coupling. Thus, connexins have been identified in mitochondria where they are contributing to the changes brought about by ischaemic preconditioning[76]. Direct mechano-sensitivity has been attributed to Cx43 hemichannels in the surface membrane of osteocytes[77], and to connexin 46 (Cx46) surface hemichannels expressed in Xenopus oocytes[78]. All these findings point to a much more complex role of connexins in cell biology than previously inferred from the traditional concept of gap junction channels solely forming relatively 'inert' high permeability channels between cells.

References

1. Gumbiner BM. Cell adhesion: the molecular basis of tissue architecture and morphogenesis. Cell 1996;**84**:345–357.
2. Fawcett DW, McNutt NS. The ultrastructure of the cat myocardium. I. Ventricular papillary muscle. J Cell Biol 1969;**42**:1–45.
3. Hoyt RH, Cohen ML, Saffitz JE. Distribution and three-dimensional structure of intercellular junctions in canine myocardium. Circ Res 1989;**64**:563–574.

4. Jansen LA, Mesnil M, Jongen WM. Inhibition of gap junctional intercellular communication and delocalization of the cell adhesion molecule E-cadherin by tumor promoters. *Carcinogenesis* 1996;**17**:1527–1531.

5. Hertig CM, Butz S, Koch S, Eppenberger-Eberhardt M, Kemler R, Eppenberger HM. N-cadherin in adult rat cardiomyocytes in culture. II. Spatio-temporal appearance of proteins involved in cell–cell contact and communication. Formation of two distinct N-cadherin/catenin complexes. *J Cell Sci* 1996;**109**:11–20.

6. Hertig CM, Eppenberger-Eberhardt M, Koch S, Eppenberger HM. N-cadherin in adult rat cardiomyocytes in culture. I. Functional role of N-cadherin and impairment of cell–cell contact by a truncated N-cadherin mutant. *J Cell Sci* 1996;**109**:1–10.

7. Kostin S, Hein S, Bauer EP, Schaper J. Spatiotemporal development and distribution of intercellular junctions in adult rat cardiomyocytes in culture. *Circ Res* 1999;**85**:154–167.

8. Zuppinger C, Schaub MC, Eppenberger HM. Dynamics of early contact formation in cultured adult rat cardiomyocytes studied by N-cadherin fused to green fluorescent protein. *J Mol Cell Cardiol* 2000;**32**:539–555.

9. Lipp P, Huser J, Pott L, Niggli E. Spatially non-uniform Ca^{2+} signals induced by the reduction of transverse tubules in citrate-loaded guinea-pig ventricular myocytes in culture. *J Physiol* 1996;**497**:589–597.

10. Ai Z, Fischer A, Spray DC, Brown AM, Fishman GI. Wnt-1 regulation of connexin 43 in cardiac myocytes. *J Clin Invest* 2000;**105**:161–171.

11. Wu JC, Tsai RY, Chung TH. Role of catenins in the development of gap junctions in rat cardiomyocytes. *J Cell Biochem* 2003;**88**:823–835.

12. Shaw RM, Fay AJ, Puthenveedu MA, von Zastrow M, Jan YN, Jan LY. Microtubule plus-end-tracking proteins target gap junctions directly from the cell interior to adherens junctions. *Cell* 2007;**128**:547–560.

13. Lim BK, Xiong D, Dorner A, *et al.* Coxsackievirus and adenovirus receptor (CAR) mediates atrioventricular-node function and connexin 45 localization in the murine heart. *J Clin Invest* 2008;**118**:2758–2770.

14. Kashimura T, Kodama M, Hotta Y, *et al.* Spatiotemporal changes of coxsackievirus and adenovirus receptor in rat hearts during postnatal development and in cultured cardiomyocytes of neonatal rat. *Virchows Arch* 2004;**444**:283–292.

15. Hunter AW, Barker RJ, Zhu C, Gourdie RG. Zonula occludens-1 alters connexin 43 gap junction size and organization by influencing channel accretion. *Mol Biol Cell* 2005;**16**:5686–5698.

16. McKoy G, Protonotarios N, Crosby A, *et al.* Identification of a deletion in plakoglobin in arrhythmogenic right ventricular cardiomyopathy with palmoplantar keratoderma and woolly hair (Naxos disease). *Lancet* 2000;**355**:2119–2124.

17. Norgett EE, Hatsell SJ, Carvajal-Huerta L, *et al.* Recessive mutation in desmoplakin disrupts desmoplakin-intermediate filament interactions and causes dilated cardiomyopathy, woolly hair and keratoderma. *Hum Mol Genet* 2000;**9**:2761–2766.

18. Sen-Chowdhry S, Syrris P, McKenna WJ. Role of genetic analysis in the management of patients with arrhythmogenic right ventricular dysplasia/cardiomyopathy. *J Am Coll Cardiol* 2007;**50**:1813–1821.

19. Sen-Chowdhry S, Syrris P, Ward D, Asimaki A, Sevdalis E, McKenna WJ. Clinical and genetic characterization of families with arrhythmogenic right ventricular dysplasia/cardiomyopathy provides novel insights into patterns of disease expression. *Circulation* 2007;**115**:1710–1720.

20. Thiene G, Corrado D, Basso C. Arrhythmogenic right ventricular cardiomyopathy/dysplasia. *Orphanet J Rare Dis* 2007;**2**:45.

21. Asimaki A, Tandri H, Huang H, *et al.* A new diagnostic test for arrhythmogenic right ventricular cardiomyopathy. *N Engl J Med* 2009;**360**:1075–1084.

22. Darrow BJ, Laing JG, Lampe PD, Saffitz JE, Beyer EC. Expression of multiple connexins in cultured neonatal rat ventricular myocytes. *Circ Res* 1995;**76**:381–387.

23. Laird DW, Puranam KL, Revel JP. Turnover and phosphorylation dynamics of connexin 43 gap junction protein in cultured cardiac myocytes. *Biochem J* 1991;**273**:67–72.

24. Laing JG, Tadros PN, Westphale EM, Beyer EC. Degradation of connexin 43 gap junctions involves both the proteasome and the lysosome. *Exp Cell Res* 1997;**236**:482–492.

25. Beardslee MA, Laing JG, Beyer EC, Saffitz JE. Rapid turnover of connexin 43 in the adult rat heart. *Circ Res* 1998;**83**:629–635.

26. Gaietta G, Deerinck TJ, Adams SR, *et al.* Multicolor and electron microscopic imaging of connexin trafficking. *Science* 2002;**296**:503–507.

27. Goodenough DA, Goliger JA, Paul DL. Connexins, connexons, and intercellular communication. *Annu Rev Biochem* 1996;**65**:475–502.

28. Lampe PD, Lau AF. Regulation of gap junctions by phosphorylation of connexins. *Arch Biochem Biophys* 2000;**384**:205–215.

29. Lau AF, Kurata WE, Kanemitsu MY, *et al.* Regulation of connexin 43 function by activated tyrosine protein kinases. *J Bioenerg Biomembr* 1996;**28**:359–368.

30. Lampe PD, TenBroek EM, Burt JM, Kurata WE, Johnson RG, Lau AF. Phosphorylation of connexin 43 on serine 368 by protein kinase C regulates gap junctional communication. *J Cell Biol* 2000;**149**:1503–1512.

31. TenBroek EM, Lampe PD, Solan JL, Reynhout JK, Johnson RG. Ser 364 of connexin 43 and the upregulation of gap junction assembly by cAMP. *J Cell Biol* 2001;**155**:1307–1318.

32. Crow DS, Beyer EC, Paul DL, Kobe SS, Lau AF. Phosphorylation of connexin 43 gap junction protein in uninfected and Rous sarcoma virus-transformed mammalian fibroblasts. *Mol Cell Biol* 1990;**10**:1754–1763.

33. Giepmans BN, Hengeveld T, Postma FR, Moolenaar WH. Interaction of c-Src with gap junction protein connexin-43. Role in the regulation of cell–cell communication. *J Biol Chem* 2001;**276**:8544–8549.

34. Lin R, Warn-Cramer BJ, Kurata WE, Lau AF. v-Src phosphorylation of connexin 43 on Tyr247 and Tyr265 disrupts gap junctional communication. *J Cell Biol* 2001;**154**:815–827.

35. Toyofuku T, Yabuki M, Otsu K, Kuzuya T, Tada M, Hori M. Functional role of c-Src in gap junctions of the cardiomyopathic heart. *Circ Res* 1999;**85**:672–681.

36. Moorman A, Webb S, Brown NA, Lamers W, Anderson RH. Development of the heart, (1) formation of the cardiac chambers and arterial trunks. *Heart* 2003;**89**:806–814.

37. Bruneau BG, Nemer G, Schmitt JP, *et al.* A murine model of Holt–Oram syndrome defines roles of the T-box transcription factor Tbx5 in cardiogenesis and disease. *Cell* 2001;**106**:709–721.

38. Kasahara H, Ueyama T, Wakimoto H, *et al.* Nkx2.5 homeoprotein regulates expression of gap junction protein connexin 43 and sarcomere organization in postnatal cardiomyocytes. *J Mol Cell Cardiol* 2003;**35**:243–256.

39. Wakimoto H, Kasahara H, Maguire CT, Moskowitz IP, Izumo S, Berul CI. Cardiac electrophysiological phenotypes in postnatal expression of Nkx2.5 transgenic mice. *Genesis* 2003;**37**:144–150.

40. Akazawa H, Komuro I. Too much Csx/Nkx2-5 is as bad as too little? *J Mol Cell Cardiol* 2003;**35**:227–229.

41. McIntyre H, Fry CH. Abnormal action potential conduction in isolated human hypertrophied left ventricular myocardium. *J Cardiovasc Electrophysiol* 1997;**8**:887–894.

42. Winterton SJ, Turner MA, O'Gorman DJ, Flores NA, Sheridan DJ. Hypertrophy causes delayed conduction in human and guinea pig myocardium, accentuation during ischaemic perfusion. *Cardiovasc Res* 1994;**28**:47–54.

43. Cooklin M, Wallis WR, Sheridan DJ, Fry CH. Changes in cell-to-cell electrical coupling associated with left ventricular hypertrophy. *Circ Res* 1997;**80**:765–771.

44. Spach MS, Dolber PC. Relating extracellular potentials and their derivatives to anisotropic propagation at a microscopic level in human

cardiac muscle. Evidence for electrical uncoupling of side-to-side fiber connections with increasing age. *Circ Res* 1986;**58**:356–371.

45. Spach MS, Josephson ME. Initiating reentry, the role of nonuniform anisotropy in small circuits. *J Cardiovasc Electrophysiol* 1994;**5**:182–209.

46. Peters NS, Coromilas J, Severs NJ, Wit AL. Disturbed connexin 43 gap junction distribution correlates with the location of reentrant circuits in the epicardial border zone of healing canine infarcts that cause ventricular tachycardia. *Circulation* 1997;**95**:988–996.

47. Luke RA, Saffitz JE. Remodeling of ventricular conduction pathways in healed canine infarct border zones. *J Clin Invest* 1991;**87**:1594–1602.

48. Peters NS New insights into myocardial arrhythmogenesis, distribution of gap-junctional coupling in normal, ischaemic and hypertrophied human hearts. *Clin Sci (Lond)* 1996;**90**:447–452.

49. Smith JH, Green CR, Peters NS, Rothery S, Severs NJ. Altered patterns of gap junction distribution in ischemic heart disease. An immunohistochemical study of human myocardium using laser scanning confocal microscopy. *Am J Pathol* 1991;**139**:801–821.

50. Kaprielian RR, Gunning M, Dupont E, *et al.* Downregulation of immunodetectable connexin 43 and decreased gap junction size in the pathogenesis of chronic hibernation in the human left ventricle. *Circulation* 1998;**97**:651–660.

51. Peters NS, Green CR, Poole-Wilson PA, Severs NJ. Reduced content of connexin 43 gap junctions in ventricular myocardium from hypertrophied and ischemic human hearts. *Circulation* 1993;**88**:864–875.

52. Petrich BG, Gong X, Lerner DL, *et al.* c-Jun N-terminal kinase activation mediates downregulation of connexin 43 in cardiomyocytes. *Circ Res* 2002;**91**:640–647.

53. Darrow BJ, Fast VG, Kleber AG, Beyer EC, Saffitz JE. Functional and structural assessment of intercellular communication. Increased conduction velocity and enhanced connexin expression in dibutyryl cAMP-treated cultured cardiac myocytes. *Circ Res* 1996;**79**:174–183.

54. Dodge SM, Beardslee MA, Darrow BJ, Green KG, Beyer EC, Saffitz JE. Effects of angiotensin II on expression of the gap junction channel protein connexin 43 in neonatal rat ventricular myocytes. *J Am Coll Cardiol* 1998;**32**:800–807.

55. Sadoshima J, Izumo S. Mechanical stretch rapidly activates multiple signal transduction pathways in cardiac myocytes, potential involvement of an autocrine/paracrine mechanism. *Embo J* 1993;**12**:1681–1692.

56. Komuro I, Katoh Y, Kaida T, *et al.* Mechanical loading stimulates cell hypertrophy and specific gene expression in cultured rat cardiac myocytes. Possible role of protein kinase C activation. *J Biol Chem* 1991;**266**:1265–1268.

57. Komuro I, Kaida T, Shibazaki Y, *et al.* Stretching cardiac myocytes stimulates protooncogene expression. *J Biol Chem* 1990;**265**:3595–3598.

58. Komuro I, Kudo S, Yamazaki T, Zou Y, Shiojima I, Yazaki Y. Mechanical stretch activates the stress-activated protein kinases in cardiac myocytes. *FASEB J* 1996;**10**:631–636.

59. Ruwhof C, van der Laarse A. Mechanical stress-induced cardiac hypertrophy, mechanisms and signal transduction pathways. *Cardiovasc Res* 2000;**47**:23–37.

60. Seko Y, Takahashi N, Tobe K, Kadowaki T, Yazaki Y. Pulsatile stretch activates mitogen-activated protein kinase (MAPK) family members and focal adhesion kinase (p125(FAK)) in cultured rat cardiac myocytes. *Biochem Biophys Res Commun* 1999;**259**:8–14.

61. Shyu KG, Chen CC, Wang BW, Kuan P. Angiotensin II receptor antagonist blocks the expression of connexin 43 induced by cyclical mechanical stretch in cultured neonatal rat cardiac myocytes. *J Mol Cell Cardiol* 2001;**33**:691–698.

62. Seko Y, Takahashi N, Shibuya M, Yazaki Y. Pulsatile stretch stimulates vascular endothelial growth factor (VEGF) secretion by cultured rat cardiac myocytes. *Biochem Biophys Res Commun* 1999;**254**:462–465.

63. Ruwhof C, van Wamel AE, Egas JM, van der Laarse A. Cyclic stretch induces the release of growth promoting factors from cultured neonatal cardiomyocytes and cardiac fibroblasts. *Mol Cell Biochem* 2000;**208**:89–98.

64. Sadoshima J, Xu Y, Slayter HS, Izumo S. Autocrine release of angiotensin II mediates stretch-induced hypertrophy of cardiac myocytes in vitro. *Cell* 1993;**75**:977–984.

65. Zhuang J, Yamada KA, Saffitz JE, Kleber AG. Pulsatile stretch remodels cell-to-cell communication in cultured myocytes. *Circ Res* 2000;**87**:316–322.

66. Pimentel RC, Yamada KA, Kleber AG, Saffitz JE. Autocrine regulation of myocyte Cx43 expression by VEGF. *Circ Res* 2002;**90**:671–677.

67. Ross RS, Pham C, Shai SY, *et al.* Beta1 integrins participate in the hypertrophic response of rat ventricular myocytes. *Circ Res* 1998;**82**:1160–1172.

68. Shanker AJ, Yamada K, Green KG, Yamada KA, Saffitz JE. Matrix-protein-specific regulation of Cx43 expression in cardiac myocytes subjected to mechanical load. *Circ Res* 2005;**96**:558–566.

69. Takahashi N, Seko Y, Noiri E, *et al.* Vascular endothelial growth factor induces activation and subcellular translocation of focal adhesion kinase (p125FAK) in cultured rat cardiac myocytes. *Circ Res* 1999;**84**:1194–1202.

70. Pham CG, Harpf AE, Keller RS, *et al.* Striated muscle-specific beta(1D)-integrin and FAK are involved in cardiac myocyte hypertrophic response pathway. *Am J Physiol* 2000;**279**:H2916–H2926.

71. Taylor JM, Rovin JD, Parsons JT. A role for focal adhesion kinase in phenylephrine-induced hypertrophy of rat ventricular cardiomyocytes. *J Biol Chem* 2000;**275**:19250–19257.

72. Eble DM, Strait JB, Govindarajan G, Lou J, Byron KL, Samarel AM. Endothelin-induced cardiac myocyte hypertrophy, role for focal adhesion kinase. *Am J Physiol* 2000;**278**:H1695–H1707.

73. Torsoni AS, Constancio SS, Nadruz W, Jr., Hanks SK, Franchini KG. Focal adhesion kinase is activated and mediates the early hypertrophic response to stretch in cardiac myocytes. *Circ Res* 2003;**93**:140–147.

74. Zhuang J, Yamada KA, Saffitz JE, Kléber AK. Pulsatile stretch remodels cell-to-cell communication in cultured myocytes. *Circ Res* 2000;**87**:316–322.

75. Yamada K, Green KG, Samarel AM, Saffitz JE. Distinct pathways regulate expression of cardiac electrical and mechanical junction proteins in response to stretch. *Circ Res* 2005;**97**:346–353.

76. Boengler K, Dodoni G, Rodriguez-Sinovas A, *et al.* Connexin 43 in cardiomyocyte mitochondria and its increase by ischemic preconditioning. *Cardiovasc Res* 2005;**67**:234–244.

77. Cherian PP, Siller-Jackson AJ, Gu S, *et al.* Mechanical strain opens connexin 43 hemichannels in osteocytes, a novel mechanism for the release of prostaglandin. *Mol Biol Cell* 2005;**16**:3100–3106.

78. Bao L, Sachs F, Dahl G. Connexins are mechanosensitive. *Am J Physiol* 2004;**287**:C1389–C1395.

The origin of fibroblasts, extracellular matrix and potential contributions to cardiac mechano-electric coupling

Troy A. Baudino and Thomas K. Borg

Background

What is a fibroblast? Over the years, the definition of a fibroblast has not changed, in that it is considered a cell of mesenchymal origin whose primary role is the production of a wide variety of extracellular matrix (ECM) components including collagens, proteoglycans, growth factors, proteolytic enzymes, such as matrix metalloproteinases (MMP), and small signalling molecules, such as cytokines[1–4]. Morphologically, fibroblasts are flat, spindle-shaped cells with numerous processes radiating off of the cell body. When active, fibroblasts display a prominent Golgi apparatus and extensive rough endoplasmic reticulum[1]. Fibroblasts are resident cells associated with the ECM and the cellular components of the parenchyma of a tissue. In the case of the heart, fibroblasts exhibit cell–cell interactions with other fibroblasts, as well as with myocytes and endothelial cells[2]. Indeed, they play a critical role in chemical, mechanical and electrical signalling in the heart.

Origin and distribution of fibroblasts

What has recently become as important as the definition of the fibroblast is the question of the origin of the fibroblast. This issue is of great importance as the fibroblast is a critical cell in the fibrotic response in disease, as well as the major contributor to the normal ECM of the heart[5]. As there is considerable heterogeneity in the fibroblast population in any given tissue, it is difficult to precisely define a fibroblast, let alone their origin. However, recent studies have helped to shed light on the potential different origins of fibroblasts. Fibroblasts can originate at various times during the developmental process, as well as during pathophysiological conditions, such as following myocardial infarction.

During embryonic development, fibroblasts originate from the mesenchyme and are intimately involved in cardiac development[4–7].

These epicardial-derived cells (EPDC) first arise from the proepicardial organ and contribute to the fibroblast population of the developing heart. In addition, these EPDC can differentiate into other cell types including smooth muscle cells and endothelial cells. Besides EPDC, cardiac fibroblasts can also originate from other sources. One source is fibrocytes, which are bone marrow-derived mesenchymal progenitor cells that make up a rare subpopulation of the leukocyte lineage[8]. Over recent years, the fibrocyte has received considerable attention for its role in contributing to fibrosis (reactive and reparative) and wound repair[8,9]. Fibrocytes are defined by specific cell surface markers, their ability to home to sites of injury and differentiate into active fibroblasts (Fig. 19.1). In addition, fibrocytes are able to deposit collagen, as well as play an important role in the immune response. This has been best documented in the lung, but a similar process is believed to be present in the heart.

Competing with the circulating fibrocyte origin of fibroblasts is the concept that epithelial–mesenchymal transformation (EMT) contributes fibroblasts to the particular organ[10]. While EMT is a fundamental process in embryological development, its role in adult tissues is less well defined, but clearly it is a contributing source of fibroblasts, especially in the adult[10]. Indeed, EMT-derived fibroblastic cells help to form the cardiac valves. Additionally, both fibroblasts and fibrocytes can further differentiate into myofibroblasts[8,10,11].

Myofibroblasts appear to be a distinct phenotypic variant of the fibroblast[11,12]. They are found in a wide array of tissues and, in general, are found in locations that are under some sort of mechanical stress. Most reports on myofibroblasts come from *in vitro* studies where myofibroblasts are easily formed from isolated fibroblasts and plating the cells at low density. As the cells spread and increase focal adhesion sites, mechanical stress increases, resulting in an

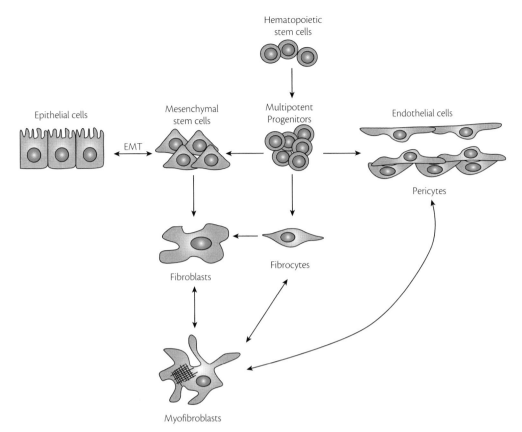

Fig. 19.1 Diagrammatic representation of potential pathways in the formation of fibroblasts and myofibroblasts in the adult heart. Fibroblasts can arise from epithelial–mesenchymal transformation (EMT), fibrocytes from the bone marrow via the vasculature and/or pericytes. The regulation of these lineages is unknown but appears to involve both local and systemic signals.

increase in the classical marker of the myofibroblasts, smooth muscle actin (sma). In addition to sma, myofibroblasts also upregulate transforming growth factor β, fibronectin and integrins[11]. A critical question, which remains controversial, concerns where the phenotypic markers of the myofibroblast are reversible when the mechanical stress is removed. *In vitro* studies seem to point to reversibility or at least downregulation of sma. *In vivo* there is some evidence that myofibroblasts undergo apoptosis[11].

The dynamic origin(s) of fibroblastic cells, which contribute to cardiac valves and other structures in the heart, are not well understood. They can come from fibrocytes, EMT or pre-existing fibroblasts, and their progeny may vary depending on the stage of development. For example, EPDC are probably the primary lineage for the initial fibroblasts of the heart[2]. With late fetal, neonatal and adult development, this paradigm shifts to bone marrow-derived EMT and fibrocytes. EMT would represent the chronic replacement of fibroblasts, whereas the fibrocytes would be an acute response to injury or abnormal pathophysiology.

Currently unanswered is the origin and function of the pericyte. Previous studies have demonstrated that pericytes are derived from the neural crest, while other studies have suggested that pericytes have a mesodermal beginning[8,13,14]. Additionally, it has been demonstrated that perivascular cells (pericytes and smooth muscle cells), as well as endothelial cells, can be derived from a common progenitor cell. As well as being derived from several cell types, pericytes themselves have the potential to differentiate into a variety of cell types. Indeed, pericytes that are associated with the vasculature have been shown to differentiate into myofibroblasts.

While fibroblasts in the parenchyma have been termed 'sentinel cells', as they receive and respond to changes in chemical and mechanical signals associated with changes in pathophysiology, it is the pericyte that would probably fill this role as a sensor directly from the vasculature[15]. Pericytes have a particular location associated with different regions of the vasculature (capillary vs venule), which may have an important regulatory effect on fluid dynamics. Pericytes also respond to a variety of chemical and mechanical signals, which results in a wide range of physiological responses[16]. These include constriction of blood vessels, contribution to the fibroblastic cell population and contribution to new blood vessel formation[8,13,14].

Relationship of fibroblasts to the ECM and the vasculature

In the early 1980s several groups reported the organization of the collagen of the heart[17–19]. These reports showed that collagen was arranged in a three-dimensional (3D) network interconnecting myocytes and the vasculature. This network exists at three different levels, the endomysium, the perimysium and the epimysium. The endomysium surrounds individual myocytes and has three main parts: (1) a weave network around the myocytes, (2) myocyte–myocyte connections and (3) myocyte–capillary connections. The perimysium consists of thick bundles of woven collagen that connect to the endomysium. Recently this system has been elegantly shown in 3D across the entire thickness of the myocardium[20]. These examinations of the ECM focused primarily on collagen and did not include the distribution of other ECM components such as proteoglycans, glycosaminoglycans (GAG) or matrikines. The distribution of these latter components is known for only focal regions of the heart.

Antibodies against the discodin domain receptor 2 (DDR2) have been shown to be specific to fibroblasts but also localize to lymphocytes[21,22]. More recently, periostin has been proposed as a marker that is not only fibroblast-specific, but also apparently near-comprehensive, labelling a majority of cardiac fibroblasts[4]. Using DDR2, it has been demonstrated that fibroblasts are interspersed within the collagen network of the heart[21,22]. Similar studies using vimentin, which stains primarily fibroblasts, have also shown the distribution of fibroblasts in several areas of the heart and their association with myocytes[23,24]. It is also important to appreciate that the fibroblasts localized within the collagenous network can apply mechanical force by contraction of the connective tissue in a manner analogous to that observed in collagen gels. Taken together, these observations demonstrated that the cardiac fibroblasts within the 3D collagen network could exhibit important mechanical, chemical and electrical properties.

Attachment of the collagen network to the various cellular components of the heart is of two principal types: (1) perpendicular to the Z line of myocytes and (2) tangential to the cell surface[17,18,25]. It is probable that both types play important mechanical roles, as they display different levels of adhesion. Perpendicular attachments of the collagen struts form lateral to the Z line in late fetal, early neonatal growth of myocytes[25]. These connections seem to form before the basement membrane is present, which may be an important point as this type of connection does not form after the basement membrane has been laid down in the adult. Fibroblasts and endothelial cells display tangential association with collagen. In the former, the fibroblast appears to lie in the collagen network and has the ability to 'contract' the collagen similar to what is observed in *in vitro* studies. While collagen does not appear to attach directly to endothelial cells, it associates with endothelial cells by weaving around the capillaries[17,25]. In this form, the collagen can provide mechanical support, as well as change shape with the peristaltic movement of the capillary. Disruption of the collagen connections has been proposed to alter the mechanical properties of the heart by altering the mechanical properties between the fibroblasts, myocyte and the ECM connections[26].

Fibroblasts are the principal cells responsible for the production of ECM components, and their distribution changes in number and signalling potential are critically associated with cardiac function[3–5]. Many of these functional interactions have been recently reviewed[3–5]. However, one area that has not been well documented is the role of the fibroblast in vascular development and remodelling.

Fibroblasts have been intimately described in association with the vasculature[28,29]. Initially, this association was portrayed as forming an elastic, stress-tolerant network between the muscle and vasculature. Fibroblasts associated with the vasculature were described as being involved in 'reactive fibrosis' by differentiating into myofibroblasts[9,11]. These studies were important as they clearly linked fibrosis with the fibroblasts and vasculature; however, identification and lineage origins of these fibroblasts remain speculative (see above discussion on what is a fibroblast).

Fibroblasts clearly play a role in angiogenesis, as fibroblasts are always seen in close proximity to the capillary during development

and hypertrophy[26,27]. In addition, *in vitro* studies have documented increased vessel formation in the presence of fibroblasts[30]. These latter studies indicated that both cell–cell interactions and chemical signalling between the fibroblasts and the endothelial cells are important for the developing capillary. Fibroblasts can produce a multitude of growth factors that are potent inducers of angiogenesis. These growth factors, such as fibroblast growth factor (FGF) and vascular endothelial growth factor (VEGF), act on endothelial cells to stimulate angiogenesis. In addition, fibroblasts can produce anti-angiogenic factors such as pigment epithelium-derived factor (PEDF). These studies indicate that a proper balance of pro- and anti-angiogenic factors secreted by the fibroblasts is important for proper vascular development and remodelling. Furthermore, a better understanding of the interactions between fibroblasts and endothelial cells is important for understanding how blood vessel formation is being controlled.

In addition to fibroblastic association with the capillary, the pericyte is also a potential player in this process. The association of the fibroblast with the capillary presents several potential applications of mechanical and chemical signalling. A cell type that is associated with the fibroblast lineage, as well as mechanical signalling, is the pericyte[11,13–16]. Pericytes are tightly associated with the capillary basement membrane and can differentiate into fibroblasts and myofibroblasts (Fig. 19.1). Additionally, the pericytes can apply mechanical force in the form of contraction to the vessel wall. Are the pericytes sensory in that they detect vascular signals? Can fibrocytes form pericytes? These are critical questions that need to be resolved in order to better understand the lineage and signalling capacity of the non-myocyte population of the heart.

Potential roles of fibroblasts in mechano-electric coupling

The role of fibroblasts in relation to electrical signalling has been a complex and controversially debated topic[31]. Evidence of structural coupling of fibroblasts shows that this can be both homotypic (fibroblast:fibroblast) and heterotypic (myocyte:fibroblast or fibroblast:endothelial cell). This coupling is mediated by a variety of molecules including connexins, cadherins and unknown proteins[32,33]. However, it is clear that since the distribution of fibroblasts is varied in different regions of the heart, fibroblasts may exhibit different functional effects. Fibroblasts express both N-cadherin and cadherin 11 (OB cadherin), but their specific roles are not well defined[2]. Connexins 40, 43 and 45 have all been observed in fibroblasts and by inference play important roles in cell–cell communication[3–5,34]. Several *in vitro* models have demonstrated the potential for fibroblasts to communicate via electrical signals between fibroblasts and myocytes[35–38].

While most studies demonstrating electrical coupling of fibroblasts and myocytes have been done *in vitro* using cell culture models, dye transfer studies done *in vivo* demonstrate the potential importance of fibroblasts in conducting electrical potentials between cardiomyocytes[24]. Especially notable are the studies in infracted regions which demonstrate that fibroblasts in the scar region dynamically change their expression patterns of connexins[23]. This may give rise to electrical coupling between healthy myocardium and infracted tissue, supporting electrical invasion of fully transmural infarcts as established in experimental animals using voltage mapping[39–44]. Clinical correlates of such fibroblast-mediated electrical impulse conduction include the 'bridging' of post-transplanatation scars observed in about 10% of donor heart recipients[45], or the re-connection of post-ablation scar tissue that is seen in the majority of atrial ablation patients[46].

Electrical interaction between fibroblasts and cardiomyocytes *in vivo* may be of relevance for cardiac mechano-electric coupling (MEC), potentially affecting normal pacemaker activity[47] and arrhythmogenesis in atrial[48] and ventricular myocardium[49]. Fibroblasts possess stretch-activated ion channels[39,40,50,51]. These mechano-sensitive ion channels are important in regulating the electrical properties of fibroblasts. Interactions between myocytes and fibroblasts appear to activate specific K^+ channels[34,35]. It has also been demonstrated that cardiac fibroblasts express several different voltage-gated channels[37].

Mechanical signalling by stretch can cause changes in the resting potential of the fibroblasts, but the pathophysiological implications of mechanical stimulations remain speculative[31,36]. It is likely that both mechanical and electrical coupling can result in paracrine signalling, as postulated for the release of cytokines and other factors[2,3]. Future studies utilizing 3D culture models will be particularly useful in analyzing these different variables[32,45]. From fluorescence-activated cell sorting (FACS) analysis, it is clear that the distribution of fibroblasts, based on DDR2 staining, varies by region of the heart[29]. For example, those in the sino-atrial node may exhibit properties different from those located in the left ventricle. In addition, the electrical signalling would be expected to vary as the numbers of cells change in association with hypertrophy or other pathophysiological conditions[29,44]. These studies clearly illustrate the potentially important roles and novel therapeutic targets related to fibroblasts in these processes[5,36].

Conclusions and outlook

Many studies have now shown that fibroblasts are important players in normal growth and in response to pathophysiological signals. It will be important for future studies to integrate mechanical, chemical and electrical activity of the fibroblasts and their interaction with cardiac myocytes. Multiscale analyses of cardiac fibroblasts as they interact with myocytes and other cell types of the heart, including computational modelling studies, will hopefully produce a new understanding of their role and purpose in maintaining normal cardiac function and in their contributions to pathogenesis[52–54].

Fibroblasts have been proposed to be potential targets for therapeutic intervention of a variety of functions including MEC, modification of the ECM and as carriers of specific gene products[45–50]. Regulation of arrhythmias by myofibroblast modification, the use of fibroblasts as promoters of angiogenesis and secretion of specific ECM components such as cytokines, growth factors and proteases[55–59] are examples of potential targets and/or manipulation in certain pathophysiological conditions. Critical to these therapeutic interventions will be a better understanding of the lineage(s), population dynamics, sensor/effector properties and dynamic interactions with other cardiac cell types.

Acknowledgements

The authors wish to apologize to all those authors who have made contributions to this field but who were not cited in the references. Special thanks to Stephanie Kidder, Colby Souders and Adam Bedenbaugh for assistance and comments. Grant support from NIH 1R01HL85847 is gratefully acknowledged.

References

1. Junqueira LC, Carneiro J (2005) *Basic Histology: Text and Atlas*. McGraw -Hill, New York.
2. Baudino TA, Carver W, Giles W, Borg TK. Cardiac fibroblasts: friend or foe? *Am J Physiol* 2006;**291**:H1015–H1026.
3. Souders C, Kidder S, Baudino TA. Cardiac fibroblasts: the renaissance cell. *Circ Res* 2009;**105**:1164–1170.
4. Snider P, Standley KN, Wang J, Azhar M, Doetschman T, Conway SJ. Origin of cardiac fibroblasts and the role of periostin. *Circ Res* 2009;**105**:934–947.
5. Porter KE, Turner NA. Cardiac fibroblasts: at the heart of myocardial remodeling. *Pharmacol Therap* 2009;**123**:255–278.
6. Moorman AF, Christoffels VM. Cardiac chamber formation: development, genes and evolution. *Physiol Rev* 2003;**83**:1223–1267.
7. Manner J, Perez-Pomares JM, Macias D, Munoz-Chapuli R. The origin, formation and developmental significance of the epicardium. *Cells Tissues Organs* 2001;**169**:89–103.
8. Strieter RM, Keeley EC, Hughes MA, Burdick MD, Mehrad B. The role of circulating mesenchymal progenitor cells (fibrocytes) in the pathogenesis of pulmonary fibrosis. *Trans Am Clin Climatol Assoc* 2009;**120**:49–59.
9. Weber KT. Fibrosis in hypertensive heart disease: focus on cardiac fibroblasts. *J Hypertension* 2004;**22**:47–50.
10. Zeisberg EM, Tarnavski O, Zeisberg M, *et al.* Endothelial-to-mesenchymal transition contributes to cardiac fibrosis. *Nat Med* 2007;**13**:952–961.
11. Hinz, B. Formation and function of the myofibroblast during tissue repair. *J Invest Dermatol* 2007;**127**:526–537.
12. Wipff PJ, Hinz B. Myofibroblasts work best under stress. *J Body Mov Ther* 2009;**1**:121–127.
13. Bellini A. Mattoli S. The role of the fibrocyte, a bone marrow-derived mesenchymal progenitor, in reactive and reparative fibroses. *Lab Invest* 2007;**87**:858–870.
14. Hirschi KK, D'Amore PA. Pericytes in the microvasculature. *Cardiovasc Res* 1996;**32**:687–698.
15. Silzle T, Randolph GJ, Kreutz M, Kunz-Schughart LA. The fibroblast: sentinel cell and local immune modulator in tumor tissue. *Int J Cancer* 2004;**108**:173–180.
16. Diaz-Flores L, Gutierrez R, Madrid JF, *et al.* Pericytes. Morphofunction, interactions and pathology in a quiescent and activated mesenchymal niche. *Histol Histopathol* 2009;**24**:909–969.
17. Caulfield JB Borg TK. The collagen network of the heart. *Lab Invest* 1979;**40**:364–372.
18. Robinson TF, Cohen-Gould L, Factor SM. Skeletal framework of mammalian heart muscle. Arrangement of inter- and pericellular connective tissue structures. *Lab Invest* 1983;**49**:482–498.
19. LeGrice IJ, Smaill BH, Chai LZ, Edgar SG, Gavin JB, Hunter PJ. Laminar structure of the heart: ventricular myocyte arrangement and connective tissue architecture in the dog. *Am J Physiol* 1995;**269**:H571–H582.
20. Pope AJ, Sands GB, Smaill BH, LeGrice IJ. Three-dimensional transmural organization of perimysial collagen in the heart. *Am J Physiol* 2008;**295**:H1243-H1252.
21. Goldsmith EC, Hoffman A, Morales MO, *et al.* Organization of fibroblasts in the heart. *Dev Dyn* 2004;**230**:787–794.
22. Morales MO, Price RL, Goldsmith EC. Expression of Discoidin Domain Receptor 2 (DDR2) in the developing heart. *Microsc Microanal* 2005;**11**:260–267.
23. Camelliti P, Devlin GP, Matthews KG, Kohl P, Green CR. Spatially and temporally distinct expression of fibroblast connexins after sheep ventricular infarction. *Cardiovasc Res* 2004;**62**:415–425.

24. Camelliti P, Green CR, LeGrice I, Kohl P. Fibroblast network in rabbit sinoatrial node: structural and functional identification of homogeneous and heterogeneous cell coupling. *Circ Res* 2004;**94**: 828–835.

25. Borg TK. Development of the connective tissue network in the neonatal hamster heart. *Am J Anat* 1982;**165**:435–443.

26. Goldsmith EC, Carver W, McFadden A, Goldsmith JG, Price RL, Sussman M, *et al.* Integrin shedding as a mechanism of cellular adaptation during cardiac growth. *Am J Physiol* 2003;**284**: H2227–H2234.

27. Banerjee I, Fuseler JW, Price RL, Borg TK, Baudino TA. Determination of cell types and numbers during cardiac development in the neonatal and adult rat and mouse. *Am J Physiol* 2007;**293**:H1883–H1891.

28. Staton CA, Reed MW, Brown NJ. A critical analysis of current in vitro and in vivo angiogenesis assays. *Int J Exp Pathol* 2009;**90**: 195–221.

29. Banerjee I, Fuseler JW, Intwala AR, Baudino TA. IL-6 loss causes ventricular dysfunction, fibrosis, reduced capillary density, and dramatically alters the cell populations of the developing and adult heart. *Am J Physiol* 2009;**296**:H1694–H1704.

30. Liu H, Chen B, Lilly B. Fibroblasts potentiate blood vessel formation partially through secreted factor TIMP-1. *Angiogenesis* 2008;**11**: 223–234.

31. McDowell KS, Trayanova NA, Kohl P. Fibroblasts and cardiac electrophysiology. In: *The Cardiac Fibroblast* (ed N Turner). Research Signpost, Kerala (India) 2011: pp. 9–27.

32. Banerjee I, Yekkala K, Borg TK, Baudino TA. Dynamic interactions between myocytes, fibroblasts, and extracellular matrix. *Ann N Y Acad Sci* 2006;**1080**:76–84.

33. Bowers SLK, Borg TK, Baudino TA. The dynamics of fibroblast-myocyte–capillary interactions in the heart. *Ann NY Acad Sci* 2010;**1188**:143–152.

34. Palatinus JA, Rhett JM, Gourdie RG. Translational lessons from scarless healing of cutaneous wounds and regenerative repair of the myocardium. *J Mol Cell Cardiol* 2010;**48**:550–557.

35. Chilton L, Ohya S. Freed D, *et al.* K+ currents regulate the resting membrane potential, proliferatin and contractile responses in ventricular fibroblasts and myofibroblasts. *Am J Physiol* 2005;**288**:H2931–H2939.

36. Rohr S. Myofibroblasts in diseased hearts: new players in cardiac arrhythmias? *Heart Rhythm* 2009;**6**:848–856.

37. Walsh KB, Zhang J. Neonatal rat cardiac fibroblasts express three types of voltage-gated K+ channels: regulation of a transient outward current by protein kinase C. *Am J Physiol* 2008;**29**: H1010–H1017.

38. Maleckar MM, Greenstein JL, Giles WR, Trayanova NA. K+ current changes account for the rate dependence of the action potential in the human atrial myocyte. *Am J Physiol* 2009;**29**:H1398–H1410.

39. Stockbridge LL, French AS. Stretch-activated cation channels in human fibroblasts. *Biophys J* 1988;**54**:187–190.

40. Kamkin A, Kiseleva I, Wagner KD, *et al.* Mechanically induced potentials in fibroblasts from human right atrium. *Exp Physiol* 1999;**84**:347–356.

41. Kohl P, Camelliti P, Burton FL, Smith GL. Electrical coupling of fibroblasts and myocytes: relevance for cardiac propagation. *J Electrocardiol* 2005;**38**:45–50.

42. Kamkin A, Kiseleva I, Isenberg G, *et al.* Cardiac fibroblasts and mechano-electric feedback mechanism in healthy and diseased hearts. *Prog Biophys Mol Biol* 2003;**82**:111–120.

43. Kamkin A, Kiseleva I, Lozinsky I, Scholz H. Electrical interaction of mechanosensitive fibroblasts and myocytes in the heart. *Basic Res Cardiol* 2005;**100**:337–344.

44. Walker NL, Burton FL, Kettlewell S, Smith GL, Cobbe MM. Mapping of epicardial activation in a rabbit model of chronic myocardial infarction: response to atrial, endocardial,and epicardial pacing. *J Cardiovasc Electrophysiol* 2007;**18**:862–868.

45. Lefroy DC, Fang JC, Stevenson LW, Hartley LH, Friedman P, Stevenson WG. Recipient-to-donor atrioatrial conduction after orthotopic heart transplantation: surface electrocardiographic features and estimated prevalence. *Am J Cardiol* 1998;**82**:444–450.

46. Gaita F, Riccardi R, Caponi D, *et al.* Linear cryoablation of the left atrium versus pulmonary vein cryoisolation in patients with permanent atrial fibrillation and valvular heart disease: correlation of electroanatomic mapping and long-term clinical results. *Circulation* 2005;**111**:136–142.

47. Pratola C, Baldo E, Notarstefano P, Toselli T, Ferrari R. Radiofrequency ablation of atrial fibrillation: is the persistence of all intraprocedural targets necessary for long-term maintenance of sinus rhythm? *Circulation* 2008;**117**:136–143.

48. Kohl P, Kamkin A, Kiseleva I, Noble D. Mechanosensitive fibroblasts in the sino-atrial node region of rat heart: interaction with cardiomyocytes and possible role. *Exp Physiol* 1994;**79**:943–956.

49. Maleckar MM, Greenstein JL, Giles WR, Trayanova NA. Electrotonic coupling between human atrial myocytes and fibroblasts alters myocyte excitability and repolarization. *Biophys J* 2009;**97**: 2179–2190.

50. Xie Y, Garfinkel A, Camelliti P, Kohl P, Weiss JN, Qu Z. Effects of fibroblast-myocyte coupling on cardiac conduction and vulnerability to reentry: a computational study. *Heart Rhythm* 2009;**6**:1641–1649.

51. Kamkin A, Kiseleva I, Wagner KD, *et al.* Characterization of stretch-activated ion currents in isolated atrial myocytes from human hearts. *Pflugers Arch* 2003; **446**:339–346.

52. Shimizu T, Sekine H, Yamato M, Okano T. Cell sheet-based myocardial tissue engineering: new hope for damaged heart rescue. *Curr Pharm Des* 2009;**15**:2807–2814.

53. Hunter PJ, Borg TK. Integration from proteins to organs: the Physiome Project. *Nat Rev Mol Cell Biol* 2003;**4**:237–243.

54. Kohl P, Noble D. Systems biology and the virtual physiological human. *Mol Syst Biol* 2009;**5**:292.

55. Trimboli JA, Cantemir-Stone CZ, Li F, *et al.* Pten in stromal fibroblasts suppresses mammary epithelial tumors. *Nature* 2009;**461**:1084–1091.

56. Santos AM, Jung J, Aziz N, *et al.* Targeting fibroblast activation protein inhibits tumor stromagenesis and growth in mice. *JCI* 2009;**119**: 3613–3625.

57. Kim JY, Rim Y, Wang J, Jackson D. A novel cell-to-cell trafficking assay indicates that the KNOX homeodomain is necessary and sufficient for intercellular protein and mRNA trafficking. *Genes Development* 2009;**19**:788–793.

58. Davis GE. Matricryptic sites control tissue injury responses in the cardiovascular system: Relationships to pattern recognition receptor regulated events. *J Mol Cell Cardiol* 2010;**48**:454–460.

59. Frangogiannis NG. The immune system and cardiac repair. *Pharmacol Res* 2008;**58**:88–111.

Advantages and pitfalls of cell cultures as model systems to study cardiac mechano-electric coupling

Leslie Tung and Susan A. Thompson

Background

Primary cultures of cardiac cells are experimental models of the physiological and pathophysiological functions of intact cardiac tissue. Originally intended for studies of isolated cells, they were initially derived from embryonic chick and newborn rat hearts and have been in use for over half a century[10,21]. The benefits of using isolated cells to investigate their physiological behaviour are well recognized[40] and include elimination of a restricted interstitial space from the free surface of the cell, ability to visualize the cell and option to select for cell type. Cells can be maintained in culture for weeks to months. Cultures of populations of cells have been subjected to chemical and mechanical stimuli to enable assays of fundamental signalling pathways, such as those involved with cardiac hypertrophy[52]. Cultured cells have been grown as confluent strands and sheets for the purpose of studying fundamental electrophysiological properties of cardiac tissue. They have been utilized to investigate normal and abnormal impulse generation and propagation, including mechano-electric coupling (MEC) in a syncytium. In this chapter we review the strengths and weakness of cell culture models (with emphasis on confluent monolayers), discuss their use and potential for studies of MEC, and conclude with a look to future cell culture models that may supplant existing models.

Cell culture models in comparison with other cardiac preparations

Cell culture models are structurally and functionally intermediate between the single cell and native tissue.

Cell cultures compared with intact tissue

Mechanical loading in the intact ventricle has a complex three-dimensional (3D) distribution within the myocardial wall that is multiscale from the organ to the cell[57]. Heterogeneous wall pressure and the twisting motion of the heart during systolic contraction produce fibre shortening, wall thickening and transverse shearing between the laminar sheets of myocardial cells. Thus, the mechanical stimulus to the cell is quite complex within the intact organ. *Ex vivo* excised tissue offers better control over the mechanical loading and other experimental conditions and facilitates the measurement of important physiological parameters such as contractile force. However, dissection involves some degree of cellular damage, and the preparation usually consists of an uncontrolled mixture of cardiac cell types (i.e. myocytes, fibroblasts, endothelial cells, vascular smooth muscle cells).

In cell culture, researchers have good control of the experimental preparation, including the morphological, biochemical, electrophysiological and mechanical characteristics of the culture and substrate. When grown as confluent monolayers, cultures contain in the order of 10^4–10^5 cells/cm^2 and retain the functional behaviour of a tissue syncytium, including cell–cell interactions that provide mechanical and electrical coupling. Cultures are a simplified tissue system and avoid irregularities in conduction arising from connective tissue, blood vessels and neural input. Unlike the intact tissue that contains many cell types, the composition and density of the cell population can be varied in cultures[1,5,43,49,77]. Detailed imaging for the purposes of detecting cell contraction or monitoring fluorescent probes in real time is feasible. Diffusional access of pharmacological agents and signalling molecules from the bathing medium to the cells is very rapid. Furthermore, the association between cell type, size, shape and junctions with the functional electrophysiology is greatly facilitated. The tissue structure (e.g. anisotropy) in culture can be controlled by various methods[7,50], making the monolayer a biological analogue to two-dimensional (2D) computational models of cardiac tissue that have been used to study cardiac arrhythmia[65]. Unlike *in silico* models with computational limitations, cell culture models can be used for dynamic studies spanning minutes, hours and days.

As with any model, the simplifications of cultures also present limitations. The physiological influences of blood flow and sympathetic and parasympathetic nervous systems are absent. The ratio of cell types has been modified from that in native tissue, and complex cell–cell interactions may be altered in cell culture. The orderly organization of cardiac tissue as fibres and sheets is greatly simplified, and the 3D microenvironment around the cells, which can influence cell function, is commonly absent (but see section 'Cell culture microenvironment').

Cell cultures compared with freshly dissociated single cells

Isolated, single cardiac cells afford precise experimental control, but several practical limitations exist in the context of MEC. First, the applied forces (e.g. by carbon fibres, indentation, suction) differ from those exerted naturally on the cell via the extracellular matrix (ECM), focal adhesions and junctional complexes. Thus, the responses to mechanical stimulation may differ from those that occur *in situ*. Second, studies on single cells are typically carried out on small numbers (tens) of cells, which may suffice if the cell behaviour is homogeneous, but not if only a minute fraction exhibits robust mechanical responses[47]. Third, it is not possible to study tissue-level electrophysiology such as conduction velocity.

Like acutely dissociated myocytes, cultured cardiac cell monolayers allow ready access to the cell membrane from the bathing medium and easy visualization of the cell. The aggregate behaviour of large numbers (10^4–10^5) of cells can be studied at once, and they can be made with controlled mixtures of cell types. Cardiac cell monolayers have been grown in investigator-designated patterns, including linear strands, curved strands, hatched patterns and islands, using methods of photolithography[50], microcontact printing[7], microfluidic patterning[9] and stenciling[56]. Culture over time permits the researcher to observe adaptive or remodelling changes in gene and protein expression in response to prolonged mechanical inputs. Cell–cell interactions via adherens junctions and gap junctions in the intercalated disk can be studied, as well as cell–matrix interactions. The latter are particularly important as the ECM acts to transmit mechanical forces to transmembrane integrin receptors and focal adhesion complexes, where various signalling molecules reside[45] and which couple to the cytoskeletal network. Mechanical signals can influence ion channel function, nuclear shape and structure, calcium binding to troponin C, and numerous other force-sensing molecules such as titin, muscle LIM protein and four-and-a-half LIM (FHL) domain protein (LIM domains are protein interaction motifs, containing two Zn^{2+} binding sites that are widely distributed in cells of both plants and animals; see Chapter 9 and review[29]). Cultured cells are useful for the study of not only intracellular signalling pathways activated by stretch, but also stretch-induced release of autocrine and paracrine factors[61], which, for example, mediate hypertrophy[67]. Cell monolayers can be cultured on selected extracellular matrices (see section 'Cell culture microenvironment'), which are important physiological regulators of cell function[17].

On the other hand, cultured cells are morphologically quite different from freshly dissociated cells, being much flatter after attaching and spreading out on a substratum. The higher surface-to-volume ratio and alteration of cytoskeletal structure have as yet unknown consequences in terms of MEC. For monolayers, cultured cells are typically drawn from embryonic, fetal or newborn cell types, because these cells are capable of remodelling to form a syncytium and may retain the ability to proliferate (but see section

'Adult cardiomyocytes'). This means, however, that the electrophysiological characteristics of the cell population can change during time in culture owing to developmental changes in ion channel expression and calcium cycling[18]. Additionally, cell phenotype is sensitive to the culture conditions and microenvironment (see sections 'Cell culture microenvironment' and 'Phenotypic changes of cells during culture').

Other considerations in the use of cell culture models

Neonatal rat cell culture model

Presently available cardiac cell culture models used in electrophysiological studies are derived primarily from the neonatal rat, and to some extent from the neonatal mouse or embryonic chick[65]. However, compared with human, neonatal rat ventricular myocyte (NRVM) action potentials are much shorter with a much less prominent plateau phase. Furthermore, the immature state of the neonatal cells is reflected in the lack of a T-tubule system and the developing electrophysiology, which affect ion channel expression and the dynamics of calcium cycling[37]. In addition, connexin 43 (Cx43) is evenly distributed around the perimeter of the cell, unlike that in normal adult cells[16].

Cell culture microenvironment

The nature of cell culture introduces variability in the preparations. The activity of dissociating enzymes, agitation, length of procedure and prepared solutions are all factors that can influence the consistency of primary cells obtained from tissue. Fetal bovine serum, a common supplement in culture media, contains growth factors, binding proteins, hormones and nutrients necessary for cell culture, but also has batch-to-batch variability and unidentified proteins which can influence the cells in unknown ways. To control for serum variability, serum-free culture conditions have been optimized for cardiomyocyte viability and provide a chemically defined system[63], although these tend to be costly and may have reduced cell viability. Other variables that affect the phenotype of the cells include the numbers of non-myocytes and the substrata on which the cells are grown[27].

Cardiac cell cultures are comprised of myocytes and non-myocytes (primarily fibroblasts). The cardiomyocyte population can be purified by exploiting the characteristics of the different cell types, such as attachment speed, cell density and proliferation rate[11], although no method exists to eliminate all non-myocyte cells from primary cell culture. On the other hand, it may be desirable to retain certain non-myocytes. The emerging importance of fibroblast–myocyte interactions in the heart[8,49] suggests that this cell type should not be underestimated, particularly in the context of MEC.

Cardiomyocytes are frequently cultured on 2D tissue culture polystyrene, or glass or polyvinyl chloride coverslips coated with a solubilized ECM protein such as collagen I, collagen III, laminin, fibronectin or vitronectin[11]. This is a far different arrangement than the natural structure within the heart. Substrates can be coated instead with ECM produced by mouse tumours (Matrigel) or by cardiac fibroblasts (Cardiogel). These contain proteins, proteoglycans and growth factors that significantly enhance the viability and calcium handling efficiency of cardiomyocytes[68]. 3D scaffolds that more closely emulate the *in situ* environment can be fabricated with controlled parameters such as elasticity, porosity, degradability and shape. Cardiomyocytes have been cultured on scaffolds made by crosslinking or electrospinning synthetic or natural polymers, on temperature-sensitive polymers that allow detachment of the monolayer as a fully transplantable cell sheet, and within injectable gels for *in situ* engineering[31]. Not surprisingly, scaffold elasticity, which can be precisely controlled by polymer concentration and crosslinking, has a significant effect on cardiomyocyte structural organization and spontaneous contraction, and is most effective when similar to that found *in vivo*[28,59].

Phenotypic changes of cells during culture

Cultured NRVM that start with rod-shapes *in vivo* become pleiomorphic after attachment to surfaces, but can reform myofibrils and sarcomeres[22]. These structural changes are likely due to the relocation and composition of focal adhesions, which are forced to adapt to the rigid 2D surface and remodel[53]. Further, unless specific techniques are used to pattern cells (see section 'Cell cultures compared with freshly dissociated single cells') into an aligned anisotropic structure, cultured cells exhibit an isotropic organization. These considerations are important because cell shape may influence the expression of ion channels[69]. Additionally, the artificial microenvironment discussed in the section on 'Cell culture microenvironment' will moderate the cellular phenotype under culture conditions.

Studies of mechano-electric coupling

MEC is the process by which a mechanical stimulus produces a change in the electrical behaviour of the cell in terms of its transmembrane potential (V_m), intracellular free calcium ($[Ca^{2+}]_i$) or some protein associated with the electrophysiological response (e.g. Cx43). Apart from V_m, $[Ca^{2+}]_i$ is often the focal point because it can influence V_m via a number of calcium-sensitive currents, including the L-type calcium current ($I_{Ca,L}$), the electrogenic Na^+/Ca^{2+} exchanger (NCX) current (I_{NCX}), or certain potassium and chloride currents. Stretch also modulates myocyte growth, apoptosis, ion channel remodelling, gene expression and secretion of bioactive molecules[61], providing additional pathways for MEC.

Electrophysiological outcomes

Early efforts to grow mammalian cardiac cells as organized tissue used monolayers of neonatal rat heart cells to study the syncytial properties of electrically coupled cells, manifested as electrotonic spread[26,32] or mutual entrainment of beating cells[33]. The introduction of patterned growth of cardiac cells to form synthetic linear strands was achieved in the early 1970s using chick embryonic cells grown in channels cut in agar, and was used with microelectrode recordings to compare the passive and active properties of the strands with those predicted by one-dimensional (1D) cable theory[39,51]. This technological advance was the first step for investigators to obtain patterns of cells without resorting to tissue dissection. In the early 1990s, arrays of NRVM were grown for the first time on photolithographically defined lines of collagen, allowing even greater freedom to define growth patterns of the cells[50]. This was soon followed by multisite optical mapping using voltage-sensitive dyes to record action potential upstrokes, impulse propagation, conduction block and arrhythmia in NRVM monolayers[48,65] and calcium dyes to measure $[Ca^{2+}]_i$ as a surrogate for

cellular voltage in embryonic chick ventricular monolayers[5]. Dual voltage and calcium recordings have been performed in NRVM monolayers for the study of responses to electric field pulses[15]. Extracellular microelectrode arrays (MEA) have also provided a means to measure impulse propagation[71] with the advantages of long-term recordings and avoidance of toxic fluorescent dyes, although these arrays are generally limited to areas of several square millimetres. The spread of contractile waves can also be followed optically[25].

Mechanically modulated expression of proteins involved in electrical activity can be studied with cell cultures. To date, studies have focused mainly on connexins (components of the gap junctions that provide electrical communication between adjoining cardiac cells).

Mechanical stimuli

Many methods have been developed to apply mechanical forces to cultured cells, as briefly discussed below (for more details see[4,29]). Of interest for cardiac cell cultures are substrate deformation, altered substrate stiffness, mechanical loading by the medium or by microspheres, fluid shear and pressure, although not all have yet been applied for the study of MEC.

With substrate deformation, a biocompatible elastic membrane (e.g. silicone) is coated with an ECM protein and cardiomyocytes are cultured on top. With a circular membrane, an indenter is pressed against the bottom surface. Deformation of the membrane by positive or negative pressure, or upward displacement of the indenter, results in a biaxial strain in the central area of the membrane. Equibiaxial strain is achieved with a circular indenter, anisotropic biaxial strain with an elliptical indenter and uniaxial strain with a rectangular bridge-shaped indenter.

A rectangular membrane can be stretched in a uniaxial or biaxial manner with mechanical actuators attached to its edges. Uniaxial strain is achieved by pulling the opposite ends of the membrane in a static or cyclic manner, whereas biaxial strain involves pulling the four sides of the membrane with two pairs of orthogonally oriented actuators. The design of a biaxial system suitable for cell cultures has been published recently[24] but has not yet been used with cardiac cells.

For 3D cultures, cardiomyocytes have been embedded in a collagen gel and cast as cylindrical strands, planar constructs or circular rings that can be stretched[76]. Planar constructs are cast with their ends around Velcro or silk suture to enable attachment. The attachment problem is avoided in ring-shaped constructs by slipping the ring over a pair of rods whose spacing can be varied statically or cyclically.

To vary the local mechanical load, the stiffness of a polymer substrate can be altered by varying the crosslinking in the material. Alternatively, the load can be varied for freely shortening cells by increasing the viscosity of the medium[35] or by attaching collagen-coated glass microspheres to the myocyte surface[2].

For fluid shear, a parallel plate flow chamber is commonly used to produce a uniform laminar flow field, while a cone and plate chamber can be used to generate laminar or turbulent flow. Alternatively, a local flow field can be generated by directing a fluid stream from a micropipette onto the surface of the cell monolayer.

Finally, pressure can be elevated around cell cultures by using compressed air[54] or hydrostatic pressure[74], achieving levels as high as 200 mmHg above ambient pressure.

Review of published studies

In an early study, NRVM were cultured on rubber membranes and stretched manually by as much as 25% using a micromanipulator[64]. Short stretches (< 10 s) initially suppressed the $[Ca^{2+}]_i$ transient but then produced a large transient increase in $[Ca^{2+}]_i$ that was unaffected by ryanodine (a blocker of the 'ryanodine receptor' [RyR] calcium release channels in the sarcoplasmic reticulum) but was inhibited by Ca^{2+}-free medium or by gadolinium (a non-specific blocker of stretch-activated channels in the plasma membrane). Ca^{2+}-free medium, but not ryanodine or gadolinium, eliminated a small sustained (5–10 min) increase in $[Ca^{2+}]_i$, suggesting another sarcolemmal pathway for the stretch response.

Using a Flexcell system (Flexcell International Corp.), a 1 Hz, 20% continuous strain of NRVM grown on silicone membranes caused a threefold increase in Cx43 mRNA levels in 2 h and Cx43 protein levels in 4 h, which lasted another 16 h[70]. These changes were attributed to activation of the Na^+/H^+ exchanger (NHE). In a different study, a 1 Hz, 20% strain of NRVM caused measurable increases in Cx43 mRNA and Cx43 protein levels in less than 2 h, which peaked at a sixfold higher level at 24 h and remained that way for another 24 h[62]. Both increases were attributed to autocrine effects of stretch-mediated release of angiotensin II.

Uniaxial cyclic stretch has been applied in customized systems to NRVM grown on silicone elastomeric membranes. A 0.5 Hz, 20% strain for 24 h resulted in an alignment of NRVM and a localization of Cx43 at the longitudinal termini of the cell in a manner that was regulated by the Rac1 signalling pathway acting downstream of N-cadherin[42]. A 3 Hz, 10% strain applied continuously to patterned strands of NRVM produced an increase in Cx43 expression after 1 h that increased further after 6 h and was maintained for at least 24 h[75]. Static stretch resulted in similar but smaller changes in Cx43 expression. The same study used optical mapping that showed a concomitant 30% increase in conduction velocity (CV) after 1 h, which increased to 37% after 6 h. In a follow-up study, the stretch-induced upregulation of Cx43 was found to be mediated by vascular endothelial growth factor (VEGF), which appeared to act downstream of stretch-mediated release of transforming growth factor-beta (TGF-β) in an autocrine manner[46]. The VEGF secretion was found, in turn, to depend on focal adhesion kinase-dependent signalling[73].

The importance of the extracellular matrix in mediating the mechano-sensitive effect was demonstrated in a study showing that the stretch-induced upregulation of Cx43 was present with type-I collagen but not with fibronectin or denatured collagen[58]. Proteins associated with intercellular junctional complexes (N-cadherin, plakoglobin, desmoplakin) were also upregulated by stretch, via integrin signalling acting downstream of src kinase[73].

Using a different approach, static, biaxial anisotropic stretch (10%:5% strain) was applied for 24 h to patterned strands of NRVM. Interestingly, Cx43 protein expression increased significantly only when the principal strain was aligned along the transverse, and not the longitudinal, axis of the cells[19]. The directional influence of strain relative to cell alignment may be related to changes in protein kinase C (PKC) expression[19]. Static or 0.2 Hz cyclic stretch up to 10% strain affected different PKC isoenzymes by varying degrees, depending on the direction of stretch, the particular isoenzyme and the phosphorylation state of the isoenzyme[6].

When biaxial, anisotropic static stretch (10%:5% strain) was applied continuously to isotropic NRVM monolayers, the action potential duration increased by 6.9% and within 10 min CV slowed by 7.5%, although longer-term changes were not measured[74]. The short duration of this experiment probably precluded the change of Cx43 protein expression observed in the study mentioned earlier[75].

The influence of substrate stiffness on electrophysiological function has also been studied. NRVM had the highest percentage of beating cells and strongest synchronized contraction patterns across the constructs after 2–4 weeks in culture on the softest gels (shear moduli from 8–340 Pa)[59]. In another study[28], the percentage of beating NRVM increased with decreasing elastic modulus of substrates on which they were cultured. With elastic moduli around 10 kPa, a stiffness a little lower than that found in vivo in normal rat myocardium, NRVM form aligned striations and had peak expression of SERCA2a (Ca^{2+}-ATPase), the highest concentrations of stored calcium, peak calcium transient concentrations and peak force generation. This substrate sensitivity appears to be mediated through RhoA (a member of the Ras homology family of small GTPases).

An unusual approach to apply mechanical loads to NRVM consists of attaching 15-μm-diameter collagen-coated glass microspheres. Their effects on conduction velocity, as measured by MEA, were compared with those of a 3 Hz, 10% cyclic strain following 24 h exposure to various drugs[2]. Similar to the stretch responses, mRNA levels of angiogenic factors (angiotensin II, TGF-β and basic fibroblast growth factor [bFGF]) increased, but unlike the case for stretch, the microspheres did not alter Cx43 expression or CV. Instead, diastolic and systolic calcium levels were elevated, while the decay rate of the calcium transient decreased. Arrhythmias in the form of triggered activity (early after-depolarizations) were also observed with the microspheres but not with cyclic stretch.

The deformation of cells in response to fluid shear may be fundamentally different from that for stretch, and may involve adhesion receptors and their associated signalling complexes[30]. NRVM monolayers subjected to low shear rates (5–50/s) responded with an immediate, graded increase in their spontaneous beating rate by up to 500%, which was reversible[41]. This response was not suppressed by 70 μM streptomycin (a non-specific blocker of stretch-activated channels), but was abolished in serum-free media and attenuated with integrin-blocking RGD peptides or by isoproterenol. These results suggest that the shear stress response is mediated by integrin activation and the β-adrenergic pathway.

Optical mapping experiments showed that anisotropic NRVM monolayers subjected to 1.1 dyn/cm^2 fluid shear stress exhibited only modest changes in CV and APD[74], perhaps because serum-containing solution is required for a robust response[41]. These changes occurred with some delay and evolved with increasing amplitude over 4–6 min, possibly because of the viscous nature of the cytoskeletal networks[12]. Among the several hundred recording sites distributed over an area 1.8 cm in diameter, a few outliers had significantly prolonged or shortened APD (Fig. 20.1), indicating that perhaps these outliers may reflect particularly highly mechano-sensitive cells[47] or locally high deformations.

Other optical mapping experiments revealed that fluid pulses from a pipette tip impinging upon an NRVM monolayer acted as a stimulus source that could activate propagating electrical wavefronts in a stochastic manner (Fig. 20.2), and in one case could

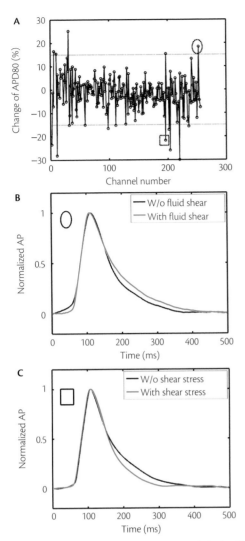

Fig. 20.1 Change in action potential duration at 80% repolarization (APD$_{80}$) measured at 231 recording sites following application of 1.0 dyn/cm^2 shear stress for ~1 min to an NRVM monolayer. Distribution of response **A** shows a small number of sites with changes exceeding ± 15%, as illustrated for sites marked by the oval and square. Individual traces are plotted in **B** with APD$_{80}$ > 15% and **C** with APD$_{80}$ < 15%. [Reproduced, with permission, from Zhang Y, Sekar RB, McCulloch AD, Tung L (2008) Cell cultures as models of cardiac mechanoelectric feedback. *Prog Biophys Mol Biol* **97**:367–382.]

initiate re-entrant activity[36]. The incidence of mechanical excitation increased with fluid jet velocity and time between pulses, and was partially suppressed by streptomycin or gadolinium, but not by nifedipine (an L-type calcium channel blocker). Action potential initiation may be the result of an inward current through stretch-activated channels or of an increase in spontaneous calcium release[38,72], which in concert with the electrogenic NCX, can depolarize the cell and cause cellular excitation.

Finally, elevation of ambient pressure has limited effect on NRVM monolayers[54]. Elevated pressure of 100 mmHg was reported to have no effect, whereas an increase of 200 mmHg resulted in an increase in cell area, a transient slowing of contraction/relaxation at 6 h without a change in spontaneous beating rate, and elevated mRNA and protein expression levels of RyR and SERCA2a. In electrophysiological experiments, static pressures of 110 mmHg above atmosphere were applied to NRVM monolayers for 5 min in a sealed pressure chamber, and action potential durations and CVs did not change significantly[74].

Future cell culture models

In the future, it would be desirable to develop new cell culture models that more closely resemble human, or even from human tissue itself.

Adult cardiomyocytes

The advantages of cultured adult cardiomyocytes as models of cardiac tissue have been known for over two decades[27], and the applications, culture methods and morphological and electrophysiological properties of cultured adult cardiomyocytes have been reviewed[44]. Unlike acutely dissociated myocytes, these cells can be used for long-term studies involving experimentally induced changes in gene and protein expression. Furthermore, a single adult heart is a bountiful source of cells, providing enough material for dozens or more of experiments. Human cardiomyocytes are available from patient biopsies and failed transplanted hearts.

In culture, freshly dissociated ventricular cardiomyocytes obtained from enzymatic dissociation of intact adult hearts undergo morphological and ultrastructural changes. In the first stage (termed **short-term culture**), cells that survive the dissociation procedure and attach to a surface are suitable for culture so long as they remain rod-shaped, clearly striated and calcium-tolerant. Such cells are useful for short-term studies[27]. Eventually they undergo dedifferentiation and lose some or all of their myotypic structure. However, after about 2 weeks (depending on the species) the surviving myocytes enter a second stage (termed **long-term culture**), undergoing redifferentiation and reacquisition of much of their lost structure and intracellular organization[27]. Long-term cultures have been obtained using cardiomyocytes (mainly ventricular) from rat, hamster, guinea pig, rabbit, cat, monkey and human, proving that the viability of these cells can be sustained. Of these, beating monolayers of cells have been reported for rat[23], guinea pig[23] and rabbit[14]. Among the challenges facing the use of these cells are possible alterations in cellular electrophysiology during long-term culture[55].

Cardiomyocytes derived from stem cells

Pluripotent stem cells, such as embryonic stem cells (ESC) and induced pluripotent stem cells (iPSC), can differentiate into cardiomyocytes and serve as *in vitro* models of monogenic and patient-specific myocardial disease[3]. Cardiomyocytes derived from human ESC and iPSC are contractile with cardiac-like action potentials, and can be cultured as a working syncytium that supports electrical propagation[34,78]. Human ESC-derived cardiomyocytes express functional integrins and produce extracellular matrix *in vitro* and after transplantation *in vivo*[66], while mechanical loading affects gene expression and promotes cell differentiation[60]. These observations promote confidence that stem cell-derived cardiomyocytes can be used to study MEC in a human model.

Tissue slices

Tissue slices derived from explanted hearts are a simplified experimental organotypic preparation that maintains the *in vivo* tissue structure as well as sympathetic and parasympathetic nerve

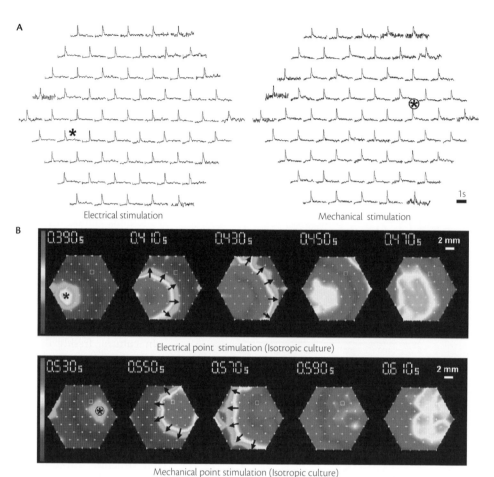

Fig. 20.2 Comparison of electrically and mechanically induced action potential propagation in the same isotropic NRVM monolayer. **A** Optical action potentials shown at 61 recording sites for electrical (left) and mechanical (right) stimulation. Asterisk indicates location of bipolar point electrode (1.2 × threshold); circled asterisk indicates location of 0.4-mm-diameter pipette (0.5 m/s, 10 ms). **B** Propagation maps. Optical signals were normalized per site to the action potential amplitude. Plus symbols indicate recording sites. Both electrical and mechanical stimulation resulted in wavefronts that spread radially from the stimulating electrode or pipette, respectively. [Reproduced, with permission, from Kong CR, Bursac N, Tung L (2005) Mechanoelectrical excitation by fluid jets in monolayers of cultured cardiac myocytes. *J Appl Physiol* **98**: 2328–2336.] (See color plate section.)

endings[13]. In principle, mounting systems used for force measurements can be used to apply stretch to the tissue slice. Although the physiological function of tissue slices is typically lost in less than a week, by adapting methods used to maintain brain slices *in vitro*, it is now possible to culture 1-mm-thick ventricular tissue slices from newborn rat and human fetus for more than a month, while preserving normal histology, rhythmic contractions, calcium transients and adrenergic response[20].

Conclusions and outlook

Confluent monolayers of cultured cardiac cells constitute a greatly simplified tissue system that nevertheless retains many of the salient functional aspects of the intact heart, including cell–cell interactions. They consist of very large numbers of cells, whose behaviour as a population surmounts the sampling issues associated with studies of small numbers of cells. Mechanical stimuli can be controlled more precisely than in the intact heart, and electrophysiological outcomes are readily accessible.

Cardiac cells can be cultured on elastic substrates coated with ECM proteins to which a prescribed deformation can be applied. Cell culture systems allow cells to be stretched biaxially or uniaxially

with controlled frequency and force magnitude. Anisotropic cultures allow the study of stretch that is applied along or transverse to the cell axis. Experimental studies have shown that stretch of cultured cells results in augmented calcium transients, prolongation of the action potential, slowing of conduction and increased expression of Cx43 mediated by activation of NHE and autocrine effects of angiotensin II and VEGF. Proteins associated with mechanical junctions and focal adhesions are upregulated by stretch and involve integrin and/or PKC signalling pathways. Shear stress affects the spontaneous beating rate but has only modest effects on action potential duration and conduction velocity. The effects on beating rate are mediated by integrin activation and the β-adrenergic pathway. Substrate stiffness affects the beating rate of cells, size of intracellular calcium transients and SERCA2a expression, and is mediated by RhoA signalling.

Finally, adult cardiomyocytes or cardiomyocytes derived from human stem cells are potentially new cell sources for cell culture experiments that can be expected to accelerate basic scientific knowledge in the cardiac field. Cell culture technology may also be applied to improve the viability and utility of tissue slices. As research continues, the ability to gain human-specific insights into MEC through cell culture will increase dramatically.

Acknowledgement

The writing of this chapter was supported by NIH grant R01 HL066239.

References

1. Abraham MR, Henrikson CA, Tung L, et al. Antiarrhythmic engineering of skeletal myoblasts for cardiac transplantation. *Circ Res* 2008;**97**:159–167.

2. Barac DY, Reisner Y, Silberman M, et al. Mechanical load induced by glass microspheres releases angiogenic factors from neonatal rat ventricular myocytes cultures and causes arrhythmias. *J Cell Mol Med* 2008;**12**:2037–2051.

3. Beqqali A, van Eldik W, Mummery C, Passier R. Human stem cells as a model for cardiac differentiation and disease. *Cell Mol Life Sci* 2009;**66**:800–813.

4. Brown TD. Techniques for mechanical stimulation of cells in vitro: a review. *J Biomech* 2000;**33**:3–14.

5. Bub G, Tateno K, Shrier A, Glass L. Spontaneous initiation and termination of complex rhythms in cardiac cell culture. *J Cardiovasc Electrophysiol* 2003;**14**:S229–S236.

6. Bullard TA, Hastings JL, Davis JM, Borg TK, Price RL. Altered PKC expression and phosphorylation in response to the nature, direction, and magnitude of mechanical stretch. *Can J Physiol Pharmacol* 2007;**85**:243–250.

7. Bursac N, Parker KK, Iravanian S, Tung L. Cardiomyocyte cultures with controlled macroscopic anisotropy: a model for functional electrophysiological studies of cardiac muscle. *Circ Res* 2002;**91**: e45–e54.

8. Camelliti P, Green CR, Kohl P. Structural and functional coupling of cardiac myocytes and fibroblasts. *Adv Cardiol* 2006;**42**:132–149.

9. Camelliti P, Gallagher JO, Kohl P, McCulloch AD. Micropatterned cell cultures on elastic membranes as an in vitro model of myocardium. *Nat Protoc* 2006;**1**:1379–1391.

10. Cavanaugh MW. Pulsation, migration and division in dissociated chick embryo heart cells in vitro. *J Exp Zool* 1955;**128**:573–589.

11. Chlopcikova S, Psotova J, Miketova P. Neonatal rat cardiomyocytes–a model for the study of morphological, biochemical and electrophysiological characteristics of the heart. *Biomed Pap Med Fac Univ Palacky Olomouc Czech Repub* 2001;**145**:49–55.

12. Cooper G. Cytoskeletal networks and the regulation of cardiac contractility: microtubules, hypertrophy, and cardiac dysfunction. *Am J Physiol* 2006;**291**:H1003–H1014.

13. de Boer TP, Camelliti P, Ravens U, Kohl P. Myocardial tissue slices: organotypic pseudo-2D models for cardiac research & development. *Future Cardiol* 2009;**5**:425–430.

14. Decker ML, Simpson DG, Behnke M, Cook MG, Decker RS. Morphological analysis of contracting and quiescent adult rabbit cardiac myocytes in long-term culture. *Anat Rec* 1990;**227**:285–299.

15. Fast VG. Simultaneous optical imaging of membrane potential and intracellular calcium. *J Electrocardiol* 2005;**38**:107–112.

16. Fast VG, Darrow BJ, Saffitz JE, Kleber AG. Anisotropic activation spread in heart cell monolayers assessed by high-resolution optical mapping. Role of tissue discontinuities. *Circ Res* 1996;**79**:115–127.

17. Goldsmith EC, Borg TK. The dynamic interaction of the extracellular matrix in cardiac remodeling. *J Card Fail* 2002;**8**:S314–S318.

18. Gomez JP, Potreau D, Raymond G. Intracellular calcium transients from newborn rat cardiomyocytes in primary culture. *Cell Calcium* 1994;**15**:265–275.

19. Gopalan SM, Flaim C, Bhatia SN, et al. Anisotropic stretch-induced hypertrophy in neonatal ventricular myocytes micropatterned on deformable elastomers. *Biotechnol Bioeng* 2003;**81**:578–587.

20. Habeler W, Pouillot S, Plancheron A, Puceat M, Peschanski M, Monville C. An in vitro beating heart model for long-term assessment of experimental therapeutics. *Cardiovasc Res* 2009;**81**:253–259.

21. Harary I, Farley B. In vitro studies of single isolated beating heart cells. *Science* 1960;**131**:1674–1675.

22. Hilenski LL, Terracio L, Borg TK. Myofibrillar and cytoskeletal assembly in neonatal rat cardiac myocytes cultured on laminin and collagen. *Cell Tissue Res* 1991;**264**:577–587.

23. Horackova M, Mapplebeck C. Electrical, contractile, and ultrastructural properties of adult rat and guinea-pig ventricular myocytes in long-term primary cultures. *Can J Physiol Pharmacol* 1989;**67**:740–750.

24. Humphrey JD, Wells PB, Baek S, Hu JJ, McLeroy K, Yeh AT. A theoretically-motivated biaxial tissue culture system with intravital microscopy. *Biomech Model Mechanobiol* 2008;**7**:323–334.

25. Hwang SM, Yea KH, Lee KJ. Regular and alternant spiral waves of contractile motion on rat ventricle cell cultures. *Phys Rev Lett* 2004;**92**:198103.

26. Hyde A, Blondel B, Matter A, Cheneval JP, Filloux B, Girardier L. Homo- and heterocellular junctions in cell cultures: an electrophysiological and morphological study. *Prog Brain Res* 1969;**31**:283–311.

27. Jacobson SL, Piper HM. Cell cultures of adult cardiomyocytes as models of the myocardium. *J Mol Cell Cardiol* 1986;**18**:661–678.

28. Jacot JG, McCulloch AD, Omens JH. Substrate stiffness affects the functional maturation of neonatal rat ventricular myocytes. *Biophys J* 2008;**95**:3479–3487.

29. Jacot JG, Raskin AM, Omens JH, McCulloch AD, Tung L. (2009). Mechanotransduction in cardiac and stem-cell derived cardiac cells. In: *Mechanosensitivity of the Heart* (eds A Kamkin, I Kiseleva). Springer, New York. 2009, pp. 99–139.

30. Janmey PA, McCulloch CA. Cell mechanics: integrating cell responses to mechanical stimuli. *Annu Rev Biomed Eng* 2007;**9**:1–34.

31. Jawad H, Ali NN, Lyon AR, Chen QZ, Harding SE, Boccaccini AR. Myocardial tissue engineering: a review. *J Tissue Eng Regen Med* 2007;**1**:327–342.

32. Jongsma HJ, van Rijn HE. Electronic spread of current in monolayer cultures of neonatal rat heart cells. *J Membr Biol* 1972;**9**: 341–360.

33. Jongsma HJ, Masson-Pevet MA, Hollander CC, de Bruyn JR. Synchronization of the beating frequency of cultured rat heart cells. In: *Developmental and Physiological Correlates of Cardiac Muscle* (eds M Lieberman, T Sano). Raven Press, New York, p. 185.

34. Kehat I, Gepstein A, Spira A, Itskovitz-Eldor J, Gepstein L. High-resolution electrophysiological assessment of human embryonic stem cell-derived cardiomyocytes: a novel in vitro model for the study of conduction. *Circ Res* 2002;**91**:659–661.

35. Kent RL, Mann DL, Urabe Y, Hisano R, Hewett KW, Loughnane M, Cooper G. Contractile function of isolated feline cardiocytes in response to viscous loading. *Am J Physiol* 1989;**257**:H1717–H1727.

36. Kong CR, Bursac N, Tung L. Mechanoelectrical excitation by fluid jets in monolayers of cultured cardiac myocytes. *J Appl Physiol* 2005;**98**:2328–2336.

37. Korhonen T, Hanninen SL, Tavi P. Model of excitation–contraction coupling of rat neonatal ventricular myocytes. *Biophys J* 2009;**96**: 1189–1209.

38. Lee S, Kim JC, Li Y, Son MJ, Woo SH. Fluid pressure modulates L-type Ca^{2+} channel via enhancement of Ca^{2+}-induced Ca^{2+} release in rat ventricular myocytes. *Am J Physiol* 2008;**294**:C966–C976.

39. Lieberman M, Sawanobori T, Kootsey JM, Johnson EA. A synthetic strand of cardiac muscle: its passive electrical properties. *J Gen Physiol* 1975;**65**:527–550.

40. Lieberman M, Hauschka SD, Hall ZW, et al. Isolated muscle cells as a physiological model. *Am J Physiol* 1987;**253**:C349–C363.

41. Lorenzen-Schmidt I, Schmid-Schonbein GW, Giles WR, McCulloch AD, Chien S, Omens JH. Chronotropic response of cultured neonatal rat ventricular myocytes to short-term fluid shear. *Cell Biochem Biophys* 2006;**46**:113–122.

42. Matsuda T, Fujio Y, Nariai T, *et al.*N-cadherin signals through Rac1 determine the localization of connexin 43 in cardiac myocytes. *J Mol Cell Cardiol* 2006;**40**:495–502.

43. McSpadden LC, Kirkton RD, Bursac N. Electrotonic loading of anisotropic cardiac monolayers by unexcitable cells depends on connexin type and expression level. *Am J Physiol* 2009;**297**:C339–C351.

44. Mitcheson JS, Hancox JC, Levi AJ. Cultured adult cardiac myocytes: future applications, culture methods, morphological and electrophysiological properties. *Cardiovasc Res* 1998;**39**:280–300.

45. Parker KK, Ingber DE. Extracellular matrix, mechanotransduction and structural hierarchies in heart tissue engineering. *Phil Trans R Soc (Lond) B* 2007;**362**:1267–1279.

46. Pimentel RC, Yamada KA, Kleber AG, Saffitz JE. Autocrine regulation of myocyte Cx43 expression by VEGF. *Circ Res* 2002;**90**:671–677.

47. Riemer TL, Tung L. Stretch-induced excitation and action potential changes of single cardiac cells. *Prog Biophys Mol Biol* 2003;**82**:97–110.

48. Rohr S. Role of gap junctions in the propagation of the cardiac action potential. *Cardiovasc Res* 2004;**62**:309–322.

49. Rohr S. Myofibroblasts in diseased hearts: new players in cardiac arrhythmias? *Heart Rhythm* 2009;**6**:848–856.

50. Rohr S, Fluckiger-Labrada R, Kucera JP. Photolithographically defined deposition of attachment factors as a versatile method for patterning the growth of different cell types in culture. *Pflugers Arch* 2003;**446**:125–132.

51. Sachs F. Electrophysiological properties of tissue cultured heart cells grown in a linear array. *J Membr Biol* 1976;**28**:373–399.

52. Sadoshima J, Izumo S. The cellular and molecular response of cardiac myocytes to mechanical stress. *Annu Rev Physiol* 1997;**59**:551–571.

53. Samarel AM. Costameres, focal adhesions, and cardiomyocyte mechanotransduction. *Am J Physiol* 2005;**289**:H2291–H2301.

54. Sato T, Ohkusa T, Suzuki S, Nao T, Yano M, Matsuzaki M. High ambient pressure produces hypertrophy and up-regulates cardiac sarcoplasmic reticulum Ca^{2+} regulatory proteins in cultured rat cardiomyocytes. *Hypertens Res* 2006;**29**:1013–1020.

55. Schackow TE, Decker RS, Ten Eick RE. Electrophysiology of adult cat cardiac ventricular myocytes: changes during primary culture. *Am J Physiol* 1995;**268**:C1002–C1017.

56. Sekar RB, Kizana E, Cho HC. *et al.* I_{K1} heterogeneity affects genesis and stability of spiral waves in cardiac myocyte monolayers. *Circ Res* 2009;**104**:355–364.

57. Sengupta PP, Korinek J, Belohlavek M, Narula J, Vannan MA, Jahangir A, Khandheria BK. Left ventricular structure and function: basic science for cardiac imaging. *J Am Coll Cardiol* 2006;**48**:1988–2001.

58. Shanker AJ, Yamada K, Green KG, Yamada KA, Saffitz JE. Matrix-protein-specific regulation of Cx43 expression in cardiac myocytes subjected to mechanical load. *Circ Res* 2005;**96**:558–566.

59. Shapira-Schweitzer K, Seliktar D. Matrix stiffness affects spontaneous contraction of cardiomyocytes cultured within a PEGylated fibrinogen biomaterial. *Acta Biomater* 2007;**3**:33–41.

60. Shimko VF, Claycomb WC. Effect of mechanical loading on three-dimensional cultures of embryonic stem cell-derived cardiomyocytes. *Tissue Eng Part A* 2008;**14**:49–58.

61. Shyu KG. Cellular and molecular effects of mechanical stretch on vascular cells and cardiac myocytes. *Clin Sci (Lond)* 2009;**116**:377–389.

62. Shyu KG, Chen CC, Wang BW, Kuan P. Angiotensin II receptor antagonist blocks the expression of connexin43 induced by cyclical mechanical stretch in cultured neonatal rat cardiac myocytes. *J Mol Cell Cardiol* 2001;**33**:691–698.

63. Suzuki T, Ohta M, Hoshi H. Serum-free, chemically defined medium to evaluate the direct effects of growth factors and inhibitors on proliferation and function of neonatal rat cardiac muscle cells in culture. *In Vitro Cell Dev Biol* 1989;**25**:601–606.

64. Tatsukawa Y, Kiyosue T, Arita M. Mechanical stretch increases intracellular calcium concentration in cultured ventricular cells from neonatal rats. *Heart Vessels* 1997;**12**:128–135.

65. Tung L, Zhang Y. Optical imaging of arrhythmias in tissue culture. *J Electrocardiol* 2006;**39**:S2–S6.

66. van Laake LW, van Donselaar EG, Monshouwer-Kloots J, *et al.* Extracellular matrix formation after transplantation of human embryonic stem cell-derived cardiomyocytes. *Cell Mol Life Sci* 2010;**67**:277–290.

67. van Wamel AJ, Ruwhof C, van der Valk-Kokshoom LE, Schrier PI, van der Laarse A. The role of angiotensin II, endothelin-1 and transforming growth factor-beta as autocrine/paracrine mediators of stretch-induced cardiomyocyte hypertrophy. *Mol Cell Biochem* 2001;**218**:113–124.

68. VanWinkle WB, Snuggs MB, Buja LM. Cardiogel: a biosynthetic extracellular matrix for cardiomyocyte culture. *In Vitro Cell Dev Biol Anim* 1996;**32**:478–485.

69. Walsh KB, Parks GE. Changes in cardiac myocyte morphology alter the properties of voltage-gated ion channels. *Cardiovasc Res* 2002;**55**:64–75.

70. Wang TL, Tseng YZ, Chang H. Regulation of connexin 43 gene expression by cyclical mechanical stretch in neonatal rat cardiomyocytes. *Biochem Biophys Res Comm* 2000;**267**:551–557.

71. Weinberg S, Lipke EA, Tung L. In vitro mapping of stem cells, in *Methods in Molecular Biology: Stem Cells for Myocardial Repair and Regeneration* (ed R Lee), Humana Press, 2010, pp. 215–237.

72. Woo SH, Risius T, Morad M. Modulation of local Ca^{2+} release sites by rapid fluid puffing in rat atrial myocytes. *Cell Calcium.* 2007;**41**:397–403.

73. Yamada K, Green KG, Samarel AM, Saffitz JE. Distinct pathways regulate expression of cardiac electrical and mechanical junction proteins in response to stretch. *Circ Res* 2005;**97**:346–353.

74. Zhang Y, Sekar RB, McCulloch AD, Tung L. Cell cultures as models of cardiac mechanoelectric feedback. *Prog Biophys Mol Biol* 2008;**97**:367–382.

75. Zhuang J, Yamada KA, Saffitz JE, Kleber AG. Pulsatile stretch remodels cell-to-cell communication in cultured myocytes. *Circ Res* 2000;**87**:316–322.

76. Zimmermann WH, Eschenhagen T. Cardiac tissue engineering for replacement therapy. *Heart Fail Rev* 2003;**8**:259–269.

77. Zlochiver S, Munoz V, Vikstrom KL, Taffet SM, Berenfeld O, Jalife J. Electrotonic myofibroblast-to-myocyte coupling increases propensity to reentrant arrhythmias in two-dimensional cardiac monolayers. *Biophys J* 2008;**95**:4469–4480.

78. Zwi L, Caspi O, Arbel G, Huber I, Gepstein A, Park IH, Gepstein L. Cardiomyocyte differentiation of human induced pluripotent stem cells. *Circulation.* 2009;**120**:1513–1523.

SECTION 3

Multi-cellular manifestations of mechano-electric coupling

21. **Activation sequence of cardiac muscle in simplified experimental models: relevance for cardiac mechano-electric coupling**   *153*
Vladimir S. Markhasin, Alexander Balakin, Yuri Protsenko and Olga Solovyova

22. **Mechanical triggers and facilitators of ventricular tachy-arrhythmias**   *160*
T. Alexander Quinn and Peter Kohl

23. **Acute stretch effects on atrial electrophysiology**   *168*
Michael R. Franz and Frank Bode

24. **Stretch effects on potassium accumulation and alternans in pathological myocardium**   *173*
Christian Bollensdorff and Max J. Lab

25. **The effects of wall stretch on ventricular conduction and refractoriness in the whole heart**   *180*
Robert W. Mills, Adam T. Wright, Sanjiv M. Narayan and Andrew D. McCulloch

26. **Mechanical triggers of long-term ventricular electrical remodelling**   *187*
Darwin Jeyaraj and David S. Rosenbaum

27. **Mechanisms of mechanical pre- and postconditioning**   *193*
Asger Granfeldt, Rong Jiang, Weiwei Shi and Jakob Vinten-Johansen

Activation sequence of cardiac muscle in simplified experimental models: relevance for cardiac mechano-electric coupling

Vladimir S. Markhasin, Alexander Balakin, Yuri Protsenko and Olga Solovyova

Background

In 1927, Carl Wiggers was the first to focus on the regional features of left ventricular (LV) wall motion during the contractile cycle[1]. He found that during the isovolumic phase of ventricular contraction, shortly before the onset of ejection, apical myocardial regions that contract earlier stretch the basal segments that contract later. He called this the 'entrant phase' of contraction and suggested that it may contribute to increasing mechanical efficiency[1]. Current experimental techniques allow one to register the detailed spatial and temporal patterns of mechanical activation in different layers and regions of LV myocardial walls caused by the spread of excitation. In this chapter we address in detail the effects of the activation sequence on regional and global functions of the LV myocardium and demonstrate that the activation sequence of the LV can be a key mechanism organizing ventricular wall motion for effective pumping. Finally, we show that the activation sequence probably contributes to cardiac remodelling via mechano-electric coupling (MEC).

Activation sequence of the left ventricle

Contraction

Mechanical activation of the ventricles is the key determinant of global systolic and diastolic function. Mechanical activation is primarily driven by electrical excitation, but both processes are linked.

Electrical excitation of heart muscle starts from the left apical region of the septum, then spreads from sub-*endo*cardium (sub-ENDO) to sub-*epi*cardium (sub-EPI) and from apex to base[2]. Mechanical activation and the onset of fibre shortening in the sub-ENDO precedes that of sub-EPI[3]. Delays between electrical and mechanical activation in different regions of the LV wall may play a role in spatial and temporal coordination between electrical excitation and contraction of the LV. The heterogeneous distribution of regional mechanical loads and sarcomere lengths produces variation in the electro-mechanical delays. Higher preloads increase end-diastolic sarcomere lengths which cause shorter electro-mechanical delays due to the length-dependent increase in the affinity of troponin C (TnC) for Ca^{2+}[4].

Recent data on the regional timing of longitudinal and circumferential shortening of the LV via high-temporal resolution sonomicrometry can be summarized as follows[5]. Both longitudinal and circumferential strains in the sub-ENDO are higher than in corresponding regions of the sub-EPI and tend to increase from apex to base. Times to reach 10, 20, 40 and 80% of longitudinal shortening are shorter in apical versus basal regions both in sub-ENDO and sub-EPI layers, which is in agreement with earlier activation of apical regions and suggests a progressive decrease in the velocity of contractions from apex to base. The onset of longitudinal shortening is earlier than the circumferential one in the apical sub-ENDO. The characteristics of circumferential shortening do not significantly differ along sub-ENDO layers. Biplane cineradiography of implanted transmural markers is consistent and shows for the first time significant heterogeneity of transmural myofibre motions even during isovolumic contractions of the LV[6]. Significant sub-ENDO shortening and sub-EPI lengthening occurred in the anterior free wall of the LV, along with opposite local circumferential strain in the transmural layers and with longitudinal shortening and thickening across the entire wall. Isovolumic contraction is a highly dynamic mechanical reconfiguration of the LV within the isovolumic constraint.

While electrical excitation of the septum precedes that of the lateral LV wall, the onset of contraction is earlier in the latter. In the lateral wall peak strain is higher and is reached later. Asynchrony in peak shortening between the lateral wall and septum in human LV is up to 120 ms, about three times higher than the asynchrony in the onset of shortening[7].

Using echocardiography we assessed regional motion of the LV wall by analyzing time-dependent changes in the areas of sectors segmenting the sub-ENDO LV contour[8]. We found significant spatial and temporal heterogeneity of LV wall motion in healthy people with a negative correlation between the amount of segmental area change and the time required for it. The biggest segmental area changes were registered in the mid regions of the LV lateral wall and septum and the time required for the change was the shortest. The minimal area change was registered in the apical region of the LV wall with the longest time to the change.

Relaxation

The onset and time to reach 20% of myocardial lengthening in the sub-ENDO LV in both longitudinal and circumferential directions is earlier in the apical sub-ENDO regions with significant delay in basal regions[5]. The patterns of sub-EPI relaxation (especially the timing of circumferential lengthening) are opposite to sub-ENDO gradients. The time of onset of circumferential lengthening was longest in the apical sub-EPI region and was delayed beyond the onset of the isovolumic relaxation phase of the LV. This delay reflects the presence of post-systolic apical sub-EPI shortening, which period correlates with the time required for reaching the lowest LV diastolic pressure ($T_{LV,min}$). Furthermore, the delay of apex-to-base circumferential lengthening linearly correlated with both the duration of isovolumic relaxation and $T_{LV,min}$[5]. The data agree with earlier reported post-systolic shortening of myofibres in healthy subjects[9]. Post-systolic shortening of the apical sub-EPI and basal sub-ENDO during the isovolumic phase of LV relaxation creates gradients of relaxation from apex to base and from sub-ENDO to sub-EPI that may facilitate an increase in the cavity of apical regions and thus accelerate the decrease in LV pressure. The prolongation of apical sub-EPI contraction beyond LV end-systole may constitute an active component of LV wall relaxation for facilitating blood suction during early diastole[5].

Twisting

In addition to radial and longitudinal regional motions of the LV wall, twisting and untwisting also occur[10,11]. If the radial and longitudinal strains correspond to preferential change in the short or long LV axes, respectively, twisting arises from shear deformations of sub-ENDO versus sub-EPI layers. During isovolumic contraction the segments of the LV wall rotate counterclockwise. During mid systole, basal regions change the direction so that the base twists against the apex[11]. As suggested in[6], delayed activation of sub-EPI versus sub-ENDO myocardial layers drives LV wall twisting. This twisting provides for effective blood wringing movements of the LV during systole. On the other hand, twisting

allows the LV to reserve potential energy which is then released for untwisting during diastole and facilitating blood suction.

According to the ventricular myocardial band (VMB) model[12], ventricular architecture consists of two spiral bands (ascending sub-EPI and descending sub-ENDO bands, crossing at the apical loop of the LV) forming the right and left ventricles as an entire double coiled helicoids. It was suggested that the ascending and descending bands interact like muscle agonists–antagonists. Specifically, according to the VMB model, contraction of the descending band contributes predominantly to ventricular systole, while contraction of the ascending band occurs with some time delay during ventricle filling, ensuring LV twisting–untwisting[13]. This prediction was substantiated using sono-micrometric crystals implanted in selected regions of intact animal heart[12].

Disturbances in activation sequence

Ectopic pacing of the LV with stimulating leads placed at different regions of the ventricular walls is widely used for studying the role of activation sequence in cardiac function[14,15]. It was shown that abnormal ventricular excitation may cause systolic dysfunction (e.g. a decrease in the ejection fraction) probably because of increased asynchrony and heterogeneity of regional wall motion[15]. Relaxation velocity of LV was shown to decrease due to disturbances in the activation sequence and the consequent regional dyskinesia[16]. Cardiac resynchronization therapy, being a standard treatment for synchronizing ventricular contractions, may create a substrate for arrhythmias by inducing an increase in transmural dispersion of repolarization[17,18].

Activation sequence and mechano-electric interactions in heterogeneous myocardium

In spite of ample evidence for the role of activation sequence in cardiac function, little is known about how the activation sequence affects the electrical and mechanical activity of interacting cardiomyocytes in myocardial tissue.

Muscle duplex approach

To address the effects of mechanical interactions between spatially distant but mechanically coupled segments of myocardial tissue we use the simplest case model – the muscle duplex[19]. Muscle segments are mechanically connected either in series or in parallel and different sequences of muscle stimulation with varying time lags (from 0 to ±100 ms) are applied for simulating excitation propagation throughout the myocardial tissue. The physiological relevance of the duplex model stems from the fact that mechanical signal transduction in cardiac tissue (at the velocity of sound in liquids, i.e. about 300 m × s^{-1}) is about three orders of magnitude faster than electrical excitation propagation (at a velocity of 0.3–0.5 m × s^{-1})[12], so the mechanical effects (e.g. stretch) from earlier activated myocardial segments are almost immediately transferred to even distant surrounding passive tissue, preconditioning it to later activation.

Our group developed six principal duplex configurations [see[19–22] for details], using either *in-series* or *in-parallel* pairs of (1) multicellular cardiac muscle preparations (*biological duplexes*), (2) two interacting samples of a computational model of cardiac muscle (*virtual duplexes*), or (3) hybrid combinations of one real and one virtual muscle (*hybrid duplexes*). The duplex model is a simple and useful tool to address the effects of activation sequence on myocardial tissue. As widely reported elsewhere [e.g. reviewed in our Chapter 22 of the 1st edition of this book[23]], cardiac muscle is structurally and functionally heterogeneous, and this heterogeneity manifests itself at all levels of functional organization: from the molecular to the whole organ. Briefly, the sub-EPI myocytes that are activated later than sub-ENDO ones have shorter action potentials (AP), faster decay of Ca^{2+} transients, and faster contractions[24–26]. All these differences are provided on the molecular level by variable expression of different isoforms of ion channels, Ca^{2+} handling and contractile proteins[25,27]. The longitudinal heterogeneity of cardiomyocytes from apex to base is less well studied[28], but in agreement with the data on transmural myocyte heterogeneity, *regional distribution of durations of AP, Ca^{2+} transient and contraction are closely, and inversely, related to the sequence of ventricular depolarization*[23].

Presented here are muscle duplexes we used to simulate interactions between transmural (in parallel) or base-to-apex (in series) ventricular segments with specific differences in their electrical and mechanical characteristics. In particular, the paired muscles (either biological or virtual ones) that we selected to mimic interactions between 'slow' sub-ENDO and 'fast' sub-EPI fibres developed nearly equal peak isometric forces but displayed a prominent

asynchrony in the time courses of force generation or shortening and showed significant differences in their length–force and force–velocity relationships [see Fig. 21.1 and refs[19,20,22]]. In the corresponding virtual muscle samples, faster contracting muscles displayed shorter AP and Ca^{2+} transients than their slower counterparts[21].

In all duplex settings (biological, virtual and hybrid), mechanical coupling of two cardiac muscles (duplex formation) causes significant changes in their mechanical behaviour[19–22]. Moreover, mechanical interactions between segments causes modulation of Ca^{2+} kinetics, and AP generation in both muscles[20–22]. The responses depended on the sequence of muscle activation, imitating possible variations in the delay and direction of the excitation wavefront.

In all configurations of **in-parallel duplexes**, individual length–force and force–velocity relations for both segments changed significantly in opposite directions compared to those obtained before mechanical coupling [see Fig. 21.1 and refs[20,22]]. Unlike high sensitivity of the elements, the overall force–velocity curve of the parallel duplex was independent of the activation sequence and time delay between element excitation (Fig. 21.1). Because the force–velocity curve is widely used to characterize cardiac muscle

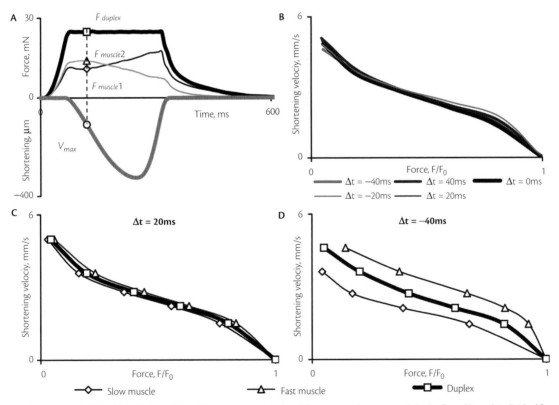

Fig. 21.1 'Contractility conservation' in a biological, parallel and heterogeneous duplex. **A** From top to bottom: total duplex force (F_{duplex}), individual forces ($F_{muscle1}$, $F_{muscle2}$) and shortening recorded in in-parallel connected 'slow' [time to peak force (TPF) = 178 ms] and 'fast' (TPF = 142 ms) papillary muscles from rat right ventricle under constant afterload imposed on the pair [20% of isometric peak force (F_0) produced by the duplex]. Dots on the traces indicate the time to maximal velocity of shortening V_{max}. Forces developed at this time (normalized by corresponding F_0 of either duplex or each muscle) are plotted vs the V_{max} to obtain force–velocity relationships for each element and entire duplex (**B-D**). **B** Overlap of the force–velocity curves is shown for the duplex with different activation sequences and time delays (Δt) between muscle excitation. Positive Δt correspond to excitation delays of the fast muscle, while negative Δt are for delays of the slow muscle. **C** and **D** Individual force–velocity relationships of coupled muscles change due to muscle interaction depending on the activation sequence. **C** Delayed activation of the fast element (which contracts/relaxes faster in isolation and its force–velocity curve lies above that of the slow element) causes the force–velocity relations of the elements to approach each other, up to a perfect overlap (here at $\Delta t = 20$ ms). **D** Delayed stimulation of the slow muscle (here at $\Delta t = -40$ ms), in contrast, causes force–velocity relationships to diverge.

contractility, its stability for the whole duplex prompted us to propose a phenomenon of 'contractility conservation' that is ensured by changes (either convergence or divergence) of individual characteristics of the mechanical activity of interacting muscle segments. This phenomenon reflects high stability and adaptation reserve of 'normal' heart muscle. On the other hand, it clearly shows that apparently normal function of the whole ventricle can hide subcritical local heterogeneities and dysfunctions which, together with disturbed blood supply, may provide a substrate for myocardial infarction.

The main feature of **in-series duplexes** is that end-to-end coupling of individual muscle segments forces the elements to switch from isometric to auxotonic mode of contraction, governed by opposite length changes in the elements under a fixed entire duplex length [see Fig. 21.2 and refs[19–22]]. The dynamical behaviour of coupled myocardial segments under isometric constraint for the whole duplex agrees well with the experimental data on the dynamical reorganization of the LV wall during isovolumic contractions with opposite directions of myofibre shortening in sub-ENDO and sub-EPI layers[6].

Mechanical interactions between fast and slow muscles stimulated simultaneously caused a decrease in the duplex peak force. In virtual duplexes, this was accompanied by an increase in the dispersion of repolarization (DR) assessed as the difference between times required for 90% repolarization of coupled muscles. In contrast, duplex performance improved when fast muscle stimulation was delayed (causing precontraction stretch by the earlier activated slow element). In all duplex configurations, isometric peak force was maintained at a maximum level or even increased over a wide range of delays (from 0 to 100 ms) in fast muscle activation (e.g. 15–20% peak force increase was registered in coupled papillary

muscles from the right ventricle of rat). In contrast to the stability of duplex force generation, the DR in virtual duplexes was very sensitive to the activation delay, and abruptly decreased with an increase in activation delay of the fast muscle from 0 to 40 ms. The inverted activation sequence (fast first, slow second) of in-series duplexes caused a pronounced decrease (more than 50%) in peak force. In virtual duplexes, the difference in action potential duration (APD) between elements increased, and the DR exceeded the sum of the original APD difference and activation delay. On the basis of these results, we suggested that the pattern of regional heterogeneity should be tightly related to the excitation sequence to ensure stable electrical and mechanical function of myocardial tissue.

Mechanical interactions cause significant changes in the functional state of duplex elements revealed in the slow force responses to muscle segment coupling[29]. In all duplex configurations, with heterogeneous pairs of fast and slow muscles, an initial drop in peak force (developed upon muscle coupling) was followed by a slow cycle-by-cycle increase in peak force, along with a gradual increase in the amplitude of individual deformations performed by the coupled elements (Fig. 21.2). In virtual duplexes, the force increase was accompanied by opposite changes in the amplitude and duration of Ca^{2+} transients in interacting segments. The changes in Ca^{2+} transient duration closely correlated with respective changes in both APD and the sarcoplasmic reticulum (SR) Ca^{2+} load[29]. The results predict that local SR Ca^{2+} load and therefore the contractile potential of myocardial tissue elements are affected by the sustained interaction with their mechanical environment. This prediction was verified by experiments on both biological and hybrid duplexes[29]. The change in the contractility of interacting muscles was clearly revealed by the pronounced force

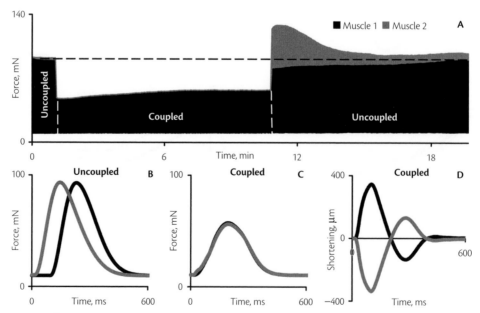

Fig. 21.2 Heterogeneity as a cause of heterometric regulation of myocardial contractility. **A** Slow force response is recorded in a pair of in-series connected papillary muscles from rat right ventricle. Overall end-to-end length of the pair is fixed (isometric constraint for the duplex), and 80 ms stimulation delay between muscles is applied with a pacing rate of 0.3 Hz. Initial drop of the peak isometric force (PF) developed by the duplex after muscle coupling is followed by a slow positive PF transient (up to 15% of the initial PF). Time-dependent isometric forces produced by the muscles before and after coupling are shown in panels **B** and **C** respectively. After muscle disconnection a significant PF transient is registered in each individual muscle (see panel **A**) which reflects changes in the functional state of muscles during the time of their dynamical interactions. The changes in muscle contractility are ensured by the dynamical deformations (dynamical heterometric regime) of coupled muscles (see panel **D**) evolved by their consequent activation.

transients registered in each of the muscles after their disconnection and return to independent isometric contractions (Fig. 21.2).

The new type of slow force response we found for in-series duplexes reflects an independent mechanism of cardiac function regulation, which we designate as 'heterogeneity caused heterometric regulation of myocardial contractility'. Thus, cardiomyocyte function within the tissue is significantly affected by mechanical loads (passive or active), including those that arise as a consequence of the activation sequence.

1D models of myocardial tissue

The basic duplex model uses only two elements, often with drastic differences in electrical and mechanical parameters. This is an extreme simplification of the complex spatio-temporal patterns of myocardial heterogeneity, and does not allow the simulation of gradual changes in spatio-temporal properties of cardiac tissue. By extending the duplex approach, we developed one-dimensional (1D) cardiac tissue models, consisting of several virtual muscle elements mechanically connected in series[29].

First we studied the effect of excitation sequence in homogeneous chains of identical fast or slow elements (Fig. 21.3A). Under external isometric constraint, internal dynamical deformations of muscle segments within the tissue transformed originally identical elements into functionally heterogeneous units. This was reflected in the gradients of mechano-electrical properties along the chain according to the activation timing: a gradual increase in individual APD from early to late activated elements with DR about twice exceeding overall stimulation delay between chain edges (Fig. 21.3A); an end-to-end decrease in the amplitude and increase in the duration of Ca^{2+} transient; and an increase in the SR Ca^{2+} loading in the interacting elements[29].

In heterogeneous 1D chains consisting of elements with gradually increasing velocity of contraction and relaxation of individual muscle segments, the deformation fields were different both *qualitatively* and *quantitatively* depending on which end of the chain was stimulated first (Fig. 21.3B,C). Excitation spreading from slow to fast elements provided the chain with stable contractile responses and tolerance to variations in activation delay of the fastest element. This mechanical stability was accompanied by a small DR ensured by the element repolarization sequence with opposite direction to that of depolarization (Fig. 21.3B), as seen in normal myocardium[30]. In contrast, in 1D models with inverted excitation sequence, the force significantly decreased and 'abnormal' repolarization sequence produced a huge increase in DR (Fig. 21.3C)[29].

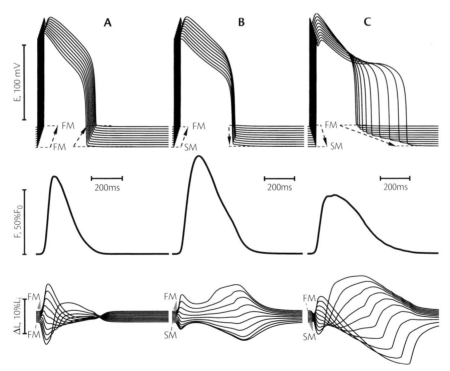

Fig. 21.3 Effects of activation sequence on the electrical and mechanical activity of 1D virtual myocardial chain composed of 10 end-to-end connected muscle segments under constant overall length of the chain. Every muscle segment has the same peak isometric force (F_0) at the same initial length ($L_i = 0.9\ L_{max}$) when contracting in isolation. Panel **A** shows the effects of activation sequence with 4 ms delay between elements in a chain composed of identical fast virtual muscles. Panels **B** and **C** show effects of oppositely directed activation sequences in a heterogeneous chain with gradual variation in individual contractile characteristics of muscle segments, with the slowest muscle (SM) on one edge and the fastest muscle (FM) on the opposite edge of the chain. From top to bottom: time-dependent changes in the membrane potential (E) in cardiomyocytes from chain segments; force (F as percentage of F_0) generated by the chain (it is identical in each in-series coupled muscle segment), and deformations (ΔL as percentage of the initial length, L_i) of muscle segments. Arrows indicate direction of depolarization and repolarization (top) and the mechanical activation sequence (bottom) in the chains. Maximal force and minimal dispersion of repolarization is produced by the heterogeneous chain with activation sequence spreading from slower to faster elements.

The effects of activation sequence in 1D models predict that disturbances in normal activation sequence of myocardial regions in intact tissue may increase the electrical heterogeneity of cardiomyocytes and produce a substrate for arrhythmias. These predictions agree with experimental findings showing that inverted activation sequence of the LV may cause ventricular electrical remodelling[31].

Underlying mechanisms

The functional state of interacting cardiomyocytes depends on their location within the tissue as this determines both the timing of element activation and the pattern of active and passive stress-strain fields. Regional mechanical deformations that evolve from the activation sequence may cause both activation of mechano-sensitive ion channels and modulation of Ca^{2+} handling via the contractile proteins. By local accumulation of Ca^{2+}, both mechanisms can also modify fluxes through Ca^{2+}-dependent currents and exchangers. The importance of the role of the contractile proteins is that one can simulate important aspects of cardiac MEC without including mechano-sensitive ion channels. Force-dependent Ca^{2+}-TnC binding can affect the AP shape and the dynamics of SR Ca^{2+} load[29]. In the complex interplay of cellular processes, *mechano-dependent Ca^{2+} kinetics play a key role in the fine adjustment of mechanical and electrical activity*. The role of mechano-sensitive ion channels has yet to be introduced.

Expanding the model to the longer time scale, myocardial mechanics can affect gene expression and protein synthesis[32]. The duration of Ca^{2+} transients is a key determinant of protein synthesis in remodelling[33]. A short-term reversal in transmural activation sequence causes electrical remodelling in myocardial tissue[34], and inverted activation sequence in the whole heart causes long-term electrical remodelling on the cellular and macroscopic levels[31]. The electrical heterogeneity produced by inverted activation sequence was shown to correlate with high gradients in the local deformations, suggesting the contribution of MEC to the electrical remodelling. These data suggest that the activation sequence is a causal factor of spatio-temporal self-organization of the myocardium[29]. These mechanisms will contribute to the selective expression of protein isoforms that determine the electrical and mechanical properties of cardiomyocytes.

Conclusions and outlook

The sequence of the activation of the ventricle ensures the requisite kinematics that optimizes systolic and diastolic LV functions. Activation sequence is inherently related to the regional heterogeneity of the myocardium. Why do heterogeneous myocardial systems benefit from such activation sequence? If the faster elements were activated before the slow ones, the peaks of their electrical and contractile activity would diverge, increasing asynchrony and reducing system performance. In contrast, delayed activation of the fast elements causes their 'pre-loading' and pre-stretching during the early phase of contraction (mechanical tuning during entrant phase) and allows myocardial elements to synchronize their activity, increasing the system's efficiency. Computational simulation results we obtained in rather simple myocardial models predict that MEC appears to play a key role in adjusting the mechanical and electrical activity of cardiomyocytes to their activation sequence within the tissue. More adequate 3D computational

models of the ventricles and the whole heart will be employed to elucidate the role of MEC in the coordination of cardiomyocyte function in the intact heart.

Acknowledgements

This work was supported by Wellcome Trust grants for a research collaboration between the Ekaterinburg group and the team of Drs D. Noble and P. Kohl at Oxford University, and by an NIH Fogarty IC award with Dr F. Sachs at the University at Buffalo. Ongoing research is supported by the Ural Branch of the RAS and Russian Foundation for Basic Research. The authors thank Dr F. Sachs for editorial help with this chapter.

References

1. Wiggers CJ. Interpretation of the intraventricular pressure curve on the basis of rapidly summated fractionate contractions. *Am J Physiol* 1927;**80**:12.

2. Liu G, Iden JB, Kovithavongs K, Gulamhusein R, Duff HJ, Kavanagh KM. In vivo temporal and spatial distribution of depolarization and repolarization and the illusive murine T-wave. *J Physiol* 2004;**555**: 267–279.

3. Ashikaga H, Coppola BA, Hopenfeld B, Leifer ES, McVeigh ER, Omens JH. Transmural dispersion of myofiber mechanics: implications for electrical heterogeneity in vivo. *J Am Coll Cardiol* 2007;**49**:909–916.

4. Konhilas JP, Irving TC, de Tombe PP. Length-dependent activation in three striated muscle types of the rat. *J Physiol* 2002;**544**:225–236.

5. Sengupta PP, Khandheria BK, Korinek J, *et al*. Apex-to-base dispersion in regional timing of left ventricular shortening and lengthening. *J Am Coll Cardiol* 2006;**47**:163–172.

6. Ashikaga H, van der Spoel TI, Coppola BA, Omens JH. Transmural myocardial mechanics during isovolumic contraction. *JACC Cardiovasc Imaging* 2009;**2**:202–211.

7. Zwanenburg JJ, Gotte MJ, Kuijer JP, Heethaar RM, van Rossum AC, Marcus JT. Timing of cardiac contraction in humans mapped by high-temporal-resolution MRI tagging: early onset and late peak of shortening in lateral wall. *Am J Physiol* 2004;**286**:H1872–H1880.

8. Chumarnaia TV, Solovyova OE, Sukhareva SV, Vargina TA, Markhasin VS. Spatio-temporal heterogeneity of human left ventricle contractions in norm and under ischemic heart disease. *Ross Fiziol Zh Im I M Sechenova* 2008;**94**:1217–1239.

9. Voigt JU, Lindenmeier G, Exner B, *et al*. Incidence and characteristics of segmental postsystolic longitudinal shortening in normal, acutely ischemic, and scarred myocardium. *J Am Soc Echocardiogr* 2003;**16**:415–423.

10. Petersen SE, Jung BA, Wiesmann F, *et al*. Myocardial tissue phase mapping with cine phase-contrast MR imaging: regional wall motion analysis in healthy volunteers. *Radiology* 2006;**238**: 816–826.

11. Jung B, Markl M, Foll D, Hennig J. Investigating myocardial motion by MRI using tissue phase mapping. *Eur J Cardiothorac Surg* 2006;**29**(Suppl 1):S150–S157.

12. Torrent-Guasp F, Kocica MJ, Corno AF, *et al*. Towards new understanding of the heart structure and function. *Eur J Cardiothorac Surg* 2005;**27**:191–201.

13. Buckberg GD, Castella M, Gharib M, Saleh S. Active myocyte shortening during the 'isovolumetric relaxation' phase of diastole is responsible for ventricular suction; 'systolic ventricular filling'. *Eur J Cardiothorac Surg* 2006;**29**(Suppl 1):S98–S106.

14. Nahlawi M, Waligora M, Spies SM, Bonow RO, Kadish AH, Goldberger JJ. Left ventricular function during and after right ventricular pacing. *J Am Coll Cardiol* 2004;**44**: 1883–1888.

15. Park RC, Little WC, O'Rourke RA. Effect of alteration of left ventricular activation sequence on the left ventricular end-systolic pressure-volume relation in closed-chest dogs. *Circ Res* 1985;**57**:706–717.

16. Zile MR, Blaustein AS, Shimizu G, Gaasch WH. Right ventricular pacing reduces the rate of left ventricular relaxation and filling. *J Am Coll Cardiol* 1987;**10**:702–709.

17. Fish JM, Brugada J, Antzelevitch C. Potential proarrhythmic effects of biventricular pacing. *J Am Coll Cardiol* 2005;**46**:2340–2347.

18. Touiza A, Etienne Y, Gilard M, Fatemi M, Mansourati J, Blanc JJ. Long-term left ventricular pacing: assessment and comparison with biventricular pacing in patients with severe congestive heart failure. *J Am Coll Cardiol* 2001;**38**:1966–1970.

19. Markhasin VS, Solovyova O, Katsnelson LB, Protsenko Y, Kohl P, Noble D. Mechano-electric interactions in heterogeneous myocardium: development of fundamental experimental and theoretical models. *Prog Biophys Mol Biol* 2003;**82**:207–220.

20. Solovyova O, Katsnelson L, Guriev S, Nikitina L, Protsenko Y, Routkevitch S, Markhasin V. Mechanical inhomogeneity of myocardium studied in parallel and serial cardiac muscle duplexes: experiments and models. *Chaos Solitons Fractals* 2002;**13**:1685–1711.

21. Solovyova O, Vikulova N, Katsnelson LB, *et al.* Mechanical interaction of heterogeneous cardiac muscle segments in silico: effects on Ca^{2+} handling and action potential. *Inter J Bifurcation Chaos* 2003;**13**:3757–3782.

22. Protsenko YL, Routkevitch SM, Gur'ev VY, *et al.* Hybrid duplex: a novel method to study the contractile function of heterogeneous myocardium. *Am J Physiol* 2005;**289**:H2733–H2746.

23. Markhasin VS, Solovyova O (2005). Mechano-electrical heterogeneity in physiological function of the heart. In: *Cardiac Mechano-Electric Feedback and Arrhythmias: From Pipette to Patient* (eds P Kohl, F Sachs, MR Franz). Saunders/Elsevier, Philadelphia, pp. 214–223.

24. Antzelevitch C. Electrical heterogeneity, cardiac arrhythmias, and the sodium channel. *Circ Res* 2000;**87**:964–965.

25. Laurita KR, Katra R, Wible B, Wan X, Koo MH. Transmural heterogeneity of calcium handling in canine. *Circ Res* 2003;**92**:668–675.

26. Wan X, Bryant SM, Hart G. A topographical study of mechanical and electrical properties of single myocytes isolated from normal guinea-pig ventricular muscle. *J Anat* 2003;**202**:525–536.

27. Nerbonne JM, Guo W. Heterogeneous expression of voltage-gated potassium channels in the heart: roles in normal excitation and arrhythmias. *J Cardiovasc Electrophysiol* 2002;**13**:406–409.

28. Ng GA, Cobbe SM, Smith GL. Non-uniform prolongation of intracellular Ca^{2+} transients recorded from the epicardial surface of isolated hearts from rabbits with heart failure. *Cardiovasc Res* 1998;**37**:489–502.

29. Solovyova O, Katsnelson LB, Konovalov P, *et al.* Activation sequence as a key factor in spatio-temporal optimization of myocardial function. *Phil Trans R Soc, (Lond) A* 2006;**364**:1367–1383.

30. Franz MR, Bargheer K, Rafflenbeul W, Haverich A, Lichtlen PR. Monophasic action potential mapping in human subjects with normal electrocardiograms: direct evidence for the genesis of the T-wave. *Circulation* 1987;**75**:379–386.

31. Jeyaraj D, Wilson LD, Zhong J, *et al.* Mechanoelectrical feedback as novel mechanism of cardiac electrical remodeling. *Circulation* 2007;**115**:3145–3155.

32. Borg TK, Goldsmith EC, Price R, Carver W, Terracio L, Samarel AM. Specialization at the Z line of cardiac myocytes. *Cardiovasc Res* 2000;**46**:277–285.

33. Berridge MJ. Cardiac calcium signalling. *Biochem Soc Trans* 2003;**31**:930–933.

34. Libbus I, Rosenbaum DS. Transmural action potential changes underlying ventricular electrical remodeling. *J Cardiovasc Electrophysiol* 2003;**14**:394–402.

Mechanical triggers and facilitators of ventricular tachy-arrhythmias

T. Alexander Quinn and Peter Kohl

Background

The heart can adjust its performance to acute changes in circulatory demand, even after transplantation, which illustrates that cardiac mechano-sensitivity is an efficient contributor to the (auto-)regulation of the heartbeat. Cardiac function involves multiple interdependent mechano-sensitive pathways, including those that feed information about the mechanical state of the myocardium to the electrical processes of excitation and conduction. This mechano-electric feedback forms part of the overall mechano-electric coupling (MEC) concept, which considers the heart as an integrated electro-mechanical organ. MEC can be observed at all levels of cardiac structural and functional integration, from (sub-)cellular and tissue levels, to whole organ and patients[1]. Perturbations of the heart's mechanical status can occur as a consequence of both intrinsic and extrinsic stimuli.

Intrinsic stimuli include changes in venous return that determine cardiac preload (e.g. Chapter 13), alterations in cardiac afterload (e.g. Chapter 37) and intracardiac stress-strain inhomogeneities that arise in normal (e.g. Chapter 21) and pathologically disturbed myocardium (e.g. Chapter 48) as a consequence of the heart's own contractile activity. The mechanisms underlying MEC are normally either 'electro-physiologically silent' or physiologically beneficial, so one should not regard MEC as arrhythmogenic *per se*. The preload-dependent modulation of cardiac Ca^{2+} handling, for example, that contributes to the Frank–Starling response of the heart is thought to act as an equalizer of cellular contractility, allowing individual cardiomyocytes to operate in mechanical balance with their neighbours. Classic Frank–Starling mechanisms allow instantaneous adaptation in contractile behaviour without changes in intracellular Ca^{2+} load. For adaptation to sustained changes in mechanical load, however, the trans-sarcolemmal Ca^{2+} flux balance must be affected. The electrophysiological consequences of mechanisms that support Na^+ and/or Ca^{2+} gain (such as stretch-activated channels, SAC) may be more apparent than SAC effects on ion balance. Therefore, mechano-electric phenomena may arise as 'side-effects' of mechanisms that support other physiological functions. This finds manifestation in pathological conditions involving inhomogeneous stress-strain distributions,

where regional mechanical modulation of Ca^{2+} handling can give rise to arrhythmogenic Ca^{2+} waves (see Chapter 16).

Extrinsic (to the myocardium) stimuli may occur in the context of invasive medical interventions (such as cardiac catheterization) or as a consequence of extra-corporeal impacts (e.g. during *Commotio cordis*, or in the context of precordial thump application for cardioversion). As in the case of intrinsic mechanical stimuli, mechanical interventions are normally electrophysiologically silent (no effect) or benign (perhaps triggering an extra beat, without causing sustained arrhythmias). Nonetheless, as illustrated by the topic of this book, MEC has clear clinical relevance, and both initiation (see Chapters 31 and 45) and termination of arrhythmias by mechanical means (see Chapter 50) have been observed.

The present chapter explores the roles of mechanical factors in the genesis of ventricular tachy-arrhythmias. Conceptually, tachy-arrhythmogenesis is thought to be a consequence of the combined action of a *trigger* event and a *sustaining mechanism* (both may be 'merged', such as when repetitive generation of a trigger [focal activity] maintains tachy-arrhythmic activity). Ventricular tachy-arrhythmias are frequently encountered in pathologies associated with volume and pressure overload, such as in patients with valve disease, ischaemia, infarction, cardiomyopathy or heart failure (e.g. Chapter 56). This is caused, at least in part, by cellular electrophysiological responses to changes in myocardial strain[2]. However, in the setting of chronic diseases it is difficult to identify causal relationships, as cardiac MEC responses occur on the background of structure–function remodelling and in the presence of changes in metabolic state, autonomic control, and responsiveness to pharmaceutical interventions.

Consideration of acute effects of changes in the mechanical environment can help to elucidate these mechanisms, even in the chronic setting. For instance, *acute removal* of ventricular volume overload by the Valsalva manoeuvre has provided one of the most impressive illustrations of the arrhythmogenicity of sustained strain: with the reduction of ventricular dimensions (a consequence of blood redistribution caused by a change in thoracico-abdominal pressure gradients), ventricular tachycardia (VT) ceases in patients[3], even after surgical denervation of the heart (transplant recipients)[4].

More commonly, however, acute *application* of mechanical stimuli is investigated, often in the healthy heart, which somewhat restricts the applicability of observations to chronic disease states. Nonetheless, acute changes in myocardial strain, whether global (e.g. increased intraventricular volume) or regional (e.g. extrinsically applied local mechanical stimulation, or intrinsic paradoxical segment lengthening during local metabolic impairment), has been shown to have pronounced effects on cardiac electrophysiology. Experimental investigations in isolated whole heart, tissue, and cellular models have provided insight into the translation of mechanical factors into triggers (ectopic excitation of myocardial tissue) and facilitators (promoting re-entry) of ventricular tachy-arrhythmias.

Effects of acute mechanical stimulation on heart rhythm: temporal aspects

General considerations

One of the major mechanisms underlying MEC is activation of specialized, mechano-sensitive ion channels. These can be divided into SAC that increase their open probability in direct response to cell deformation and cell-volume activated channels (VAC) that respond, usually with some delay in cardiomyocytes, to an increase in cytosolic volume. Acute mechanical stimulation of the heart is assumed to not be associated with changes in cell volume (for information on VAC and their roles in settings such as ischaemia, reperfusion and hypertrophy, see Chapters 4 and 51).

Interestingly, most of the *acute* cardiac electrophysiological responses to mechanical stimulation can be explained by considering effects mediated via sarcolemmal SAC, although non-sarcolemmal SAC (Chapter 5), changes in cellular Ca^{2+} handling (Chapter 10), effects on other messenger systems (Chapter 11) or interaction with non-cardiomyocytes (Chapter 19) are undoubtedly important contributors to MEC. In addition, the open probability of many ion channels that are not customarily regarded as SAC is sensitive to the mechanical environment (see Chapter 6), highlighting the multitude of possible pathways underlying cardiac MEC.

Since the discovery of SAC in cardiac cells over two decades ago[5,6], their properties and contribution to arrhythmogenesis have been important targets of basic and applied research. Two categories of SAC can be distinguished, based on their ion selectivity: cation non-selective SAC (SAC_{NS}), with a reversal potential somewhere half-way between peak action potential (AP) and resting potential levels (usually around –20 to 0 mV), and K^+ selective SAC (SAC_K), with a reversal potential that is negative to cardiomyocyte resting potential (i.e. near the potassium equilibrium potential, usually between –90 and –95 mV)[7–9].

The reversal potential is an important determinant of acute SAC effects on cardiac myocytes as it acts like a sink-hole towards which, if opened, the cell's membrane potential will be drawn. Thus, direct activation of SAC_{NS} can be sufficient to trigger an AP in isolated cardiomyocytes at rest[10]. However, as cardiomyocyte membrane potential changes during the cardiac cycle, electrophysiological effects of acute mechanical stimulation depend on timing relative to the cardiac cycle (see also Chapter 14).

In this chapter we use the terms 'systole' and diastole' to distinguish key phases of the cardiac cycle. More specifically, and even though the terms were originally designated to describe mechanical behaviour, we follow the prevailing trend and use these terms to

refer to the period of time during which ventricular cardiomyocytes are either at resting membrane potential (diastole) or inside the AP (systole).

Mechanical stimulation during diastole

If large enough to cause any change in potential at all, diastolic strain depolarizes the resting membrane of ventricular myocytes (Fig. 22.1). This has been demonstrated in isolated cells[11], tissue[12] and whole heart preparations[13].

In one of the classic MEC illustrations, Franz *et al.* showed in 1989 that transient increases in the volume of an intraventricular balloon cause diastolic depolarizations in isolated canine hearts[14]. The amplitude of these mechanically induced depolarizations correlates with the magnitude of volume changes applied. If sufficiently large, mechanically induced depolarizations can trigger premature ventricular contractions (PVC)[13] or short runs of VT[15]. This response has been attributed to SAC_{NS}, as their pharmacological block eliminates MEC responses in ventricular[16] and atrial[17] tissue (for more detail regarding acute stretch effects on atrial electrophysiology, see Chapter 23). Interestingly, the change in intraventricular volume required for arrhythmia induction is remarkably consistent between experiments in the same species, while the associated changes in intraventricular pressure show high variability. This suggests that myocardial strain (material deformation) may be a more important, though not exclusive, mediator of cardiac MEC responses compared to stress (force inside the material)[15].

Local ventricular mechanical stimulation, such as by finger-tapping of the epicardium in open heart surgery or by external impacts to the precordium, can be used to pace the asystolic heart via diastolic depolarization-mediated MEC effects (see Chapter 50). As with changes in intraventricular volume, there is a threshold for

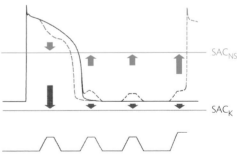

Fig. 22.1 Schematic representation of transient stretch effects on whole cell membrane potential and indication of contributions by cation non-selective and potassium-selective stretch-activated channels (SAC_{NS} and SAC_K, respectively). SAC_{NS} (red) have a reversal potential about half-way between action potential (AP) peak and resting potential (black curve). Depending on the timing of mechanical stimulation (bottom curve), their activation may shorten AP duration (grey dashed curve), cause behaviour reminiscent of early or delayed after-depolarizations (EAD and DAD, respectively; black dashed curves) or – if strong enough – trigger a new AP (red dashed curve). The reversal potential of SAC_K (grey) is negative to the resting membrane potential. Their activation during *any* part of the cardiac cycle would tend to re- or hyperpolarize cardiac cells, in particular during the AP plateau when their electrotonic driving force is largest (compare lengths of arrows indicating SAC effects on membrane potential). [Reproduced, with permission, from Kohl P (2009) Cardiac stretch-activated channels and mechano-electric transduction. In: *Cardiac Electrophysiology: From Cell to Bedside* (eds D P Zipes, J Jalife). Saunders, Philadelphia, pp. 115–126.]

mechanical PVC induction, which has been established in healthy adult volunteers by defibrillation pioneer Paul Zoll as 0.04–1.50 J for precordial impacts[18]. For comparison, 0.1 J is equivalent to the impact energy of a 40 g glue stick dropped from a height of just under 30 cm (i.e. from your hand with the elbow resting on the table). This illustrates the exquisite mechano-sensitivity of the healthy, resting heart.

Mechanical stimulation during systole

The effects of systolic mechanical stimulation on cardiac electrophysiology are more varied (Fig. 22.1). During the AP plateau, activation of either SAC$_{NS}$ or SAC$_K$ will have a repolarizing effect on the cell. As a consequence, AP shortening has frequently been observed[19]. However, as the cell membrane repolarizes, it approaches, and eventually passes, the reversal potential of SAC$_{NS}$. This can give rise to prolongation of the AP[20], in particular at near-complete AP repolarization levels, and may find an expression in cross-over of the repolarization curve[21]. Furthermore, acute axial strain can cause early after-depolarization (EAD)-like events in isolated cardiomyocytes[22], which may underlie similar responses in multicellular experimental preparations[13,23]. Mechanically induced EAD-like depolarizations have also been reported in patients during balloon valvuloplasty, an intervention where the ventricular outflow tract is temporarily blocked, causing an increase in intraventricular pressure that can give rise to PVC[24].

Strain maintained beyond the end of the AP (and therefore acting somewhere at the cross-roads of electrical systole and diastole, according to the definition used in this chapter) can cause delayed after-depolarization (DAD)-like behaviour. This may also serve as a source of PVC induction which, in the presence of a suitably arrhythmogenic background (such as experimentally induced prolongation of the QT segment of the electrocardiogram, ECG), can contribute to the initiation of sustained arrhythmias (e.g. *torsades de pointes* in the anaesthetized dog)[25].

In addition to the variable effects of mechanical stimulation on the AP of individual cells, it must be noted that at the whole organ level 'electrical systole' is associated with significant spatial non-uniformity in membrane potential across the ventricular myocardium. This means that timing of a mechanical stimulus 'relative to the AP' will be different in different parts of the heart (Fig. 22.2). While the ventricular activation wave-front is steep and fast (leaving comparatively little room for regionally differing responses to mechanical stimulation; see narrow QRS complex of the ECG in Fig. 22.2), repolarization is a more graded process (broader and lower ECG T-wave). This gives rise to an additional temporal component at the organ level: a vulnerable window for mechanical induction of tachy-arrhythmias, which conceptually is very similar to the vulnerable window for electrical stimulation that was systematically established in the 1930s[26].

The vulnerable window for mechanical induction of ventricular fibrillation (VF) has been identified by Link *et al.* in an anaesthetized pig model of *Commotio cordis* to occur 15–30 ms before the peak of the ECG T-wave[27] (see Chapter 45). This behaviour can be linked to SAC$_{NS}$ (Fig. 22.2). Their activation may give rise to DAD-like events (in cells that have regained excitability) or EAD-like behaviour (in cells that are repolarizing). If supra-threshold, these depolarizations can cause ectopic foci, potentially providing a trigger for arrhythmogenesis. SAC$_{NS}$ activation in cells at more

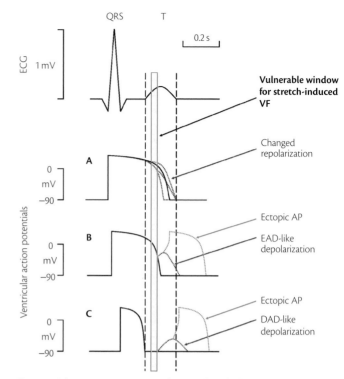

Fig. 22.2 Schematic representation of potentially arrhythmogenic SAC$_{NS}$ effects during early repolarization (upstroke of the T-wave, see red box and electrocardiogram, ECG, at top). Regionally differing effects would be determined by locally differing stages of AP repolarization and include: **A** changes in AP duration such as shortening, prolongation or crossover of repolarization; **B** EAD-like behaviour; **C** DAD-like events. Both EAD- and DAD-like events may trigger ectopic excitation, while sub-threshold changes increase heterogeneity in the electrophysiological background behaviour, potentially contributing to arrhythmia sustenance. VF, ventricular fibrillation. [Reproduced, with permission, from Kohl P, Nesbitt AD, Cooper PJ, Lei M (2001) Sudden cardiac death by *Commotio cordis*: role of mechano-electric feedback. *Cardiovasc Res* **50**:280–289.]

positive membrane potentials may affect the time-course of repolarization, increasing electrophysiological heterogeneity in affected areas of the myocardium, which could contribute to the formation of an arrhythmia-sustaining substrate for re-entry.

Computational modelling has been helpful in assessing the quantitative *plausibility* of this concept. Using a two-dimensional (2D) model of ventricular tissue, Garny and Kohl[28] demonstrated that sustained re-entry is observed only if the mechanical stimulus (1) encounters excitable tissue (giving rise to an ectopic focus by cellular depolarization), (2) overlaps with the repolarization wave end (giving rise to an area of functional block by AP prolongation) and (3) extends into tissue with membrane potentials above the SAC$_{NS}$ reversal potential (giving rise to an arrhythmia-sustaining substrate by regional AP shortening). In the model, this can occur during the second quarter of the T-wave (Fig. 22.3A). Impacts timed earlier or later in the cardiac cycle either are inefficient in triggering PVC or result in a single ectopic activation only, without sustained re-entry (Fig. 22.3B and C, respectively). While the situation will be more complex in a three-dimensional (3D) substrate such as the whole heart, similar results have been obtained using an anatomically detailed whole-ventricular model[29].

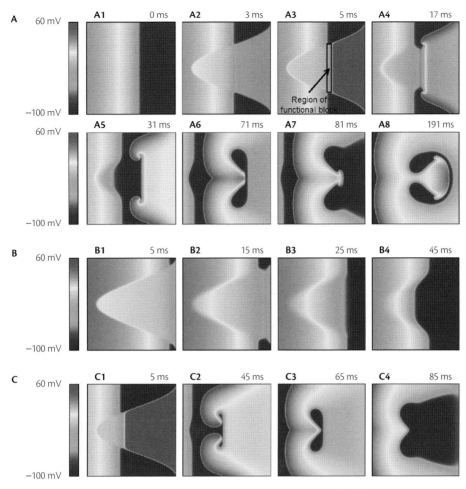

Fig. 22.3 Computer simulation of epicardial impact effects on ventricular electrophysiology. Impacts are simulated by 5 ms activation of SAC$_{NS}$ in the area highlighted in A2 and applied at different stages of ventricular repolarization (i.e. during different times of the ECG T-wave). **A** Development of a mechanically induced sustained ventricular arrhythmia, following a simulated impact at 40% repolarization. Arrhythmia sustenance depends on supra-threshold mechanical stimulation that triggers an extra AP in tissue that has recovered from inactivation, and on overlap of the mechanically stimulated tissue region with the trailing wave of repolarization, where an area of functional block gives rise to wave-split. Arrhythmia sustenance is further favoured by partial repolarization of near-endocardial myocardium from AP plateau towards membrane potentials closer to the reversal potential of SAC$_{NS}$. **B** Lack of arrhythmogenic effect of impacts applied too early during repolarization (< 10% repolarization). **C** Single ectopic AP without subsequent re-entry, caused by later impacts (here at 60% repolarization). [Reproduced, with permission, from Garny A, Kohl P (2004) Mechanical induction of arrhythmias during ventricular repolarization: modeling cellular mechanisms and their interaction in two dimensions. *Ann N Y Acad Sci* **1015**:133–143.] (See color plate section.)

Even though the electrophysiological response to mechanical stimulation appears to be dominated, in healthy myocardium, by SAC$_{NS}$ activation, there is experimental evidence in support of a contribution by certain SAC$_K$. In particular, a role for the mechano-sensitive[30,31] adenosine triphosphate-sensitive K$^+$ channel (K$_{ATP}$) has been demonstrated in the context of arrhythmias induced by precordial impact. Interestingly, mechanical and ischaemic activation of K$_{ATP}$ channels has been reported to act co-operatively, helping to explain why some of the changes in electrocardiographic parameters after precordial impact (like ECG ST-segment elevation) mimic those commonly associated with myocardial ischaemia, even though there does not appear to be significant disturbance of coronary flow[27]. Equally, reduced K$_{ATP}$ channel activation may be one of the mechanisms by which mechanical *prevention* of 'ischaemic bulging' can help to reduce extracellular potassium accumulation in the ischaemic

myocardium (see Chapter 24). In whole animal studies of *Commotio cordis*, application of glibenclamide, a non-specific inhibitor of K$_{ATP}$ channels, was found to significantly reduce VF induction, as well as ST segment elevation[32]. As impacts during the previously established vulnerable window still triggered PVC in the anaesthetized pig, the contribution of this particular SAC$_K$ population is likely to support sustenance, rather than induction, of arrhythmias (it is also possible that their pharmacological block shifted the vulnerable window for VF induction).

Interestingly, application of streptomycin (an efficient blocker of SAC$_{NS}$ in isolated cells)[33] had no effect on VF inducibility in the same model[34]. This raises the question as to what causes the impact-induced depolarization that underlies PVC, not only in diastole, but also during the T-wave (such as unmasked in the presence of glibenclamide). PVC arise in consequence of supra-threshold depolarization and may thus be caused either by mechanical activation of a depolarizing SAC (such as SAC_{NS}) or by mechanical reduction of a hyperpolarizing SAC (such as SAC_K) in the presence of sufficient background depolarizing currents. Given that there is little evidence in support of the latter scenario, the question remains why streptomycin had no effect on mechanical VF induction *in vivo*. Potential explanations include contributions by a streptomycin-insensitive form of SAC_{NS}, or limited efficacy of streptomycin as an acute SAC blocker in the whole animal. The latter would seem plausible, based on the absence of acutely impeded mechano-reception in patients receiving the antibiotic (side effects on inner ear function, for example, are usually seen only after prolonged exposure to the antibiotic). Limited efficacy of streptomycin for acute SAC_{NS} block *in situ* has also been documented in previous experiments on sino-atrial node tissue, in which stretch responses were unaffected by high doses of the antibiotic, yet abolished by the peptide SAC_{NS} blocker *Grammostola spatulata* mechano-toxin 4 (GsTMx-4)[35]. Thus, further studies are required to elucidate the contribution of different SAC types to mechanical induction of ventricular tachy-arrhythmias.

Mechanically induced VF probability further depends on impact site, contact area, and projectile stiffness. Impacts in an area of close approximation between precordium and heart are more likely to initiate VF than others, smaller contact areas are more arrhythmogenic, and projectile stiffness is correlated with propensity to induce VF. All these observations highlight the importance of localized mechanical energy transfer, first noted in the 1930s by Schlomka, who reported that precordial impacts in larger animals held in supine position (where the heart is relieved of its intimate mechanical coupling to the chest wall) do not readily induce arrhythmias[36].

In addition to local effects, arrhythmogenic precordial impacts are also associated in whole animal studies with large, but brief, surges in intraventricular pressure. These could give rise to a mechanical stimulus that affects ventricular tissue in a more global manner. Indeed, studies by Link *et al.* demonstrate a Gaussian relationship between the amplitude of intraventricular pressure surges and VF probability, which was greatest at pressure levels between 250 and 450 mmHg, reaching 68% at ~ 350 mmHg[37]. An interesting aspect of these data is that amplitude and *duration* of pressure surges are likely to be correlated; whether there is an independent contribution of the duration of intraventricular pressure changes remains to be investigated. Equally, the individual importance of global vs regional mechanical effects on cardiac electrical activity deserves more detailed consideration.

Effects of acute mechanical stimulation on heart rhythm: spatial aspects

General considerations

Increases in intraventricular volume or pressure, whether induced by intrinsic mechanisms that affect pre- or afterload or by causes extrinsic to the cardiovascular system such as intraventricular balloon inflation, can give rise to global strain of the ventricular tissue. However, myocardial compliance varies throughout the ventricles, due to the anisotropy of structural, active contractile, and passive viscoelastic properties. Therefore, 'globally uniform' mechanical stimulation can result in 'regionally heterogeneous' MEC effects. At the same time, more localized interventions such as precordial impact are associated with an increase in ventricular pressure,

which may induce more globally acting responses. Thus, in many settings, global and regional MEC effects will coincide, making identification of their individual contributions to arrhythmogenesis difficult.

Global mechanical stimulation

Some of the earliest *ex situ* whole heart investigations into the effects of mechanical stimulation on electrical behaviour used intraventricular balloons to apply global ventricular volume loads[14]. More recently, intraventricular balloons have been used in Langendorff-perfused hearts to simulate the pressure surges seen in whole animal models of *Commotio cordis*. Bode *et al.* found that large changes in intraventricular volume can induce VF in isolated rabbit hearts, in a magnitude- and (ECG) timing-dependent manner[38]. Pressure pulses between 209 and 289 mmHg were capable of inducing VF in 11% of cases where the stimulus was applied within a vulnerable window that was phenomenologically similar to that described for precordial impact[37].

The biophysical characteristics of pressure surges during precordial impact (ultra-fast pressure transients that occur in the absence of causal intraventricular volume alterations, with optimal VF induction at a peak-rate of ventricular pressure change, dP/dt_{max}, of 50 mmHg $\times$ ms^{-1})[37] are not easily reproduced by volume-pulsing of isolated hearts. Conceptually, the former may be regarded as an intervention where local stress (or strain) causes a global change in mechanics (pressure surge), while the latter is based on a global intervention (more slowly occurring volume pulse) which is translated into regionally heterogeneous stress-strain patterns. During volume loading, heterogeneity of myocardial structure and viscoelasticity will result in regional variation of tissue strain, giving rise to spatio-temporal dissociation between the globally uniform stimulus and its regional representation.

The response of cardiac muscle to ultra-fast pressure surges (few milliseconds duration) in the absence of volume loading may be even more complex, as such short-lived pressure surges may be too brief to cause effective tissue strain (buffered by myocardial viscosities). This may create peak stress levels that cause local tissue damage, even at pressure levels that would be tolerated in steady-state conditions, and should be assessed in future research.

The importance of regionally heterogeneous effects of global stimulation *in vivo* is supported by the observation that diastolic increases in intraventricular volume yield non-uniform depolarization, with the origin of ectopic AP induction most often in the postero-lateral region of the left ventricle, typically a region of high compliance[13]. More recently, Seo *et al.* have shown that stretch, applied across a flap of right ventricular tissue, gives rise to focal excitation at the point of the largest differences in strain, resulting in sustained tachy-arrhythmias[39]. Thus, regional heterogeneity of globally uniform mechanical stimulation appears to be a key contributor to arrhythmogenesis. In fact, in the computational model by Garny and Kohl[28], simultaneous activation of SAC_{NS} in the entire tissue block does not result in re-entry. If it captures all tissue that has regained excitability, a single ectopic beat, forming a planar wave, is caused (data not shown). So, in the absence of heterogeneity beyond the already pre-existing repolarization-related regional differences, mechanical stimulation is much less arrhythmogenic compared to scenarios where either the mechanical stimulus or its effects at the tissue level differ across the heart.

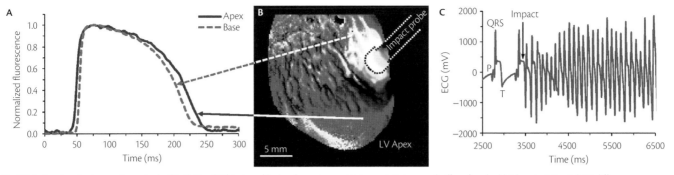

Fig. 22.4 Focal activation and ventricular fibrillation (VF) induced by local non-traumatic impacts in Langendorff-perfused rabbit hearts. **A** Spatial AP differences, visualized by epicardial optical voltage mapping, illustrate apico-basal activation delay during normal sinus rhythm and progression of the repolarization wave in the opposite direction. **B** Diastolic impact using a precision-controlled probe at energy levels < 1 mJ cause focal activation, followed by ectopic excitation of the ventricles. **C** Impact during the early T-wave causes focal excitation, followed by VF. This behaviour occurs when there is spatio-temporal overlap of the repolarization wave and mechanically stimulated tissue. [Reproduced, with permission, from Quinn TA, Lee P, Bub G, Epstein A, Kohl P (2010) Regional impact-induced arrhythmia in isolated rabbit heart visualised by optical mapping. *Heart Rhythm* **7**:S353.] (See color plate section.)

Regional mechanical stimulation

Regional mechanical stimulation may play an important role for arrhythmogenesis in diseases that involve heterogeneous changes in ventricular compliance, such as regional ischaemia[40] and infarction[41]. In both settings there is an increase in the probability of excitation in areas of particularly high strain gradients, such as via paradoxical segment lengthening of ischaemic tissue or at the scar–myocardial tissue interface of infarcts. In fact, the degree of dilation of an ischaemic region is a strong predictor of arrhythmia probability, including VF[42]. 3D computational modelling suggests that premature ventricular excitation originates, in this setting, from the ischaemic border zone, where mechanically induced depolarizations may contribute to the formation of ectopic foci (if supra-threshold) or to the slowing and block of conduction (if sub-threshold)[43]. Similarly, in VF, localized strain increases the complexity of activation maps in the affected region, with more areas of conduction block and transmural excitation breakthrough sites[44]. These results support the hypothesis that local strain gradients, whether applied regionally or resulting from heterogeneous translation of global mechanical perturbations, play important roles in the initiation and sustenance of re-entrant arrhythmias.

Still, quantitative discrimination between MEC effects of mechanical stimulation with primarily global or primarily local character remains a challenging task for further research. One published endocardial activation sequence, recorded in a single pig experiment during precordial impact-induced VF, shows focal excitation of the ventricle directly underneath the site of impact[45] (see Fig. 46.3). This might suggest that local effects are relevant even in the setting of *Commotio cordis*. Our own preliminary optical mapping studies demonstrate focal activation during non-traumatic epicardial impacts[46], applied to Langendorff-perfused rabbit hearts using a local impactor[47] (Fig. 22.4). In this setting, ectopic ventricular excitation can induce VF when there is spatio-temporal overlap of the mechanically stimulated tissue with the receding wave of previous excitation[46], confirming experimentally prior modelling-based predictions.

Conclusions and outlook

Acute mechanical stimulation can cause ventricular tachy-arrhythmias, by providing a trigger (ectopic excitation) and by creating or enhancing arrhythmia-sustaining mechanisms. The molecular substrates of this behaviour are believed to include SAC, and SAC$_{NS}$ in particular are contenders for the mechanism underlying mechanical AP induction. Additional activation of SAC$_K$ is likely to form one of the mechanisms that help to sustain tachyarrhythmic responses. Further examination of the precise contributions of different SAC populations call for studies in which global *versus* regional ventricular strain effects can be controlled, or at least monitored, and where the activity of SAC$_{NS}$ and SAC$_K$ can be pharmacologically manipulated with confirmed efficacy and specificity in native tissue. Novel non-invasive imaging approaches, combined with individualized quantitative computational modelling, will increasingly allow one to link the characterization of 'global' descriptors of cardiac mechano-electric activity (e.g. intraventricular volume or pressure changes or ECG) to 'regional' behaviour (e.g. transmural stress-strain distributions or high-resolution endo- or epicardial electrical activation and repolarization maps)[48]. This will be an important step towards linking cellular and sub-cellular MEC responses to spatio-temporal variations in ventricular stress-strain patterns, identifying molecular mechanisms that underlie ventricular function in three-dimensions and time.

References

1. Kohl P, Hunter P, Noble D. Stretch-induced changes in heart rate and rhythm: clinical observations, experiments and mathematical models. *Prog Biophys Mol Biol* 1999;**71**:91–138.
2. Lab MJ. Contraction–excitation feedback in myocardium. Physiological basis and clinical relevance. *Circ Res* 1982;**50**:757–766.
3. Waxman MB, Wald RW, Finley JP, Bonet JF, Downar E, Sharma AD. Valsalva termination of ventricular tachycardia. *Circulation* 1980;**62**:843–851.
4. Ambrosi P, Habib G, Kreitmann B, Faugere G, Metras D. Valsalva manoeuvre for supraventricular tachycardia in transplanted heart recipient. *Lancet* 1995;**346**:713.

5. Craelius W, Chen V, el-Sherif N. Stretch activated ion channels in ventricular myocytes. *Biosci Rep* 1988;**8**:407–414.

6. Sigurdson WJ, Morris CE, Brezden BL, Gardner DR. Stretch activation of a potassium channel in molluscan heart cells. *J Exp Biol* 1987;**127**:191–210.

7. Sachs F. Mechanical transduction by membrane ion channels: a mini review. *Mol Cell Biochem* 1991;**104**:57–60.

8. Sackin H. Stretch-activated ion channels. *Kidney Int* 1995;**48**: 1134–1147.

9. Morris CE. Mechanosensitive ion channels. *J Membr Biol* 1990;**113**: 93–107.

10. Craelius W. Stretch-activation of rat cardiac myocytes. *Exp Physiol* 1993;**78**:411–423.

11. White E, Boyett MR, Orchard CH. The effects of mechanical loading and changes of length on single guinea-pig ventricular myocytes. *J Physiol* 1995;**482**:93–107.

12. Lab MJ. Depolarization produced by mechanical changes in normal and abnormal myocardium [proceedings]. *J Physiol* 1978;**284**(Suppl):143P–144P.

13. Franz MR, Cima R, Wang D, Profitt D, Kurz R. Electrophysiological effects of myocardial stretch and mechanical determinants of stretch-activated arrhythmias. *Circulation* 1992;**86**:968–978.

14. Franz MR, Burkhoff D, Yue DT, Sagawa K. Mechanically induced action potential changes and arrhythmia in isolated and in situ canine hearts. *Cardiovasc Res* 1989;**23**:213–223.

15. Hansen DE, Craig CS, Hondeghem LM. Stretch-induced arrhythmias in the isolated canine ventricle. Evidence for the importance of mechanoelectrical feedback. *Circulation* 1990;**81**:1094–1105.

16. Hansen DE, Borganelli M, Stacy GP, Taylor LK. Dose-dependent inhibition of stretch-induced arrhythmias by gadolinium in isolated canine ventricles. Evidence for a unique mode of antiarrhythmic action. *Circ Res* 1991;**69**:820–831.

17. Bode F, Sachs F, Franz MR. Tarantula peptide inhibits atrial fibrillation. *Nature* 2001;**409**:35–36.

18. Zoll PM, Belgard AH, Weintraub MJ, Frank HA. External mechanical cardiac stimulation. *N Engl J Med* 1976;**294**:1274–1275.

19. White E, Le Guennec JY, Nigretto JM, Gannier F, Argibay JA, Garnier D. The effects of increasing cell length on auxotonic contractions; membrane potential and intracellular calcium transients in single guinea-pig ventricular myocytes. *Exp Physiol* 1993;**78**: 65–78.

20. Zeng T, Bett GC, Sachs F. Stretch-activated whole cell currents in adult rat cardiac myocytes. *Am J Physiol* 2000;**278**:H548–H557.

21. Zabel M, Koller BS, Franz MR. Amplitude and polarity of stretch-induced systolic and diastolic voltage changes depend on the timing of stretch: a means to characterize stretch-activated channels in the intact heart. *Pacing Clin Electrophysiol* 1993;**16**:886.

22. Kohl P (2009). Cardiac stretch-activated channels and mechano-electric transduction. In: *Cardiac Electrophysiology: From Cell to Bedside* (eds D.P. Zipes, J. Jalife). Saunders, Philadelphia, pp. 115–126.

23. Nazir SA, Lab MJ. Mechanoelectric feedback in the atrium of the isolated guinea-pig heart. *Cardiovasc Res* 1996;**32**:112–119.

24. Levine JH, Guarnieri T, Kadish AH, White RI, Calkins H, Kan JS. Changes in myocardial repolarization in patients undergoing balloon valvuloplasty for congenital pulmonary stenosis: evidence for contraction–excitation feedback in humans. *Circulation* 1988;**77**: 70–77.

25. Gallacher DJ, Van de Water A, van der Linde H, *et al.* In vivo mechanisms precipitating torsades de pointes in a canine model of drug-induced long-QT1 syndrome. *Cardiovasc Res* 2007;**76**: 247–256.

26. Wiggers CJ, Wégria R. Ventricular fibrillation due to single, localized induction and condenser shocks applied during the vulnerable phase of ventricular systole. *Am J Physiol* 1940;**128**:500–505.

27. Link MS, Wang PJ, Pandian NG, *et al.* An experimental model of sudden death due to low-energy chest-wall impact (*Commotio cordis*). *N Engl J Med* 1998;**338**:1805–1811.

28. Garny A, Kohl P. Mechanical induction of arrhythmias during ventricular repolarization: modeling cellular mechanisms and their interaction in two dimensions. *Ann N Y Acad Sci* 2004;**1015**: 133–143.

29. Li W, Kohl P, Trayanova N. Induction of ventricular arrhythmias following mechanical impact: a simulation study in 3D. *J Mol Histol* 2004;**35**:679–686.

30. Van Wagoner DR. Mechanosensitive gating of atrial ATP-sensitive potassium channels. *Circ Res* 1993;**72**:973–983.

31. Van Wagoner DR, Lamorgese M. Ischemia potentiates the mechanosensitive modulation of atrial ATP-sensitive potassium channels. *Ann N Y Acad Sci* 1994;**723**:392–395.

32. Link MS, Wang PJ, VanderBrink BA, *et al.* Selective activation of the K_{ATP} channel is a mechanism by which sudden death is produced by low-energy chest-wall impact (*Commotio cordis*). *Circulation* 1999;**100**:413–418.

33. Belus A, White E. Streptomycin and intracellular calcium modulate the response of single guinea-pig ventricular myocytes to axial stretch. *J Physiol* 2003;**546**:501–509.

34. Garan AR, Maron BJ, Wang PJ, Estes NA, 3rd, Link MS. Role of streptomycin-sensitive stretch-activated channel in chest wall impact induced sudden death (*Commotio cordis*). *J Cardiovasc Electrophysiol* 2005;**16**:433–438.

35. Cooper PJ, Kohl P. Species- and preparation-dependence of stretch effects on sino-atrial node pacemaking. *Ann N Y Acad Sci* 2005;**1047**:324–335.

36. Schlomka G. *Commotio cordis* und ihre Folgen. Die Einwirkung stumpfer Brustwandtraumen auf das Herz. *Ergebn Inn Med Kinderheilkd* 1934;**47**:1–91.

37. Link MS, Maron BJ, Wang PJ, VanderBrink BA, Zhu W, Estes NA, 3rd. Upper and lower limits of vulnerability to sudden arrhythmic death with chest-wall impact (*Commotio cordis*). *J Am Coll Cardiol* 2003;**41**:99–104.

38. Bode F, Franz M, Wilke I, Bonnemeier H, Schunkert H, Wiegand U. Ventricular fibrillation induced by stretch pulse: implications for sudden death due to *Commotio cordis*. *J Cardiovasc Electrophysiol* 2006;**17**:1011–1017.

39. Seo K, Inagaki M, Nishimura S, *et al.* Structural heterogeneity in the ventricular wall plays a significant role in the initiation of stretch-induced arrhythmias in perfused rabbit right ventricular tissues and whole heart preparations. *Circ Res* 2010;**106**:176–184.

40. Parker KK, Lavelle JA, Taylor LK, Wang Z, Hansen DE. Stretch-induced ventricular arrhythmias during acute ischemia and reperfusion. *J Appl Physiol* 2004;**97**:377–383.

41. Fu L, Cao JX, Xie RS, *et al.* The effect of streptomycin on stretch-induced electrophysiological changes of isolated acute myocardial infarcted hearts in rats. *Europace* 2007;**9**:578–584.

42. Barrabes JA, Garcia-Dorado D, Padilla F, *et al.* Ventricular fibrillation during acute coronary occlusion is related to the dilation of the ischemic region. *Basic Res Cardiol* 2002;**97**: 445–451.

43. Jie X, Gurev V, Trayanova N. Mechanisms of mechanically induced spontaneous arrhythmias in acute regional ischemia. *Circ Res* 2010;**106**:185–192.

44. Chorro FJ, Trapero I, Guerrero J, *et al.* Modification of ventricular fibrillation activation patterns induced by local stretching. *J Cardiovasc Electrophysiol* 2005;**16**:1087–1096.

45. Alsheikh-Ali AA, Akelman C, Madias C, Link MS. Endocardial mapping of ventricular fibrillation in *Commotio cordis*. *Heart Rhythm* 2008;**5**:1355–1356.

46. Quinn TA, Lee P, Bub G, Epstein A, Kohl P. Regional impact-induced arrhythmia in isolated rabbit heart visualised by optical mapping. *Heart Rhythm* 2010;**7**(5S):S353.

47. Cooper PJ, Epstein A, Macleod IA, *et al.* Soft tissue impact characterisation kit (STICK) for ex situ investigation of heart rhythm responses to acute mechanical stimulation. *Prog Biophys Mol Biol* 2006;**90**:444–468.

48. Plank G, Burton RA, Hales P, *et al.* Generation of histo-anatomically representative models of the individual heart: tools and application. *Phil Trans R Soc (Lond.) A* 2009;**367**:2257–2292.

23

Acute stretch effects on atrial electrophysiology

Michael R. Franz and Frank Bode

Background

Electrophysiological changes in response to mechanical perturbations or changes in haemodynamic loading have been well established in ventricular myocardium, in isolated heart preparations[1–3], in in-situ hearts[4,5], and in man[6,7]. Ventricular stretch leads to a shortening of action potential duration (APD)[3,5,8,9] and effective refractory period (ERP)[2,3,10,11]. Acute ventricular dilatation may induce premature depolarizations and triggered activity[7,12,13]. Critically timed ventricular stretch pulses may even lead to the induction of ventricular fibrillation[14].

In the atrium, shortening of atrial repolarization and of the associated refractory period (ERP), and in particular their non-uniform alteration, has been suggested as an arrhythmia substrate because it may shorten the re-entrant wavelength and favour functional block[15]. Recent data suggest that atrial stretch can provoke these electrophysiological changes and might be directly responsible for the induction or sustenance of atrial arrhythmias. This chapter focuses on the evidence showing that atrial dilatation promotes atrial fibrillation (AF) and that block of stretch-activated channels (SAC) suppresses AF during stretch.

Evidence for atrial mechano-electrical coupling

The prevalence of AF increases with age and is mostly associated with haemodynamic or mechanical disorders of the heart (i.e. hypertension, mitral valve disease, cardiac failure). Atrial dilatation assessed by echocardiography is found in the majority of patients with AF, implicating mechanical strain of the myocardium. It also has been suggested that AF itself could lead to atrial dilatation, thereby further increasing AF probability. Due to these clinical observations it has long been assumed that atrial stretch plays an important role in AF.

The presence of mechano-electrical coupling (MEC) has been proven at the atrial level in humans. Pulsatile atrial stretch caused by ventricular contraction modulates the atrial flutter cycle length in man[16]. The effect of sustained stretch on the atrial myocardium was investigated by several teams by ERP measurements and has offered differing results. Some groups[17–20] reported shortening of ERP, while others[21] reported ERP lengthening. This discrepancy may be explained by several factors. For example, the repolarization

level at which APD is determined is crucial because there may be shortening at early repolarization levels (APD20, APD50 or APD70) while APD90 may have increased duration. After-depolarizations caused by stretch may further prolong APD90 measurement. ERP measurements may depict APD near the 50% or 70% level, or at the 90% level, depending not only on stimulus timing but also on the stimulus strength. This is further complicated by the fact that atrial loading may produce wall stretch in a spatially non-uniform manner, where shortening and lengthening of atrial repolarization may occur in the same heart[22].

Arrhythmogenic effects of atrial stretch have been investigated in the Langendorff-perfused rabbit heart[18,23]. Differently from the normal rabbit atrium, which showed no sustained atrial arrhythmia, the stretched rabbit atria exhibited a variety of atrial arrhythmias, including rapid repetitive responses, atrial flutter and AF. The inducibility of AF by rapid burst pacing was measured at increasing atrial pressures (Fig. 23.1) and correlated to the refractory period. AF inducibility increased from 0% at low pressures to 100% at

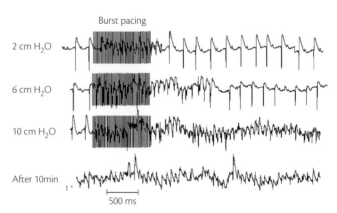

Fig. 23.1 Effect of step-wise increases in atrial pressure on inducibility and sustainability of atrial fibrillation (AF). The high-amplitude bursts at the left of each tracing are high-frequency electrical stimuli applied to induce AF. The lower amplitude high frequency deflections represent AF recorded by a monophasic action potential probe. [Reproduced, with permission, from Ravelli F, Allessie M (1997) Effects of atrial dilatation on refractory period and vulnerability to atrial fibrillation in the isolated Langendorff-perfused rabbit heart. *Circulation* **96**: 1686–1695.]

pressures > 10 cm H_2O. This vulnerability was attributed to concurrent reductions in APD and ERP (see below)[18], resulting in decreased atrial excitation wavelength[24–26]. Changes were completely reversible after release of atrial stretch, which terminated AF[18].

Stretch has also been shown to significantly decrease conduction velocity in atrial tissue (Fig. 23.2). In the isolated rabbit heart, acute dilatation of the atrium resulted in slowing of conduction and an increase in the amount of intra-atrial conduction block[27]. Conduction properties were assessed using a rectangular mapping array of 240 electrodes with a spatial resolution of 0.5 mm. The right atrium was paced from four different sites (Fig. 23.2A). At normal atrial pressure (2 cm H_2O), conduction was uniform in all directions. Increasing the pressure to 9 cm H_2O decreased the normalized conduction velocity during rapid pacing by 18%. The incidence of areas of slow conduction and conduction block increased from 6.6% and 1.6% to 10.2% and 3.3%. At 14 cm H_2O, conduction velocity decreased by 31% and the percentage of slow conduction and block further increased to 11.5% and 6.6% ($p < 0.001$)[27] (Fig. 23.2B). In the left atrium, an increase in atrial pressure to 14 cm H_2O also increased the amount of intra-atrial conduction block threefold to fourfold. Dependent on the pacing site, lines of intra-atrial block occurred which were oriented parallel to the major trabeculae and the crista terminalis[27,28]. Thus, the interception of thin, membranous-like atrial tissue with thicker pectinate muscles may, during atrial dilatation, provide a substrate for heterogeneous conduction slowing and partial block, promoting functional re-entry arrhythmias (Fig. 23.2C).

The role of pulmonary veins and the left atrium

The generation of ectopic electrical trigger activity in the pulmonary veins (PV) and the maintenance of re-entrant waves have evolved as crucial factors in promoting AF in man[29]. Ablation of the tissue surrounding the exits of PV into the left atrium has proven to often limit recurrence of AF in patients with paroxysmal AF and, to a lesser extent, in patients with chronic AF. Several experimental studies have explored the effects of stretch on PV tissue, which has led to increases of spontaneous PV 'firing' and the increased rate of such depolarizations.

In isolated perfused sheep hearts, optical mapping studies using potentiometric dye compared dominant frequencies (DF) in the left atrial free wall and the left superior PV junction[30]. Below 10 cm H_2O, the maximal dominant frequency during induced AF was similar in both locations (10.8±0.3 versus 10.2±0.3 Hz). At intra-atrial pressures > 10 cm H_2O, the maximal dominant frequency was significantly higher in the left superior PV junction than in the left atrial free wall (12.0±0.2 and 10.5±0.2 Hz, respectively; $p < 0.001$). Thus, intra-atrial pressure increase seems to particularly enhance the ability of the PV junction to sustain re-entry and/or to induce focal activity. For further detail see Chapters 15 and 29.

The role of SAC in AF inducibility

Experimental evidence has shown that SAC play an important role in promoting arrhythmias during stretch (see Chapter 14). Gadolinium (Gd^{3+}), a potent blocker of stretch-activated cation

channels, suppressed the occurrence of stretch-induced depolarizations in ventricular myocardium[12] and atrial tissue[31]. We performed studies to further explore the influence of SAC-block on the intact atrium and on the propensity of stretch to facilitate AF. The first aim was to evaluate in an isolated heart model whether the SAC-blocker Gd^{3+} influences the inducibility and maintenance of AF during acute stretch.

Effect of Gd^{3+} on AF inducibility

In the non-dilated atrium at a pressure of 0 cm H_2O, burst pacing induced no AF response. With increase in atrial pressure, AF could be induced in each preparation[19] (similar to Fig. 23.1)[23]. The initial AF response seen during a step-wise pressure increase was predominantly non-sustained, while sustained AF responses emerged at greater pressure levels. On average, intra-atrial pressure needed to be raised to 8.8±0.2 cm H_2O to enable perpetuation of AF after cessation of burst pacing. A further increase of intra-atrial pressure to 11.6±0.6 cm H_2O ($p < 0.01$) was required to induce sustained AF that lasted longer than 60 s. The increase in AF inducibility in response to pressure increase followed a sigmoidal curve.

Upon exposure to successively increased doses of Gd^{3+} (12.5, 25 and 50 µM), the vulnerability to AF progressively decreased (Fig. 23.3). After application of Gd^{3+} 50 µM, the lowest atrial pressure that had enabled AF induction during baseline was no longer sufficient to maintain AF. The average atrial pressure for AF inducibility was shifted from 8.8±0.2 to 19.0±0.5 cm H_2O ($p < 0.001$) and to 21.9±0.4 cm H_2O to obtain sustained AF ($p < 0.001$). The intra-arterial pressure providing a 50% probability of AF induction (P50) showed a linear correlation ($r = 0.99$; $p < 0.005$) with Gd^{3+} concentration for the 0–50 µM dose range, with reversibility upon washout[19].

Effect of verapamil on vulnerability to AF

Gd^{3+} has been reported to block calcium channels. To rule out that calcium channel block interferes with AF vulnerability during stretch, the effect of specific L-type calcium channel block was studied. Verapamil 1 µM did not inhibit AF induction during acute dilatation. The average atrial pressure for AF induction was 6.3±0.1 cm H_2O at baseline and 4.9±0.2 cm H_2O after application of verapamil (not significant)[19].

Effect of GsMTx-4 on vulnerability to AF

The clinical use of Gd^{3+} as an SAC-blocker (in concentrations required for this blocking action) is hampered by non-specific side effects and its tendency to precipitate in physiological buffers. Novel substances will therefore be required to provide effective and non-harmful SAC blockade in vivo. A peptide from the spider venom (GsMTx-4) of the tarantula *Grammostola spatulata* has been reported to exert specific block of SAC in myocardial cells[33]. We therefore evaluated in the isolated rabbit heart whether GsMTx-4 influences the inducibility and maintenance of AF during acute stretch[19,20].

In the presence of 170 µM GsMTx-4, induction of AF was possible only at significantly higher atrial pressures of 18.5±0.5 cm H_2O. Sustained AF was obtained at 24.8±0.6 cm H_2O after GsMTx-4, representing an increase of 13.2±0.6 cm H_2O compared to baseline ($p < 0.001$). Similar to Gd^{3+} the dose-response curve for GsMTx-4 was sigmoidal (Fig. 23.4).

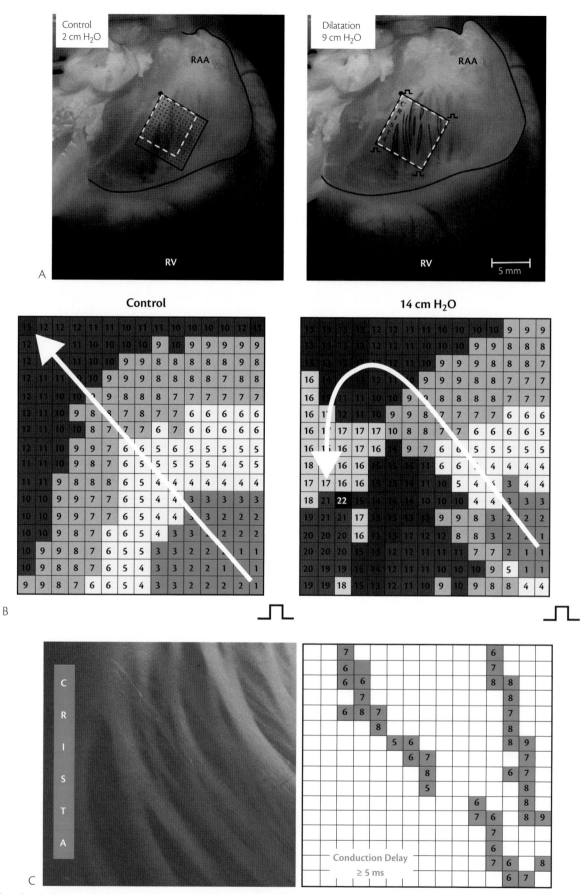

Fig. 23.2 Effect of atrial dilatation of isolated rabbit heart on conduction properties. **A** High-density mapping set-up superimposed on normal (control) and dilated right atrium. **B** Disruption of smooth conduction from site of electrical stimulus (control) to a heterogeneous and pivoting conduction pattern during atrial dilatation. **C** Alignment of conduction delays along the anatomical structures of the crista terminalis. RAA, right atrial appendage; RV, right ventricle. [Reproduced, with permission, from Eijsbouts SC, Majidi M, van Zandvoort M, Allessie MA (2003) Effects of acute atrial dilation on heterogeneity in conduction in the isolated rabbit heart. *J Cardiovasc Electrophysiol* **14**:269–278.]

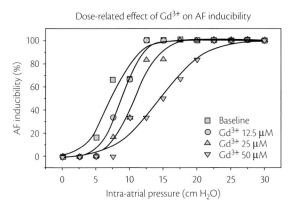

Fig. 23.3 Sigmoidal response curves of AF inducibilty to step-wise increased atrial pressure, and rightward shifts with increasing doses of Gd^{3+}. [Reproduced, with permission, from Bode F, Katchman A, Woosley RL, Franz MR (2000) Gadolinium decreases stretch-induced vulnerability to atrial fibrillation. *Circulation* **101**: 2200–2205.]

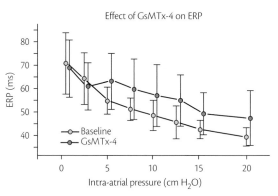

Fig. 23.5 Right atrial effective refractory period (ERP) measured at different atrial pressures (mean ± SD). ERP progressively decreased with a rise in atrial pressure during control. ERP was not significantly changed after GsMtx-4. [Reproduced, with, permission, from Bode F, Katchman A, Woosley RL, Franz MR (2000) Gadolinium decreases stretch-induced vulnerability to atrial fibrillation. *Circulation* **101**:2200–2205.]

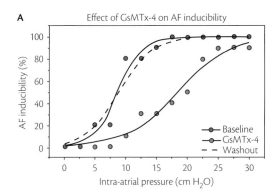

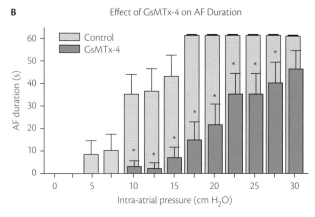

Fig. 23.4 GsMTx-4 effects on AF duration and effective refractory period (ERP). **A** Effect of GsMTx-4 on AF inducibility at increasing atrial pressures during baseline and after GsMTx-4 170 μM. **B** Duration of AF during control and in the presence of GsMTx-4.

Effect of stretch and SAC-blockade on atrial refractoriness

Atrial ERP shortened with increasing intra-atrial pressure regardless of the presence of either Gd^{3+} or GsMTx-4. During GsMTx-4 ERP decreased from 73±3 ms at 0.5 cm H_2O to 54±2 ms at 20 cm

H_2O, with only a non-significant tendency towards longer ERP at atrial pressures above 2.5 cm H_2O (Fig. 23.5)[19,20]. Thus, stretch-induced ERP decrease alone cannot be the main mechanism of stretch-induced AF vulnerability. Other factors must play a role and need further investigation. While in our model the standard error of ERP regardless of site was similar before and during SAC blockade, this finding does not support a significant role of ERP dispersion in this acute stretch model. However, other more detailed mapping studies suggest a significant role of spatial heterogeneity of atrial electrophysiology and conduction properties in linkage to anatomical features[27,28,34].

Conclusions and outlook

In summary, experiments in isolated hearts have shown that acute sustained atrial dilatation facilitates the induction and maintenance of AF. The experimental data support the hypothesis that SAC play an important role in facilitating AF induction and AF maintenance during acute dilatation of the atrial myocardium. Further, SAC block greatly reduces the susceptibility to AF of atria undergoing dilatation. Conforming to most previous studies, atrial stretch decreased the atrial ERP in a linear correlation with the degree of stretch. Stretch-induced decrease in ERP has been implicated in stretch-induced AF because of its excitation wavelength-shortening effect. Yet, the AF-preventing action of either Gd^{3+} or GsMTx-4 was not associated with a prevention of stretch-induced shortening of atrial ERP. While SAC block appears to be a novel and promising anti-arrhythmic approach to AF under conditions of elevated atrial pressure or volume, it may not be 'the one for all' solution. Besides, GsMTx-4 is not yet available in the quantities required for research in large animals.

Stretch has been shown to significantly decrease conduction velocity in myocardial tissue and to enhance spatial heterogeneity in conduction that may be related to the diverse anatomic and anisotropic properties of the atrial wall[27,28,34]. The pectinate muscle organization of atrial structure with thin membranes in between lends itself to be both a filling reservoir and a modest contractile apparatus. It is, however, not well suited for smooth electrical processes.

Effects of a possible protective effect of SAC block on dispersion of atrial ERP and conduction properties have not yet been investigated. This may be an important challenge for new drug development and will need to take into account the various forms and stages of substrate remodelling, including fibrosis in atrial myocardium in aging hearts.

References

1. Reiter MJ, Synhorst DP, Mann DE. Electrophysiological effects of acute ventricular dilatation in the isolated rabbit heart. *Circ Res* 1988;**62**: 554–562.

2. Calkins H, Maughan WL, Kass DA, Sagawa K, Levine JH. Electrophysiological effect of volume load in isolated canine hearts. *Am J Physiol* 1989;**256**:H1697–H1706.

3. Lerman BB, Burkhoff D, Yue DT, Franz MR, Sagawa K. Mechanoelectrical feedback: independent role of preload and contractility in modulation of canine ventricular excitability. *J Clin Invest* 1985;**76**:1843–1850.

4. Dean JW, Lab MJ. Effect of changes in load on monophasic action potential and segment length of pig heart in situ. *Cardiovasc Res* 1989;**23**:887–896.

5. Franz MR, Burkhoff D, Yue DT, Sagawa K. Mechanically induced action potential changes and arrhythmia in isolated and in situ canine hearts. *Cardiovasc Res* 1989;**23**:213–223.

6. Taggart P, Sutton PM, Treasure T, *et al*. Monophasic action potentials at discontinuation of cardiopulmonary bypass: evidence for contraction–excitation feedback in man. *Circulation* 1988;**77**: 1266–1275.

7. Levine JH, Guarnieri T, Kadish AH, White RI, Calkins H, Kan JS. Changes in myocardial repolarization in patients undergoing balloon valvuloplasty for congenital pulmonary stenosis: evidence for contraction–excitation feedback in humans. *Circulation* 1988;**77**: 70–77.

8. Dean JW, Lab MJ. Arrhythmia in heart failure: role of mechanically induced changes in electrophysiology. *Lancet* 1989;**1**:1309–1312.

9. Avitall B, Naimi S, Levine HJ. Prolongation of the conduction time of early premature beats: a marker of ventricular action potential duration. *Am Heart J* 1988;**116**:1247–1252.

10. Reiter MJ, Landers M, Zetelaki Z, Kirchhof CJ, Allessie MA. Electrophysiological effects of acute dilatation in the isolated rabbit heart: cycle length-dependent effects on ventricular refractoriness and conduction velocity. *Circulation* 1997;**96**:4050–4056.

11. Zabel M, Portnoy S, Franz MR. Effect of sustained load on dispersion of ventricular repolarization and conduction time in the isolated intact rabbit heart. *J Cardiovasc Electrophysiol* 1996;**7**:9–16.

12. Hansen DE, Borganelli M, Stacy G, Jr., Taylor LK. Dose-dependent inhibition of stretch-induced arrhythmias by gadolinium in isolated canine ventricles. Evidence for a unique mode of antiarrhythmic action. *Circ Res* 1991;**69**:820–831.

13. Franz MR, Cima R, Wang D, Profitt D, Kurz R. Electrophysiological effects of myocardial stretch and mechanical determinants of stretch-activated arrhythmias [published erratum appears in *Circulation* 1992;**86**:1663]. *Circulation* 1992;**86**:968–978.

14. Bode F, Franz MR, Wilke I, Bonnemeier H, Schunkert H, Wiegand UK. Ventricular fibrillation induced by stretch pulse: implications for sudden death due to *Commotio cordis*. *J Cardiovasc Electrophysiol* 2006;**17**:1011–1017.

15. Wijffels MC, Kirchhof CJ, Dorland R, Power J, Allessie MA. Electrical remodeling due to atrial fibrillation in chronically instrumented conscious goats: roles of neurohumoral changes, ischemia, atrial stretch, and high rate of electrical activation. *Circulation* 1997;**96**: 3710–3720.

16. Ravelli F, Disertori M, Cozzi F, Antolini R, Allessie MA. Ventricular beats induce variations in cycle length of rapid (type II) atrial flutter in humans. Evidence of leading circle reentry. *Circulation* 1994;**89**: 2107–2116.

17. Solti F, Szatmary L, Vecsey T, Szabolcs Z. Effect of the infusion of magnesium sulfate during atrial pacing on ECG intervals, serum electrolytes, and blood pressure. *Am Heart J* 1989;**117**:1278–1283.

18. Ravelli F, Allessie M. Effects of atrial dilatation on refractory period and vulnerability to atrial fibrillation in the isolated Langendorff-perfused rabbit heart. *Circulation* 1997;**96**:1686–1695.

19. Bode F, Katchman A, Woosley RL, Franz MR. Gadolinium decreases stretch-induced vulnerability to atrial fibrillation. *Circulation* 2000;**101**:2200–2205.

20. Bode F, Sachs F, Franz MR. Tarantula peptide inhibits atrial fibrillation. *Nature* 2001;**409**:35–36.

21. Kaseda S, Zipes DP. Contraction–excitation feedback in the atria: a cause of changes in refractoriness. *J Am Coll Cardiol* 1988;**11**: 1327–1336.

22. Satoh T, Zipes DP. Unequal atrial stretch in dogs increases dispersion of refractoriness conducive to developing atrial fibrillation. *J Cardiovasc Electrophysiol* 1996;**7**:833–842.

23. Ravelli F, Allessie M. Effects of atrial dilatation on refractory period and vulnerability to atrial fibrillation in the isolated Langendorff-perfused rabbit heart. *Circulation* 1997;**96**:1686–1695.

24. Lammers WJ, Kirchhof C, Bonke FI, Allessie MA. Vulnerability of rabbit atrium to reentry by hypoxia. Role of inhomogeneity in conduction and wavelength. *Am J Physiol* 1992;**262**: H47–H55.

25. Smeets JL, Allessie MA, Lammers WJ, Bonke FI, Hollen J. The wavelength of the cardiac impulse and reentrant arrhythmias in isolated rabbit atrium. The role of heart rate, autonomic transmitters, temperature, and potassium. *Circ Res* 1986;**58**:96–108.

26. Wijffels MC, Kirchhof CJ, Dorland R, Allessie MA. Atrial fibrillation begets atrial fibrillation. A study in awake chronically instrumented goats. *Circulation* 1995;**92**:1954–1968.

27. Eijsbouts SC, Majidi M, van Zandvoort M, Allessie MA. Effects of acute atrial dilation on heterogeneity in conduction in the isolated rabbit heart. *J Cardiovasc Electrophysiol* 2003;**14**:269–278.

28. Eijsbouts SC, Houben RP, Blaauw Y, Schotten U, Allessie MA. Synergistic action of atrial dilation and sodium channel blockade on conduction in rabbit atria. *J Cardiovasc Electrophysiol* 2004;**15**: 1453–1461.

29. Barold S, Shah D, Jais P, Takahashi A, Lamaison D, Haissaguerre M, Clementy J. Intermittent VA conduction block in junctional reentrant tachycardia: true or false? *Pacing Clin Electrophysiol* 1997;**20**: 2989–2991.

30. Kalifa J, Jalife J, Zaitsev AV, *et al*. Intra-atrial pressure increases rate and organization of waves emanating from the superior pulmonary veins during atrial fibrillation. *Circulation* 2003;**108**:668–671.

31. Tavi P, Laine M, Weckstrom M. Effect of gadolinium on stretch-induced changes in contraction and intracellularly recorded action- and afterpotentials of rat isolated atrium. *Br J Pharmacol* 1996;**118**:407–413.

32. Lacampagne A, Gannier F, Argibay J, Garnier D, Le Guennec JY. The stretch-activated ion channel blocker gadolinium also blocks L-type calcium channels in isolated ventricular myocytes of the guinea-pig. *Biochim Biophys Acta* 1994;**1191**:205–208.

33. Hu H, Sachs F. Mechanically activated currents in chick heart cells. *J Membr Biol* 1996;**154**:205–216.

34. Neuberger HR, Schotten U, Blaauw Y, Vollmann D, Eijsbouts S, van Hunnik A, Allessie M. Chronic atrial dilation, electrical remodeling, and atrial fibrillation in the goat. *J Am Coll Cardiol* 2006;**47**: 644–653.

Stretch effects on potassium accumulation and alternans in pathological myocardium

Christian Bollensdorff and Max J. Lab

Background

There is a pathophysiological enigma concerning the relationships between sudden arrhythmic death during myocardial pathology and the diversity of their cardiac correlates. Electrophysiological correlates include late potentials, dispersion in the QT segment duration of the electrocardiogram (ECG) and alternans, while mechanical/haemodynamic indices include ejection fraction and blood pressure. Non-linear dynamics ('chaos') and heart rate variability also provide indices, as do psychosocial factors and autonomic imbalance. Explanatory mechanisms in more focused experimental observations in regional ischaemia are also diverse, and include, beside imbalances of Ca^{2+} and $pH^{(1,2)}$, extracellular potassium $([K^+]_o)$ accumulation[3]. The latter is the focus of this chapter. The pathway as to how K^+ leaves the cell is still not completely understood, but there is evidence that the Na^+/K^+ pump[4,5] and the Na^+/Ca^{2+} and Na^+/H^+ exchangers[6–8] contribute (directly or indirectly) to an increase in $[K^+]_o$, as well as the adenosine triphosphate (ATP)-sensitive K^+ (K_{ATP}) channel[9].

A unified hypothesis, mechano-electric coupling (MEC), is emerging [see previous reviews[10,11] which cover mechanisms of MEC, including stretch activated channels[12]]. This chapter focuses on three characteristic observations and departs from familiar explanations contending that a major contributor is regional variation in cardiac load. The chapter refers to laboratory experiments detailed by Max Lab in the first edition of this book[13] and mainly centres on $[K^+]_o$, pathological amplification of MEC and alternans.

The question posed is: can the diverse electrophysiological factors relating to arrhythmias relate to mechano-electric mechanisms at the cellular level?

Brief methodology

Basic model and electrical measurements

Studies on MEC centre on heart preparations with a mechanical input (e.g. changes in length, force, pressure) that produce an electrophysiological change [e.g. membrane current, action potential (AP)].

This chapter draws on studies of intact heart during acute regional ischaemia and on simulated ischaemia in single isolated cardiomyocytes from guinea pig exposed to axial stretch under ATP depletion. This induces current through the K_{ATP} channel, as during ischaemic conditions.

In the whole heart experiments described here, large mammals were premedicated with ketamine or azaparone, deeply anaesthetized and their hearts exposed. For a detailed description see[13].

In brief, we measured end-diastolic epicardial segment length (coinciding with AP upstroke) and maximum length excursion (end-diastolic length minus the greatest deviation from this value; see Fig. 24.1 for instrumentation overview). In the healthy control area, this had a positive value, indicating tissue shortening during systole. In the ischaemic area, it was negative, indicating systolic lengthening. The integral of pressure and length for each beat gives an index of regional work. For measurement of $[K^+]_o$, a flexible PVC-valinomycin electrode [after[3]] was inserted mid-myocardially in the ischaemic region[3]; unwanted side effects of the device itself were excluded as described in[13].

Whole heart in vivo studies

For the $[K^+]_o$ study, after recording control regional electromechanical signals, a device for later regional restraint was applied to the affected area and pre-ischaemic signals recorded. On occlusion of a selected branch of the coronary artery, changes in $[K^+]_o$ and electromechanical signals were recorded. The area was reperfused to re-attain control values. The same area was then restrained and the protocol repeated [for detail see[13]].

To see if MEC amplified signals, the aorta was snared (with or without coronary occlusion).

For alternans, the pacing rate was increased to determine the pacing threshold for pulsus alternans. The selected coronary artery was ligated and 10–15 seconds of burst pacing applied at the cycle length required to produce alternans at 5 min intervals after the coronary tie, up to a total of 30 min.

Alternans was simulated by placing a pneumatically driven snare around the proximal aorta and activated on alternate beats during steady-state right atrial pacing to produce beat-to-beat fluctuations

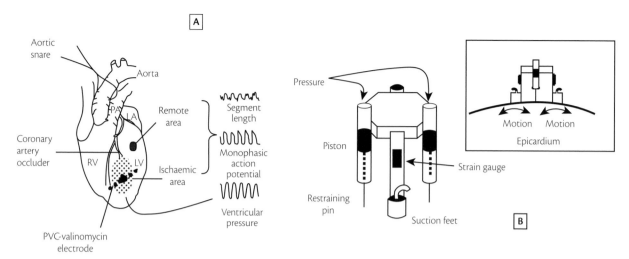

Fig. 24.1 Diagrams of whole heart *in vivo* experimental setup (**A**) and tripodal recording device with regions of measurements (**B**). Three faces of the hexagonal recording device platform have suction feet, which incorporate strain gauges to record motion when sucked onto the epicardium. One of the feet can record a monophasic action potential (MAP) or segment length from the left ventricular epicardium. The other three platform faces have pressure-operated pistons driving the restraining pins into the myocardium. (Inset: diagram of device on epicardium.)

in peak intraventricular pressure that are qualitatively similar to those seen during pacing-induced pulsus alternans.

Single cell study

Cardiomyocytes were enzymatically isolated from Langendorff perfused hearts of female guinea pigs and exposed to axial stretch using the two carbon fibre (CF) technique[15,16]. To provoke the K_{ATP} current ($I_{K, ATP}$), carbonyl cyanide p-(trifluoromethoxy) phenylhydrazone (FCCP) was used to uncouple oxidative phosphorylation in mitochondria, to reduce cytosolic ATP concentration $[ATP]_i$. At body temperature it takes about half a minute to lower $[ATP]_i$ before K_{ATP} channels open. The cells were exposed to axial stretch before and after $I_{K,ATP}$ increases[16].

MEC and $[K^+]_o$ in ischaemia

Can MEC provide an alternative mechanism for the well-known changes in the AP and accumulation of $[K^+]_o$ in ischaemic areas? Acute regional ischaemia raises regional $[K^+]_o$ with a defined time course, which contributes to arrhythmogenesis[14]. For example, the AP duration (APD) changes, which have been described in the present experimental model increase $[K^+]_o$[3]. This accumulation results from altered transport and/or a reduction in extracellular space. The precise mechanisms by which this accumulation occurs have yet to be finally elucidated. It seems that none of the currently proposed mechanisms for this accumulation, implicated in the genesis of lethal arrhythmia, seem entirely satisfactory. These mechanisms include partial inhibition of the Na^+/K^+ pump (an ATPase), cellular loss of anions as a consequence of intracellular metabolic acidification and opening of K_{ATP} channels[17].

The question posed in the previous edition of this book[13] was: does the regional dyskinesia (stretch during systole – 'bulging') observed in the acutely ischaemic area open mechano-sensitive channels to contribute to $[K^+]_o$ accumulation? To test this hypothesis, one has to use an experimental model in which regional ischaemia reliably produces dyskinesia (stretch during systole)[18], and then manipulate the model to test the hypothesis.

Results and discussion

In the whole heart *in vivo* studies, the device's pin insertion produced minimal myocardial damage and pressure/length loops were normal, inscribing an 'upright' roughly rectangular clockwise loop, with shortening during systole (active contraction). The restraining device, applied in diastole, reduced systolic shortening and reduced the inscribed area (Fig. 24.2A). In regional ischaemia it also reduced the passive (segment is non-contractile) systolic stretch – that is, the loops usually lean to the right and can go clockwise – not shown. In the presence of the restraining device, all observed loops were anticlockwise.

Acute regional ischaemia reduced APD in a time-dependent manner (e.g. Fig 24.3)[19]. Ten minutes of mechanically unrestrained ischaemia reduced the monophasic AP duration at 50% repolarization (MAPD50; Fig. 24.2B)). After reperfusion and recovery, mechanical restraints reduced this change in MAPD50 in a subsequent period of 10 min ischaemia.

Ischaemia with the affected area unrestrained produced clear dyskinetic myocardium, showing systolic bulging (loops clockwise)[19]. End-systolic length increased (Fig. 24.2C). Concomitantly, $[K^+]_o$ rose. After recovery, repeated transient ischaemia while mechanically restraining of the ischaemic tissue curtailed the increase in end-systolic length. With the restraint, $[K^+]_o$ increased less than with no restraint (Fig. 24.2C). Longer ischaemia (20 min) produced comparable results (not shown). All the above effects were fully reversible (on reperfusion and/or removal of restraint). Myocardial preconditioning may confound the interpretation of these results (for review see[20]; see also chapter 27). Preconditioning with a transient episode of ischaemia reduces damage from a second episode, so changes in the second episode of ischaemia may relate to preconditioning, not the presence of a mechanical restraint. However, in some experiments the restraint was applied during the first period of ischaemia, with no effect on the outcome.

One of the molecular targets of extracellular K+ accumulation, the K_{ATP} channel, opens during the early phase of ischaemia due to ATP depletion[3]. Interestingly, the set-point of ATP levels at

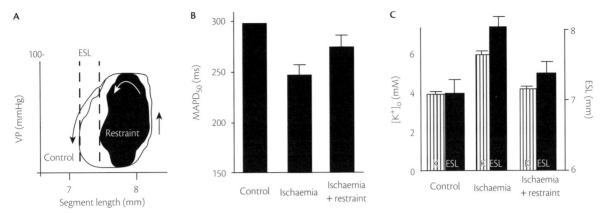

Fig. 24.2 Recorded and derived data from whole heart *in vivo* studies. **A** Pressure-segment length loops. **B** Bar chart showing monophasic action potential duration changes measured at 50% repolarization (MAPD$_{50}$) in control tissue, acute regional ischaemia, and ischaemia together with myocardial restrain. The latter curtailed the shortening of MAPD$_{50}$ found in unrestrained tissue. **C** Bar chart showing changes in [K$^+$]$_o$ (striped columns) and end-systolic segment length (ESL, black columns). Both rise in unrestrained ischaemia and this rise is curtailed by mechanically restraining the ischaemic area VP, Ventricular pressure.

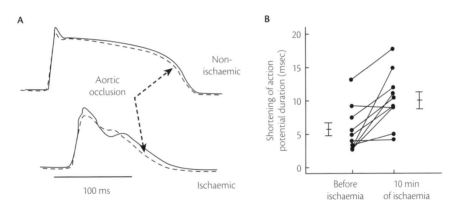

Fig. 24.3 Effects of aortic occlusion on action potential (AP) configuration, with and without ischaemia. **A** AP recordings: aortic occlusion reduced AP duration (dashed lines) in the control non-ischaemic situation (upper traces) and under ischaemic conditions (lower traces). However, the effect was greater during ischaemia as illustrated in **B**. [Modified, with permission, from Horner SM, Lab MJ, Murphy CF, Dick DJ, Zhou B, Harrison FG (1994) Mechanically induced changes in action potential duration and left ventricular segment length in acute regional ischaemia in the in situ porcine heart. *Cardiovasc Res* **28**:528–534.]

which K$_{ATP}$ channels open seems significantly lower when studied in mechanically unrestrained isolated cells compared to (always mechanically loaded) ventricular cardiomyocytes *in situ*. Measurements of the K$_{ATP}$ channel in isolated atrial cells have shown that their open probability (P$_o$) increases during mechanical stimulation[21]. If this was the case also for ventricular cells, it could explain some of the above discrepancy. In addition, it is well known that the K$_{ATP}$ channels show a fast rundown after activation[22], which should stop the K$^+$ efflux in the early phase of ischaemia. Figure 24.4 shows that axial stretch, applied to ventricular cardiomyocytes after the activation of K$_{ATP}$ channels by FCCP, during both early and descending phase (rundown of the current), increases I$_{K,ATP}$[16]. Due to the high numbers of K$_{ATP}$ channels in the sarcolemma, the mechanically induced increase in P$_o$ could significantly increase the K$^+$ efflux. At the same time, axial stretch before ATP depletion (i.e. when the K$_{ATP}$ channel is normally closed) does not increase I$_{K,ATP}$[16].

This points to a plausible explanation of the above *in vivo* data: stretch of the ischaemic area may contribute to opening of (stretch-sensitive) K$_{ATP}$ channels[23], increasing K$^+$ efflux. These results also point to a potential therapeutic avenue in ischaemic

arrhythmias, perhaps explaining how blockers of K$_{ATP}$ channels are antiarrhythmic[24].

Interestingly, clinical hypokalaemia can be arrhythmogenic[25] and, experimentally, low K$^+$ enhances mechanically induced arrhythmias, as reviewed elsewhere[10,11].

MEC, electrophysiology and regional ischaemia

Regional amplification of MEC

MEC, induced by aortic occlusion in the intact heart *in situ*, shortens APD during normal coronary perfusion (Fig. 24.5A, upper traces). During regional ischaemia, aortic occlusion also shortens the APD (Fig. 24.5A, lower traces). However, the net effect is enhanced, compared to control, particularly after 10 min of ischaemia (Fig. 24.5B). This difference varies over the first 30 min of ischaemia[19], with an initial increase peaking at 10 min and then decaying to virtually zero at 30 min. The enhanced contribution of MEC, compared with controls, is in keeping with other studies conducted in the context of heart failure [as reviewed in[10,11]].

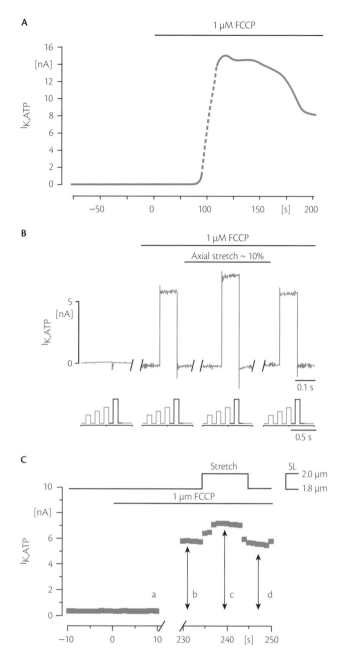

Fig. 24.4 Stretch-induced increase of $I_{K,ATP}$ in single ventricular cardiomyocytes from guinea pig. **A** Time course of whole-cell K_{ATP} current ($I_{K,ATP}$) before and after application of FCCP at body temperature (control measurement, without stretch). **B** Whole-cell $I_{K,ATP}$ raw data at 40 mV pulse, showing $I_{K,ATP}$ increase during stretch applied at the descending phase of $I_{K,ATP}$ (lower panel: voltage clamp protocol – depolarizing pulses from –80 mV to –40, –20, 0 and 40 mV'; only the 40 mV trace is shown). **C** Axial stretch applied after FCCP-induced activation of $I_{K,ATP}$. Metabolic uncoupling causes a significant increase in whole-cell $I_{K,ATP}$ (compare a and b), which is enhanced by axial stretch (c) in a fully reversible manner (d). [Modified, with permission, from Kohl P, Bollensdorff C, Garny A (2006) Effects of mechanosensitive ion channels on ventricular electrophysiology: experimental and theoretical models. *Exp Physiol* **91**:307–321.]

The increased expression of MEC corresponds in time with the occurrence of phase IA arrhythmias and with the increase in arrhythmias following acute regional ischaemia in this pig model[26].

Does ischaemia change the expression or sensitivity of MEC, or are the effects simply related to altered passive mechanical properties? Although there are compliance changes, their nature and time course are different from that of the APD changes seen, for example, in the experiments by Horner *et al.*[19]. There is an immediate decrease in stiffness with coronary occlusion, followed by a progressive monotonic stiffening over the next 2 h. At the same time, AP responses are biphasic, despite the systolic stretches in controls and the ischaemia being comparable. Thus, the variation in the expression of MEC cannot be easily attributed to changes in tissue mechanical properties.

The potentiating effects of ischemia on MEC could be explained by: (1) sympathetic stimulation which increases early in ischaemia[27] [β receptor antagonism can modulate load-induced changes in electrical restitution and arrhythmia, as reviewed in[10,11]]; (2) cell swelling, seen in acute ischaemia, which could activate mechano-sensitive channels [see Chapter 4 and ref[28]]; (3) changes in intracellular Ca^{2+} handling[29] (see also Chapters 10 and 21); or (4) changes in $[K^+]_o$, as described above.

The conduction velocity in ischaemic myocardium may be reduced, delaying activation and repolarization (Fig. 24.3A – compare timing of upstrokes). Nonetheless, ischaemic myocardium usually repolarizes before non-ischaemic myocardium, and this dispersion is pro-arrhythmic. The enhanced shortening of the ischaemic AP by MEC would increase electrical dispersion and this could be deleterious. In addition, APD and refractory period shorten heterogeneously in this preparation, and the decreased conduction velocity[10,11] promotes re-entry.

Heterogeneous alternans

Alternans describes alternate beat-to-beat changes in derived measures from the myocardium at a steady heart rate. It may be electrical, mechanical or both simultaneously. Electromechanical alternans may be discordant in the relationship between systolic pressure and APD (small pressure/long AP – e.g. Fig. 24.5A) or concordant (small pressure/short AP – e.g. Fig. 24.5B, middle panel). In addition, when comparing one region of the ventricular wall with another, alternans may be in phase (e.g. both regions big/small/big) or out of phase (e.g. one region big/small/big, the other small/big/small – see Fig. 24.5A,B). There is also beat-to-beat regional heterogeneity.

In the whole heart *in vivo* preparation, rapid atrial pacing of control hearts induced global pulsus alternans in all experiments, with a persistent discordant relationship (Fig. 24.5A). But regional ventricular wall motion shows a highly heterogeneous regional contraction pattern[30].

Acute regional ischaemia produced characteristic changes in the morphology of the MAP – reduction of APD (Figs 24.4A and 24.5B) and a failure of regional contraction, with systolic bulging or dyskinesia[14]. Pressure-length loops (cf. Fig. 24.2A), indices of regional work, were either reduced or showed 'negative' work (i.e. external work conducted 'on' the affected tissue). Instead of a clockwise loop, as in perfused myocardium (Fig. 24.2A), the loop was anticlockwise (not shown).

The control areas always showed a discordant relationship between peak systolic pressure and APD (Fig. 24.5A), while the ischaemic areas could initially display concordant alternans, but

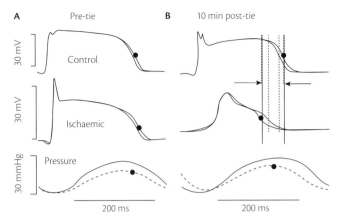

Fig. 24.5 Electromechanical relationship in whole heart *in situ* during alternans before and after regional ischaemia (upper traces: control areas remote from ischaemic area; middle traces: from ischaemic or denoted ischaemic area; lower traces: intraventricular pressures). **A** Before ischaemia (pre-tie) discordant electromechanical relationships are observed in both areas (longer AP with small pressure). **B** After ischaemia (post-tie). Control area still shows discordant electromechanical relationship (right vertical line), but ischaemic tissue now shows a concordant electromechanical relationship (left vertical line) (short AP with small pressure). [Modified, with permission, from Murphy CF, Lab MJ, Horner SM, Dick DJ, Harrison FG (1994) Regional electromechanical alternans in anesthetized pig hearts: modulation by mechanoelectric feedback. *Am J Physiol* **267**:H1726–H1735.]

after 10 min alternans became discordant (Fig. 24.5B). After 20 min the MAP degenerated or showed no alternans[31,32].

Simulating *pulsus alternans* using a pneumatically driven snare programmed to occlude the aorta on alternate beats (during steady-state pacing without evidence of alternans), faithfully simulated discordant alternans in control areas. Alternate beat occlusion produced an alternate shortening and lengthening of MAPD on clamped and unclamped beats respectively[30]. In the ischaemic areas, alternate beat occlusion produced either no discernable AP alternans or a concordant alternans that was out of phase with the simultaneous discordant alternans in the control area: a regional beat-to-beat dispersion of repolarization comparable to that found in spontaneous or pacing-induced alternans[31].

MEC and arrhythmic mechanisms

Electrophysiological heterogeneity

The results above show that MEC can induce electrophysiological heterogeneity (dispersion of repolarization, excitability/refractoriness). Dispersion of repolarization promotes abnormal current flow between areas of the myocardium that are at different membrane potentials. This current can initiate abnormal depolarizations, particularly in pathological hearts[33].

Spatial electrophysiological heterogeneity and re-entry are crucial aspects of arrhythmic pathology. The major factors involved in re-entry are reductions in conduction velocity and refractory period, and increased excitability. As reviewed earlier[10,11], mechanical events can induce changes in myocardial refractoriness and excitability, although some studies find less convincing data. The latter may be related to where the recordings were taken – heterogeneity of the expression of MEC. Fully activated (refractory)

cells recover full excitability over time, and this is termed electrical restitution. Changes in the restitution curve (supernormality and steepening) which could theoretically produce fibrillation (and chaos), and mechanical load can produce analogous changes via MEC[10,11].

Electrophysiological alternans

Electrophysiological alternans in experimental and clinical ischaemia[31,34,35] can precede ventricular fibrillation, and cardiac failure can modulate or produce electromechanical alternans[36]. Importantly, mechano-electric alternans, as demonstrated above, can be heterogeneous[30,32]. In this setting, MEC would be heterogeneous and potentially pro-arrhythmic.

Triggered after-depolarizations are a well-recognized way of producing arrhythmias. Mechanically induced after-depolarization-like events, which have been described in several preparations of myocardium and isolated cells, appear able to reach threshold to initiate premature beats.

Correlates between experimental MEC and clinical conditions

Many cardiac pathologies have both electrical and mechanical alterations as part of the syndrome. The conventional dogma is that the electric changes produce the load changes, or that some aetiological factors produce both. Table 24.1 shows that many of the experimental loading conditions producing electrophysiological changes have correlates in clinical conditions. This raises the possibility that the initiating cause of the electrical observation, at least in some of the clinical conditions, is the mechanical change.

Cell mechanisms

Is there some commonality between the well-established diverse aetiologies and mechanisms for arrhythmias? Stretch-activated channels, as reviewed by Hu and Sachs[12], appear to be a major mechanism for mechano-electric transduction. Stretch opens the channels, moving the membrane potential closer towards the relevant equilibrium potential. This alters the cell's electrophysiology. In addition, we[34] and others[37–39] have shown a form of MEC that involves myofibrils and intracellular calcium during systole (see also Chapter 16).

Changes in intracellular calcium may have a pivotal role in the generation of arrhythmias. This component of MEC was reviewed by White's group[40]. Importantly, calcium alternans features in both mechanical[41] and electrical alternans, and recent findings suggest that even ryanodine receptor channel opening may be mechanically modulated[42]. It is unquestionably the case, one way or another, that calcium changes contribute to the electrophysiological consequences of MEC.

MEC, clinical correlates and arrhythmia

The experiments described above fit within the context of arrhythmic mechanism, but do they have any context in patient populations? Possible candidates are summarized in Table 24.1. The clinical correlates that show possible consequences of MEC-related arrhythmic mechanisms are: a prolonged APD if, for example, a normal segment contracts against a weaker (say ischaemic) segment and shortens more, or in the case of the weaker stretched segment the AP (and refractory period) abbreviates. The stretched segment may

Table 24.1 MEC measures, interventions and clinical correlates. Overview of mechano-electrical interrelations observed in experimental and clinical conditions

Measures	MEC	Clinical correlation	Pathology/comment
Mechanical	Increased force/length alters electrophysiology	Dyskinesia, arrhythmia[43,44] – poor ejection	Patchy remodelling
Systemic load	Peripheral vasodilators, e.g. nitroprusside	Good for arrhythmia (ACE inhibitors)	Reduce wall stress/strain
	Aortic occlusion	Hypertension, aortic stenosis	Relate to arrhythmia
Electrophysiology	ME alternans in experimental ischaemia	Mechano-electric alternans in clinical ischaemia	Heralds VF
	Can produce EAD and U-wave.[45,46]	Abnormal U-wave[47] (also low K+)	EAD, arrhythmia
Autonomic – ANS	β agonists/blockers modify MEC[48–50]	β blockers reduce arrhythmic death	Load changes/ANS coexist
	Bretylium tosylate curtails ME arrhythmia[51]	Similarly bretilium tosylate (acute)	Depletes catecholamines
Hypokalaemia	Low K+ enhances MEC arrhythmia	Diuretic therapy andlow K+ are arrhythmogenic	Patients need K+ supplements
Chronic load	Stretch alters early genes and AP[52]	Chronic stretch, hypertrophy, remodelling	Mechano-electric heterogeneity

ACE, angiotensin-converting enzyme; ME, mechano-electric; EAD, early after-depolarization; VF, ventricular fibrillation; ANS, autonomic nervous system.

also trigger an after-depolarization and premature ventricular contractions. For more detail see[11,13] and Chapter 21.

In keeping with the observations reviewed and presented above, 'MEC begets MEC'. Pathological situations appear to amplify MEC, and one could predict an increased likelihood of mechanically induced arrhythmia in these situations.

Conclusions and outlook

It is beyond question that there are multiple contributors to arrhythmic mechanisms and their clinical correlates, including sudden arrhythmic death. However, the essence of the presented data proposes that many clinical and electrophysiological correlates of lethal arrhythmias may involve a causal contribution by MEC: that is, they are accompanied by pathological mechanical changes, which would produce or amplify electrical changes. At one extreme, this would be ischaemically induced dyskinesia or infarction, with gross mechano-electric dispersion. At the other end, remodelling, with very patchy MEC, could produce less uniform mechano-electric dispersion, but nonetheless a potentially grave one. Moreover, there is an extensive reach for interaction with other apparently unrelated clinical correlates, for example electrolyte and autonomic imbalances. The altered stress and strain could summon after-depolarizations, electrical dispersion, changes in wavelength and re-entry, all of which play a part in arrhythmic mechanisms. In addition, MEC, perhaps acting as a homeostatic feedback control system in the normal situation[10], is amplified in cardiac pathology. The feedback is now a destabilizing mechanism.

The tentative argument is that the common factor in many of the known arrhythmic mechanisms and clinical correlates, or risk factors in arrhythmic death, is a patchy but lethal expression of MEC. If this ultimately proves to be the case, it means that the philosophy behind current therapeutic targeting will have to be reappraised, concentrating on mechanical initiators and their downstream cell signalling consequences.

References

1. Shine KI. Myocardial ischemia: ionic events in ischemia and anoxia. *Am J Pathol* 1981;**102**:256–261.

2. Stamm C, Friehs I, Choi YH, Zurakowski D, McGowan FX, del Nido PJ. Cytosolic calcium in the ischemic rabbit heart: assessment by pH- and temperature-adjusted rhod-2 spectrofluorometry. *Cardiovasc Res* 2003;**59**:695–704.

3. Hill JL, Gettes LS. Effect of acute coronary artery occlusion on local myocardial extracellular K+ activity in swine. *Circulation* 1980;**61**: 768–778.

4. Egger M, Niggli E. Paradoxical block of the Na+-Ca2+ exchanger by extracellular protons in guinea-pig ventricular myocytes. *J Physiol* 2000;**523**:353–366.

5. Swift F, Tovsrud N, Enger UH, Sjaastad I, Sejersted OM. The Na+/K+-ATPase alpha2-isoform regulates cardiac contractility in rat cardiomyocytes. *Cardiovasc Res* 2007;**75**:109–117.

6. Dennis SC, Coetzee WA, Cragoe EJ, Jr., Opie LH. Effects of proton buffering and of amiloride derivatives on reperfusion arrhythmias in isolated rat hearts. Possible evidence for an arrhythmogenic role of Na+-H+ exchange. *Circ Res* 1990;**66**:1156–1159.

7. Karmazyn M, Gan XT, Humphreys RA, Yoshida H, Kusumoto K. The myocardial Na+-H+ exchange: structure, regulation, and its role in heart disease. *Circ Res* 1999;**85**:777–786.

8. Schaefer S, Ramasamy R. Short-term inhibition of the Na-H exchanger limits acidosis and reduces ischemic injury in the rat heart. *Cardiovasc Res* 1997;**34**:329–336.

9. Bollensdorff C, Knopp A, Biskup C, Zimmer T, Benndorf K. Na+ current through KATP channels: consequences for Na+ and K+ fluxes during early myocardial ischemia. *Am J Physiol* 2004;**286**: H283–H295.

10. Lab MJ. Mechanosensitivity as an integrative system in heart: an audit. *Prog Biophys Mol Biol* 1999;**71**:7–27.

11. Lab MJ. Mechanoelectric transduction/feedback: prevalence and pathophysiology. In: *Cardiac Electrophysiology from Cell to Bedside*, 4th edn, 2004; (eds DP Zipes, J Jalife). WB Saunders, Philadelphia, pp. 242–253.

12. Hu H, Sachs F. Stretch-activated ion channels in the heart. *J Mol Cell Cardiol* 1997;**29**:1511–1523.

13. Lab MJ. Regional stretch effects in pathological myocardium. In *Cardiac mechano-electric feedback and arrhythmias: from pipette to patient.* 2005 (eds P Kohl, F Sachs, MR Franz), Michael Franz, Elsevier, Philadelphia:108–118.

14. Kleber AG. Resting membrane potential, extracellular potassium activity, and intracellular sodium activity during acute global ischemia in isolated perfused guinea pig hearts. *Circ Res* 1983;**52**: 442–450.

15. Iribe G, Helmes M, Kohl P. Force-length relations in isolated intact cardiomyocytes subjected to dynamic changes in mechanical load. *Am J Physiol* 2007;**292**:H1487–H1497.

16. Kohl P, Bollensdorff C, Garny A. Effects of mechanosensitive ion channels on ventricular electrophysiology: experimental and theoretical models. *Exp Physiol* 2006;**91**:307–321.

17. Wilde AA, Escande D, Schumacher CA, *et al.* Potassium accumulation in the globally ischemic mammalian heart. A role for the ATP-sensitive potassium channel. *Circ Res* 1990;**67**:835–843.

18. Lab MJ, Woollard KV. Monophasic action potentials, electrocardiograms and mechanical performance in normal and ischaemic epicardial segments of the pig ventricle in situ. *Cardiovasc Res* 1978;**12**:555–565.

19. Horner SM, Lab MJ, Murphy CF, Dick DJ, Zhou B, Harrison FG. Mechanically induced changes in action potential duration and left ventricular segment length in acute regional ischaemia in the in situ porcine heart. *Cardiovasc Res* 1994;**28**:528–534.

20. Lawson CS, Downey JM. Preconditioning: state of the art myocardial protection. *Cardiovasc Res* 1993;**27**:542–550.

21. Van Wagoner DR. Mechanosensitive gating of atrial ATP-sensitive potassium channels. *Circ Res* 1993;**72**:973–83.

22. Takano M, Qin DY, Noma A. ATP-dependent decay and recovery of K^+ channels in guinea pig cardiac myocytes. *Am J Physiol* 1990;**258**: H45–H50.

23. Van Wagoner DR, Lamorgese M. Ischemia potentiates the mechanosensitive modulation of atrial ATP-sensitive potassium channels. *Ann N Y Acad Sci* 1994;**723**:392–395.

24. D'Alonzo AJ, Sewter JC, Darbenzio RB, Hess TA. Effects of cromakalim or glibenclamide on arrhythmias and dispersion of refractoriness in chronically infarcted in anesthetized dogs. *Naunyn Schmiedebergs Arch Pharmacol* 1995;**352**:222–228.

25. Podrid PJ. Potassium and ventricular arrhythmias. *Am J Cardiol* 1990;**65**:33E–44E; discussion 52E.

26. Dilly SG, Lab MJ. Changes in monophasic action potential duration during the first hour of regional myocardial ischaemia in the anaesthetised pig. *Cardiovasc Res* 1987;**21**:908–915.

27. Sakai K, Abiko Y. Acute changes of myocardial norepinephrine and glycogen phosphorylase in ischemic and non-ischemic areas after coronary ligation in dogs. *Jpn Circ J* 1981;**45**:1250–1255.

28. Clemo HF, Stambler BS, Baumgarten CM. Persistent activation of a swelling-activated cation current in ventricular myocytes from dogs with tachycardia-induced congestive heart failure. *Circ Res* 1998;**83**:147–157.

29. Steenbergen C, Murphy E, Levy L, London RE. Elevation in cytosolic free calcium concentration early in myocardial ischemia in perfused rat heart. *Circ Res* 1987;**60**:700–707.

30. Murphy CF, Lab MJ, Horner SM, Dick DJ, Harrison FG. Regional electromechanical alternans in anesthetized pig hearts: modulation by mechanoelectric feedback. *Am J Physiol* 1994;**267**:H1726–H1735.

31. Dilly SG, Lab MJ. Electrophysiological alternans and restitution during acute regional ischaemia in myocardium of anaesthetized pig. *J Physiol* 1988;**402**:315–333.

32. Murphy CF, Horner SM, Dick DJ, Coen B, Lab MJ. Electrical alternans and the onset of rate-induced pulsus alternans during acute regional ischaemia in the anaesthetised pig heart. *Cardiovasc Res* 1996;**32**: 138–147.

33. Janse MJ, van Capelle FJ, Morsink H, *et al.* Flow of 'injury' current and patterns of excitation during early ventricular arrhythmias in acute regional myocardial ischemia in isolated porcine and canine hearts. Evidence for two different arrhythmogenic mechanisms. *Circ Res* 1980;**47**:151–165.

34. Janse MJ, Kleber AG, Capucci A, Coronel R, Wilms-Schopman F. Electrophysiological basis for arrhythmias caused by acute ischemia. Role of the subendocardium. *J Mol Cell Cardiol* 1986;**18**:339–355.

35. Rosenbaum DS, Jackson LE, Smith JM, Garan H, Ruskin JN, Cohen RJ. Electrical alternans and vulnerability to ventricular arrhythmias. *N Engl J Med* 1994;**330**:235–241.

36. Cannon RO, 3rd, Schenke WH, Bonow RO, Leon MB, Rosing DR. Left ventricular pulsus alternans in patients with hypertrophic cardiomyopathy and severe obstruction to left ventricular outflow. *Circulation* 1986;**73**:276–285.

37. Tavi P, Han C, Weckstrom M. Mechanisms of stretch-induced changes in $[Ca^{2+}]i$ in rat atrial myocytes: role of increased troponin C affinity and stretch-activated ion channels. *Circ Res* 1998;**83**:1165–1177.

38. ter Keurs HE, Shinozaki T, Zhang YM, Zhang ML, Wakayama Y, Sugai Y, *et al.* Sarcomere mechanics in uniform and non-uniform cardiac muscle: a link between pump function and arrhythmias. *Prog Biophys Mol Biol* 2008;**97**:312–331.

39. Wakayama Y, Miura M, Sugai Y, *et al.* Stretch and quick release of rat cardiac trabeculae accelerates Ca^{2+} waves and triggered propagated contractions. *Am J Physiol* 2001;**281**:H2133–H2142.

40. Calaghan SC, White E. The role of calcium in the response of cardiac muscle to stretch. *Prog Biophys Mol Biol* 1999;**71**:59–90.

41. Lab MJ, Lee JA. Changes in intracellular calcium during mechanical alternans in isolated ferret ventricular muscle. *Circ Res* 1990;**66**: 585–595.

42. Iribe G, Ward CW, Camelliti P, *et al.* Axial stretch of rat single ventricular cardiomyocytes causes an acute and transient increase in Ca^{2+} spark rate. *Circ Res* 2009;**104**:787–795.

43. Perticone F, Ceravolo R, Maio R, Cosco C, Giancotti F, Mattioli PL. [Mechano-electric feedback and ventricular arrhythmias in heart failure. The possible role of permanent cardiac stimulation in preventing ventricular tachycardia]. *Cardiologia* 1993;**38**: 247–252.

44. Siogas K, Pappas S, Graekas G, Goudevenos J, Liapi G, Sideris DA. Segmental wall motion abnormalities alter vulnerability to ventricular ectopic beats associated with acute increases in aortic pressure in patients with underlying coronary artery disease. *Heart* 1998;**79**: 268–273.

45. Choo MH, Gibson DG. U waves in ventricular hypertrophy: possible demonstration of mechano-electrical feedback. *Br Heart J* 1986;**55**: 428–433.

46. Lepeschkin E. Role of myocardial temperature; electrolyte and stress gradients in the genesis of the normal T-wave. In: *Advances in Electrocardiography* 1976 (eds RC Schlant, JW Hurst); Grune + Stratton.

47. el-Sherif N, Bekheit SS, Henkin R. Quinidine-induced long QTU interval and torsade de pointes: role of bradycardia-dependent early afterdepolarizations. *J Am Coll Cardiol* 1989;**14**: 252–257.

48. Horner SM, Murphy CF, Coen B, Dick DJ, Lab MJ. Sympathomimetic modulation of load-dependent changes in the action potential duration in the in situ porcine heart. *Cardiovasc Res* 1996;**32**:148–157.

49. Lab MJ, Dick D, Harrison FG. Propranolol reduces stretch arrhythmia in isolated rabbit heart. *J Physiol* 1992;**446**:P538–P538.

50. Lab MJ. Contraction-excitation feedback in myocardium. Physiological basis and clinical relevance. *Circ Res* 1982;**50**:757–766.

51. Dick DJ, Lab MJ, Harrison FG, Green S, Gruber PC. Cardiac and smooth muscle: a possible role of endogenous catecholamines in stretch induced premature ventricular beats in the isolated rabbit heart. *J Physiol* 1994;**479**:133P.

52. Meghji P, Nazir SA, Dick DJ, Bailey ME, Johnson KJ, Lab MJ. Regional workload induced changes in electrophysiology and immediate early gene expression in intact in situ porcine heart. *J Mol Cell Cardiol* 1997;**29**:3147–3155.

The effects of wall stretch on ventricular conduction and refractoriness in the whole heart

Robert W. Mills, Adam T. Wright, Sanjiv M. Narayan and Andrew D. McCulloch

Background

Many studies have linked volume overload or increased myocardial strain (wall stretch) with atrial and ventricular arrhythmias[1]. Although the mechanisms for these mechanical load-induced rhythm disturbances remain unclear, they generally involve either triggered activity or re-entrant conduction[2]. Though both of these mechanisms may contribute, re-entry is the predominant mechanism underlying ventricular arrhythmias associated with mechanical dysfunction[3]. Stability of a re-entrant circuit depends on the constant presence of excitable tissue ahead of the activation wavefront. Slowed conduction and decreased refractoriness can therefore promote and sustain re-entry, while increased dispersion of conduction velocity and refractoriness can provide a substrate for its initiation[4]. Observations on the acute effects of myocardial strain on conduction velocity have varied widely with experimental preparation, mechanical loading conditions and measurement techniques, while findings on the stretch-dependence of effective refractory period have been somewhat more consistent. Given the inherent difficulties in measuring regional myocardial mechanics and conduction velocity in the whole heart without disturbing mechanical or electrical properties, many of the discrepancies between experimental reports are probably attributable to differences in experimental methods or definitions.

The effects of myocardial stretch on conduction velocity

Factors influencing speed and path of conduction

Intracellular conduction is determined by passive membrane capacitance, longitudinal resistances and voltage-dependent membrane conductances[5]. Membrane capacitance is a function of the dielectric properties of the membrane and the membrane surface area to cell volume ratio. Increasing membrane capacitance slows the initial depolarization from resting potential to threshold and reduces conduction velocity. Intracellular and extracellular longitudinal resistances determine how rapidly ions travel in the direction of conduction, and are affected by the effective internal and external cross-sectional areas available for ion transport.

The voltage-gated fast sodium current usually determines how rapidly the local membrane depolarizes (action potential phase 0), creating the electrochemical gradient that drives longitudinal ion diffusion. The conductance of these channels is influenced by channel kinetics and other regulatory processes, such as ligand gating and autonomic stimulation[6]. Altering resting membrane potential influences conduction speed in a biphasic manner[7]. Model studies suggest that this effect acts through membrane excitability[8], as depolarization of the resting membrane potential decreases the charge required to reach threshold, but increases sodium channel inactivation, decreasing conduction velocity.

Intercellular conduction is primarily regulated by the conductance of gap junction. Gap junction open probability is sensitive to ischaemia, pH, intracellular cation concentrations and transjunctional voltage[9]. Activation wavefront curvature also affects propagation speed; a convex wavefront must stimulate an expanding volume of resting tissue, imposing a greater electrical load and slowing conduction[10].

The path of conduction through the myocardium is a function of gap junction distributions, myocyte branching, fibre angle dispersion, the laminar sheet organization of the myofibres and the presence of connective tissue septa within the interstitium. The direction of fastest propagation follows the myocardial fibre direction due to the distribution of gap junctions within the cell[9], with fibre conduction speed typically being two- to tenfold faster than the cross-fibre direction. Within the ventricle, fibre angles follow a left-handed helix in the epicardium and smoothly transition to a right-handed helix in the endocardium. Therefore, as activation spreads transmurally the principal axis of fastest in-plane propagation rotates and the wave front changes shape. Transverse to the fibre direction, cardiomyocytes are stacked into branching laminar sheets about 4–6 cells thick surrounded by a perimysial collagen fascia. A model reconstruction of tissue microarchitecture showed that this organization results in conduction across the sheet planes being slowed by 40% compared with cross-fibre conduction within the sheets[11].

Determinants of regional wall stress and strain

Myocardium and single myocytes are viscoelastic at rest, with a time constant for stress relaxation of about 1,000 s, and exhibit mechanical preconditioning behaviour and strain softening during repeated loading cycles[12]. Myofilament activation also causes stress and strain to vary phasically throughout the cardiac cycle[13]. In studies of the effects of mechano-electric feedback on conduction velocity in the normal heart, diastolic mechanics are the most important determinant as electrical activation precedes systolic contraction, but may be influenced by myofilament interactions when relaxation is incomplete at high heart rates. At lower heart rates, afterload alterations have little direct influence on conduction velocity, but may significantly affect repolarization and refractoriness. Finally, cardiac geometry and fibre architecture results in significant mechanical anisotropy and heterogeneity[13]. Changes in conduction path are determined by strain, but whether cellular responses are determined primarily by stress or strain depends fundamentally on the relative compliance of the molecular mechanotransducer, such as a stretch-activated ion channel.

Measuring conduction velocity during myocardial stretch

Conduction velocity in one direction is usually calculated as the distance between recording electrodes aligned perpendicular to the wavepath divided by the interelectrode conduction time. In this case, the distance between recording sites and the number of myocytes per unit physical length can change during loading. Therefore, conduction velocity has been defined with both a spatial and material reference. Spatial conduction velocity is defined with a constant interelectrode distance before and during stretch. Material conduction velocity is defined between the same two physical points on the myocardium; thus material conduction velocity describes mechano-electric coupling effects over a constant segment of tissue.

However, to account for potential changes in conduction path with stretch in studies of two- or three-dimensional conduction, a highly resolved spatial description is most appropriate. In practice, to determine the two-dimensional conduction direction, the conduction time is sampled from an array of positions, and the gradients of activation time are used to calculate local conduction velocities[14]. High spatial resolution sampling is achieved using contact electrode arrays or high speed optical mapping of action potential propagation with a fluorescent voltage-sensitive dye. An advantage of optical mapping being that it is non-contact, diminishing the chance of mechanical artifacts during measurement.

Effects of stretch on conduction velocity in the heart

Early investigations into the effects of myocardial stretch on conduction speed were limited to one-dimensional propagation. In studies of ventricular and atrial strips of myocardium from various species, stretching from slack length to the length of maximal developed tension caused a proportionate increase in spatial conduction velocity while material conduction velocity remained nearly unchanged, but additional stretch caused slowing of both measures[15]. A similar biphasic relationship between spatial conduction velocity and stretch has been observed in more recent studies in isolated rabbit papillary muscle[16]. Faster spatial conduction during stretch was also observed in sheep Purkinje fibres[17,18]. In canine Purkinje fibres, both spatial and material conduction velocity initially increased with stretch and then decreased, but conduction in cat trabeculae was not similarly affected[19]. Conversely, spatial conduction velocity in rat papillary muscle decreased with stretch, while papillary muscle from several other species showed no effect[20]. Despite the varied effects of stretch across different structures, tissue types and species, most of these studies imply that conduction velocity may increase with stretch. However, these studies mostly concentrated on specialized structures, and after being excised these tissues were not subject to the same multiaxial constraints as in vivo.

Other studies have focused on the effect of physiological loading on whole chamber activation times. In the dog heart in vivo, QRS duration correlated with acute increases in left ventricular pressure[21], while left atrial dilation increased atrial activation time[22], and ventricular volume inflation in isolated rabbit hearts increased maximal activation times[23]. In contrast, one study of volume load in canine ventricle in vivo reported no change in spatial conduction time[24], while cellular conduction velocity increased during volume load of rat atrium[25]. These whole chamber studies indicate that stretch slows material conduction; however, they do not directly compare measures of conduction speed or path.

More recent studies have investigated the effects of stretch on two-dimensional epicardial surface conduction using electrode arrays, in order to directly study the path of propagation. In volume-loaded left ventricle of isolated rabbit hearts after ventricular cryoablation of all but a thin epicardial layer, neither graded load nor changes in pacing cycle length significantly alter fibre or cross-fibre conduction velocities[26]. The authors acknowledged that the cryoablation procedure stiffened the ventricle, possibly protecting the viable layer from mechanical stimulus. Conversely, studies in the isolated rabbit atria displayed decreased spatial conduction velocity[27,28] as well as increased dispersion of conduction velocity, altered direction of propagation and increased occurrence of local conduction block[28] during myocardial stretch.

Sung et al.[29] used non-contact optical mapping during left ventricular volume loading in isolated rabbit heart, and employed a model-based analysis technique[30] that accounted for epicardial curvature and changes in conduction path and allowed comparison of conduction velocity with local fibre direction. An increase of intraventricular pressure from 0 to 30 mmHg resulted in heterogeneous epicardial fibre and cross-fibre strains on the order of 3% and 1.5%, respectively, and a 16% decrease in transverse spatial conduction velocity[29]. Figure 25.1 shows an example of the increase in activation times due to ventricular volume loading and the resulting velocity vector field. It also illustrates that application

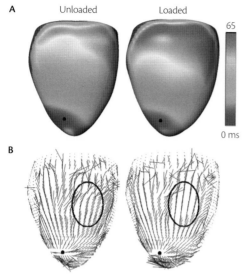

Fig. 25.1 Activation time fields (**A**) and conduction velocity vector fields (**B**) before and during application of 30 mmHg ventricular volume load in isolated rabbit heart, using methods from Sung and colleagues[29]. The small solid circle indicates the approximate position of pacing. The circled areas outline a region in which the apparent direction of conduction has been changed by application of load. (See color plate section.)

of stretch can alter the path of conduction. Conduction velocity returned to baseline when load was removed. Similar results were obtained by our group in a more recent study in the isolated rabbit ventricle[31]. Additionally, we see comparable conduction slowing in the freely beating isolated mouse heart during pressure loading of the left ventricle. In an alternative preparation, optical mapping revealed a 7.5% slowing of conduction velocity in monolayers of neonatal rat ventricular cardiomyocytes cultured on an elastic membrane during stretch[32] (see Chapter 20 for more details on mechano-electric coupling in cell cultures). These two-dimensional studies that also include changes in conduction path more consistently show conduction slowing due to stretch.

Potential interactions of stretch with factors that influence conduction velocity

Myocardial stretch may affect conduction speed in a number of ways. Stretch has been reported to depolarize the resting membrane potential[33], and this may be sufficient to slow conduction through fast sodium channel inactivation. Inward current through cation non-selective stretch-activated channels (SAC_{NS}) may depolarize the resting membrane during stretch. Several of the effects of mechano-electric coupling in myocardial preparations have been seen to be blocked by non-specific inhibitors of SAC_{NS}, including gadolinium inhibition of increased cellular conduction velocity during stretch in rat atria[25], and reduction of peak conduction velocity increase in stretched papillary muscle by streptomycin[34]. However, Mills and colleagues found that conduction slowing during ventricular filling was likely not due to changes in excitability and not attenuated in the presence of gadolinium[31] or streptomycin[29]. Sustained stretch may also increase resting membrane potential through altered cellular calcium handling[35]. Myofilament binding sensitivity to calcium increases with stretch, and prolonged

stretch results in a slow increase in the calcium transient, which subsequently interacts with other currents. However, increased resting potential should lower pacing threshold, but ventricular filling has been reported to have no effect on[23,36] or to increase threshold[26]. SAC_{NS}, altered calcium handling or stretch-sensitive cellular signalling could also regulate the conductances associated with phase 0 of the action potential, thus decreasing the maximum rate of rise of membrane potential[6].

Alternatively, stretch may result in changes in tissue and cell geometry, changing path of conduction or altering distributed electrical properties of the myocardium. Penefsky and Hoffman[15] postulated that increased one-dimensional spatial conduction velocity was the result of increased fibre alignment during stretch. Rosen et al.[19] observed that stretch caused significant membrane unfolding, decreased cell diameter and slightly increased packing of the extracellular space. Unfolding of 'slack' membrane and integration of caveolae to the surface sarcolemma has also been observed in the loaded intact rabbit ventricle in a more recent study[37]. Cell stretch would result in an increased surface area to volume ratio and a reduced cell cross-sectional area, increasing the effective longitudinal intracellular resistance. Others suggested stretch might result in a decrease in specific membrane capacitance (capacitance/area)[17,18], possibly due to membrane unfolding, accounting for increased spatial conduction velocity during moderate stretch. However, recent data indicate that increased membrane tension results in an increase in capacitance[38].

Myocardial stretch might also alter conduction through changes in intercellular coupling. Gap junction permeability is regulated by several factors that might be regulated by stretch, including intracellular cation concentrations and cell signalling pathways (primarily through connexin phosphorylation)[9]. Additionally, it has been demonstrated that connexin hemichannel permeability is sensitive to both shear strain[39] and membrane stretch[40], so mechanical forces at cell–cell junctions might directly affect gap junction conductance. However, it has been shown that rate of propagation is not very sensitive to changes in intercellular conductance at normal levels of cellular coupling[41].

Mills et al. implemented a bidomain model analysis of the membrane potential response to a non-excitatory stimulus to investigate changes in these myocardial electrical properties during ventricular volume loading[31]. The results suggested that wall stretch resulted in a 21% increase in cross-fibre space constant, indicating reduced intercellular resistance that would increase conduction velocity, and a 56% increase in membrane capacitance, which would slow conduction (Fig. 25.2). Computational simulations implementing these counteracting changes were consistent with experimental findings of a 15% slowing of conduction during ventricular loading. This explanation of stretch-induced changes in conduction velocity might account for the varying results obtained in different experimental preparations if the interaction between these two changes in tissue electrical properties varies in different tissue preparations and loading conditions. Further studies are required to investigate the cellular mechanisms behind these changes in passive electrical properties of the myocardium and the resulting change in conduction velocity. Development of similar experimental techniques in the isolated mouse heart provides a platform to conduct such studies, taking advantage of the availability of genetically modified murine models.

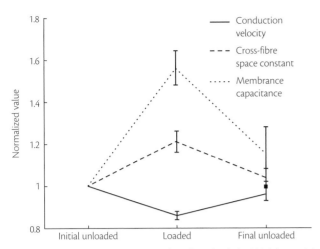

Fig. 25.2 Conduction velocity slowing in the volume loaded rabbit left ventricle is associated with an increase in space constant and an increase in membrane capacitance, as observed by Mills and colleagues[31]. Space constant and capacitance were measured with a bidomain model analysis of the potential response to a non-excitatory point stimulus. Values returned to baseline when load was removed. All values are normalized by initial unloaded values.

Summary

Conduction speed is functionally dependent on the distribution of heterogeneous properties including membrane excitability and cellular coupling, as well as activation wavefront curvature, while conduction path is functionally dependent upon regionally heterogeneous cellular and myocardial architectures. Evidence suggests that stretch effects on conduction speed are variable in various cardiac tissue types, but more consistently results in slowed conduction in the intact heart. Conduction could be slowed due to decreased excitability through SAC_{NS} activation or length-dependent calcium handling, but investigations implementing SAC_{NS} blockers have been inconsistent. Altered conduction velocity may also be due to simple geometric and structural changes, membrane unfolding and altered intercellular coupling.

The effect of myocardial stretch on effective refractory period

Determinants and measurement of effective refractory period

Effective refractory period (ERP) is the time interval following activation during which tissue is unable to activate again in response to the same stimulus, and thus is a measure of late-repolarization membrane excitability. ERP is determined by the voltage-regulated transition of fast sodium channels from the inactivated to the resting state, and is thus dependent on the time course of repolarization. Consequently, ERP is closely related to action potential duration (APD) and is also cycle-length dependent. One study observed that the ratio of ERP to monophasic APD at 90% repolarization (APD_{90}) remains nearly constant despite a 60% decrease in APD as cycle length decreases[36].

ERP is typically measured after continuous pacing at a single cycle length to minimize dynamic variations in APD and other cellular kinetics. After this stabilization period, a stimulus is delivered at a shortened time delay (coupling interval). ERP is typically defined as the longest possible coupling interval that does not elicit a propagating action potential. Experimentally, action potentials are recorded directly with microelectrodes using a contact monophasic action potential electrode, or optically with a potentiometric fluorescent probe.

Effects of stretch on effective refractory period in whole heart

A number of studies have investigated the effect of stretch on ERP and APD in the atria. *In vivo* studies have had varied results, primarily attributed to differences in timing and duration of stretch, as seen in model studies[42]. In isolated preparations, ERP more consistently decreases with acute myocardial stretch[27,43–46], but insignificantly increased in the isolated canine right atrium[47]. Despite these variations, studies have consistently shown that acute atrial stretch increases the dispersion of effective refractory periods (mechano-electric coupling in the atria is covered more thoroughly in Chapter 23 and in the review by Ravelli[4]).

Studies on the effects of stretch on ventricular ERP have been more consistent across different species and experimental methods. In swine heart *in vivo*, an increase in afterload caused a greater decrease in ERP at the apex than the base, thus increasing dispersion of refractoriness[48]. Similarly, left ventricular loading in isolated rabbit[23,49] and guinea pig[50] hearts also decreased ERP. Increased preload decreased ERP in a manner that correlated better with increased diastolic wall stress, as estimated from end diastolic pressure and ventricular geometry, than with increased systolic wall stress or diastolic circumference. Dilation also shortened ERP more significantly on the endocardial than epicardial surface[36]. This indicates that ERP may correlate better with cross-fibre than fibre stress or strain, since myocardial residual stress and torsion during filling allow a more uniform transmural distribution of fibre strain[13] under load at the expense of cross-fibre strain gradients.

In rabbit, ventricular stretch caused by increasing preload also caused greater shortening of ERP as the drive cycle length decreased[26]. This finding was later corroborated in isovolumically contracting rabbit ventricles[36]. Reiter *et al.*[26] suggest that this rate dependency may follow dependency on the stretch-sensitive delayed rectifier potassium current.

Those studies that also examined the effect of stretch on APD observed that mechano-electric feedback on late APD (typically analyzing APD_{90}) reflected the observed effects on ERP, decreasing with stretch in the ventricles[23,36,48,50], and did not alter the ratio of ERP to late APD[36]. Several other studies have reported a decrease in late APD with stretch in various species including lamb, swine, guinea pig, rabbit, rat and human. However, some investigators report an increase in APD during stretch, primarily at late repolarization levels. Volume loading of the isolated rabbit ventricle caused an increase in both APD_{20} and APD_{80} (APD at 20% and 80% repolarization, respectively), suggesting ERP may increase with stretch[29]. Left ventricular APD_{90} increased during loading of the *in situ* canine heart[24] and the isolated rat heart[51]. Chen *et al.* reported a regional decrease in APD_{25}, APD_{50} and APD_{70} (APD at 25%, 50% and 70% repolarization, respectively) with increased local sarcomere length in the loaded right ventricle of sheep, but heterogeneously increased APD_{90} and incidence of early after-depolarizations[52]. Similarly, several studies by Franz and colleagues also observe late APD lengthening in canine and rabbit, but see shortening at earlier levels of recovery[33]. Franz suggests that depending on the stimulus strength used, mechano-electric feedback on ERP may simply reflect changes in APD at varying levels; thus ERP could shorten during stretch reflecting shortening of early APD or lengthen with late APD (the effect of stretch on APD is covered in more detail in Chapter 37.)

Potential interactions of stretch with factors that influence effective refractory period

SAC_{NS} and altered calcium handling have both been implicated in stretch-induced APD shortening[4], and consequently could influence ERP. Model studies indicate that the effect of stretch can have various influences on action potential shape depending on the relative contributions of SAC_{NS} and calcium handling, both of which are sensitive to timing and intensity of stretch[42,53]. Zabel et al.[53] showed that including a length-dependent non-specific cationic conductance with a reversal potential near −30 mV could reproduce several experimental observations including early APD shortening and late APD lengthening during stretch, while Kohl et al.[42] showed that a more moderate stretch can lead to an overall shortening of APD. Kohl further showed that stretch in a model that included sarcomere length-dependent calcium handling would produce an overall prolongation of APD if applied early or sustained throughout the action potential, but an overall shortening if applied during late repolarization.

Investigations into the mechanisms of stretch-induced ERP shortening by pharmacological interventions have yielded inconsistent results. The non-specific SAC_{NS} blockers streptomycin and gadolinium attenuated[31] or had a limited effect[36,51] on acute stretch-induced changes in ERP and APD in some studies, but had no effect in others[29,50,54]. The more specific SAC_{NS} blocker GsMtx-4 did not block stretch-induced shortening of rabbit atrial ERP[45]. This may be due to resistance of the potassium-selective SAC_{NS} to these compounds, or conductance changes of other mechano-sensitive channels during load. Zarse et al.[44] found that the L-type calcium channel blocker verapamil inhibited stretch-induced shortening of atrial ERP, suggesting the contribution of a length-dependent calcium handling mechanism[35], but others have observed no effect of verapamil on guinea pig[50] and rabbit[36] ventricular ERP shortening.

Increased dispersion of effective refractory period with stretch may follow inhomogeneous stress or strain distributions. A ventricular model study that coupled physiological fibre and cross-fibre strains to a stretch-dependent current within an action potential model predicted a near doubling of the dispersion of late APD[55]. Finally, changes in electrotonic coupling could alter heterogeneity of repolarization in the myocardium, so changes in tissue architecture and gap junction conductivities may play a role in these arrhythmogenic effects of stretch on ERP.

Summary

Increased preload, afterload or sustained load typically decrease ERP; however, ERP follows APD, and some have observed APD prolongation at all levels of recovery. How stretch affects ERP is likely a result of the balance of several competing effects including SAC_{NS}, altered calcium handling and the timing and intensity of stretch, which could have varying levels of activation in different species and manners of stretch.

Conclusions and outlook

Recent evidence provides a basis to explain why stretch is associated with arrhythmias, particularly re-entrant forms. Both atrial and ventricular stretch slow spatial conduction, while atrial stretch increases conduction velocity dispersion and increases the occurrence of local functional conduction block, all of which promote re-entrant arrhythmias. These stretch effects may correlate with the application of diastolic mechanical load, but correlation with stress or strain is less clear owing to regionally heterogeneous cardiac geometry, structure and time-dependent material properties. Stretch may affect conduction velocity through altered effective cellular coupling, tissue and cellular level geometric changes, changes in intracellular resistance and membrane capacitance or alterations in excitability, particularly an increase in resting membrane potential due to the activity of SAC_{NS} or altered calcium handling.

In general, both atrial and ventricular stretch decrease ERP, but stretch consistently increases dispersion of ERP, both of which are associated with increased incidence of re-entrant arrhythmias. The effects of stretch on refractoriness parallel effects on APD, which may vary as a function of the relative activation of competing mechanisms, SAC_{NS} and altered calcium handling. Future studies should aim to identify the exact underlying cellular mechanisms responsible for these arrhythmogenic stretch-induced changes in conduction velocity and refractoriness. New experimental techniques and development of genetically modified animal models can provide a platform for these investigations in hopes of identifying potential therapeutic targets to prevent arrhythmias associated with mechanical dysfunction.

Acknowledgements

The authors acknowledge the research support of the National Science Foundation (BES-0086482), the National Institutes of Health (RR08605), the National Space Biomedical Research Institute (CA00216) and the American Heart Association (02651208Y).

References

1. Stevenson WG, Stevenson LW. Prevention of sudden death in heart failure. *J Cardiovasc Electrophysiol* 2001;**12**:112–114.
2. Taggart P, Sutton PM. Cardiac mechano-electric feedback in man: clinical relevance. *Prog Biophys Mol Biol* 1999;**71**:139–154.
3. Kuo CS, Munakata K, Reddy CP, Surawicz B. Characteristics and possible mechanism of ventricular arrhythmia dependent on the dispersion of action potential durations. *Circulation* 1983;**67**: 1356–1367.
4. Ravelli F. Mechano-electric feedback and atrial fibrillation. *Prog Biophys Mol Biol* 2003;**82**:137–149.
5. Kootsey JM (1991) Electrical propagation in distributed cardiac tissue. In: *Theory of Heart: Biomechanics, Biophysics, and Nonlinear Dynamics of Cardiac Function* (eds L Glass, P Hunter, AD McCulloch). Springer, New York, pp. 391–403.
6. Roden DM, Balser JR, George AL, Jr., Anderson ME. Cardiac ion channels. *Annu Rev Physiol* 2002;**64**: 431–475.
7. Rohr S, Kucera JP, Kleber AG. Slow conduction in cardiac tissue, I: effects of a reduction of excitability versus a reduction of electrical coupling on microconduction. *Circ Res* 1998;**83**:781–794.

8. Nygren A, Giles WR. Mathematical simulation of slowing of cardiac conduction velocity by elevated extracellular [K+] in a human atrial strand. *Ann Biomed Eng* 2000;**28**:951–957.

9. Dhein S (1998). Cardiac Gap Junctions, Karger, New York

10. Cabo C, Pertsov AM, Baxter WT, Davidenko JM, Gray RA, Jalife J. Wave-front curvature as a cause of slow conduction and block in isolated cardiac muscle. *Circ Res* 1994;**75**:1014–1028.

11. Hooks DA, Tomlinson KA, Marsden SG, et al. Cardiac microstructure: implications for electrical propagation and defibrillation in the heart. *Circ Res* 2002;**91**:331–338.

12. Emery JL, Omens JH, McCulloch AD. Strain softening in rat left ventricular myocardium. *J Biomech Eng* 1997;**119**:6–12.

13. McCulloch AD, Omens JH (1991). Factors Affecting the Regional Mechanics of the Diastolic Heart, *Theory of Heart: Biomechanics, Biophysics, and Nonlinear Dynamics of Cardiac Function*, (eds L Glass, PJ Hunter, AD McCulloch) . Springer-Verlag, New York; pp.87–119.

14. Bayly PV, KenKnight BH, Rogers JM, Hillsley RE, Ideker RE, Smith WM. Estimation of conduction velocity vector fields from epicardial mapping data. *IEEE Trans Biomed Eng* 1998;**45**:563–571.

15. Penefsky ZJ, Hoffman BF. Effects of stretch on mechanical and electrical properties of cardiac muscle. *Am J Physiol* 1963;**204**: 433–438.

16. Sachse FB, Steadman BW, JH BB, Punske BB, Taccardi B. Conduction velocity in myocardium modulated by strain: measurement instrumentation and initial results. *Conf Proc IEEE Eng Med Biol Soc* 2004;**5**:3593–3596.

17. Deck KA. [Changes in the Resting Potential and the Cable Properties of Purkinje Fibers During Stretch]. *Pflugers Arch* 1964;**280**: 131–140.

18. Dominguez G, Fozzard HA. Effect of stretch on conduction velocity and cable properties of cardiac Purkinje fibers. *Am J Physiol* 1979;**237**:C119–C124.

19. Rosen MR, Legato MJ, Weiss RM. Developmental changes in impulse conduction in the canine heart. *Am J Physiol* 1981;**240**:H546–H554.

20. Spear JF, Moore EN. Stretch-induced excitation and conduction disturbances in the isolated rat myocardium. *J Electrocardiol* 1972;**5**:15–24.

21. Sideris DA, Toumanidis ST, Kostopoulos K, et al. Effect of acute ventricular pressure changes on QRS duration. *J Electrocardiol* 1994;**27**:199–202.

22. Solti F, Vecsey T, Kekesi V, Juhasz-Nagy A. The effect of atrial dilatation on the genesis of atrial arrhythmias. *Cardiovasc Res* 1989;**23**:882–886.

23. Zabel M, Portnoy S, Franz MR. Effect of sustained load on dispersion of ventricular repolarization and conduction time in the isolated intact rabbit heart. *J Cardiovasc Electrophysiol* 1996;**7**:9–16.

24. Zhu WX, Johnson SB, Brandt R, Burnett J, Packer DL. Impact of volume loading and load reduction on ventricular refractoriness and conduction properties in canine congestive heart failure. *J Am Coll Cardiol* 1997;**30**:825–833.

25. Tavi P, Laine M, Weckström M. Effect of gadolinium on stretch-induced changes in contraction and intracellularly recorded action- and afterpotentials of rat isolated atrium. *Br J Pharmacol* 1996;**118**:407–413.

26. Reiter MJ, Landers M, Zetelaki Z, Kirchhof CJ, Allessie MA. Electrophysiological effects of acute dilatation in the isolated rabbit heart: cycle length-dependent effects on ventricular refractoriness and conduction velocity. *Circulation* 1997;**96**:4050–4056.

27. Chorro FJ, Egea S, Mainar L, et al. [Acute changes in wavelength of the process of auricular activation induced by stretching. Experimental study]. *Rev Esp Cardiol* 1998;**51**:874–883.

28. Eijsbouts SC, Majidi M, van Zandvoort M, Allessie MA. Effects of acute atrial dilation on heterogeneity in conduction in the isolated rabbit heart. *J Cardiovasc Electrophysiol* 2003;**14**:269–278.

29. Sung D, Mills RW, Schettler J, Narayan SM, Omens JH, McCulloch AD. Ventricular filling slows epicardial conduction and increases action potential duration in an optical mapping study of the isolated rabbit heart. *J Cardiovasc Electrophysiol* 2003;**14**:739–749.

30. Sung D, Omens JH, McCulloch AD. Model-based analysis of optically mapped epicardial activation patterns and conduction velocity. *Ann Biomed Eng* 2000;**28**:1085–1092.

31. Mills RW, Narayan SM, McCulloch AD. Mechanisms of conduction slowing during myocardial stretch by ventricular volume loading in the rabbit. *Am J Physiol* 2008;**295**:H1270–H1278.

32. Zhang Y, Sekar RB, McCulloch AD, Tung L. Cell cultures as models of cardiac mechanoelectric feedback. *Prog Biophys Mol Biol* 2008;**97**: 367–382.

33. Franz MR. Mechano-electrical feedback in ventricular myocardium. *Cardiovasc Res* 1996;**32**:15–24.

34. McNary TG, Sohn K, Taccardi B, Sachse FB. Experimental and computational studies of strain-conduction velocity relationships in cardiac tissue. *Prog Biophys Mol Biol* 2008;**97**:383–400.

35. Calaghan SC, Belus A, White E. Do stretch-induced changes in intracellular calcium modify the electrical activity of cardiac muscle? *Prog Biophys Mol Biol* 2003;**82**:81–95.

36. Eckardt L, Kirchhof P, Monnig G, Breithardt G, Borggrefe M, Haverkamp W. Modification of stretch-induced shortening of repolarization by streptomycin in the isolated rabbit heart. *J Cardiovasc Pharmacol* 2000;**36**:711–721.

37. Kohl P, Cooper PJ, Holloway H. Effects of acute ventricular volume manipulation on in situ cardiomyocyte cell membrane configuration. *Prog Biophys Mol Biol* 2003;**82**:221–227.

38. Suchyna TM, Besch SR, Sachs F. Dynamic regulation of mechanosensitive channels: capacitance used to monitor patch tension in real time. *Physical Biology* 2004;**1**:1–18.

39. Cherian PP, Siller-Jackson AJ, Gu S, et al. Mechanical strain opens connexin 43 hemichannels in osteocytes: a novel mechanism for the release of prostaglandin. *Mol Biol Cell* 2005;**16**:3100–3106.

40. Bao L, Sachs F, Dahl G. Connexins are mechanosensitive. *Am J Physiol* 2004;**287**:C1389–C1395.

41. Thomas SP, Kucera JP, Bircher-Lehmann L, Rudy Y, Saffitz JE, Kleber AG. Impulse propagation in synthetic strands of neonatal cardiac myocytes with genetically reduced levels of connexin43. *Circ Res* 2003;**92**:1209–1216.

42. Kohl P, Day K, Noble D. Cellular mechanisms of cardiac mechano-electric feedback in a mathematical model. *Can J Cardiol* 1998; **14**:111–119.

43. Ravelli F, Allessie M. Effects of atrial dilatation on refractory period and vulnerability to atrial fibrillation in the isolated Langendorff-perfused rabbit heart. *Circulation* 1997;**96**:1686–1695.

44. Zarse M, Stellbrink C, Athanatou E, Robert J, Schotten U, Hanrath P. Verapamil prevents stretch-induced shortening of atrial effective refractory period in langendorff-perfused rabbit heart. *J Cardiovasc Electrophysiol* 2001;**12**:85–92.

45. Bode F, Sachs F, Franz MR. Tarantula peptide inhibits atrial fibrillation. *Nature* 2001;**409**:35–36.

46. Qi J, Xiao J, Zhang Y, et al. Effects of potassium channel blockers on changes in refractoriness of atrial cardiomyocytes induced by stretch. *Exp Biol Med (Maywood)* 2009;**234**:779–784.

47. Huang JL, Tai CT, Chen JT, et al. Effect of atrial dilatation on electrophysiologic properties and inducibility of atrial fibrillation. *Basic Res Cardiol* 2003;**98**:16–24.

48. Dean JW, Lab MJ. Regional changes in ventricular excitability during load manipulation of the in situ pig heart. *J Physiol* 1990;**429**: 387–400.

49. Halperin BD, Adler SW, Mann DE, Reiter MJ. Mechanical correlates of contraction-excitation feedback during acute ventricular dilatation. *Cardiovasc Res* 1993;**27**:1084–1087.

50. Wang XX, Chen JZ, Cheng LX, Zhou LL. [Effect of tetradrine on electrophysilogic changes caused by rising of left ventricular preload in guinea pigs]. *Zhongguo Zhong Yao Za Zhi* 2003;**28**:1054–1056.

51. Fu L, Cao JX, Xie RS, *et al.* The effect of streptomycin on stretch-induced electrophysiological changes of isolated acute myocardial infarcted hearts in rats. *Europace* 2007;**9**:578–584.

52. Chen RL, Penny DJ, Greve G, Lab MJ. Stretch-induced regional mechanoelectric dispersion and arrhythmia in the right ventricle of anesthetized lambs. *Am J Physiol* 2004;**286**: H1008–H1014.

53. Zabel M, Koller BS, Sachs F, Franz MR. Stretch-induced voltage changes in the isolated beating heart: importance of the timing of stretch and implications for stretch-activated ion channels. *Cardiovasc Res* 1996;**32**:120–130.

54. Bode F, Katchman A, Woosley RL, Franz MR. Gadolinium decreases stretch-induced vulnerability to atrial fibrillation. *Circulation*, 2000;**101**:2200–2205.

55. Vetter FJ, McCulloch AD. Mechanoelectric feedback in a model of the passively inflated left ventricle. *Ann Biomed Eng* 2001;**29**:414–426.

Mechanical triggers of long-term ventricular electrical remodelling

Darwin Jeyaraj and David S. Rosenbaum

Background

Ventricular electrical remodelling (VER) is a persistent change in the electrophysiological properties of myocardium in response to a variety of physiological or pathological perturbations such as altered electrical activation, heart rate and mechanical or chemical stimuli. This chapter focuses on VER triggered by altered electrical activation, which is commonly associated with heart disease or therapeutic ventricular pacing. Pathological changes in the structure and/or function of the cardiac conduction system are a common manifestation of a wide variety of disease processes including ischaemia, hypertrophy and heart failure. Further, therapy for major disorders of the conduction system, i.e. external pacing, is also an important cause of altered activation. It has been known for several decades that changing the rate or sequence of ventricular activation triggers remarkable changes in the polarity of the T-wave [1]. This was initially described as 'T-wave memory' by Mauricio Rosenbaum [2]. These profound changes in the T-wave polarity are indicative of remodelling of myocardial repolarization and illustrate dynamic changes in repolarization triggered by abnormal depolarization. In this chapter we aim to provide an overview of pathophysiological implications, cellular electrophysiological changes and mechanisms that drive the remodelling response.

Pathophysiological consequences of VER

The pathophysiological consequences of VER are primarily related to adverse mechanical and electrical remodelling, but these have been largely unrecognized until the last decade. In the MADIT-II trial (Multicenter Automatic Defibrillator Implantation Trial II), patients randomized to defibrillator therapy had better survival; however, they were also hospitalized more often for heart failure, presumably due to adverse mechanical remodelling from ventricular pacing [3]. This clinical observation was reaffirmed in the DAVID trial (Dual Chamber and VVI Implantable Defibrillator Trial) which was designed to test the hypothesis that beta-blockade therapy aided by ventricular pacing to maintain physiological heart rates would improve survival in heart failure [4]. However, patients in the DAVID trial with back-up ventricular pacing had greater morbidity and mortality.

The adverse electrical consequences of altered activation came to clinical attention long before the mechanical side effects. This was first observed in patients who underwent atrioventricular-node ablation for rapid atrial fibrillation (AF), and subsequently had increased susceptibility to ventricular arrhythmias and sudden death [5,6]. In these subjects, long periods of rapid erratic heart rates during atrial fibrillation followed by a slow ventricular paced rhythm created a substrate favourable for development of malignant ventricular rhythms. In addition, short-term epicardial ventricular pacing, i.e. bi-ventricular pacing, in certain subjects was demonstrated to increase dispersion of repolarization and increase susceptibility to arrhythmias [7]. Increased repolarization heterogeneity was also reported in a clinical study that examined ventricular pacing for sick-sinus syndrome [8]. These clinical observations illustrate that altered activation is not 'benign' and has deleterious consequences.

The pattern of impulse conduction in the heart during sinus activation is through the His-Purkinje network, resulting in synchronous mechanical activation and efficient ejection of blood from the ventricle. In contrast, during pacing, impulse propagation occurs almost exclusively via conduction between working myocytes, causing dyssynchronous activation which reduces mechanical efficiency. This has led to development of cardiac resynchronization therapy with biventricular pacing which aims to synchronize electrical activation and improve efficiency of left ventricular (LV) contraction. Initial clinical studies using biventricular pacing (MIRACLE [myocardial ischaemia reduction with acute cholesterol lowering] and COMPANION [comparison of medical, pacing, and defibrillation therapies in heart failure]) demonstrated an improvement in morbidity [9,10]. However, in the Care-HF trial (Cardiac Resynchronization in Heart Failure Trial), synchronous LV activation improved not only symptoms but also survival in patients with heart failure [11]. This has led to the widespread use of biventricular pacing as an important clinical tool in heart failure therapy.

Electrocardiographic changes associated with VER

The classical electrocardiogram (ECG) manifestation of VER is significant change in T-wave polarity following cessation of abnormal activation when normal activation resumes. The first clinical evaluation of this problem was conducted by Chatterjee et al. in 1969, who identified that abnormal depolarization was a key element in triggering T-wave changes following altered activation[12]. Mauricio Rosenbaum in 1982 reported that altered activation was a more important trigger for VER than change in heart rate. He also coined the term 'memory,' because the polarity of the T-wave following cessation of altered activation was in the direction of QRS during altered activation, i.e. the T-wave vector following altered activation remembers the vector of the QRS during altered activation[22]. The duration and frequency of altered activation also predict how long the T-wave changes persist after cessation of altered activation, and this phenomenon is also referred to as 'accumulation'. A recent clinical study quantitatively demonstrated accumulation in patients who developed T-wave memory following dual-chamber pacing[13]. Therefore, short-term memory is used to describe T-wave changes lasting minutes to hours, commonly observed after brief episodes of tachyarrhythmias or ventricular pacing. In contrast, long-term memory lasting hours to days is noted in patients after His-Purkinje activation is restored following long periods of altered ventricular activation, such as with temporary cessation of permanent pacing or after ablation of accessory pathway for Wolff–Parkinson–White (WPW) syndrome[14,15].

Before delving into the details of basis for T-wave changes in VER, it is important to review the electrophysiological basis for the normal T-wave, which has been somewhat controversial. In normal hearts, the myocytes that span the transmural surface of the left ventricle exhibit the largest ventricular repolarization gradient[16]. This gradient arises because endocardial and mid-myocardial (M) cell action potential duration (APD) is significantly longer than epicardial myocyte APD[17]. Consequently, there is a repolarization gradient between epicardial and mid-myocardial layers, which is opposite to the direction of depolarization. Hence, the normal T-wave is upright with respect to the QRS. Recently, we demonstrated that similar transmural gradients existed in myocardium obtained from multiple (anterior, lateral and posterior) regions of the canine LV[18]. In contrast, the difference in APD[17] between the different regions of LV was minimal. These data reaffirm that the most prominent repolarization gradients that underlie the normal T-wave arise from the transmural surface of the left ventricle. However, repolarization measured in vivo from activation recovery interval (ARI) revealed greater regional dispersion of repolarization compared to transmural dispersion[19]. So controversy remains regarding the origin of the normal T-wave.

Cellular electrophysiological changes induced by VER

In order to understand the pathophysiology and mechanisms inducing VER, it is important to examine the cellular electrophysiological changes that occur following VER. In sharp contrast to atrial electrical remodelling that is characterized by APD shortening,

action potential prolongation underlies VER. This was first illustrated from monophasic action potential (MAP) studies conducted in isolated rabbit hearts[20]. Ventricular pacing induced action potential prolongation in ventricular regions adjacent to the pacing site, and progressive shortening was noted in distal regions that followed the direction of propagation. Subsequent studies from Michael Rosen's laboratory have identified several important components of the action potential remodelling response[21]. Utilizing a canine epicardial tissue model of remodelling they first identified that altered activation caused significant attenuation of the action potential phase 1 notch following altered activation[22]. Further, administration of 4-aminopyridine (pharmacological blocker of transient outward potassium current (I_{to}) – the ionic current responsible for phase 1 notch) inhibits development of short-term memory, indicating an important role for I_{to} in this process. Subsequent studies in long-term pacing models have clearly illustrated that APD prolongation and attenuation of epicardial phase 1 notch are essential components of the remodelling response[23]. However, the mechanistic link between cellular electrophysiological remodelling and marked changes on the surface ECG was poorly understood.

In order to determine the global LV remodelling following altered activation and to elucidate the electrophysiological basis for T-wave memory, we developed a pacing-induced model of VER[18]. Further, we aimed to study the isolated role of altered activation without changing the intrinsic heart rate. Therefore, we employed a canine model of epicardial LV pacing triggered by atrial sensing utilizing short AV-delay for 4 weeks. This resulted in progressive and persistent change in T-wave polarity indicative of successful induction of VER. Following VER, we utilized high-resolution transmural optical imaging to measure action potentials from wedge preparations isolated from the anterior, lateral and posterior LV regions. Interestingly, when compared to control hearts, minimal changes were observed in transmural repolarization gradients. This raised the suspicion of whether changes in other repolarization gradients could account for T-wave changes in VER. We then examined regional repolarization gradients, i.e. repolarization gradients between different LV regions. As illustrated in Fig. 26.1 (top panel), the APD was homogenous across multiple LV regions in control hearts, indicating that transmural gradients were the major repolarization gradients in the normal heart. In sharp contrast, following VER, there was marked enhancement of regional LV repolarization gradients. Consistent with previous studies[23], we observed prolongation of APD in myocardial regions proximal to the site of pacing (early-activated). Paradoxically, the most significant APD prolongation occurred in the myocardial region that was most distal to the site of pacing (late-activated) (Fig. 26.1). Interestingly, the segment between the early- and late-activated had modest APD shortening likely due to electrotonic mechanisms discussed later in this chapter (Fig. 26.1). These regional APD changes greatly enhanced regional repolarization gradients following VER. Utilizing ECG calculations we identified that the enhanced regional repolarization gradients underlie the electrophysiological basis for T-wave memory[18].

Ionic changes underlying VER

The most obvious abnormality in epicardial APD from the early-activated region was attenuation of the epicardial phase 1 notch due

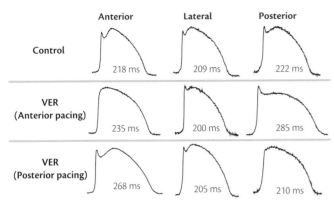

Fig. 26.1 Action potential changes following VER. Top panel illustrates epicardial action potentials from anterior, lateral and posterior LV region of control hearts. In contrast to control hearts with homogenous action potentials (top panel), VER induced by anterior LV pacing causes heterogeneous regional action potential remodelling (middle panel). Specifically, significant attenuation of action potential phase 1 notch is noted in the early-activated anterior region and the most significant action potential remodelling is observed in the late-activated posterior region. The converse is noted when VER was induced by pacing the posterior LV (lower panel). [Reproduced, with permission, from Jeyaraj D, Wilson LD, Zhong J, et al. (2007) Mechanoelectrical feedback as novel mechanism of cardiac electrical remodeling. *Circulation* **115**:3145–3155.]

to reduced expression of I_{to}[22]. This is due to reduced expression of Kv4.3 (α subunit) and KChIP2 (β subunit) responsible for I_{to}[21]. Interestingly, as illustrated in Fig. 26.1, following VER induced by anterior LV pacing, attenuation of the phase 1 notch was limited to the myocardial region adjacent to the site of pacing[18]. The action potential phase 1 notch amplitude gradually increased and reached normal levels in the late-activated posterior region. The converse occurs when VER was induced by posterior LV pacing; therefore I_{to} remodelling in VER possibly accounts for APD prolongation in the early- but not in the late-activated region.

In addition to I_{to}, the early-activated region exhibits changes in L-type calcium current ($I_{Ca,L}$), reduced expression of rapid component of the delayed rectifier K^+ current (I_{Kr}) and reduced connexin 43 (Cx43)[24,25]. Pharmacological blockade of $I_{Ca,L}$ attenuates development of both long- and short-term memory. Reduced Cx43 expression in the early-activated region causes local reduction in conduction velocity and could increase repolarization gradients following VER.[26] In the late-activated region of the dyssynchronous model of heart failure (rapid atrial pacing with left bundle branch block [LBBB]) there was reduced conduction due to redistribution of Cx43 to the sides of the myocyte instead of the intercalated disc, termed 'lateralization'[27]. Further, recent study in the dyssynchronous model of heart failure identified a plethora of ionic current changes in the late-activated region[28]. However, electrophysiological changes in this model are potentially caused by both heart failure and altered activation, and therefore the primary changes caused by altered activation in the late-activated region remain to be elucidated. Future studies to fully evaluate ionic remodelling in the early- and late-activated regions will provide important insights into the ionic processes that cause heterogeneous action potential remodelling following altered activation.

Signalling mechanisms underlying VER

An important consequence of ectopic ventricular pacing is altered pattern of electrotonic flow, where the region around the pacing electrode serves as the source and distal regions from the sink. This causes changes in the membrane potential whereby fully depolarized myocytes downstream of the site of altered activation extend the action potential plateau of upstream cells. Consequently, there is APD prolongation in the early-activated region, which gradually shortens in the direction of propagation (Fig. 26.1)[20]. In addition, electronic load-dependent changes in membrane potential were demonstrated to regulate the expression of I_{to}[29].

An important signalling pathway implicated in VER is angiotensin II (AT-II)[30]. AT-II regulates sarcolemmal expression of Kv4 channels and the stability of its messenger ribonucleic acid (mRNA)[31,32]. Interestingly, AT-II blockade inhibits development of short-term memory; however, its role in attenuating long-term VER was not as robust[24]. Therefore, AT-II-dependent I_{to} remodelling may play an important role in short-term VER.

Mechano-electrical feedback as a mechanism for triggering VER

As illustrated in Fig. 26.2 (top panel), following VER we observed the most prominent action potential remodelling in the late-activated segment[18]. This paradoxical effect could not be explained by traditional biophysical principles that govern impulse propagation and repolarization. To examine this further, we reversed the pattern of activation by pacing the posterior LV instead of the anterior LV. Interestingly, as illustrated in Fig. 26.2 (top panel), the most prominent action potential remodelling occurred in the late-activated anterior region. This confirmed the role of altered activation as a primary trigger in establishing specific remodelling responses in the early- and late-activated regions.

Another important effect of altered activation is change in myocardial strain[33]; therefore we utilized tagged magnetic resonance (MR) imaging to measure myocardial strain during altered activation. As illustrated in Fig. 26.2 (middle panel), during sinus rhythm there was a similar pattern of myocardial strain in all myocardial regions. In contrast, during altered activation, there was a marked increase in strain in the late-activated region irrespective of pacing from the anterior or posterior LV. The altered mechanical strain directly correlated with APD remodelling (Fig. 26.2, lower panel), linking strain-induced changes to VER. A recent rabbit model of short-term memory also demonstrated similar effects with electrical remodelling following mechanical perturbations[34]. In contrast to our studies that are induced by chronic mechanical perturbations, acute stretch as occurs with acute arterial occlusion causes action potential shortening[35].

The final common pathway in transducing mechanical signals to electrophysiological and structural remodelling is likely through a variety of signalling pathways including: protein kinase A, protein kinase C, protein kinase G, AT-II, calmodulin activated kinase, calcineurin, mitogen-activated protein kinase and focal adhesion kinase[36–38]. These pathways activate a number of key transcription factors (MEF2, GATA4, etc.) that regulate myocyte growth and function. The following provides an outline of mechano-sensors

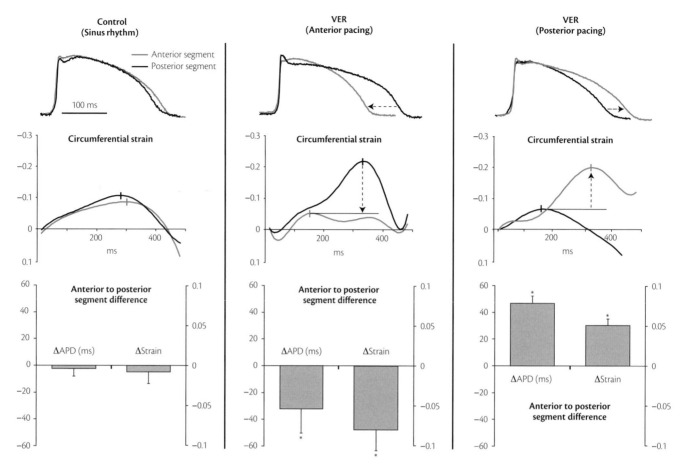

Fig. 26.2 Mechano-electrical feedback as a mechanism for VER. The top panel illustrates action potentials from control and VER hearts. The middle panel illustrates MR strain tracings from anterior and posterior LV regions during sinus rhythm, anterior or posterior LV pacing. During sinus activation, the anterior and posterior regions have similar magnitude and temporal occurrence of peak circumferential strain. In contrast, during anterior LV pacing, circumferential strain is increased in the late-activated posterior region, and the converse occurs during posterior LV pacing (middle panel). The lower panel illustrates the mechanistic link between altered mechanical strain and action potential remodelling. [Modified, with permission, from Jeyaraj D, Wilson LD, Zhong J, *et al.* (2007) Mechanoelectrical feedback as novel mechanism of cardiac electrical remodeling. *Circulation* **115**:3145–3155.]

that are present in the sarcolemmal membrane, sarcomere, sarcoplasmic reticulum and the extracellular matrix/cytoskeleton:

1. Stretch-activated ion channels: these are specialized ion channels which are activated by mechanical stretch that conduct non-selective cations. These ionic currents are expressed at higher levels following hypertrophy and could play a role in changing intracellular calcium or sodium[39].

2. Sarcomere length and myofilament calcium sensitivity: an important consequence of altered myocyte stretch is changes in sarcomere length; this principle underlies the basis for the Frank–Starling mechanism. In addition, changes in sarcomere length also change myofilament sensitivity to calcium, which over time could cause myocyte calcium overload[40].

3. Sarcoplasmic reticulum (SR) changes in calcium handling: calcium release from the SR directly corresponds to myocyte force generation, i.e. the larger the release the greater the force generated. Hypertrophy and heart failure are characterized by a myriad of changes in SR calcium handling. Changes in SR reuptake or release of calcium due to mechanical perturbations

could lead to changes in myocyte calcium load and action potential remodelling[41,42].

4. Extracellular matrix/cytoskeleton: integrins and the extracellular matrix proteins play a key role in transducing mechanical strain. Genetic loss-of-function studies have established an important role for extracellular matrix proteins in activating signalling pathways, force development, fibrosis and myocyte hypertrophy[43].

Conclusions and outlook

In contrast to atrial electrical remodelling, VER induced by an alteration in activation sequence is characterized by prolongation of the cardiac action potential in ventricular myocytes. However, myocytes localized to regions most distal to the site of pacing (i.e. late-activated) undergo much more substantial VER than myocytes proximal to the site of pacing, producing a spatial gradient in repolarization which accounts for the electrocardiographic T-wave changes ascribed to 'T-wave memory'. The mechanism for triggering VER in late-activated myocytes appears to be regional mechanical strain. Hence, rather than being a direct electrophysiological mechanism, VER involves mechano-electrical feedback mechanisms. A variety of signalling pathways have been implicated to respond to a stretch trigger and lead to ionic remodelling in these myocytes. Since pacing therapies and heart disease itself are often characterized by alterations in activation sequence, VER may play a significant role in modulating electrical heterogeneity and, hence, electrical stability in the heart.

The current paradigm of electrical remodelling assumes that electrical remodelling is secondary to structural remodelling; i.e. hypertrophy or heart failure. Interestingly, in our recent study we observed marked action potential remodelling in the absence of histological or gross pathological evidence of cardiac hypertrophy[18]. This begs the question whether electrical remodelling that precedes onset of structural remodelling could play a role in the development of structural remodelling. Future studies that identify signalling cascades activated by altered activation are needed to understand the molecular mechanisms that link altered stretch to pathological electrical and structural remodelling.

Acknowledgements

This study was supported by National Institutes of Health grants RO1-HL54807 (David S. Rosenbaum) and KO8-HL094660 (Darwin Jeyaraj).

References

1. Campbell M. Inversion of T waves after long paroxysms of tachycardia. *Br Heart J* 1942; **4**:49–56.

2. Rosenbaum MB, Blanco HH, Elizari MV, Lazzari JO, Davidenko JM. Electrotonic modulation of the T-wave and cardiac memory. *Am J Cardiol* 1982;**50**:213–222.

3. Moss AJ, Zareba W, Hall WJ, et al. Prophylactic implantation of a defibrillator in patients with myocardial infarction and reduced ejection fraction. *New Engl J Med* 2002;**346**:877–883.

4. Wilkoff BL, Cook JR, Epstein AE, et al. Dual-chamber pacing or ventricular backup pacing in patients with an implantable defibrillator: the Dual Chamber and VVI Implantable Defibrillator (DAVID) Trial. *JAMA* 2002;**288**:3115–3123.

5. Geelen P, Brugada J, Andries E, Brugada P. Ventricular fibrillation and sudden death after radiofrequency catheter ablation of the atrioventricular junction. *Pacing Clin Electrophysiol* 1997;**20**: 343–348.

6. Darpo B, Walfridsson H, Aunes M, et al. Incidence of sudden death after radiofrequency ablation of the atrioventricular junction for atrial fibrillation. *Am J Cardiol* 1997;**80**:1174–1177.

7. Medina-Ravell VA, Lankipalli RS, Yan GX, et al. Effect of epicardial or biventricular pacing to prolong QT interval and increase transmural dispersion of repolarization: does resynchronization therapy pose a risk for patients predisposed to long QT or torsade de pointes? *Circulation* 2003;**107**:740–746.

8. Wecke L, Rubulis A, Lundahl G, Rosen MR, Bergfeldt L. Right ventricular pacing-induced electrophysiological remodeling in the human heart and its relationship to cardiac memory. *Heart Rhythm* 2007;**4**:1477–1486.

9. Bristow MR, Saxon LA, Boehmer J, et al. Cardiac-resynchronization therapy with or without an implantable defibrillator in advanced chronic heart failure. *New Engl J Med* 2004;**350**: 2140–2150.

10. Abraham WT, Fisher WG, Smith AL, et al. Cardiac resynchronization in chronic heart failure. *New Engl J Med* 2002;**346**:1845–1853.

11. Cleland JG, Daubert JC, Erdmann E, et al. The effect of cardiac resynchronization on morbidity and mortality in heart failure. *New Engl J Med* 2005;**352**:1539–1549.

12. Chatterjee K, Harris AM, Davies JG, Leatham A. T-wave changes after artificial pacing. *Lancet* 1969;**293**:759–760.

13. Wecke L, Gadler F, Linde C, Lundahl G, Rosen MR, Bergfeldt L. Temporal characteristics of cardiac memory in humans: vectorcardiographic quantification in a model of cardiac pacing. *Heart Rhythm* 2005;**2**:28–34.

14. Takada Y, Inden Y, Akahoshi M, et al. Changes in repolarization properties with long-term cardiac memory modify dispersion of repolarization in patients with Wolff-Parkinson-White syndrome. *J Cardiovasc Electrophysiol* 2002;**13**:324–330.

15. Helguera ME, Pinski SL, Sterba R, Trohman RG. Memory T waves after radiofrequency catheter ablation of accessory atrioventricular connections in Wolff-Parkinson-White syndrome. *J Electrocardiol* 1994;**27**:243–249.

16. Antzelevitch C, Fish J. Electrical heterogeneity within the ventricular wall. *Basic Res Cardiol* 2001;**96**:517–527.

17. Yan GX, Shimizu W, Antzelevitch C. Characteristics and distribution of M cells in arterially perfused canine left ventricular wedge preparations. *Circulation* 1998;**98**:1921–1927.

18. Jeyaraj D, Wilson LD, Zhong J, et al. Mechanoelectrical feedback as novel mechanism of cardiac electrical remodeling. *Circulation* 2007;**115**:3145–3155.

19. Janse MJ, Sosunov EA, Coronel R, et al. Repolarization gradients in the canine left ventricle before and after induction of short-term cardiac memory. *Circulation* 2005;**112**:1711–1718.

20. Costard-Jackle A, Goetsch B, Antz M, Franz MR. Slow and long-lasting modulation of myocardial repolarization produced by ectopic activation in isolated rabbit hearts. Evidence for cardiac "memory". *Circulation* 1989;**80**:1412–1420.

21. Ozgen N, Rosen MR. Cardiac memory: a work in progress. *Heart Rhythm* 2009;**6**:564–570.

22. del Balzo U, Rosen MR. T wave changes persisting after ventricular pacing in canine heart are altered by 4-aminopyridine but not by lidocaine. Implications with respect to phenomenon of cardiac 'memory'. *Circulation* 1992;**85**:1464–1472.

23. Shvilkin A, Danilo P, Jr., Wang J, et al. Evolution and resolution of long-term cardiac memory. *Circulation* 1998;**97**:1810–1817.

24. Plotnikov AN, Yu H, Geller JC, et al. Role of L-type calcium channels in pacing-induced short-term and long-term cardiac memory in canine heart. *Circulation* 2003;**107**:2844–2849.

25. Obreztchikova MN, Patberg KW, Plotnikov AN, et al. I_{kr} contributes to the altered ventricular repolarization that determines long-term cardiac memory. *Cardiovasc Res* 2006;**71**:88–96.

26. Patel PM, Plotnikov A, Kanagaratnam P, et al. I_{kr} Altering ventricular activation remodels gap junction distribution in canine heart. *J Cardiovasc Electrophysiol* 2001;**12**:570–577.

27. Spragg DD, Akar FG, Helm RH, Tunin RS, Tomaselli GF, Kass DA. Abnormal conduction and repolarization in late-activated myocardium of dyssynchronously contracting hearts. *Cardiovasc Res* 2005;**67**:77–86.

28. Aiba T, Hesketh GG, Barth AS, et al. Electrophysiological consequences of dyssynchronous heart failure and its restoration by resynchronization therapy. *Circulation* 2009;**119**:1220–1230.

29. Libbus I, Wan X, Rosenbaum DS. Electrotonic load triggers remodeling of repolarizing current Ito in ventricle. *Am J Physiol* 2004;**286**:H1901–H1909.

30. Ricard P, Danilo P, Jr., Cohen IS, Burkhoff D, Rosen MR. A role for the renin-angiotensin system in the evolution of cardiac memory. *Cardiovasc Electrophysiol* 1999;**10**:545–551.

31. Yu H, Gao J, Wang H, et al. Effects of the renin-angiotensin system on the current I_{to} in epicardial and endocardial ventricular myocytes from the canine heart. *Circ Res* 2000;**86**:1062–1068.

32. Zhou C, Ziegler C, Birder LA, Stewart AF, Levitan ES. Angiotensin II and stretch activate NADPH oxidase to destabilize cardiac Kv4.3 channel mRNA. *Circ Res* 2006;**98**:1040–1047.

33. Prinzen FW, Hunter WC, Wyman BT, McVeigh ER. Mapping of regional myocardial strain and work during ventricular pacing: experimental study using magnetic resonance imaging tagging. *J Am Coll Cardiol* 1999;**33**:1735–1742.

34. Sosunov EA, Anyukhovsky EP, Rosen MR. Altered ventricular stretch contributes to initiation of cardiac memory. *Heart Rhythm* 2008;**5**: 106–113.

35. Chen RL, Penny DJ, Greve G, Lab MJ. Stretch-induced regional mechanoelectric dispersion and arrhythmia in the right ventricle of anesthetized lambs. *Am J Physiol* 2004;**286**:H1008–H1014.

36. Heineke J, Molkentin JD. Regulation of cardiac hypertrophy by intracellular signalling pathways. *Nat Rev Mol Cell Biol* 2006;**7**: 589–600.

37. Romer LH, Birukov KG, Garcia JG. Focal adhesions: paradigm for a signaling nexus. *Circ Res* 2006;**98**:606–616.

38. Sadoshima J, Izumo S. The cellular and molecular response of cardiac myocytes to mechanical stress. *Annu Rev Physiol* 1997;**59**:551–571.

39. Watanabe H, Murakami M, Ohba T, Takahashi Y, Ito H. TRP channel and cardiovascular disease. *Pharmacol Ther* 2008;**118**: 337–351.

40. Hanft LM, Korte FS, McDonald KS. Cardiac function and modulation of sarcomeric function by length. *Cardiovasc Res* 2008;**77**:627–636.

41. Iribe G, Ward CW, Camelliti P, *et al.* Axial stretch of rat single ventricular cardiomyocytes causes an acute and transient increase in Ca^{2+} spark rate. *Circ Res* 2009;**104**:787–795.

42. Iribe G, Kohl P. Axial stretch enhances sarcoplasmic reticulum Ca^{2+} leak and cellular Ca^{2+} reuptake in guinea pig ventricular myocytes: experiments and models. *Prog Biophys Mol Biol* 2008;**97**:298–311.

43. Brancaccio M, Hirsch E, Notte A, Selvetella G, Lembo G, Tarone G. Integrin signalling: the tug-of-war in heart hypertrophy. *Cardiovasc Res* 2006;**70**:422–433.

Mechanisms of mechanical pre- and postconditioning

Asger Granfeldt, Rong Jiang, Weiwei Shi and Jakob Vinten-Johansen

Background

Although timely reperfusion salvages myocardium, reperfusion contributes to the overall extent of cell death by necrosis and apoptosis. This 'reperfusion injury' reduces the therapeutic advantage of timely reperfusion from what was intended, and most importantly for what is achievable with appropriate therapies. Studies recently have demonstrated convincingly that reperfusion injury is initiated in the first minutes of reperfusion, but can continue and be amplified over time. In its practical application, this observation implies that therapies have to be administered within the early moments of reperfusion, or the reperfusion salvage window may close and the opportunity to salvage myocardium and function and reduce arrhythmias may be lost.

The three temporal windows during which therapeutics can be applied to salvage myocardium are (1) before the ischaemic event occurs (i.e. preconditioning) (2) during ischaemia (i.e. 'perconditioning') and (3) at onset of reperfusion (i.e. postconditioning). In 1986 a report from Murry et al.[1] showed that short periods of ischaemia imposed before the ischaemic event occurs could salvage myocardium. This 'ischaemic preconditioning' (I-precon) set into play metabolic and molecular adaptations exerted before and during ischaemia that made the heart more resilient to ischaemia. It was later found that some mechanisms of I-precon were also exerted at reperfusion[2], again highlighting the importance of reperfusion in the aetiology of post-ischaemic injury. The third window of opportunity to deliver cardioprotection is at the onset of reperfusion. Studies in 2003 from the laboratory of Vinten-Johansen introduced postconditioning (postcon) as a strategy that targets the complex mechanisms of reperfusion injury[3]. Postcon, also referred to as 'stutter reperfusion', is defined as brief periods of reperfusion interrupted by similarly brief periods of ischaemia applied at the onset of reperfusion (Fig. 27.1). Later studies reported that this stuttering pattern of reperfusion could be applied to a remote organ at the time when the coronary artery was reperfused (remote postcon)[4]. Interestingly, certain aspects of the protection afforded by short periods of ischaemia can also be induced using mechanical stimuli. This chapter reviews the mechanisms involved in protection afforded by ischaemic pre- and postcon, explores what is known about mechanical contributions to conditioning and highlights the relevance of both for post-ischaemic arrhythmias and contractile function.

Preconditioning

Infarct size (necrosis and apoptosis)

Measurement of infarct size (IS) is regarded as the ultimate endpoint of myocardial salvage and was the original endpoint of the first I-precon study reported by Murry et al.[1] A reduction of IS by I-precon has been confirmed in every animal species tested including rat, rabbits, canine, pig and monkeys.

Following reperfusion injury cardiomyocytes undergo cell death by either necrosis or apoptosis. Both processes are accelerated by reperfusion and extend over time, with necrosis peaking after 24 h and apoptosis increasing for up to 72 h. Consistent with the robust reduction in IS, accumulating evidence supports that I-precon attenuates apoptosis in addition to necrosis[5]. The mechanisms of the anti-apoptotic effect of I-precon have not been fully clarified but may involve an attenuation of reactive oxygen species (ROS) – a known trigger of apoptosis – and altered apoptotic and intracellular signaling[5].

Stunning and contractile function

While IS reduction by I-precon is well established, the question of whether I-precon improves contractile function is not totally resolved. One reason for this discrepancy may be different experimental conditions of the models used, i.e. (1) in vitro models in which global ischaemia is imposed in buffer perfused isolated hearts vs models in which regional ischaemia is imposed and (2) global contractile function vs contractile function in the region at risk. In models of global ischaemia, the recovery of contractile function is related to IS since necrosis is globally distributed unlike the regional ischaemia counterpart.

Short durations of index ischaemia (less than 20 min) result in reversible myocardial injury, also known as 'stunning' since cells are viable yet dysfunctional. Several studies have found that I-precon has no salubrious effect on myocardial stunning[6,7]. With longer periods of ischaemia, irreversible injury occurs in the form of necrosis and apoptosis; hence in acute models post-ischaemic contractile dysfunction is a combination of both necrotic and stunned viable myocardium[8]. Improved myocardial function with I-precon is observed after 72 h and 21 days, respectively[8,9]. The improved mechanical function is consistent with improved remodelling of the heart secondary to a reduction in IS rather than

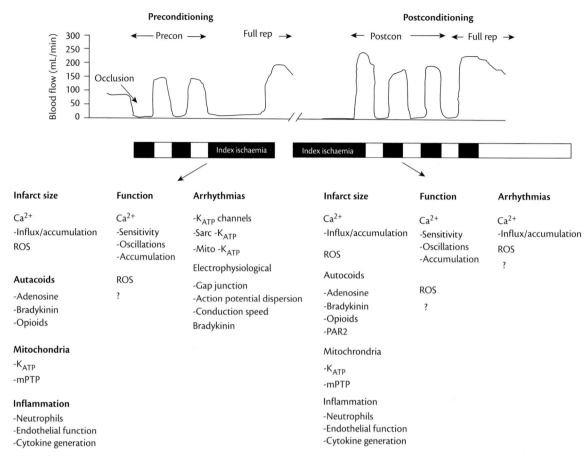

Fig. 27.1 A schematic diagram of pre- and postconditioning and the mechanisms involved in their cardioprotective effects. Preconditioning is initiated before index ischaemia while postconditioning is initiated immediately at the onset of reperfusion. Both manoeuvres share similarities with regards to end-points (infarct size, function and arrhythmias) and physiological and molecular mechanisms involved. In contrast to I-postcon, pacing-induced preconditioning (P-precon) and pacing-induced postconditioning (P-postcon) do not involve changes in blood flow, thereby suggesting involvement of different mechanisms, e.g. SAC (P-postcon) versus adenosine and K_{ATP} channels, etc. (I-postcon). The questionmark indicates that the mechanism is not clear. ROS, reactive oxygen species; mPTP, mitochondrial permeability transition pore; Sarc, sarcolemmal; Mito, mitichondrial; PAR2, protease-activated receptor.

attenuation of stunning *per se* that is normally reversed after 72 h[6].

Arrhythmias

An anti-arrhythmic effect of I-precon was first demonstrated by Shiki and Hearse[10] and later confirmed in the mouse, rabbit and dog. However, Ovize *et al.*[11] reported an accelerated time to ventricular fibrillation (VF) and a lowered VF threshold during ischaemia after I-precon using a porcine model, while Przyklenk and Kloner[12] failed to demonstrate an effect on the incidence of arrhythmias in dogs. The precise mechanisms involved in the anti-arrhythmic effect of I-precon remain elusive, but data suggest the involvement of adenosine triphosphate (ATP)-sensitive K^+ channel (K_{ATP}) channels, adrenergic stimulation, bradykinin and changes in electrophysiological properties[13–19]. Some of these mechanisms are also involved in the anti-necrotic effect of I-precon, while other triggers like phosphatidylinositol-3,4,5-trisphosphate (PIP_3) kinase (PIP_3K) are only involved in the anti-necrotic effect of I-precon[20,21]. Whether I-precon elicits sarcolemmal K_{ATP} ($K_{ATP,sarc}$) channel or mitochondrial K_{ATP} ($K_{ATP,mito}$) channel activation is not clear. The only study demonstrating $K_{ATP,sarc}$

channel activation uses a model of low flow ischaemia in which K_{ATP} channel blockers are administered during the entire study protocol[22], while studies demonstrating $K_{ATP,mito}$ use no-flow ischaemia and only infuse the antagonists for a limited period[15,16,23].

I-precon also induces electrophysiological changes in the ischaemic myocardium including changes to both active and passive electrical properties. Cinca *et al.*[24] demonstrated that I-precon delays changes in tissue resistivity and sharp phase-angle deviation. Papp *et al.* confirmed and extended these findings to show that I-precon reduces electrical uncoupling and closure of gap junctions[25]. I-precon is also associated with a reduction in conduction slowing[14], a reduction in QT dispersion[26] and a reduction in dispersion of monophasic action potentials between the epicardium and endocardium[18].

Pacing/stretch-induced preconditioning

Pacing-induced preconditioning (P-precon) was first introduced by Vegh *et al.* in 1991[27]. In anaesthetized dogs, two periods of 2 min at 300 beats per minute (bpm) reduced ST segment elevation and the incidence of ventricular arrhythmias during ischaemia.

Numerous studies confirmed the anti-arrhythmic effect of rapid pacing, and demonstrated that rapid pacing also decreased IS and attenuated ST segment elevation[28,29]. Vegh *et al.* suggested that rapid pacing induces global ischaemia accompanied by a release of protective substances. Whether rapid pacing induces ischaemia is debated and depends on the animal model, the pacing protocol and how ischaemia is defined, e.g. by lactate dehydrogenase (LDH) release, lactate release or electrocardiogram (ECG) changes. Several studies report that pacing is associated with an increase in ST segment elevation and left ventricular end diastolic pressure[30,31]. In addition, an increase in coronary effluent lactate, an indicator of ischaemia, was reported using an *in vitro* rat model with a pacing rate at 300—600 bpm[32]. However, in another *in vitro* (blood-perfused) rat study, 3 min of rapid pacing at 600–720 bpm did not affect high-energy phosphate levels, whereas I-precon decreased creatine phosphate and ATP levels[33]. These findings of a non-ischaemic effect of P-precon have been confirmed in several large *in vivo* animal studies[28,29], which suggests the existence of a mechanism different from that of I-precon. Rapid pacing increases oxygen consumption and oxygen demand, which may cause relative ischaemia (i.e. in the subendocardium) and a release of autacoids such as adenosine, bradykinin and nitric oxide[29,31,34]. Ferdinandy *et al.*[30] were the first to demonstrate involvement of K_{ATP} channels and this was later confirmed by Macho *et al.*[35] using a specific $K_{ATP,mito}$ channel blocker.

However, local stretch within a region of the heart may also be a mechanism of protection. Local pacing promotes alterations in regional myocardial stretch and loading which are known cardioprotective stimuli. Vanagt *et al.*[36] demonstrated that three periods of posterior ventricular pacing at a physiological heart rate before the ischaemic insult decreased infarct size, and this effect was mediated by local myocardial stretch and not ischaemia. Ventricular pacing at the posterior wall increases mechanical loading and stretch remote from the pacing site, since the normal electrical activation pathway by the Purkinje network is not activated. Myocardial stretch without concomitant ischaemia serving as a cardioprotective stimulus was discovered in the early 1990s. Brief occlusions of the circumflex artery increased end-diastolic segment length and reduced infarct size in the left anterior descending artery bed, and the concept of stretch-induced cardioprotection was further demonstrated by an infarct size reduction through an acute volume overload[37,38]. Subsequent studies revealed that administration of gadolinium – a blocker of stretch-activated ion channels (SAC) – abolished the protective effect, suggesting a putative role of SAC in stretch-induced protection. Gysembergh *et al.*[39] confirmed the involvement of SAC and demonstrated that blockade of adenosine receptors, protein kinase C and K_{ATP} channels also abolished the protective effect, while later studies revealed that it is $K_{ATP,sarc}$ channels and not $K_{ATP,mito}$ channels that are involved[40]. Interestingly, $K_{ATP,sarc}$ channels are mechano-sensitive, in that they respond with an increase in open probability to both ischaemia-induced ATP reduction and stretch, both in atrial[41] and ventricular[42] cardiomyocytes. Whether $K_{ATP,mito}$ channels are also affected by the mechanical environment is currently unknown (for mechanical modulation of non-sarcolemmal ion channels, see also Chapter 5).

Clinical data

Yellon and colleagues[43] were the first to demonstrate the feasibility of I-precon in the human heart. In patients undergoing coronary artery bypass grafting (CABG) two periods of brief aortic cross-clamping, applied prior to a longer cross-clamp, preserved myocardial ATP levels. In 2008 Walsh *et al.*[44] performed a systematic review and meta-analysis of all randomized clinical trials on I-precon in surgery. The majority of studies can be regarded as small proof-of-concept studies not powered for clinical endpoints. However, one study demonstrated a reduction in the incidence of myocardial infarction and renal impairment[45]. According to the meta-analysis, I-precon is associated with significant reductions in ventricular arrhythmias, requirement of inotropic support and length of stay in the intensive care unit. Regarding arrhythmias, an anti-arrhythmic effect was revealed in the clinical setting despite the somewhat conflicting animal studies. In chronic angina patients undergoing balloon angioplasty, the occurrence of ventricular ectopy and tachycardia was reduced during the second balloon occlusion when compared to the first occlusion[46]. Furthermore, Wu *et al.*[47] were the first to demonstrate that I-precon by transient aorta cross-clamping in stable and unstable angina patients reduced the incidence of VF and ventricular tachycardia after CABG surgery. These findings were later extended to include off-pump CABG patients, patients with three vessel disease and recent unstable angina. However, inducing I-precon by aortic cross-clamping has made clinicians resistant to adopt I-precon as an intervention. Furthermore, the prerequisite that the mechanical stimulus has to be performed prior to ischaemia has restricted its clinical use to various cardiovascular surgical procedures where the onset of ischaemia is predictable.

Postconditioning

Infarct size and apoptosis

Postcon has been shown to reduce both major cell pathways leading to cell death – necrosis and apoptosis. The robust reduction in IS by postcon as first demonstrated by Zhao *et al.*[48] was confirmed later by many investigators in *in vitro* and *in vivo* models in a wide range of species including mice, rats, rabbits, canines, pigs, monkeys and humans. Whether postcon provides cardioprotection as powerful as I-precon is unclear and is dependent on the species investigated. In mice, rabbits and dogs I-precon and postcon are equally protective, while in the rat I-precon is found to be more protective[48]. More research needs to be conducted to resolve the issue of the optimal algorithm and the comparative efficacy of I-precon versus postcon.

Arrhythmias

In contrast to I-precon that protects against arrhythmias during both ischaemia and reperfusion, postcon, by definition, affects only reperfusion arrhythmias. To date all studies exploring a possible anti-arrhythmic effect of postcon support it as a potential anti-arrhythmic intervention. In a study using an *in vivo* rat model postcon protected against reperfusion-induced arrhythmias[49]. Kloner and colleagues[50] later confirmed that cardioprotection was maintained in the senescent heart, but the mechanism by which postcon protects from reperfusion arrhythmias remains unclear. The anti-arrhythmic effect of postcon was not abolished by infusion of inhibitors of PI-3Kinase, adenosine or $K_{ATP,mito}$ channels, all of which are known to be involved in the anti-necrotic effect of postcon. In contrast to I-precon, a consensus emerges for anti-arrhythmic effects of postcon in large animal models.

Mykytenko et al. using a 24-h canine model reported decreased incidence of VT and VF in the postcon group when compared to the control group, and the protective effect was not blocked by either a $K_{ATP,sarc}$ or a $K_{ATP,mito}$ channel blocker[51]. The mechanisms by which postcon exerts an anti-arrhythmic effect remain speculative, but may involve atttenuation of intracellular calcium accumulation and ROS production, factors known to influence arrhythmogenesis[3,52,53].

Stunning and contractile function

The effect of postcon on myocardial stunning has been studied in rats, rabbits and dogs[54–56]. All three aforementioned studies reported that postcon did not reduce contractile stunning despite an IS limiting effect. However, other studies report improved post-ischaemic function when postcon was applied in models of global ischaemia[57,58]. Kin et al.[57] reported that hearts in which reperfusion was initiated using postcon algorithms showed a greater recovery of systolic and diastolic function compared to control hearts in which buffer perfusion was abruptly started. In the original study by Zhao et al.[3] post-ischaemic function was evaluated by implanting ultrasonic crystals in the area at risk to measure regional contractile function. No effect of postcon on contractile function was observed after 3 h of reperfusion; Mykytenko et al. observed similar findings with 24 h of reperfusion[59]. In in vivo models of regional (coronary artery occlusion) 'stunning' postcon does not attenuate post-ischaemic contractile 'stunning'[60]. In global models the improved function may simply be a consequence of IS reduction. However, in global ischaemia models, the protection may also be related to preservation of calcium handling. Sun et al.[53] reported that postcon reduced cytosolic and mitochondrial calcium accumulation in isolated cardiomyocytes after hypoxia and postcon reoxygenation ('hypoxic postcon'). The sarcoplasmic reticulum is important in the pathogenesis of necrosis, contractile dysfunction and arrhythmias because the sarcoplasmic/endoplasmatic reticulum calcium ATP-ase (SERCA) is activated by transient recovery of ATP, which sequesters cytosolic calcium. This is followed by repetitive cycles of release through the ryanodine receptor calcium release channel and sequestration by the sarcoplasmic reticulum. This cycling leads to calcium oscillations and high peak cytosolic calcium concentrations that can cause hypercontracture and calcium-induced opening of the mitochondrial permeability transition pore (mPTP), all of which have been associated with cell death. Although a reduction in cardiomyocyte injury and suppression of calcium overload would predict recovery of function, this has not been shown in the existing experimental models. However, experiments have not looked beyond the acute reperfusion phase to determine whether contractile function is improved in later phases of reperfusion. The clinical studies on effects of postcon, summarized below, have shown recovery of global function, but with no mechanistic explanation.

Pacing-induced dyssynchrony as a form of postconditioning

The protective effect of rapid pacing involves ischaemia, whereas ventricular pacing at physiological heart rates causes ventricular dyssynchrony and local stretch of the myocytes. In 2007 Vanagt et al.[61] introduced the concept of inducing postcon by applying intermittent pacing-induced dyssynchrony at the onset of reperfusion.

In the first study, pacing-induced postconditioning (P-postcon) was tested in an isolated rabbit heart and in an anaesthetized pig model of regional ischaemia. During the onset of reperfusion an algorithm of alternating cycles of 30 s ventricular epicardial pacing, each followed by 30 s of right atrial pacing, was repeated 10 times. In the isolated ejecting rabbit heart model and in the porcine model, both P-precon and P-postcon reduced IS. Intermittent ischaemia reperfusion is not induced in this variant of postcon as demonstrated by the lack of change in lactate release. Vanagt et al.[61] postulated that dyssynchronous activation of the left ventricular myocardium leads to regional differences in ventricular stretch and reductions in regional stroke work, which are known stimulators of P-precon[37]. A subsequent study by Babiker[62] showed that P-postcon does not produce alterations in reperfusion such as graded reperfusion, and does not involve the trigger phase mediated by adenosine as observed with 'ischaemic postcon'. However, the reduction in infarct size with pacing-induced postcon did involve mitochondrial K_{ATP} channel activation and molecular pathways such as protein kinase C and PI-3 kinase. This pacing-induced variant of postcon clearly deserves further investigation.

Clinical data

Postcon has enjoyed a remarkably rapid translational trajectory from bench to bedside. The first clinical study appeared in 2005[63], just 2 years after the first publication of the original studies by Zhao et al.[3] Clinical experience has now been reported for percutaneous coronary intervention (PCI), paediatric and adult cardiac surgery[64,65] and hepatic surgery[66], and the procedures include conventional (ischaemic) postcon, remote postcon and pharmacological postcon. The first investigation in PCI was conducted in patients undergoing PCI for ST-segment elevation acute myocardial infarction who were admitted within 6 h of symptoms onset[63]. Staat et al.[63] randomized to postcon with four alternating cycles of 60 s balloon deflation followed by 60 s balloon inflation or a control group receiving standard care for PCI. Postcon reduced the 72 h plasma creatine kinase (CK) activity curve by 36% vs control PCI. Notably, these patients had significant comorbidities. Subsequent studies confirmed the infarct sparing effect of postcon, but also showed an improvement in blood flow and ejection fraction as long as 6 months to a year after revascularization[67–69]. All clinical studies are remarkably consistent in the degree of IS reduction in PCI patients. A recently published meta-analysis of clinical studies[70] confirms the consistency of outcomes despite often differing postcon algorithms. Larger clinical trials are warranted by the preliminary clinical data.

Conclusions and outlook

Pre- and postconditioning are examples of the innate ability of the heart to protect itself from adverse stresses such as ischaemia-reperfusion. That these endogenous responses marshall a complex array of physiological, cellular and molecular responses to combat an equally complex array of adverse elements in ischaemia and reperfusion is testament to evolutionary adaptation. As effective as preconditioning and postconditioning are at countering ischaemia reperfusion injury in experimental models, they may be overwhelmed in the clinical situation. The early data on postconditioning in small groups of patients in particular indicate that this strategy may be clinically effective, but efficacy needs to be demonstrated in a larger population of patients. In addition, the efficacy of postconditioning should be determined for isolated as well as clustered comorbidities. Since most of the studies on postconditioning have centered on infarct sparing, more studies are needed on its effects on the pathophysiology of systolic and diastolic dysfunction, as well as on the inhibition of arrhythmias. Studies have not investigated the salient causes of reduction in arrhythmias or recovery of function in contra-distinction to preconditioning. Notably, it must be determined whether the reduction in either intracellular calcium accumulation or oxidant release is related to global or regional functional recovery as observed in clinical studies. How postcon reduces reperfusion arrhythmias is also ripe for investigation.

Mechanical postconditioning in the experimental setting has gained increasing attention since its introduction in 2007. However, the mechanisms of this endogenous response specifically evoked by mechanical postconditioning remain unidentified. Future studies confirming the existence of mechanical postconditioning induced by pacing or stretch of cardiomyocytes are necessary to understand the mechanisms. Experiments can be performed in isolated cardiomyocytes under different preload conditions to determine if the fundamental mechanics (force–frequency relationship, length–tension relationship) of the contractile apparatus is changed. Furthermore, isolated cell preparations can be used to determine if P-postcon preserves sensitivity to calcium or adrenergic agents that alter contractility. Whether P-postcon, or conventional postcon, alters excitation–contraction coupling on a cellular level requires further exploration. In addition, whether P-postcon alters the biomechanics of actin–myosin interactions is an interesting question. Other forms of mechanical stimuli beyond P-postcon have not been identified, but may include post-extrasystolic potentiated beats. The intriguing question of whether stretch itself, as observed in the paradoxically bulging ischaemic area at risk, is cardioprotective during either conventional postcon or P-postcon should be studied. It is of particular interest to investigate whether signalling pathways modified by comorbidities are involved and whether the response by mechanical postcon is blunted in animal models of comorbidities. Changes in blood flow during reperfusion or involvement of molecular triggers normally found to be involved in ischaemic postcon are not involved in the response to mechanical postconditioning such as P-postcon, which suggests that the combination of ischaemic and mechanical postconditioning as well as a 'triple play' regimen comprised of ischaemic, mechanical and pharmacologically induced postconditioning is a potentially beneficial intervention that demands further proof of concept exploration. Of course, all these physiological and mechanical topics require studies in the clinical scenario demonstrating feasibility and safety if mechanical postconditioning is going to be a therapeutic option in the future.

References

1. Murry CE, Jennings RB, Reimer KA. Preconditioning with ischemia: a delay of lethal cell injury in ischemic myocardium. *Circulation* 1986;**74**:1124–1136.
2. Hausenloy DJ, Wynne AM, Yellon DM Ischemic preconditioning targets the reperfusion phase. *Basic Res Cardiol* 2007;**102**:445–452.
3. Zhao ZQ, Corvera JS, Halkos ME, *et al.* Inhibition of myocardial injury by ischemic postconditioning during reperfusion: comparison with ischemic preconditioning. *Am J Physiol* 2003;**285**:H579–H588.
4. Kerendi F, Kin H, Halkos ME, *et al.* Remote postconditioning. Brief renal ischemia and reperfusion applied before coronary artery reperfusion reduces myocardial infarct size via endogenous activation of adenosine receptors. *Basic Res Cardiol* 2005;**100**:404–412.
5. Zhao ZQ, Vinten-Johansen J. Myocardial apoptosis and ischemic preconditioning. *Cardiovasc Res* 2002;**55**:438–455.
6. Bolli R, Marban E. Molecular and cellular mechanisms of myocardial stunning. *Physiol Rev* 1999;**79**:609–634.
7. Ovize M, Przyklenk K, Hale SL, Kloner RA. Preconditioning does not attenuate myocardial stunning. *Circulation* 1992;**85**:2247–2254.
8. Cohen MV, Yang XM, Neumann T, Heusch G, Downey JM. Favorable remodeling enhances recovery of regional myocardial function in the weeks after infarction in ischemically preconditioned hearts. *Circulation* 2000;**102**:579–583.
9. Cohen MV, Yang XM, Downey JM. Smaller infarct after preconditioning does not predict extent of early functional improvement of reperfused heart. *Am J Physiol* 1999;**277**: H1754–H1761.
10. Shiki K, Hearse DJ. Preconditioning of ischemic myocardium: reperfusion-induced arrhythmias. *Am J Physiol* 1987;**253**: H1470–H1476.
11. Ovize M, Aupetit JF, Rioufol G, *et al.* Preconditioning reduces infarct size but accelerates time to ventricular fibrillation in ischemic pig heart. *Am J Physiol* 1995;**269**:H72–H79.
12. Przyklenk K, Kloner RA. Preconditioning: a balanced perspective. *Br Heart J* 1995;**74**:575–577.
13. Parikh V, Singh M. Possible role of adrenergic component and cardiac mast cell degranulation in preconditioning-induced cardioprotection. *Pharmacol Res* 1999;**40**:129–137.
14. Shome S, Lux RL, Punske BB, MacLeod RS. Ischemic preconditioning protects against arrhythmogenesis through maintenance of both active as well as passive electrical properties in ischemic canine hearts. *J Electrocardiol* 2007;**40**:S150–S159.
15. Gross GJ. The role of mitochondrial K_{ATP} channels in the antiarrhythmic effects of ischaemic preconditioning in dogs. *Br J Pharmacol* 2002;**137**:939–940.
16. Vegh A, Parratt JR. The role of mitochondrial K_{ATP} channels in antiarrhythmic effects of ischaemic preconditioning in dogs. *Br J Pharmacol* 2002;**137**:1107–1115.
17. Driamov SV, Bellahcene M, Butz S, Buser PT, Zaugg CE. Bradykinin is a mediator, but unlikely a trigger, of antiarrhythmic effects of ischemic preconditioning. *J Cardiovasc Electrophysiol* 2007;**18**:93–99.
18. Botsford MW, Lukas A. Ischemic preconditioning and arrhythmogenesis in the rabbit heart: effects on epicardium versus endocardium. *J Mol Cell Cardiol* 1998;**30**:1723–1733.
19. Ravingerova T, Pancza D, Ziegelhoffer A, Styk J. Preconditioning modulates susceptibility to ischemia-induced arrhythmias in the rat heart: the role of alpha-adrenergic stimulation and K_{ATP} channels. *Physiol Res* 2002;**51**:109–119.
20. Ravingerova T, Matejikova J, Neckar J, Andelova E, Kolar F. Differential role of PIP3K/Akt pathway in the infarct size limitation and antiarrhythmic protection in the rat heart. *Mol Cell Biochem* 2007;**297**:111–120.
21. Ravingerova T, Matejikova J, Pancza D, Kolar F. Reduced susceptibility to ischemia-induced arrhythmias in the preconditioned rat heart is independent of PI3-kinase/Akt. *Physiol Res* 2009;**58**:443–447.
22. Driamov S, Bellahcene M, Ziegler A, *et al.* Antiarrhythmic effect of ischemic preconditioning during low-flow ischemia. The role of bradykinin and sarcolemmal versus mitochondrial ATP-sensitive K^+ channels. *Basic Res Cardiol* 2004;**99**:299–308.
23. Matejikova J, Kucharska J, Pinterova M, Pancza D, Ravingerova T. Protection against ischemia-induced ventricular arrhythmias and myocardial dysfunction conferred by preconditioning in the rat heart: involvement of mitochondrial K_{ATP} channels and reactive oxygen species. *Physiol Res* 2009;**58**:9–19.

24. Cinca J, Warren M, Carreno A, *et al.* Changes in myocardial electrical impedance induced by coronary artery occlusion in pigs with and without preconditioning: correlation with local ST-segment potential and ventricular arrhythmias. *Circulation* 1997;**96**:3079–3086.

25. Papp R, Gonczi M, Kovacs M, Seprenyi G, Vegh A. Gap junctional uncoupling plays a trigger role in the antiarrhythmic effect of ischaemic preconditioning. *Cardiovasc Res* 2007;**74**:396–405.

26. Okishige K, Yamashita K, Yoshinaga H, *et al.* Electrophysiologic effects of ischemic preconditioning on QT dispersion during coronary angioplasty. *J Am Coll Cardiol* 1996;**28**:70–73.

27. Vegh A, Szekeres L, Parratt JR. Transient ischaemia induced by rapid cardiac pacing results in myocardial preconditioning. *Cardiovasc Res* 1991;**25**:1051–1053.

28. Koning MM, Gho BC, van Klaarwater E, Opstal RL, Duncker DJ, Verdouw PD. Rapid ventricular pacing produces myocardial protection by nonischemic activation of K_{ATP}^+ channels. *Circulation* 1996;**93**:178–186.

29. Domenech RJ, Macho P, Velez D, Sanchez G, Liu X, Dhalla N. Tachycardia preconditions infarct size in dogs: role of adenosine and protein kinase C. *Circulation* 1998;**97**:786–794.

30. Szilvassy Z, Ferdinandy P, Bor P, Jakab I, Lonovics J, Koltai M. Ventricular overdrive pacing-induced anti-ischemic effect: a conscious rabbit model of preconditioning. *Am J Physiol* 1994;**266**:H2033–H2041.

31. Kaszala K, Vegh A, Papp JG, Parratt JR. Modification by bradykinin B2 receptor blockade of protection by pacing against ischaemia-induced arrhythmias. *Eur J Pharmacol* 1997;**328**:51–60.

32. Takeda S, Satoh T, Osada M, Komori S, Mochizuki S, Tamura K. Protective effect of pacing on reperfusion-induced ventricular arrhythmias in isolated rat hearts. *Can J Cardiol* 1995;**11**:573–579.

33. Hearse DJ, Ferrari R, Sutherland FJ. Cardioprotection: intermittent ventricular fibrillation and rapid pacing can induce preconditioning in the blood-perfused rat heart. *J Mol Cell Cardiol* 1999;**31**:1961–1973.

34. Kis A, Vegh A, Papp J, Parratt J. Pacing-induced delayed protection against arrhythmias is attenuated by aminoguanidine, an inhibitor of nitric oxide synthase. *Br J Pharmacol* 1999;**127**:1545–1550.

35. Macho P, Solis E, Sanchez G, Schwarze H, Domenech R. Mitochondrial ATP dependent potassium channels mediate non-ischemic preconditioning by tachycardia in dogs. *Mol Cell Biochem* 2001;**216**:129–136.

36. Vanagt WY, Cornelussen RN, Poulina QP, *et al.* Pacing-induced dys-synchrony preconditions rabbit myocardium against ischemia/reperfusion injury. *Circulation* 2006;**114**:1264–1269.

37. Ovize M, Kloner RA, Przyklenk K. Stretch preconditions canine myocardium. *Am J Physiol* 1994;**266**:H137–H146.

38. Przyklenk K, Bauer B, Ovize M, Kloner RA, Whittaker P. Regional ischemic 'preconditioning' protects remote virgin myocardium from subsequent sustained coronary occlusion. *Circulation* 1993;**87**:893–899.

39. Gysembergh A, Margonari H, Loufoua J, *et al.* Stretch-induced protection shares a common mechanism with ischemic preconditioning in rabbit heart. *Am J Physiol* 1998;**274**:H955–H964.

40. Mosca SM. Cardioprotective effects of stretch are mediated by activation of sarcolemmal, not mitochondrial, ATP-sensitive potassium channels. *Am J Physiol* 2007;**293**:H1007–H1012.

41. Van Wagoner DR, Lamorgese M. Ischemia potentiates the mechanosensitive modulation of atrial ATP-sensitive potassium channels. *Ann N Y Acad Sci* 1994;**72**:392–395.

42. Kohl P, Bollensdorff C, Garny A. Effects of mechanosensitive ion channels on ventricular electrophysiology: experimental and theoretical models. *Exp Physiol* 2006;**91**:307–321.

43. Yellon DM, Alkhulaifi AM, Pugsley WB. Preconditioning the human myocardium. *Lancet* 1993;**342**:276–277.

44. Walsh SR, Tang TY, Kullar P, Jenkins DP, Dutka DP, Gaunt ME. Ischaemic preconditioning during cardiac surgery: systematic review and meta-analysis of perioperative outcomes in randomised clinical trials. *Eur J Cardiothorac Surg* 2008;**34**:985–994.

45. Ali ZA, Callaghan CJ, Lim E, *et al.* Remote ischemic preconditioning reduces myocardial and renal injury after elective abdominal aortic aneurysm repair: a randomized controlled trial. *Circulation* 2007;**116**:I98–I105.

46. Edwards RJ, Redwood SR, Lambiase PD, Tomset E, Rakhit RD, Marber MS. Antiarrhythmic and anti-ischaemic effects of angina in patients with and without coronary collaterals. *Heart* 2002;**88**:604–610.

47. Wu ZK, Iivainen T, Pehkonen E, Laurikka J, Tarkka MR. Ischemic preconditioning suppresses ventricular tachyarrhythmias after myocardial revascularization. *Circulation* 2002;**106**:3091–3096.

48. Granfeldt A, Lefer DJ, Vinten-Johansen J. Protective Ischemia in Patients: Preconditioning and Postconditioning. *Cardiovasc Res* 2009;**83**:234–246.

49. Galagudza M, Kurapeev D, Minasian S, Valen G, Vaage J. Ischemic postconditioning: brief ischemia during reperfusion converts persistent ventricular fibrillation into regular rhythm. *Eur J Cardiothorac Surg* 2004;**25**:1006–1010.

50. Dow J, Bhandari A, Kloner RA. Ischemic postconditioning's benefit on reperfusion ventricular arrhythmias is maintained in the senescent heart. *J Cardiovasc Pharmacol Ther* 2008;**13**:141–148.

51. Mykytenko J, Reeves JG, Kin H, *et al.* Persistent beneficial effect of postconditioning against infarct size: role of mitochondrial K_{ATP} channels during reperfusion. *Basic Res Cardiol* 2008;**103**:472–484.

52. Manning AS, Hearse DJ. Reperfusion-induced arrhythmias: mechanisms and prevention. *J Mol Cell Cardiol* 1984;**16**:497–518.

53. Sun HY, Wang NP, Kerendi F, *et al.* Hypoxic postconditioning reduces cardiomyocyte loss by inhibiting ROS generation and intracellular Ca^{2+} overload. *Am J Physiol* 2005;**288**:H1900–H1908.

54. Penna C, Tullio F, Merlino A, *et al.* Postconditioning cardioprotection against infarct size and post-ischemic systolic dysfunction is influenced by gender. *Basic Res Cardiol* 2009;**104**:390–402.

55. Vinten-Johansen J, Zhao ZQ, Jiang R, Zatta AJ, Dobson GP. Preconditioning and postconditioning: innate cardioprotection from ischemia-reperfusion injury. *J Appl Physiol* 2007;**103**:1441–1448.

56. Couvreur N, Lucats L, Tissier R, Bize A, Berdeaux A, Ghaleh B. Differential effects of postconditioning on myocardial stunning and infarction: a study in conscious dogs and anesthetized rabbits. *Am J Physiol* 2006;**291**:H1345–H1350.

57. Kin H, Zatta AJ, Lofye MT, *et al.* Postconditioning reduces infarct size via adenosine receptor activation by endogenous adenosine. *Cardiovasc Res* 2005;**67**:124–133.

58. Tawa M, Fukumoto T, Yamashita N, *et al.* Postconditioning improves post ischemic cardiac dysfunction independently of norepinephrine overflow after reperfusion in rat hearts: comparison with preconditioning. *J Cardiovasc Pharmacol* 2010;**55**:6–13.

59. Mykytenko J, Kerendi F, Reeves JG, *et al.* Long-term inhibition of myocardial infarction by postconditioning during reperfusion. *Basic Res Cardiol* 2007;**102**:90–100.

60. Vinten-Johansen J, Zhao ZQ, Jiang R, Zatta AJ, Dobson GP. Preconditioning and postconditioning: innate cardioprotection from ischemia-reperfusion injury. *J Appl Physiol* 2007;**103**:1441–1448.

61. Vanagt WY, Cornelussen RN, Baynham TC, *et al.* Pacing-induced dyssynchrony during early reperfusion reduces infarct size. *J Am Coll Cardiol* 2007;**49**:1813–1819.

62. Babiker FA, Vanagt WY, Delhaas T, Waltenberger J, Cleutjens J, Prinzen F. Exploration of the mechanisms of pacing postconditioning. *Circulation* 2009;**120**:S870.

63. Staat P, Rioufol G, Piot C, *et al.* Postconditioning the human heart. *Circulation* 2005;**112**:2143–2148.

64. Luo W, Li B, Lin G, Huang R. Postconditioning in cardiac surgery for tetralogy of Fallot. *J Thorac Cardiovasc Surg* 2007;**133**:1373–1374.

65. Luo W, Li B, Chen R, Huang R, Lin G. Effect of ischemic postconditioning in adult valve replacement. *Eur J Cardiothorac Surg* 2008;**33**:203–208.

66. Sadat U, Varty K. Preconditioning or postconditioning in hepatic surgery. *Arch Surg* 2008;**143**:1026.

67. Thibault H, Piot C, Staat P, *et al.* Long-Term Benefit of Postconditioning. *Circulation.* 2008;**117**:1037–1044.

68. Iliodromitis EK, Zoga A, Vrettou A, *et al.* The effectiveness of postconditioning and preconditioning on infarct size in hypercholesterolemic and normal anesthetized rabbits. *Atherosclerosis* 2006;**188**:356–362.

69. Yang XC, Liu Y, Wang LF, *et al.* Reduction in myocardial infarct size by postconditioning in patients after percutaneous coronary intervention. *J Invasive Cardiol* 2007;**19**:424–430.

70. Hansen PR, Thibault H, Abdulla J. Postconditioning during primary percutaneous coronary intervention: A review and meta-analysis. *Int J Cardiol* .2010;**144**:22–25.

SECTION 4

Integrated model systems to study specific cases of cardiac MEC and arrhythmias

28. **Mechano-electric coupling in chronic atrial fibrillation** 203
Ulrich Schotten

29. **Mechanically induced pulmonary vein ectopy: insight from animal models** 212
Omer Berenfeld

30. **Regional variation in mechano-electric coupling: the right ventricle** 217
Ed White, David Benoist and Olivier Bernus

31. **Mechanical induction of arrhythmia in the *ex situ* heart: insight into *Commotio cordis*** 223
Frank Bode and Michael R. Franz

32. **Arrhythmias in murine models of the mechanically impaired heart** 227
Larissa Fabritz and Paulus Kirchhof

33. **Studying cardiac mechano-sensitivity in man** 234
Flavia Ravelli and Michela Masè

34. **Mathematical models of cardiac structure and function: mechanistic insights from models of heart failure** 241
Vicky Y. Wang, Martyn P. Nash, Ian J. LeGrice, Alistair A. Young, Bruce H. Smaill and Peter J. Hunter

35. **Mathematical models of human atrial mechano-electric coupling and arrhythmias** 251
Elizabeth M. Cherry

36. **Mathematical models of ventricular mechano-electric coupling and arrhythmia** 258
Natalia A. Trayanova, Viatcheslav Gurev, Jason Constantino and Yuxuan Hu

Mechano-electric coupling in chronic atrial fibrillation

Ulrich Schotten

Background

Ever since atrial fibrillation (AF) was first described as a clinical entity by Arthur Cushny in 1907, it was recognized that AF has a tendency to become more stable with time[1]. In most patients, both frequency and duration of AF episodes increase until the arrhythmia becomes persistent. During the last two decades the self-perpetuating and progressive nature of AF have attracted the attention of an increasing number of researchers. They have tried to understand how AF is initiated, how it is sustained and why it progresses from paroxysmal to persistent.

In 1995, two groups reported changes of the atrial electrophysiological properties as a consequence of AF. In a dog model of prolonged rapid atrial pacing Morillo *et al.* found that the atrial refractory period was reduced by about 15%[2]. In goats with artificially maintained AF, atrial refractoriness shortened from ~150 to ~80 ms (−45%)[3]. More importantly, in both studies a pronounced increase of the stability of AF was found which, at first glance, might be attributed to the shortening of the wavelength due to the abbreviated refractory period[3].

However, since shortening of the refractory period and the time course of AF to become persistent did not run parallel we suggested the existence of additional positive feedback loops in AF (Fig. 28.1)[4]. In this scheme atrial stretch and dilatation play a crucial role. On the one hand, atrial stretch and dilatation are the consequence of a loss of atrial contractility induced by AF; on the other hand, they serve as a trigger to start a deleterious structural remodelling process which leads to atrial connective tissue formation, fibrosis and conduction disturbances which stabilize the arrhythmia. Today, many researchers regard atrial dilatation as the most likely candidate to serve as a 'second factor'.

In clinical trials a relationship between atrial size and AF was established 50 years ago. In 1955 Fraser and Turner showed that left and right atrial enlargement correlated with the incidence of AF in patients with mitral valve disease[5]. Large prospective trials established left atrial enlargement as an independent risk factor for the development of AF[6,7]. Psaty *et al.* included about 5000 participants who were all in sinus rhythm in the Cardiovascular Health Study[8]. Left atrial size at baseline was strongly and independently associated with the incidence of AF during the follow-up of 3 years. In a recent study, left atrial size was (apart from age) even the only predictive parameter for the occurrence of AF in patients with mitral regurgitation. The data suggest that atrial dilatation may be a cause of AF, and it was proposed that 'interventions that maintain left atrial size may be important in the prevention of AF'[8].

On the other hand, atrial enlargement can also be a consequence of AF. Sanfilippo *et al.* performed in 1990 a small but prospective echocardiographic study in patients with AF, a normal atrial size at baseline and no evidence of other cardiac abnormalities[9]. After an average time of 20.6 months, left and right atrial volume was significantly increased.

None of these studies can establish a causal relationship between atrial dilatation and AF, but they convincingly demonstrate the mutual dependency of AF and atrial dilatation.

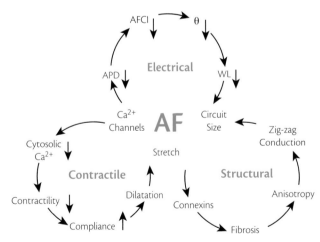

Fig. 28.1 Three proposed positive feedback loops of atrial remodelling on AF. Downregulation of the L-type Ca^{2+} channels is considered to be the primary cause for electrical and contractile remodelling. The loss of atrial contractility leads to an increase in compliance of the fibrillating atria which in turn facilitates atrial dilatation. The resulting stretch acts as a stimulus for structural remodelling of the enlarged atria. The combination of electrical and structural remodelling allows intra-atrial re-entrant circuits of a smaller size, due to a reduction in wavelength (shortening of refractoriness and slowing of conduction) and increased non-uniform tissue anisotropy (zig-zag conduction)[4]. AFC1, atrial fibrillation cycle length; APD, action potential duration; WL, wave length; θ, conduction speed. [Reproduced, with permission, from Allessie M, Ausma J, Schotten U (2002) Electrical, contractile and structural remodeling during atrial fibrillation. *Cardiovasc Res* **54**:230–246.]

Why do fibrillating atria dilate?

Atrial dilatation frequently occurs in patients with valve diseases, hypertension, coronary artery disease and heart failure. In these patients, atrial dilatation is mostly caused by increased mechanical load due to AV-valve regurgitation or increased end-diastolic ventricular pressures. Depending on the severity of the heart disease, up to 50% of these patients will develop AF. Once the atria fibrillate further dilatation might reflect progression of the underlying heart disease or the dilatation might be caused by AF itself. AF-related increase in atrial size is caused by several mechanisms. Two of them, loss of atrial contractility and changes in ventricular rate, are particularly important.

In chronically instrumented goats, we studied the effects of AF on atrial contractility, compliance and size using ultrasonic piezoelectric crystals to measure the mediolateral diameter of the atrium and with a tip pressure transducer in the right atrium. After 5 days of AF the amplitude of the pressure waves, and the atrial wall excursions during AF, were reduced to less than 15% of control, indicating that atrial contractility was nearly completely abolished. To study the effect of this loss of atrial contractility on the compliance of the fibrillating atrium, pressure and diameter were measured after unloading the atria with a fast-acting loop diuretic and after loading the atria with 1 L of saline infused within 10 min (Fig. 28.2)[10]. During the first days of AF, the compliance curve flattened, indicating that the compliance of the atrium increased. This caused a rightward shift of the working point and the mean atrial diameter increased by ~10%. The mean atrial pressure did not change throughout the experiment. The changes in atrial compliance and size followed the same time course as the loss of contractility of the fibrillating atria and were fully reversible within 2 days of sinus rhythm (SR) recovery. These data suggest that atrial dilatation during the first days of AF is a direct consequence of the loss of atrial contractility.

Echocardiographic studies have shown that atrial dilatation during AF is a progressive process which may continue for months to years[9]. In contrast, in our experimental studies, atrial contractile function was already almost completely abolished after a couple of days. Obviously, apart from the loss of atrial contractility, additional mechanisms are operative which cause the atria to dilate during prolonged AF. The loss of atrial contractility will transfer atrial stretch more to the passive elements of the atrial wall, which might lead to elongation of collagen fibres. Synthesis of connective tissue and cellular hypertrophy could also produce a slow increase in atrial dimensions.

An additional mechanism by which AF may induce atrial dilatation is the increase in ventricular rate. In most patients the ventricular rate during AF is higher than during sinus rhythm. It was suggested that inadequate ventricular rate response might result in reduced ventricular pump function which might explain impaired exercise tolerance both during AF as well as after cardioversion. While some authors suggested that decreased exercise capacity is due to the loss of atrial systole, van Gelder et al. demonstrated that reduced ventricular pump function is likely to underlie the poor exercise capacity that follows cardioversion of AF[11]. In patients without valvular heart disease, ejection fraction and exercise capacity significantly improved between 1 week and 1 month postcardioversion, whereas the atrial systole improved by week 1 and remained unchanged thereafter. This discrepancy in time course of

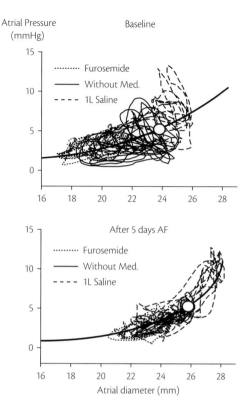

Fig. 28.2 Representative right atrial compliance curves during acute AF and after 3 or 5 days of AF in goat. The compliance was measured by unloading the atria with a rapidly acting loop-diuretic and loading by infusion of 1 L saline in 10 min. Due to an increase in atrial compliance at low atrial diameters (flattening of the compliance curve) the working point during AF shifted to the right (black circle)[10]. [Reproduced, with permission, from Schotten U, de Haan S, Neuberger HR, et al. (2004) Loss of atrial contractility is primary cause of atrial dilatation during first days of atrial fibrillation. Am J Physiol **287**:H2324–H2331.]

recovery suggests that an intrinsic left ventricular cardiomyopathy was present in these patients which gradually subsided after cardioversion. Elevated end-diastolic pressures might significantly contribute to the slow atrial dilatation process during AF.

Recent experimental data support an important role of ventricular rate in the modulation of atrial size. Both high and low ventricular rates can produce significant atrial dilatation (Fig. 28.3). In goats undergoing 4 weeks of rapid AV-sequential pacing at a cycle length of 250 ms, Schoonderwoerd et al. demonstrated pronounced atrial dilatation (+50%)[12]. This increase in atrial size was not due to the high atrial rate. In a control group the AV-node was ablated and the ventricles were paced at a cycle length of 750 ms. In this group, rapid atrial pacing alone did not change atrial size throughout 4 weeks. It rather appeared that progressive ventricular dysfunction was the cause of atrial dilatation in this model. When the ventricular rate is low, atrial dilatation probably results from the accumulation of blood in the atria during the long diastolic pauses. This applies cyclic stretch stimuli to the atria. In goats with chronic AV block (cycle length ~1,200 ms), Neuberger et al. reported atrial dilatation of ~12% in 4 weeks[13]. Regardless of whether atrial dilatation was produced by too high or too low ventricular rates, the increased atrial size went along with a pronounced increase in the stability of AF in both studies.

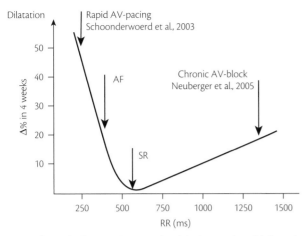

Fig. 28.3 Relationship between RR-interval and the increase in atrial dimensions in goats. Ventricular rates, both too high and too low, result in progressive atrial dilatation. High ventricular rates cause a tachycardiomyopathy with ventricular dilatation and elevated end diastolic pressures[12]. Slow rates result in cyclic stretch stimuli during the long diastolic pauses[16]. The slow atrial dilatation during AF might in part be due to the fact that the ECG cycle (assessed by RR-interval) during AF is shorter than during sinus rhythm (SR).

Animal models of chronic atrial dilatation

Numerous studies have addressed the effect of atrial enlargement on atrial electrophysiology during the past two decades. In most of these investigations, the effect of acute atrial dilatation on atrial refractoriness and conduction was studied. These studies, however, had conflicting results. Acute atrial dilatation in isolated rabbit hearts or in open-chest dogs resulted in a shortening of atrial refractoriness. Others described no change, or even a prolongation, of the refractory period during acute stretch. The only common finding in most of these studies was an increase in the inducibility and persistence of AF.

The first experiments on chronic enlargement of the atria were performed in the early 1980s by Boyden *et al.* In eight dogs with tricuspid regurgitation and stenosis of the pulmonary artery, the right atrial volume increased by 40 % during ~100 days of follow-up[14]. Atrial arrhythmias did not occur spontaneously. However, the inducibility and the duration of artificially induced atrial tachyarrhythmias increased significantly. Atrial refractoriness was not measured, but the duration of action potentials recorded *in vitro* was not different compared to control. Histological and ultrastructural analysis revealed cardiac hypertrophy and an increase in connective tissue content. In another study in dogs with spontaneous mitral valve fibrosis (MVF) and left atrial enlargement, the authors also found no change in transmembrane potentials[15]. In the MVF dogs, left atrial volume was six to eight times that of control dogs. A large amount of connective tissue was found in between these hypertrophied atrial myocytes (17 vs 10 μm in diameter). Most MVF animals had spontaneous atrial arrhythmias, but the underlying mechanism could not be defined. The authors speculated that atrial conduction could be impaired.

To describe the chronological sequence of progressive atrial dilatation and its correlation with alterations in atrial electrophysiology, we studied goats with chronic complete AV block[16,17]. Within 4 weeks after the ablation, the atrial diameter was increased

by ~12%. Together with atrial dilatation, the duration of AF paroxysms increased from a few seconds during control to several hours. Since the atrial refractory period and the AF cycle length kept constant throughout 4 weeks of complete AV block, the increased persistence of AF could not be explained by a shortening of refractoriness. Instead, high density activation mapping revealed local conduction disturbances which most likely underlie enhanced persistence of AF in this model (Fig. 28.4). Interestingly, the extracellular matrix was not altered in this model, suggesting that atrial fibrosis does not form a necessary condition for increased AF vulnerability in dilated atria. Also, the expression of connexin 40 (Cx40) and connexin 43 (Cx43) did not show marked alterations. Rather, conduction disturbances were related to the degree of cellular hypertrophy.

Animal models of rapid-pacing-induced heart failure with atrial dilatation demonstrated either a prolongation of refractoriness[18,19] or no change[20]. In dogs with cardiomyopathy and pronounced atrial dilatation, AF paroxysms were prolonged and discrete regions of slow atrial conduction were found. The atrial myofibres were separated by thick layers of connective tissue, which may cause local conduction block during AF (Fig. 28.5)[20].

In dogs with mitral valve regurgitation produced by partial mitral valve avulsion, the left atria dilated by ~25% within 4 weeks after the operation[21]. Sustained AF (> 1 h) was not observed in control dogs but was inducible in 10 of 19 dogs with mitral regurgitation. In the left atria, pronounced atrial tissue fibrosis and inflammatory changes were found. In high resolution optical

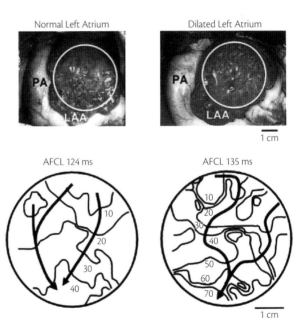

Fig. 28.4 Activation mapping in dilated atria of goats with 4 weeks of chronic complete AV block. After 4 weeks of AV block the atria are enlarged (25% increase in atrial volume). In the AV block goats, the conduction pattern is more complex and the incidence of slow conduction and conduction block is increased. LAA=left atrial appendage, AFCL= atrial fibrillation cycle length [Reproduced, with permission, from Neuberger HR, Schotten U, Blaauw Y, *et al.* (2006) Chronic atrial dilation, electrical remodeling, and atrial fibrillation in the goat. *J Am Coll Cardiol* **47**:644–653.]

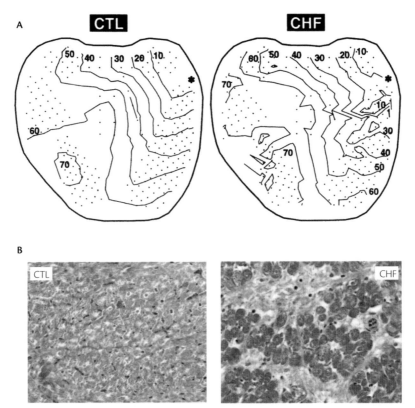

Fig. 28.5 A Activation map of the left atrium in dogs with (right) and without (left) tachycardiomyopathy induced by rapid ventricular pacing for 6 weeks. Crowding of isochrones indicates local slowing of conduction in the congestive heart failure (CHF) dog (lines represent 10 ms isochrones). **B** Light microscopy of atrial specimen in the same dogs as in **A**. Note cellular hypertrophy and accumulation of collagen in the CHF dog. Magnification ×1,250. CTL, control. [Reproduced, with permission, from Li D, Fareh S, Leung TK, Nattel S (1999) Promotion of atrial fibrillation by heart failure in dogs: atrial remodeling of a different sort. *Circulation* **100**:87–95.] (See color plate section.)

mapping experiments, AF was more complex than in control dogs[22]. Wavefronts occupied less of the field of view and there were large areas of slow conduction or block.

In a rabbit model, an arteriovenous shunt led to chronic overload with an estimated increase in left atrial surface area of 112%[23]. Atrial conduction velocity was significantly decreased by about 30%. The inducibility of AF was increased, and in the majority of cases the arrhythmias arose from the posterior left atrium, with either a focal pattern of origin or a single re-entrant circuit. In this model, the expression levels of both Cx40 and Cx43 protein were significantly reduced[24].

In summary, animal models have demonstrated that chronic atrial dilatation increases AF stability without shortening of refractoriness. The contribution of increased tissue mass is also probably limited. Atrial tissue fibrosis occurs in most but not all models of atrial dilatation. Cellular hypertrophy appears to be the only structural alteration all models of atrial dilatation have in common.

Cellular mechanisms of structural remodelling in chronically dilated atria

Acute stretch induces various changes of the atrial electrophysiology which are all transient and rapidly reversible. These changes include a shortening of the action potential duration, a depolarization of the resting membrane potential, the occurrence of early after-depolarizations and the generation of ectopic beats[25]. They are probably mediated by the activation of mechano-sensitive channels. Activation might provoke stretch-induced arrhythmias

through changes in excitability and refractoriness, or the occurrence of ectopic activity.

Chronic stretch not only induces changes in shape and duration of the atrial action potential, but also activates various intracellular signalling pathways in both myocytes and fibroblasts. This has a significant impact on atrial anatomy and structure at the microscopic and the macroscopic scale. These structural changes are often irreversible.

An overview of some of the pathways probably involved in atrial connective tissue formation and structural remodelling in fibrillating atria is shown in Fig. 28.6. An important step of structural remodelling of the atria caused by mechanical load is the induction of paracrine activity of the cardiomyocytes. In adult myocytes, stretch stimulates secretion of angiotensin II, endothelin-1 and atrial natriuretic peptide (ANP). These hormones activate the mitogen-activated protein kinase (MAPK) pathway, the janus kinase/signal transducers and activators of transcription pathway (JAK/STAT) as well as Ca^{2+}/calmodulin-dependent pathways[26]. Some MAPK activate extracellular signal regulated kinases (ERK-1 and ERK-2). All these pathways are known to promote cellular hypertrophy, to stimulate fibroblast proliferation and to activate matrix protein synthesis leading to tissue fibrosis[27]. Interestingly, activation of the local rennin–angiotensin system and ERK occurs within hours of the onset of rapid ventricular pacing indicating that stretch-induced signalling occurs much faster than the development of the structural damage in the atria (Fig. 28.7).

Pacing-induced ventricular failure also increased atrial transforming growth factor β (TGF-β) and platelet-derived growth

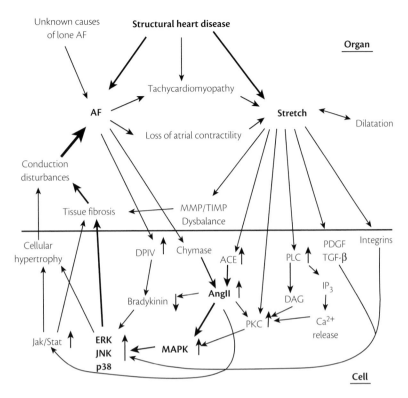

Fig. 28.6 Complexity of the pathophysiological network underlying structural remodelling caused by or finally resulting in AF. Blockade of a single pathway may not be sufficient to effectively and permanently prevent structural remodelling of the atria. See text for details and abbreviations.

factor (PDGF) levels. Atrial fibroblasts are activated significantly faster than ventricular fibroblast in the chronic heart failure (CHF) models, explaining the rapid and more severe degree of interstitial fibrosis in the atria[28]. PDGF appeared to play a particularly important role. The elimination of atrial-ventricular fibroblast response differences to TGF-β suggests that a substantial part of the differential cell type-specific response is mediated by PDGF, probably because of preferential atrial expression of both PDGF and the PDGF receptor.

Studies clearly suggest that oxidative stress contributes to atrial remodelling in CHF models[29]. The peroxisome proliferator-activated receptor-γ (PPAR-γ) activator pioglitazone antagonizes angiotensin II actions and possesses anti-inflammatory and anti-oxidant properties. Pioglitazone attenuated CHF-induced atrial structural remodelling and AF vulnerability[30]. In the same study, both pioglitazone and candesartan reduced TGF-β, TNF-α and MAPK, but neither affected p38-kinase or c-Jun N-terminal kinase activation. In contrast, ω-3 polyunsaturated fatty acids attenuate CHF-related phosphorylation of the MAPK, ERK and p38[31].

Stretch also stimulates phospholipase C directly, and via angiotensin II[32]. Phospholipase C generates inositol-1,4,5-triphosphate (IP3) and diacylglycerol (DAG). IP3-induced release of Ca^{2+} from intracellular stores and DAG stimulate protein kinase C. Protein kinase C in turn activates ERKs.

There is increasing evidence that the renin–angiotensin system and its downstream signalling pathways are activated in atrial myocardium of patients with chronic AF. The protein expression of angiotensin converting enzyme (ACE) and ERK-1 and 2 is upregulated[33]. Fibroblasts seem to be the source of increased amounts of ERK in the atrial tissue of AF patients. The angiotensin II type 1

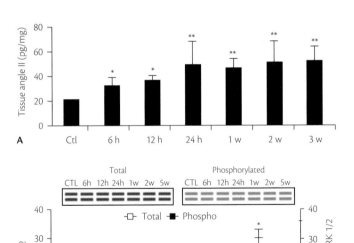

Fig. 28.7 Time course of angiotensin II elevation (**A**) and ERK activation (**B**) after the onset of rapid ventricular pacing in dogs. The local rennin–angiotensin system becomes activated within 24 h resulting in rapid activation of ERK[34].
[Reproduced, with permission, from Cardin S, Li D, Thorin-Trescases N, Leung TK, Thorin E, Nattel S (2003) Evolution of the atrial fibrillation substrate in experimental congestive heart failure: angiotensin-dependent and -independent pathways. *Cardiovasc Res* **60**:315–325.]

receptor (AT-I) is downregulated, whereas the angiotensin II type 2 receptor (AT-II) is upregulated, both probably reflecting feedback mechanisms to prevent excessive stimulation of the angiotensin system[33]. In dogs with heart failure, the amount of activated ERK could be significantly reduced by blockade of the angiotensin system[34]. Both ACE and DPIV, a serine protease, catalyze the release of N-terminal dipeptides. This contributes to the degradation of bradykinin. Bradykinin has cardioprotective effects, by which it diminishes the development of interstitial fibrosis. DPIV activity has been shown to be enhanced in fibrillating atrial tissue[35]. The increase in atrial ACE activity acts synergistically with increased DPIV activity to lower atrial bradykinin levels, which further stimulates atrial connective tissue formation[27].

Stretch can also activate ERK-1 and ERK-2 independent of angiotensin II by stimulation of integrins[27]. Integrins are stretch-sensitive trans-membrane adhesion molecules that are anchored in the extracellular matrix. A short cytoplasmic tail binds to adaptor proteins which interact with intracellular kinases and cytoskeleton proteins. Integrins can transfer stretch stimuli to the cytosol of the cardiomyocytes resulting in activation of focal adhesion kinases (FAK), which in turn activate ERKs. Thus, angiotensin II and stretch-induced activation of integrins stimulate common downstream signalling cascades. Also, angiotensin II upregulates integrin expression and FAK activity, indicating close cross-talk between these pathways. It has been suggested that membrane-bound metalloproteinases called ADAM (A desintegrin and metalloprotease) interact with integrins in atrial tissue. The desintegrin activity of these enzymes loosens the tight junctions of cardiomyocytes to the surrounding extracellular matrix. In patients with chronic AF, ADAM-10 and ADAM-15 are upregulated[36]. Progressive loss of integrins might therefore enhance sliding and slippage of cells and contribute to dilatation of fibrillating atria. Whether the signalling function of integrins is altered in fibrillating or dilated atria is not known[36].

Atrial stretch is also associated with an altered expression of matrix metalloproteinases (MMP). MMP are a large group of enzymes that function to break down the extracellular matrix. Patients with persistent AF show decreased atrial expression/activity of MMP-1 and increased tissue inhibitor of metalloproteinase (TIMP)-1 levels[37,38]. In AF patients with congestive heart failure, an increased collagen I fraction appears to be associated with upregulation of MMP-2 and downregulation of TIMP-1[39,40]. These apparent discrepancies could be explained by temporal changes in MMP function and the presence of concomitant cardiac diseases (valvular regurgitation, heart failure, etc.), which have a substantial effect on atrial MMP expression[41].

How does atrial dilatation promote AF?

Atrial dilatation *per se* might promote AF because more re-entrant circuits can co-exist on the atrial surface area. Since in many animal models the degree of atrial dilatation is modest but AF vulnerability and stability are significantly increased, it does not seem likely that the larger mean surface area contributes much to the increased stability of AF. The consensus is that stretch-induced tissue fibrosis promotes AF in dilated atria. In fibrotic myocardium, the macroscopic conduction velocity is slowed by microscopic zigzagging circuits or depressed propagation in branching muscle bundles[42]. This electro-anatomical substrate permits multiple small re-entrant circuits that can stabilize the arrhythmia[43]. Multiple entry and exit points, and multiple sites at which unidirectional block occurs, will shift the balance between generation and extinction of wavelets to favour the generation of new wavefronts. Also, fibrosis will tend to increase electrophysiological dispersion[44]. While the scarred matrix will transfer stretch primarily to the adjacent atrial myocardium, other regions might even become shielded by surrounding strands of connective tissue. Unequal atrial stretch has been shown to differentially affect the local refractory period depending on the degree of elongation of the atrial muscle fibres[45]. Therefore, tissue fibrosis will increase not only anisotropy in conduction but also the dispersion in refractoriness. Cellular hypertrophy increases the complexity of the substrate even more, since in hypertrophied myocytes, smaller mechanical stimuli are sufficient to activate stretch-activated channels[46]. Also, conduction transverse to the cell orientation might be slowed by cellular hypertrophy[47].

Chronic atrial stretch might also contribute to initiation and perpetuation of AF by enhancing triggered activity in the atria. In dogs with congestive heart failure, focal atrial tachycardia was inducible by rapid atrial pacing[48,49]. This atrial tachycardia showed repetitive focal spread of activation from the crista terminalis in both endocardial and epicardial mapping experiments. In a comparable model, congestive heart failure produced changes of the Ca^{2+} homeostasis which are expected to favour triggered activity. The load of the sarcoplasmic reticulum was enhanced and spontaneous Ca^{2+} release from the sarcoplasmic reticulum was more frequently observed than in control dogs[50]. Radial spread of activation indeed occurs more often in structurally remodelled atria. However, this phenomenon might also reflect dyssynchronous activation of the epicardial layer and the endocardial bundle network, occasionally resulting in transmural conduction of fibrillation wavefronts[51].

Finally, the development of such an electro-anatomical substrate would also explain the loss of efficacy of drugs to cardiovert AF. In discontinuous tissue the safety factor for conduction is higher than in normal tissue[52]. Thus, a higher degree of fast sodium current () blockade is required to terminate AF. Anatomical obstacles might widen the excitable gap during AF, making drugs that prolong atrial refractoriness less effective[53]. Also, multiple sites at which unidirectional block occurs might facilitate reinduction of AF immediately after cardioversion by early premature beats.

Therefore, new experimental strategies put more emphasis on the prevention of structural remodelling. During past years, a variety of compounds interacting with the described signalling pathways have been shown to prevent or delay the development of a substrate of AF in different animal models. Among these compounds are ACE inhibitors[34,54,55], AT-I-receptor antagonists[56], spironolactone[57], statins[58] and ω-3 polyunsaturated fatty acids[31]. Clinical trials are in favour of a beneficial effect of 'upstream therapy' targets on atrial remodelling and AF in patients with and without structural heart disease[59–64].

Of note, ACE-independent pathways exist in the heart that convert angiotensin I to angiotensin II. In the human heart, a considerable percentage of angiotensin II is formed by tissue chymase. In patients undergoing cardiac transplantation, tissue chymase even accounts for up to 75% of total cardiac angiotensin II-forming enzyme activity. Inhibition of cardiac chymase has been demonstrated to suppress collagen synthesis and to reduce the degree of fibrosis in human failing myocardium. Thus, the mechanisms finally resulting in tissue fibrosis and hypertrophy form a complex network involving parallel intracellular cascades and a variety of neurohumoral pathways. The observation that ACE inhibitors do not necessarily prevent atrial fibrosis in patients with chronic AF[65], or in dogs with heart failure[34], possibly reflects the complexity of the mechanisms that control connective tissue formation. The results also suggest that blockade of single pathways may not be sufficient to prevent, or delay, structural remodelling in dilated atria.

Conclusions and outlook

Numerous clinical investigations as well as recent experimental studies have demonstrated that AF is a progressive arrhythmia. With time, paroxysmal AF becomes persistent and the success rate of cardioversion of persistent AF declines. Electrical remodelling (shortening of atrial refractoriness) develops within the first days of AF and contributes to the increase in stability of the arrhythmia. However, 'domestication of AF' must also depend on other mechanisms since the persistence of AF continues to increase after electrical remodelling has been completed. Atrial dilatation is a promising candidate to serve as such a 'second factor'. Loss of atrial contractility during AF enhances atrial dilatation by increasing the compliance of the fibrillating atrium. Alternatively, the increase of the ventricular rate during AF might compromise left ventricular pump function and thus promote atrial dilatation in some patients with AF. Chronic atrial stretch induces activation of numerous signalling pathways leading to cellular hypertrophy, fibroblast proliferation and tissue fibrosis. The resulting electro-anatomical substrate in dilated atria is characterized by increased non-uniform anisotropy and macroscopic slowing of conduction, promoting re-entrant circuits in the atria. Prevention of electro-anatomical remodelling by blockade of pathways activated by chronic atrial stretch therefore has become the focus of research on future strategies for the management of AF.

References

1. Cushny AR, Edmunds CW. Paroxysmal irregularity of the heart in auricular fibrillation. *Am J Med Sci* 1907;**133**:66–77.
2. Morillo CA, Klein GJ, Jones DL, Guiraudon CM. Chronic rapid atrial pacing. Structural, functional, and electrophysiological characteristics of a new model of sustained atrial fibrillation. *Circulation* 1995;**91**:1588–1595.
3. Wijffels MC, Kirchhof CJ, Dorland R, Allessie MA. Atrial fibrillation begets atrial fibrillation. A study in awake chronically instrumented goats. *Circulation* 1995;**92**:1954–1968.
4. Allessie M, Ausma J, Schotten U. Electrical, contractile and structural remodeling during atrial fibrillation. *Cardiovasc Res* 2002;**54**:230–246.
5. Fraser HR, Turner RW. Auricular fibrillation; with special reference to rheumatic heart disease. *Br Med J* 1955;**2**:1414–1418.
6. Vasan RS, Larson MG, Levy D, Evans JC, Benjamin EJ. Distribution and categorization of echocardiographic measurements in relation to reference limits: the Framingham Heart Study: formulation of a height- and sex-specific classification and its prospective validation. *Circulation* 1997;**96**:1863–1873.
7. Vaziri SM, Larson MG, Benjamin EJ, Levy D. Echocardiographic predictors of nonrheumatic atrial fibrillation. The Framingham Heart Study. *Circulation* 1994;**89**:724–730.
8. Psaty BM, Manolio TA, Kuller LH, *et al.* Incidence of and risk factors for atrial fibrillation in older adults. *Circulation* 1997;**96**:2455–2461.

9. Sanfilippo AJ, Abascal VM, Sheehan M, *et al.* Atrial enlargement as a consequence of atrial fibrillation. A prospective echocardiographic study. *Circulation* 1990;**82**:792–797.
10. Schotten U, de Haan S, Neuberger HR, Eijsbouts S, Blaauw Y, Tieleman R, Allessie M. Loss of atrial contractility is primary cause of atrial dilatation during first days of atrial fibrillation. *Am J Physiol* 2004;**287**:H2324–H2331.
11. Van Gelder IC, Crijns HJ, Blanksma PK, *et al.* Time course of hemodynamic changes and improvement of exercise tolerance after cardioversion of chronic atrial fibrillation unassociated with cardiac valve disease. *Am J Cardiol* 1993;**72**:560–566.
12. Schoonderwoerd BA, Van Gelder IC, van Veldhuisen DJ, *et al.* Electrical remodeling and atrial dilation during atrial tachycardia are influenced by ventricular rate: role of developing tachycardiomyopathy. *J Cardiovasc Electrophysiol* 2001;**12**:1404–1410.
13. Neuberger HR, Schotten U, Ausma J, *et al.* Atrial remodeling in the goat due to chronic complete atrioventricular block. *Eur Heart J* 2002;**23**:136.
14. Boyden PA, Hoffman BF. The effects on atrial electrophysiology and structure of surgically induced right atrial enlargement in dogs. *Circ Res* 1981;**49**:1319–1331.
15. Boyden PA, Tilley LP, Pham TD, Liu SK, Fenoglic JJ, Jr., Wit AL. Effects of left atrial enlargement on atrial transmembrane potentials and structure in dogs with mitral valve fibrosis. *Am J Cardiol* 1982;**49**:1896–1908.
16. Neuberger HR, Schotten U, Verheule S, Eijsbouts S, Blaauw Y, van Hunnik A, Allessie M. Development of a substrate of atrial fibrillation during chronic atrioventricular block in the goat. *Circulation* 2005;**111**:30–37.
17. Neuberger HR, Schotten U, Blaauw Y, Vollmann D, Eijsbouts S, van Hunnik A, Allessie M. Chronic atrial dilation, electrical remodeling, and atrial fibrillation in the goat. *J Am Coll Cardiol* 2006;**47**:644–653.
18. Power JM, Beacom GA, Alferness CA, Raman J, Farish SJ, Tonkin AM. Effects of left atrial dilatation on the endocardial atrial defibrillation threshold: a study in an ovine model of pacing induced dilated cardiomyopathy. *Pacing Clin Electrophysiol* 1998;**21**:1595–1600.
19. Power JM, Beacom GA, Alferness CA, *et al.* Susceptibility to atrial fibrillation: a study in an ovine model of pacing-induced early heart failure. *J Cardiovasc Electrophysiol* 1998;**9**:423–435.
20. Li D, Fareh S, Leung TK, Nattel S. Promotion of atrial fibrillation by heart failure in dogs: atrial remodeling of a different sort. *Circulation* 1999;**100**:87–95.
21. Verheule S, Wilson E, Everett Tt, Shanbhag S, Golden C, Olgin J. Alterations in atrial electrophysiology and tissue structure in a canine model of chronic atrial dilatation due to mitral regurgitation. *Circulation* 2003;**107**:2615–2622.
22. Everett THt, Verheule S, Wilson EE, Foreman S, Olgin JE. Left atrial dilatation resulting from chronic mitral regurgitation decreases spatiotemporal organization of atrial fibrillation in left atrium. *Am J Physiol* 2004;**286**:H2452–H2460.
23. Hirose M, Takeishi Y, Miyamoto T, Kubota I, Laurita KR, Chiba S. Mechanism for atrial tachyarrhythmia in chronic volume overload-induced dilated atria. *J Cardiovasc Electrophysiol* 2005;**16**:760–769.
24. Haugan K, Miyamoto T, Takeishi Y, Kubota I, Nakayama J, Shimojo H, Hirose M. Rotigaptide (ZP123) improves atrial conduction slowing in chronic volume overload-induced dilated atria. *Basic Clin Pharmacol Toxicol* 2006;**99**:71–79.
25. Franz MR. Mechano-electrical feedback. *Cardiovasc Res* 2000;**45**:263–266.
26. Ruwhof C, van der Laarse A. Mechanical stress-induced cardiac hypertrophy: mechanisms and signal transduction pathways. *Cardiovasc Res* 2000;**47**:23–37.

27. Goette A, Lendeckel U, Klein HU. Signal transduction systems and atrial fibrillation. *Cardiovasc Res* 2002;**54**:247–258.

28. Burstein B LE, Calderone A, Nattel S. Differential behaviors of atrial versus ventricular fibroblasts: a potential role for platelet-derived growth factor in atrial-ventricular remodeling differences. *Circulation* 2008;**117**:1630–1641.

29. Cha YM DP, Shen WK, Jahangir A, Hart CY, Terzic A, Redfield MM. Failing atrial myocardium: energetic deficits accompany structural remodeling and electrical instability. *Am J Physiol* 2003;**284**: H1313–H1320.

30. Shimano M TY, Inden Y, Kitamura K, Uchikawa T, Harata S, Nattel S, Murohara T. Pioglitazone, a peroxisome proliferator-activated receptor-gamma activator, attenuates atrial fibrosis and atrial fibrillation promotion in rabbits with congestive heart failure. *Heart Rhythm* 2008;**5**:451–459.

31. Sakabe M, Shiroshita-Takeshita A, Maguy A, Dumesnil C, Nigam A, Leung TK, Nattel S. Omega-3 polyunsaturated fatty acids prevent atrial fibrillation associated with heart failure but not atrial tachycardia remodeling. *Circulation* 2007;**116**:2101–2109.

32. Sadoshima J, Izumo S. The cellular and molecular response of cardiac myocytes to mechanical stress. *Annu Rev Physiol* 1997;**59**: 551–571.

33. Goette A, Staack T, Rocken C, et al. Increased expression of extracellular signal-regulated kinase and angiotensin-converting enzyme in human atria during atrial fibrillation. *J Am Coll Cardiol* 2000;**35**:1669–1677.

34. Cardin S, Li D, Thorin-Trescases N, Leung TK, Thorin E, Nattel S. Evolution of the atrial fibrillation substrate in experimental congestive heart failure: angiotensin-dependent and -independent pathways. *Cardiovasc Res* 2003;**60**:315–325.

35. Lendeckel U, Arndt M, Wrenger S, et al. Expression and activity of ectopeptidases in fibrillating human atria. *J Mol Cell Cardiol* 2001;**33**:1273–1281.

36. Arndt M, Lendeckel U, Rocken C, et al. Altered expression of ADAMs (A Disintegrin And Metalloproteinase) in fibrillating human atria. *Circulation* 2002;**105**:720–725.

37. Goette ARC, Nepple K, Lendeckel U (2003) Proteases and arrhythmias. In: *Proteases in Tissue Remodelling of Lung and Heart* (ed. UHN Lendeckel). Kluwer Academic, Plenum Publishers, Dordrecht, pp. 191–218.

38. Marin F RV, Climent V, Garcia A, Marco P, Lip GYH. Is thrombogenesis in atrial fibrillation related to matrix metalloproteinase-1 and ist inhibitor, TIMP-1? *Stroke* 2003;**34**:1181–1186.

39. Xu J, Cui G, Esmailian F, et al. Atrial extracellular matrix remodeling and the maintenance of atrial fibrillation. *Circulation* 2004;**109**: 363–368.

40. Cooradi D CS, Benussi S, Nascimbene S, et al. Regional left atrial interstitial remodeling in patients with chronic atrial fibrillation undergoing mitral-valve surgery. *Virchows Arch* 2004;**445**: 498–505.

41. Anne W, Willems R, Roskams T, et al. Matrix metalloproteinases and atrial remodeling in patients with mitral valve disease and atrial fibrillation. *Cardiovasc Res* 2005;**67**:655–666.

42. de Bakker JM, van Capelle FJ, Janse MJ, Tasseron S, Vermeulen JT, de Jonge N, Lahpor JR. Slow conduction in the infarcted human heart. 'zigzag' course of activation. *Circulation* 1993;**88**:915–926.

43. Spach MS, Josephson ME. Initiating reentry: the role of nonuniform anisotropy in small circuits. *J Cardiovasc Electrophysiol* 1994;**5**: 182–209.

44. Allessie MA, Boyden PA, Camm AJ, et al. Pathophysiology and prevention of atrial fibrillation. *Circulation* 2001;**103**:769–777.

45. Satoh T, Zipes DP. Unequal atrial stretch in dogs increases dispersion of refractoriness conducive to developing atrial fibrillation. *J Cardiovasc Electrophysiol* 1996;**7**:833–842.

46. Kamkin A, Kiseleva I, Isenberg G. Stretch-activated currents in ventricular myocytes: amplitude and arrhythmogenic effects increase with hypertrophy *Cardiovasc Res* 2000;**48**:409–420.

47. Spach MS, Heidlage JF, Dolber PC, Barr RC. Changes in anisotropic conduction caused by remodeling cell size and the cellular distribution of gap junctions and Na+ channels. *J Electrocardiol* 2001;**34** Suppl: 69–76.

48. Fenelon G, Shepard RK, Stambler BS. Focal origin of atrial tachycardia in dogs with rapid ventricular pacing-induced heart failure. *J Cardiovasc Electrophysiol* 2003;**14**:1093–1102.

49. Ryu K, Shroff SC, Sahadevan J, Martovitz NL, Khrestian CM, Stambler BS. Mapping of atrial activation during sustained atrial fibrillation in dogs with rapid ventricular pacing induced heart failure: evidence for a role of driver regions. *J Cardiovasc Electrophysiol* 2005;**16**:1348–1358.

50. Yeh YH, Wakili R, Qi XY, et al. Calcium-handling abnormalities underlying atrial arrhythmogenesis and contractile dysfunction in dogs with congestive heart failure. *Circ Arrhythm Electrophysiol* 2008;**1**: 93–102.

51. Eckstein J, Verheule S, de Groot NM, Allessie M, Schotten U. Mechanisms of perpetuation of atrial fibrillation in chronically dilated atria. *Prog Biophys Mol Biol* 2008;**97**:435–451.

52. Shaw RM, Rudy Y. Ionic mechanisms of propagation in cardiac tissue. Roles of the sodium and L-type calcium currents during reduced excitability and decreased gap junction coupling. *Circ Res* 1997;**81**: 727–741.

53. Girouard SD, Pastore JM, Laurita KR, Gregory KW, Rosenbaum DS. Optical mapping in a new guinea pig model of ventricular tachycardia reveals mechanisms for multiple wavelengths in a single reentrant circuit. *Circulation* 1996;**93**:603–613.

54. Li D, Shinagawa K, Pang L, Leung TK, Cardin S, Wang Z, Nattel S. Effects of angiotensin-converting enzyme inhibition on the development of the atrial fibrillation substrate in dogs with ventricular tachypacing-induced congestive heart failure. *Circulation* 2001;**104**:2608–2614.

55. Li Y, Li W, Yang B, Han W, Dong D, Xue J, Li B, Yang S, Sheng L. Effects of Cilazapril on atrial electrical, structural and functional remodeling in atrial fibrillation dogs. *J Electrocardiol* 2007;**40**:100 e101–e106.

56. Kumagai K, Nakashima H, Urata H, Gondo N, Arakawa K, Saku K. Effects of angiotensin II type 1 receptor antagonist on electrical and structural remodeling in atrial fibrillation. *J Am Coll Cardiol* 2003;**41**:2197–2204.

57. Milliez P, Deangelis N, Rucker-Martin C, et al. Spironolactone reduces fibrosis of dilated atria during heart failure in rats with myocardial infarction. *Eur Heart J* 2005;**26**:2193–2199.

58. Shiroshita-Takeshita A, Brundel BJ, Burstein B, Leung TK, Mitamura H, Ogawa S, Nattel S. Effects of simvastatin on the development of the atrial fibrillation substrate in dogs with congestive heart failure. *Cardiovasc Res* 2007;**74**:75–84.

59. Pedersen OD, Bagger H, Kober L, Torp-Pedersen C. Trandolapril reduces the incidence of atrial fibrillation after acute myocardial infarction in patients with left ventricular dysfunction. *Circulation* 1999;**100**:376–380.

60. Vermes E TJ, Bourassa MG, Racine N, Levesque S, White M, Guerra PG, Ducharme A. Enalapril decreases the incidence of atrial fibrillation in patients with left ventricular dysfunction: insight from the Studies Of Left Ventricular Dysfunction (SOLVD) trials. *Circulation* 2003;**107**:2926–2931.

61. Hansson L LL, Niskanen L, Lanke J, et al. Effect of angiotensin-converting-enzyme inhibition compared with conventional therapy on cardiovascular morbidity and mortality in hypertension: the Captopril Prevention Project (CAPPP) randomised trial. *Lancet* 1999;**353**: 611–616.

62. Young-Xu Y JS, Goldberg R, Blatt CM, Graboys T, Bilchik B, Ravid S. Usefulness of statin drugs in protecting against atrial fibrillation in patients with coronary artery disease. *Am J Cardiol* 2003;**92**: 1379–1383.

63. Marín F PD, Roldán V, Arribas JM, *et al.* Statins and postoperative risk of atrial fibrillation following coronary artery bypass grafting. *Am J Cardiol* 2006;**97**:55–60.

64. Lertsburapa K WC, Kluger J, Faheem O, Hammond J, Coleman CI. Preoperative statins for the prevention of atrial fibrillation after cardiothoracic surgery. *J Thorac Cardiovasc Surg* 2008;**135**:405–411.

65. Hirayama Y, Atarashi H, Kobayashi Y, Takano T. Angiotensin-converting enzyme inhibitors are not effective at inhibiting further fibrous changes in the atria in patients with chronic atrial fibrillation: speculation from analysis of the time course of fibrillary wave amplitudes. *Jpn Heart J* 2004;**45**:93–101.

Mechanically induced pulmonary vein ectopy: insight from animal models

Omer Berenfeld

Background

The pulmonary veins (PV) and the anatomical region surrounding their entrance into the left atrium were found to play an important role in the initiation and maintenance of atrial fibrillation (AF), which is the most common sustained arrhythmia. High-resolution mapping data and Fourier power spectrum analysis with its dominant frequency (DF) recently published by our group support the hypothesis that acute AF in the structurally normal sheep heart[1–6] and in some patients[7] is not a totally random phenomenon. These data are consistent with the widely accepted notion that paroxysmal AF in patients is initiated by focal triggers localized in one or more PV[8] and is accessible to catheter-based ablation procedures[9]. On the other hand, in persistent AF the prevailing theory is that multiple random wavelets of activation coexist to create a chaotic cardiac rhythm[10], and that AF ablative therapy is more challenging[11–14].

Our studies on the cholinergic AF in isolated sheep hearts show the importance of the left atrium and particularly the PV as the site with highest DF and source of the arrhythmia maintenance[4,5,15]. Mandapati et al. analyzed the DF distribution across the atria in 35 episodes of AF and found that in 66% of all those episodes, ≥ 2 sites had the highest DF[4]. As shown in Fig. 29.1, in the 35 AF episodes analyzed, the region surrounding the PV ostium had the highest DF in 80% of AF episodes. Other sites having the highest DF in a particular AF episode decreased in their percentage toward the right atrium free wall (only 4%). Our findings of the PV activity during acute cholinergic AF in sheep isolated hearts were consistent with the study of Wu et al.[16] who recorded electrical activity from the atria, the ligament of Marshall and the PV in the canine model of AF. In that study it was found that the mean cycle length during sustained AF induced in dogs subjected to chronic rapid pacing was shorter in the PV compared with those in the left atrial free wall (LAFW)[16].

Increased intra-atrial pressure and atrial fibrillation dynamics

Atrial dilation has been found to be an independent risk factor for the development of AF[17–19], maybe through mechano-electric feedback[20]. To get a mechanistic insight into the role of stretch in AF we employed yet another sheep model of sustained AF under conditions of acutely increased intra-atrial pressure (IAP) to explore the AF dynamics and to test the hypothesis that dilation induces arrhythmogenic sources at the superior PV during AF[21]. A pressure of 10 cm H_2O was found to be the lower limit to obtain sustained AF episodes. In comparison, below 10 cm H_2O AF usually terminates after 10–20 min[21].

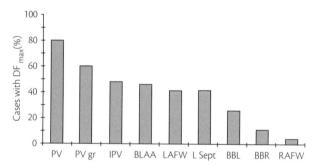

Fig. 29.1 Spatial distribution of highest DF (DF$_{max}$) expressed as a percentage of AF episodes ($n = 35$). PV, pulmonary veins; PV gr, groove between LA and PV ostium; IPV, region inferior to PV ostium; BLAA, base of LA appendage; LAFW, pseudo-electrogram calculated from LA free wall fluorescence imaging data; L Sept, left septum; BBL, left side of Bachmann's bundle; BBR, right side of Bachmann's bundle; RAFW, right atrium free wall. [Reproduced, with permission, from Mandapati R, Skanes A, Chen J, Berenfeld O, Jalife J (2000) Stable microreentrant sources as a mechanism of atrial fibrillation in the isolated sheep heart. *Circulation* **101**:194–199.]

As in our studies on cholinergic AF presented above, frequency analysis was used to characterize the organization of activity during AF[2,6] and to establish the likelihood of localizing sources maintaining the AF from which propagation is originating[5]. Figure 44.1 (see Chapter 44) clearly illustrates the strong dependence of AF frequency in the LAFW and the LA superior PV junction (JPV) on IAP. Below 10 cm H_2O, the difference between the maximum dominant frequency (DF_{Max}) in the JPV and LAFW was not significant (10.8 ± 0.3 vs 10.2 ± 0.3; $P = 0.6$; Fig. 44.1C). However, at pressures > 10 cm H_2O, DF_{Max} in the JPV was significantly higher than that in LAFW (12.0 ± 0.2 and 10.5 ± 0.2 Hz, respectively; mean $\pm$ SEM; $n = 9$; $P < 0.001$; see also representative single-pixel recordings in Fig. 44.1D). At all pressures, DF_{Max} in both JPV and LAFW was significantly higher than the largest frequency recorded in the right atrial free wall (7.8 ± 0.3 Hz; $P < 0.001$).

Propagation of waves in AF may be highly periodic, both spatially and temporally[1]. Such spatio-temporal periodicities (STP) may take various forms, including periodic waves emerging from the edge of the recording field, breakthroughs occurring at constant frequencies and, in some cases, stable rotors[1]. We found similar STP waves in high IAP-associated AF. In Fig. 44.1E we show quantification of directionality of STP electrical activation as a function of the IAP during AF. Clearly, the direction of propagation from left superior PV (LSPV) to LAFW (grey symbols) was very consistent. In all experiments the directionality of local excitation in the JPV area that corresponded to the highest frequencies correlated strongly with IAP ($r = 0.79$, $P = 0.02$; Fig. 44.1E). In contrast, the directionality of LAFW to LSPV had a negative and statistically non-significant correlation with pressure ($r = 0.54$, $P = 0.09$). These data are particularly valuable when one considers that there is evidence that in patients with paroxysmal AF, the diameters of the superior PV ostia are markedly dilated compared with the inferior PV ostia[22], particularly when considered as arrhythmogenic PV[23]. Our data demonstrate that the sources of rapid atrial activation during stretch-related AF are located in the PV region and that their level of spatio-temporal organization correlates with pressure.

The structure and function of the pulmonary veins

The PV are composed of a variety of tissues, including cardiomyocyte sleeves along with an outermost covering connective tissue that surrounds the veins (tunica adventitia), a middle layer (media) and an innermost layer (intima). In humans, myocardial continuity from the left atrial wall extending to the outer surface of the pulmonary venous walls is well recognized[24]. In guinea pigs the middle layer of the pulmonary vein is made up of cardiac muscle at the proximal end joining the atria and smooth muscle at the distal intrapulmonary end[25]. At the atrial muscle–smooth muscle junction located about 4 mm intrapulmonarily, there is a drastic reduction in vessel diameter from more than 0.8 mm at the cardiac portion to about 0.4 mm at the smooth muscle portion. Brunton and Fayrer first reported in 1876 that independent pulsation of the PV (suggestive of electrical activity) occurred in cats and rabbits even after activity of the heart had ceased[26].

Using intracellular micro-electrode recordings in isolated preparations of the PV and the adjacent atrial tissue from guinea pigs, Cheung showed in 1981 heterogeneous electrophysiology with different resting membrane potentials, responses to stimuli and automaticity between these two regions[25,27]. Spontaneous pulsative beating of the atrial PV synchronous with atrial contraction was observed when a guinea pig thoracic wall was opened up and when the lungs were removed together with the heart for experimentation[25].

In 7 out of 17 isolated guinea pig PV studied by Cheung[25], spontaneous activity was observed (Fig. 29.2; see also Chapter 15). The frequency of the spontaneous activity was variable but was usually maintained at about 0.5 Hz, which is significantly lower than the normal heart rate of that species at 230–380 beats per minute (about 3.8–4.7 Hz). The origin of spontaneous activity was observed at the distal end of the atrial PV. Cells at this region displayed prominent pace-making activity (Fig. 29.2B). The maximal diastolic potential was 66.36 ± 3.2 mV ($n = 22$) and the action potentials had small depolarization overshoots. The transition from diastolic depolarization to the upstroke of action potential (i.e. the foot of the action potential) was smooth and slow. There was a gradual change in the electrical characteristics in cells from the distal region to cells more proximal to the atria. Figure 29.2C demonstrates the activity of a cell 1.6 mm from the cell in panel B. This cell had a higher membrane potential as well as a larger overshoot. Small diastolic depolarization was still present between action potentials. However, the transition from pace-making potential to action potential was more abrupt, suggesting that this cell was a bystander to a propagating action potential originating

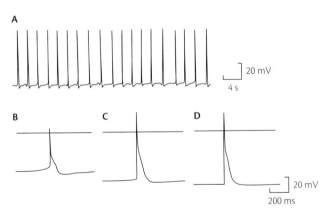

Fig. 29.2 A Spontaneous electrical activity of the isolated pulmonary vein. Some small membrane oscillations were present between action potentials in this cell. **B–D** show spontaneous activity recorded at three different sites in the same preparation. **B** was recorded at the distal end of the cardiac PV. Note the small overshoot of the action potential and the low and unstable membrane potential. **C** was recorded 1–6 mm from **B**. The membrane potential of **C** was higher although diastolic depolarization was still present. The transition from diastolic depolarization to the upstroke of the action potential was abrupt, unlike that of **B**. The overshoot of the action potential was over 25 mV. **D** was 4 mm from **B**. The membrane potential was stable between action potentials with little diastolic depolarization. [Reproduced, with permission, from Cheung DW (1981) Electrical activity of the pulmonary vein and its interaction with the right atrium in the guinea-pig. *J Physiol* **314**:445–456.]

from other sites. Cells further away from the pace-making region showed little diastolic depolarization between action potentials (Fig. 29.2D). The maximal diastolic potential of cells proximal to the atria averaged at 72.5±2.34 mV ($n = 20$).

Chen et al.[28] studied isolated canine and rabbit PV and also found initially very rapid and low amplitude spiking activity of unknown mechanism in tissue beyond the end of the cardiomyocyte sleeve. In a subsequent study Chen et al.[29] showed that cardiomyocytes isolated from normal canine and rabbit PV can manifest automaticity, as well as after-depolarizations, which are enhanced by recognized atrial profibrillatory manoeuvres such as chronic atrial tachy-pacing and in vitro exposure to thyroid hormone by unknown mechanisms[30,31]. Miyauchi et al.[32] showed that heterogeneous PV repolarization properties are associated with the propensity to early after-depolarizations and triggered activity initiation by isoproteranol and rapid pacing. These observations add to the possible mechanisms rendering the PV vulnerable to arrhythmogenesis, such as marked tissue anisotropy[33], Ca^{2+}-handling[34,35] and arrhythmogenic response to local autonomic activity[36]. Indeed, compared with LA myocytes, PV sleeve cardiomyocytes display distinct electrophysiological properties including differences in the expression of several ionic currents[37], including potassium channels[38]. As AF in the clinical setting has been associated with atrial dilation Seol et al.[39] characterized stretch-activated currents in cardiomyocytes isolated from rabbit PV (see Chapter 15). This study found distinct currents induced by swelling versus axial mechanical stretching of the myocytes. Both types of stretching induced anionic and non-selective cationic currents obeying a positive monotonic current–voltage (I–V) relationship, although the cationic currents activated faster than the anionic currents and were likely mediated through different channels[39].

Stretch and ectopic activity in the pulmonary veins

From the foregoing it is evident that under acute stretch in sheep isolated hearts AF displays an increasing number of waves originating at the junction of the posterior LA wall and the LSPV[21] which may be explained in part by increased incidence of ectopic activity in the PV. Chang et al.[40] investigated this proposition by studying the effect of stretch on preparations of rabbit PV tissue isolated from rabbits. One end of the preparation (about 10 mm long), consisting of the LA–PV junction, was pinned to the bottom of a tissue bath. The other end was connected to a force transducer with silk thread[40]. To investigate the effects of different tensions on the PV, the trans-membrane action potentials were recorded before and after successive stretch by microelectrodes at more than 20 sites in the PV myocardial sleeve[28,40].

In 23 isolated pulmonary vein preparations, 5 showed spontaneous activity before the stretch. After exposure to a 100 mg load, 11 PV developed spontaneous activity, while a 300 mg stretch initiated spontaneous activity in 19 PV[40]. Figure 29.3A shows an example of such stretch-induced occurrences of the spontaneous activity. Elevating the tension across the PV preparation from 0 to 300 mg resulted in the induction of spontaneous electrical activation concomitantly with transient mechanical twitches. Figure 29.3B shows another example in which the stretch force increased the firing rates in a PV. While in this case even in the absence of

tension spontaneous firing was observed, the increase in tension to 100 and further to 300 mg induced a clear monotonic increase in the frequency of the spontaneous firing. In Fig. 29.3C cumulative data show that on average the frequency of the spontaneous firing was about 1.75 Hz in the absence of stretch and that that frequency increased significantly to about 2 and 3 Hz with increasing tension to 100 and 300 mg, respectively. The overall percentage of activity was also shown to increase monotonically with tension (Fig. 29.3D). When single action potentials in PV preparations were studied Chang et al. found that their amplitude and duration decreased with increasing stretch; however, the incidence of early and delayed after-depolarizations in the PV increased with tension force, which may explain the stretch-induced increase in the occurrence of their spontaneous firing[40].

To further elucidate on the possible role of stretch in the occurrence of the spontaneous firing non-selective stretch-activated channel (SAC_{NS})blockers gadolinium and streptomycin were used to study the electrical activity in the veins and compared with the L-type calcium channel blocker verapamil effect[41–43]. The only specific SAC_{NS} blocker, GsMTx-4, found in the venom of the tarantula Grammostola spatulata, effectively reverses the effects of stretch on burst-pacing-induced AF[44]. In the study of Chang et al.[40], both gadolinium and streptomycin could inhibit the stretch-induced automaticity in the PV and triggered activity in a dose-dependent manner (see also Chapter 65). The reversal of stretch-induced shortening of the duration of the action potential by gadolinium may also prevent the genesis of micro-re-entrant circuits in the PV. Although gadolinium also inhibits the L-type calcium channel, the relatively lesser effects of verapamil on the stretch-induced electrical activity of the PV compared with gadolinium and streptomycin indicate that these results are mainly caused by the SAC_{NS} blockade[40]. This mechanism is also suggested by the findings that gadolinium did not suppress the electrical activity of the PV before the stretch.

Conclusions and outlook

There is experimental evidence that increasing stretch increases the dominance of the PV during AF in isolated hearts[4,21] and ectopic activity in the isolated PV[40], but the ionic mechanisms underlying such effect are not clear and the ability of the PV to favourably host functional re-entry during stretch cannot be excluded[4,21]. In single cardiomyocytes isolated from the PV of rabbits Seol et al. recently found stretch-induced anionic and cationic currents[39]; however, it is not clear whether the dominance of the PV in the initiation and maintenance of AF depends on spatial heterogeneity in the distribution of those currents, or alternatively in the relative increase in stretch due to the relatively thinner myocardial wall in the PV sleeve compared with the walls of the atria[39,45]. In view of the high propensity of normal PV as assessed by these studies for generating ectopic activity an important question that arises is what prevents paroxysmal AF from being even more commonly present in the population compared with its already high rate. It is possible that additional insults or specific clinical pathology are needed to unmask that latent vulnerability under in vivo conditions[46]. Thus the manner by which the mechano-electric coupling effects in the PV become important in the initiation and maintenance of AF will require further detailed investigation.

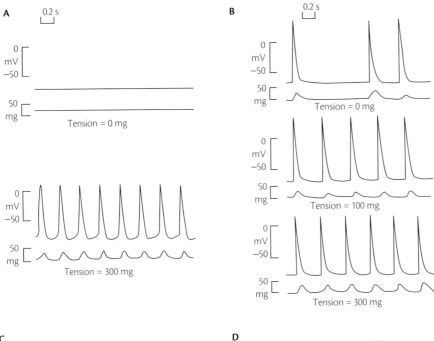

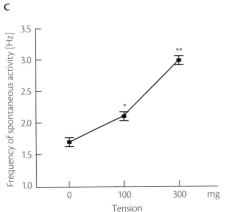

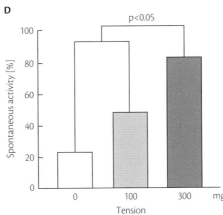

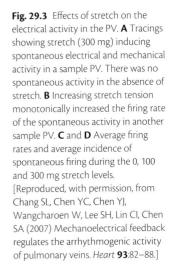

Fig. 29.3 Effects of stretch on the electrical activity in the PV. **A** Tracings showing stretch (300 mg) inducing spontaneous electrical and mechanical activity in a sample PV. There was no spontaneous activity in the absence of stretch. **B** Increasing stretch tension monotonically increased the firing rate of the spontaneous activity in another sample PV. **C** and **D** Average firing rates and average incidence of spontaneous firing during the 0, 100 and 300 mg stretch levels. [Reproduced, with permission, from Chang SL, Chen YC, Chen YJ, Wangcharoen W, Lee SH, Lin CI, Chen SA (2007) Mechanoelectrical feedback regulates the arrhythmogenic activity of pulmonary veins. *Heart* **93**:82–88.]

References

1. Skanes AC, Mandapati R, Berenfeld O, Davidenko JM, Jalife J. patiotemporal periodicity during atrial fibrillation in the isolated sheep heart. *Circulation* 1998;**98**:1236–1248.

2. Berenfeld O, Mandapati R, Dixit S, *et al.* Spatially distributed dominant excitation frequencies reveal hidden organization in atrial fibrillation in the Langendorff-perfused sheep heart. *J Cardiovasc Electrophysiol* 2000;**11**:869–879.

3. Chen J, Mandapati R, Berenfeld O, Skanes AC, Gray RA, Jalife J. Dynamics of wavelets and their role in atrial fibrillation in the isolated sheep heart. *Cardiovasc Res* 2000;**48**:220–232.

4. Mandapati R, Skanes A, Chen J, Berenfeld O, Jalife J. Stable microreentrant sources as a mechanism of atrial fibrillation in the isolated sheep heart. *Circulation* 2000;**101**:194–199.

5. Mansour M, Mandapati R, Berenfeld O, Chen J, Samie FH, Jalife J. Left-to-right gradient of atrial frequencies during acute atrial fibrillation in the isolated sheep heart. *Circulation* 2001;**103**:2631–2636.

6. Berenfeld O, Zaitsev AV, Mironov SF, Pertsov AM, Jalife J. Frequency-dependent breakdown of wave propagation into fibrillatory conduction across the pectinate muscle network in the isolated sheep right atrium. *Circ Res* 2002;**90**:1173–1180.

7. Sanders P, Berenfeld O, Hocini M, *et al.* Spectral analysis identifies sites of high-frequency activity maintaining atrial fibrillation in humans. *Circulation* 2005;**112**:789–797.

8. Haissaguerre M, Jais P, Shah DC, *et al.* Spontaneous initiation of atrial fibrillation by ectopic beats originating in the pulmonary veins. *N Eng J Med* 1998;**339**:659–666.

9. Haissaguerre M, Shah DC, Jais P, *et al.* Mapping-guided ablation of pulmonary veins to cure atrial fibrillation. *Am J Cardiol* 2000;**86**: 9K–19K.

10. Moe GK, Abildskov JA. Atrial fibrillation as a self-sustaining arrhythmia independent of focal discharges. *Am Heart J* 1959;**58**: 59–70.

11. Haissaguerre M, Jais P, Shah DC, *et al.* Catheter ablation of chronic atrial fibrillation targeting the reinitiating triggers. *J Cardiovasc Electrophysiol* 2000;**11**:2–10.

12. Benussi S, Pappone C, Nascimbene S, *et al.* A simple way to treat chronic atrial fibrillation during mitral valve surgery: the epicardial radiofrequency approach. *Europ J Cardio-Thoracic Surg* 2000;**17**:524–529.

13. Knight BP, Weiss R, Bahu M, *et al.* Cost comparison of radiofrequency modification and ablation of the atrioventricular junction in patients with chronic atrial fibrillation. *Circulation* 1997;**96**:1532–1536.

14. Oral H, Pappone C, Chugh A, *et al.* Circumferential pulmonary-vein ablation for chronic atrial fibrillation. *N Engl J Med* 2006;**354**:934–941.

15. Jalife J, Berenfeld O, Mansour M. Mother rotors and fibrillatory conduction: a mechanism of atrial fibrillation. *Cardiovasc Res* 2002;**54**:204–216.

16. Wu TJ, Ong JJC, Chang CM, *et al.* Pulmonary veins and ligament of Marshall as sources of rapid activations in a canine model of sustained atrial fibrillation. *Circulation* 2001;**103**:1157–1163.

17. Vaziri SM, Larson MG, Benjamin EJ, Levy D. Echocardiographic predictors of nonrheumatic atrial fibrillation. The Framingham Heart Study. *Circulation* 1994;**89**:724–730.

18. Psaty BM, Manolio TA, Kuller LH, *et al.* Incidence of and risk factors for atrial fibrillation in older adults. *Circulation* 1997;**96**: 2455–2461.

19. Vasan RS, Larson MG, Levy D, Evans JC, Benjamin EJ. Distribution and categorization of echocardiographic measurements in relation to reference limits: the Framingham Heart Study: formulation of a height- and sex-specific classification and its prospective validation. *Circulation* 1997;**96**:1863–1873.

20. Schotten U, Neuberger HR, Allessie MA. The role of atrial dilatation in the domestication of atrial fibrillation. *Prog Biophys Mol Biol* 2003;**82**:151–162.

21. Kalifa J, Jalife J, Zaitsev AV, *et al.* Intra-atrial pressure increases rate and organization of waves emanating from the superior pulmonary veins during atrial fibrillation. *Circulation* 2003;**108**:668–671.

22. Lin WS, Prakash VS, Tai CT, *et al.* Pulmonary vein morphology in patients with paroxysmal atrial fibrillation initiated by ectopic beats originating from the pulmonary veins: implications for catheter ablation. *Circulation* 2000;**101**:1274–1281.

23. Yamane T, Shah DC, Jais P, *et al.* Dilatation as a marker of pulmonary veins initiating atrial fibrillation. *J Intervent Cardiac Electrophysiol* 2002;**6**:245–249.

24. de Bakker JMT, Ho SY, Hocini M. Basic and clinical electrophysiology of pulmonary vein ectopy. *Cardiovasc Res* 2002;**54**:287–294.

25. Cheung DW. Electrical activity of the pulmonary vein and its interaction with the right atrium in the guinea-pig. *J Physiol* 1981;**314**:445–456.

26. Brunton TL, Fayrer J. Note on independent pulsation of the pulmonary veins and vena cava. *Proc R Soc Lond* 1876;**25**:174–176.

27. Cheung DW. Pulmonary vein as an ectopic focus in digitalis-induced arrhythmia. *Nature* 1981;**294**:582–584.

28. Chen YJ, Chen SA, Chang MS, Lin CI. Arrhythmogenic activity of cardiac muscle in pulmonary veins of the dog: implication for the genesis of atrial fibrillation. *Cardiovasc Res* 2000;**48**:265–273.

29. Chen YJ, Chen SA, Chen YC, Yeh HL, Chan P, Chang MS, Lin CI. Effects of rapid atrial pacing on the arrhythmogenic activity of single cardiomyocytes from pulmonary veins - Implication in initiation of atrial fibrillation. *Circulation* 2001;**104**:2849–2854.

30. Cha TJ, Ehrlich JR, Zhang L, Chartier D, Leung TK, Nattel S. Atrial Tachycardia Remodeling of Pulmonary Vein Cardiomyocytes: Comparison With Left Atrium and Potential Relation to Arrhythmogenesis. *Circulation* 2005;**111**:728–735.

31. Chen YC, Chen SA, Chen YJ, Chang MS, Chan P, Lin CI. Effects of thyroid hormone on the arrhythmogenic activity of pulmonary vein cardiomyocytes. *J Am Coll Cardiol* 2002;**39**:366–372.

32. Miyauchi Y, Hayashi H, Miyauchi M, Okuyama Y, Mandel WJ, Chen PS, Karagueuzian HS. Heterogeneous pulmonary vein myocardial cell repolarization implications for reentry and triggered activity. *Heart Rhythm* 2005;**2**:1339–1345.

33. Hocini M, Ho SY, Kawara T, *et al.* Electrical conduction in canine pulmonary veins - Electrophysiological and anatomic correlation. *Circulation* 2002;**105**:2442–2448.

34. Honjo H, Boyett MR, Niwa R, *et al.* Pacing-induced spontaneous activity in myocardial sleeves of pulmonary veins after treatment with ryanodine. *Circulation* 2003;**107**:1937–1943.

35. Patterson E, Lazzara R, Szabo B, *et al.* Sodium-calcium exchange initiated by the Ca^{2+} transient: an arrhythmia trigger within pulmonary veins. *J Am Coll Cardiol* 2006;**47**:1196–1206.

36. Patterson E, Po SS, Scherlag BJ, Lazzara R. Triggered firing in pulmonary veins initiated by in vitro autonomic nerve stimulation. *Heart Rhythm* 2005;**2**:624–631.

37. Ehrlich JR, Cha TJ, Zhang LM, Chartier D, Melnyk P, Hohnloser SH, Nattel S. Cellular electrophysiology of canine pulmonary vein cardiomyocytes: action potential and ionic current properties. *J Physiol* 2003;**551**:801–813.

38. Melnyk P, Ehrlich JR, Pourrier M, Villeneuve L, Cha TJ, Nattel S. Comparison of ion channel distribution and expression in cardiomyocytes of canine pulmonary veins versus left atrium. *Cardiovasc Res* 2005;**65**:104–116.

39. Seol CA, Kim WT, Ha JM, *et al.* Stretch-activated currents in cardiomyocytes isolated from rabbit pulmonary veins. *Prog Biophys Mol Biol* 2008;**97**:217–231.

40. Chang SL, Chen YC, Chen YJ, Wangcharoen W, Lee SH, Lin CI, Chen SA. Mechanoelectrical feedback regulates the arrhythmogenic activity of pulmonary veins. *Heart* 2007;**93**:82–88.

41. Bode F, Katchman A, Woosley RL, Franz MR. Gadolinium decreases stretch-induced vulnerability to atrial fibrillation. *Circulation* 2000;**101**: 2200–2205.

42. Tavi P, Laine M, Weckstrom M. Effect of gadolinium on stretch-induced changes in contraction and intracellularly recorded action- and afterpotentials of rat isolated atrium. *Br J Pharmacol* 1996;**118**: 407–413.

43. Gannier F, White E, Lacampagne A, Garnier D, Le Guennec JY. Streptomycin reverses a large stretch induced increases in $[Ca^{2+}]i$ in isolated guinea pig ventricular myocytes. *Cardiovasc Res* 1994;**28**: 1193–1198.

44. Bode F, Sachs F, Franz MR. Tarantula peptide inhibits atrial fibrillation. *Nature* 2001;**409**:35–36.

45. Nathan H, Eliakim M. The junction between the left atrium and the pulmonary veins. An anatomic study of human hearts. *Circulation* 1966;**34**:412–422.

46. Nattel S. Pulmonary vein cellular electrophysiology and atrial fibrillation: does basic research help us understand clinical pulmonary-vein arrhythmogenesis? *Heart Rhythm* 2005;**2**:1346.

Regional variation in mechano-electric coupling: the right ventricle

Ed White, David Benoist and Olivier Bernus

Background

The right ventricle (RV) is thinner walled and operates at lower pressures than the left ventricle (LV). Despite the fact that, according to the US National Institutes of Health, 1 in 20 may suffer from RV failure (RV failure is a common consequence of LV failure), it remains the case that the American Heart Association/American College of Cardiology practice guidelines offer no guidance for management of either acute or chronic RV failure, and no clinically orientated professional society has a published guideline specializing in RV failure[1]. Our knowledge of the role of mechanical stimulation in the normal and diseased right heart is less developed than for the left heart. This chapter describes how mechanical stimulation differs between the RV and LV and discusses relatively unexplored aspects of RV physiology that may play important roles in the response of the RV to stress and strain.

The right ventricle: a substrate for mechanically induced arrhythmias?

Right ventricular structure and function

The RV is understudied compared to the LV although the RV is both anatomically and functionally distinct from the LV and works under very different mechanical conditions. Specialized investigation of the RV is needed[2].

During embryonic development the RV is derived from the anterior or second heart field while the LV is derived from the first[3]. Within the chest cavity the RV is anteriorly positioned relative to the LV (see below). In the adult heart the RV has three distinct regions: the inlet region; the apical myocardium, which is highly trabecularized; and the RV outflow tract (RVOT), which is also referred to as the *conus* or *infundibulum*. This is a smooth region that connects to the pulmonary artery. The orientation of the RV myocardial fibres tends to be oblique in the sub-epicardial regions and longitudinal in the sub-endocardium[4]. The contraction of the RV has less of a twisting motion than the LV[5].

While the LV is ellipsoid in shape, the RV is crescent shaped in cross-section. This shape has important implications regarding the ratio of surface area to volume during filling and ejection, and because of this the Frank–Starling mechanism plays a significant role. The RV undergoes a larger change in volume for a given change in surface area than the LV. It ejects blood to the lungs in an almost continuous manner at low pressure, in contrast to the high pressure pulsatile flow generated by the LV. Typical RV ventricular pressures are 25/4 mmHg compared to 130/80 mmHg in the LV. Consistent with these lower operating pressures the RV is thin walled (2–5 mm) compared to the LV (7–11 mm). Although the end diastolic volume of the RV tends to be larger than the LV, its mass is much less[5–7].

The normal RV produces a pressure–volume (P–V) relationship that tends to be triangular. The RV isovolumic contraction and relaxation phases are much less prominent than in the LV which has a more rectangular P–V loop[8] (Fig. 30.1). In normal tissue the RV is sensitive to loading, showing a steeper fall in stroke volume with increasing afterload than the LV[9]. In pathological conditions associated with pulmonary hypertension the P–V loop of the RV becomes more LV-like (rectangular) with a reduction in the ejection of blood during pressure decline and a prominent isovolumic relaxation[10].

Evidence of mechano-electric coupling in the right ventricle

The thin wall of the RV makes it sensitive to acute changes in end diastolic volume[6] and it would not be surprising if mechano-electric coupling (MEC) had some distinguishing features from that in the LV, but a comparison is difficult due to lack of data. However, MEC has been demonstrated in the RV. Indeed, there is an important body of evidence relating to the effects of myocardial stretch upon the regulation of contraction, intracellular Ca^{2+} ($[Ca^{2+}]_i$) and electrical activity. Papillary muscles and free running trabeculae are convenient and useful experimental preparations. RV preparations have frequently been chosen over those in the LV because of the highly trabecularized nature of the RV and the relatively long, narrow and thin RV papillary muscles of some species (e.g. ferret). These are ideal characteristics for an externally superfused (rather than a coronary perfused) preparation used in experiments

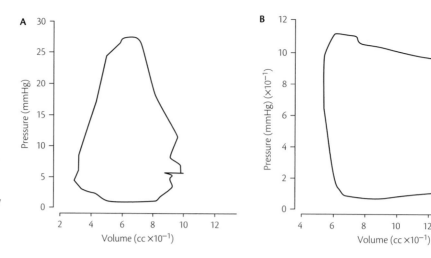

Fig. 30.1 Pressure volume loops from (**A**) a normal human right ventricle and (**B**) a normal human left ventricle (note that the scales on the y axes are different). The right ventricular loop is triangular and lacks prominent isovolumic phases of pressure increase and decrease. [Reproduced, with permission, from Redington AN, Gray HH, Hodson ME, Rigby ML, Oldershaw PJ (1988) Characterisation of the normal right ventricular pressure-volume relation by biplane angiography and simultaneous micromanometer pressure measurements. *Br Heart J* **59**:23–30.]

that manipulate length. Therefore seminal works, such as those by Allen and colleagues[11,12], were performed on RV papillary muscle. These studies showed that changes in length could alter electrical activity via the manipulation of $[Ca^{2+}]_i$ and the consequential effect of this upon Ca^{2+}-activated currents.

Although few studies have deliberately targeted the RV for study of MEC in the intact heart, acute distension of the RV can induce arrhythmias in a manner similar to that described in the LV (Fig. 30.2).

Work by Lab and colleagues showed that (*in situ*) occlusion of the pulmonary artery in lambs distended the RV and shortened the monophasic action potential duration (MAPD) measured at 25% and 75% repolarization. It also generated early after-depolarizations

(EAD, elevation of the MAP profile late in repolarization that can develop into extra systoles) and extra systoles (Fig. 30.3)[13]. RV distension may cause desynchronization of the electrical activity in the RV, resulting in an increased electrical and mechanical dispersion and increased susceptibility to arrhythmia[14]. If this is correct then a substrate that becomes more inhomogeneous, as occurs in disease, should be more susceptible to mechanically induced arrhythmias (see below).

Potential clinical importance of mechano-electric coupling in the right ventricle

Mechanical stimulation of the RV may be important in the acute induction of dysrhythmia. *Commotio cordis* is a rare but dramatic

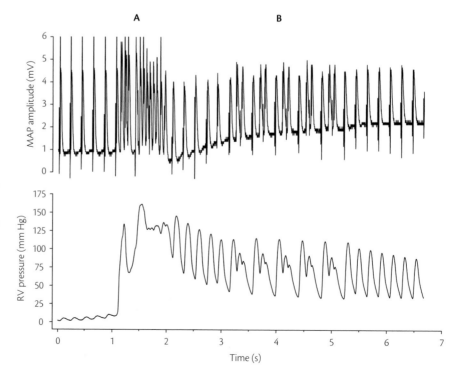

Fig. 30.2 Monophasic action potentials (MAP) recorded from the right ventricular epicardial surface of a Langendorff-perfused rat heart paced at 5 Hz (upper panel) and right ventricular pressure in an indwelling balloon (lower panel). Stretch of the right ventricle by increasing the volume increases pressure and generates arrhythmias, first in the form of tachycardia (**A**) and then in the form of an extra systole paired with a triggered MAP (**B**). The interbeat interval pre-stretch was 199.9 ± 0.2 ms (mean ± standard deviation) and post-stretch was 192.6 ± 22.2 ms. The rhythm of the heart is disturbed as indicated by the significant increase in the standard deviation of the interbeat interval following stretch ($p < 0.001$, $n = 15$ hearts).

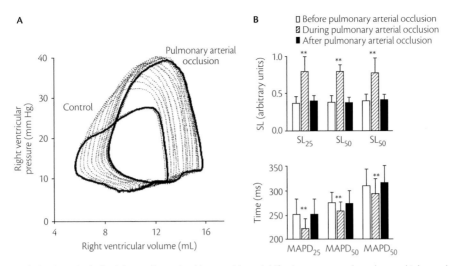

Fig. 30.3 **A** Pulmonary artery occlusion in an *in situ* lamb heart dilates the right ventricle and shifts the pressure–volume loop to higher end diastolic volumes and end systolic pressures. **B** Pulmonary artery occlusion caused a reversible increase in segment length (SL, an index of stretch) and (**C**) a decrease in the duration of the monophasic action potential (MAPD) at various points of repolarization. [Reproduced, with permission, from Greve G, Lab MJ, Chen R, *et al.* (2001) Right ventricular distension alters monophasic action potential duration during pulmonary arterial occlusion in anaesthetised lambs: evidence for arrhythmogenic right ventricular mechanoelectrical feedback. *Exp Physiol* **86**:651–657.]

event that describes the mechanical triggering of cardiac arrhythmias of varying severity, including sudden cardiac death, by a non-damaging blow to the chest area above the heart (see also Chapter 45). This accounts for the death of about 20 young athletes a year in the USA[15]. This event may be highly relevant to the RV when one considers that the RV is anteriorly situated in the chest cavity and may therefore be directly beneath the site of pre-cordial impact.

Second, pulmonary regurgitation and RV dilatation can occur as a consequence of tetralogy of Fallot repair, and abnormal RV mechanics have been implicated in the generation of arrhythmias[16]. A study of long-term survivors of tetralogy of Fallot repair revealed a strong correlation between RV mechanics and electrical activity, with RV dilatation positively correlated with QRS duration and the incidence of sustained ventricular tachycardia[17]. Subsequently, a sheep model of pulmonary regurgitation revealed that although the MAP shortening, observed in response to pulmonary artery occlusion, was not altered by regurgitation, there was a significant increase in the dispersion of activation times and a decrease in conduction velocity, possibly leading to an increase in the number of EAD and extra systoles in response to pulmonary artery occlusion[18].

The third example, pulmonary artery hypertension (PAH), is a disease characterized by elevated pulmonary arterial pressure but not mean arterial pressure; thus the RV is subjected to increased loading while the LV is not. There is no cure for this condition, current treatments target the vasculature[19] and RV failure is a common outcome. Studies by Guyton *et al.*[20] showed that initial increases in proximal pulmonary arterial pressure and right ventricular pressure have little effect upon systemic arterial pressure until RV compensatory mechanisms are exhausted, at which point catastrophic collapse of both pulmonary and systemic pressure occurs. The disease can therefore be unpredictable and is linked to LV failure[2,21]. Mechanical stimuli, such as increased stress due to

elevated afterload and strain due to diastolic chamber dilation, are predicted to be important factors in the progression to RV failure.

It has been shown in animal models of pressure (but not volume) overload that the transition from compensated to failing states is associated with a proliferation of the microtubule cytoskeleton[22–24] and contractile dysfunction. Depressed ejection fraction and elevated levels of cellular tubulin occur in whole hearts[25]. Microtubules are load-bearing and load-modulated (stress-polymerized) components of the cytoskeleton[26]. They are hollow protein cylinders of α and β-tubulin heterodimers about 25 nm in diameter aligned predominantly along the longitudinal axis. Roughly 25% of tubulin is in the polymerized form in a state of dynamic stability with constant addition or loss of sub-units. Associated with microtubules are guanosine-5′-triphosphatase (GTP)-binding proteins such as G_i and G_s and also microtubule-associated proteins, which promote microtubule stability [predominantly MAP4 in cardiac muscle; see[23,24,26]]. In tissue from human sufferers of heart failure where wall stress is enhanced there is evidence of increased mRNA and protein levels for tubulin, e.g.[27,28].

The mechanism whereby increased wall stress triggers microtubule proliferation does not appear to be chamber specific. It occurs in the RV in response to pulmonary artery banding[22] or pulmonary hypertension induced by monocrotaline (MCT)[29] and in the LV in response to aortic stenosis[30] or in spontaneously hypertensive rats[31]. However, the microtubule proliferation is not seen in all LV studies[32]. It appears that microtubule proliferation occurs when compensatory growth to normalize wall stress reaches its limit. Thus in the LV of some animals where LV growth continued, proliferation did not occur[23,24,30]. It may be that microtubule proliferation is more utilized in the thin-walled RV as a strategy to combat increasing wall stress.

There is limited evidence concerning the effect of microtubules on stretch-induced arrhythmias and the studies have all been

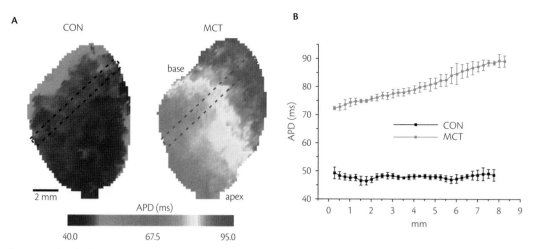

Fig. 30.4 A Optically measured and colour-coded action potential durations (APD) at (80% repolarization) from the epicardial surface of a normal rat right ventricle (CON) and a pulmonary hypertensive rat with right ventricular failure induced by monocrotaline (MCT). **B** APD was recorded in the region marked by the dotted lines. The APD and its dispersion is greater in the MCT animals. (See color plate section.)

performed on the LV. The probability of triggering such arrhythmias in the isolated rabbit heart increased following exposure to taxol (a microtubule stabilizer) but was unaffected by colchicine (a microtubule disruptor)[33]. These data suggest a pro-arrhythmic substrate in the pressure overloaded and failing RV where a proliferated microtubule cytoskeleton is expected to exist. However, the incidence of ventricular fibrillation in a swine model of *Commotio cordis* was increased by colchicine[34], perhaps because of negative effects on the mechanical buffering capacity of the pre-cordial tissue.

There are conflicting theories about the effect that cytoskeletal changes might have upon mechano-sensitive channels (MSC). The cytoskeleton may reinforce the lipid membrane, and in this scenario disruption would increase MSC activation. Conversely if the cytoskeleton acts as a tether transferring stress to MSC, proliferation would increase MSC activation [see[26,35]]. With specific reference to MEC and hypertension, it is interesting to note that transient receptor potential channel (TRPC)1 currents (a putative non-specific cationic mechano-sensitive current) are reported to be upregulated in systemic hypertension[36], as are protein levels of the mechano-sensitive K[+] channel (TWIK-related K[+] channel, TREK)-1[37]. In contrast, in the MCT model of RV failure we found a decreased expression of mRNA for both TREK-1 and TRPC-1.

Heterogeneity in the right ventricle

Heterogeneity, or variation, in the electrical, mechanical and structural properties of the myocardium between different regions of the heart is recognized as an important factor in the functioning of the heart. The role of heterogeneity has been derived almost exclusively from studies in the LV. When the properties of LV and RV myocytes have been compared, the RV is usually treated as homogenous[38,39]. There is limited information to suggest that gradients in ion channel function exist in both human[40] and animal[41] RV, but in the failing rat RV there is evidence for substantial electrical remodelling, including lengthening and dispersion of APD consistent with the idea that the diseased RV is pro-arrhythmic (Fig. 30.4).

A body of evidence is developing for an important role for RV heterogeneity in the generation of human arrhythmias. The Brugada syndrome is particularly prominent in south-east Asian males [see[42]] and is associated with sudden cardiac death. It is thought that alterations in sodium channel densities and the interaction of sodium current and transient outward potassium currents result in shortened APD in some RV sub-epicardial myocytes and lengthened APD in others. The sub-endocardial APD is unaltered and the enhanced APD dispersion makes the myocardium more susceptible to fibrillation. Interestingly, recent studies have suggested that the heterogeneity of repolarization and arrhythmias in patients and in induced isolated canine preparations come from heterogeneity within the RVOT and/or heterogeneity between the RVOT and the rest of the RV. The sub-epicardial region of the RVOT may be the arrhythmic source[43–45]. A slowing of conduction across the RVOT may also be involved[46].

Conclusions and outlook

Given the very different mechanical environments of the RV and LV it is likely that the response of the RV to mechanical stimulation is different from that of the LV. MEC may play a role in RV arrhythmias associated with pulmonary regurgitation. There may be an enhanced involvement of microtubules in the RV response to hypertension and the RVOT may be a particular source of arrhythmias. The gap in our knowledge regarding RV physiology and pathology is well summarized by Voelkel *et al.*[2]: '*right ventricular failure cannot be understood simply by extrapolating data and experience from left ventricular failure*'.

References

1. Greyson CR. Pathophysiology of right ventricular failure. *Crit Care Med* 2008;**36**:S57–S65.
2. Voelkel NF, Quaife RA, Leinwand LA, *et al.* Right ventricular function and failure: report of a National Heart, Lung, and Blood Institute working group on cellular and molecular mechanisms of right heart failure. *Circulation* 2006;**14**:1883–1891.

3. Boukens BJ, Christoffels VM, Coronel R, Moorman AF. Developmental basis for electrophysiological heterogeneity in the ventricular and outflow tract myocardium as a substrate for life-threatening ventricular arrhythmias. *Circ Res* 2009;**104**:19–31.

4. Ho SY, Nihoyannopoulos P. Anatomy, echocardiography, and normal right ventricular dimensions. *Heart* 2006;**92**:i2–i13.

5. Haddad F, Hunt SA, Rosenthal DN, Murphy DJ. Right ventricular function in cardiovascular disease, part I: anatomy, physiology, aging, and functional assessment of the right ventricle. *Circulation* 2008;**117**:1436–1448.

6. Bristow MR, Zisman LS, Lowes BD, et al. The pressure-overloaded right ventricle in pulmonary hypertension. *Chest* 1998;**114**:101S–106S.

7. Mebazaa A, Karpati P, Renaud E, Algotsson L. Acute right ventricular failure–from pathophysiology to new treatments. *Intensive Care Med* 2004;**30**:185–196.

8. Redington AN, Gray HH, Hodson ME, Rigby ML, Oldershaw PJ. Characterisation of the normal right ventricular pressure-volume relation by biplane angiography and simultaneous micromanometer pressure measurements. *Br Heart J* 1988;**59**:23–30.

9. MacNee W. Pathophysiology of cor pulmonale in chronic obstructive pulmonary disease. *Am J Respir Crit Care Med* 1994;**150**:833–852.

10. Redington AN, Rigby ML, Shinebourne EA, Oldershaw PJ. Changes in the pressure-volume relation of the right ventricle when its loading conditions are modified. *Br Heart J* 1990;**63**:45–49.

11. Allen DG, Kurihara S. The effects of muscle length on intracellular calcium transients in mammalian cardiac muscle. *J Physiol* 1982;**327**:79–94.

12. Lab MJ, Allen DG, Orchard CH. The effects of shortening on myoplasmic calcium concentration and on the action potential in mammalian ventricular muscle. *Circ Res* 1984;**55**:825–829.

13. Greve G, Lab MJ, Chen R, et al. Right ventricular distension alters monophasic action potential duration during pulmonary arterial occlusion in anaesthetised lambs: evidence for arrhythmogenic right ventricular mechanoelectrical feedback. *Exp Physiol* 2001;**86**:651–657.

14. Chen RL, Penny DJ, Greve G, Lab MJ. Stretch-induced regional mechanoelectric dispersion and arrhythmia in the right ventricle of anesthetized lambs. *Am J Physiol* 2004;**286**:H1008–H1014.

15. Maron BJ, Estes NA, 3rd, Link MS. Task Force 11: *Commotio cordis*. *J Am Coll Cardiol* 2005;**45**:1371–1373.

16. Chaturvedi RR, Redington AN. Pulmonary regurgitation in congenital heart disease. *Heart* 2007;**93**:880–889.

17. Gatzoulis MA, Till JA, Somerville J, Redington AN. Mechanoelectrical interaction in tetralogy of Fallot. QRS prolongation relates to right ventricular size and predicts malignant ventricular arrhythmias and sudden death. *Circulation* 1995;**92**:231–237.

18. Gray R, Greve G, Chen R, et al. Right ventricular myocardial responses to chronic pulmonary regurgitation in lambs: disturbances of activation and conduction. *Pediatr Res* 2003;**54**:529–535.

19. Lee SH, Rubin LJ. Current treatment strategies for pulmonary arterial hypertension. *J Intern Med* 2005;**258**:199–215.

20. Guyton AC, Lindsey AW, Gilluly JJ. The limits of right ventricular compensation following acute increase in pulmonary circulatory resistance. *Circ Res* 1954;**2**:326–332.

21. Haddad F, Doyle R, Murphy DJ, Hunt SA. Right ventricular function in cardiovascular disease, part II: pathophysiology, clinical importance, and management of right ventricular failure. *Circulation* 2008;**117**:1717–1731.

22. Tsutsui H, Tagawa H, Kent RL, et al. Role of microtubules in contractile dysfunction of hypertrophied cardiocytes. *Circulation* 1994;**90**:533–555.

23. Cooper G. Cardiocyte cytoskeleton in hypertrophied myocardium. *Heart Fail Rev* 2000;**5**:187–201.

24. Cooper G. Cytoskeletal networks and the regulation of cardiac contractility: microtubules, hypertrophy, and cardiac dysfunction. *Am J Physiol* 2006;**291**:H1003–H1014.

25. Koide M, Hamawaki M, Narishige T, et al. Microtubule depolymerization normalizes in vivo myocardial contractile function in dogs with pressure-overload left ventricular hypertrophy. *Circulation* 2000;**102**:1045–1052.

26. Calaghan SC, Le Guennec JY, White E. Cytoskeletal modulation of electrical and mechanical activity in cardiac myocytes. *Prog Biophys Mol Biol* 2004;**84**:29–59.

27. Heling A, Zimmermann R, Kostin S, et al. Increased expression of cytoskeletal, linkage, and extracellular proteins in failing human myocardium. *Circ Res* 2000;**86**:846–853.

28. Zile MR, Green GR, Schuyler GT, Aurigemma GP, Miller DC, Cooper G. Cardiocyte cytoskeleton in patients with left ventricular pressure overload hypertrophy. *J Am Coll Cardiol* 2001;**37**:1080–1084.

29. Stones R, Drinkhill M, Benoist D, White E. ECG alterations and microtubule proliferation following monocrotaline induced right ventricular heart failure in rats. *Proc Physiol Soc* 2009;**15**:C25.

30. Tagawa H, Koide M, Sato H, Zile MR, Carabello BA, Cooper G. Cytoskeletal role in the transition from compensated to decompensated hypertrophy during adult canine left ventricular pressure overloading. *Circ Res* 1998;**82**:751–761.

31. Tsutsui H, Ishibashi Y, Takahashi M, et al. Chronic colchicine administration attenuates cardiac hypertrophy in spontaneously hypertensive rats. *J Mol Cell Cardiol* 1999;**31**:1203–1213.

32. Collins JF, Pawloski-Dahm C, Davis MG, Ball N, Dorn GW, Walsh RA. The role of the cytoskeleton in left ventricular pressure overload hypertrophy and failure. *J Mol Cell Cardiol* 1996;**28**:1435–1443.

33. Parker KK, Taylor LK, Atkinson JB, Hansen DE, Wikswo JP. The effects of tubulin-binding agents on stretch-induced ventricular arrhythmias. *Eur J Pharmacol* 2001;**417**:131–140.

34. Madias C, Maron BJ, Supron S, Estes NA, 3rd Link MS. Cell membrane stretch and chest blow-induced ventricular fibrillation: *Commotio cordis*. *J Cardiovasc Electrophysiol* 2008;**19**:1304–1309.

35. White E. Mechanosensitive channels:therapeutic targets in the myocardium? *Curr Pharm Des* 2006;**12**:3645–3664.

36. Seth M, Zhang ZS, Mao L, et al. TRPC1 Channels Are Critical for Hypertrophic Signaling in the Heart. *Circ Res* 2009;**10**:1023–1030.

37. Cheng L, Su F, Ripen N, et al. Changes of expression of stretch-activated potassium channel TREK-1 mRNA and protein in hypertrophic myocardium. *J Huazhong Univ Sci Technolog Med Sci* 2006;**26**:31–33.

38. Sathish V, Xu A, Karmazyn M, Sims SM, Narayanan N. Mechanistic basis of differences in Ca^{2+}-handling properties of sarcoplasmic reticulum in right and left ventricles of normal rat myocardium. *Am J Physiol* 2006;**291**:H88–H96.

39. Kondo RP, Dederko DA, Teutsch C, et al. Comparison of contraction and calcium handling between right and left ventricular myocytes from adult mouse heart: a role for repolarization waveform. *J Physiol* 2006;**571**:131–146.

40. Li GR, Feng J, Yue L, Carrier M. Transmural heterogeneity of action potentials and Ito1 in myocytes isolated from the human right ventricle. *Am J Physiol* 1998;**275**:H369–H377.

41. Wan X, Bryant SM, Hart G. A topographical study of mechanical and electrical properties of single myocytes isolated from normal guinea-pig ventricular muscle. *J Anat* 2003;**202**:525–536.

42. Chen PS, Priori SG. The Brugada syndrome. *J Am Coll Cardiol* 2008 25;**51**:1176–1180.

43. Morita H, Zipes DP, Morita ST, Wu J. Differences in arrhythmogenicity between the canine right ventricular outflow tract

and anteroinferior right ventricle in a model of Brugada syndrome. *Heart Rhythm* 2007;**4**:66–74.

44. Morita H, Zipes DP, Fukushima-Kusano K, *et al.* Repolarization heterogeneity in the right ventricular outflow tract: correlation with ventricular arrhythmias in Brugada patients and in an in vitro canine Brugada model. *Heart Rhythm* 2008;**5**:725–733.

45. Nagase S, Kusano KF, Morita H, *et al.* Longer repolarization in the epicardium at the right ventricular outflow tract causes type 1

electrocardiogram in patients with Brugada syndrome. *J Am Coll Cardiol* 2008;**51**:1154–1161.

46. Coronel R, Casini S, Koopmann TT, *et al.* Right ventricular fibrosis and conduction delay in a patient with clinical signs of Brugada syndrome: a combined electrophysiological, genetic, histopathologic, and computational study. *Circulation* 2005;**112**:2769–2777.

Mechanical induction of arrhythmia in the *ex situ* heart: insight into *Commotio cordis*

Frank Bode and Michael R. Franz

Background

Commotio cordis is defined as rhythm disturbance including sudden cardiac death resulting from a blunt and often innocent-appearing blow to the chest wall[1]. It has become apparent that *Commotio cordis* is not associated with any structural heart disease but is primarily a mechanically induced electrical event. Young athletes struck by baseballs, hockey pucks or lacrosse balls are most at risk. Death is instantaneous and resuscitation is often not successful. Where electrocardiogram (ECG) recordings have been obtained after the arrest, the presenting rhythm most often is ventricular fibrillation (VF). Precordial impacts are not usually of sufficient magnitude to cause any significant damage to overlying thoracic structures (except from superficial bruising), and autopsy is notable for the absence of any obvious structural injury to the heart[2]. Over the last decade, an intact anaesthetized porcine model of low energy chest impact replicated the clinical scenario of *Commotio cordis*[3] (see also Chapter 45). This experimental model has provided substantial insights into mechanisms underlying sudden death after pre-cordial impact. In anaesthetized juvenile swine, induction of VF can be instantaneous following chest impacts. Critical variables include impact velocity and location and the hardness of the projectile. These determine the ventricular pressure spike generated by the impact, whose amplitude can be correlated with the risk of VF. Importantly, precordial impacts result in VF only when timed to occur just before the peak of the T-wave[4,5]. Impacts, timed to coincide with the early T-wave of the ECG, were capable of triggering short runs of VF in the isolated perfused guinea pig heart[6]. The T-wave marks a period when cardiac electrical activity is inhomogeneous, due to dispersion of repolarization[7,8]. This dispersion leaves the heart vulnerable to VF induction by an electrical stimulus. In the setting of *Commotio cordis*, the mechanical stimulus may be translated into an electrical current to induce VF during the vulnerable period.

Langendorff model of sudden ventricular stretch

To further investigate the electrophysiological basis of VF induction during *Commotio cordis*, isolated rabbit hearts were perfused in a modified Langendorff apparatus. Five epicardial bipolar contact electrodes were evenly spread over the LV circumference to record monophasic action potentials (MAP). Constant contact pressure between electrodes and the heart was maintained by a spring-loading mechanism[9]. A volume-conducted ECG was obtained by means of ten unipolar electrodes flanking the tissue chamber in an approximate Einthoven and Wilson configuration[10]. A latex balloon was inserted into the left ventricle (LV) and connected to a piston pump. By application of abrupt volume pulses to the balloon, sudden intraventricular pressure pulses between 94 and 355 mmHg were produced during sinus rhythm[11]. Intra-ventricular pressure increases were designed to mimic the pressure spike that had been observed in the porcine model of *Commotio cordis* following chest impact.

Pressure amplitudes that exceeded 138±29 mmHg were able to trigger action potentials during diastole. In six isolated hearts, ten episodes of sustained VF were induced by sudden pressure application. VF was consecutively terminated by defibrillation. Pressure amplitudes of VF-inducing pulses ranged from 208 to 289 mmHg (mean 252±30 mmHg), defining an upper and lower limit of vulnerability. VF-inducing stretch pulses had coupling intervals of 35–88 ms (mean 63±16 ms) after the onset of spontaneous activation (Fig. 31.1A). This vulnerable window was characterized by an increase in intrinsic dispersion of repolarization, i.e. a growing spatial disparity of excitability.

Repolarization dispersion during VF induction was based on two components: (1) intrinsic dispersion of repolarization typical for the T-wave and (2) stretch-induced dispersion of repolarization. Intrinsic dispersion of repolarization between different LV sites could be detected during sinus rhythm and was reflected by the occurrence of the T-wave in the surface ECG. Intrinsic dispersion was 18±8 ms, measured as the latency between the first and the last MAP to reach 70% repolarization (Fig. 31.2A). Application of a global stretch pulse influenced local repolarization, thereby enhancing repolarization dispersion. During the pressure pulse that induced VF, dispersion of repolarization increased to 26±8 ms ($p < 0.01$, Fig. 31.2A). Thus, a vulnerable period for VF induction existed based on intrinsic dispersion of repolarization. Pressure pulses further increased repolarization dispersion while at the same time inducing depolarizations. During VF induction, a stretch

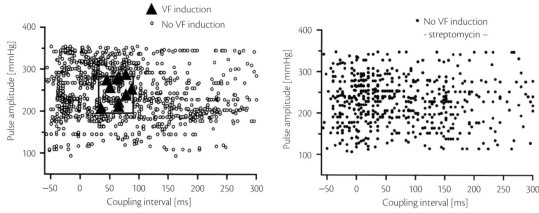

Fig. 31.1 Left ventricular stretch pulses (o) applied in the isolated rabbit heart, according to their coupling interval after onset of spontaneous activation during the cardiac cycle and according to the pressure amplitude. **A** Ten episodes of ventricular fibrillation (VF) were induced (▲). The inducing pressure pulses occurred in a window (□) that was confined by coupling intervals of 35–88 ms after onset of activation and by intermediate pressure amplitudes of 208–289 mmHg. **B** Stretch pulses applied after perfusion with 200μM streptomycin induced no VF. [Reproduced, with permission, from Bode F, Franz MR, Wilke I, Bonnemeier H, Schunkert H, Wiegand UK (2006) Ventricular fibrillation induced by stretch pulse: implications for sudden death due to *Commotio cordis*. *J Cardiovasc Electrophysiol* **17**:1011–1017.]

pulse initiated an action potential at a site that had regained excitability. Adjacent LV sites with longer repolarization were not excited by the global stretch pulse. Instead, we observed a spread of activation from a site with earlier repolarization to sites with later repolarization. As compared to the small activation delay of 8±3 ms between sites during sinus rhythm, a stretch-induced depolarization that initiated VF exhibited a prominent activation delay of 23±10 ms between LV sites (*p* <0.01; Fig. 31.2B). Non-uniform

excitability and conduction slowing were indicative of functional block, forming the substrate of VF induction.

Potential cellular mechanisms

Human victims of *Commotio cordis* collapse quickly after impact[2]. In the porcine model of *Commotio cordis*, VF occurred immediately after precordial impact during the critical time window[3].

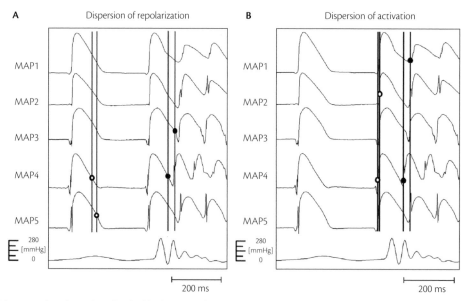

Fig. 31.2 Induction of VF by a stretch-pulse in the isolated rabbit heart. Simultaneous recordings of five monophasic action potentials (MAP) from the left ventricle and the intracavitary pressure. Two evaluation schemes are illustrated. **A** Repolarization dispersion measured as the delay between the earliest and the latest action potential to reach the 70% repolarization level. Measurements were performed during two cardiac cycles: at baseline (o) for the sinus beat before the pressure pulse and for the beat during pressure pulse application that induced VF (•). As compared to baseline, a pressure impulse that induced VF significantly increased repolarization dispersion (18±8 vs 26±8 ms; mean ± SEM; *p* < 0.01). This could be attributed to local changes in the repolarization process during the pressure pulse. **B** Activation dispersion measured at baseline for the sinus beat before the pressure pulse (o) and for the beat induced by pressure pulse application that initiated VF (•). As compared to baseline, dispersion of activation between LV sites increased significantly upon induction of VF (8±3 vs 23±10 ms; *p* < 0.01). The earliest, stretch-induced *depolarization* was detected at the LV site with the shortest *repolarization*. Adjacent LV sites showed delayed *depolarization* due to pre-existing or stretch-induced prolongation of *repolarization*. Early, stretch-induced activation and adjacent slow or blocked activation may form the substrate for functional re-entry. [Reproduced, with permission, from Bode F, Franz MR, Wilke I, Bonnemeier H, Schunkert H, Wiegand UK (2006) Ventricular fibrillation induced by stretch pulse: implications for sudden death due to *Commotio cordis*. *J Cardiovasc Electrophysiol* **17**:1011–1017.]

In the isolated heart, VF also commenced instantaneously upon pressure application, supporting the notion of an immediate electrical event induced by sudden myocardial stretch. The observations do not support a VF genesis secondary to myocardial ischaemia, haemorrhage or heart block[12,13] but suggest a primary electrical event due to mechanical force. Mechanical stimuli have been recognized to produce electrical effects in myocardium, including arrhythmias[10].

The phenomenon of mechano-electric coupling has been attributed to the existence of stretch-activated ion channels (SAC)[14,15] and/or other ion channels that exhibit non-specific mechano-sensitivity (see also Chapter 6)[16]. SAC can be divided into cation non-selective channels (SAC_{NS}; reversal potential between 0 and –30 mV) or potassium-selective channels (SAC_K; reversal potential negative to cardiomyocyte resting potentials). Activation of SAC_{NS} will lead to depolarization by generation of inward cation currents. Block of SAC_{NS} suppresses stretch-induced depolarization[17] and arrhythmias[18,19] in isolated hearts. Quantitative modelling studies of isolated rabbit heart impacts support a role of SAC_{NS} in VF genesis[20] (see also Chapter 36). *In vivo* experiments in the porcine model of *Commotio cordis* indicate a role of mechano-sensitive adenosine triphosphate (ATP)-sensitive K$^+$ (K_{ATP}) channels for arrhythmia sustenance[21]. Glibenclamide, a blocker of K_{ATP} channels, inhibited the occurrence of VF during chest wall impact by a firm object. In the same model, streptomycin, a non-selective blocker of cationic SAC_{NS}, did not prevent VF[22]. The lack of streptomycin effects may mean that either SAC_{NS} are not involved in the initiation of *Commotio cordis*, or streptomycin did not efficiently block these channels, perhaps because of sub-inhibitory plasma concentrations, or that the lack of specificity altered compensating elements of the electrophysiological response.

In the isolated rabbit heart model, no mechanically induced episodes of VF were inducible after addition of streptomycin (200 µM) to the perfusate (Fig. 31.1B), suggesting involvement of SAC_{NS} in the initiation of VF. At the same time, MAP recordings revealed no specific changes in the myocardial activation sequence during streptomycin perfusion, suggesting that the drug had no effect on background electrical activity (i.e. it only affected the mechanically induced component). However, VF was not readily reproducible in the isolated heart, even during baseline conditions, as only 11% of pressure pulses applied within the vulnerable window induced VF.

Therefore, the role of mechano-sensitive channels in *Commotio cordis* remains to be further elucidated. The investigation into different mechanisms, be it stretch of the sarcolemmal membrane or other cellular elements or pressure changes in the intracellular cytoplasm, will shed additional light on mechano-electrical coupling.

Conclusions and outlook

Commotio cordis arises from blunt chest impacts which give rise to an abrupt intra-ventricular pressure. During a short vulnerable period, this may give rise to VF, whose induction depends on intrinsic repolarization dispersion. Isolated heart experiments suggest that critically timed stretch pulses can augment repolarization dispersion via mechano-electric coupling. Rapid left ventricular pressure rises, following chest impact, are believed to activate SAC. During early repolarization, the generation of an inward current may lead to non-uniform depolarization, triggering ectopic excitation in the presence of increased spatial dispersion of repolarization. This facilitates non-uniform activation and may induce VF. Repolarization dispersion may therefore play an important role in the generation of fatal tachyarrhythmias during *Commotio cordis*. Utilization of more specific SAC blockers might help to further elucidate the contribution of SAC to mechanically induced VF.

References

1. Nesbitt AD, Cooper PJ, Kohl P. Rediscovering *Commotio cordis*. *Lancet* 2001;**357**:1195–1197.
2. Maron BJ, Poliac LC, Kaplan JA, Mueller FO. Blunt impact to the chest leading to sudden death from cardiac arrest during sports activities. *N Engl J Med* 1995;**333**:337–342.
3. Link MS, Wang PJ, Pandian NG, *et al*. An experimental model of sudden death due to low-energy chest-wall impact (*Commotio cordis*). *N Engl J Med* 2003;**338**:1805–1811.
4. Link MS, Maron BJ, Wang PJ, VanderBrink BA, Zhu W, Estes NA, 3rd. Upper and lower limits of vulnerability to sudden arrhythmic death with chest-wall impact (*Commotio cordis*). *J Am Coll Cardiol* 2003;**41**:99–104.
5. Madias C, Maron BJ, Weinstock J, Estes NA, 3rd, Link MS. *Commotio cordis* – sudden cardiac death with chest wall impact. *J Cardiovasc Electrophysiol* 2007;**18**:115–122.
6. Cooper PJ, Epstein A, Macleod IA, *et al*. Soft tissue impact characterisation kit (STICK) for ex situ investigation of heart rhythm responses to acute mechanical stimulation. *Prog Biophys Mol Biol* 2006;**90**:444–468.
7. Franz MR, Bargheer K, Rafflenbeul W, Haverich A, Lichtlen PR. Monophasic action potential mapping in human subjects with normal electrocardiograms: direct evidence for the genesis of the T-wave. *Circulation* 1987;**75**:379–386.
8. Yue AM, Paisey JR, Robinson S, Betts TR, Roberts PR, Morgan JM. Determination of human ventricular repolarization by noncontact mapping: validation with monophasic action potential recordings. *Circulation* 2004;**110**:1343–1350.
9. Franz MR, Cima R, Wang D, Profitt D, Kurz R. Electrophysiological effects of myocardial stretch and mechanical determinants of stretch-activated arrhythmias. *Circulation* 1992;**86**:968–978.
10. Zabel M, Portnoy S, Franz MR. Electrocardiographic indexes of dispersion of ventricular repolarization: an isolated heart validation study. *J Am Coll Cardiol* 1995;**25**:746–752.
11. Bode F, Franz MR, Wilke I, Bonnemeier H, Schunkert H, Wiegand UK. Ventricular fibrillation induced by stretch pulse: implications for sudden death due to *Commotio cordis*. *J Cardiovasc Electrophysiol* 2006;**17**:1011–1017.
12. Louhimo I. Heart injury after blunt thoracic trauma: an experimental study on rabbits. *Acta Chir Scand Suppl* 1968;**380**:1–60.
13. Pringle SD, Davidson KG. Myocardial infarction caused by coronary artery damage from blunt chest injury. *Br Heart J* 1987;**57**:375–376.
14. Hu H, Sachs F. Stretch-activated ion channels in the heart. *J Mol Cell Cardiol* 1997;**29**:1511–1523.
15. Kohl P, Nesbitt AD, Cooper PJ, Lei M. Sudden cardiac death by *Commotio cordis*: role of mechano-electric feedback. *Cardiovasc Res* 2001;**50**:280–289.
16. Van Wagoner DR. Mechanosensitive gating of atrial ATP-sensitive potassium channels. *Circ Res* 1993;**72**:973–983.
17. Hansen DE, Borganelli M, Stacy GP, Jr., Taylor LK. Dose-dependent inhibition of stretch-induced arrhythmias by gadolinium in isolated canine ventricles. Evidence for a unique mode of antiarrhythmic action. *Circ Res* 1991;**69**:820–831.
18. Bode F, Sachs F, Franz MR. Tarantula peptide inhibits atrial fibrillation. *Nature* 2001;**409**:35–36.

19. Bode F, Katchman A, Woosley RL, Franz MR. Gadolinium decreases stretch-induced vulnerability to atrial fibrillation. *Circulation* 2000;**101**:2200–2205.

20. Li W, Kohl P, Trayanova N. Induction of ventricular arrhythmias following mechanical impact: a simulation study in 3D. *J Mol Histol* 2004;**35**:679–686.

21. Link MS, Wang PJ, VanderBrink BA, *et al.* Selective activation of the K^+_{ATP} channel is a mechanism by which sudden death is produced by low-energy chest-wall impact (*Commotio cordis*). *Circulation* 1999;**100**:413–418.

22. Garan AR, Maron BJ, Wang PJ, Estes NA, 3rd, Link MS. Role of streptomycin-sensitive stretch-activated channel in chest wall impact induced sudden death (*Commotio cordis*). *J Cardiovasc Electrophysiol* 2005;**16**:433–438.

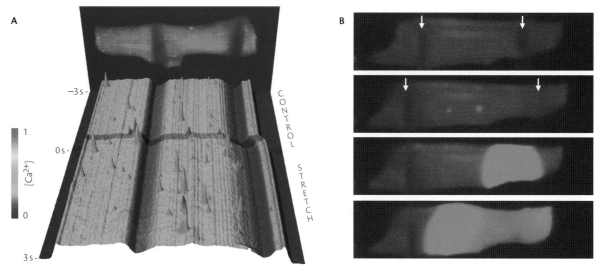

Fig. 5.3 A Acute stretch-induced increase in Ca²⁺ spark rate. Stretch (8%) was applied, at time 0 s, to the right half of the cell only, using carbon fibres attached to centre of the cell (anchor) and the right cell-end (low signal intensity regions on cell image panel at rear and 'canyons' in space–time plot at front). Spark rate increased after stretch only at the stretched part of the cell. **B** Acute application of large whole-cell axial stretch (> 20%, compare first and second row) increases spark rate (see bright spots in second row) and gives rise to a mechanically induced full Ca²⁺ wave (third and fourth rows). (See pg. 37)

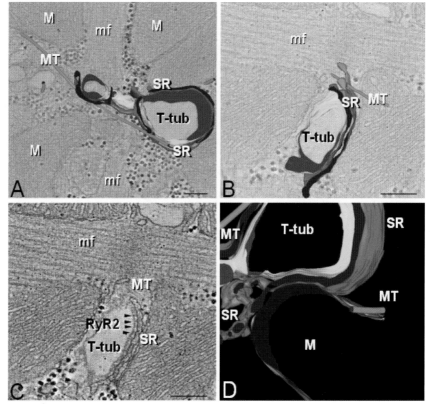

Fig. 5.4 Electron microscopic tomography (EMT) images of an SR–t-tubular membrane complex with associated microtubules from a rat ventricular cardiomyocyte. **A** and **B** Three-dimensional (3D) reconstructions, superimposed on single EMT sections. **C** Single EMT X–Y plane with outline of relevant structures. **D** Detail of 3D reconstruction showing close approximation of SR–t-tubular membrane complex, mitochondria and microtubules. Microtubules approach ryanodine receptor locations to within ~10 nm. T-tub, t-tubular membrane (yellow outline); SR, sarcoplasmic reticulum (red); MT, microtubule (green); M, mitochondria (blue); mf, myofilaments; RyR2, ryanodine receptor. Scale bars: 200 nm. (See pg. 38)

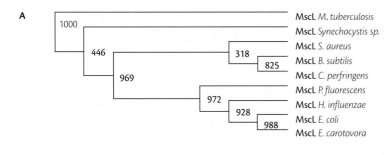

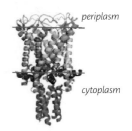

periplasm

cytoplasm

A

1000	MscL *M. tuberculosis*
	MscL *Synechocystis sp.*
446	MscL *S. aureus*
318 825	MscL *B. subtilis*
969	MscL *C. perfringens*
972	MscL *P. fluorescens*
928	MscL *H. influenzae*
988	MscL *E. coli*
	MscL *E. carotovora*

B

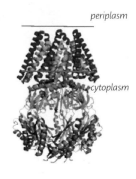

periplasm

cytoplasm

TRICHOTOMY

YF46 *A. fulgidus*
YBDG *E. coli*
600 — Q9LXA1 *A.thaliana*
1000 — Q9C731 *A. thaliana*
998 — Q9C6RO *A. thaliana*
1000 — CAA21091 *S. pombe*
1000 — CAB16377 *S. pombe*
580
951 — Y812 *A. aeolicus*
1000 — Q9K9G4 *B.halodurans*
785 — YHDY *B.subtilis*
683 — 1000 MscMJ *M.jannaschii*
MscMJLR *M.jannaschii*
488 — 1000 Y415 *H.pylori*
YNAI *E.coli*
976 — YJEP *E.coli*
1000 — AEFA *E.coli*
YJEP *H. influenzae*
807 — Q9KR91 *V. cholerae*
992 — Y639 *syechocystis sp.*
1000 — MscS *E .ictaluri*
MscS *E. coli*

Fig. 1.1 Families of prokaryotic SAC. **A** A subfamily of MscL-like proteins found in bacteria. The structure of the MscL homopentamer from *Mycobacterium tuberculosis*[22,85] is shown on the right. The position of the lipid bilayer relative to the channel protein is indicated by red lines. The most divergent members of the MscL subfamily, the archaeal and fungal proteins, most closely resemble those of Gram-positive bacteria[26]. **B** A representative phylogenetic tree of MscS homologues found in three kingdoms of living organisms. The structure of the MscS heptamer from *E. coli*[24,85] is shown on the right. The position of the lipid bilayer relative to the channel protein is indicated by red lines. MscS-like proteins of bacteria are shown in black, those of *Archaea* are shown in red, whereas MscS homologues found in fungi and plants are shown in green. [Adapted, with permission from Elsevier, from Martinac B, Kloda A (2003) Evolutionary origins of mechanosensitive ion channels. *Prog Biophys Mol Biol* **82**:11–24.] (See pg. 5)

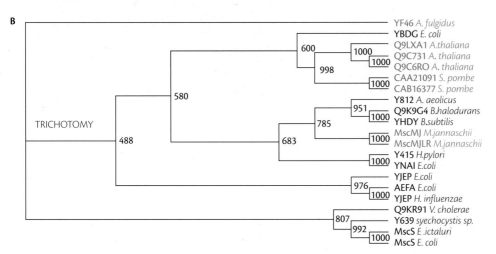

Anaesthetics
Lipids

Heat

Stretch   Stretch

Voltage

pH$_i$

COOH   NH$_2$ COOH

PKA/PKC   Cytoskeleton

Fig. 3.1 Polymodal activation of TREK-1 by physical and chemical stimuli. TREK-1 is opened by stretch, heat, intracellular acidosis, depolarization, lipids and volatile general anaesthetics, but closed by protein kinase A (PKA) and protein kinase C (PKC) phosphorylation pathways. TREK-1 is tonically inhibited by the actin cytoskeleton. The cytosolic carboxy terminal domain plays a key role in the regulation of TREK-1 activity. Phosphorylation of S333 by PKA and phosphorylation of both S333 and S300 by PKC in this region inhibit TREK-1 opening. PIP$_2$ as well as AKAP interact with a cluster of positive charges (overlapping with E306) in the carboxy terminal domain. Protonation of E306 induces channel opening. (See pg. 21)

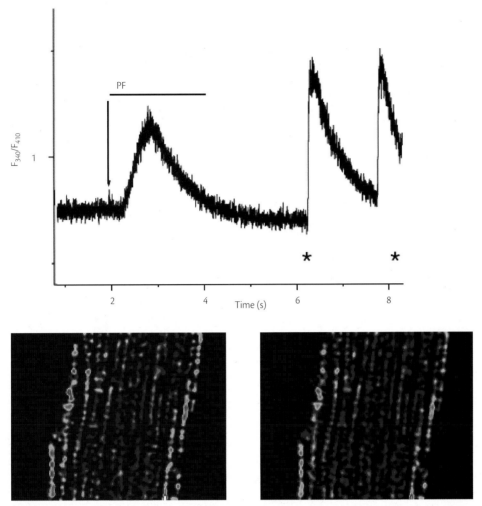

Fig. 5.5 Pressure flow (PF)-induced slow $[Ca^{2+}]_i$ transient (top: ratiometric measurement using Fura 2) and mitochondrial Ca signal (rhod-2) before applying PF (bottom left) and 6 s after applying PF in permeabilized ventricular myocytes (bottom right). PF-induced Ca^{2+} transients are accompanied by a reduction in mitochondrial $[Ca^{2+}]$. [Reproduced, with permission, from Belmonte S, Morad M (2008) 'Pressure-flow'-triggered intracellular Ca^{2+} transients in rat cardiac myocytes: possible mechanisms and role of mitochondria. *J Physiol* **586**:1379–1397.] (See pg. 39)

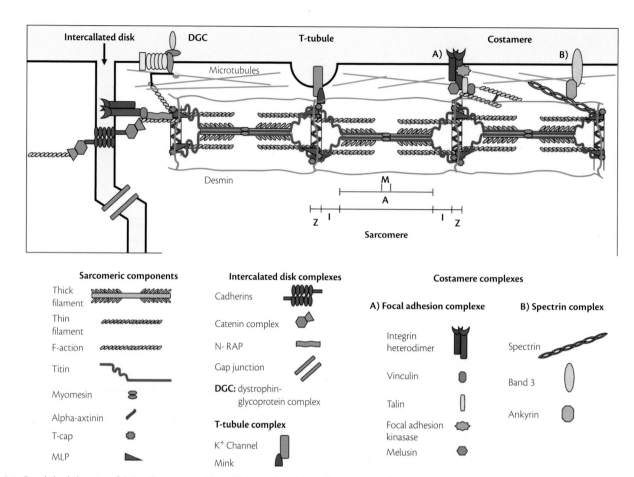

Fig. 9.1 Cytoskeletal elements of the cardiac myocyte. Microtubules are found throughout the cytoplasm and are most dense near the nuclei. Desmin forms intermediate filaments that connect myofibrils laterally at the level of the Z-disk and M-line and that connect successive Z-disks longitudinally. They also link myofibrils to nuclei and cell membranes. F-actin filaments are part of the sarcomeric thin filaments and constitute various linking systems that connect Z-disks to the plasma membrane and intercalated disk. They are linked to the cadherins of the intercalated disks by interacting with catenins and to the dystrophin–glycoprotein complex (DGC) via binding to dystrophin. Titin spans half-sarcomeres, with its terminal ends overlapping in the Z-disk and at the M-line. Titin is associated with the other parts of the cytoskeleton at various locations. T-cap interacts with the Z-disk end of titin and with MLP, forming part of an MLP-dependent stretch sensing complex. MLP interacts with N-RAP, a protein that may be involved in mediating interactions between myofibrils and the cell membrane at adherens junctions through its possible interactions with cadherin-based protein complexes and/or integrin-associated vinculin. T-cap also interacts with the potassium channel subunit minK at t-tubules, forming a complex that may be involved in the stretch-dependent regulation of potassium flux. (See pg. 67)

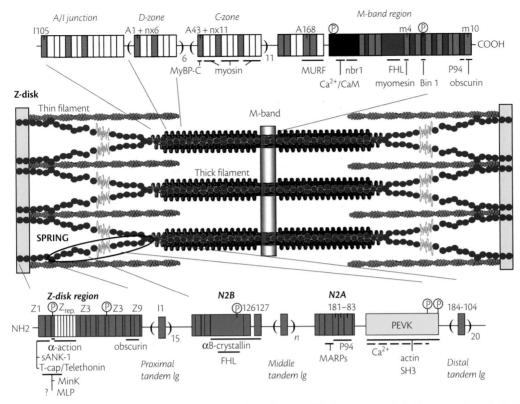

Fig. 9.2 Schematic of titin in sarcomere. The sarcomere contains thin, thick and titin filaments. Titin filaments span the half sarcomere from the Z-disk to the M-band. The domain composition of the various regions of the titin molecule is shown (red: Ig-like, white: Fn3-like, blue: unique, yellow: PEVK domains). The various known titin-binding proteins and their bindings sites are also shown. P, phosphorylation sites. See text for details. (See pg. 68)

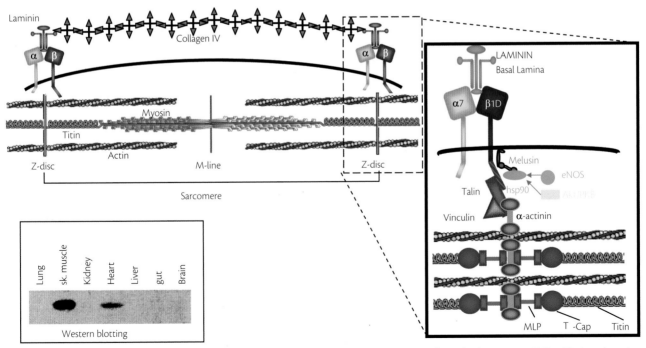

Fig. 11.1 Representation of the sarcomeric structure and its junction with the plasma membrane. The contractile unit lies between two Z-discs. The boxed area is magnified to illustrate the junctional complex connecting the Z-disc structure to integrins at the plasma membrane[60]. Melusin acts as a co-chaperone with Hsp90. Stretch-dependent signalosome assembly results in Akt activation and subsequent eNOS phosphorylation. Insert: muscle-specific expression of melusin in newborn mouse tissue[61]. [Reproduced, with permission, from Tarone G, Lembo G (2003) Molecular interplay between mechanical and humoral signalling in cardiac hypertrophy. *Trends Mol Med* **9**:376–382.] (See pg. 82)

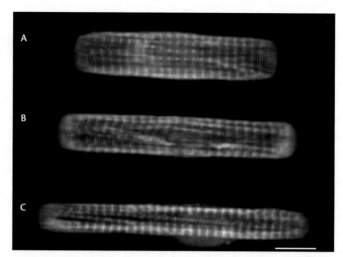

Fig. 12.2 Neonatal rat ventricular myocytes cultured on microcontact printed fibronectin islands with aspect rations of 5:1 (**A**), 7:1 (**B**) and 10:1 (**C**) and stained for DNA [using 4′,6-diamidino-2-phenylindole (DAPI), staining nucleus blue], F-actin (phalloidin, staining inter-Z-disc space of sarcomeres green) and sarcomeric α-actinin (red, thin striations that appear red, or yellow in co-stained areas; see full-colour insert). Scale bar is 10 μm. (See pg. 90)

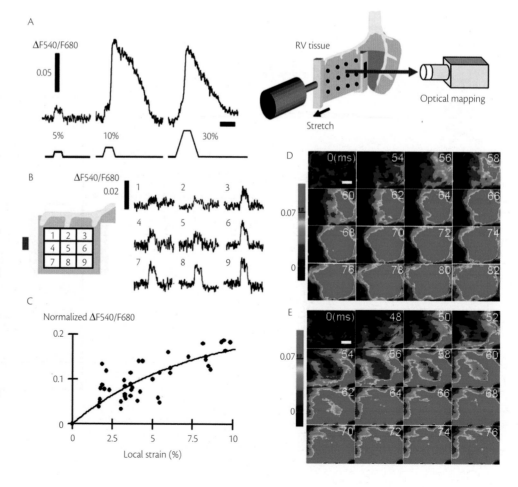

Fig. 14.8 Alterations in the electrical response in right-ventricular (RV) tissue from isolated perfused rabbit heart. **A** Ratiometric optical signals in response to 5%, 10% and 30% stretches (from left to right; scale bar: 100 ms). **B** Spatiotemporal pattern of the depolarizations in response to a 5% stretch. **C** Relationship between the changes in the normalized optical signals and the local strain under the excitation threshold (*n* = 5). **D** and **E** Representative action potentials and optical maps in response to 10% and 30% stretches. [Reproduced, with permission, from Seo K, Inagaki M, Nishimura S, *et al.* (2010) Structural heterogeneity in the ventricular wall plays a significant role in the initiation of stretch-induced arrhythmias in perfused rabbit right ventricular tissues and whole heart preparations. *Circ Res* **106**:176–184.] (See pg. 108)

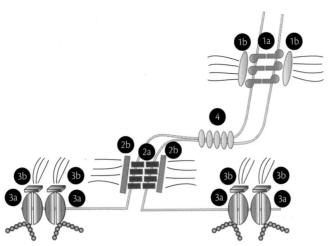

Fig. 18.1 The cell membranes of two adjacent cardiomyocytes are connected by fascia adherens junctions(1), desmosomes(2) and gap junctions(4). The surface membranes are connected to extracellular matrix proteins via cell adherens molecules(3). Fascia adherens junctions consist of the transmembrane spanning Ca^{2+}-dependent adherens proteins [N-cadherins (1a)] that are anchored in a submembranous scaffold (1b) consisting of several proteins (plakoglobin, catenins). The submembranous complex binds to the microfilaments of the cytoskeleton (actin). Desmosomes are formed by the transmembrane spanning proteins desmocollin and desmoglein (2a), anchored in a submembranous scaffold of plakoglobin and desmoplakin (2b). The latter proteins are bound to intermediate filaments (desmin). Gap junctions(4) consist of clustered gap junction channels each formed by two juxtaposed hemichannels (each formed by six connexin proteins). The extracellular matrix is connected to integrin (3a) via fibronectin. Intracellularly, integrins bind to cytoskeletal proteins via a number of intermediate proteins (3b) that cluster intergrin molecules and can induce intracellular signals when activated by extracellular mechanical stimuli. (See pg. 133)

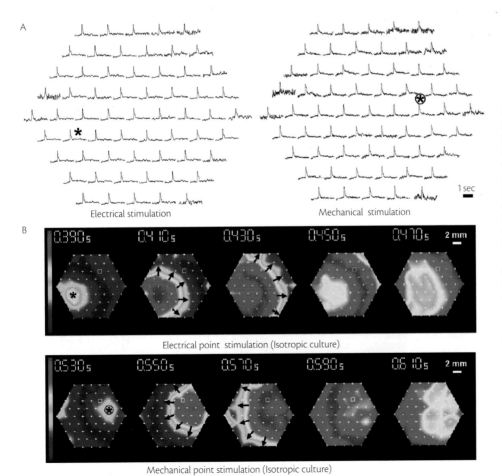

Fig. 20.2 Comparison of electrically and mechanically induced action potential propagation in the same isotropic NRVM monolayer. **A** Optical action potentials shown at 61 recording sites for electrical (left) and mechanical (right) stimulation. Asterisk indicates location of bipolar point electrode (1.2X threshold); circled asterisk indicates location of 0.4-mm-diameter pipette (0.5 m/s, 10 ms). **B** Propagation maps. Optical signals were normalized per site to the action potential amplitude. Colour bar at *left* indicates resting potential (in blue) and peak of action potential (in red). Plus symbols indicate recording sites. Both electrical and mechanical stimulation resulted in wavefronts that spread radially from the stimulating electrode or pipette, respectively. [Reproduced, with permission, from Kong CR, Bursac N, Tung L (2005) Mechanoelectrical excitation by fluid jets in monolayers of cultured cardiac myocytes. *J Appl Physiol* **98**:2328–2336.] (See pg. 148)

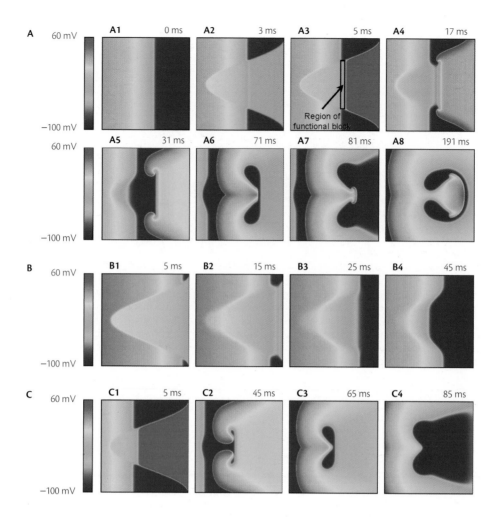

Fig. 22.3 Computer simulation of epicardial impact effects on ventricular electrophysiology. Impacts are simulated by 5 ms activation of SAC$_{NS}$ in the area highlighted in A2 and applied at different stages of ventricular repolarization (i.e. during different times of the ECG T-wave). **A** Development of a mechanically induced sustained ventricular arrhythmia, following a simulated impact at 40% repolarization. Arrhythmia sustenance depends on supra-threshold mechanical stimulation that triggers an extra AP in tissue that has recovered from inactivation, and on overlap of the mechanically stimulated tissue region with the trailing wave of repolarization, where an area of functional block gives rise to wave-split. Arrhythmia sustenance is further favoured by partial repolarization of near-endocardial myocardium from AP plateau towards membrane potentials closer to the reversal potential of SAC$_{NS}$. **B** Lack of arrhythmogenic effect of impacts applied too early during repolarization (< 10% repolarization). **C** Single ectopic AP without subsequent re-entry, caused by later impacts (here at 60% repolarization). [Reproduced, with permission, from Garny A, Kohl P (2004) Mechanical induction of arrhythmias during ventricular repolarization: modeling cellular mechanisms and their interaction in two dimensions. *Ann N Y Acad Sci* **1015**:133–143.] (See pg. 163)

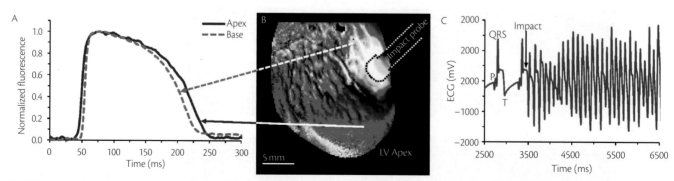

Fig. 22.4 Focal activation and ventricular fibrillation (VF) induced by local non-traumatic impacts in Langendorff-perfused rabbit hearts. **A** Spatial AP differences, visualized by epicardial optical voltage mapping, illustrate apico-basal activation delay during normal sinus rhythm and progression of the repolarization wave in the opposite direction. **B** Diastolic impact using a precision-controlled probe at energy levels < 1 mJ cause focal activation, followed by ectopic excitation of the ventricles. **C** Impact during the early T-wave causes focal excitation, followed by VF. This behaviour occurs when there is spatio-temporal overlap of the repolarization wave and mechanically stimulated tissue. [Reproduced, with permission, from Quinn TA, Lee P, Bub G, Epstein A, Kohl P (2010) Regional impact-induced arrhythmia in isolated rabbit heart visualised by optical mapping. *Heart Rhythm* **7**:S353.] (See pg. 165)

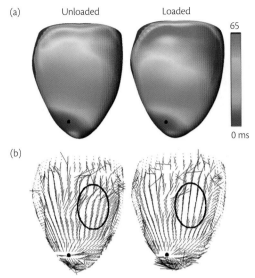

Fig. 25.1 Activation time fields (**A**) and conduction velocity vector fields (**B**) before and during application of 30 mmHg ventricular volume load in isolated rabbit heart, using methods from Sung and colleagues[29]. The small solid circle indicates the approximate position of pacing. The circled areas outline a region in which the apparent direction of conduction has been changed by application of load. (See pg. 182)

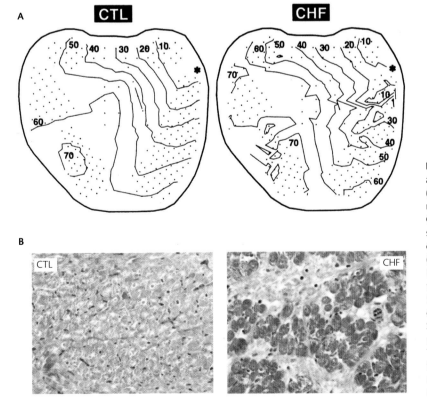

Fig. 28.5 A Activation map of the left atrium in dogs with (right) and without (left) tachycardiomyopathy induced by rapid ventricular pacing for 6 weeks. Crowding of isochrones indicates local slowing of conduction in the congestive heart failure (CHF) dog (lines represent 10 ms isochrones). **B** Light microscopy of atrial specimen in the same dogs as in **A**. Note cellular hypertrophy and accumulation of collagen in the CHF dog. Magnification ×1,250. CTL, control. [Reproduced, with permission, from Li D, Fareh S, Leung TK, Nattel S (1999) Promotion of atrial fibrillation by heart failure in dogs: atrial remodeling of a different sort. *Circulation* **100**:87–95.] (See pg. 206)

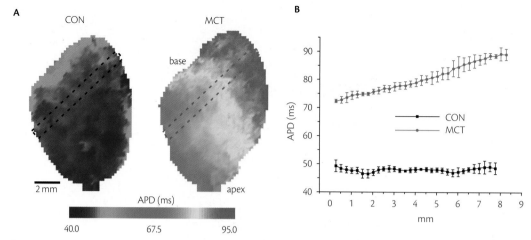

Fig. 30.4 A Optically measured and colour-coded action potential durations (APD) at (80% repolarization) from the epicardial surface of a normal rat right ventricle (CON) and a pulmonary hypertensive rat with right ventricular failure induced by monocrotaline (MCT). **B** APD was recorded in the region marked by the dotted lines. The APD and its dispersion is greater in the MCT animals. (See pg. 220)

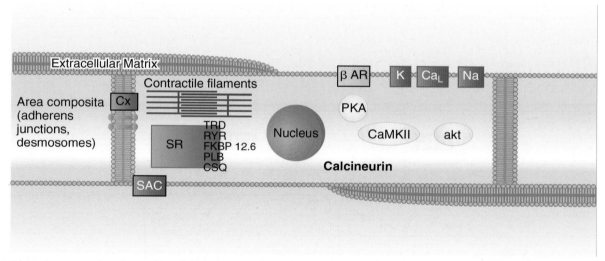

Fig. 32.3 Schematic representation of some of the cellular components that mediate the interaction between electrical and contractile function in cardiomyocytes. CSQ, calsequestrin; PLB, phospholamban; TRD, triadin. [Modified, with permission, from Kirchhof P (2009) New antiarrhythmic drugs and new concepts for old drugs. In: *Cardiac Electrophysiology – From Cell to Bedside* (eds DP Zipes, J Jalife). 5th edition, Saunders (Elsevier), New York, pp. 975–982.] (See pg. 231)

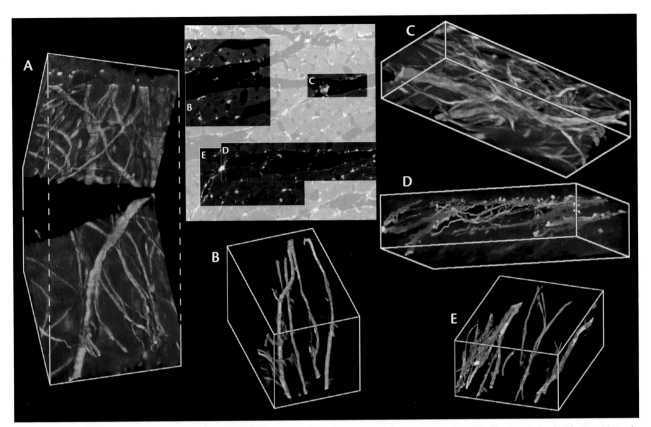

Fig. 34.2 High-resolution sub-volumes reveal the nature of perimysial collagen. A midwall segment from a 12-month WKY control rat stained with picrosirius red was imaged using extended-volume confocal imaging at 0.4 µm voxel size and representative sub-volumes were extracted. The sub-volume in **A** has been opened to show the detail of the meshwork on two opposing laminar surfaces. Long intralaminar collagen cords have been segmented from the tissue volumes using connectivity-based thresholding (**B**, **E**) and show the relationship between the axial cords, as well as small tethering branches which extend into the neighbouring tissue. In **D**, collagen spanning the cleavage plane separating adjacent layers is highlighted, and such collagen sometimes fuses to form larger collagen tendons near the edges of the laminae (**C**). [Reproduced, with permission, from Pope A, Sands GB, Smaill BH, LeGrice IJ (2008) Three dimensional transmural organization of perimysial collagen in the rat heart. *Am J Physiol* **295**:H1243–H1252.] (See pg. 243)

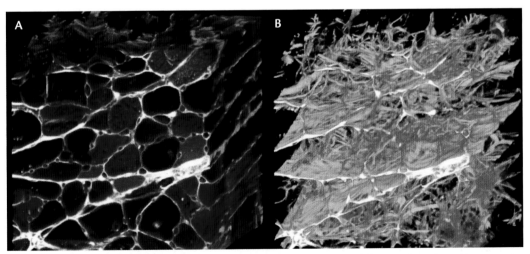

Fig. 34.3 High resolution images of LV midwall (block size 200×200×50 µm) from a 12-month spontaneously hypertensive rat heart. Myocytes and capillaries as well as perimysial and endomysial collagen are evident in **A**, although myocytes are stained with variable intensity. **B** shows collagen structures segmented from **A**. Compared with age-matched WKY controls (Fig. 34.2D), perimysial collagen has fused between adjacent muscle layers and the endomysial collagen surrounding myocytes has thickened. (See pg. 243)

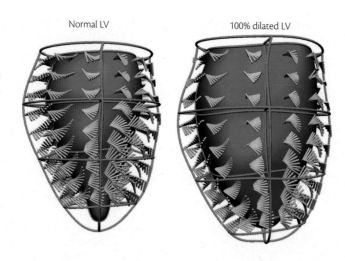

Fig. 34.5 Finite element models of the normal LV (left) and the 100% dilated LV (right). The LV free walls of each model are in view, with anterior and posterior walls at the left and right, respectively, of each panel. Ventricular dilatation is accompanied by a more spherical shape of the LV and relative wall thinning. LV endocardial surfaces are shaded with lines outlining the epicardial surface. The groups of rotating rods show the transmural variation in fibre orientation across the LV wall. (See pg. 245)

Normal LV   100% dilated LV

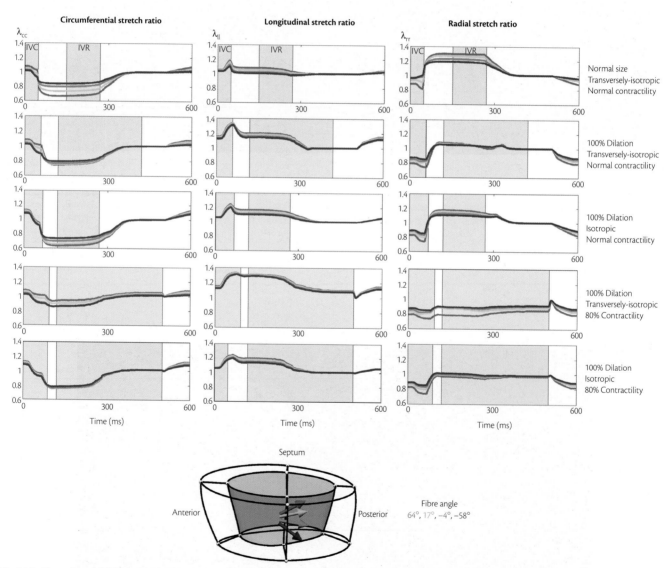

Fig. 34.8 Circumferential (left), longitudinal (centre) and radial (right) stretch ratios (λ) in the equatorial free wall of the LV during the cardiac cycle, with shading indicating the isovolumic contraction (IVC) and isovolumic relaxation (IVR) phases. The normal LV simulation (top) is compared to four pathological cases (see text for details). The inset below shows the equatorial slice of the LV, with arrows indicating the transmural locations at which the components of stretch were analyzed. The fibre angles relative to the LV's short axis plane are also indicated (counter-clockwise positive). Stretch ratios for subendocardial (red), midwall (yellow and green) and subepicardial (blue) locations are plotted. (See pg. 248)

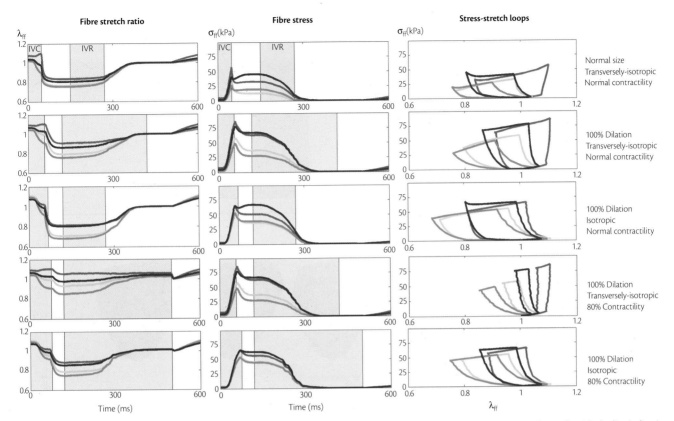

Fig. 34.9 Fibre stretch ratio (left), fibre stress (centre) and fibre stress-stretch loops in the equatorial free wall of the LV during the cardiac cycle, with shading indicating the isovolumic contraction (IVC) and isovolumic relaxation (IVR) phases. The normal LV (top) is compared to the four pathological cases (see text for details). Analysis locations and trace colours are the same as those described in the legend of Fig. 34.8. (See pg. 249)

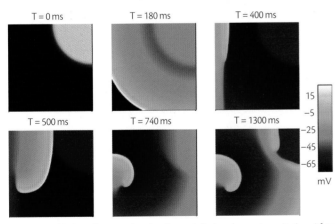

Fig. 35.6 Initiation of re-entry by a local stretch-induced ectopic excitation. After a pause in pacing, local stretch in the upper right corner gave rise to a DAD (0 ms) that produced focal activity which interfered with propagation of a subsequent normal beat (400 ms). Re-entry resulted (500 ms) and the dispersion of refractoriness that occurred could lead to subsequent wave breaks as well (1,300 ms); in this case these wave breaks were not sustained. Prior to induction, the tissue was paced for 3 s at a CL of 300 ms. (See pg. 256)

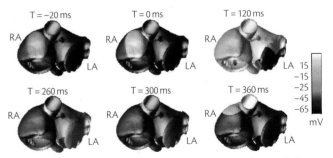

Fig. 35.7 Complex wave interactions in a realistic human atrial anatomical model. A region of local stretch in the right atrium (RA) near the right atrial appendage produced a spontaneous depolarization (−20 ms) that developed into a DAD that acted as an ectopic focus (0 ms). After the beat propagated to the left atrium (LA) (120 ms), a normal sinus beat arose at 240 ms (not shown). Because of the repolarization gradient set up by the ectopic beat, the beat was able to propagate toward the superior *vena cava* (260 ms) but initially was blocked in the region of the ectopic beat (300 ms). This gave rise to a re-entrant wave in the RA; in this case, the re-entry was not sustained. (See pg. 256)

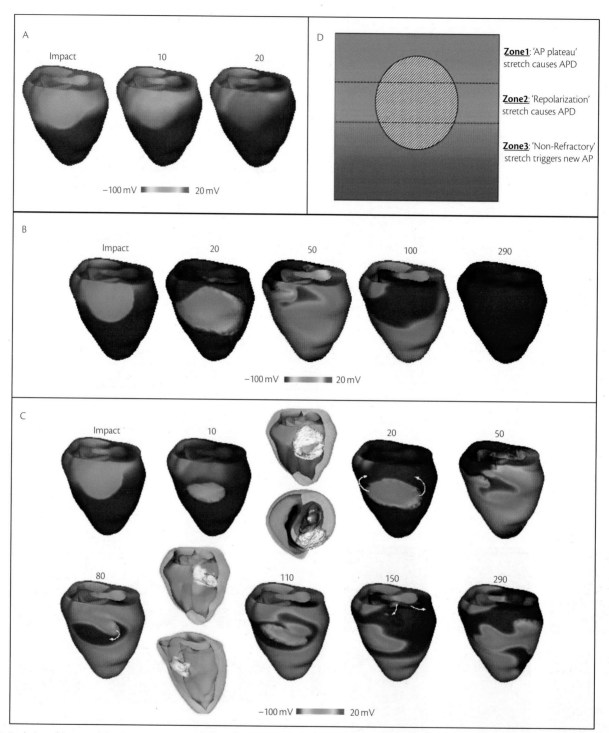

Fig. 36.2 Evolution of the spatial distribution of trans-membrane potential in a rabbit ventricular model following a mechanical impact delivered at coupling intervals (CI) of 135 ms (**A**) and 155 ms (**B**). Both CI are outside the vulnerable window; the impact does not result in re-entry. **C** Evolution of the spatial distribution of trans-membrane potential in the rabbit ventricular model at a CI of 145 ms. Mechanical stimulation results in re-entry. Time is counted since the onset of the impact and is denoted by the numbers above each image with 'impact' referring to the trans-membrane potential distribution at the end of impact. The smaller images are semi-transparent renditions of the trans-membrane potential distribution in the ventricular volume, and represent anterior, basal or side views of the ventricles; they refer to the couplings shown in the images to their left. In the semi-transparent images, the propagating wavefront is shown as a white surface. White arrows in 20, 80 and 150 ms panels indicate direction of propagation. **D** Schematic representation of trans-membrane potential distribution in and around the impact zone prior to mechanical stimulation. [Reproduced, with permission, from Li W, Kohl P, Trayanova N (2004) Induction of ventricular arrhythmias following mechanical impact: a simulation study in 3D. *J Mol Histol* **35**:679–686.] (See pg. 260.)

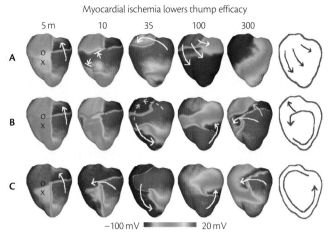

Myocardial ischemia lowers thump efficacy

Fig. 36.3 Evolution of post-impact trans-membrane potential distribution on the epicardial surface (anterior view) in a simulation of rabbit ventricles under normal (**A**) and ischaemic (**B**, **C**) conditions. In all cases, the pre-impact ventricles were in VT. Time, counted from impact onset, is shown above each column. Right-most images are schematics of post-impact electrical activity with re-entrant patterns shown in red. The beginning of each red line marks the location of unidirectional block that led to the establishment of the corresponding post-thump re-entry; its arrow indicates the direction of rotation. Grey arrows show direction of propagation of post-impact wavefronts that did not lead to establishment of re-entry. Colour scale as in Fig. 36.2. [Reproduced from Li W, Kohl P, Trayanova N (2006) Myocardial ischemia lowers precordial thump efficacy: an inquiry into mechanisms using three-dimensional simulations. *Heart Rhythm* **3**:179–186.] (See pg. 262)

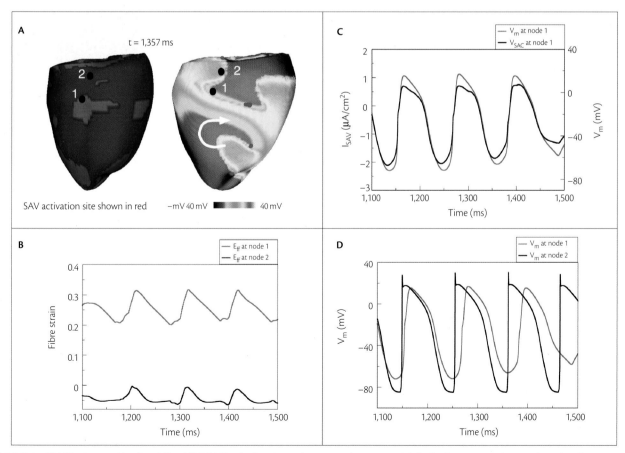

Fig. 36.4 Role of SAC in the transition from VT to VF. **A** SAC activation sites and trans-membrane potential distribution maps on the posterior epicardium at $t = 1{,}357$ ms from the onset of VT. The white arrow shows the direction of spiral wave rotation. Two nodes, marked 1 and 2, denote the locations at which the current, voltage and strain traces were taken from. **B** Fibre strain at nodes 1 and 2. **C** Stretch-activated current and trans-membrane potential at node 1. **D** Trans-membrane potentials at nodes 1 and 2. (See pg. 263)

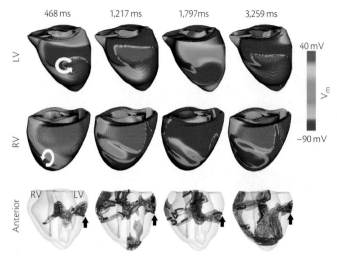

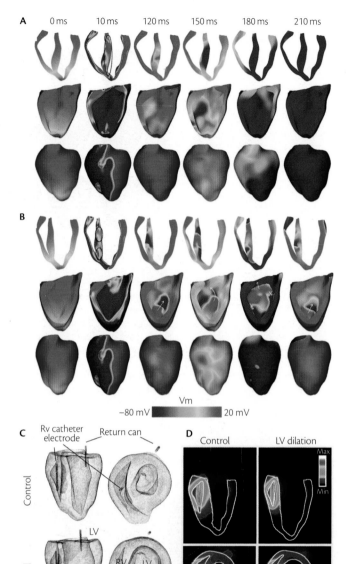

Fig. 36.5 Epicardial trans-membrane potential distribution maps on the LV (top) and RV (middle). The white arrows denote the direction of wave propagation. Anterior semi-transparent view of the ventricles (bottom) showing the filament distribution (blue) and the activation wavefronts (red). Small black arrows indicate the filament of the stable spiral wave on LV. $t = 0$ ms corresponds to the instant at which re-entry was induced. (See pg. 263)

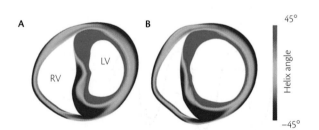

Fig. 36.6 Short axis view of ventricular geometry and fibre helix angle for the undeformed (**A**) and the dilated (**B**) ventricles. The most prominent changes are seen in the septum. (See pg. 264)

Fig. 36.7 Distributions of trans-membrane potential in: a ventricular long axis cross-section view; a view towards the septum with the RV free wall removed; and an epicardial view at shock end (0 ms) and for post-shock activation at 10, 120, 150, 180 and 210 ms in the undeformed (**A**) and dilated (**B**) ventricles.
C Ventricular geometry of the control (top) and dilated ventricles (bottom) with ICD-like electrode configuration in anterior (left) and basal (right) views. RV catheter (red) was inserted into the RV cavity and the active can (blue) was positioned in the bath near the posterior LV wall. **D** Distribution of electrical field magnitude in the control and dilated ventricles. (See pg. 264)

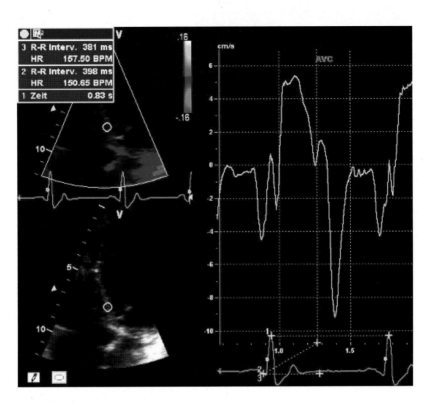

Fig. 38.3 Tissue Doppler echocardiography recording in a patient with short QT syndrome. Tissue velocity (yellow line, right) with sample volume positioned in the basal interventricular septum in the apical four chamber view (yellow circle, left lower view without and left upper view with colour Doppler imaging). Aortic valve closure (AVC, vertical green dotted lines) and beginning of isovolumic relaxation is correlating with beginning of the U wave. Left upper corner timings with corresponding blue dotted markers in ECG (bottom right): (1) RR interval (831 ms); (2) interval from Q wave to beginning of the U wave (398 ms, transferred timing from 12-lead ECG); (3) interval from Q wave to aortic valve closure (381 ms). Bottom right single-lead ECG (speed 50 mm/s). [Reproduced, with permission, from Schimpf R, Antzelevitch C, Haghi D, *et al.* (2008) Electromechanical coupling in patients with the short QT syndrome: further insights into the mechanoelectrical hypothesis of the U wave. *Heart Rhythm* **5**:241–245.] (See pg. 278)

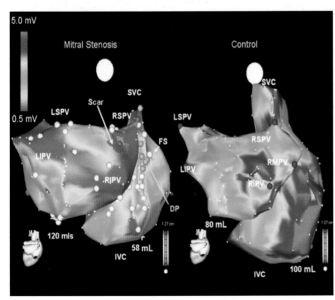

Fig. 40.1 Electroanatomical map of a patient with mitral stenosis (MS; left) and a representative control (right) (for voltage colour coding see scale bar in color plate section). The MS patient has an enlarged left atrium with extended regions of low voltage, inexcitable scar tissue and evidence of conduction abnormalities such as fractionated signals (FS) and double potentials (DP). [Reproduced, with permission, from John B, Stiles MK, Kuklik P, *et al.* (2008) Electrical remodelling of the left and right atria due to rheumatic mitral stenosis. *Eur Heart J* **29**: 2234–2243.] (See pg. 292)

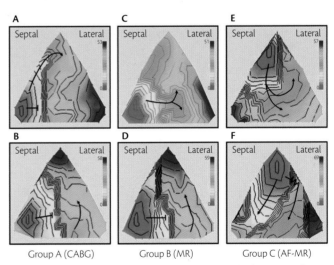

Group A (CABG)   Group B (MR)   Group C (AF-MR)

Fig. 40.3 Activation patterns on the posterior left atrium (LA) in patients from three different groups. Activation proceeds from *red* to *blue* with pacing from a corner of the plaque. Patients in group A (sinus rhythm, undergoing coronary artery bypass grafting, CABG) and group B (mitral regurgitation, MR) had one line of slow conduction, running vertically down the posterior LA between the pulmonary veins (**A–D**). Activation proceeded either around the line of conduction delay (**B, D**), through a gap in the line (**C**), or slowly across the line. Patients in group C (MR plus atrial fibrillation, AF) showed two (**E**) or more (**F**) lines of conduction delay with more complex patterns of activation across the LA. [Reproduced, with permission, from Roberts-Thomson K, Sanders P, Kalman J (2009) The role of chronic atrial stretch and atrial fibrillation on posterior left atrial wall conduction. *Heart Rhythm* **6**:1109–1117.] (See pg. 293)

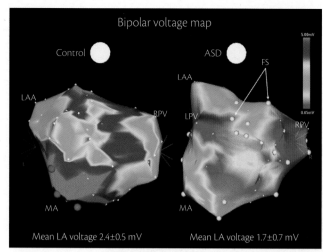

Fig. 40.7 Bipolar voltage maps of the left atrium (LA) projected in the posterior–anterior view. On the right is a representative map of a patient with ASD, and on the left a control patient. The ASD patient shows significantly lower voltages, particularly on the posterior LA, associated with fractionated signals (FS). [Reproduced, with permission, from Roberts-Thomson K, Sanders P, Kalman J (2009) Left atrial remodeling in patients with atrial septal defects. *Heart Rhythm* **6**:1000–1006.] (See pg. 295)

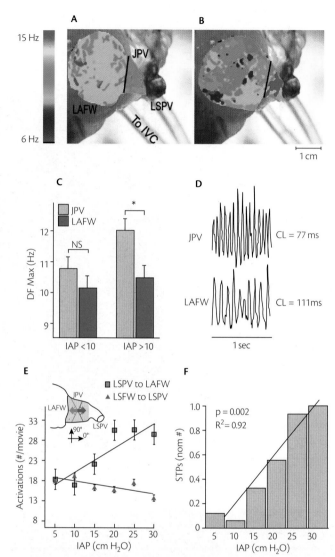

Fig. 44.1 **A** and **B** Dominant frequency (DF) maps from one heart at intra-atrial pressures of 5 and 18 cm H_2O, respectively. DF maps are superimposed on colour picture of a heart for illustrative purposes. **C** Bar graph showing DF_{max} (mean ± SEM) in the JPV (blue) and LAFW (red) at IAp < 10 and > 10 cm H_2O (*p < 0.001). **D** Single-pixel recordings from JPV and LAFW at 30 cm H_2O. IVC, inferior *vena cava*; CL, cycle length. **E** Number of activations (mean ± SEM) moving from LSPV to LAFW and from LAFW to LSPV (*p < 0.01 compared with LAFW to LSPV). Left inset: directionality of activity from the PV to LAFW (grey arrow) and from the LAFW to LSPV (red arrow) assessed at the JPV region. **F** Relation between the normalized number of STP wavefronts by episode and the level of pressure. [Reproduced, with permission, from Kalifa J, Jalife J, Zaitsev AV, *et al.* (2003) Intra-atrial pressure increases rate and organization of waves emanating from the superior pulmonary veins during atrial fibrillation. *Circulation* **108**:668–671.] (See pg. 319)

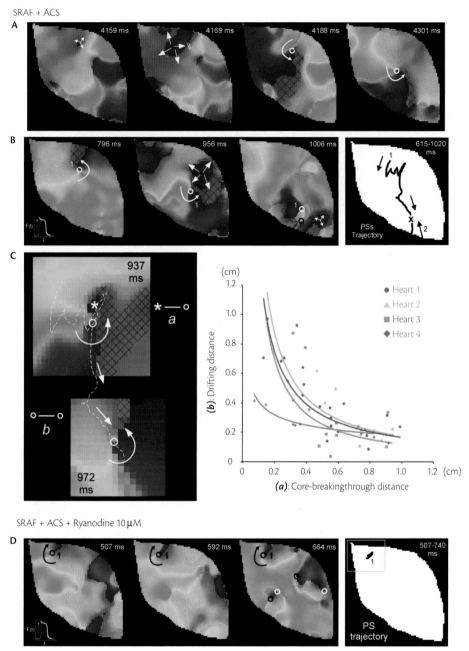

Fig. 44.3 Interaction between rotors and spontaneous breakthroughs in the setting of adrenocholinergic stimulation (ACS). **A** Representative phase maps during ACS; repeated breakthroughs gave rise to rotor formation after wavebreak. **B** Left: a breakthrough induced substantial rotor drift. Right: the corresponding PS trajectory is shown for rotor 1, which was forced to drift inferiorly and terminate after collision with counter-rotating rotor 2; both rotors mutually annihilated. **C** Quantification of breakthrough-induced-rotor drift. Left: example of measurements between PS and breakthrough centre (distance a: asterisk to open circle) and breakthrough-induced rotor drifting (distance b: between open circles) in the presence of ACS. Right: relationship between (a) and (b). We added a trend line to fit a line according to a power function $y = x^n$. A black shaded area depicts the excitable gap for the rotors presented. **D** Representative example of phase maps and corresponding rotor PS trajectory in the setting of ACS in the presence of RYA. A long-lasting and stable rotor (left) with a stationary PS trajectory (right) was visualized. Notably, a decrease in the number of breakthroughs was also noted. This re-entry showed the fastest atrial frequency of activation (12.2 Hz). SRAF stretch-related AF; PS, phase singularity. [Reproduced, with permission, from Yamazaki M, Vaquero LM, Hou L, *et al.* (2009) Mechanisms of stretch-induced atrial fibrillation in the presence and the absence of adrenocholinergic stimulation: interplay between rotors and focal discharges. *Heart Rhythm* **6**:1009–1017.] (See pg. 320)

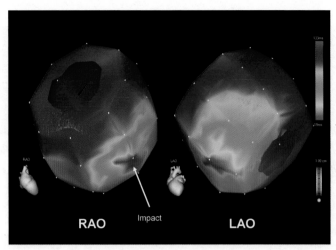

Fig. 45.3 A three-dimensional electrical activation map of the LV in a swine. The earliest ventricular depolarization occurs at the site of impact on the myocardium. This depolarization initiates a continuing re-entry circuit which then anchors in the septum. RAO, right anterior oblique view; LAO, left anterior oblique view. [Reproduced, with permission from, Alsheikh-Ali AA, Akelman C, Madias C, Link MS (2008) Endocardial mapping of ventricular fibrillation in *Commotio cordis*. *Heart Rhythm* **5**:1355–1356.] (See pg. 328)

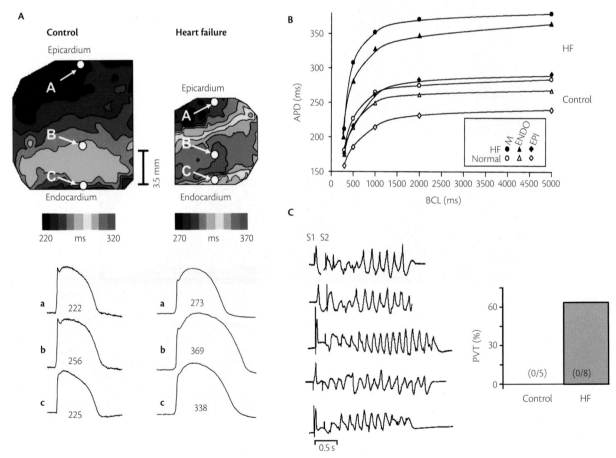

Fig. 46.1 Heart failure (HF) induced transmural dispersion of repolarization. **A** Upper panel: representative APD contour maps recorded from the transmural surfaces of a control (left) and canine tachypacing HF wedge (right). APD was heterogeneously prolonged across all layers in HF. Lower panel: representative action potentials from sub-epicardial (EPI; a), mid-myocardial (M; b) and sub-endocardial (ENDO; c) layers of the control (left) and HF wedges (right). **B** HF wedges exhibited a significant prolongation of APD, which was associated with a marked increase in arrhythmia inducibility (**C**) with a single premature stimulus. PVT, polymorphic ventricular arrhythmia; BCL, basic cycle length. [Modified, with permission, from Akar FG, Rosenbaum DS (2003) Transmural electrophysiological heterogeneities underlying arrhythmogenesis in heart failure. *Circ Res* **93**:638–645.]. (See pg. 331)

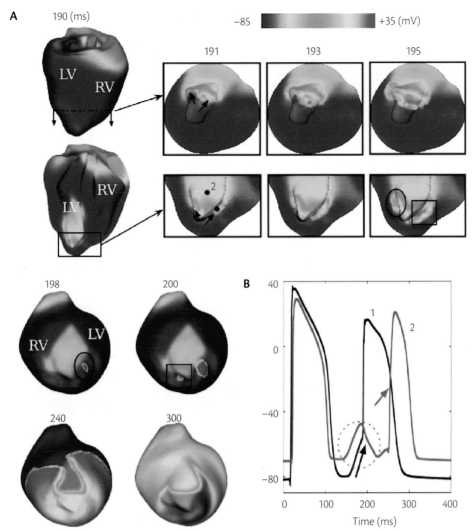

Fig. 49.7 A Evolution of the mechanically induced ventricular premature beat (VPB) for regional ischaemia stage I. The 191- to 195-ms insets present both short and long axis views of the apical region. The 198- to 300-ms insets present a tilted anterior view of the ventricles for better observation of epicardial activation. Arrows in the 191-ms inset indicate locations of earliest spontaneous firing. Ellipse and rectangle in the bottom 195-ms inset indicate the parts of the wavefront that make the earliest epicardial breakthrough at the locations encircled with an ellipse in the 198-ms inset and a rectangle in the 200-ms inset, respectively. **B** Traces of trans-membrane potential (V$_m$) recorded at site 1 [black, border zone (BZ)] and 2 [red, central ischaemic zone (CIZ)] marked in the bottom 191-ms inset in **A**. Black arrow and red dashed circle denote mechanically induced depolarization at sites 1 and 2, respectively. Red arrow indicates activation at site 2 by the propagation of the mechanically induced VPB. [Reproduced, with permission, from Jie X, Gurev V, Trayanova N (2010) Mechanisms of mechanically-induced spontaneous arrhythmias in acute regional ischemia. *Circ Res* **106**:185–192.] (See pg. 356)

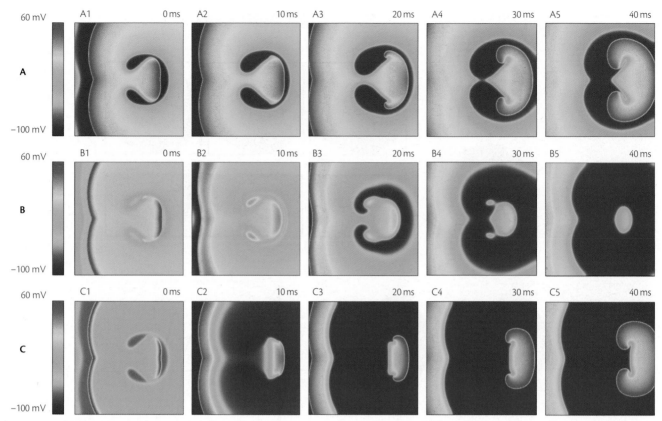

Fig. 50.5 Two-dimensional model (2.5 x 2.5 cm) of ventricular myocardium, consisting of 251 x 251 Noble'98[58] single cell models (trans-membrane voltage is colour coded; for mesh implementation see[59]). **A** Control figure-of-eight re-entry activity. **B** Mechanical stimulation, modelled by activation for 5 ms of SACNS (reversal potential −10 mV), causes depolarization of tissue in the excitable gap and terminates re-entry. **C** Mechanical stimulation of tissue after simulated ischaemic sensitization of SAC_K to stretch shifts net mechanically induced reversal potential to more negative levels (here −35 mV), which (1) prevents depolarization of resting tissue and (2) shortens action potential duration, rendering mechanical stimulation incapable of instantaneously terminating re-entry. [Figure by Dr Alan Garny.] (See pg. 366)

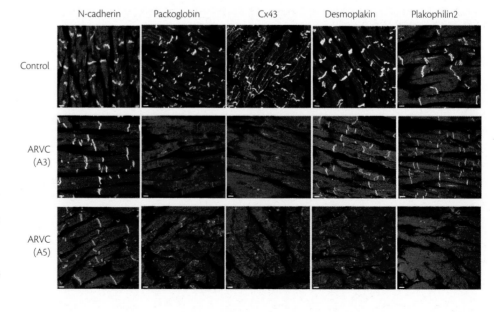

Fig. 57.1 Representative images showing that immunoreactive signal for plakoglobin at intercalated disks is reduced in subjects with ARVC compared with normal control subjects. [Reproduced, with permission, from Asimaki A, Tandri H, Huang H, Halushka MK, Gautam S, Basso C, *et al.* (2009) A new diagnostic test for arrhythmogenic right ventricular cardiomyopathy. *New Engl J Med* **360**:1075–1084, © Massachusetts Medical Association, all rights reserved.] (See pg. 408)

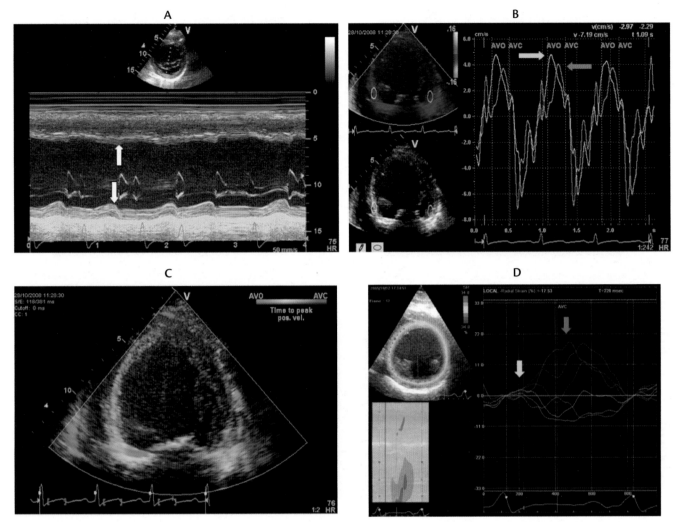

Fig. 58.2 Echocardiographic parameters of intraventricular dyssynchrony. **A** The septal to posterior wall motion delay (SPWMD) measurement by M-mode echocardiography obtained from the short-axis view. A delay of 150 ms between the maximal systolic excursion of the septum and posterior walls (arrows) indicates significant intraventricular dyssynchrony. **B** Dyssynchrony assessment by measuring the time difference between the peak myocardial systolic velocities of the septal (yellow) and lateral (green) wall on colour-coded tissue Doppler images; aortic valve opening (AVO) and closure (AVC) are indicated to facilitate identification of systolic peak velocities (arrows). **C** Automated measurement of time to peak myocardial systolic velocities by tissue synchronization imaging (TSI). Timings are translated in a colour scheme, green indicating early activation and orange late activation. **D** Short-axis slice of the left ventricle at the level of the papillary muscles, with reconstruction of six LV segments. Separate 2D strain time curves for each individual segment are depicted (the colours of the individual curves correspond to the individual segments). In this example severe baseline intraventricular dyssynchrony was present as expressed by the delay in time to peak systolic radial 2D strain > 130 ms between the anterior (yellow) and posterior wall (purple) peak strain. (See pg. 414)

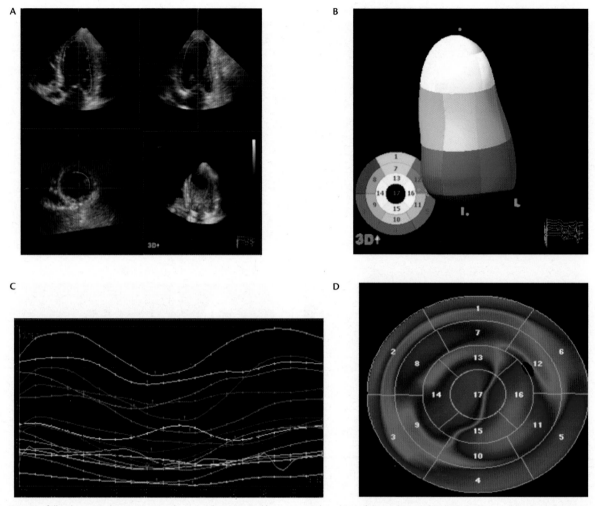

Fig. 58.3 **A** From a full-volume 3D dataset, an LV volume can be generated by automated tracking of the endocardial wall. **B** The LV model is divided into 17 segments. **C** From each of the 17 LV segments a time/volume curve is derived. **D** Time to peak minimal volume of the segments is presented in a bull's eye plot. Colour-coding allows quick visual identification of the area of latest mechanical activation: red segments are activated latest, green segments are activated earlier. (See pg. 416)

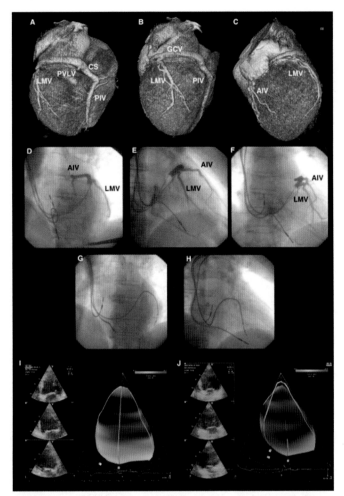

Fig. 58.5 Case example of an 85-year-old patient with idiopathic dilated cardio-myopathy, NYHA class III HF and wide QRS complex (157 ms, LBBB-configuration). MSCT shows a large left marginal vein with prominent side branches (A, B, C). These findings are confirmed by invasive venography (D, E, F). In the 3D LV dyssynchrony assessment with TSI (I), the late mechanical activation (yellow) is located in the lateral wall. The LV lead is positioned in the left marginal vein (G, H), resulting in synchronous activation of the LV, represented (green) on TSI, obtained immediately after CRT (J). In addition, a reduction of LV end-systolic volume from 191 to 153 ml was observed, with an increase in LV ejection fraction from 13% to 28%. [Reproduced, with permission, from Van de Veire NR, Marsan NR, Schuijf JD, *et al.* (2008) Noninvasive imaging of cardiac venous anatomy with 64-slice multi-slice computed tomography and noninvasive assessment of left ventricular dyssynchrony by 3-dimensional tissue synchronization imaging in patients with heart failure scheduled for cardiac resynchronization therapy. *Am J Cardiol* **101**:1023–1029.] (See pg. 417)

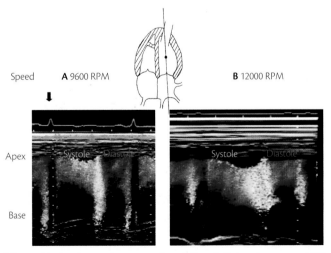

Fig. 59.2 Colour M-mode recording of the left ventricle showing continuous systolic and diastolic flow at the apex at a VAD-speed of 9,600 RPM (**A**) and 12,000 RPM (**B**). The continuous pump may result in discontinuous flow. The distortions in the ventricular wall induced by the VAD might alter a number of functional properties in the myocardium including the heart rhythm. The colour scale is a visual representation of the blood flow. Blue represents flow away from the probe and red represents flow towards the probe. [Reproduced, with permission, from Henein M, Birks EJ, Tansley PD, Bowles CT, Yacoub MH (2002) Images in cardiovascular medicine. Temporal and spatial changes in left ventricular pattern of flow during continuous assist device "HeartMate II". *Circulation* **105**:2324–2325.] (See pg. 423)

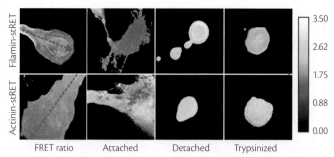

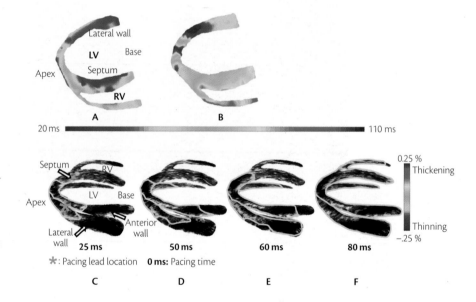

Fig. 60.4 stFRET detects resting strain in living cells. Dashed arrows in the left panels show the migrating directions. The cells show decreasing FRET (higher stress) at the front of the cell. Filamin and actinin in attached cells showed lower stress and local domains with stress gradients. Naturally rounded cells (Detached) and cells detached with trypsin (Trypsinized) displayed higher energy transfer as the stress in filamin and actinin was released. The FRET ratio calibration bar is given on the right. (See pg. 433)

Fig. 63.2 Experimental canine heart EWI isochrones during (**A**) normal sinus rhythm and (**B**) apical pacing. In **A**, 0 ms is the onset of the QRS complex, and in **B** it is equivalent to the pacing stimulus application time. **C–F** Propagation of the EMW (delineated in yellow) during pacing from the apical region of the antero-lateral wall in a normal canine heart. Propagation is initiated at the pacing lead location close to the apex and continues towards the base. (See pg. 453)

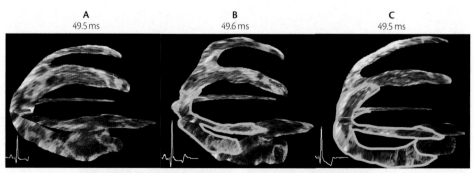

Fig. 63.3 Bi-plane (two-chamber and four-chamber) view of the same heart under different LAD coronary artery flow occlusion levels. Red, white and green arrows indicate the propagation of the EMW in the septal, anterior and lateral wall, respectively. **A** Without any occlusion, i.e. normal coronary flow, radial thinning is visible up to regions where the axial direction of the ultrasound beam coincides with the longitudinal direction of the cardiac geometry, where shortening is expected (in blue). **B** At 60% flow occlusion, this behaviour is reversed in the presence of ischaemia: a region (delimited with a yellow line) containing radial thinning (blue) and longitudinal lengthening (red) is observed. **C** At complete occlusion this region increases in size. The ischaemia is visible in the anterior, posterior and lateral wall near the apex at 60% flow occlusion and in the anterior, posterior, lateral and septal wall at 100% flow occlusion. Colour coding as in Fig. 63.2, bottom row. (See pg. 453)

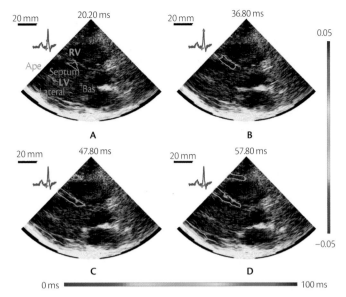

Fig. 63.4 Propagation of the EMW (delineated in yellow) overlayed on the echocardiogram of a healthy human subject. The EMW is initiated at the mid-septum (**A**) and propagates toward the apex (not shown) and the base (**B**). Activation of the lateral wall and right-ventricular wall follow approximately 10 ms later (**C**). **D** Propagation in the right-ventricular wall occurs from the apex to the base. The time shown denotes time lapsing after the onset of the QRS complex (green cross on the ECG; top left on images). Red denotes contraction (i.e. thickening). (See pg. 454)

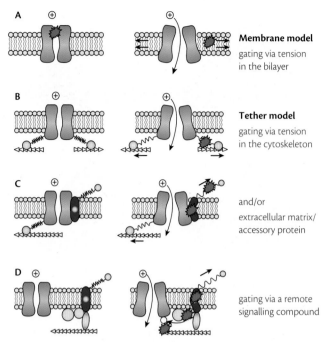

Fig. 65.1 Gating models of MSC. **A** The membrane model: increased tension in the lipid bilayer favours occupancy of the open state as a result of the open channel having a larger in-plane area and a contribution of hydrophobic mismatch. **B** The tether model: the MSC is gated by tension in the cytoskeleton linked to the channel and by (**C**) the extracellular matrix which keeps the channel from being pulled through the bilayer. Accessory proteins close to the channel may be involved. **D** Force may be transmitted remotely to the MSC and/or a signalling pathway is activated that results in an intracellular second messenger gating the channel. Possible sites of action for pharmacological agents are shown (flashes). It is apparent that MSC need not be the site of action of agents. [Modified, with permission, from Christensen AP, Corey DP (2007) TRP channels in mechanosensation: direct or indirect activation? *Nat Rev Neurosci* **8**:510–521.] (See pg. 463)

Arrhythmias in murine models of the mechanically impaired heart

Larissa Fabritz and Paulus Kirchhof

Background

Heart failure (HF) is a severe condition that can provoke premature deaths due to haemodynamic dysfunction or ventricular arrhythmias[1]. Sudden and presumably arrhythmic death causes approximately half of the HF-related deaths and haemodynamic failure the other half. There is a marked inter-individual difference in the time course during which haemodynamic and/or electrical dysfunction develop in HF patients: some patients with compromised left ventricular (LV) function fare well for a long time, while others die within a short time after the initial diagnosis. Clinical, genetic and genomic analyses suggest that genetic predisposition may render some patients prone to contractile and/or electrical dysfunction of the heart, while others may be genetically protected. In the majority of such patients, electrical and mechanical dysfunction of the heart concur[2].

Heart failure may be caused or accompanied by thinning or thickening (hypertrophy) of LV walls and enlargement of the cardiac chambers (dilatation). Cardiac hypertrophy or dilation may temporarily compensate for increased work or increased volume needs, but may convert to 'pathological' hypertrophy associated with worsening of HF or with arrhythmias. Alterations in cardiac structure, contractile function and rhythm can appear separately but are usually interrelated. In some patients they may also all be due to the same molecular cause.

Transgenic murine models with defined genetic abnormalities allow us to characterize the functional relevance of specific genetic abnormalities (Fig. 32.1). For their work on introducing specific gene modifications in mice, using embryonic stem cells, Mario R. Capecchi, Sir Martin J. Evans and Oliver Smithies were jointly awarded the Nobel Prize for Medicine in 2007. Thousands of murine models carrying specific mutations are available today. Transgenic models allow us to study cardiac function at the cellular and organ level and *in vivo*. For the study of arrhythmias, experiments in the beating heart and *in vivo* are invaluable, as single cells can provide only surrogates for arrhythmias. Although mice differ from men in many physiological aspects, e.g. heart rate and action potential duration, most aspects of cardiac physiology are remarkably similar to humans. The propensity for triggered arrhythmias

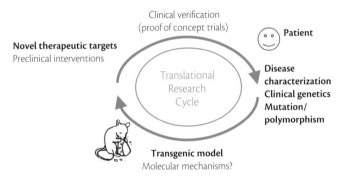

Fig. 32.1 Position of transgenic mouse models in a 'translational research cycle'. Such an integrative approach to cardiovascular research projects has been proposed by several scientists in the past. The entry into such a research cycle may be a new genetic alteration or an altered protein expression or function of a given protein that is identified in patients with a given disease. The gene encoding for that protein is then altered in a transgenic model to test its functional relevance. Established disease models can then be used to study disease-specific or gene-specific mechanisms of electrical and contractile dysfunction. Furthermore, such models can be used to assess new therapeutic interventions prior to their application in patients.

in wild-type murine hearts is influenced by age, weight and experimental conditions, and also genetic background[3]. Many differences can be compensated for by comparing age- and sex-matched pairs of genetically altered and wild-type littermate mice.

With these precautions in mind, studies of cardiac function in transgenic models have given novel insights into molecular and genetic determinants of contractile and electrical dysfunction in the hypertrophied and failing heart. This chapter reviews insights into mechano-electrical coupling gained from the study of transgenic mice.

Angiotensin, atrial natriuretic peptide, cardiac hypertrophy and sudden death

Approximately half of patients with HF suffer from diastolic (filling) defects rather than systolic (contractile) defects. LV hypertrophy, often the myocardial response to arterial hypertension, is one of the common clinical findings in patients with HF and preserved LV systolic function. LV hypertrophy is associated with sudden death in this population[4], and antihypertensive therapy may prevent sudden death in patients with LV hypertrophy[5]. Expression of angiotensin II, one of the most potent known stimuli for hypertrophy and hypertension, provokes LV hypertrophy and may also prolong the ventricular action potential due to altered expression of inward rectifier K^+ current (I_{K1})[6]. Interestingly, locally enhanced expression of angiotensin II in the heart also causes sudden death and atrial fibrillation[7].

Atrial natriuretic peptide (ANP) is the main signalling molecule generated by angiotensin II. Interestingly, increased levels of ANP correlate with clinical outcomes in patients with HF and hypertrophy, suggesting that cardiac ANP signalling may be relevant for arrhythmias in hypertrophied hearts. In mice with a global deletion of the ANP receptor, guanylyl cyclase A, polymorphic ventricular arrhythmias develop during periods of bradycardia in the beating heart[8]. Electrophysiological changes include prolongation of cardiac repolarization and increased dispersion of repolarization, Ca^{2+} transient amplitude and expression of calmodulin-dependent kinase II (CaMKII)[8].

Calmodulin, CaMKII, regulation of ion channels, cardiac hypertrophy and arrhythmias

CaMKII is one of the main kinases that regulate protein function in cardiomyocytes. It is activated by ß-adrenoreceptor stimulation through the Ca^{2+}-binding protein calmodulin[9]. Evidence from other transgenic models including models with enhanced activation of CaMKII and calmodulin-dependent kinase IV (CaMKIV) supports the arrhythmogenic effects of this signalling cascade by demonstrating a crucial role of calmodulin, CaMKII and CaMKIV for normal function of L-type Ca^{2+} channels and the cardiac Na^+ channel[10-12]. Interestingly, CaMKII also alters the function of Na^{+}[10] and K^+ channels[13], suggestive of an involvement of CaMKII in mechano-electric coupling in cardiac hypertrophy[14,15]. In addition, calmodulin interacts with the Ca^{2+} release channel in the sarcoplasmic reticulum (SR), the so-called ryanodine receptor (RyR). Genetic inhibition of the interaction between the RyR and calmodulin causes premature LV hypertrophy and sustained intracellular Ca^{2+} release in cardiomyocytes[14].

Altered function of other kinases and arrhythmias

Chronic activation of protein kinase A (PKA), one of the main mediators of catecholaminergic stimulation in cardiomyocytes, also provokes 'abnormal' LV hypertrophy, reduced LV function and sudden death[16]. Activation of other kinases such as c-Jun-activated N-terminal kinases (JNK)[17] may also favour ventricular hypertrophy and arrhythmias. In addition to prolonged repolarization and increased and defective myocellular Ca^{2+} release, disturbed electrical activation may play a key role in the generation of arrhythmias in such models. JNK7 expression reduces expression of connexin (Cx) 43, the main Cx between ventricular cardiomyocytes, and slows ventricular conduction[17]. The phenotype of reduced QRS complex amplitude and defective electrical cell–cell

coupling is also found when integrin 5K is transiently reduced in the heart[18]. In this context, it is worth noting that Cx lateralization and reduction is found in patients with LV hypertrophy induced by aortic stenosis[19] in experimental models of myocardial infarction[20] and in models of arrhythmogenic right ventricular cardiomyopathy (ARVC; see below).

Similarly, activation of the ras–raf pathway causes ventricular hypertrophy and arrhythmias in transgenic mice, again associated with prolongation of the ventricular action potential, reduced transient outward current (I_{to}) and increased systolic Ca^{2+} release from the SR[21]. In this model, pharmacological modulation of intracellular G-proteins prevents the development of hypertrophy and arrhythmias[21], suggesting that G-proteins can mediate the intracellular signal that provokes hypertrophy and arrhythmias.

Role of phosphatases in hypertrophy, dilatation and heart failure

Protein phosphorylation is the main mechanism by which kinases regulate protein function, and therefore dephosphorylation should be equally important. Protein dephosphorylation mainly occurs through specialized proteins called protein phosphatases. Lack of protein phosphatase 2b, or calcineurin, causes marked premature hypertrophy in mice. Calsarcin deletion has similar effects[22,23]. In these models, hypertrophy appears to be mediated by an altered nuclear genetic program and subsequent alteration in cardiac protein expression[22,23]. Two additional cardiac phosphatases that appear to regulate cardiac protein function more directly are protein phosphatase 2A (PP2A) and protein phosphatase 1 (PP1). In HF, expression of protein phosphatases is increased. Both dilatation and HF are found in mice with enhanced expression of PP2A[24]. Mice with enhanced expression of PP1 develop cardiac hypertrophy[25].

The function of PP2A and PP1 is regulated by inhibitors of phosphatases. The main inhibitors of phosphatases in the heart are called inhibitor 2 (I2) and inhibitor 1 (I1). Cardiac hypertrophy induced by enhanced expression of PP1 can be rescued by overexpression of I2[25]. Enhanced expression of I2, however, was not able to protect from pressure overload by transaortic constriction, but may even exacerbate progression of HF[26]. Enhanced expression of I1 leads to temporary increase in cardiac contractility, but, similar to chronic ß-adrenergic stimulation, may have deleterious chronic effects and predisposes to arrhythmias upon catecholamine excess or physiological stress[27]. These data suggest that altered expression or function of cardiac kinases, protein phosphatases and their inhibitors may provide molecular links between cardiac hypertrophy and arrhythmias.

Dysfunction of Sarcoplasmic reticulum proteins, calcium leaks and arrhythmias

The SR is the main Ca^{2+} store in cardiomyocytes. Each action potential triggers Ca^{2+} release from the SR through the RyR. Contraction ends when the SR Ca^{2+} ATP-ase resorbs Ca^{2+} from the cytosol. Increased Ca^{2+} transient release and altered intracellular Ca^{2+} homeostasis can be provoked by many different molecular processes: altered IP3 Ca^{2+} receptor[28] as well as mutations in the RyR[29] or reduced expression of calstabin (FKBP 12.6,[30]), an accessory protein to the RyR. Some of these mouse models develop HF, while others have normal cardiac contractile function.

SR protein mutations are found in patients with catecholaminergic ventricular tachycardias, substantiating the hypothesis that SR Ca^{2+} release confers arrhythmias[31]. Mice carrying mutations in calsequestrin or the RyR show similar ventricular arrhythmias associated with abnormal Ca^{2+} release from the SR[29,32,33]. Such primary abnormalities of intracellular Ca^{2+} homeostasis may also provoke atrial arrhythmias[34,35].

Defective calmodulin binding to RyR can cause hypertrophy[14]. Models of genetically determined dysfunction of the SR show arrhythmias and HF[36]. Altered function of other SR proteins reproduces a phenotype of arrhythmias in hypertrophy associated with prolongation of ventricular repolarization and increased and prolonged cardioymocyte Ca^{2+} release[37,38], and these effects are correlated with decreased contractile reserve upon catecholamine stimulation when calsequestrin is reduced[36]. Reduction in calsequestrin causes a 'leaky' SR, similar to reduced FKBP 12.6 expression. Impaired Ca^{2+} homeostasis across the sarcolemmal membrane may also provoke ventricular arrhythmias in failing hearts, e.g. altered function of cardiac Na^+/Ca^{2+} exchanger (NCX)[39]. Dysfunction of SR proteins is also intricately linked to contractile dysfunction of the heart[40], suggesting that abnormal SR function could be a molecular link to explain simultaneous electrical and contractile dysfunction in the heart. Furthermore, altered Ca^{2+} binding to the contractile filaments (see next paragraph) is also sufficient to cause intracellular Ca^{2+} imbalance and ventricular arrhythmias[41].

In summary, an altered function of intracellular Ca^{2+} homeostasis and its regulation can be a 'downstream' consequence of molecular and functional changes in several central cellular compartments of the cardiomyocyte, and these changes are found in different disease models associated with arrhythmias and/or HF. Ca^{2+} release and re-uptake are central to normal electrical and contractile function in the heart. Any therapeutic target involving alterations in intracellular Ca^{2+} homeostasis may become a 'double-edged sword' in the therapy of arrhythmias in the mechanically impaired heart.

Complex arrhythmia mechanisms in models of hypertrophic cardiomyopathy

Hypertrophic cardiomyopathy (HCM) is one of the most common inherited cardiomyopathies[2] and is characterized by mutations in sarcomeric proteins associated with LV hypertrophy and sudden death[2]. As Ca^{2+} binding to the contractile filaments is a main modifying factor of intracellular Ca^{2+} homeostasis and contraction, altered function of sarcomeres may contribute to mechano-electric coupling. Deletion of troponin[42] or mutations of myosin[43] in rodents cause abnormal LV hypertrophy and arrhythmias. In a large study of two transgenic lines carrying a classical HCM mutation, the degree of LV hypertrophy was associated with ventricular arrhythmias[44], thereby reproducing findings in patients[45]. In patients, slow and inhomogeneous activation of excitation is found in markedly hypertrophic septa[46], consistent with myocardial disarray and reduced Cx43 expression in a transgenic rabbit model[47].

Some patients with HCM may, however, die suddenly in the absence of LV hypertrophy. In a model carrying a troponin I mutation (I79N), reduced Ca^{2+} binding to the sarcomere caused exercise-induced arrhythmias which were associated with a shortening of early repolarization and abnormal release of Ca^{2+} from the sarcomeres[41]. Mice carrying a mutated troponin T show a similar susceptibility to cardiac arrhythmia that may be conferred by myofilament sensitization to Ca^{2+}[48]. It is hence likely that a combination of myocardial dysarray, LV hypertrophy, altered metabolic state, abnormal cardiomyocyte Ca^{2+} handling and abnormal cardiac repolarization causes arrhythmias in this condition.

Arrhythmogenesis in right ventricular cardiomyopathy – conduction slowing as a consequence of altered mechano-electric coupling?

ARVC is a genetically conferred cardiomyopathy that often manifests in athletes and is characterized by predominantly right ventricular (RV) contractile dysfunction, and arrhythmias originating from the right heart that may lead to sudden death. Genetic studies have identified mutations in genes that express proteins required for normal mechanical cell–cell connections (desmosomes, adherens junctions[49]). Reduced myocardial expression of plakoglobin may be a final common pathway in the development of ARVC[50]. Several transgenic models with targeted deletions[51,52] or mutations[53] of these proteins replicate the development of several features of ARVC, thereby demonstrating that the genetic alterations found are sufficient to generate the disease. Hence, ARVC can be regarded as a defect of mechanical cardiomyocyte–cardiomyocyte contacts. In light of the high sudden death rate in ARVC, this condition may provide a paradigm for arrhythmogenesis linked to mechano-electric coupling.

Mice with heterozygous deletion of the plakoglobin gene develop selective dysfunction of the right ventricle (RV), RV conduction slowing, and arrhythmias of RV origin with old age. Chronic endurance training accelerates development of these pathological changes. Surprisingly, the typical morphological findings of ARVC, fibro-fatty infiltration of the RV myocardium, do not develop in this model, suggesting that the functional phenotype of ARVC can develop without morphological changes[52].

Deletion of desmoplakin in mice replicates fibro-fatty replacement, biventricular hypertrophy and HF[51]. The authors suggest that this phenotype is due to nuclear translocation of plakoglobin and activation of the wnt signalling pathway[51]. As plakoglobin connects cardiomyocytes mechanically, reducing plakoglobin may confer slower conduction (including effects mediated via mechanical modulation of connexion expression and function; see also Chapter 18), contributing to RV dysfunction and arrhythmias in ARVC. In the desmoplakin-deficient model, translocation of plakoglobin from the mechanical cell–cell contacts to the cytosol and subsequent nuclear accumulation of plakoglobin may confer fibro-fatty replacement, e.g. when mutations in other area composita proteins reduce adhesion of plakoglobin to its partners. Mutations in desmoglein, in addition, may confer cardiomyocyte necrosis in ARVC[53].

Atrial brady-cardiomyopathy – another phenotypic facet of mechano-electric coupling?

Enhanced expression of adenosine receptors has been suggested as a means to protect the heart against ischaemic damage[54].

This genetic intervention also confers bradycardia[55,56]. Enhanced expression of A3 adenosine receptors generates relatively severe bradycardia with structural consequences reminiscent of a 'brady-cardiomyopathy': A3 adenosine receptor transgenic hearts develop atrial enlargement, atrial fibrosis and even ventricular fibrosis and enlargement over time[56] (Fig. 32.2). In this 'brady-cardiomyopathy', atrial structural changes precede ventricular alterations.

Therapeutic perspectives derived from transgenic models relate to mechano-electrical coupling

Increasing contractile force may increase arrhythmias; this is an old dilemma in heart failure therapy. Therapeutic interventions that target intracellular Ca^{2+} homeostasis in the heart, e.g. by reducing CaMKII function, have profound effects on cardiac contraction and on arrhythmias that may be beneficial[9,57] or deleterious[14]. In general, it appears difficult to interfere with cardiomyocyte Ca^{2+} regulation without unpredictable unwanted effects. Selective interruption of gene regulation inflicted in cardiac hypertrophy, in contrast, may be possible without altering 'normal'

cardiac function: inhibition of nab1 protects mice against pathological cardiac hypertrophy without inducing overt dysfunction in the heart[58]. Selective deletion of the cyclic adenosine monophosphate (cAMP)-responsive element modulator (CREM) protects the heart against pathological hypertrophy induced by chronically increased ß-adrenoceptor activity[59]. These potentially attractive new therapeutic targets are, however, buried deep within cardiac cells and hence are still difficult to reach *in vivo* with currently available drugs.

Reduced expression of Cx43 is one of the molecular paradigms conferring inducible arrhythmias after a myocardial infarction[20,60]. Genetically conferred reduction in Cx43 expression is sufficient to render the heart susceptible to inducible ventricular arrhythmias[61]. Conversely, mobilization of bone marrow-derived cells into the myocardium[62] or direct 'cell transfer' of progenitor cells with enhanced Cx43 expression into infarcted myocardium[63] may help to prevent arrhythmias after a myocardial infarction through increased expression of Cx43 in the border zone of the infarction[62,63], i.e. the area where slow conduction generates re-entrant circuits. Whether mechanical factors – e.g. a modified response to mechanical load in the border zone – contribute to this beneficial effect of progenitor cells remains to be tested.

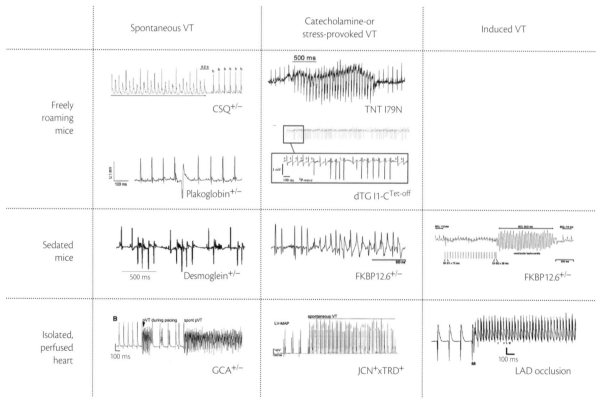

Fig. 32.2 Examples for ventricular arrhythmias observed in genetically altered mouse models. Shown are arrhythmias recorded in freely roaming mice using telemetric ECG monitoring (first row of ECG examples), in sedated mice using conventional limb lead ECG recordings (second row) and arrhythmias observed in the isolated, perfused heart instrumented with electrophysiological catheters (third row). Arrhythmias were observed under different conditions, i.e. spontaneously (first column), after physiological stress tests or pharmacological challenge with catecholamines (second column) or during programmed electrical stimulation (third column) via an electrophysiological intracardiac catheter. Spontaneous arrhythmias and the majority of provoked and induced arrhythmias are polymorphic with the exception of repetitive monomorphic ventricular tachycardias (VT) provoked by stress in JCN × TRD-transgenic mice and in mice expressing the constitutively active phosphatase inhibitor I1, and the exception of induced monomorphic VT in an isolated mouse heart in the chronic healing phase after an anterior myocardial infarction. Arrhythmia morphology and provocation conditions give first suggestions for potential arrhythmia mechanisms. [Recordings are reproduced, with permission, from[36,52] and[41] (first row),[53,30] and[27] (second row) and[8,37] and[62] (third row, all from left to right).] Abbreviations indicate the respective genotypes. LAD, left anterior descending coronary artery.

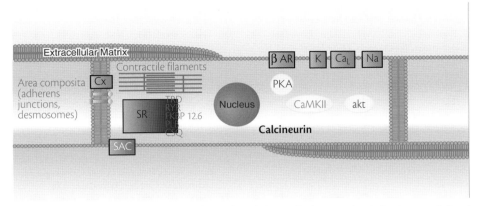

Fig. 32.3 Schematic representation of some of the cellular components that mediate the interaction between electrical and contractile function in cardiomyocytes CSQ, calsequestrin; PLB, phospholamban; TRD, triadin. [Modified, with permission, from Kirchhof P (2009) New antiarrhythmic drugs and new concepts for old drugs. In: *Cardiac Electrophysiology – From Cell to Bedside* (eds DP Zipes, J Jalife). 5th edition, Saunders (Elsevier) Futura, Armonk, New York, pp. 975–982.] (See color plate section.)

Transgenic models have been used to test therapeutic interventions in inherited arrhythmogenic cardiomyopathies. Interestingly, a load-reducing therapy using approved, clinically available substances can prevent ARVC in genetically susceptible animals[64]. Comparably, 'de-training' reduced the incidence of ventricular arrhythmias in athletes[65]. Reducing RV load thus may emerge as a novel way to prevent arrhythmias in ARVC.

Rabbits carrying a classical HCM mutation in the ß-myosin heavy chain (Q403) show signs of metabolic depletion early in the development of the disease[47]. Long-term therapy with high doses of acetylcysteine, an antioxidant, prevents arrhythmias and LV dysfunction in this model, demonstrating that early metabolic changes contribute to HF and arrhythmias in HCM[66].

Conclusions and outlook

Heart rhythm, cardiac contraction, and myocardial morphology are closely interrelated. Electrical dysfunction can cause contractile dysfunction of the heart and vice versa. Genetically altered mouse models allow one to study the functional and molecular consequences of defined genetic alterations *in vivo*, in the intact heart and at the cellular and subcellular level. To address current shortcomings in insight, care should be taken to look at problems from all sides. However, understanding of these complex mechanisms will most likely require a mosaic of insights from functional and molecular studies rather than a focussed study of a single molecular 'mosaic stone'.

Studies in transgenic models suggest several 'molecular links' between electrical and contractile dysfunction, i.e. proteins that affect electrical *and* contractile function of the heart (Fig. 32.3). The available data in transgenic models suggest that arrhythmias may be more closely related to cardiac hypertrophy than to heart failure. Transgenic models can also be applied to study the effects of therapeutic interventions in genetically determined cardiomyopathies, diseases that usually affect electrical and contractile function of the heart.

Targeted genetic alterations also exemplify that even the most selective modulation of a single protein confers complex regulatory and counter-balancing effects in other proteins and cell compartments, e.g. when genetic modification of one Ca^{2+} handling protein affects expression and function of other genes and proteins. It is a very fragile balance that conveys normal electrical and

contractile function of the heart, and therapeutic targets need to be chosen carefully.

Acknowledgements

Support for this chapter came from from the Interdisziplinäres Zentrum für Klinische Forschung (IZKF) Münster (Core unit CarTel), Deutsch Forschungsgemeinschaft (DFG Ki 731/1-1, FA 413/3-1, SFB 656-A8). We thank Tonja Fabritz for help with the figures.

References

1. Dickstein K, Cohen-Solal A, Filippatos G, *et al.* ESC Guidelines for the diagnosis and treatment of acute and chronic heart failure 2008: the Task Force for the Diagnosis and Treatment of Acute and Chronic Heart Failure 2008 of the European Society of Cardiology. Developed in collaboration with the Heart Failure Association of the ESC (HFA) and endorsed by the European Society of Intensive Care Medicine (ESICM). *Eur Heart J* 2008;**29**:2388–2442.
2. Maron BJ, Towbin JA, Thiene G, *et al.* Contemporary definitions and classification of the cardiomyopathies: an American Heart Association Scientific Statement from the Council on Clinical Cardiology, Heart Failure and Transplantation Committee; Quality of Care and Outcomes Research and Functional Genomics and Translational Biology Interdisciplinary Working Groups; and Council on Epidemiology and Prevention. *Circulation* 2006;**113**:1807–1816.
3. Waldeyer C, Fabritz L, Fortmueller L, *et al.* Regional, age-dependent, and genotype-dependent differences in ventricular action potential duration and activation time in 410 Langendorff-perfused mouse hearts. *Bas Res Cardiol* 2009;**104**:523–533.
4. Haider AW, Larson MG, Benjamin EJ, Levy D. Increased left ventricular mass and hypertrophy are associated with increased risk for sudden death. *J Am Coll Cardiol* 1998;**32**:1454–1459.
5. Kirchhof P, Breithardt G, Eckardt L. Primary prevention of sudden cardiac death. *Heart* 2006;**92**:1873–1878.
6. Domenighetti AA, Boixel C, Cefai D, Abriel H, Pedrazzini T. Chronic angiotensin II stimulation in the heart produces an acquired long QT syndrome associated with IK1 potassium current downregulation. *J Mol Cell Cardiol* 2007;**42**:63–70.
7. Xiao HD, Fuchs S, Campbell DJ, *et al.* Mice with cardiac-restricted angiotensin-converting enzyme (ACE) have atrial enlargement, cardiac arrhythmia, and sudden death. *Am J Pathol* 2004;**165**:1019–1032.
8. Kirchhof P, Fabritz L, Begrow F, Kilic A, Breithardt G, Kuhn M. Ventricular arrhythmias, increased cardiac calmodulin kinase II expression, and altered repolarization kinetics in ANP-receptor deficient mice. *J Mol Cell Cardiol* 2004;**36**:691–700.

9. Zhang R, Khoo MS, Wu Y, et al. Calmodulin kinase II inhibition protects against structural heart disease. Nat Med 2005;11:409–417.

10. Wagner S, Dybkova N, Rasenack E, et al. Ca/calmodulin-dependent protein kinase II regulates cardiac Na channels. J Clin Invest 2006;116:3127–3138.

11. Zuhlke RD, Pitt GS, Deisseroth K, Tsien RW, Reuter H. Calmodulin supports both inactivation and facilitation of L-type calcium channels. Nature 1999;399:159–162.

12. Wu Y, Temple J, Zhang R, et al. Calmodulin kinase II and arrhythmias in a mouse model of cardiac hypertrophy. Circulation 2002;106: 1288–1293.

13. Wagner S, Hacker E, Grandi E, et al. Ca/calmodulin kinase II differentially modulates potassium currents. Circ Arrhythm Electrophysiol 2009;2:285–294.

14. Yamaguchi N, Takahashi N, Xu L, Smithies O, Meissner G. Early cardiac hypertrophy in mice with impaired calmodulin regulation of cardiac muscle Ca release channel. J Clin Invest 2007;117:1344–1353.

15. Zhang T, Maier LS, Dalton ND, Miyamoto S, Ross J, Jr., Bers DM, Brown JH. The deltaC isoform of CaMKII is activated in cardiac hypertrophy and induces dilated cardiomyopathy and heart failure. Circ Res 2003;92:912–919.

16. Antos CL, Frey N, Marx SO, et al. Dilated cardiomyopathy and sudden death resulting from constitutive activation of protein kinase A. Circ Res 2001;89:997–1004.

17. Petrich BG, Gong X, Lerner DL, Wang X, Brown JH, Saffitz JE, Wang Y. c-Jun N-terminal kinase activation mediates downregulation of connexin43 in cardiomyocytes. Circ Res 2002;91:640–647.

18. Valencik ML, Zhang D, Punske B, Hu P, McDonald JA, Litwin SE. Integrin activation in the heart: a link between electrical and contractile dysfunction? Circ Res 2006;99:1403–1410.

19. Kostin S, Dammer S, Hein S, Klovekorn WP, Bauer EP, Schaper J. Connexin 43 expression and distribution in compensated and decompensated cardiac hypertrophy in patients with aortic stenosis. Cardiovasc Res 2004;62:426–436.

20. Yao JA, Hussain W, Patel P, Peters NS, Boyden PA, Wit AL. Remodeling of gap junctional channel function in epicardial border zone of healing canine infarcts. Circ Res 2003;92:437–443.

21. Ruan H, Mitchell S, Vainoriene M, et al. Gi alpha1-mediated cardiac electrophysiological remodeling and arrhythmia in hypertrophic cardiomyopathy. Circulation 2007;116:596–605.

22. Molkentin JD, Lu JR, Antos CL, et al. A calcineurin-dependent transcriptional pathway for cardiac hypertrophy. Cell 1998;93:215–228.

23. Frey N, Barrientos T, Shelton JM, et al. Mice lacking calsarcin-1 are sensitized to calcineurin signaling and show accelerated cardiomyopathy in response to pathological biomechanical stress. Nat Med 2004;10:1336–1343.

24. Gergs U, Boknik P, Buchwalow I, et al. Overexpression of the catalytic subunit of protein phosphatase 2A impairs cardiac function. J Biol Chem 2004;279:40823–40834.

25. Bruchert N, Mavila N, Boknik P, et al. Inhibitor-2 prevents phosphatase 1 induced cardiac hypertrophy and mortality. Am J Physiol 2008;295:H1539–H1546.

26. Grote-Wessels S, Baba HA, Boknik P, et al. Inhibition of protein phosphatase 1 by inhibitor-2 exacerbates progression of cardiac failure in a model with pressure overload. Cardiovasc Res 2008;79:464–471.

27. Wittkopper K, Fabritz L, Neef S, et al. (2010) Constitutively active phosphatase inhibitor-1 improves cardiac contractility in young mice but is deleterious after catecholaminergic stress and with aging. J Clin Invest 120:617–626.

28. Harzheim D, Movassagh M, Foo RS, et al. (2009) Increased InsP3Rs in the junctional sarcoplasmic reticulum augment Ca2+ transients and arrhythmias associated with cardiac hypertrophy. Proc Natl Acad Sci USA 106:11406–11411.

29. Rizzi N, Liu N, Napolitano C, et al. Unexpected structural and functional consequences of the R33Q homozygous mutation in cardiac calsequestrin. A complex arrhythmogenic cascade in a knock in mouse model. Circ Res 2008;103:298.

30. Wehrens XH, Lehnart SE, Reiken SR, et al. Protection from cardiac arrhythmia through ryanodine receptor-stabilizing protein calstabin2. Science 2004;304:292–296.

31. Leenhardt A, Lucet V, Denjoy I, Grau F, Ngoc DD, Coumel P. Catecholaminergic polymorphic ventricular tachycardia in children. A 7-year follow-up of 21 patients. Circulation 1995;91:1512–1519.

32. Liu N, Colombi B, Memmi M, et al. Arrhythmogenesis in catecholaminergic polymorphic ventricular tachycardia: insights from a RyR2 R4496C knock-in mouse model. Circ Res 2006;99:292–298.

33. Postma AV, Denjoy I, Hoorntje TM, et al. Absence of calsequestrin 2 causes severe forms of catecholaminergic polymorphic ventricular tachycardia. Circ Res 2002;91:e21–e26.

34. Kirchhefer U, Baba HA, Jones LR, Kirchhof P, Schmitz W, Neumann J. Age-dependent biochemical and contractile properties in atrium of transgenic mice overexpressing junctin. Am J Physiol 2004;287: H2216–H2225.

35. Chelu MG, Satyam S, Sood S, et al. Calmodulin kinase II-mediated sarcoplasmatic reticulum Ca2+ leak promotes atrial fibrillation in mice. J Clin Invest 2009;119:1940–1951.

36. Knollmann BC, Chopra N, Hlaing T, et al. Casq2 deletion causes sarcoplasmic reticulum volume increase, premature Ca2+ release, and catecholaminergic polymorphic ventricular tachycardia. J Clin Invest 2006;116:2510–2520.

37. Kirchhof P, Klimas J, Fabritz L, et al. Stress and high heart rate provoke ventricular tachycardia in mice expressing triadin. J Mol Cell Cardiol 2007;42:962–971.

38. Viatchenko-Karpinski S, Terentyev D, Gyorke I, et al. Abnormal calcium signaling and sudden cardiac death associated with mutation of calsequestrin. Circ Res 2004;94:471–477.

39. Pott C, Goldhaber JI, Philipson KD. Genetic manipulation of cardiac Na+/Ca2+ exchange expression. Biochem Biophys Res Commun 2004;322:1336–1340.

40. Terentyev D, Cala SE, Houle TD, et al. Triadin overexpression stimulates excitation-contraction coupling and increases predisposition to cellular arrhythmia in cardiac myocytes. Circ Res 2005;96:651–658.

41. Knollmann BC, Kirchhof P, Sirenko SG, et al. Familial hypertrophic cardiomyopathy-linked mutant troponin T causes stress-induced ventricular tachycardia and Ca2+-dependent action potential remodeling. Circ Res 2003;92:428–436.

42. Frey N, Franz WM, Gloeckner K, et al. Transgenic rat hearts expressing a human cardiac troponin T deletion reveal diastolic dysfunction and ventricular arrhythmias. Cardiovasc Res 2000;47:254–264.

43. Vikstrom KL, Factor SM, Leinwand LA. Mice expressing mutant myosin heavy chains are a model for familial hypertrophic cardiomyopathy. Mol Med 1996;2:556–567.

44. Wolf CM, Moskowitz IP, Arno S, et al. Somatic events modify hypertrophic cardiomyopathy pathology and link hypertrophy to arrhythmia. Proc Natl Acad Sci USA 2005;102:18123–18128.

45. Spirito P, Bellone P, Harris KM, Bernabo P, Bruzzi P, Maron BJ. Magnitude of left ventricular hypertrophy and risk of sudden death in hypertrophic cardiomyopathy. N Engl J Med 2000;342:1778–1785.

46. Schumacher B, Gietzen FH, Neuser H, et al. Electrophysiological characteristics of septal hypertrophy in patients with hypertrophic obstructive cardiomyopathy and moderate to severe symptoms. Circulation 2005;112:2096–2101.

47. Ripplinger CM, Li W, Hadley J, et al. Enhanced transmural fiber rotation and connexin 43 heterogeneity are associated with an increased upper limit of vulnerability in a Transgenic rabbit model of human hypertrophic cardiomyopathy. Circ Res 2007;101: 1049–1057.

48. Baudenbacher F, Schober T, Pinto JR, et al. Myofilament Ca2+ sensitization causes susceptibility to cardiac arrhythmia in mice. J Clin Invest 2008;118:3893–3903.

49. Gerull B, Heuser A, Wichter T, *et al*. Mutations in the desmosomal protein plakophilin-2 are common in arrhythmogenic right ventricular cardiomyopathy. *Nat Genet* 2004;**36**:1162–1164.

50. Asimaki A, Tandri H, Huang H, *et al*. A new diagnostic test for arrhythmogenic right ventricular cardiomyopathy. *N Engl J Med* 2009;**360**:1075–1084.

51. Garcia-Gras E, Lombardi R, Giocondo MJ, Willerson JT, Schneider MD, Khoury DS, Marian AJ. Suppression of canonical Wnt/beta-catenin signaling by nuclear plakoglobin recapitulates phenotype of arrhythmogenic right ventricular cardiomyopathy. *J Clin Invest* 2006; **116**:2012–2021.

52. Kirchhof P, Fabritz L, Zwiener M, *et al*. Age- and training-dependent development of arrhythmogenic right ventricular cardiomyopathy in heterozygous plakoglobin-deficient mice. *Circulation* 2006;**114**:1799–1806.

53. Pilichou K, Remme CA, Basso C, *et al*. Myocyte necrosis underlies progressive myocardial dystrophy in mouse dsg2-related arrhythmogenic right ventricular cardiomyopathy. *J Exp Med* 2009;**206**:1787–1802.

54. Guo Y, Bolli R, Bao W, *et al*. Targeted deletion of the A3 adenosine receptor confers resistance to myocardial ischemic injury and does not prevent early preconditioning. *J Mol Cell Cardiol* 2001;**33**:825–830.

55. Kirchhof P, Fabritz L, Fortmüller L, *et al*. Decreased chronotropic response to exercise and atrio-ventricular nodal conduction delay in mice overexpressing the A1-adenosine receptor. *Am J Physiol* 2003;**285**:H145–H153.

56. Fabritz L, Kirchhof P, Fortmüller L, *et al*. Gene dose-dependent atrial arrhythmias, heart block and atrial brady-cardiomyopathy in mice overexpressing the A3 -adenosine receptor. *Cardiovasc Res* 2004; **62**:500–508.

57. Ling H, Zhang T, Pereira L, *et al*. Requirement for Ca^{2+}/calmodulin-dependent kinase II in the transition from pressure overload-induced cardiac hypertrophy to heart failure in mice. *J Clin Invest* 2009;**119**: 1230–1240.

58. Buitrago M, Lorenz K, Maass AH, *et al*. The transcriptional repressor Nab1 is a specific regulator of pathological cardiac hypertrophy. *Nat Med* 2005;**11**:837–844.

59. Lewin G, Matus M, Basu A, *et al*. Critical role of transcription factor cyclic AMP response element modulator in beta1-adrenoceptor-mediated cardiac dysfunction. *Circulation* 2009;**119**:79–88.

60. Peters NS, Coromilas J, Severs NJ, Wit AL. Disturbed connexin43 gap junction distribution correlates with the location of reentrant circuits in the epicardial border zone of healing canine infarcts that cause ventricular tachycardia. *Circulation* 1997;**95**:988–996.

61. van Rijen HV, Eckardt D, Degen J, *et al*. Slow conduction and enhanced anisotropy increase the propensity for ventricular tachyarrhythmias in adult mice with induced deletion of connexin43. *Circulation* 2004;**109**:1048–1055.

62. Kuhlmann MT, Kirchhof P, Klocke R, *et al*. G-CSF/SCF reduces inducible arrhythmias in the infarcted heart potentially via increased connexin43 expression and arteriogenesis. *J Exp Med* 2006;**203**: 87–97.

63. Roell W, Lewalter T, Sasse P, *et al*. Engraftment of connexin 43-expressing cells prevents post-infarct arrhythmia. *Nature* 2007; **450**:819–824.

64. Fabritz L, Hoogendijk M, Scicluna BP, Van Amersfoorth SC, Fortmueller L, Wolf S, *et al*. Preload-reducing therapy prevents expression of arrhythmogenic right ventricular cardiomyopathy in plakoglobin-deficient mice. *J Am Coll Cardiol* 2011 (in press).

65. Biffi A, Maron BJ, Verdile L, *et al*. Impact of physical deconditioning on ventricular tachyarrhythmias in trained athletes. *J Am Coll Cardiol* 2004;**44**:1053–1058.

66. Lombardi R, Rodriguez G, Chen SN, *et al*. Resolution of established cardiac hypertrophy and fibrosis and prevention of systolic dysfunction in a transgenic rabbit model of human cardiomyopathy through thiol-sensitive mechanisms. *Circulation* 2009;**119**:1398–1407.

67. Kirchhof P. New antiarrhythmic drugs and new concepts for old drugs. In: *Cardiac Electrophysiology – From Cell to Bedside* (eds DP Zipes, J Jalife). 5th edition, Saunders (Elsevier), New York, 2009: pp. 975–982.

Studying cardiac mechano-sensitivity in man

Flavia Ravelli and Michela Masè

Background

The human heart performs its function in a constantly changing mechanical environment, due to the action of both intrinsic and extrinsic mechanical stimuli. The cardiac cycle itself, alternating between filling and emptying of the cardiac chambers, involves conditions of muscle distension and shortening. Changes in intrathoracic pressure, venous return to the heart and peripheral resistance, associated with respiration, constitute additional sources of mechanical variability of the heart.

Changes in the mechanical state of the heart are known to affect the behaviour of pacemaker cells as well as the conductive and refractory properties of the cardiac tissue via mechano-electrical coupling (MEC). These variations are mirrored by changes in the variability of heart beat interval series, determined from electrocardiogram (ECG) or endocardial signals, which allows in principle a non-invasive assessment of MEC effects in humans. The ability to determine mechanical modulation of cardiac performance and its resulting electrical variations depends on both the availability of suitable signal analysis methods (allowing to associate rhythm variations to their physiological correlates) and the choice of human models where mechanical effects are not overridden by other prevalent factors, such as autonomic modulation.

This chapter reviews the evidence supporting the contribution of non-neural mechanical mechanisms in the modulation of sinus rhythm as well as the mechanical origin of atrial rate variability during re-entrant arrhythmias, such as atrial flutter.

Studying heart rate and rhythm in man

Beat-by-beat cardiovascular time series with their particular oscillations mirror the complexity of their underlying physiological functions, including mechanical variations, and thus their characterization may offer a unique insight into the integrated control of the cardiovascular system.

Since physiological control mechanisms and neural regulatory activities appear to be coded in different modalities such as amplitude and frequency, spectral and cross-spectral parameters[1] may be used to track and determine the relative contributions of the various mechanisms that influence heart rate variability. Indeed, spectral analysis that involves the decomposition of a time series into its oscillatory components has identified the existence of two

primary oscillations in inter-beat interval (established from RR duration on the ECG) variability in humans: a high-frequency component (hF, 0.15–0.4 Hz) which is respiratory-related and largely seen as representative of vagal tone, and a low-frequency component (lF, 0.03–0.15 Hz) which is attributed to both vagal and sympathetic innervations of the heart[1–3]. Indices from cross-spectral analysis can be used to identify correlations between couples of variability series at different frequencies. Specifically, the coherence function has been used to assess the strength of linear coupling between spontaneous fluctuations of heart period, systolic pressure and respiration in different frequency bands, while the phase spectrum, quantifying the delay by which rhythms propagate, has provided information about time delays associated with transmission over fast/slow reflex pathways[1,4].

Since the complexity of the relations between haemodynamical, electrophysiological and humoral variables questions the assumption of pure linear dynamics in the genesis of cardiovascular event fluctuations, linear descriptors have been integrated with tools from non-linear dynamics and phase synchronization theory[5], allowing us to model, characterize and predict synchronization and modulation in multivariate cardiovascular series. Indeed the stroboscopic observation of coupled time series[5], as provided by synchrograms and phase-response curves, has revealed the existence of synchronized states of different orders in the cardiorespiratory system[5], as well as the correlation between atrial flutter variability and atrial volume changes during the cardiac cycle[6].

Mechanical modulation of sinus rhythm: the non-neural component of respiratory sinus arrhythmia

From observations in animal experiments it has long been known that the heart responds to an increase in right-atrial filling pressure with an increase in heart rate[7]. Although evidence of a positive chronotropic response to stretch has been observed in the human heart, mechanical effects are usually overridden by other regulatory mechanisms that may mask their physiological significance. One example of this entanglement of multiple mechanisms is represented by respiratory sinus arrhythmia (RSA). RSA is the modulation of heart rate that occurs in phase with the respiratory cycle, generally recognized to reflect fluctuations in cardiac parasympathetic efferent activity to the sinoatrial node (SAN) pacemaker[3]. However, the presence of residual RSA in denervated hearts[8,9] and during autonomic blockade[10,11] has suggested the existence of additional non-neural regulatory mechanisms that could affect heart rate via periodic alteration in the extent of SAN pacemaker tissue strain, in synchrony with respiratory changes in venous return. Clinical and experimental evidence has thus been provided for a relevant role of non-neural mechanisms in conditions associated with reduced cardiac vagal tone, such as exercise[10,12] and heart failure[11].

Respiratory sinus arrhythmia in heart-transplanted patients

Heart transplant recipients represent a unique model to evaluate mechanical contributions to rhythm regulation, since donor hearts are fully denervated during the operation and autonomic reinnervation is unlikely to occur in the first year after operation[8,9].

Respiratory mechanical effects on heart rate series were studied by spectral and cross-spectral analysis in cardiac allograft transplant recipients, in resting conditions and during specific respiratory manoeuvres[8]. Although the amplitude of the oscillation was markedly reduced in heart transplant recipients (1.7–7.9% of that seen in normal subjects), an hF peak synchronous with respiration was found in the RR spectrum of all patients (Fig. 33.1). RSA in transplant patients presented peculiar features, which differed from those typically observed in normal subjects, and were suggestive of a mechanical origin of the phenomenon. Indeed the respiratory modulation of heart rate involved short time delays with respect to normal RSA[12], and its amplitude was markedly influenced by tidal volume and respiratory rate and magnified by respiratory manoeuvres (such as single deep breaths) involving sudden changes in intrathoracic pressure[8].

Respiratory sinus arrhythmia in exercise and heart failure

Although negligible in healthy humans at rest, intrinsic mechanisms can make relevant contributions to heart rate regulation in conditions where cardiac vagal control and responsiveness are greatly reduced, as during exercise or in severe heart failure.

During exercise at lower loads, normal subjects exhibited a progressive increase in heart rate, decrease of hF heart rate variability and relative increase in lF variability, which are generally interpreted as markers of sympathetic tone prevalence. Nevertheless at peak exercise the relative proportion of lF and hF was subverted, with the hF oscillations accounting for the majority of heart rate variability[12]. The increase of RSA at peak exercise was consistent with a non-neural mechanism, which became evident when autonomic modulation was very low due to or in coincidence with tachycardia, and when the changes in intrathoracic pressure were maximal, as typically occurs at peak exercise. A similar behaviour at peak exercise was indeed observed not only in normal subjects, but also in heart transplant recipients[9,12], who displayed a progressive increase of hF power from beginning to peak exercise, showing a direct correlation between RSA and the increase of ventilation with exercise. Moreover, experiments in healthy subjects before and during ganglion blockade showed non-neural modulation to account for one third of RSA amplitude during mild exercise, while being negligible (1%) at rest[10].

Non-neural mechanisms have been suggested to play a significant role in heart rate regulation in patients with congestive heart failure (CHF)[11,13]. CHF is associated with a reduction in cardiac vagal responsiveness and a decrease of absolute hF and lF powers with disease progression. Nonetheless, hF oscillations, accounting for most heart rate variability, have been shown to persist even in the most advanced stages of the disease, suggesting that RSA in severe CHF might be entirely mediated by intrinsic mechanisms[11,13].

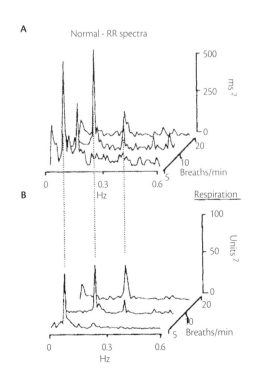

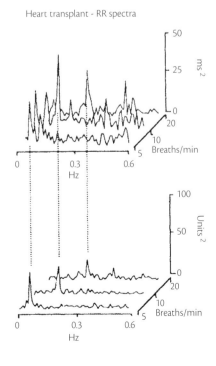

Fig. 33.1 Respiratory component of heart rate variability in a heart transplant patient compared with a normal subject. RR interval (**A**) and respiratory (**B**) power spectra during controlled breathing at varying respiratory rate. [Reproduced, with permission, from Bernardi L, Keller F, Sanders M, *et al.* (1989) Respiratory sinus arrhythmia in the denervated human heart. *J Appl Physiol* **67**: 1447–1455.]

Indeed small heart rate fluctuations synchronous with breathing persisted after ganglion blockade in patients with mild CHF and age-matched healthy subjects[11], with similar magnitude in the two populations. However, the relative contribution of non-neural oscillations was relevant only in CHF patients (15% vs 3% in controls), due to the decreased value of RSA with the disease.

Mechanisms of non-neural respiratory sinus arrhythmia

The peculiar features of non-neural RSA during sinus rhythm are consistent with a mechano-sensitive mechanism, intrinsic to the heart itself, which would affect heart rate in response to changes in venous return associated with the respiratory cycle. Specifically, during inspiration, venous return from the lower part of the body towards the right atrium is favoured, which increases right-atrial preload and promotes diastolic distension of the right atrial wall and SAN pacemaker[14]. As stretch of the pacemaker is known to increase heart rate, even in isolated tissue[15], this chronotropic mechanism may play a role in RSA generation. Indeed mechano-electrical modulation has been shown to operate on a beat-to-beat basis and to occur rapidly[16], which is consistent with the small time delays observed between respiratory and heart rate oscillations[12]. Additionally, the mechanical origin of non-neural RSA is supported by the strong dependence of its amplitude on factors affecting the magnitude of right atrial pressure changes, such as tidal volume, respiratory rate and body position[9,10,12]; for a discussion of transmural atrial pressure, see Chapter 39.

Although the positive chronotropic effect of stretch on heart rate has been known for almost a century, the specific cellular mechanisms by which stretch would induce a variation in the SAN beating frequency are still under investigation. Stretch may directly affect the behaviour of myocardial cells, modulating ion-channel activity[17] and cellular calcium handling[18], or its effect may be mediated by second messengers [such as nitric oxide (NO)[19]] and other cell populations [e.g. fibroblasts[7,20]]. Indeed current-clamp

and voltage-clamp experiments during application of moderate longitudinal stretch to isolated, spontaneously beating rabbit SAN cells showed that stretch-activation of cation non-selective ion channels could produce the observed increase in beating rate and associated reductions in maximum diastolic and systolic potentials[17]. Moreover the correlation between stretch and NO release from endothelial cells[19] points to an additional NO-mediated pathway, which may increase heart rate both by stimulation of the hyperpolarization-activated inward current (If) and facilitation of Ca^{2+} release from the sarcoplasmic reticulum[7]. Finally, although functionally assessed only in mathematical models, direct electrotonic interaction of SAN cells with mechano-sensitive cardiac fibroblasts[20] could additionally contribute to the positive chronotropic effect of stretch[7].

Mechanical modulation of re-entrant rhythms: the atrial flutter case

Mechanical events of the heart may also influence cardiac arrhythmias. Evidence has been reported that documents the mechanical modulation of atrial flutter (AFL) a common supraventricular arrhythmia based on a re-entrant mechanism[21]. Despite the stability of the re-entrant circuit underlying the arrhythmia, several observations have indicated that AFL is not a strictly regular rhythm[6,22–24] but displays small variations in the length of intra-auricular cycles, with an average of about 5 ms (Fig. 33.2). The nature of these fluctuations, unknown for so long, has been demonstrated recently to be of mechanical origin[6,24–27].

Ventricular contraction and respiration: two sources of AFL cycle length variability

The small spontaneous beat-to-beat variability of AFL cycle length is not random, but composed of periodic patterns. Indeed spectral analysis and power band interpretation applied to AFL interval series identified two main oscillatory components which correlated

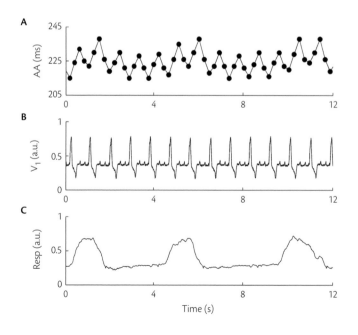
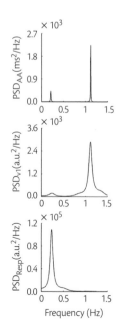

Fig. 33.2 Ventricular and respiratory origin of atrial flutter (AFL) cycle length variability. Signals (left) and corresponding power spectra (right) in a representative patient: atrial cycle length series (**A**), ECG (**B**) and respiratory signal (Resp.) (**C**). a.u., arbitrary units. [Reproduced, with permission, from Ravelli F, Masè M, Disertori M (2008) Mechanical modulation of atrial flutter cycle length. *Prog Biophys Mol Biol* **97**: 417–434.]

with ventricular and respiratory activities[25]. The ventricular contraction-related oscillation was predominant, comprising 54% of the total spectral power, and was shifted by ventricular pacing in line with changing frequency, while the respiratory-related oscillation represented 22% of the power and followed respiratory rate changes under controlled breathing (Fig. 33.2).

Modulation of AFL cycle length by ventricular activity

The strict coupling between atrial interval fluctuations and the timing of ventricular activation has been disclosed both in animals and humans by phase-response curves[6,24,28], in which AFL cycle length was displayed against the time after the previous ventricular activation complex. Indeed in typical AFL, the atrial interval gradually increased after the onset of the QRS complex, reached a maximum value after about 400 ms and decreased until the next ventricular beat occurred (Fig. 33.3). The critical role of ventricular contraction in the modulation of AFL interval variability was also evidenced by applying carotid sinus massage. Indeed ventricular asystole, caused by the massage, markedly reduced or even abolished variations in AFL rate[6].

Modulation of AFL cycle length by respiratory activity

The dependence of AFL rate on respiratory phase was first investigated by Waxman et al.[29], who observed the shortening of AFL cycle length during respiratory manoeuvres that reduced cardiac volume, such as the strain phase of the Valsalva manoeuvre or expiration. A quantitative and thorough characterization of the cardio-respiratory interactions during AFL was provided in a recent study[27], which revealed the reverse and frequency-independent nature of the modulation. Cross-spectral analysis showed AFL cycle lengths to oscillate in phase with respiration for all respiratory frequencies in the range of 0.1–0.4 Hz, with small temporal delay (0.40 ± 0.15 s) between coupled oscillations, resulting in paradoxically longer atrial intervals during inspiration than expiration (Fig. 33.4). These features distinguish respiratory variations

in AFL cycle length from normal RSA, which is characterized at typical breathing frequencies (around 0.25 Hz) by the lengthening of heart period during expiration and its shortening during inspiration, by longer temporal delays (1.5 s) and by frequency-dependent behaviours, with both amplitude and phase relations strongly affected by the respiratory rate[3,4,30].

Evidence for a mechanical origin of AFL cycle length variability

Although various mechanisms may account for oscillations in AFL cycle length, the available evidence supports an intrinsic, mechano-sensitive mechanism, which affects AFL rate on a beat-by-beat basis by atrial volume changes.

Evidence against a neurally mediated origin of AFL cycle length variability

Autonomic nervous reflexes caused by haemodynamic variations associated with ventricular and respiratory activities may hypothetically cause the observed changes in AFL cycle length. Changes in arterial pressure, atrial and lung volume associated with ventricular contraction and/or respiration may stimulate arterial baroreceptors, atrial mechanoreceptors and lung receptors, which could in turn cause reflex responses[31,32]. Although changes in autonomic nervous activity are known to influence the electrophysiological properties of atrial muscle[33], sound evidence has been reported which excludes a role of neural mechanisms in the generation of AFL interval variability. Studies in humans and animals showed the persistence of AFL cycle length oscillations after pharmacological autonomic blockade by combined muscarinic and beta-adrenergic receptor blockers[25,28,29] and in denervated hearts[34]. Additional evidence against an autonomic involvement in AFL variability is represented by the small temporal delays between the onset of ventricular contraction and the initial lengthening of the flutter cycle [about 50 ms[6]] and between respiratory events and the related AFL interval oscillations[27].

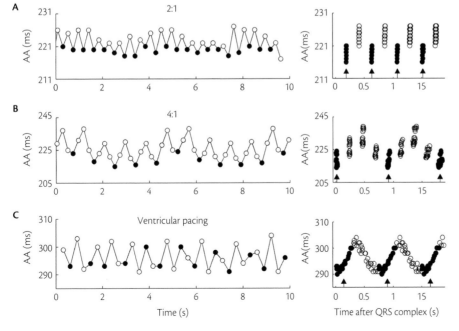

Fig. 33.3 Ventricular modulation of AFL cycle length. Atrial cycle length series (left) and corresponding phase-response curves (right) in AFL patients with 2:1 (**A**) and 4:1 (**B**) AV conduction and during ventricular pacing (**C**). Intervals in which a ventricular beat occurs are marked by filled circles and vertical arrows. [Reproduced, with permission, from Lammers WJEP, Ravelli F, Disertori M, Antolini R, Furlanello F, Allessie MA (1991) Variations in human atrial flutter cycle length induced by ventricular beats: evidence of a reentrant circuit with a partially excitable gap. *J Cardiovasc Electrophysiol* **2**:375–387.]

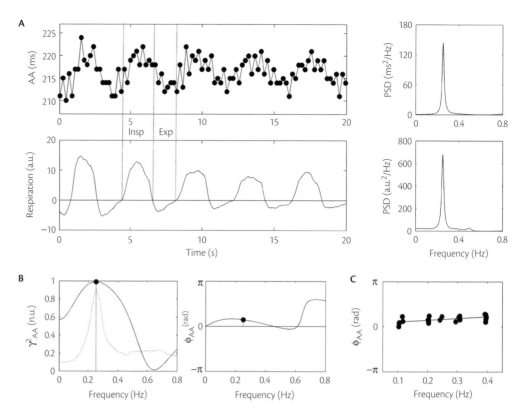

Fig. 33.4 Respiratory modulation of AFL cycle length. **A** Atrial cycle length series (top) and respiratory signal (bottom) with corresponding power spectra in a representative patient. **B** Coherence (left) and phase (right) functions between atrial cycle length and respirogram series. Full dots represent the frequency of respiration. **C** Phase between atrial cycle length and respiration at changing respiratory rate during controlled respiration in the overall population. insp, Inspiration; exp, expiration. [Reproduced, with permission, from Masè M, Disertori M, Ravelli F (2009) Cardiorespiratory interactions in patients with atrial flutter. *J Appl Physiol* **106**:29–39.]

Correlation between atrial volume changes and AFL variability patterns

Evidence for a straight correlation between the variability pattern of AFL cycle length and changes in atrial volume, induced by ventricular and respiratory activity, supports a mechanical origin of these interval oscillations.

The existence of a relationship between atrial size and AFL rate was shown many decades ago, when acute or chronic atrial enlargement were found to slow the rate of experimentally induced AFL in dogs[35]. Similarly, AFL patients displayed a strong correlation between atrial size and the average atrial cycle length[36,37]. Consistent experimental evidence of the direct effect of atrial volume/pressure on AFL circuit and rate was provided by the studies of Waxman *et al.*[29,38]. Passive upright tilting, the strain phase of the Valsalva manoeuvre, and expiration, three interventions that reduced cardiac size, were shown to increase AFL rate in patients, independently of autonomic tone[29]. In addition, occlusion of the inferior *vena cava* increased AFL rate in dogs[38]. Interestingly, development of 1:1 AV conduction in patients with atrial flutter slowed AFL rate by increasing atrial pressure[38].

Likewise, a correlation between the variability pattern of AFL cycle length and spontaneous alterations in atrial volume subsequent to ventricular systole has been demonstrated[24]. As shown in Fig. 33.5, the phase-response curve of AFL cycle length was found to be synchronous with changes in atrial pressure and/or volume occurring during the ventricular cycle, concomitant with closure/opening of the atrio-ventricular (AV) valves [6,24,28]. Although not directly proven by simultaneous measurements, a causal relationship between the respiratory variability of AFL and atrial volume changes, induced by respiration, was suggested by

the similar time course of the paradoxical increase/decrease of AFL cycle length during inspiration/expiration (Fig. 33.4) and the increase/decrease of venous return to the heart associated with the two respiratory phases[14]. Additional evidence supporting a mechanical origin of AFL cycle length variability has been recently provided by a closed-loop mathematical model of AFL variability, including a MEC branch, whose dynamical predictions were experimentally validated in AFL variability patterns in patients[26].

Mechanical modulation of re-entry: the MEC hypothesis for AFL cycle length variability

The persistence of AFL variability after pharamacological denervation and the striking correlation between changes in AFL cycle length and variations in atrial volume suggest a direct influence of atrial volume on atrial flutter re-entry.

The specific mechanisms by which stretch may modulate the atrial flutter re-entrant circuit, thus provoking the described changes in AFL cycle length, are still hypothetical. Different parameters determine AFL rate, depending on the kind of re-entrant mechanism underlying the arrhythmia[21,39]. Specifically, the rate of typical AFL, which is based on a macro-re-entry with large excitable gap, is governed by both conduction velocity and circuit length, while moderate changes in refractory period are not expected to produce rate variations[21,39]. Deformations of the re-entrant circuit associated with changes in atrial volume during ventricular and respiratory phases, as well as a stretch-induced slowing of conduction, may theoretically account for AFL cycle length variability. Experimental and clinical studies have shown that changes in mechanical loading conditions may affect electrophysiological properties of the atria, including refractoriness and

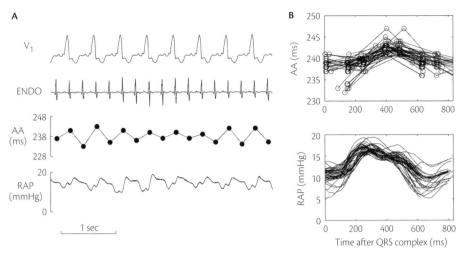

Fig. 33.5 Synchronism between AFL cycle length variations and atrial pressure changes during ventricular cycle. **A** ECG (V$_1$), endocardial atrial electrogram (ENDO), atrial cycle length series (AA) and right atrial pressure (RAP) signal during atrial flutter in a patient with 2:1 AV conduction. **B** Comparison between AFL cycle length variations and changes in atrial pressure after the onset of the QRS in a patient with variable AV conduction. [Reproduced, with permission, from Ravelli F, Disertori M, Cozzi F, Antolini R, Allessie MA (1994) Ventricular beats induce variations in cycle length of rapid (type II) atrial flutter in humans. Evidence of leading circle reentry. *Circulation* **89**:2107–2116.]

conduction velocity[40–42]. Different effects of strain on conduction velocity have been experimentally and computationally observed in various species and tissue types. Studies of atrial conduction in the isolated rabbit heart[41] and humans[42] indicate depressed conduction velocity in the presence of atrial stretch. Consistent with experimental data, computer simulations by Kuijpers *et al.*[43] showed a stretch-induced conduction slowing in atrial fibres, acting via depolarization of resting membrane potential.

All this evidence supports the MEC paradigm for AFL cycle length oscillations[25] schematized in Fig. 33.6. According to this, the observed increase in AFL cycle length during ventricular systole and inspiration may be explained by the corresponding increase in atrial volume and stretch. Stretch may produce the prolongation of the revolution time of the re-entry, both via lengthening of the anatomical pathway of the circuit and via a decrease in conduction velocity along the circuit. Opposite effects are expected during ventricular diastole and expiration, when atrial volume decreases, thus producing the shortening of AFL cycle length.

Conclusions and outlook

Mechano-sensitive mechanisms play a role in the generation of cardiac rhythm fluctuations. MEC is important in the determination of heart rate variability in heart transplant recipients. Similarly, fluctuations in heart rate, elicited by breathing-induced changes in right atrial volume, significantly contribute to RSA in conditions of reduced vagal tone, such as seen in exercise or heart failure. While MEC contributions to respiratory heart rate variability are small during sinus rhythm at rest, they increase with respiratory effort during exercise. Additional evidence supports a mechanical origin of the variability in cycle length of re-entrant arrhythmias, such as AFL. Indeed the spontaneous phasic variations of AFL cycle length are closely related to atrial volume changes caused by ventricular and respiratory activities, and are independent of autonomic tone.

This has led to the formulation of the MEC paradigm, according to which atrial volume changes directly affect AFL cycle length by modifying the conduction properties of the circulating impulse in the atrium.

While a causal link between stretch and rhythm modulation in humans is well supported by clinical evidence, the actual cellular mechanisms through which stretch affects pacemaker activity and re-entrant circuit properties are still under investigation. Thus further computational, experimental and clinical studies are required to bridge the gap between the microscopic changes induced by

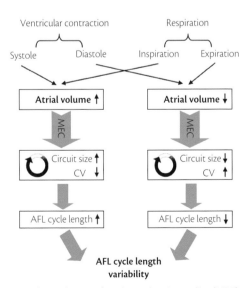

Fig. 33.6 Potential contribution of mechano-electric coupling (MEC) to cycle length variability of typical atrial flutter. CV, conduction velocity. [Modified, with permission from Ravelli F, Masè M, Disertori M (2008) Mechanical modulation of atrial flutter cycle length. *Prog Biophys Mol Biol* **97**:417–434.]

stretch and the macroscopic responses observed in human heart rhythm modulation.

References

1. Baselli G, Cerutti S, Civardi S, *et al.* Spectral and cross-spectral analysis of heart rate and arterial blood pressure variability signals. *Comput Biomed Res* 1986;**19**:520–534.

2. Malliani A, Pagani M, Lombardi F, Cerutti S. Cardiovascular neural regulation explored in the frequency domain. *Circulation* 1991;**84**: 482–492.

3. Eckberg DL. Human sinus arrhythmia as an index of vagal cardiac outflow. *J Appl Physiol* 1983;**54**:961–966.

4. Saul JP, Berger RD, Chen MH, Cohen RJ. Transfer function analysis of autonomic regulation. II. Respiratory sinus arrhythmia. *Am J Physiol* 1989;**256**:H153–H161.

5. Pikovsky A, Rosenblum MG, Kurths J (2003) *Synchronization. A Universal Concept in Nonlinear Sciences.* Cambridge University Press, New York.

6. Lammers WJEP, Ravelli F, Disertori M, Antolini R, Furlanello F, Allessie MA. Variations in human atrial flutter cycle length induced by ventricular beats: evidence of a reentrant circuit with a partially excitable gap. *J Cardiovasc Electrophysiol* 1991;**2**:375–387.

7. Kohl P, Hunter P, Noble D. Stretch-induced changes in heart rate and rhythm: clinical observations, experiments and mathematical models. *Prog Biophys Mol Biol* 1999;**71**:91–138.

8. Bernardi L, Keller F, Sanders M, *et al.* Respiratory sinus arrhythmia in the denervated human heart. *J Appl Physiol* 1989;**67**:1447–1455.

9. Radaelli A, Valle F, Falcone C, *et al.* Determinants of heart rate variability in heart transplanted subjects during physical exercise. *Eur Heart J* 1996;**17**:462–471.

10. Casadei B, Moon J, Johnston J, Caiazza A, Sleight P. Is respiratory sinus arrhythmia a good index of cardiac vagal tone in exercise? *J Appl Physiol* 1996;**81**:556–564.

11. El Omar M, Kardos A, Casadei B. Mechanisms of respiratory sinus arrhythmia in patients with mild heart failure. *Am J Physiol* 2001; **280**:H125–H131.

12. Bernardi L, Salvucci F, Suardi R, *et al.* Evidence for an intrinsic mechanism regulating heart rate variability in the transplanted and the intact heart during submaximal dynamic exercise? *Cardiovasc Res* 1990;**24**:969–981.

13. Guzzetti S, Cogliati C, Turiel M, *et al.* Sympathetic predominance followed by functional denervation in the progression of chronic heart failure. *Eur Heart J* 1995;**16**:1100–1107.

14. Robotham JL, Lixfeld W, Holland L, *et al.* Effects of respiration on cardiac performance. *J Appl Physiol* 1978;**44**:703–709.

15. Deck KA. Dehnungseffekte am spontanschlagenden, isolierten Sinusknoten. *Pflugers Arch* 1964;**280**:120–130.

16. Kaufmann RL, Lab MJ, Hennekes R, Krause H. Feedback interaction of mechanical and electrical events in the isolated mammalian ventricular myocardium (cat papillary muscle). *Pflugers Arch* 1971;**324**:100–123.

17. Cooper PJ, Lei M, Cheng LX, Kohl P. Selected contribution: axial stretch increases spontaneous pacemaker activity in rabbit isolated sinoatrial node cells. *J Appl Physiol* 2000;**89**:2099–2104.

18. Arai A, Kodama I, Toyama J. Roles of Cl$^-$ channels and Ca^{2+} mobilization in stretch-induced increase of SA node pacemaker activity. *Am J Physiol* 1996;**270**:H1726–H1735.

19. Pinsky DJ, Patton S, Mesaros S, *et al.* Mechanical transduction of nitric oxide synthesis in the beating heart. *Circ Res* 1997;**81**:372–379.

20. Camelliti P, Green CR, LeGrice I, Kohl P. Fibroblast network in rabbit sinoatrial node: structural and functional identification of homogeneous and heterogeneous cell coupling. *Circ Res* 2004;**94**: 828–835.

21. Waldo AL. Treatment of atrial flutter. *Heart* 2000;**84**:227–232.

22. Lewis T. Observations upon flutter and fibrillation. I. The regularity of clinical auricolar flutter. *Heart* 1920;**7**:127–130.

23. Wells JL, MacLean WA, James TN, Waldo AL. Characterization of atrial flutter. Studies in man after open heart surgery using fixed atrial electrodes. *Circulation* 1979;**60**:665–673.

24. Ravelli F, Disertori M, Cozzi F, Antolini R, Allessie MA. Ventricular beats induce variations in cycle length of rapid (type II) atrial flutter in humans. Evidence of leading circle reentry. *Circulation* 1994;**89**:2107–2116.

25. Ravelli F, Masè M, Disertori M. Mechanical modulation of atrial flutter cycle length. *Prog Biophys Mol Biol* 2008;**97**:417–434.

26. Masè M, Glass L, Ravelli F. A model for mechano-electrical feedback effects on atrial flutter interval variability. *Bull Math Biol* 2008;**70**: 1326–1347.

27. Masè M, Disertori M, Ravelli F. Cardiorespiratory interactions in patients with atrial flutter. *J Appl Physiol* 2009;**106**:29–39.

28. Yamashita T, Oikawa N, Murakawa Y, *et al.* Contraction–excitation feedback in atrial reentry: role of velocity of mechanical stretch. *Am J Physiol* 1994;**267**:H1254–H1262.

29. Waxman MB, Yao L, Cameron DA, Kirsh JA. Effects of posture, Valsalva maneuver and respiration on atrial flutter rate: an effect mediated through cardiac volume. *J Am Coll Cardiol* 1991;**17**: 1545–1552.

30. Angelone A, Coulter NA. Respiratory sinus arrhythmia: a frequency dependent phenomenon. *J Appl Physiol* 1964;**19**:479–482.

31. Baertschi AJ, Gann DS. Responses of atrial mechanoreceptors to pulsation of atrial volume. *J Physiol* 1977;**273**:1–21.

32. Triedman JK, Saul JP. Blood pressure modulation by central venous pressure and respiration. Buffering effects of the heart rate reflexes. *Circulation* 1994;**89**:169–179.

33. Liu L, Nattel S. Differing sympathetic and vagal effects on atrial fibrillation in dogs: role of refractoriness heterogeneity. *Am J Physiol* 1997;**273**:H805–H816.

34. Stambler BS, Ellenbogen KA. Elucidating the mechanisms of atrial flutter cycle length variability using power spectral analysis techniques. *Circulation* 1996;**94**:2515–2525.

35. Hayden WG, Hurley EJ, Rytand DA. The mechanism of canine atrial flutter. *Circ Res* 1967;**20**:496–505.

36. Rytand DA, Onesti SJ, Bruns DL. The atrial rate in patients with flutter; a relationship between atrial enlargement and slow rate. *Stanford Med Bull* 1958;**16**:169–202.

37. Vulliemin P, Del Bufalo A, Schlaepfer J, Fromer M, Kappenberger L. Relation between cycle length, volume, and pressure in type I atrial flutter. *PACE* 1994;**17**:1391–1398.

38. Waxman MB, Kirsh JA, Yao L, Cameron DA, Asta JA. Slowing of the atrial flutter rate during 1:1 atrioventricular conduction in humans and dogs: an effect mediated through atrial pressure and volume. *J Cardiovasc Electrophysiol* 1992;**3**:544–557.

39. Allessie MA, Lammers WJEP, Rensma PL, Bonke FIM. Flutter and fibrillation in experimental models: what has been learned that can be applied to humans? In: *Cardiac Arrhythmias: Where to Go From Here?* (eds P Brugada, HJJ Wellens). Futura, Mount Kisco, New York, 1987, pp. 67–82.

40. Ravelli F. Mechano-electric feedback and atrial fibrillation. *Prog Biophys Mol Biol* 2003;**82**:37–149.

41. Eijsbouts S, Van Zandvoort M, Schotten U, Allessie M. Effects of acute atrial dilation on heterogeneity in conduction in the isolated rabbit heart. *J Cardiovasc Electrophysiol* 2003;**14**:269–278.

42. Ravelli F, Masè M, Del Greco M, Marini M, Disertori M. Acute Atrial Dilatation Slows Conduction and Increases AF Vulnerability in the Human Atrium. *J Cardiovasc Electrophysiol* 2011;(in press; doi: 10.1111/j.1540-8167.2010.01939.x).

43. Kuijpers NH, ten Eikelder HM, Bovendeerd PH, *et al.* Mechanoelectric feedback leads to conduction slowing and block in acutely dilated atria: a modeling study of cardiac electromechanics. *Am J Physiol* 2007;**292**: H2832–H2853.

Mathematical models of cardiac structure and function: mechanistic insights from models of heart failure

Vicky Y. Wang, Martyn P. Nash, Ian J. LeGrice, Alistair A. Young, Bruce H. Smaill and Peter J. Hunter

Background

Heart failure (HF) is defined as the inability of the heart to meet the body's requirements for blood flow as a result of impaired function of one or both ventricles (see Chapters 47 and 56). The majority of patients with congestive HF exhibit systolic failure in which ejection fraction is reduced[1]. However, in at least one third of congestive HF cases, ejection fraction is normal or near-normal at rest[2]. These patients have diastolic HF. Left ventricular (LV) distensibility is markedly reduced during diastole resulting in elevated LV end-diastolic and pulmonary venous pressures.

The pumping performance of the heart is influenced by the passive and active mechanical properties of ventricular myocardium and by the geometry of the ventricles (chamber size, shape and wall thickness). HF is associated with substantial and characteristic changes in ventricular geometry and myocardial tissue architecture. Diastolic failure is linked with ventricular wall thickening, whereas systolic HF is correlated with progressive ventricular dilatation (increased ventricular mass and relative wall thinning). In both cases there is considerable structural remodelling at the cell and tissue levels, including proliferation of interstitial fibrosis.

In this chapter we outline our current understanding of myocardial tissue structure in the normal heart and describe the structural remodelling that occurs during the progression from diastolic dysfunction to decompensated HF in spontaneously hypertensive rats (SHR), an established model of hypertensive heart disease. We present a kinematic analysis of the role of ventricular geometry and myocardial architecture in normal cardiac mechanics and speculate on how this is affected by the structural remodelling that occurs in HF. Finally, we analyze the relative contributions of material properties and ventricular geometry to HF using anatomically detailed finite element models of ventricular mechanics. These models are based on large deformation elasticity theory and include mechanical properties related to tissue microstructure. LV mechanics and myocardial stress-strain distributions during the cardiac cycle are presented for normal and dilated LV geometries, including a loss of tissue anisotropy and/or reduced contractility, in order to investigate the relative effects of these pathological disturbances during HF.

Myocardial structure in the normal and failing heart

Key features of ventricular tissue architecture in the normal heart are shown in Fig. 34.1. Cardiac myocytes have a well-defined orientation at all points within the myocardium and this so-called fibre direction varies relatively smoothly across the ventricular wall (note that, strictly speaking, cardiac muscle does not contain muscle fibres; the term, borrowed from skeletal muscle morphology, is nonetheless used widely). In the LV free wall, fibre orientation is about −60° with respect to the circumferential direction at the epicardial surface (Fig. 34.1C), and it rotates through 0° in the midwall to around +90° in the subendocardial region[3,4].

Detailed morphometric investigation of three-dimensional (3D) cardiac tissue architecture[6,7] has shown that ventricular myocytes are arranged in layers or sheets three to five cells thick. Within layers, neighbouring myocytes are tightly coupled electrically and mechanically, but adjacent layers are separated by clefts across which there is little direct cell-to-cell electrical or mechanical coupling. Neighbouring layers branch and interconnect, but this occurs at an intermediate scale (Fig. 34.1C). At any point within the ventricular wall, therefore, it is possible to define three distinct structural axes of the myocardial tissue: the fibre axis v_1, the sheet axis v_2 and the sheet-normal v_3 (Fig. 34.1A). The sheet axis is near radial through much of the ventricular wall, but rotates to become

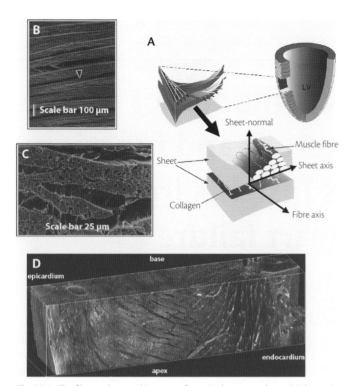

Fig. 34.1 The fibrous-sheet architecture of ventricular myocardium. **A** Schematic of the laminar arrangement of myocytes in a transmural LV segment. Muscle layers are three to five cells thick and are oriented approximately radially through the LV wall. They are aligned with the myofibre direction parallel to the epicardial tangent plane and adjacent layers are separated by substantial cleavage planes, but branch and interconnect. The transmural variation of myofibre orientation is indicated by the white rods. The lower inset of **A** illustrates how myocytes are tightly coupled within layers, which gives rise to a natural set of orthotropic material axes as indicated. **B** Scanning electron micrograph of midwall segment from the LV free wall in a dog heart viewed parallel to the epicardial tangent plane. Branching between adjacent layers is indicated by the arrowhead. **C** Scanning electron micrograph of a midwall segment from the LV free wall in a dog heart viewed approximately transverse to the local myofibre axis. **D** 3D reconstruction using extended volume confocal microscopy of myocyte arrangement and collagen organization in a transmural segment from the LV free wall of a normal rat heart. This specimen was fixed with Bouin's solution, stained with picrosirius red and embedded in epoxy resin. Dimensions are 4.3×1.1×0.9 [mm] and the image volume consists of 2.3×10^9 voxels at 1.2 μm resolution. Collagen is brightly stained, but the laminar arrangement of myocytes is also clear.

approximately tangential to the endocardial surface[8]. Such laminar organization has been reported consistently in fresh and fixed tissues for a wide range of species, employing microscopic techniques, and in hearts using diffusion tensor magnetic resonance imaging (DT-MRI)[7,9]. The laminar architecture of ventricular myocardium affects its electrical[5,10] and mechanical properties[11,12].

Collagen is the main structural component of the cardiac extracellular matrix (ECM), which is described using a classification defined initially for skeletal muscle[13]. Epimysium is the connective tissue surrounding the entire muscle, while the endomysium is

the reticular network that surrounds and interconnects individual myocytes and capillaries. The perimysium surrounds and interconnects groups of myocytes and therefore determines the organization of muscle layers. We have used extended-volume confocal microscopy[14] to reconstruct 3D perimysial collagen organization and associated myocyte arrangement across the LV free wall in the normal rat heart at higher resolution than has previously been reported[7]. This reveals three forms of perimysial collagen. In addition to the meshwork of collagen fibres and bundles that surrounds muscle layers (Fig. 34.2A), long cords aligned approximately with the fibre axis also run within the muscle layers and appear to originate and terminate in the surface mesh (Fig. 34.2B and C). Taken together, these two forms of perimysial collagen provide a collagenous skeleton that organizes the ventricular myocardium into tightly coupled laminar units. The third form of perimysium is the network of long convoluted collagen fibres that cross cleavage planes and connect into the surface meshwork on adjacent layers (Fig. 34.2D).

We believe that these different forms of perimysial collagen meet a range of functional requirements. Muscle layers are the structural units that enable local myocyte rearrangement or shearing to occur, while the dense array of longitudinal cords distributed throughout the LV myocardium (along with titin – see Chapter 9) limits passive extension along the myocyte axis. Finally, the 3D assembly of these connective tissue components accommodates transmural myofibre rotation and provides mechanical coupling across the ventricular wall. This laminar arrangement does not extend to the subepicardial region, where perimysial collagen is mainly in the form of longitudinal cords. Note that a longitudinal study in our laboratory, using the SHR animal model, has shown that age-related perimysial connective tissue remodelling is associated with impaired cardiac performance[15] and that SHR replicate many of the features of human hypertensive heart disease[16].

Proliferation of interstitial fibrosis occurs throughout the progression from diastolic dysfunction to decompensated HF. However, there are striking changes in the organization and extent of perimysial collagen throughout this period (with associated remodelling of the endomysium). At 3 months, no difference was evident in the arrangement of perimysial components in SHR or Wistar Kyoto (WKY) controls. By 12 months, perimysial collagen surrounding adjacent muscle layers and the long perimysial cords that connect those layers fuse to form thick sheets in SHR and the endomysial collagen surrounding individual myocytes appears much thicker (Fig. 34.3). Subsequently, laminar structure is disrupted and associated perimysial collagen components are reduced. Throughout this process there is a progressive increase in the extent and thickness of endomysial collagen (as well as continuing accumulation of replacement fibrosis and perivascular fibrosis). These observations in SHR are consistent with those of others researchers[16] and closely match the *post mortem* observations of Rossi[17] in failing human hearts. It seems evident that the perimysial scarring at 12 months increases transmural mechanical coupling, but constrains the shearing of adjacent layers. Furthermore, proliferation and thickening of the endomysium, and its incorporation of the longitudinal collagen cords that are a characteristic element of the perimysial network in the normal heart, will likely further impair the capacity of myocytes to increase their cross-sectional dimension during systole.

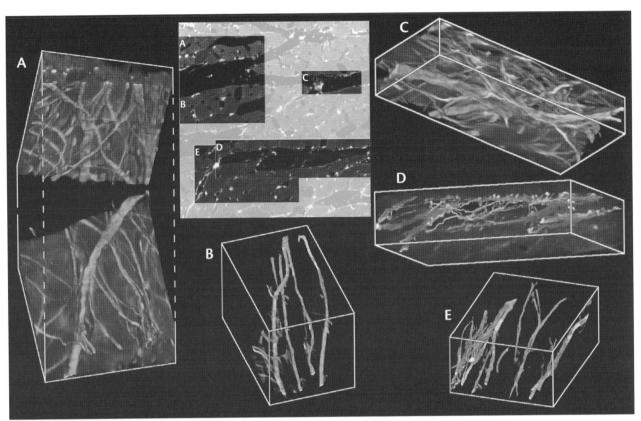

Fig. 34.2 High-resolution sub-volumes reveal the nature of perimysial collagen. A midwall segment from a 12-month WKY control rat stained with picrosirius red was imaged using extended-volume confocal imaging at 0.4 μm voxel size and representative sub-volumes were extracted. The sub-volume in **A** has been opened to show the detail of the meshwork on two opposing laminar surfaces. Long intralaminar collagen cords have been segmented from the tissue volumes using connectivity-based thresholding (**B**, **E**) and show the relationship between the axial cords, as well as small tethering branches which extend into the neighbouring tissue. In **D**, collagen spanning the cleavage plane separating adjacent layers is highlighted, and such collagen sometimes fuses to form larger collagen tendons near the edges of the laminae (**C**). [Reproduced, with permission, from Pope A, Sands GB, Smaill BH, LeGrice IJ (2008) Three dimensional transmural organization of perimysial collagen in the rat heart. *Am J Physiol* **295**:H1243–H1252.] (See color plate section.)

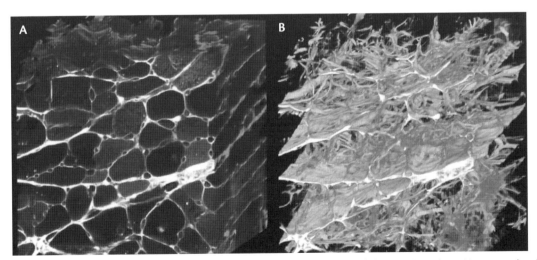

Fig. 34.3 High resolution images of LV midwall (block size 200×200×50 μm) from a 12-month spontaneously hypertensive rat heart. Myocytes and capillaries as well as perimysial and endomysial collagen are evident in **A**, although myocytes are stained with variable intensity. **B** shows collagen structures segmented from **A**. Compared with age-matched WKY controls (Fig. 34.2D), perimysial collagen has fused between adjacent muscle layers and the endomysial collagen surrounding myocytes has thickened. (See color plate section.)

Cardiac mechanics in the normal and failing heart: a kinematic analysis

Detailed information about 3D wall motion, deformation and strain in the normal heart has been obtained using a variety of imaging modalities and across a wide range of species including human, dog, pig and rat. There are consistent transmural gradients of 3D strain in the LV and strains during both systole and diastole are normally greatest close to the endocardial surface. In general, circumferential strain exceeds longitudinal strain[13,18,19]. Maximum principal strains in systole and diastole are oriented at around −20° with respect to the circumferential direction and therefore do not coincide with myofibre orientation in the inner ventricular wall[18,20]. Despite these substantial gradients in 3D strain, myofibre extension across the LV wall is remarkably uniform in both systole and diastole[11,18–20].

These findings frame an important question. Because sarcomere length relations for ventricular myocytes are highly length-dependent, the length range over which they can develop force and shorten is much more limited than for skeletal muscle. In cardiac muscle, little force is generated at a sarcomere length of 1.6 μm, whereas skeletal muscle generates around 80% of peak force at this sarcomere length[21]. Moreover, the cardiac ECM (along with intracellular titin) limits passive sarcomere extension to around 2.3 μm, thereby preventing operation on the descending limb of the force–sarcomere length relationship. In the normal heart, LV ejection fraction is approximately 60% at rest and greater than this during exercise. As a result, the inner wall of the LV undergoes very large deformations throughout the cardiac cycle. These are much larger than can be accounted for by local myocyte strains in the fibre direction, which are on the order of 15–20%.

A simple kinematic analysis provides some insights into the ways in which LV geometry and transmural myofibre rotation contribute to efficient mechanical function in the normal heart. In Fig. 34.4, we present individual MR short- and long-axis views of the normal human heart at end-diastole and end-systole. When referred to end-diastole, the relative change in circumferential LV cavity dimension (short-axis view) during systole is substantial, whereas the corresponding change at the outer surface of the LV (free wall and interventricular septum) is much less. Corresponding dimensional changes in the longitudinal direction (long-axis view) are also greatest at the LV cavity, but are less in the longitudinal than the circumferential plane.

These observations can be related to two factors. First, throughout the cardiac cycle the LV approximates a thick-walled ellipsoid of revolution, in which the circumferential radius of curvature is smaller than the longitudinal radius of curvature. Thus, mean circumferential strain is greater than mean longitudinal strain. Second, ventricular myocardium is approximately incompressible. Therefore, circumferential and axial shortening are accompanied by wall thickening, and strains are substantially greater near the LV endocardial surface compared to its outer surface.

Within this context, transmural fibre rotation plays a crucial role in ensuring that sarcomere shortening and extension remains within the appropriate functional range. Thus, while circumferential strain may be as high as 40% near the LV endocardium, myocytes in this region have a longitudinal orientation and are subject to axial strains of only 15–20%. In the LV midwall, fibre orientation is approximately circumferential, but because of the rapid

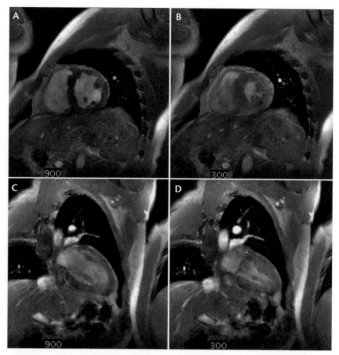

Fig. 34.4 Short- (top) and long- (bottom) axis MR views of a normal human heart at end-diastole (**A** and **C**) and end-systole (**B** and **D**). The deformation of the LV cavity during systole is substantial as is LV wall thickening. Relative changes in LV cavity dimension during systole are greater in the circumferential plane (short-axis views **A** and **B**) than in the longitudinal plane (long-axis views **C** and **D**).

drop in circumferential strain across the LV wall, myocytes are still subjected to strains within the appropriate range. On the basis of kinematic modelling that incorporates these features[22], it has been argued that the transmural fibre rotation in the normal heart ensures maximum uniformity of sarcomere length across the LV wall throughout the cardiac cycle.

While such kinematic analysis provides a satisfyingly simple framework for relating ventricular geometry and tissue structure to heart mechanics, it fails to resolve a key observation. The wall thickening observed in the subendocardial region during systole is much greater than can be accounted for by local myocyte shortening. These dimensional changes have been related to altered myocyte arrangement in the inner wall of the LV[23]. Three-dimensional strain analysis reveals substantial shearing between adjacent subendocardial layers during systole[11,19,24] and diastole[19]. It has been shown both experimentally[24] and theoretically[25] that myocyte layers coincide with planes of maximum shear deformation. In addition, the LV undergoes significant torsional deformation during systole, which also contributes to the effectiveness of ejection. The apex twists counter-clockwise relative to the base (as viewed from the apex) during systole, and then rapidly uncoils in early diastole[26], which is associated with a marked ascent of the ventricular valve plane away from the apex contributing to the efficient transfer of blood from atria to ventricles during early diastole. Torsional deformation occurs in the same direction across the LV, but is greater at the endocardium than the epicardium.

We have identified a number of factors that support relatively complete ejection in the normal LV, despite the restricted sarcomere length range over which myocytes develop force and shorten. These include: the ellipsoid geometry of the LV; the transmural rotation of myofibres; slippage or shearing of adjacent muscle layers; strain locking mechanisms that prevent overextension of myocytes; and finally torsional deformations that occur throughout the cardiac cycle. The perimysial collagen network provides an integrated load-bearing framework that meets these functional requirements[7]. Myolaminae provide structural units that enable local myocyte rearrangement or shearing, while the dense array of longitudinal cords distributed throughout the LV myocardium limits passive extension along the myocyte axis. The 3D assembly of these connective tissue components accommodates transmural myofibre rotation and provides mechanical coupling across the ventricular wall. The fact that laminar structure is not evident in the outer 10–20% of the rat LV may reflect the relatively low shear strains in this subepicardial region.

This analysis provides a conceptual framework for understanding ways in which remodelling at the tissue and organ levels contributes to the progression of cardiac mechanical dysfunction as HF develops. It is evident that the fusion of perimysial collagen between adjacent muscle layers early in hypertensive heart disease will increase transmural mechanical coupling, compromise local shearing and increase passive LV stiffness. This results in diastolic dysfunction, but ejection fraction is maintained because increased torsion initially offsets the reduction in other modes of deformation[26,27]. The subsequent development of decompensated HF is associated with geometric and tissue remodelling, which certainly contribute to impaired mechanical performance. Ventricular dilatation is accompanied by a more spherical shape of the LV and relative wall thinning. This is associated with substantial further changes in the organization and character of the cardiac tissue hierarchy. These include progressive loss of the ordered laminar arrangement of myocytes, the disappearance of perimysial ECM components linked with this organization, and proliferation and thickening of the endomysial network. All modes of deformation, including torsion[28], are reduced in systolic HF. However, these structural changes are also accompanied by impaired contractile function due to apoptosis, sarcomere disarray, altered calcium homeostasis and electrical dyssynchrony. The relative roles of these different factors remain unclear and to address this issue more experimental work combined with continuum mechanical modelling is required.

Measuring and modelling *in vivo* ventricular mechanics

To date, some of the most detailed non-invasive information on LV mechanics has been obtained from magnetic resonance imaging (MRI) of canine hearts obtained at the National Institutes of Health in collaboration with Johns Hopkins University[29]. High-resolution *in vivo* MRI tissue tagging (resolution: 384 × 128 × 32 voxels spanning 180 mm × 180 mm × 128 mm; 5 mm slice thickness; 5 voxel MR tag spacing) and concurrent LV pressure recordings were obtained, together with *ex vivo* DT-MRI (resolution: 128 × 128 × 96 voxels spanning 100 mm × 100 mm × 86.4 mm; voxel size 780 μm × 780 μm × 900 μm) from the same hearts.

MRI tissue tagging enables quantitative evaluation of cardiac tissue displacement and strain throughout the cardiac cycle. Reconstruction of the 3D motion of the heart from the tag positions during the cardiac cycle requires specialized image processing and mathematical techniques[30]. DT-MRI quantifies the preferred orientations of the local self-diffusion of water molecules in biological tissues. The direction of maximum diffusion (the primary eigenvector) has been shown to correlate well with the local myofibre orientation observed from histological studies, and therefore can be used for mapping the 3D orientation of the myocardial fibres throughout the myocardium[31,32].

We have developed an integrative modelling framework to enable us to investigate the factors that contribute to LV dysfunction in HF. We used this framework to combine displacement and motion information from *in vivo* MRI tagging with the concurrent pressure recordings and the *ex vivo* DT-MRI data using a finite element model of LV mechanics. Full details of the modelling process are published elsewhere[33,34]. Briefly, LV epicardial and endocardial surface data (excluding the papillary muscles) were segmented from the MRI tagging data at diastasis, and a reference finite element model of the LV was constructed using non-linear least squares fitting. Primary eigenvectors derived from the DT-MRI were used to define a spatial distribution of fibre orientations embedded within the reference LV model (Fig. 34.5). Due to the lack of sheet orientation data for this heart, we chose to represent the myocardial mechanical response using an exponential constitutive relation representing transversely isotropic (i.e. isotropic in the plane perpendicular to the fibre direction) mechanical response, with parameters estimated to best match to the MRI tagging and simultaneous LV pressure data[34].

For all simulations, the end-diastolic LV cavity pressure (preload) was 1 kPa and a constant afterload of 12 kPa was specified. Whilst endocardial pressures are known to vary both spatially and temporally, as well as due to pathological changes during HF, such variations were considered to have insignificant effects on the results and were beyond the scope of this study. A time-dependent description of the active contractile stress[35] was used to drive the

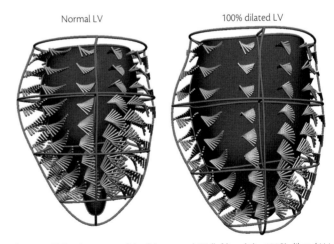

Fig. 34.5 Finite element models of the normal LV (left) and the 100% dilated LV (right). The LV free walls of each model are in view, with anterior and posterior walls at the left and right, respectively, of each panel. Ventricular dilatation is accompanied by a more spherical shape of the LV and relative wall thinning. LV endocardial surfaces are shaded with lines outlining the epicardial surface. The groups of rotating rods show the transmural variation in fibre orientation across the LV wall. (See color plate section.)

deformation throughout the systolic phases of the cycle, reaching a peak contractile stress of 65 kPa at end-systole. The contractile stress (applied along the fibre axis only) was linearly superimposed onto the passive mechanical response to construct the total Lagrangian stress tensor, which appears in the equations that govern mechanical equilibrium (derived from the physical laws of momentum conservation). The resulting system of non-linear equations was solved using standard finite element techniques[12].

For the normal LV model, the relationship between the LV cavity pressure and volume is illustrated in Fig. 34.6. Following diastolic filling, the LV pressure rapidly increased during isovolumic contraction until the afterload pressure was reached, representing the opening of the aortic valve, after which the LV contracted against the afterload pressure. End-systole was determined when the peak contractile tension was reached, and the subsequent isovolumic relaxation phase ended when the cavity pressure returned to zero. The LV subsequently returned to its stress-free state, after which all of the elastic energy had been released.

Myocardial mechanical modelling of heart failure

Using the normal canine LV model as a control, we then varied basic biomechanical properties to simulate the known physiological changes that occur during HF in order to investigate the influence of these factors on LV mechanical function. Here, we considered the following pathological variations:

(1) Dilated LV, mimicked by increasing the size of the LV cavity by 25%, 50%, 75% and 100% (Fig. 34.5), whilst the resting sarcomere length remained unchanged.

(2) Isotropic passive myocardial properties, for which the constitutive parameters were altered to represent the tighter coupling between fibres (i.e. increased cross-fibre stiffness) due to collagen reorganization. For this case, the overall LV (organ) stiffness was held constant by matching the global diastolic PV relation with that of the normal model.

(3) Reduced contractility, where the maximum contractile stress was decreased from 65 kPa to 52 kPa (80% contractility), without a change in its timing.

For the range of dilations, the following variations were compared to investigate HF-related factors:

- Case 1: Transversely isotropic stiffness and normal contractility.
- Case 2: Isotropic stiffness and normal contractility.
- Case 3: Transversely isotropic stiffness + reduced contractility.
- Case 4: Isotropic stiffness + reduced contractility.

In each case, we investigated the following indices of LV mechanics: ejection fraction [EF (%)], stroke volume [SV (ml)], average fractional shortening (FS) in the short-axis plane [AFSS (%)] and average wall thickening [AWT (%)]. Eq. (1) defines FS, which is a common clinical index to examine changes in LV dimension throughout the cardiac cycle. FS values in the short-axis (Y-Z) plane at the equator were calculated using the distances between diametrically opposite endocardial model nodes spanning the Y- and Z-axes, and averaged to calculate the AFSS. To study the changes in wall thickness throughout the cardiac cycle, the Euclidean distances between adjacent endocardial and epicardial nodes at four locations around the equatorial LV (anterior, free-wall, posterior and septum) were determined at end-diastole (ED) and end-systole (ES). Eq. (1) was then used to calculate the systolic wall thickness at each region, and these four values were used to calculate the AWT.

$$FS = \frac{(LVEDD - LVESD)}{LVEDD} \qquad WT = \frac{(ESWT - EDWT)}{EDWT} \qquad (1)$$

where LVEDD is the LV end-diastolic dimension, and LVESD is the LV end-systolic dimension, and WT is wall thickness.

Effect of dilation

As the reference LV was dilated, the EF decreased in a non-linear manner (Fig. 34.7). Dilating the LV by 100% reduced the EF by 25%, 11%, 46% and 34% for Cases 1, 2, 3 and 4, respectively. Unlike the EF, the effect of dilation on SV was independent of muscle contractility. Under conditions of normal contractility, dilation increased stroke volume, whilst the observed reduction in EF was due to the greater end-diastolic cavity volume. On the other

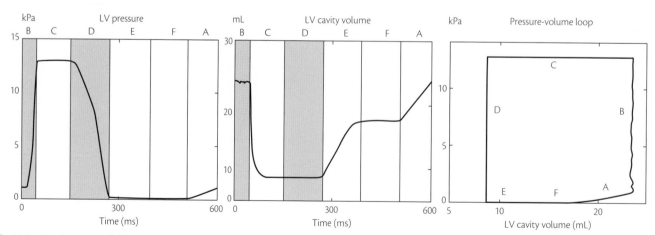

Fig. 34.6 LV cavity pressure (left), volume (centre) and pressure–volume loop (right) during the cardiac cycle for the normal LV simulation. The individial phases are: A passive inflation by atrial contraction; B (shaded) isovolumic contraction; C ejection; D (shaded) isovolumic relaxation; E rapid filling; and F diastasis.

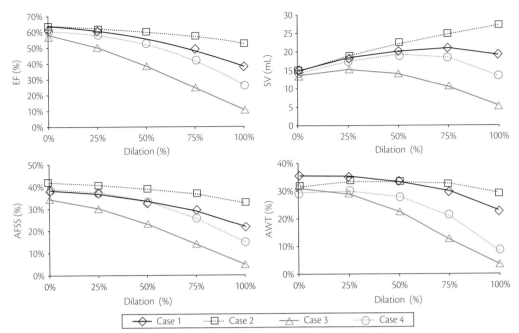

Fig. 34.7 Changes in cardiac indices: ejection fraction (EF); stroke volume (SV); average fractional shortening in the short-axis plane (AFSS); and average wall thickening (AWT) with changes in LV dilation. Case 1 (black diamonds): transversely isotropic elasticity, normal contractility; Case 2 (black squares): isotropic elasticity, normal contractility; Case 3 (red triangles): transversely isotropic elasticity, 80% contractility; Case 4 (red circles): isotropic elasticity, 80% contractility. Solid lines represent transversely isotropic cases, whereas dotted lines represent the isotropic cases.

hand, when the myocardial contractility was compromised (i.e. Cases 3 and 4), the decreased mechanical performance of the dilated LV ultimately lead to a dramatic decrease of both SV and EF. Average fractional shortening in the short-axis plane and average wall thickening both markedly reduced with LV dilation, particularly when combined with reduced contractility.

Effect of tissue remodelling (loss of anisotropy)

The loss of fibre structure did not significantly affect global pump function (i.e. EF and SV) for the normal LV (Fig. 34.7). Average wall thickening slightly decreased (–4%), whilst the short-axis FS was slightly elevated (4%). On the other hand, in the dilated LV, the increased EF (14%) and SV (8 ml) for the isotropic model indicates that the mechanical behaviour was significantly improved compared with the transversely isotropic case. This was also supported by the increase in the AFSS (11%) and AWT (6%). This paradoxical increase in mechanical performance associated with a loss of fibre anisotropy in the dilated LV may be a driver for the microstructural remodelling that is known to occur during HF.

Effect of reduced contractility

For the normal LV, reduced contractility affected most cardiac indices for both the isotropic and transversely isotropic cases (Fig. 34.7; note that the impact on the latter was greater than that on the former). For transversely isotropic tissue, the combination of dilation and reduced contractility caused a significant reduction in EF, SV, AFFS and AWT. These effects were diminished by a loss of fibre anisotropy, which again may help to explain the remodelling observed during HF.

Analysis of myocardial fibre stretch and stress

To investigate the effects of the HF case studies at the localized scale, we analyzed myocardial stretch and stress throughout the cardiac cycle. We extracted the circumferential (λ_{cc}), longitudinal (λ_{ll}) and radial (λ_{rr}) stretch ratios at four material points across the free wall LV equator (Fig. 34.8). In all cases, circumferential stretch moderately increased during diastolic filling; then rapidly decreased (to a greater extent in the subendocardium compared to the subepicardium) during the isovolumic contraction and ejection phases, before returning to resting length following isovolumic relaxation and rapid filling. Conversely, radial stretch followed the opposite trend, with a reversed transmural gradient. The transmural heterogeneity in the stretch ratios predicted for in the normal LV was reduced by LV dilation and, in particular, when combined with reduced contractility.

Longitudinal stretch increased during diastolic filling and continued to increase during isovolumic contraction, which is contrary to clinical observations. The constitutive relation used in these computations was transversely isotropic, which could have been a significant factor. However, preliminary simulations using fully orthotropic constitutive properties have in fact shown little effect on base-to-apex length changes. On the other hand, further pilot simulations using the same geometric LV model embedded with an idealized uniform transmural fibre rotation (epicardium –60° to endocardium +90°), which was spatially homogeneous around the entire LV, exhibited the expected apex-to-base shortening during systolic contraction.

We also computed the fibre stretch ratio (λ_{ff}) and stress ratio (σ_{ff}) in the equatorial LV free wall during the cardiac cycle (Fig. 34.9). In the normal LV, fibre stretch increased during inflation and isovolumic contraction and then rapidly decreased by approximately

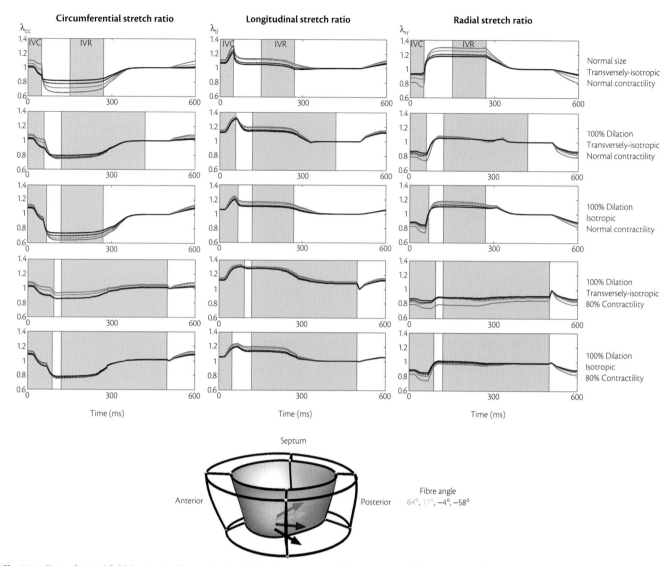

Fig. 34.8 Circumferential (left), longitudinal (centre) and radial (right) stretch ratios (λ) in the equatorial free wall of the LV during the cardiac cycle, with shading indicating the isovolumic contraction (IVC) and isovolumic relaxation (IVR) phases. The normal LV simulation (top) is compared to four pathological cases (see text for details). The inset below shows the equatorial slice of the LV, with arrows indicating the transmural locations at which the components of stretch were analyzed. The fibre angles relative to the LV's short axis plane are also indicated (counter-clockwise positive). Stretch ratios for subendocardial (solid red), midwall (dashed red and dashed black) and subepicardial (solid black) locations are plotted. (See color plate section.)

20% following the onset of ejection, before gradually recovering during isovolumic relaxation and rapid filling. Myocardial fibre stress increased significantly during isovolumic contraction and remained relatively constant during a large portion of ejection, although significant transmural gradients were predicted with lowest stresses in the midwall. LV dilation again reduced the transmural stress gradients, particularly when combined with loss of anisotropic stiffness. LV dilation also decreased energetic performance, as indicated by the area decrease of the local stress-stretch loops. In particular, the combination of dilation and reduced contractility substantially reduced myocardial efficiency, which was primarily due to the marked reduction in stroke volume (Fig. 34.7). Reduced contractility led to a substantial lengthening of the durations of isovolumic contraction and relaxation, which is attributed to the fact that active tension trace was unchanged for all

case studies. Changes in the active tension transients that are known to occur during HF will likely elucidate further effects underpinning the compromised ventricular mechanical function.

Conclusions and outlook

In this chapter, we have reviewed our current understanding of the 3D structure of myocardial tissue, based on studies in normal and diseased hearts from several species using a variety of imaging methods including confocal microscopy. We have also summarized the results of research carried out in our laboratory using a rat model of hypertensive heart disease. In this time-course study, changes in both cardiac structure and function that occur during the progression to decompensated heart failure have been systematically characterized.

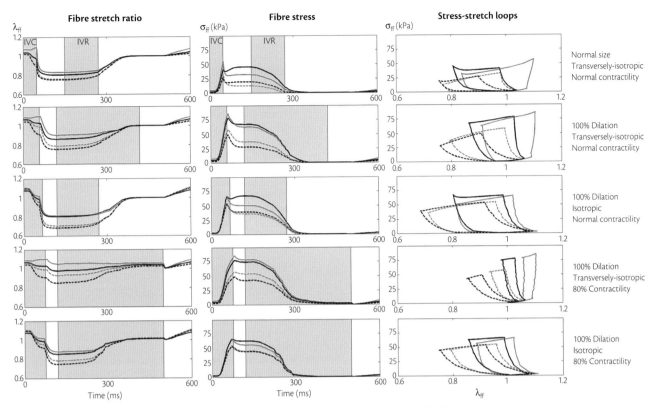

Fig. 34.9 Fibre stretch ratio (left), fibre stress (centre) and fibre stress-stretch loops in the equatorial free wall of the LV during the cardiac cycle, with shading indicating the isovolumic contraction (IVC) and isovolumic relaxation (IVR) phases. The normal LV (top) is compared to the four pathological cases (see text for details). Analysis locations and trace colours are the same as those described in the legend of Fig. 34.8. (See color plate section.)

It is possible to develop kinematic analyses that provide considerable insight into the ways in which the progressive tissue and geometric remodelling that occur in the failing heart impact on its mechanical function. However, the origins of cardiac dysfunction are multifactorial and include alterations in contractility at the cellular level and electrical dyssynchrony. Coupled multiscale models of ventricular electrical activation and mechanics are required in order to better understand the mechanisms involved.

Despite considerable effort over a number of years, we are only now getting to the point where we can address this problem in a meaningful way. Finite element models that accurately represent the geometry and the 3D microstructure of the whole heart are now available. Computational power has developed to the extent where solution of sophisticated cardiac mechanics problems is certainly tractable. Finally, the technology exists to acquire high resolution data on heart wall motion and regional deformation using cine MR imaging techniques and to simultaneously record cavity pressures. The modelling framework described here demonstrates the power and the limitations of this approach. The present LV model reproduces many aspects of ventricular mechanics, but does not predict the apparent degree of base-to-apex shortening during systole. Future developments will examine the effects of spatial heterogeneities in fibre orientation (e.g. as quantified by DT-MRI) as well as the role of other factors such as the right ventricle, papillary muscles and pericardium, and the coupling of wall mechanics to ventricular fluid mechanics, which all affect the global mechanical function of the heart. Whilst there is still much to learn, mathematical modelling, as illustrated in this chapter, is capable of providing insight into the functional implications of tissue structure in normal hearts and how changes in tissue structure in heart disease alter the mechanical behaviour of the intact failing heart.

Acknowledgements

This research was supported by the Health Research Council (HRC) of New Zealand. V.Y.W. received funding from the New Zealand Institute of Mathematics & Its Applications (NZIMA). M.P.N. was supported by a James Cook Fellowship administrated by the Royal Society of New Zealand on behalf of the New Zealand Government. We gratefully acknowledge Assistant Professor Daniel Ennis from the University of California, Los Angeles, and Professor McVeigh and Dr Helm from National Institutes of Health and Johns Hopkins University for providing the MRI data.

References

1. Jessup M, Brozena S. Heart failure. *N Engl J Med* 2003;**348**:2007–2018.
2. Gaasch WH, Zile MR. Left ventricular diastolic dysfunction and diastolic heart failure. *Annu Rev Med* 2004;**55**:373–394.
3. Hunter PJ, Smaill BH. The analysis of cardiac function: a continuum approach. *Prog Biophys Mol Biol* 1989;**52**:101–164.
4. Nielsen P, LeGrice I, Smaill BH, Hunter PJ. Mathematical model of geometry and fibrous structure of the heart. *Am J Physiol* 1991; **260**:H1365–H1378.

5. Hunter PJ, Pullan AJ, Smaill BH. Modeling total heart function. *Annu Rev Biomed Eng* 2003;**5**:147–177.

6. LeGrice I, Smaill B, Chai L, Edgar S, Gavin J, Hunter P. Laminar structure of the heart : ventricular myocyte arrangment and connective tissue architecture in the dog. *Am J Physiol* 1995;**269**:H571–H582.

7. Pope A, Sands GB, Smaill BH, LeGrice IJ. Three dimensional transmural organization of perimysial collagen in the rat heart. *Am J Physiol* 2008; **295**:H1243–H1252.

8. LeGrice I, Hunter P, Smaill B. Laminar structure of the heart: a mathematical model. *Am J Physiol* 1997;**272**:H2466–H2476.

9. Gilbert SH, Benson AP, Li P, Holden AV. Regional loacalisation of left ventricular sheet structure: integration with current models of cardiac fibre, sheet and band structure. *Eur J Cardiothorac Surg* 2007;**32**: 231–249.

10. Caldwell BJ, Trew ML, Sands GB, Hooks DA, LeGrice IJ, Smaill BH. Three distinct directions of intramural activation reveal nonuniform side-to-side electrical coupling in ventricular myocytes. *Circ Arrhythmia Electrophysiol* 2009;**2**:433–440.

11. Costa K, Takayama Y, McCulloch AD, Covell JW. Laminar fiber architecture and three-dimensional systolic mechanics in canine ventricular myocardium. *Am J Physiol* 1999;**283**:H2650–H2659.

12. Nash MP, Hunter PJ. Computational mechanics of the heart: From tissue structure to ventricular function. *J Elasticity* 2000;**61**: 113–141.

13. Robinson TF, Cohen-Gould L, Factor SM. The skeletal framework of mammalian heart muscle: Arrangement of inter- and pericellular connective tissues structures. *Lab Invest* 1983;**49**:482–498.

14. Sands GB, Gerneke DA, Hoks DA, Green CR, Smaill BH, LeGrice IJ. Automated imaging of extended tissue volumes. *Microsc Rese Tech* 2005;**67**:227–239.

15. Pope AJ. *Characterising myocardial remodelling in hypertensive heart disease: Structural and functional changes in the spontaneously hypertensive rat.* PhD Thesis, University of Auckland, 2011.

16. Bing OHL, Conrad CH, Boluyt MO, Robinson KG, Brooks WW. Studies of prevention, treatment and mechanisms of heart failure in the aging spontaneously hypertensive rat. *Heart Failure Rev* 2002;**7**: 71–88.

17. Rossi MA. Pathologic fibrosis and connective tissue matrix in left ventricular hypertrophy due to chronic arterial hypertension in humans. *J Hypertension* 1998;**16**:1031–1041.

18. Waldman LK, Nossan D, Villarreal FP, Covell JW. Relation between transmural deformation and local myofiber direction in canine left ventricle. *Circ Res* 1988;**63**:550–562.

19. Takayama Y, Costa KD, Covell JW. Contribution of laminar myofiber archiecture to load-dependent changes in mechanics of LV myocardium. *Am J Physiol* 2001;**282**:H1510–H1520.

20. Omens JH, May KD, McCulloch AD. Transmural distribution of three-dimensional strain in the isolated arrested canine left ventricle. *Am J Physiol* 1991;**261**:H918–H928.

21. Allen DG, Kentish JC. The cellular basis of the of the length-tension relation in cardiac muscle. *J Mol Cell Cardiol* 1985;**17**: 821–840.

22. Bovendeerd PHM, Arts T, Huyghe JM, van Campen DH, Reneman RS. Dependence of left ventricular wall mechanics on myocardial fiber orientation: a model study. *J Biomech* 1992;**25**:1129–1140.

23. Spotnitz HM, Spotnitz WD, Cottrell TS, Spiro D, Sonnenblick EH. Cellular basis for volume related wall thickness changes in the rat left ventricle. *J Mol Cell Cardiol* 1974;**6**:317–331.

24. LeGrice IJ, Takayama Y, Covell JW. Transverse shear along myocardial cleavage planes provides a mechanism for normal systolic wall thickening. *Circ Res* 1995;**77**:182–193.

25. Arts T, Costa KC, Covell, JW, McCulloch AD. Relating myocardial architecture to shear strain and muscle fiber orientation. *Am J Physiol* 2001;**280**:H2222–H2229.

26. Phan TT, Shivu GN, Abozguia K, Gnandevan M, Ahmed I, Frenneaux M. Left ventricular torsion and strain patterns in heart failure are similar to age-related changes. *Eu J Echocardiog* 2009;**10**:793–800.

27. Cingolani OH, Yang XP, Cavasin MA, Carretero OA. Increased systolic performance with diastolic dysfunction in adult spontaneously hypertensive rats. *Hypertension* 2003;**41**:249–254.

28. Tibayan FA, Lai DTM, Timek TA, Dagum P, Daughters GT, Ingels NB, Miller DC. Alterations in left ventricular torsion in tachycardia-induced dilated cardiomyopathy. *J Thorac Cardiovasc Surg* 2002; **124**:43–49.

29. Ennis DB. *Assessment of myocardial structure and function using magnetic resonance imaging.* PhD Thesis. John Hopkins University, Baltimore, 2004.

30. Young AA, Kraitchman DL, Dougherty L, Axel L. Tracking and finite element analysis of stripe deformation in magnetic resonance tagging. *IEEE Trans Med Imaging* 1995;**14**:413–421.

31. Le Bihan D, Mangin JF, Poupon C, Clark CA, Pappata S, Molko N, Chabriat H. Diffusion tensor imaging: concepts and applications. *J Magn Reson Imaging* 2001;**13**:534–546.

32. Douek P, Turner R, Pekar J, Patronas NJ, Le Bihan D. MR color mapping of myelin fibre orientation. *J Comput Assist Tomogr* 1991; **15**:923–929.

33. Wang VY, Lam HI, Ennis DB, Young AA, Nash MP. Passive ventricular mechanics modelling using MRI of structure and function. *Lect Notes Comp Sci (MICCAI-2008)* 2008;**5242**:814–821.

34. Wang VY, Lam HI, Ennis DB, Cowan BR, Young AA, Nash MP. Modelling passive diastolic mechanics with quantative MRI of cardiac structure and function. *Med Image Anal* 2009;**13**:773–784.

35. Hunter PJ, McCulloch A, ter Keurs HEDJ. Modelling the mechanical properties of cardiac muscle. *Prog Biophys Mol Biol* 1998;**69**: 289–331.

Mathematical models of human atrial mechano-electrical coupling and arrhythmias

Elizabeth M. Cherry

Background

The role of mechano-sensitive channels (MSC) in cardiac tissue has been examined extensively, in particular in the context of arrhythmia induction and sustenance[1]. Given that MSC blockers can prevent or terminate stretch-induced atrial arrhythmias[2], they also form a therapeutically interesting target. However, projection from the single channel level to organ or patient behaviour is often difficult, in particular since specific pharmacological tools to target individual MSC in an organ-specific manner are still missing.

Mathematical modelling can be a powerful tool for understanding the mechanisms responsible for cardiac arrhythmogenesis, both in interpreting experimental results and in positing and testing new hypotheses[3,4]. Understanding the role of MSC in human atrial arrhythmias may be furthered by appropriate modelling and simulations. In this chapter, we describe how atrial tissue, including MSC, can be modelled and show the potential utility of such models for explaining the potentially arrhythmogenic effects of atrial mechanical stimulation, such as described in the context of atrial fibrillation in Chapter 28.

Modelling human atrial tissue

Human atrial cell models

Two primary mathematical models describing the electrophysiology of human atrial cells have been developed: the Nygren et al. model[5] (and a subsequent update[6]) and the Courtemanche et al. model[7]. The two models include the same 12 trans-membrane currents, including two Na$^+$ currents (fast current I_{Na} and background current $I_{b,Na}$), two Ca^{2+} currents (L-type current $I_{Ca,L}$ and background current $I_{b,Ca}$) and five K$^+$ currents (transient outward current I_{to}, slow and fast delayed rectifier currents I_{Kr} and I_{Ks}, inward rectifier I_{K1} and sustained or ultra-rapid rectifier I_{sus} or I_{Kur}), as well as three pump or exchanger currents (Na$^+$/Ca^{2+} exchanger current I_{NCX}, Na$^+$/K$^+$ pump I_{NaK} and sarcolemmal pump Ca^{2+} current I_{pCa}). The two models have different representations of ion concentrations and intracellular calcium dynamics. The Nygren et al. model builds on the formulation of Lindblad et al.[8], which features separate cytoplasmic, restricted sub-sarcolemmal, and junctional and non-junctional sarcoplasmic reticulum (SR) calcium concentrations; dyadic cleft ionic concentrations; and detailed calcium buffering. The Courtemanche et al. model follows the formulation of Luo and Rudy[9], which includes separate cytoplasmic, junctional SR and non-junctional SR calcium concentrations along with buffering.

The two models, despite being developed largely from the same experimental data, have many differences in behaviour[10,11]. The most immediately obvious difference is in action potential (AP) morphology. The Nygren et al. model assumes a triangular morphology for all pacing rates, whereas the Courtemanche et al. model features a spike-and-dome morphology at slow rates that transitions at faster rates to a triangular shape[10,11]. The rate dependence of the two models is also different: the Nygren et al. model adapts to faster rates primarily through increasing resting membrane potential (RMP), whereas the Courtemanche et al. model adapts primarily through AP shortening[11].

In tissue simulations, the models display additional dissimilarities. Thus, in two-dimensional (2D) sheet models, re-entrant waves induced for the Nygren et al. model remain stable[10], with a circular core measuring about 1.5 cm[12]. In contrast, spirals in the Courtemanche et al. model are quasi-stable, with hypermeandering paths measuring about 5 cm across and occasional longer excursions, with periods of (usually transient) break-up in larger domains[12] (in smaller domains, spiral wave activity usually self-terminates)[10].

Taking multicellular models a step further by using a representative three-dimensional (3D) human atrial anatomy causes drift of otherwise stable re-entry patterns for both models and thus usually results in termination at a physical boundary[12].

Mechano-electrical coupling

Modelling mechano-electrical coupling usually focuses on the inclusion of MSC as a first target. Both atrial and ventricular cells have ion channels whose open probability is affected by the mechanical environment. Because K+-selective MSC have a much more negative reversal potential and therefore cannot be a trigger for AP generation, models usually focus on incorporating expression of the non-selective cation channel that is permeable to K+, Na+ and, in some cells, Ca2+. Although early models represented this current by increasing background conductances[13], MSC currents are generally formulated separately now, in one of two ways. One common approach is to express MSC simply as an Ohmic conductance, where the product of a stretch-dependent conductance term and the difference between the membrane potential and the reversal potential determines the current[14–20]. Parameters needed for this expression include the maximum conductance, degree of stretch, relation between stretch and conductance and MSC reversal potential. Evidence suggests that the reversal potential for non-selective MSC in the atria is around 0 mV or slightly negative to that[21,22], which is at the high end of values reported for cardiac tissue (between −50 and 0 mV[23]). Another formulation uses the Goldman–Hodgkin–Katz equation with a stretch-dependent conductance term[24]. For this type of equation, necessary parameters include the maximum conductance, degree of stretch, coupling between stretch and permeability changes and relative permeabilities of K+, Na+ and Ca2+ ions. The stretch-dependent conductance term often takes the form $(1 + a\exp(-b\Delta S))^{-1}$ [14,15,21,24,25], where a governs the amount of current in the absence of stretch, b controls the sensitivity to stretch and ΔS is a measure of stretch such as the change in sarcomere length[14,21,24,25], isometric tension[25] or strain[15] relative to a reference value. Other forms of stretch-dependent conductance can be used as well[16,17].

Other types of mechano-electric coupling effects also have been modelled. Iribe and Kohl[26] incorporated stretch-induced changes in intracellular calcium handling, including SR Ca2+ leak through the ryanodine receptor (RyR) channels, modified SR Ca2+ uptake and altered Ca2+ influx. Furthermore, Kohl et al.[27] modelled interactions of cardiomyocytes with coupled mechano-sensitive fibroblasts. Kuijpers et al.[24] incorporated variations in the diffusion coefficient resulting from stretch-induced changes in cell length and cross-sectional area.

Several computational studies have investigated how MSC can facilitate initiation of arrhythmias. Rice et al.[18] used a cross-field protocol in a 2D sheet designed to simulate local regions of 'paradoxical segment lengthening', as seen in ischaemic tissue. In this condition, certain regions of myocardium stretch rather than contract during systole. This spatially localized stretch can give rise to re-entry. Kohl et al.[23] similarly demonstrated that a local ischaemic region can induce re-entry in a 2D sheet. In this case, a localized region of ischaemia that is unable to conduct a normal impulse experiences passive distention as surrounding tissue contracts. This stretch, in turn, activates MSC that are then able to promote ectopic excitation; under the right conditions, this can induce re-entry. Kohl et al. also showed that such stretch-mediated ectopic foci could be initiated in an anatomically realistic model of canine ventricular anatomy[23].

In the simulations described below, we utilize the Nygren et al. and Courtemanche et al. human atrial cell models with additional

non-selective MSC currents following the Goldman–Hodgkin–Katz expressions in Kuijpers et al.[24] for Na+, K+ and Ca2+ contributions. Parameter values are set as indicated in Table 35.1, with the relative permeabilities of Na+, K+ and Ca2+ assigned using the values of Youm et al.[21] Stretch values (ratio of the stretched cell length to the reference length) are varied between 0 and 20%[15].

Human atrial anatomical models

Although re-entrant arrhythmias can be demonstrated readily in a simple rectangular 2D tissue sheets, the complex anatomy of the atria offers a very different structural substrate with additional opportunities for potentially arrhythmogenic wave interactions. Whereas human atrial cell electrophysiological models are essentially limited to the Nygren et al. (with its subsequent update[6]) and Courtemanche et al. models, several efforts to obtain detailed models of human atrial anatomy have been made. The first detailed 3D model of atrial anatomy for computational purposes was developed by Harrild and Henriquez[28] and was used to investigate normal and arrhythmic activation sequences. The model consisted of about 250,000 elements and its anatomical features included structures such as the superior and inferior Venae cavae, pulmonary veins, Bachmann's bundle, Crista terminalis and pectinate muscles in the right atrium. Regionally varying conductivities were assigned to obtain appropriate conduction velocities for the bulk tissue, rapidly conducting bundles and poorly conducting regions. The model later was interpolated to a uniform mesh and was extended to include a portion of the coronary sinus with electrical connections to the left atrium[12].

Vigmond et al.[29] developed an idealized 3D atrial model that incorporated similar anatomical features, including the coronary sinus, along with anisotropic conduction. The model was discretized using the cable approach[30] with 350,000 segments and was used to investigate the role of anatomical structure on re-entrant arrhythmia pathways. Virag et al.[31] constructed a curved 2D shell structure in 3D space for investigating long-duration arrhythmias and, subsequently, ablation strategies[32]. The model was based on MRI data and included similar anatomical structures, with the

Table 35.1 Parameter values used for MSC with the two human atrial cell models. G_{SAC}, maximum stretch-activated channel conductance; K_{SAC}, baseline stretch-activated current parameter in the absence of stretch; α_{SAC}, sensitivity of stretch-activated current to stretch; P_{Na}, permeability to Na+ ions; P_K, permeability to K+ ions; P_{Ca}, permeability to Ca2+ ions. Because the Nygren et al. model is already susceptible to delayed after-depolarizations (DAD), it requires a smaller conductance than the Courtemanche et al. model to produce arrhythmogenic behaviour.

Parameter (μm/s)	Value used with Nygren et al. model	Value used with Courtemanche et al. model
G_{SAC}	1e-8	2.35e-5
K_{SAC}	100	100
α_{SAC}	20	20
P_{Na}	1.0	1.0
P_K	1.32	1.32
P_{Ca}	0.7	0.7

exception of pectine muscles, which were not incorporated. Anisotropy was not used. In most cases, a mesh of 100,000 vertices, corresponding to a spatial resolution of about 0.4 mm, was used.

Zemlin et al.[33] developed another 2D surface model of the human atria using data from the Visible Human Project, which included the features of the Virag et al. model along with pectinate muscles and anisotropy. The mesh included 600,000 triangles whose average side length was 0.28 mm. Seemann et al.[34] also derived their model from the Visible Human Project, but in their case a full 3D model was developed and used to study normal conduction and, later, arrhythmias and ablation strategies[35]. The model contained approximately 1.7 million elements with a spatial resolution of 0.33 mm[35].

Effects of MSC in atrial models

Isolated cells

In isolated cells, models of MSC are able to reproduce important experimentally observed AP changes. Among the most important effects are increased (less negative) RMP and AP prolongation (although early AP duration may be shortened, particularly at long cycle lengths[36]). As shown in Fig. 35.1, inclusion of a non-selective MSC current raised RMP and increased AP duration (APD) in both the Nygren et al. and Courtemanche et al. models, with the magnitude of the changes related to the degree of stretch. Within the Courtemanche et al. model, increased stretch also altered AP morphology from spike-and-dome to triangular, and especially large stretch produced pronounced diastolic (or phase 4) depolarization.

The changes in RMP and APD can be important arrhythmogenic factors. Less negative RMP can facilitate the development of delayed after-depolarizations (DAD), and prolonged APD can extend the range of cycle lengths at which phenomena like DAD or conduction block occur. This arrhythmogenic behaviour can be reproduced by the models. The Nygren et al. model is already susceptible to DAD development upon cessation of stimulation following a period of rapid pacing[11]. However, inclusion of MSC current makes DAD easier to elicit by reducing the extent to which the pacing cycle length must be shortened before DAD can be induced (or by increasing the number of DAD that arise for a given cycle length). Figure 35.2 shows how increases in stretch affected

the development of DAD in the Nygren et al. model at two different cycle lengths. At a longer cycle length of 1,000 ms (Fig. 35.2A), stretch induced a DAD where none arose without the inclusion of MSC. At a shorter cycle length (Fig. 35.2B), even the case without stretch displayed DAD; however, DAD activity began sooner and lasted longer with more extra beats as stretch was increased.

One-dimensional cables

In single cells, DAD can be induced relatively easily with the inclusion of stretch. Importantly, this arrhythmogenic mechanism remains viable in tissue, as DAD can continue to arise and to propagate. Figure 35.3 shows examples of propagating DAD using the Nygren et al. model in a one-dimensional (1D) cable using the monodomain approach. Although DAD were elicited without stretch, during a 6-s window additional DAD were elicited with 15 and 20% stretch, with the time elapsing before the first DAD decreasing as stretch increased. In all cases, the DAD were able to propagate, and in many cases DAD arose away from the stimulus site and propagated bidirectionally. As shown in Fig. 35.4, DAD activity also increased with increased pacing rate (because of increased intracellular calcium, which facilitates transient inward current via I_{NCX}). For a fixed stretch value of 20%, the number and frequency of DAD increased as the cycle length at which the tissue was paced decreased.

Propagating DAD also could be elicited using the Courtemanche et al. model. Figure 35.5 shows examples of DAD activity that arose along a 1D cable with 20% stretch. With cessation of pacing (Fig. 35.5A), DAD activity quickly became coordinated at all sites along the cable. When pacing was continued (Fig. 35.5B), dyssynchrony arose between the pacing site and other sites along the cable, as some paced beats were blocked or delayed. Such dispersion itself may be arrhythmogenic.

Re-entrant waves

Stretch-induced DAD can lead to the formation of re-entrant waves by dispersion of repolarization. A local region of stretch can interact with normal waves to produce re-entry. Figure 35.6 shows an example of the induction of re-entry in a 2D sheet using the Nygren et al. model. In this case, a locally stretched region (top right corner) produced a DAD (0 ms) upon cessation of several seconds of rapid pacing to condition the model. The DAD propagated (180 ms), causing dispersion of repolarization, which then interacted with a subsequent normal wave originating from the left edge of the tissue. Because the tissue farther from the area of local stretch had not fully repolarized, the tissue in that region was refractory during the normal beat. Closer to the stretch-induced ectopic focus, the tissue had recovered and propagation was successful (400 ms). The repolarization gradient thus fostered development of a re-entrant wave from the normal beat (500 ms) that could become sustained in the tissue and might even lead to further wave breaks (1,300 ms).

Even more complex wave interactions can be induced in 3D atrial geometries. Figure 35.7 shows a region of local stretch near the right atrial appendage in the extended[12] human atrial anatomical model of Harrild and Henriquez[28] using the Nygren et al. model. This region produced a DAD that served as an ectopic focus. As the wave propagated, it caused dispersion of refractoriness that interfered with a subsequent sinus node beat. Partial conduction block initially occurred within the right atrium (300 ms), which gave rise to a re-entrant wave within the right atrium.

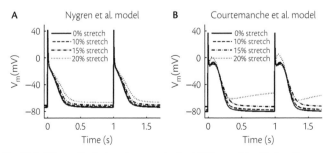

Fig. 35.1 Effects of inclusion of a non-selective MSC in models of isolated human atrial cells by Nygren et al. (**A**) and Courtemanche et al. (**B**). For both models, stretch raised the RMP and prolonged APD. For pronounced stretch in the Courtemanche et al. model (**B**), diastolic depolarization occurred. AP were elicited here and in subsequent simulations by applying a stimulus current twice diastolic threshold for 3 ms. Pacing was applied for 30 s at a cycle length of 1,000 ms. V_m, trans-membrane potential.

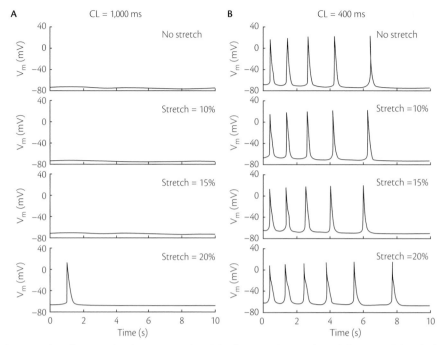

Fig. 35.2 Delayed after-depolarizations (DAD) generated in the Nygren *et al.* model with varying degrees of stretch for two cycle lengths (CL). Although the model generated DAD even without stretch at fast pacing rates, increased stretch facilitated DAD induction. For example, with greater stretch, the frequency and, in some cases, the number of DAD increased. Panels show DAD induced during an interval without pacing following 10 s of pacing at the indicated CL.

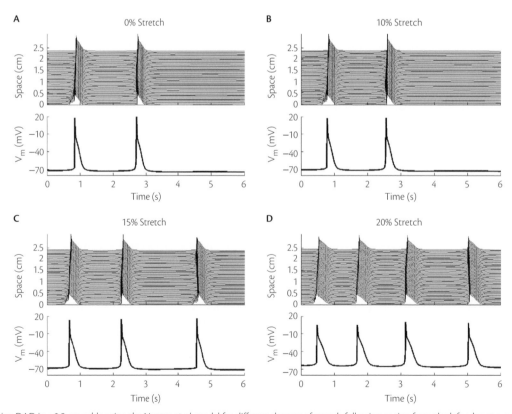

Fig. 35.3 Propagating DAD in a 2.5 cm cable using the Nygren *et al.* model for different degrees of stretch following pacing from the left edge at a cycle length of 600 ms. In all cases, the DAD were able to propagate. Although the initial DAD always began near the site of stimulation, subsequent DAD sometimes originated from other locations. Upper panels: space-time plots. Lower panels: voltage traces at the centre point of the cable. Here and in subsequent cable simulations, the spatial resolution was 0.025 cm, the value of the monodomain diffusion coefficient was 0.001 cm²/ms and the stimulus was applied to the leftmost 0.1 cm of the cable.

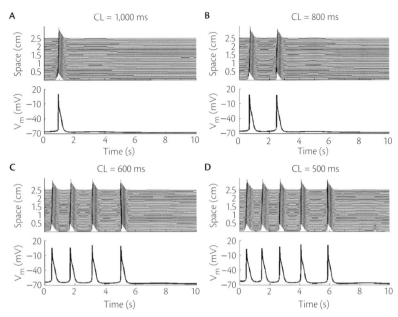

Fig. 35.4 Increased DAD activity as a function of initial pacing CL for the Nygren *et al.* model with 20% stretch (2.5 cm cable). Activity resulted after pacing for 10 s at CLs of **A** 1,000 ms, **B** 800 ms, **C** 600 ms and **D** 500 ms. Upper panels: space–time plots. Lower panels: voltage traces at the centre point of the cable.

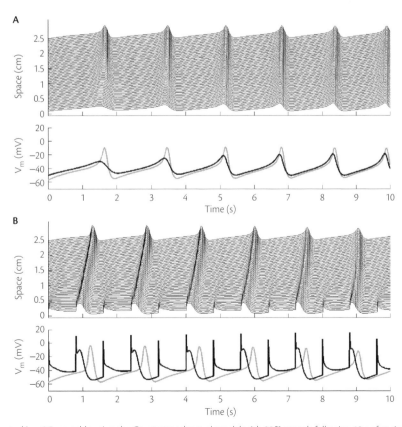

Fig. 35.5 Propagating DAD generated in a 2.5 cm cable using the Courtemanche *et al.* model with 20% stretch following 10 s of pacing at a CL of 800 ms. Upper panels: space–time plots. Lower panels: voltage traces at the bottom edge (black) and 1.875 cm away (grey). **A** DAD appearing during 10 s without pacing. **B** DAD appearing during 10 s with continued pacing at the same CL. Not all paced beats were able to propagate, resulting in variable degrees of synchrony along the cable.

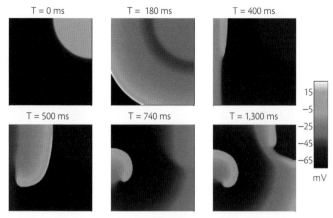

Fig. 35.6 Initiation of re-entry by a local stretch-induced ectopic excitation. After a pause in pacing, local stretch in the upper right corner gave rise to a DAD (0 ms) that produced focal activity which interfered with propagation of a subsequent normal beat (400 ms). Re-entry resulted (500 ms) and the dispersion of refractoriness that occurred could lead to subsequent wave breaks as well (1,300 ms); in this case these wave breaks were not sustained. Prior to induction, the tissue was paced for 3 s at a CL of 300 ms. (See color plate section.)

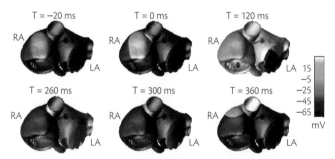

Fig. 35.7 Complex wave interactions in a realistic human atrial anatomical model. A region of local stretch in the right atrium (RA) near the right atrial appendage produced a spontaneous depolarization (−20 ms) that developed into a DAD that acted as an ectopic focus (0 ms). After the beat propagated to the left atrium (LA) (120 ms), a normal sinus beat arose at 240 ms (not shown). Because of the repolarization gradient set up by the ectopic beat, the beat was able to propagate toward the superior *vena cava* (260 ms) but initially was blocked in the region of the ectopic beat (300 ms). This gave rise to a re-entrant wave in the RA; in this case, the re-entry was not sustained. (See color plate section.)

Conclusions and outlook

Mathematical modelling of MSC can help to elucidate how stretch can affect the origin and spread of excitation. Although MSC give rise to heterogeneity in their own right through increased RMP and AP duration changes, their primary contribution to arrhythmogenesis is likely to be through the generation of DAD. This may be facilitated by altered calcium handling[26], which may arise with greater propensity in specific regions like the pulmonary veins (see also Chapter 15)[37]. Within models, MSC activation can lead to development of DAD, which are subsequently able to propagate. In higher dimensions, these DAD can interact with normal sinus node beats or with other ectopic foci to produce localized conduction block and re-entry.

It is as yet unclear how MSC contribute to the induction and maintenance of chronic AF. In the acute setting, stretch promotes extopic excitation and sustenance of burst-pacing-induced AF[37,38]. However, MSC currents may be transient, rather than sustained[21,39]. Furthermore, adding typical AF-induced electrophysiological remodelling[40] to the Courtemanche *et al.* and Nygren *et al.* models of human atrial cells reduces the propensity of MSC to cause DAD (not shown). This reduction may arise because of decreased L-type Ca^{2+} current, which in turn suppresses Ca^{2+} overload and the subsequent involvement of I_{NCX} as a transient inward current. Other types of effects that are not modelled or known likely will be of relevance in explaining the role of MSC in chronic AF. These include alterations in intracellular calcium cycling, changes in cell coupling, the possible involvement of cell swelling-activated Cl^- currents[37], substrate modification through fibrosis and fibroblast proliferation that may lead to electrotonic dissociation of epicardium and endocardium[41], or other underlying pathophysiological conditions[18,23,42].

Acknowledgements

This work was supported by the National Science Foundation through TeraGrid resources provided by the Pittsburgh Supercomputing Center.

References

1. Kohl P, Noble D. Life and mechanosensitivity. *Prog Biophys Mol Biol* 2008;**97**:159–162.
2. Franz MR, Bode F. Mechano-electrical feedback underlying arrhythmias: the atrial fibrillation case. *Prog Biophys Mol Biol* 2003;**82**:163–174.
3. Fenton FH, Cherry EM. Models of cardiac cell. *Scholarpedia* 2008;**3**: 1868.
4. Cherry EM, Fenton FH. Visualization of spiral and scroll waves in simulated and experimental cardiac tissue. *N J Phys* 2008;**10**:125016.
5. Nygren A, Fiset C, Firek L, *et al.* Mathematical model of an adult human atrial cell: the role of K^+ currents in repolarization. *Circ Res* 1998;**82**:63–81.
6. Maleckar MM, Greenstein JL, Trayanova NA, Giles WR. Mathematical simulations of ligand-gated and cell-type specific effects on the action potential of human atrium. *Prog Biophys Mol Biol* 2008;**98**:161–170.
7. Courtemanche M, Ramirez RJ, Nattel S. Ionic mechanisms underlying human atrial action potential properties: insights from a mathematical model. *Am J Physiol* 1998;**275**:H301–H321.
8. Lindblad DS, Murphey CR, Clark JW, Giles WR. A model of the action potential and underlying membrane currents in a rabbit atrial cell. *Am J Physiol* 1996;**271**:H1666–H1696.
9. CH, Rudy Y. A dynamic model of the cardiac ventricular action potential. I. Simulations of ionic currents and concentration changes. *Circ Res* 1994;**74**:1071–1096.
10. Nygren A, Leon LJ, Giles WR. Simulations of the human atrial action potential. *Phil Trans R Soc Lond A* 2001;**359**:1111–1125.
11. Cherry EM, Hastings HM, Evans SJ. Dynamics of human atrial cell models: restitution, memory, and intracellular calcium dynamics in single cells. *Prog Biophys Mol Biol* 2008;**98**:24–37.
12. Cherry EM, Evans SJ. Properties of two human atrial cell models in tissue: restitution, memory, propagation, and reentry. *J Theor Biol* 2008;**254**:674–690.
13. Gannier F, White E, Lacampagne A, Garnier D, Le Guennec JY. Streptomycin reverses a large stretch induced increases in $[Ca^{2+}]_i$ in isolated guinea pig ventricular myocytes. *Cardiovasc Res* 1994;**28**: 1193–1198.

14. Kohl P, Sachs F. Mechanoelectric feedback in cardiac cells. *Phil Trans R Soc (Lond) A* 2001;**359**:1173–1185.

15. Cherubini C, Filippi S, Nardinocchi P, Teresi L. An electromechanical model of cardiac tissue: constitutive issues and electrophysiological effects. *Prog Biophys Mol Biol* 2008;**97**:562–573.

16. Panfilov AV, Keldermann RH, Nash MP. Drift and breakup of spiral waves in reaction-diffusion-mechanics systems. *Proc Natl Acad Sci USA* 2007;**104**:7922–7926.

17. Li W, Gurev V, McCulloch AD, Trayanova NA. The role of mechanoelectric feedback in vulnerability to electric shock. *Prog Biophys Mol Biol* 2008;**97**:461–478.

18. Rice JJ, Winslow RL, Dekanski J, McVeigh E. Model studies of the role of mechano-sensitive currents in the generation of cardiac arrhythmias. *J Theor Biol* 1998;**190**:295–312.

19. Noble D, Varghese A, Kohl P, Noble P. Improved guinea pig ventricular cell model incorporating a diadic space, I_{Kr} and I_{Ks}, and length- and tension-dependent processes. *Can J Cardiol* 1998;**14**:123–134.

20. Vetter FJ, McCulloch AD. Mechanoelectric feedback in a model of the passively inflated left ventricle. *Ann Biomed Eng* 2001;**29**:414–426.

21. Youm JB, Han J, Kim N, *et al*. Role of stretch-activated channels on the stretch-induced changes of rat atrial myocytes. *Prog Biophys Mol Biol* 2006;**90**:186–206.

22. Zhang YH, Youm JB, Sung HK, *et al*. Stretch-activated and background non-selective cation channels in rat atrial myocytes. *J Physiol* 2000;**523**:607–619.

23. Kohl P, Hunter P, Noble D. Stretch-induced changes in heart rate and rhythm: clinical observations, experiments and mathematical models. *Prog Biophys Mol Biol* 1999;**71**:91–138.

24. Kuijpers NHL, ten Eikelder HMM, Bovendeerd PHM, *et al*. Mechanoelectric feedback leads to conduction slowing and block in acutely dilated atria: a modeling study of cardiac electromechanics. *Am J Physiol* 2007;**292**:H2832–H2853.

25. Kohl P, Day K, Noble D. Cellular mechanisms of cardiac mechano-electric feedback in a mathematical model. *Can J Cardiol* 1998;**14**: 111–119.

26. Iribe G, Kohl P. Axial stretch enhances sarcoplasmic reticulum Ca^{2+} leak and cellular Ca^{2+} reuptake in guinea pig ventricular myocytes: experiments and models. *Prog Biophys Mol Biol* 2008;**97**:298–311.

27. Kohl P, Kamkin AG, Kiseleva IS, Noble D. Mechanosensitive fibroblasts in the sino-atrial node region of rat heart: interaction with cardiomyocytes and possible role. *Exp Physiol* 1994;**79**:943–956.

28. Harrild D, Henriquez C. A computer model of normal conduction in the human atria. *Circ Res* 2000;**87**:E25–E36.

29. Vigmond EJ, Ruckdeschel R, Trayanova N. Reentry in a morphologically realistic atrial model. *J Cardiovasc Electrophysiol* 2001;**12**:1046–1054.

30. Vigmond EJ, Leon LJ. Computationally efficient model for simulating electrical activity in cardiac tissue with fiber rotation. *Ann Biomed Eng* 1999;**27**:160–170.

31. Virag N, Jacquemet V, Henriquez CS, *et al*. Study of atrial arrhythmias in a computer model based on magnetic resonance images of human atria. *Chaos* 2002;**12**:754–763.

32. Rotter M, Dang L, Jacquemet V, *et al*. Impact of varying ablation patterns in a simulation model of persistent atrial fibrillation. *Pacing Clin Electrophysiol* 2007;**30**:314–321.

33. Zemlin CW, Herzel H, Ho SY, Panfilov AV. A realistic and efficient model of excitation propagation in the human atria. In: *Computer Simulation and Experimental Assessment of Cardiac Electrophysiology*. (eds. N Virag, O Blanc, L Kappenberger), New York, NY: Wiley-Blackwell; 2001:29–34.

34. Seemann G, Höper C, Sachse FB, *et al*. Heterogeneous three-dimensional anatomical and electrophysiological model of human atria. *Phil Trans R Soc (Lond) A* 2006;**364**:1465–1481.

35. Reumann M, Bohnert J, Seemann G, Osswald B, Dössel O. Preventive ablation strategies in a biophysical model of atrial fibrillation based on realistic anatomical data. *IEEE Trans Biomed Eng* 2008;**55**: 399–406.

36. Taggart P, Lab M. Cardiac mechano-electric feedback and electrical restitution in humans. *Prog Biophys Mol Biol* 2008;**97**:452–460.

37. Seol CA, Kim WT, Ha JM, *et al*. Stretch-activated currents in cardiomyocytes isolated from rabbit pulmonary veins. *Prog Biophys Mol Biol* 2008;**97**:217–231.

38. Bode F, Katchman A, Woosley RL, Franz MR. Gadolinium decreases stretch-induced vulnerability to atrial fibrillation. *Circulation* 2000;**101**:2200–2205.

39. Niu W, Sachs F. Dynamic properties of stretch-activated K^+ channels in adult rat atrial myocytes. *Prog Biophys Mol Biol* 2003;**82**:121–135.

40. Courtemanche M, Ramirez RJ, Nattel S. Ionic targets for drug therapy and atrial fibrillation-induced electrical remodeling: insights from a mathematical model. *Cardiovasc Res* 1999;**42**:477–489.

41. Eckstein J, Verheule S, de Groot NM, *et al*. Mechanisms of perpetuation of atrial fibrillation in chronically dilated atria. *Prog Biophys Mol Biol* 2008;**97**:435–451.

42. Ninio DM, Saint DA. The role of stretch-activated channels in atrial fibrillation and the impact of intracellular acidosis. *Prog Biophys Mol Biol* 2008;**97**:401–416.

Mathematical models of ventricular mechano-electric coupling and arrhythmia

Natalia A. Trayanova, Viatcheslav Gurev,
Jason Constantino and Yuxuan Hu

Background

Mechano-electric coupling (MEC), the study of which this book is dedicated to, remains a very active and dynamic area of research. A large body of experimental and clinical research has demonstrated that the mechanical environment of the heart, in health and disease, is capable of exerting influence on cardiac electrophysiology[1]. Temporal changes in strain take place during all phases of the cardiac cycle, and additional spatial heterogeneity in strain can result from cardiac disease such as ischaemia, infarction and heart failure. The mechanisms that contribute to strain-dependent modulation of normal or abnormal electrical wave propagation in the heart arise from abnormal deformations of cardiac tissue and from cellular mechanisms of MEC. In the context of ventricular arrhythmogenesis, which the present chapter examines, MEC mechanisms combine with other factors, whether dynamical or those associated with remodelling in disease, to give rise to a new emergent behaviour at the level of the intact heart, through which the role of MEC in the origin, maintenance and possible termination of ventricular tachycardia (VT) and fibrillation (VF) is manifested.

At least three MEC mechanisms at the cellular level have been identified as potential contributors to the generation or exacerbation of the arrhythmogenic substrate in the heart. The first is the effect of stretch on intracellular calcium (Ca^{2+}) handling (see Chapter 10). Overall, MEC can affect the magnitude, duration and dynamics of the intracellular Ca^{2+} transient and alter the action potential duration (APD). Recently, altered Ca^{2+} handling, together with instabilities in APD, has been identified as an important mechanism underlying the dynamic formation of spatially discordant alternans and thus arrhythmogenicity[2,3]; see also Chapters 16 and 17.

The second cellular mechanism of MEC could take place through the participation of non-myocyte cell population in the heart. Every cardiomyocyte is in close proximity to multiple fibroblasts, which deposit collagen and elastin fibres, forming the extracellular matrix of the heart. Cardiac fibroblasts have been found to be mechano-sensitive (see Chapter 19). The coupling of myocytes and fibroblasts is well established in cell culture and in some *in vivo* studies, confirmed by the presence of functional gap junctions[4,5]. Depolarization of cardiac fibroblasts by stretch (via mechano-sensitive ion channels) may therefore affect both the resting potential and APD of the coupled myocyte[6,7], leading to electrophysiological heterogeneities and possibly creating an arrhythmogenic substrate.

The third, and perhaps most prominent, mechanism of MEC at the cellular level is the existence of sarcolemmal channels that are activated by mechanical stimuli. A variety of ionic channels activated by changes in cell volume or cell stretch have been identified in cardiac tissue (see Chapters 2–6). Of these, stretch-activated channels (SAC) have long been suspected as important contributors to the pro-arrhythmic substrate in the heart. The non-uniform distribution of positive myofibre strain (stretching) during mechanical contraction under a variety of pathological conditions could potentially, via SAC, produce dispersion in electrophysiological properties, shown previously to be pro-arrhythmic[8,9]. Indeed, at the cellular level SAC has been shown to shorten or lengthen APD or produce ectopic beats depending on the timing of the mechanical stimulus application relative to the phase of the AP[10]. Uncovering, however, the mechanisms by which SAC contribute to ventricular arrhythmogenesis under a variety of pathological conditions is hampered by the lack of experimental methodologies that can record the three-dimensional (3D) electrical and mechanical activity simultaneously and with high spatiotemporal resolution. The current optical mapping technique, the most powerful tool in the study of the spatiotemporal organization in the heart during arrhythmias, can only record electrical activity from the surface layers of the heart and often necessitates either physically constraining the heart or the application of pharmacological agents to block mechanical contraction[11]. Furthermore, the more readily available pharmacological agents that block SAC lack selectivity and efficacy[2,12,13], while the peptide-blocker GsMTx-4 suffers from limited availability and high cost. Thus, computer simulations have emerged as a valuable tool to dissect the mechanisms by which SAC contribute to the ventricular arrhythmogenic substrate, exacerbating arrhythmias and rendering the heart more difficult to defibrillate. Below we present an overview of the computer simulations of the role of MEC in arrhythmogenesis and defibrillation, illustrating our discussion with examples from physiologically realistic whole heart simulations.

Modelling SAC

Despite the diversity in SAC, these channels share a number of properties. The current–voltage relationship of both the cation non-selective SAC (SAC_{NS}) and the K^+-selective SAC (SAC_K) is typically linear. Furthermore, SAC are associated with fast activation and inactivation times, much faster than the time course of a physiologically relevant mechanical stimulus[14]. Thus, SAC are typically modelled as instantaneously activating linear currents[15–21]. The reversal potentials of SAC_{NS} and SAC_K are in the range of −10 mV and −90 mV, respectively[22,23]. Thus, the common reversal potential of whole-cell stretch-activated currents varies from −90 to −10 mV, depending on the fractional expression of both types of SAC. Values in this range have been widely used in simulation studies[15–17,24], and the effects of SAC on electrophysiology are strongly dependent on this reversal potential. The conductances of the two SAC currents are typically assumed to be dependent on strain rather than stress due to the limited capabilities of current experimental techniques to track changes in stress and are chosen accordingly to match experimental results[1,20,25].

During sustained stretch, the SAC current can have a significant impact on cardiac electrophysiological properties. The effects of a constant, time-independent current via SAC on general electrophysiological properties was studied by Trayanova *et al.*[26]. SAC opening progressively depolarized resting cells, caused reduction in the magnitude of the trans-membrane potential during early repolarization and often prolonged APD at 90% repolarization (APD90): APD90 increased when the SAC reversal potential was above −20 mV. Figure 36.1 shows the effect of SAC activation on the electrophysiological properties of cardiac tissue at different cycle lengths[26]. The study found that SAC caused (1) a decrease in resting membrane potential (from −85 mV to −75 mV); (2) increased APD at short cycle lengths; (3) flattening of the restitution curve; (4) a slight increase in the effective refractory period; (5) an increase in conduction velocity and wavelength for cycle lengths longer than 115 ms, and a decrease for cycle lengths smaller than 115 ms; and (6) an increase in the activation threshold. These findings[26] are broadly consistent with experimental results[20,21,25].

Studies[16,20] have also investigated the effects of SAC recruitment on AP dynamics during different phases of the AP. Different responses were found, determined by the timing of the stretch and its magnitude. If stretch is applied during the plateau phase of the AP, it changed the time course of repolarization, resulting in either shortening or lengthening of the AP. If SAC were activated when the cell was already repolarized, it resulted in a new AP if the magnitude of the SAC current was sufficient for that.

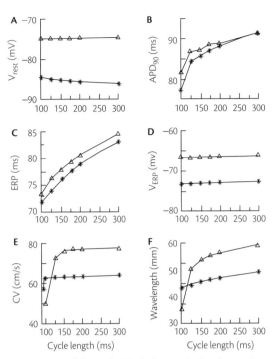

Fig. 36.1 Comparison of electrophysiological properties in a tissue strip model with SAC (lines with triangles) and without SAC (lines with stars; SAC reversal potential −20 mV). All variables are depicted as functions of cycle length. **A** Resting membrane potential (V_{rest}). **B** APD at the level of 90% repolarization (APD90). **C** Effective refractory period (ERP). **D** Trans-membrane potential at the end of ERP (V_{ERP}). **E** Conduction velocity along the tissue strip (CV). **F** Wavelength, the product of CV and ERP. [Reproduced, with permission, from Trayanova N, Li W, Eason J, Kohl P (2004) Effect of stretch-activated channels on defibrillation efficacy. *Heart Rhythm* 1:67–77.]

Modelling *Commotio cordis*: effects of mechano-electric coupling

A substantial body of research has demonstrated that moderate mechanical impact to the pre-cordial region of the chest (*Commotio cordis*) can lead to serious cardiac arrhythmias without corresponding morphological damage to the heart or other organs of the chest (see Chapter 45). A computational study by Li *et al.*[16] examined the mechanisms by which mechanical stimulation via the recruitment of SAC can result in the initiation of VT in the rabbit heart, given that impact coincides with the T-wave of electrical repolarization. The study used a purely electrophysiological model, in which mechanical impact was assumed to open SAC. The mechanical impact was delivered to the anterior epicardium of the rabbit ventricular model. The area in which SAC were activated by the mechanical intervention was assumed circular on the cardiac surface and of 16 mm diameter (scaled from baseball impacts in man or pig models to rabbit dimensions). A similar study in 2D was conducted by Garny and Kohl[27].

In the study by Li *et al.*[16], the vulnerable window was found to have duration of 10–20 ms, consistent with experimental findings[28,29]. Figure 36.2 presents several examples of mechanical impacts, corresponding to coupling intervals either outside or inside the vulnerable window. Figure 36.2A and B portray two

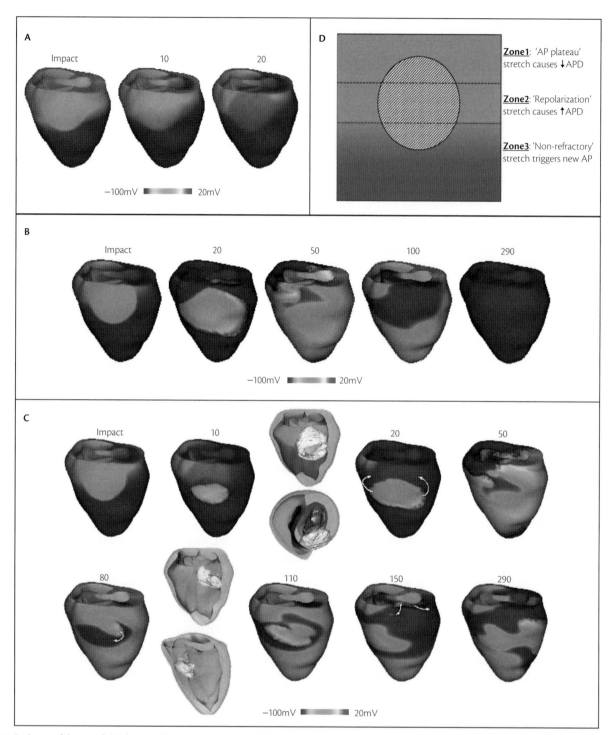

Fig. 36.2 Evolution of the spatial distribution of trans-membrane potential in a rabbit ventricular model following a mechanical impact delivered at coupling intervals (CI) of 135 ms (**A**) and 155 ms (**B**). Both CI are outside the vulnerable window; the impact does not result in re-entry. **C** Evolution of the spatial distribution of trans-membrane potential in the rabbit ventricular model at a CI of 145 ms. Mechanical stimulation results in re-entry. Time is counted since the onset of the impact and is denoted by the numbers above each image with 'impact' referring to the trans-membrane potential distribution at the end of impact. The smaller images are semi-transparent renditions of the trans-membrane potential distribution in the ventricular volume, and represent anterior, basal or side views of the ventricles; they refer to the CI shown in the image to their left. In the semi-transparent images, the propagating wavefront is shown as a white surface. White arrows in 20, 80 and 150 ms panels indicate direction of propagation. **D** Schematic representation of trans-membrane potential distribution in and around the impact zone prior to mechanical stimulation. [Reproduced, with permission, from Li W, Kohl P, Trayanova N (2004) Induction of ventricular arrhythmias following mechanical impact: a simulation study in 3D. *J Mol Histol* **35**:679–686.] (See color plate section.)

examples of mechanical impact that did not induce re-entry. The coupling intervals are before and after the vulnerable window. At the time of impact in Fig. 36.2A, the tissue within and around the impact zone was largely refractory; the impact did not, therefore, trigger an ectopic AP. Mechanical impact also failed to induce re-entry in Fig. 36.2B; however, an ectopic focus of excitation was elicited in a large proportion of the impact region, forming a figure-of-eight re-entry pattern, but not giving rise to sustained re-entry. Figure 36.2C presents a case of mechanically induced sustained re-entry within the vulnerable window. The 50 ms panel depicts the ventricles at the end of the first re-entrant cycle, when the ectopic wavefront was entering the region of impact. The activation still managed to propagate through the original zone of impact. The second cycle of the re-entry started in the epicardial layers of the LV and then continued mostly as a figure-of-eight re-entrant circuit, later deteriorating into VF.

Figure 36.2D is a schematic representation of the transmembrane potential distribution in and around the impact zone at the time of mechanical stimulation; it is presented here to provide a mechanistic explanation of the observed phenomena. The propagating wavefront has travelled from bottom to top, and the wave tail is near the middle of the tissue [equivalent to the electrocardiogram (ECG) T-wave]. The circle represents a projection of the impact profile on the epicardial surface. Three different types of responses can be induced within the region of impact. Where the circle overlaps with zone 1, the APD in mechanically stimulated tissue is shortened. Where circle and zone 2 overlap, APD is prolonged. In the mechanically stimulated tissue of zone 3, a new AP is elicited. Both the size of the impact region and its location relative to the trailing repolarization wave determine which responses will be induced by a mechanical stimulus. In Fig. 36.2A, mechanical stimulation occurs at a coupling interval prior to the onset of the vulnerable window. The trailing end of the repolarization wave would, at that point in time, be located closer to the bottom of the scheme in Fig. 36.2D, so that only zone 1, or zones 1 and 2, would appear inside the circle depicting the impact area. In the corresponding simulation (Fig. 36.2A), the impact failed to initiate a new AP. For a coupling interval past the vulnerable window, such as shown in Fig. 36.2B, the trailing wave would have moved further up towards the top and only zones 2 and 3, or zone 3 alone, would appear in the circle representing the impact site. In the corresponding simulation (Fig. 36.2B), AP was elicited by the mechanical stimulus, but the ectopic excitation propagated towards the region of lengthened APD (zone 2, located at the top of the impact region) where propagation was blocked. In the case presented in Fig. 36.2C, all three zones were present inside the impact area. A new wavefront was initiated at the lower portion of the impact region. The wavefront propagated slower than the one elicited by the impact in Fig. 36.2B since mechanical stimulation took place earlier and the ventricles had not completely recovered from the preceding paced beat. On the return pathway, upon reaching the original region of impact, the propagating wavefront encountered first a fully recovered tissue (zone 1; APD was shortened there). The next zone on the way of the re-entering wavefront was zone 2 where APD was extended. However, in contrast to Fig. 36.2B, the tissue had already recovered from the impact by the time the ectopic wavefront arrived at zone 2; the activation successfully traversed the original region of impact and arrhythmia was established.

Despite the simplified representation of the mechanical impact, the study of Li et al.[16] uncovered important mechanisms by which mechanical impact in *Commotio cordis* leads to the establishment of ventricular arrhythmias in a narrow time interval during the T-wave.

Modelling the termination of VT by precordial thump

As an arrhythmia can be initiated by a mechanical impact, it can also be terminated by it. An early study by Bierfeld et al.[30] suggested that the mechanism of mechanical conversion of VT or VF into sinus rhythm might be that the mechanical stimulus interrupted re-entrant pathways or depressed ectopic foci, thus allowing the normal sinoatrial rhythm to emerge. The goal of a simulation study by Li et al.[17] was to elucidate the mechanisms for termination of an arrhythmia by precordial thump (PT) under normal and ischaemic conditions and to determine the reasons for the decreased efficacy of PT in ischaemia. The study hypothesized that one manifestation of SAC_K could be the ATP-sensitive K+ channels (K_{ATP}); reduction in ATP content under ischaemic conditions sensitizes this channel to mechanical stimulation[31,32]. Using the same purely electrophysiological model of the whole heart as in the previous section, the study delivered PT to different cases of VT to examine how SAC activation interacts with the 3D pre-thump scroll wavefronts in the normoxic and ischaemic ventricles and to identify the determinants of PT success rate. PT was assumed to cause activation of SAC current in the right ventricular (RV) free wall and the septum only; indeed, research has demonstrated that since PT is administered directly to the chest, it causes an increase mostly in RV pressure[33]. The timing of PT delivery was chosen randomly within the re-entrant cycle of a given VT.

In accordance with the hypothesis proposed by Kohl et al.[34], the simulation results demonstrated that the increased mechano-sensitivity of the K_{ATP} channels in ischaemia lowers PT efficacy: in the normoxic heart, PT succeeds in terminating VT with a rate of 60%, while success decreased to 30% in ischaemia. As shown in Fig. 36.3A, PT succeeded in terminating VT in the normal heart following an extra beat. PT caused excited tissue in the RV to repolarize, while RV tissue at rest became depolarized. Therefore, propagation of the pre-thump wavefronts was blocked in the RV; propagation proceeded through the LV, resulting in VT termination. Figure 36.3B and C display post-thump activity under ischaemic conditions. Both PT failed to terminate VT; however, the established post-thump re-entries were different from each other and from the pre-thump one. As illustrated in Fig. 36.3B, PT under mild ischaemic conditions, which recruited a mechano-sensitive outward current of reversal potential −45 mV, depolarized resting tissue. Repolarization of excited cells was much greater than in normoxia (5 ms panel). The immediate post-thump activity (35 ms panel) gave rise to a new re-entrant circuit (see schematic, red arrow). Figure 36.3C presents post-thump activity in the case of increased degree of ischaemia severity (ischaemia case 2), where PT caused a mechano-sensitive current of −65 mV reversal potential. The increased contribution of ATP-dependent potassium current ($I_{K,ATP}$) greatly repolarized excited tissue in the RV (5 ms panel). Post-thump activity originated from undisturbed excitation in the LV (10 and 35 ms panels), which invaded the repolarized RV.

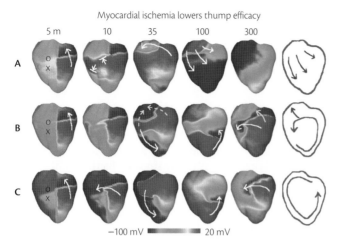

Myocardial ischemia lowers thump efficacy

Fig. 36.3 Evolution of post-impact trans-membrane potential distribution on the epicardial surface (anterior view) in a simulation of rabbit ventricles under normal (**A**) and ischaemic (**B**, **C**) conditions. In all cases, the pre-impact ventricles were in VT. Time, counted from impact onset, is shown above each column. Right-most images are schematics of post-impact electrical activity with re-entrant patterns shown in red. The beginning of each red line marks the location of unidirectional block that led to the establishment of the corresponding post-thump re-entry; its arrow indicates the direction of rotation. Grey arrows show direction of propagation of post-impact wavefronts that did not lead to establishment of re-entry. Colour scale as in Fig. 36.2. [Reproduced, with permission, from Li W, Kohl P, Trayanova N (2006) Myocardial ischemia lowers precordial thump efficacy: an inquiry into mechanisms using three-dimensional simulations. *Heart Rhythm* **3**:179–186.] (See color plate section.)

A new re-entrant circuit was established that encompassed the entire ventricles. Similar observations regarding reduced PT efficacy under ischaemic conditions were found in a 2D sheet study by Kohl *et al.*[35].

The simulation studies presented in the last two sections of this chapter employed purely electrophysiological models, representing mechanical stimuli via their effect on SAC. In the two sections below, coupled electromechanical models were used to examine the contribution of MEC in arrhythmias and defibrillation.

Role of mechano-electric coupling in the decay of VT into VF

The non-uniform distribution of positive myofibre strain (stretching) during mechanical contraction could potentially, via SAC, produce dispersion in electrophysiological properties, which might result in the degradation of VT into VF. The study by Panfilov *et al.*[19] demonstrated, in a 2D electromechanical model, that recruitment of SAC could induce spiral wave breakup. The simulation study of Hu *et al.*[36] examined the role of MEC in the transition from VT to VF in the rabbit heart model using an electromechanical model, consisting of coupled electrical and mechanical components. Tissue depolarization in the electrical component triggered the generation of active tension in the mechanical component, which led to ventricular deformation. The positive fibre strain from mechanical deformation determined the magnitude of the current through SAC.

In the trans-membrane potential map in Fig. 36.4A, spiral wave breakup occurred near the LV–RV border on the posterior wall,

which was further confirmed by the formation of phase singularities there. In the corresponding SAC activation site map (map of positive fibre strain), non-uniform distribution of SAC activation sites on the epicardial surface was observed. Two nodes were selected so that their fibre strain, SAC currents and voltage traces could be compared. Fibre strain at node 1 oscillated between 0.2 and 0.35, whereas the fibre strain at node 2 never exceeded 0 (Fig. 36.4B). As a result of the high positive strain, there was a large SAC current at node 1 (Fig. 36.4C), whereas SAC at node 2 was never activated (Fig. 36.4A). When the myocyte at node 1 was repolarizing, there was a significant inward current through SAC that caused elevation of resting potential from −85 to −60 mV and consequently Na⁺ channel inactivation, which did not occur at node 2 (Fig. 36.4D). In addition, SAC currents also caused extended refractoriness at node 1, which again did not occur at node 2 (Fig. 36.4D). The above analysis demonstrates that the heterogeneity in strain gives rise to a dispersion of electrophysiological properties, such as elevated resting potential and extended refractoriness at various locations, which leads to spiral wave breakup.

The authors also hypothesized that the pro-arrhythmic effect of SAC could be further exacerbated by the haemodynamic changes resulting from the arrhythmia itself. Diminished contractile function of the LV during arrhythmia results in a shift of blood volume to the venous side of the circulatory system, which, in turn, increases end-diastolic RV pressure and volume[37]. The resultant RV dilation could give rise to a gradient of refractoriness between LV and RV through SAC, which could further increase heterogeneity in electrophysiological properties and therefore conceivably exacerbate the deterioration of VT into VF.

Figure 36.5 presents in detail how RV dilation affects the degeneration of VT to VF. Epicardial trans-membrane potential distribution maps for the LV and RV are shown in the top and middle panels. Two scroll waves existed initially in LV and RV. The scroll wave in the LV lasted throughout 3 s of observation (top panels), whereas the one in RV remained stable for only 0.5 s (middle panel: 468 ms) and after that broke up into multiple waves (middle panels: 1,217, 1,797 and 3,259 ms). This is further demonstrated by the spatiotemporal behaviour of the filaments, the 3D organizing centres of re-entrant activity (bottom panels). Initially there was only one filament in the LV lateral wall and another in the RV lateral wall (bottom panel: 468 ms). However, after 0.5 s following re-entry induction, there were multiple filaments formed in the RV, while still only one filament existed in the LV lateral wall (bottom panels: 1,217, 1,797 and 3,259 ms).

This is the first study in which a fully coupled electromechanical model of the whole heart was used to study the dynamical mechanisms by which MEC contributed to the degradation of VT into VF [for simulations of the role of MEC in the generation of premature ventricular contractions under the conditions of acute regional ischaemia, see Chapter 49; the simulation study by Jie *et al.* is reference[38]].

Abnormal mechanical deformation and its role in vulnerability to electric shocks and defibrillation

Clinical studies have demonstrated that patients with dilated, volume or pressure overloaded hearts have elevated defibrillation

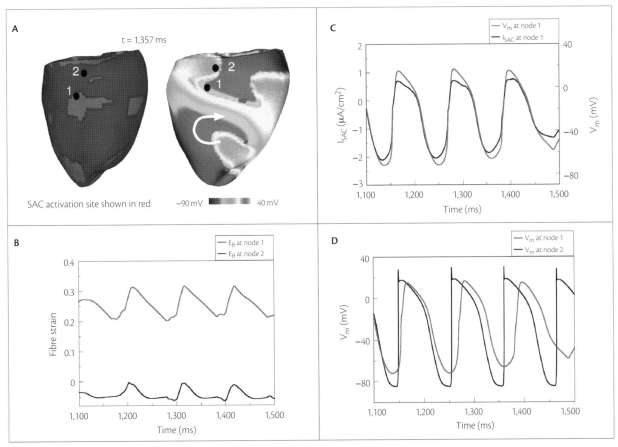

Fig. 36.4 Role of SAC in the transition from VT to VF. **A** SAC activation sites and trans-membrane potential distribution maps on the posterior epicardium at $t = 1{,}357$ ms from the onset of VT. The white arrow shows the direction of spiral wave rotation. Two nodes, marked 1 and 2, denote the locations at which the current, voltage and strain traces were taken from. **B** Fibre strain at nodes 1 and 2. **C** Stretch-activated current and trans-membrane potential at node 1. **D** Trans-membrane potentials at nodes 1 and 2. (See color plate section.)

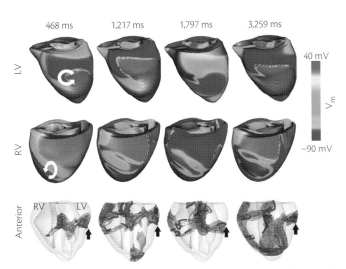

Fig. 36.5 Epicardial trans-membrane potential distribution maps on the LV (top) and RV (middle). The white arrows denote the direction of wave propagation. Anterior semi-transparent view of the ventricles (bottom) showing the filament distribution (blue) and the activation wavefronts (red). Small black arrows indicate the filament of the stable spiral wave on LV. $t = 0$ ms corresponds to the instant at which re-entry was induced. (See color plate section.)

thresholds (DFT). The mechanisms underlying this are not well understood (see Chapter 52). Here, we present simulations of vulnerability to strong shocks and defibrillation under the conditions of LV dilation, and present the mechanisms by which mechanical deformation may lead to increased vulnerability and elevated DFT.

Ventricular geometry and fibre orientation determine the large-scale distribution and magnitude of the virtual electrode polarization (VEP) induced by a strong shock[39–41]. Thus, ventricular dilation may affect VEP through changes in ventricular geometry and fibre architecture, leading to changes in the upper limit of vulnerability and DFT. A simulation study by Gurev *et al.*[42] tested this hypothesis using the rabbit ventricular electromechanics model described in the previous section. Short-axis views of the undeformed and of the dilated rabbit ventricles from this study are presented in Fig. 36.6. The figure shows that LV dilatation leads to a rounded LV chamber short-axis contour and decreased thickness of the LV wall and septum. Note that the most prominent change in fibre orientation in the dilated ventricles occurs in the septum.

To investigate the effect of LV dilation on the vulnerability to electrical shocks, the shock was applied at different timings after the last pacing stimulus. Monophasic truncated-exponential shocks of 10 ms duration were given through plate electrodes, as in the

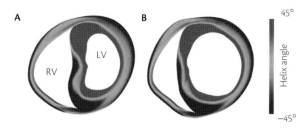

Fig. 36.6 Short axis view of ventricular geometry and fibre helix angle for the undeformed (**A**) and the dilated (**B**) ventricles. The most prominent changes are seen in the septum. (See color plate section.)

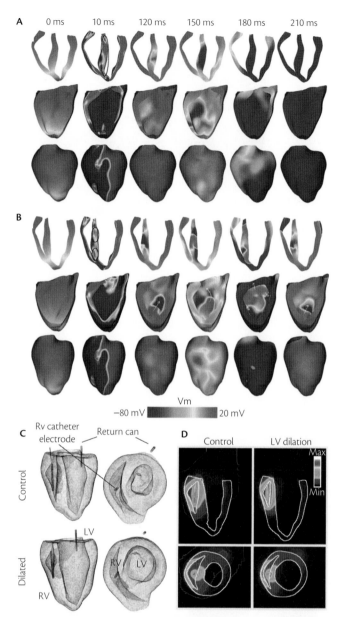

Fig. 36.7 Distributions of trans-membrane potential in: a ventricular long axis cross-section view; a view towards the septum with the RV free wall removed; and an epicardial view at shock end (0 ms) and for post-shock activation at 10, 120, 150, 180 and 210 ms in the undeformed (**A**) and dilated (**B**) ventricles. **C** Ventricular geometry of the control (top) and dilated ventricles (bottom) with ICD-like electrode configuration in anterior (left) and basal (right) views. RV catheter (red) was inserted into the RV cavity and the active can (blue) was positioned in the bath near the posterior LV wall. **D** Distribution of electrical field magnitude in the control and dilated ventricles. (See color plate section.)

study by Ashihara *et al.*[43] This electrode configuration results in a uniform electrical field; thus VEP formation depends only on ventricular geometry and fibre orientation. Trans-membrane voltage maps following shock application at a 120 ms coupling interval are shown in Fig. 36.7A,B. At the end of the shock (Fig. 36.7: 10 ms), no significant differences in VEP were detected at the surface of the ventricles. However, in the bulk of the myocardium the polarization was different in the septal region marked by black ovals. There was a larger excitable gap in the septum of the deformed ventricles following the shock. Consequently, while no re-entrant activity was observed in the undeformed ventricles, a sustained re-entry was formed on the RV side of the septum in the deformed ventricles. The re-entry had a figure-of-eight pattern (Fig. 36.7B: 120, 150 and 180 ms) and its circuit remained fully intramural until the activation made a breakthrough on the anterior (Fig. 36.7B; 180 ms) and posterior (not shown) epicardial surfaces.

The most pronounced difference in VEP took place in the ventricular septum, which was not accidental. Rabbit ventricular geometry is associated with larger changes of fibre direction at the septum as compared to the LV and RV walls. Therefore, even small mechanical deformations have large impact on fibre architecture at the septum. This finding suggests that not just the ventricular geometry but rather the rearrangement of fibre architecture in the deformed ventricles underlies the increased vulnerability upon dilatation of the rabbit LV ventricle.

The simulations found that LV dilation resulted in increase in the upper limit of vulnerability by 11%. Although this increase is significant, it is less than that reported in experimental studies[44,45]; this discrepancy could result from the choice of uniform electric field. Therefore, Gurev *et al.*[42] conducted additional simulations with an implantable cardioverter-defibrillator (ICD) electrode configuration (Fig. 36.7C), and modelled defibrillation rather than vulnerability. Fibrillation in the rabbit model was induced by a cross-field stimulation protocol. DFT was determined as described previously[46].

DFT in the dilated ventricles was found to be 38 ± 20% (581 vs 802 ± 52 V) higher than that in the normal ventricles, which was in good agreement with experimental findings. This result showed that the change in the electric field in the dilated ventricles, as compared to the normal ventricles, also played a major role in decreased defibrillation efficacy. The electrical field magnitude in the two cases is shown in Fig. 36.7D. The regions characterized with a weak electrical field are located at the LV apex and the anteriolateral LV wall in both the normal and the dilated ventricles; these regions have weaker field magnitudes in the dilated ventricles. These are also the locations where post-shock phase singularities formed after a near-DFT failed shock. Due to the dilation, the LV wall moved away from the electrodes, decreasing the electric field there, which in turn lowered the magnitude of VEP and allowed the re-entrant circuits to survive.

In conclusion, the changes in ventricular geometry and fibre orientation following dilation explain the reduced defibrillation efficacy in the dilated heart.

Conclusions and outlook

This chapter presents the use of advanced computer simulations to uncover the mechanisms by which MEC may contribute to the generation, maintenance and acceleration of ventricular arrhythmias, as well as in the mechanisms for ventricular vulnerability to electric shocks and defibrillation. The studies presented here demonstrate the power of computer models and simulations to probe mechanisms where experimentation, due to limitations in experimental techniques, fails to do so. From the chronological exposition of the studies in this chapter it is clear that models of MEC have undergone major development. They have moved from the realm of the purely electrophysiological models, which represent MEC via the opening of SAC at pre-assigned locations, to sophisticated models of coupled electro-mechanics, where mechanical deformation can exert a multitude of stretch-related effects.

Simulations of cardiac arrhythmias will increasingly become multi-physics, representing the consequences of not only soft tissue mechanics but also fluid dynamics to cardiac electrophysiological behaviours. To fully represent the role of MEC, heart models of the future will need to also incorporate, in a comprehensive manner, the relationship between structure and function at the various levels of structural complexity in the heart, allowing us to model various disease conditions. Multi-physics models that incorporate electrophysiological and structural remodelling in cardiac disease will serve as the first line of screening of new anti-arrhythmia therapies and approaches, including pharmacological interventions, and will provide new approaches to patient screening and diagnosis. As imaging modalities are becoming more prevalent in patient evaluation, a wealth of patient-specific cardiac structural and functional data are rapidly becoming available. Today, we stand at the threshold of a new era in cardiac modelling and simulation: anatomically detailed, tomographically reconstructed models of the heart and even the whole body are beginning to be developed that have the potential to integrate patient-specific information from the ion channel to the electromechanical interactions in the intact heart. The use of models in tailor-made diagnosis, treatment planning and prevention of sudden cardiac death will ultimately become a reality in the integrated healthcare of tomorrow.

References

1. Kohl P, Hunter P, Noble D. Stretch-induced changes in heart rate and rhythm: clinical observations, experiments and mathematical models. *Prog Biophys Mol Biol* 1999;**71**:91–138.
2. Hu H, Sachs F. Stretch-activated ion channels in the heart. *J Mol Cell Cardiol* 1997;**29**:1511–1523.
3. Xie LH, Sato D, Garfinkel A, Qu Z, Weiss JN. Intracellular Ca alternans: coordinated regulation by sarcoplasmic reticulum release, uptake, and leak. *Biophys J* 2008;**95**:3100–3110.
4. Gaudesius G, Miragoli M, Thomas SP, Rohr S. Coupling of cardiac electrical activity over extended distances by fibroblasts of cardiac origin. *Circ Res* 2003;**93**:421–428.
5. Pedrotty DM, Klinger RY, Kirkton RD, Bursac N. Cardiac fibroblast paracrine factors alter impulse conduction and ion channel expression of neonatal rat cardiomyocytes. *Cardiovasc Res* 2009;**83**:688–697.
6. Miragoli M, Gaudesius G, Rohr S. Electrotonic modulation of cardiac impulse conduction by myofibroblasts. *Circ Res* 2006;**98**: 801–810.
7. Rohr S. Myofibroblasts in diseased hearts: new players in cardiac arrhythmias? *Heart Rhythm* 2009;**6**:848–856.
8. Akar FG, Laurita KR, Rosenbaum DS. Cellular basis for dispersion of repolarization underlying reentrant arrhythmias. *J Electrocardiol* 2000;**33**(Suppl):23–31.
9. Kuo CS, Munakata K, Reddy CP, Surawicz B. Characteristics and possible mechanism of ventricular arrhythmia dependent on the dispersion of action potential durations. *Circulation* 1983;**67**: 1356–1367.
10. Zabel M, Koller BS, Sachs F, Franz MR. Stretch-induced voltage changes in the isolated beating heart: importance of the timing of stretch and implications for stretch-activated ion channels. *Cardiovasc Res* 1996;**32**:120–130.
11. Efimov IR, Nikolski VP, Salama G. Optical imaging of the heart. *Circ Res* 2004;**95**:21–33.
12. Docherty RJ. Gadolinium selectively blocks a component of calcium current in rodent neuroblastoma x glioma hybrid (NG108-15) cells. *J Physiol* 1988;**398**:33–47.
13. Lacampagne A, Gannier F, Argibay J, Garnier D, Le Guennec JY. The stretch-activated ion channel blocker gadolinium also blocks L-type calcium channels in isolated ventricular myocytes of the guinea-pig. *Biochim Biophys Acta* 1994;**1191**:205–208.
14. Sachs F. Modeling mechanical-electrical transduction in the heart. In: *Cell Mechanics and Cellular Engineering* (eds V.C. Mow, F. Guliak, R. Trays-Son-Tray, R.M. Hochmuth). Springer, New York, 1994, pp. 308–328.
15. Li W, Gurev V, McCulloch AD, Trayanova NA. The role of mechanoelectric feedback in vulnerability to electric shock. *Prog Biophys Mol Biol* 2008;**97**:461–478.
16. Li W, Kohl P, Trayanova N. Induction of ventricular arrhythmias following mechanical impact: a simulation study in 3D. *J Mol Histol* 2004;**35**:679–686.
17. Li W, Kohl P, Trayanova N. Myocardial ischemia lowers precordial thump efficacy: an inquiry into mechanisms using three-dimensional simulations. *Heart Rhythm* 2006;**3**:179–186.
18. Panfilov AV, Keldermann RH, Nash MP. Self-organized pacemakers in a coupled reaction-diffusion-mechanics system. *Phys Rev Lett* 2005;**95**:258104.
19. Panfilov AV, Keldermann RH, Nash MP. Drift and breakup of spiral waves in reaction-diffusion-mechanics systems. *Proc Natl Acad Sci USA* 2007;**104**:7922–7926.
20. Riemer TL, Sobie EA, Tung L. Stretch-induced changes in arrhythmogenesis and excitability in experimentally based heart cell models. *Am J Physiol* 1998;**275**:H431–H442.
21. Riemer TL, Tung L. Stretch-induced excitation and action potential changes of single cardiac cells. *Prog Biophys Mol Biol* 2003;**82**:97–110.
22. Morris CE. Mechanosensitive ion channels. *J Membr Biol* 1990;**113**: 93–107.
23. Li W, Eason JC, Kohl P, Trayanova N. The influence of stretch-activated channels on defibrillation. *Proc Ann Intnl Conf IEEE EMBS* 2002;**2**:1434–1435.
24. Gurev V, Maleckar MM, Trayanova NA. Cardiac defibrillation and the role of mechanoelectric feedback in postshock arrhythmogenesis. *Ann N Y Acad Sci* 2006;**1080**:320–333.
25. Lab M. Transient depolarization and action potential alterations following mechanical changes in isolated myocardium. *Cardiovasc Res* 1980;**14**:624–637.
26. Trayanova N, Li W, Eason J, Kohl P. Effect of stretch-activated channels on defibrillation efficacy. *Heart Rhythm* 2004;**1**:67–77.
27. Garny A, Kohl P. Mechanical induction of arrhythmias during ventricular repolarization: modeling cellular mechanisms and their interaction in two dimensions. *Ann N Y Acad Sci* 2004;**1015**: 133–143.
28. Link MS, Maron BJ, VanderBrink BA, *et al.* Impact directly over the cardiac silhouette is necessary to produce ventricular fibrillation in an experimental model of *Commotio cordis*. *J Am Coll Cardiol* 2001; **37**:649–654.

29. Link MS, Maron BJ, Wang PJ, VanderBrink BA, Zhu W, Estes NA, 3rd. Upper and lower limits of vulnerability to sudden arrhythmic death with chest-wall impact (*Commotio cordis*). *J Am Coll Cardiol* 2003;**41**:99–104.

30. Bierfeld J, Rodriguez-Viera V, Aranda J, Castellanos AJ, Lazzara R, Befeler B. Terminating ventricular fibrillation by chest thump. *Angiology* 1979;**30**:703–707.

31. Van Wagoner DR, Lamorgese M. Ischemia potentiates the mechanosensitive modulation of atrial ATP-sensitive potassium channels. *Ann N Y Acad Sci* 1994;**723**:392–395.

32. Van Wagoner DR. Mechanosensitive gating of atrial ATP-sensitive potassium channels. *Circ Res* 1993;**72**:973–983.

33. Zeh E, Rahner E. The manual extrathoracal stimulation of the heart. Technique and effect of the precordial thump (in German). *Z Kardiol* 1978;**67**:299–304.

34. Kohl P, Nesbitt AD, Cooper PJ, Lei M. Sudden cardiac death by *Commotio cordis*: role of mechano-electric feedback. *Cardiovasc Res* 2001;**50**:280–289.

35. Kohl P, Bollensdorff C, Garny A. Effects of mechanosensitive ion channels on ventricular electrophysiology: experimental and theoretical models. *Exp Physiol* 2006;**91**:307–321.

36. Hu Y, Gurev V, Constantino J, Trayanova N. Roles of mechano-electric feedback and right ventricular dilation in the degeneration of ventricular tachycarida into ventricular fibrillation. *Heart Rhythm* (submitted).

37. Mashiro I, Cohn JN, Heckel R, Nelson RR, Franciosa JA. Left and right ventricular dimensions during ventricular fibrillation in the dog. *Am J Physiol* 1978;**235**:H231–H236.

38. Jie X, Gurev V, Trayanova N. Mechanisms of mechanically-induced spontaneous arrhythmias in acute regional ischemia. *Circ Res* 2010;**106**:185–192.

39. Entcheva E, Trayanova NA, Claydon FJ. Patterns of and mechanisms for shock-induced polarization in the heart: a bidomain analysis. *IEEE Trans Biomed Eng* 1999;**46**:260–270.

40. Rodriguez B, Trayanova NA. Upper limit of vulnerability in a defibrillation model of the rabbit ventricles. *J Electrocardiol* 2003;**36** (Suppl):51–56.

41. Rodriguez B, Li L, Eason J, Efimov I, Trayanova NA. Differences between left and right ventricular chamber geometry affect cardiac vulnerability to electric shocks. *Circ Res* 2005;**97**:168–175.

42. Gurev V, Li W, Constantino J, Hu Y, Trayanova N. Effect of changes in ventricular geometry induced by mechanical deformation on virtual electrode polarization and defibrillation threshold. *Am J Physiol* (submitted).

43. Ashihara T, Constantino J, Trayanova NA. Tunnel propagation of postshock activations as a hypothesis for fibrillation induction and isoelectric window. *Circ Res* 2008;**102**:737–745.

44. Strobel JS, Kay GN, Walcott GP, Smith WM, Ideker RE. Defibrillation efficacy with endocardial electrodes is influenced by reductions in cardiac preload. *J Interv Card Electrophysiol* 1997;**1**:95–102.

45. Ott P, Reiter MJ. Effect of ventricular dilatation on defibrillation threshold in the isolated perfused rabbit heart. *J Cardiovasc Electrophysiol* 1997;**8**:1013–1019.

46. Long Y, Constantino J, Ashihara A, Trayanova N. Tunnel propagation following defibrillation with ICD shocks: hidden postshock activations in the left ventricular wall underlie isoelectric window. *Heart Rhythm* 2010;**7**:953–961.

SECTION 5

Pathophysiology of cardiac mechano-electric coupling: general aspects

37. **Load dependence of ventricular repolarization** *269*
   Peter Taggart and Peter Sutton

38. **Is the U wave in the electrocardiogram a mechano-electrical phenomenon?** *274*
   Rainer Schimpf and Martin Borggrefe

39. **Mechanical modulation of cardiac function: role of the pericardium** *281*
   John V. Tyberg

40. **Mechanically induced electrical remodelling in human atrium** *290*
   Geoffrey Lee, Prashanthan Sanders, Joseph B. Morton and Jonathan M. Kalman

41. **Drug effects and atrial fibrillation: potential and limitations** *298*
   Jurren M. van Opstal, Yuri Blaauw and Harry J.G.M Crijns

42. **Stretch as a mechanism linking short- and long-term electrical remodelling in the ventricles** *305*
   Eugene A. Sosunov, Evgeny P. Anyukhovsky and Michael R. Rosen

43. **Volume and pressure overload and ventricular arrhythmogenesis** *313*
   Michiel J. Janse and Ruben Coronel

44. **Stretch effects on fibrillation dynamics** *318*
   Masatoshi Yamazaki and Jérôme Kalifa

Load dependence of ventricular repolarization

Peter Taggart and Peter Sutton

Background

It is now established that mechanical stress/strain within the heart alters the electrophysiology and influences the behaviour of the electrical wavefronts in the heart during the cardiac cycle. Alteration in the volume within the cardiac chambers, the atria and ventricles alters the degree of stretch on the cardiac fibres. This has been shown to affect the timing of electrical recovery, i.e. repolarization, following activation in a wide variety of laboratory models and humans. The time of repolarization at a given location within the heart is a function of the time for the activation wavefront to reach that site plus action potential duration (APD) at that site. Changes in mechanical loading have been shown to exert either relatively little or no effect on the speed of conduction in the heart[1–4] but to alter APD. Thus the effect of altered load on repolarization is mainly if not entirely due to effects on APD.

Laboratory models

Following activation, cardiac muscle cells cannot usually be re-excited until sufficient time has elapsed for the recovery of membrane currents and voltage changes to resting conditions. This period of inexcitability is termed the effective refractory period (ERP). Under normal circumstances ERP approximates to the APD. The overall result of experiments investigating the effect of increased ventricular volume loading has been a shortening of APD and ERP (Fig. 37.1). For example, it has been shown in isolated canine ventricles contracting isovolumically that increased preload shortened ERP[5,6] (Fig. 37.2). In isolated rabbit heart an increase in left ventricular volume resulted in shortening of the ERP on the left ventricular epicardium[1,7]. Studies also in isolated rabbit hearts showed a shortening of both APD and ERP during left ventricular volume increase[2]. Similar results have been obtained in whole animals[6,8,9]. In general these studies have demonstrated that increased load shortens APD and refractoriness. It has been shown that these effects do not depend on circulating catecholamines, autonomic reflexes or acute ischaemia[1].

Studies in humans

Several studies have recorded monophasic action potentials (MAP) as a measure of APD in humans during changes in ventricular pressure and/or volume. In a study by Levine and colleagues, MAP recordings were obtained from the right ventricle in patients undergoing balloon valvuloplasty for congenital pulmonary stenosis[10]. In this condition the narrowed pulmonary valve orifice creates obstruction to right ventricular outflow resulting in a chronic increase in intracavity pressure and volume. Relieving the obstruction resulted in lengthening of the right ventricular MAP duration coincident with a fall in intracavity pressure and volume. The QT interval of the electrocardiogram (ECG) which reflects APD prolonged in parallel with the MAP duration prolongation. Subsequent reversal of conditions by transient occlusion of the right ventricular outflow tract with the balloon catheter resulted in a rise in intracavity pressure and shortening of MAP duration and QT interval[10]. Thus these studies demonstrated that decreasing intracavity pressure/volume (i.e. decreasing stretch) lengthened APD and vice versa.

Another study used the haemodynamic changes during the process of initiating and discontinuing cardiopulmonary bypass in patients undergoing cardiac surgery as a 'model' for studying load changes in humans. Venous blood flow returning to the heart is interrupted and siphoned from a canula placed in the right atrium to a pump/oxygenator. Oxygenated blood is then retuned to the circulation through a canula in the ascending aorta, thereby bypassing the

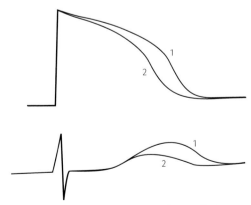

Fig. 37.1 Diagrammatic illustration of the effect of volume loading on APD and the QT interval of the ECG. Increased loading shortens APD and the QT interval from control (1) to the loaded state (2).

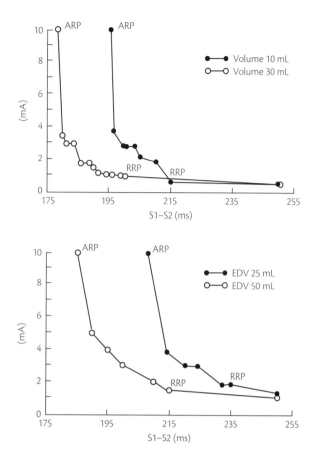

Fig. 37.2 Effect of volume loading on the ERP in the canine left ventricle. In the isovolumic beating heart increased volume loading from 10 to 30 mL shortened ERP, shifting the strength interval relation to the left (top panel). A similar effect was obtained in the ejecting heart in response to increasing volume load from 25 to 50 mL (bottom panel). S1–S2, interval between 'first' and 'second' stimulus; RRP, relative refractory period; EDV, end-diastolic volume. [Reproduced, with permission, from Lerman BB, Burkhoff D, Yue DT, Sagawa K (1985) Mechanoelectrical feedback: independent role of preload and contractility in modulation of canine ventricular excitability. *J Clin Invest* **76**:1843–1850.]

heart and lungs. Under these conditions the ventricles are unloaded, partly empty and not supporting the circulation. When the coronary artery grafts are completed the circulation is restored to normal and bypass is discontinued progressively over a period of 30–40 s. During this phase the ventricles fill, ventricular pressures rise and the heart is converted from a non-working state to a working heart supporting the circulation. MAP recordings from the left ventricular epicardium during this phase of reloading showed APD shortening as left ventricular pressure and volume increased (Fig. 37.3)[11].

It is not uncommon for patients undergoing cardiopulmonary bypass surgery to receive infusions of 100 – 200 mL administered as a bolus over 10–15 s in order to rectify the haemodynamic appearance of the heart. The increase in circulating volume as a result of the bolus infusion is accompanied by an increase in ventricular loading. In the same study, increasing the volume load by bolus infusions resulted in a progressive increase in radial artery pressure and shortening of APD[11].

Beat to beat changes in response to altered loading have been studied in animal models by recording MAP or ERP from the left ventricular epicardium and transiently occluding the ascending aorta, thereby preventing outflow from the left ventricle[6,8,9,12,13]. This technique was adapted for patients undergoing cardiac surgery such that the ascending aorta was occluded abruptly during diastole and maintained for between one and three beats[14]. The first occluded beat, i.e. non-ejecting, was therefore purely afterloaded. The subsequent occluded beats were both preloaded and afterloaded due to the combination of being non-ejecting with the addition of diastolic filling. Aortic occlusion resulted in increase in left ventricular pressure and APD shortening (Fig. 37.4). The majority of the effect was observed on the first occluded beat, i.e. in response to afterload. The effect of abrupt load change on APD was fully reversible on release of the aortic occlusion and reproducible when the occlusion was repeated.

Overall effect: added complexity

Although the overall effect of the studies reported above is for stretch to shorten APD and ERP, stretch may also lengthen APD. *In vitro* studies have shown that stretch occurring early during the course of action potential repolarization shortens APD, whereas stretch occurring late in the repolarization phase prolongs APD[15]. Thus stretch may shorten or lengthen APD depending on the timing. Several studies *in vivo* in animal and human hearts have demonstrated depolarizations in the late repolarization phase, resembling early after-depolarizations (EAD), which result in APD lengthening. It is possible that the type of stretch, including the abruptness and rapidity, as well as the timing may influence the development of after-depolarizations.

Regional heterogeneity

Most of the foregoing studies have measured APD or refractoriness at a single site. Information on the spatial characteristics of ventricular loading on APD in humans is awaited. Measurements of ERP at several sites on left ventricular epicardium in an isolated rabbit heart model showed that an increase in left ventricular volume decreased refractoriness in a markedly heterogeneous manner[1]. In the *in situ* pig heart a 33% increase in systolic pressure was achieved by aortic cross-clamping. This was accompanied by a reduction in ERP, with a greater change at the apex compared to the base[12]. In another isolated rabbit heart model up to six MAP were recorded from the left ventricular epicardium. During a sustained increase in left ventricular volume APD and ERP shortened inhomogeneously[2].

Interaction with cycle length

The effect of load on APD is cycle length-dependent. Information on the effects of ventricular loading on the cycle length dependence of APD in humans is also awaited. In a study in pigs epicardial MAP were recorded. The APD of a premature beat is dependent on the length of time elapsed following the preceding AP. During steady-state pacing test, pulses with progressively shorter interbeat intervals were introduced. Under control conditions APD of the test beats decreased monotonically as the interbeat interval was shortened. When each test beat was loaded by transient aortic

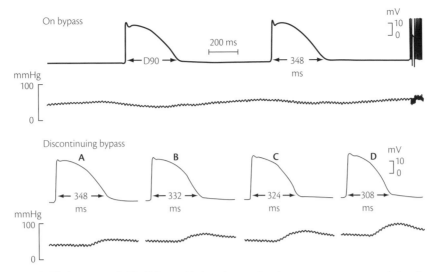

Fig. 37.3 Effect of change from an underfilled to a normally filled left ventricle in patients undergoing coronary artery surgery during discontinuing cardiopulmonary bypass. Top: ventricular epicardial MAP with radial artery pressure during bypass showing stable MAP and the slow sine wave of the pump pressure. Bottom: progressive increase in radial artery pressure as bypass is discontinued and ventricular pressure and volume are restored, accompanied by a progressive shortening of MAP duration (A to D). [Reproduced, with permission, from Taggart P, Sutton PMI, Treasure T, *et al.* (1988) Monophasic action potentials at discontinuation of cardiopulmonary bypass: evidence for contraction–excitation feedback in man. *Circulation* **77**:1266–1275.]

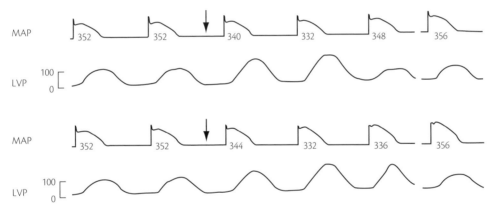

Fig. 37.4 Effect of an abrupt increase in left ventricular loading in patients undergoing coronary artery surgery. Left ventricular epicardial MAP and direct left ventricular pressures (LVP) were recorded during transient occlusion of the ascending aorta for between 1 and 3 beats. Two consecutive occlusions are shown. Arrows mark the onset of occlusion which was accompanied by an increase in LVP and shortening of MAP duration. The effect was similar for both occlusions. [Reproduced, with permission, from Taggart P, Sutton P, Lab M, Runnalls ME, O'Brien W, Treasure T (1992) Effect of abrupt changes in ventricular loading on repolarisation induced by transient aortic occlusion in man. *Am J Physiol* **263**:H816–H823.]

occlusion APD at the long interbeat intervals was shortened and APD at the short interbeat intervals was lengthened. In addition the maximum slope of the curve relating APD to the preceding interval, referred to as the restitution curve, was steepened by 32 ms/100 ms[16].

In an isolated rabbit heart model, balloon dilatation of the left ventricle increased the normal cycle length-dependent shortening of refractoriness at rapid rates[3]. For example, at a steady-state pacing cycle length of 1,000 ms an increase in left ventricular volume of 1.0 mL shortened the ERP by 1.0%, whereas at a basic drive cycle length of 250 ms the same 1.0 mL left ventricular volume increase shortened the ERP by 21% (Fig. 37.5).

The atrium

Mechano-electric coupling (MEC) has been demonstrated in the atrium in both animal models and humans. An increase in atrial pressure in an isolated rabbit heart model decreased atrial ERP and MAP duration[17]. However, a study in canines found that an increase in atrial pressure was associated with an increase in atrial ERP[18]. In isolated guinea-pig hearts atrial stretch was shown to shorten APD at 50% repolarization and to lengthen APD at 90% repolarization due to the development of EAD[19].

In humans it has been shown that very short or very long atrio-ventricular (AV) coupling intervals were associated with an increase in atrial pressure, atrial size and an *increase* in atrial ERP[20].

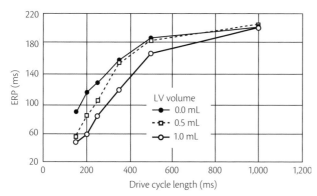

Fig. 37.5 Cycle length dependence of the influence of ventricular loading on refractoriness. In an isolated rabbit heart preparation, increasing left ventricular volume shortened ERP. This effect was more pronounced at shorter basic cycle lengths. [Reproduced, with permission, from Reiter MJ, Landers M, Zetelaki Z, Kirchhof CJ, Allessie MA (1997) Electrophysiologic effects of acute dilatation in the isolated rabbit heart: cycle length-dependent effects on epicardial refractoriness and conduction velocity. *Circulation* **96**:4050–4056.]

Proarrhythmic effect of altered loading

There is little doubt that increased loading is potentially proarrhythmic. In isolated hearts a transient stretch in diastole produced by volume loading pulses may induce a depolarization which, if it attains sufficient amplitude, may initiate an AP. As these diastolic depolarizations do not impinge on repolarization they are discussed elsewhere in this book. Transient stretch during the AP may result in depolarization during the repolarization phase resembling an EAD (Fig. 37.6). Again, if these attain sufficient amplitude they

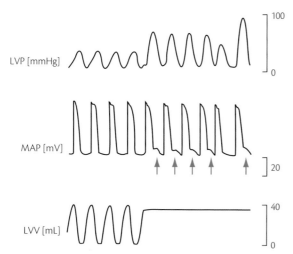

Fig. 37.6 Transient dilatation or stretch may induce depolarizations during repolarization of the AP resembling 'early after-depolarizations' (EAD). An example is shown in an *in situ* canine heart preparation during transient aortic occlusion. During occlusion left ventricular pressure rises abruptly (top trace). The MAP trace (bottom) shows the development of depolarizations occurring late in the repolarization phase (arrows). LVP, left ventricular pressure; LVV, left ventricular volume. [Reproduced, with permission, from Franz MR, Burkhoff D, Yue DT, Sagawa K (1989) Mechanically induced action potential changes and arrhythmia in isolated and *in situ* canine hearts. *Cardiovasc Res* **23**:213–223.]

may give rise to an AP. The majority of such observations have been made using MAP recordings and as a result these EAD-like deflections have been treated with some reservations on account of the susceptibility of MAP recordings to artefact. However, their reproducibility and association with premature ventricular contractions make it highly likely that at least in the majority of cases they do truly represent EAD. Several studies have provided convincing evidence for stretch-induced EAD generating single or repetitive AP; e.g. using transient occlusion of the ascending aorta to produce abrupt stretch in *in situ* canine hearts[6], *in situ* pig hearts[21] and in humans[14] and during occlusion of the right ventricular outflow tract in humans during pulmonary valvuloplasty[10].

Sustained stretch increased the inducibility of ventricular tachycardia (VT) and fibrillation (VF) in isolated rabbit hearts[1,22] and in isolated blood-perfused canine ventricles[23]. Left ventricular dilatation in isolated rabbit hearts decreases the fibrillation threshold[24].

Pathological hearts

There is evidence to suggest that the arrhythmogenic potential of MEC may be enhanced in pathological hearts. In isolated perfused canine hearts with infarction an increase in ventricular volume resulted in more pronounced shortening of ERP in the region of infarction compared to the non-infarcted area and an increase in inducibility of arrhythmias. It was suggested that the differential stretch between the normal and infarcted regions exerted an inhomogeneous effect on the electrophysiology, resulting in an enhanced dispersion of refractoriness and hence an enhanced susceptibility to arrhythmia[25].

During the ventricular pressure volume changes associated with the Valsalva manoeuvre, patients with regional wall motion abnormality frequently demonstrated changes in MAP duration that were different or even opposite in direction to subjects with normal wall motion[26]. This could be explained by regional differences in stretch forces occurring between normally and abnormally contracting segments. This would be expected to result in an increased heterogeneity of repolarization, which is a well-known substrate for arrhythmia[27].

Ventricular tachycardia is in general more unstable in patients with heart failure and more readily degenerates to ventricular fibrillation[28]. While several possible mechanisms may be involved, one possibility is an effect of MEC resulting from the interaction of ventricular dilatation and tachycardia.

Conclusions and outlook

Experiment and theory suggest that MEC may play a significant role in arrhythmogenesis in humans. As indicated earlier, deflections during repolarization resembling EAD giving rise to one or a series of premature AP in response to increased loading have been demonstrated in several animal models and in humans. Stretch could therefore be a cause of focal tachycardias due to the development of after-depolarizations. Increased loading and stretch have also been shown to shorten APD and ERP, which is well known to facilitate re-entrant arrhythmias. Nevertheless proof that mechanical factors are a direct cause of either focal tachycardias or re-entrant rhythms in patients is still awaited. The not infrequent anecdotal accounts of ventricular arrhythmia on discontinuing cardiopulmonary bypass which is resistant to cardioversion but responds on unloading the heart by re-establishing bypass is worthy of mention. Several therapeutic interventions such as pharmacological unloading and ventricular unloading using a balloon assist device may be associated with a lessening or termination of arrhythmia. However, several other factors may be influenced by these manoeuvres which make it difficult to attribute an antiarrhythmic effect directly to a mechanical action. A major difficulty in this respect is the current lack of a stretch-activated channel blocker suitable for clinical use. The stretch-activated channel blocker gadolinium has been shown to block stretch-induced premature ventricular contractions in the dog, which is promising[29]. It is to be hoped that the development of a non-toxic blocker suitable for clinical use will help to define the role of MEC in arrhythmogenesis in humans and possibly at the same time provide a therapeutic option.

References

1. Reiter MJ, Synhorst DP, Mann DE. Electrophysiologic effects of acute ventricular dilatation in the isolated rabbit heart. *Circ Res* 1988;**62**:554–562.

2. Zabel M, Portnoy S, Franz MR. Effect of sustained load on dispersion of ventricular repolarisation and conduction time in the isolated rabbit heart. *J Cardiovasc Electrophysiol* 1996;**7**:9–16.

3. Reiter MJ, Landers M, Zetelaki Z, Kirchhof CJ, Allessie MA. Electrophysiologic effects of acute dilatation in the isolated rabbit heart: cycle length-dependent effects on epicardial refractoriness and conduction velocity. *Circulation* 1997;**96**:4050–4056.

4. Reiter MJ, Zetelaki Z, Kirchhof CJ, Boersma L, Allessie MA. Interaction of acute ventricular dilatation and d-sotalol during sustained reentrant ventricular tachycardia around a fixed obstacle. *Circulation* 1994;**89**:423–431.

5. Lerman BB, Burkhoff D, Yue DT, Sagawa K. Mechanoelectrical feedback: independent role of preload and contractility in modulation of canine ventricular excitability. *J Clin Invest* 1985;**76**:1843–1850.

6. Franz MR, Burkhoff D, Yue DT, Sagawa K. Mechanically induced action potential changes and arrhythmia in isolated and *in situ* canine hearts. *Cardiovasc Res* 1989;**23**:213–223.

7. Hansen DE. Mechanoelectrical feedback effects of altering preload, afterload, and ventricular shortening. *Am J Physiol* 1993;**264**:H423–H432.

8. Dean JW, Dilly SG, Lab MJ. Increased afterload shortens the absolute refractory period *in situ* ventricle of anaesthetised pig. *J Physiol* 1987;**387**:7P.

9. Benditt DG, Kriett JM, Tobler HG, Gornick CC, Detloff BLS, Anderson RW. Electrophysiological effects of transient aortic occlusion in intact canine hearts. *Am J Physiology* 1985;**249**:H1017–H1023.

10. Levine JH, Guarnieri T, Kadish AH, White RI, Calkins H, Khan JS. Changes in myocardial repolarisation in patients undergoing balloon valvuloplasty for congenital pulmonary stenosis: Evidence for contraction excitation feedback in humans. *Circulation* 1988;**77**:70–77.

11. Taggart P, Sutton PMI, Treasure T, *et al.* Monophasic action potentials at discontinuation of cardiopulmonary bypass: evidence for contraction–excitation feedback in man. *Circulation* 1988;**77**:1266–1275.

12. Dean JW, Lab MJ. Regional changes in ventricular excitability during load manipulation of the *in situ* pig heart. *J Physiol* 1990;**429**:387–400.

13. Tobler HG, Gornick CC, Anderson RW, Benditt DG. Electrophysiology properties of the myocardial infarction border zone: effects of transient aortic occlusion. *Surgery* 1986;**100**:150–156

14. Taggart P, Sutton P, Lab M, Runnalls ME, O'Brien W, Treasure T. Effect of abrupt changes in ventricular loading on repolarisation induced by transient aortic occlusion in man. *Am J Physiol* 1992;**636**:H816–H823.

15. Kohl P, Day K, Noble D. Cellular mechanisms for cardiac mechano-electric feedback in a mathematical model. *Can J Cardiol* 1978;**14**:111–119.

16. Horner SM, Dick DJ, Murphy CF, Lab MJ. Cycle length dependence of the electrophysiological effects of increased load on the myocardium. *Circulation* 1996;**94**:1131–1136.

17. Ravelli F, Allessie MA. Effects of atrial dilatation on refractory period and vulnerability to atrial fibrillation in isolated Langendorff-perfused rabbit heart. *Circulation* 1997;**96**:1686–1695.

18. Kaseda S, Zipes DP. Contraction–excitation feedback in the atria: a cause of changes in refractoriness. *J Am Coll Cardiol* 1988;**11**:1327–1336.

19. Nazir SA, Lab MJ. Mechanoelectric feedback in the atrium of the isolated guinea-pig heart. *Cardiovasc Res* 1996;**32**:112–119.

20. Klein LS, Miles WM, Zipes DP. Effect of atrioventricular interval during pacing or reciprocating tachycardia on atrial size, pressure and refractory period: contraction-excitation feedback in human atrium. *Circulation* 1990;**82**:60–68.

21. Lab MJ. Contribution of mechano-electric coupling to ventricular arrhythmias during reduced perfusion. *Int J Microcirc Clin Exp* 1989;**8**:433–442.

22. Reiter MJ, Mann DE, Williams GR. Interaction of hypokalaemia and ventricular dilatation in isolated rabbit hearts. *Am J Physiol* 1993;**265**:H1544–H1550.

23. Hansen DE, Craig CS, Hondeghem LM. Stretch-induced arrhythmias in the isolated canine ventricle: Evidence for the importance of mechanoelactrical feedback. *Circulation* 1990;**81**:1094–1105.

24. Jalal S, Williams GR, Mann DE, Reiter MJ. Effect of ventricular dilatation on fibrillation thresholds in the isolated rabbit heart. *Am J Physiol* 1992;**263**:H1306–H1310.

25. Calkins H, Maughan WL, Weisman HF, *et al.* Effect of acute volume load on refractoriness and arrhythmia development in isolated chronically infarcted canine hearts. *Circulation* 1989;**79**:687–697.

26. Taggart P, Sutton P, John R, Lab M, Swanton H. Monophasic action potential recordings during acute changes in ventricular loading induced by the Valsalva manoeuvre. *Br Heart J* 1992;**67**:221–229.

27. Kuo CS, Munkata K, Reddy P, Surawicz B. Characteristics and possible mechanisms of ventricular arrhythmia dependant on the dispersion of action potential durations. *Circulation* 1983;**67**:1356–1367.

28. Pratt CM, Eaton T, Francis M, Woolbert S, Mahmarian J, Roberts R, Young JB. The inverse relationship between baseline left ventricular ejection fraction and outcome of antiarrhythmic therapy: A dangerous imbalance in the risk-benefit ratio. *Am Heart J* 1989;**118**:433–440.

29. Hansen DE, Borganelli M, Stacey GP, Taylor LK. Dose-dependent inhibition of stretch-induced arrhythmias by gadolinium in isolated canine ventricles: evidence for a unique mode of antiarrhythmic action. *Circ Res* 1991;**69**:820–831.

Is the U wave in the electrocardiogram a mechano-electrical phenomenon?

Rainer Schimpf and Martin Borggrefe

Background

The existence of the U wave as a distinct wave separated from the T-wave in the electrocardiogram (ECG) was reported by Willem Einthoven in 1906[1]. Lewis and Gilder observed in 1912 that the U wave is present in 75% of all ECG, with an amplitude of approximately 0,1 mV and a duration of 0.16 s[2]. Lewis and Gilder regarded the U wave as an early diastolic event, because they observed that closure of the semilunar valves and the second heart sound coincide with the start of the U wave[2].

Up to now, the small deflection in the ECG was not thought to contribute significant diagnostic information, and the U wave has therefore rarely been included in routine ECG analysis. Recently, investigations using computer simulation, echocardiographic examination and high resolution ECG, together with increased knowledge about the cellular basis of cardiac repolarization, have led to new insights into the genesis of the U wave[3–6].

The characteristics of the U wave

The U wave represents a deflection of the ECG, following the T-wave. The T-wave reflects ventricular repolarization. Termination of the T-wave usually coincides with the closure of the aortic valve and termination of mechanical systole. The U wave follows the T-wave as a separate wave under physiological conditions and begins with the second heart sound, i.e. at the beginning of ventricular relaxation[7].

The morphology of the U wave is predominantly monophasic positive or negative, but can be biphasic. The interval from the end of the T-wave to the U wave measures 90–110 ms[7]. The U wave is usually best seen in the precordial leads, at heart rates between 50 and 100 beats/min, but its timing is identical in all leads. The maximal amplitude of the U wave in leads V2–V3 ranges from 3–24% of the T-wave, and rarely exceeds 0.2 mV in human[8,9].

Unlike the QT interval, the interval from the end of the T-wave to the apex of the U wave is nearly rate independent, regardless of whether rate is decreased (e.g. during atrial fibrillation or following premature ventricular contractions) or increased (e.g. due to digitalis or hypercalcaemia)[10,11]. However, if the QT interval increases by > 100 ms, the U wave is no longer discernible[9]. Thus, the U wave can be difficult to differentiate from the T-wave under pathophysiological conditions such as the long QT syndrome (LQTS) or following administration of class III antiarrhythmic drugs.

Hypotheses for the origin of the U wave

Given its timing during the normal cardiac cycle, the U wave is the only component of the ventricular complex of the ECG that cannot be derived clearly from the ventricular action potential (AP) dynamics. This may explain why there have been many competing hypotheses on the origin of the U wave since the initial description 100 years ago. Controversy persists to the present day as to whether the U wave is a purely electrical or a mechano-electrical phenomenon.

There are three major hypotheses to explain the origin of the U wave:

1) Delayed repolarization of the His-Purkinje system[12].

2) Delayed repolarization of certain regions of the ventricular myocardium such as the papillary muscle or mid-myocardial (M) cells[13].

3) Stretch-induced delayed after-depolarizations, caused by distension of the ventricular wall during diastole (the so-called mechano-electrical hypothesis)[10,14–17].

Hypothesis 1: delayed repolarization of the His-Purkinje system

The first theory, delayed repolarization of the intraventricular conduction system and/or the Purkinje fibres, was introduced by Hoffman and Cranefield in 1960[12]. It was suggested since AP durations in these fibres are the longest for any cells in the heart.

The authors suggested that the surface record of repolarization of the intraventricular conducting system or Purkinje fibre T-wave is represented by the U wave. This conclusion was based on the electrophysiological properties of the Purkinje system as studied by microelectrode techniques. In an experimental canine model, Watanabe conducted a comparison of the AP of Purkinje and ventricular muscle fibres under conditions accentuating the U wave[18]. Trans-membrane potentials of Purkinje fibres and ventricular muscle were simultaneously recorded from canine tissue preparations, and various factors causing prominent U waves such as bradycardia, low potassium concentrations, hypothermia and quinidine were studied. The duration of phase 3 was markedly increased, while the slope of phase 3 was significantly decreased by all of these factors. The difference between Purkinje fibre and ventricular AP duration increased significantly. These comparisons revealed a good temporal correlation between phase 3 repolarization in Purkinje fibres and the electrocardiographic U wave.

Arguments against the His-Purkinje hypothesis include the fact that the involved tissue mass is too small to be recorded on the surface ECG[19]. Moreover, the interval between the end of the T-wave and apex of the U wave is constant at different heart rates, whereas Purkinje fibre AP duration is heart rate dependent[20]. Furthermore, in patients with right bundle branch block the timing of the U wave correlates better with the presence of right myocardial hypertrophy than with timing of intraventricular conduction[21]. Furthermore, amphibia can have a U wave but no Purkinje fibres[22]. Additionally, the morphology of the U wave does not fit the repolarization pattern of Purkinje fibres. The ascending limb of the T-wave is longer than its descending limb, which is similar to the repolarization pattern of ventricular and Purkinje fibres, whereas the U wave rises faster than it decays[10].

A longer duration of the T-wave to the apex of the U wave in patients with a left bundle branch block favours the Purkinje hypothesis for the generation of the U wave, as Watanabe argued[18]. The U wave most likely represents a delayed or inhomogeneous repolarization process in the ventricles. The AP duration of the Purkinje fibres is longer than that of the ventricular fibres and therefore the U wave follows the T-wave and has the same polarity. The authors found a significantly prolonged Q–T and Q–aU interval (time interval of Q wave until apex of U wave) in patients with a left bundle branch block in comparison to patients with a right bundle branch block despite no difference in the ECG RR interval. The delayed Purkinje activation led to a delayed appearance of the U wave.

However, the delayed appearance of the U wave in relation to timing of ventricular repolarization did not prove the mechanism of U wave genesis due to Purkinje fibre activation because the finding could be explained either by delayed repolarization of the Purkinje fibres or by delayed relaxation of the left ventricle. Therefore a clear link to a single mechanism responsible for the generation of the U wave is not possible[20].

Moreover, a strong argument against the Purkinje repolarization theory is the long duration of the U wave. Differences between the functional refractory period of the His-Purkinje system and ventricular muscle in humans (reflecting the differences between AP duration of the these structures) are not sufficient to explain the normal duration of a U wave (160–230 ms)[10]. Yanowitz *et al.* argued that certain AP terminate after the end of the T-wave but do not generate deflection, because they end simultaneously and

undergo cancellation[23]. Autenrieth *et al.* had no evidence of silent repolarization in dogs as all monophasic AP recorded from the surface of the left ventricle terminated during the T-wave[24]. The T-wave has the same polarity as the QRS complex, although at the cellular level depolarization and repolarization represent changes of opposite polarity. Franz *et al.* demonstrated a transmural gradient of repolarization, with earlier repolarization occurring at the epicardium, and they showed that the duration of the AP correlated with the duration of the QT interval in surface ECG recordings without evidence of a post-AP electrical activity responsible for the generation of the U wave[25].

Hypothesis 2: delayed repolarization of mid-myocardial layers

The ventricular myocardium is not as homogeneous as previously thought, as it is comprised of electrically and functionally distinct cell types. Cardiomyocytes differ with respect to currents that contribute to the early repolarization phase (phase 1). AP of epicardial and M cells display a prominent transient outward K^+ current (I_{to})-mediated phase 1, which is largely absent in endocardial cells. The principal feature of M cells is their ability to prolong AP duration during heart rate reduction much more than epicardial or endocardial cardiomyocytes.

Where present, M cells are more abundant in terms of tissue mass than Purkinje fibres, and their delayed repolarization could be sufficient to give rise to the U wave, particularly the pathological U wave appearing in LQTS or drug-induced QT prolongations[26]. In contrast, experimental findings suggest that M cells may give rise to a second component of the T-wave, often confused as an accentuated or inverted U wave[27,28]. Antzelevitch and co-workers suggested the use of the terms T1 and T2 to describe the two contiguous repolarization waves, or bifurcated T-wave, which is distinct from the U wave[28–30].

The fact that the T-wave and U wave are separate deflections was also shown in patients with acute myocardial ischaemia, where the monophasic transformed ventricular complex is independent of the shape and timing of the U wave[10].

Hypothesis 3: mechano-electric coupling

The concept of mechano-electrical coupling as a cause for, or contributor to, the U wave was suggested by Lepeschkin in 1957[31]. As the end of the T-wave coincides with the second heart sound, the mechano-electrical hypothesis suggests that after-potentials, caused by stretching of the circular muscle layers of the left ventricle, give rise to the U wave[2,7]. The existence of mechano-sensitive ion channels that transduce changes in the cardiomyocytes' mechanical environment into electrical signals has been amply documented[32–34]. Conclusive proof for the mechano-electrical hypothesis is lacking, however. Support for this hypothesis derives principally from the correlation between U wave timing and ventricular relaxation[20].

The U wave in patients with the short QT syndrome

The short QT syndrome (SQTS) represents a primary electrical disease, characterized by a substantial shortening of the QT interval and shortening of atrial and ventricular effective refractory periods[35–37]. The clear separation of the T and U waves in patients with SQTS provides a unique opportunity to obtain further insights into the origin of the U wave, either by echocardiography or by high resolution ECG imaging, including data relevant to the mechano-electrical hypothesis[5,6]. The clinical characteristics of SQTS patients have previously been described in detail and compared to healthy controls in Gaita et al.[36]. Haemodynamic parameters of ventricular mechanical systole and diastole were determined echocardiographically and correlated to electrical repolarization using precordial leads V2/V3/(V4). Haemodynamic parameters included the duration of isovolumic contraction (IVC, the interval from closure of the mitral valve to opening of the aortic valve), ejection period, end-systolic and end-diastolic volumes, ejection fraction and duration of isovolumic relaxation (IVR, the interval from closure of the aortic valve to opening of the mitral valve).

QT intervals were significantly shorter in SQTS patients (268 ± 18 ms, QTc 285 ± 28 ms) compared to controls (386 ± 20 ms, QTc 420 ± 22 ms, $p < 0.005$). The interval between the Q wave and the beginning of the U wave was 388 ± 27 ms in SQTS patients, and the interval from the end of the T-wave to the onset of the U wave was 106 ± 17 ms (vs 389 ± 20 ms and 3 ± 12 ms in controls, respectively; see Fig. 38.1).

Accordingly, in healthy controls the aortic valve closed prior to the end of the T-wave (–12 ± 11 ms), while in SQTS patients this occurred well after the end of the T-wave (111 ± 30 ms; Fig. 38.2).

Ejection fraction, end-systolic and end-diastolic volumes were all normal in SQTS patients and controls, and both groups displayed similar heart rates, IVC, IVR and systolic ejection times, suggesting minor, if any, systematic differences in cardiac mechanical performance between groups. In addition, neither the interval between the Q wave and aortic valve closure nor the time between aortic valve closure and the beginning of the U wave differed between the two groups. Thus, the timing of the U wave did not correlate with ECG indicators of ventricular repolarization, but coincided with the timing of aortic valve closure and the beginning of IVR (Fig. 38.3), lending support to the mechano-electrical hypothesis for the origin of the U wave. How IVR may give rise to an electrical phenomenon visible in the surface ECG is still unresolved, however.

These results further show that the marked abbreviation of ventricular AP durations in LQTS patients has little effect on the time-course of ventricular contraction. A similar independence of mechanical and 'electrical' systole has also been reported for LQTS patients, where the time-course of mechanical systole is similar to that of controls in spite of prolonged ventricular AP durations[38].

In patients with SQTS, electrical repolarization terminates before mechanical contraction (Fig. 38.2). This phenomenon has previously been described in an animal study of O'Rourke et al.[39] and was confirmed by Sugishita and co-workers[40].

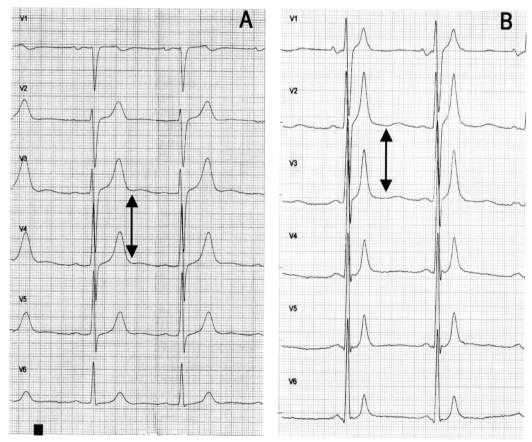

Fig. 38.1 Precordial ECG recordings from a control and SQTS patient. Onset of U wave is indicated by arrows. **A** Control (QT 360 ms, corrected QT [QTc] 397 ms): time difference between end of T-wave and onset of U wave 10 ms. **B** SQTS patient (QT 270 ms, QTc 392 ms): time difference between end of T-wave and onset of U wave 110 ms (paper speed 50 mm/s, amplitude gain 20 mm/mV). [Reproduced, with permission, from Schimpf R, Antzelevitch C, Haghi D, et al. (2008) Electromechanical coupling in patients with the short QT syndrome: further insights into the mechanoelectrical hypothesis of the U wave. *Heart Rhythm* **5**:241–245.]

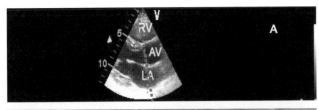

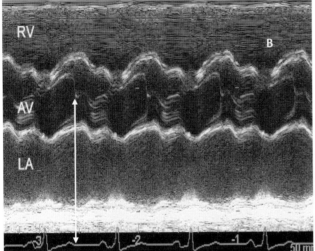

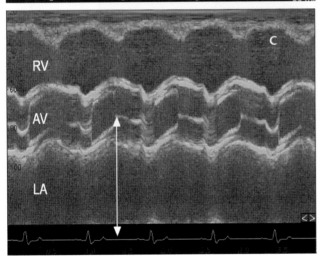

Fig. 38.2 Echocardiography of control and SQTS patient with simultaneous single-lead ECG recording (bottom line, **B** and **C**, paper speed 50 mm/s). **A** Echocardiographic sector of the parasternal long axis view with alignment of the M mode cursor (dotted line) through the aortic valve (AV) before collection of M mode echocardiography data. The right ventricle (RV) (top of each panel) is close to the transducer probe, whereas the left atrium (LA) is the most distant structure. **B** M mode echocardiography of the aortic valve in a healthy volunteer. Opening and closure of the aortic valve is visible by the rhombus-like echogenic reflections generated by abrupt movements of the anterior and posterior cusps towards and away from the transducer. The termination of electrical repolarization (end of T-wave) coincided with the end of mechanical systole (closure of aortic valve, see arrow). **C** M mode echocardiography of the aortic valve in a patient with a short QT syndrome. Termination of electrical repolarization (end of T-wave) preceded end of mechanical systole (closure of aortic valve) by 115 ms (arrow). [Reproduced, with permission, from Schimpf R, Antzelevitch C, Haghi D, *et al.* (2008) Electromechanical coupling in patients with the short QT syndrome: further insights into the mechanoelectrical hypothesis of the U wave. *Heart Rhythm* **5**:241–245.]

Interestingly, kangaroos exhibit a short QT interval. In these animals a striking disparity between mechanical systole und electrical repolarization has been demonstrated (QT interval 214 ± 50 ms; Q wave to aortic valve closure time of 393 ± 70 ms). Furthermore, the authors showed that with the occurrence of extrasystoles, the myocardium of kangaroos could be excited even though contraction was not complete, resulting in a type of 'incomplete tetanus' otherwise only associated with skeletal muscle[39,40].

In patients with SQTS, atrial and ventricular effective refractory periods are significantly reduced, so that very short coupled ventricular premature beats are capable of inducing ventricular tachyarrhythmias[36,41]. Whether an 'incomplete tetanus' may be observed in humans with SQTS remains to be investigated.

Linking IVR and the U wave

Mechanically, the cardiac cycle is traditionally divided into IVC, ejection, IVR and diastole[42]. IVC and IVR are not periods of haemodynamic stasis, as during these phases there is marked intracavitary redistribution of blood, and the shape of the ventricles changes. Initial invasive studies with analysis of left ventricular ventriculograms described a change in the shape of the left ventricle with an outward and anterior and/or apical movement during IVR[43]. An animal study with implantation of ultrasonic crystals in the myocardium to detect strain rate changes of the left ventricle demonstrated that IVR is initiated by subepicardial fibre lengthening, with consecutive asynchronous motion and deformation of the subepicardial myocardium, where cells are arranged in a left-handed helix[44]. Echocardiographic evaluation of intracavitary blood flow during isovolumic periods, using high-resolution Doppler and ultrasonic digital particle imaging velocimetry[45], showed that intracavitary flow briskly reverses direction from apex-to-base towards base-to-apex upon aortic valce closure, followed by a brief apex-to-base flow. This substantial intracavitary blood flow during the isovolumic phase is caused by ventricular morphology changes. It is conceivable, therefore, that myocardial mechano-electric coupling could underlie the ECG U wave, as it occurs at comparable timing. Stretch activates mechano-sensitive ion channels which transform changes in stretch or pressure into electrical signals through changes in membrane ion channel permeability[25–27]. Thus, regional stretch during the isovolumic phase may induce local membrane repolarization, generating a voltage gradient in the left ventricular myocardium that may be detected in the surface ECG.

Intracellular calcium dynamics and the U wave

Alternatively, changes in cardiomyocyte calcium handling, and related after-depolarizations, may be relevant for the U wave. Wu and coworkers performed studies in Langendorff-perfused rabbit hearts to determine the relationship between AP duration and the duration of the intracellular calcium transient[4]. Pincacidil, an adenosine triphosphate (ATP)-sensitive K^+ channel (K_{ATP}) channel opener, was used to simulate SQTS. This shortened significantly the QT interval. However, the effect on the duration of the intracellular calcium transient was much less pronounced. The authors concluded that a persistent increase in intracellular calcium, and after-depolarizations, underlie the U wave. Intracellular calcium

Fig. 38.3 Tissue Doppler echocardiography recording in a patient with short QT syndrome. Tissue velocity (grey line, right) with sample volume positioned in the basal interventricular septum in the apical four chamber view (bright circle, left lower view without and left upper view with colour Doppler imaging). Aortic valve closure (AVC, vertical green dotted lines) and beginning of isovolumic relaxation is correlating with beginning of the U wave. Left upper corner timings with corresponding dotted markers in ECG (bottom right): (1) RR interval (831 ms); (2) interval from Q wave to beginning of the U wave (398 ms, transferred timing from 12-lead ECG); (3) interval from Q wave to aortic valve closure (381 ms). Bottom right single-lead ECG (speed 50 mm/s). [Reproduced, with permission, from Schimpf R, Antzelevitch C, Haghi D, *et al.* (2008) Electromechanical coupling in patients with the short QT syndrome: further insights into the mechanoelectrical hypothesis of the U wave. *Heart Rhythm* **5**:241–245.] (See color plate section.)

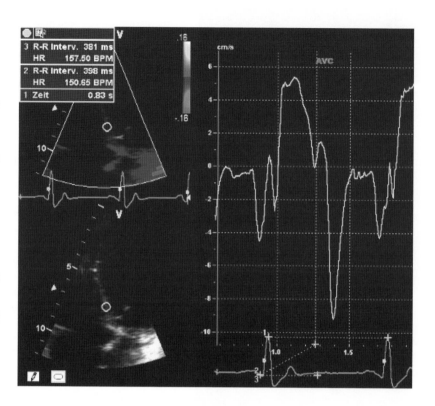

dynamics are essential for mechanical contraction, and the above discrepancy in AP duration changes and calcium transients may explain the sustained contractile activity in patients with SQTS[46]. Interestingly, the K_{ATP} channel is mechano-sensitive in atrial and ventricular cells, as are trans-sarcolemmal calcium uptake and intracellular calcium handling (see Chapters 10 and 16). Clearly, insight into the molecular links between cardiac mechano-electrical activity and the ECG U wave is required. One such molecular link has recently been proposed in the shape of the inward rectifier K^+ current (I_{K1})[34,47].

I_{K1} as modulator of the U wave

Postema and coworkers recently presented the hypothesis that the U wave is modulated by either a decrease of I_{K1} or an increase of I_{K1} with corresponding changes in the amplitude of the U wave[6]. The authors performed high resolution ECG sampling (fiducial segment averaging) focusing on the low frequency U wave signal at the end of the T-wave in patients with SQTS (SQTS-1, SQTS-3). They found that the deflection in the precordial leads V2—V3 that is referred to as the U wave seems to start 105 ms after the end of the T-wave and has its peak about 100 ms later. However, in the extremity leads II–III a positive deflection could be already observed immediately after the end of the T-wave. Following the definition that all variations of the potential after the T-wave are part of the U wave, the authors concluded that the T and U waves are parts of a single long repolarization process. The different appearances of the U wave in various leads were attributable to the varying projections on different lead vector axes. There were no differences in the effect on the amplitude of the U wave comparing

I_{Ks} (slow component of the delayed rectifier K^+ current) or I_{Kr} (rapid component of the delayed rectifier K^+ current) gain of function mutations. However, I_{K1} which regulates membrane potential differences in the late phase 3 and phase 4 of the cardiac AP may explain the genesis of the U wave. The U wave seems to be modulated by increase or decrease of I_{K1}. The authors demonstrated an influence of I_{K1} loss of function in six patients with an Anderson–Tawil syndrome (LQTS-7), in comparison to I_{K1} gain of function mutations in two patients with SQTS (SQTS-3). The resultant changes in the ECG show a modest attenuation of the T-wave and a decreased or increased amplitude of the U wave (Fig. 38.4).

The discovery of extended U waves in high resolution ECG, and their modulation by I_{K1}, is not incompatible with the theory that mechano-electrical coupling is a causal contributor to the U wave. If and how both hypotheses may be reconciled will be determined in future.

Conclusions and outlook

One hundred years after the initial description of the U wave, the mechanistic origin of this last wave in the ECG is still a matter of debate. Findings from SQTS patients have focused new attention on the theories for the origin of the U wave, due to the clear separation between the T and U waves in this cohort. Furthermore, evidence has been presented to show that intrinsic differences in the late phase of the AP are modulated by I_{K1}, which affects U wave morphology. A better understanding of the links between surface potentials and mechano-electrical coupling at the cellular level may emerge from novel approaches to optical mapping, combining multiparametric assessment of stress, strain, calcium and voltage.

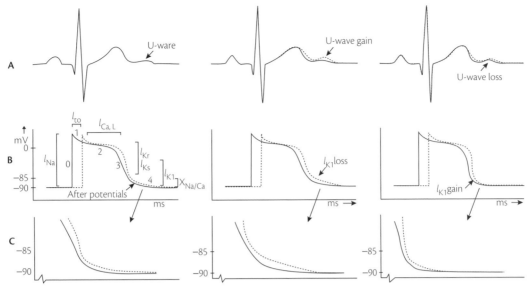

Fig. 38.4 I_{K1} and the U wave. Simplified presentation of the ECG (**A**) and the action potential with key ionic currents (**B** and **C**). The effects of either loss or gain of function of I_{K1} are illustrated in the terminal phase of the action potential (dotted lines) and the ECG. Loss of I_{K1} function (here LQTS-7) gives rise to an increase in action potential duration and U wave amplitude; gain of I_{K1} function (here SQTS-3) had the opposite effect. [Reproduced, with permission, from Postema PG, Ritsema van Eck HJ, Opthof T, *et al.* (2009) I_{K1} modulates the U-wave: insights in a 100-year-old enigma. *Heart Rhythm* **6**:393–400.]

References

1. Einthoven W Le telecardiogramme. *Arch Int Physiol* 1906;**4**:132–164.

2. Lewis T, Gilder M. The human electrocardiogram: a preliminary investigation of young male adults, to form a basis for pathological study. *Phil Trans R Soc Lond B* 1912;**202**:351–376.

3. Ritsema van Eck HJ, Kors JA, van Herpen G. The U wave in the electrocardiogram: a solution for a 100-year-old riddle. *Cardiovasc Res* 2005;**67**:256–262.

4. Wu S, Hayashi H, Lin SF, Chen PS. Action potential duration and QT interval during pinacidil infusion in isolated rabbit hearts. *J Cardiovasc Electrophysiol* 2005;**16**:872–878.

5. Schimpf R, Antzelevitch C, Haghi D, *et al.* Electromechanical coupling in patients with the short QT syndrome: Further insights into the mechanoelectrical hypothesis of the U wave. *Heart Rhythm* 2008;**5**:241–245.

6. Postema PG, Ritsema van Eck HJ, Opthof T, *et al.* I_{K1} modulates the U-wave: insights in a 100-year-old enigma. *Heart Rhythm* 2009;**6**: 393–400.

7. Lepeschkin E, Surawicz B. The duration of the Q–U interval and its components in electrocardiograms of normal persons. *Am Heart J* 1953;**46**:9–20.

8. Lepeschkin E. The U wave of the electrocardiogram. *AMA Arch Intern Med* 1955;**96**:600–617.

9. Surawicz B. U wave emerges from obscurity when the heart pumps like in a kangaroo. *Heart Rhythm* 2008;**5**:246–247.

10. Surawicz B. U wave: facts, hypotheses, misconceptions, and misnomers. *J Cardiovasc Electrophysiol* 1998;**9**:1117–1128.

11. Surawicz B. Bradycardia-dependent long QT syndrome, sudden death and late potentials. *J Am Coll Cardiol* 1992;**19**:550–551.

12. Hoffman BF, Cranefield PF (1960) Electrophysiology of the Heart. McGraw-Hill, New York.

13. Bufalari A, Furbetta D, Santucci F, Solinas P. Abnormality of the U wave and of the T–U segment of the electrocardiogram; the syndrome of the papillary muscles. *Circulation* 1956;**14**:1129–1137.

14. Brun P, Tribouilloy C, Duval AM, *et al.* Left ventricular flow propagation during early filling is related to wall relaxation: a color M-mode Doppler analysis. *J Am Coll Cardiol* 1992;**20**:420–432.

15. Fioretti P, Brower RW, Meester GT, Serruys PW. Interaction of left ventricular relaxation and filling during early diastole in human subjects. *Am J Cardiol* 1980;**46**:197–203.

16. Antzelevitch C, Nesterenko VV. Contribution of electrical heterogeneity of repolarization to the ECG. In: *Cardiac Repolarization.* (eds I Gussak, C Antzelevitch), Humana Press, Totowa, NJ, 2003, pp. 111–126.

17. Antzelevitch C. Cellular basis for the repolarization waves of the ECG. In: *Dynamic Electrocardiography*, (eds. M Malik, AJ Camm), Futura, New York, 2004, pp. 291–300.

18. Watanabe Y. Purkinje repolarization as a possible cause of the U wave in the electrocardiogram. *Circulation* 1975;**51**:1030–1037.

19. Surawicz B. Electrophysiologic substrate of torsade de pointes: dispersion of repolarization or early afterdepolarizations? *J Am Coll Cardiol* 1989;**14**:172–184.

20. Surawicz B. Is the U wave in the electrocardiogram a mechano-electric phenomenon. In: *Cardiac Mechano-Electric Feedback and Arrhythmias: from Pipette to Patient*, (eds P Kohl, F Sachs, MR Franz), Elsevier (Saunders), Philadelphia, 2005, pp. 179–190.

21. Ferrero C, Maeder M. Diagnostic de la hypertrophie ventriculaire droite par la chronologie de Lónde U. *Schweiz Med Wochenschr* 1970;**100**:190–192.

22. Lepeschkin E. Physiologic basis of the U-wave. In: *Advances in Electrocardiography* (eds. RC Schlant, JW Hurst), Grune & Stratton, New York, 1972, pp. 431–447.

23. Yanowitz F, Preston JB, Abildskov JA. Functional distribution of right and left stellate innervation to the ventricles. Production of neurogenic electrocardiographic changes by unilateral alteration of sympathetic tone. *Circ Res* 1966;**18**:416–428.

24. Autenrieth G, Surawicz B, Kuo CS. Sequence of repolarization on the ventricular surface in the dog. *Am Heart J* 1975;**89**:463–469.

25. Franz MR, Bargheer K, Rafflenbeul W, Haverich A, Lichtlen PR. Monophasic action potential mapping in human subjects with normal electrocardiograms: direct evidence for the genesis of the T-wave. *Circulation* 1987;**75**:379–386.

26. Antzelevitch C, Nesterenko VV, Yan GX. Role of M cells in acquired long QT syndrome, U waves, and torsade de pointes. *J Electrocardiol* 1995;**28**(Suppl):131–138.

27. Shimizu W, Antzelevitch C. Sodium channel block with mexiletine is effective in reducing dispersion of repolarization and preventing torsade des pointes in LQT2 and LQT3 models of the long-QT syndrome. *Circulation* 1997;**96**:2038–2047.

28. Yan GX, Antzelevitch C. Cellular basis for the normal T-wave and the electrocardiographic manifestations of the long-QT syndrome. *Circulation* 1998;**98**:1928–1936.

29. Antzelevitch C, Fish J. Electrical heterogeneity within the ventricular wall. *Basic Res Cardiol* 2001;**96**:517–527.

30. Antzelevitch C. Cellular basis for the repolarization waves of the ECG. *Ann N Y Acad Sci* 2006;**1080**:268–281.

31. Lepeschkin E. Genesis of the U wave. *Circulation* 1957;**15**:77–81.

32. Guharay F, Sachs F. Stretch-activated single ion channel currents in tissue-cultured embryonic chick skeletal muscle. *J Physiol* 1984;**352**:685–701.

33. Lab MJ. Contraction-excitation feedback in myocardium. Physiological basis and clinical relevance. *Circ Res* 1982;**50**:757–766.

34. Kohl P, Bollensdorff C, Garny A. Effects of mechanosensitive ion channels on ventricular electrophysiology: experimental and theoretical models. *Exp Physiol* 2006;**91**:307–321.

35. Gussak I, Brugada P, Brugada J, *et al*. Idiopathic short QT interval: a new clinical syndrome? *Cardiology* 2000;**94**:99–102.

36. Gaita F, Giustetto C, Bianchi F, *et al*. Short QT Syndrome: a familial cause of sudden death. *Circulation* 2003;**108**:965–970.

37. Brugada R, Hong K, Dumaine R, *et al*. Sudden death associated with short-QT syndrome linked to mutations in HERG. *Circulation* 2004;**109**:30–35.

38. Vincent GM, Jaiswal D, Timothy KW. Effects of exercise on heart rate, QT, QTc and QT/QS2 in the Romano-Ward inherited long QT syndrome. *Am J Cardiol* 1991;**68**:498–503.

39. O'Rourke MF, Avolio AP, Nichols WW. The kangaroo as a model for the study of hypertrophic cardiomyopathy in man. *Cardiovasc Res* 1986;**20**:398–402.

40. Sugishita Y, Iida K, O'Rourke MF, *et al*. Echocardiographic and electrocardiographic study of the normal kangaroo heart. *Aust NZ J Med* 1990;**20**:160–165.

41. Schimpf R, Bauersfeld U, Gaita F, Wolpert C. Short QT syndrome: successful prevention of sudden cardiac death in an adolescent by implantable cardioverter-defibrillator treatment for primary prophylaxis. *Heart Rhythm* 2005;**2**:416–417.

42. Wiggers C. Studies on the consecutive phases of the cardiac cycle. I. The duration of the consecutive phases of the cardiac cycle and the criteria for their precise determination. *Am J Physiol* 1921;**56**:415–438.

43. Ruttley MS, Adams DF, Cohn PF, Abrams HL. Shape and volume changes during "isovolumetric relaxation" in normal and asynergic ventricles. *Circulation* 1974;**50**:306–316.

44. Sengupta PP, Khandheria BK, Korinek J, Wang J, Belohlavek M. Biphasic tissue Doppler waveforms during isovolumic phases are associated with asynchronous deformation of subendocardial and subepicardial layers. *J Appl Physiol* 2005;**99**:1104–1111.

45. Sengupta PP, Khandheria BK, Korinek J, *et al*. Left ventricular isovolumic flow sequence during sinus and paced rhythms: new insights from use of high-resolution Doppler and ultrasonic digital particle imaging velocimetry. *J Am Coll Cardiol* 2007;**49**:899–908.

46. Chen PS, Lin SF. Electromechanical coupling in patients with the short QT syndrome: further insights into the mechanoelectrical hypothesis of the U wave. *Heart Rhythm* 2008;**5**:1091.

47. Van Wagoner DR. Mechanosensitive gating of atrial ATP-sensitive potassium channels. *Circ Res* 1993;**72**:973–983.

Mechanical modulation of cardiac function: role of the pericardium

John V. Tyberg

Background

Perhaps because it contains no muscle and seems to be a passive structure, little attention was paid to the role of the pericardium for many years, except to conclude that it prevents excessive cardiac dilation and somehow maintains equality between the outputs of the right ventricle (RV) and left ventricle (LV)[1]. However, without a thorough understanding of the biophysical relevance of the pericardium, it is difficult to assess effects of mechano-electric coupling (MEC) *in situ* and impossible to project from cell-level insight and *ex situ* models to whole body behaviour.

Transmural pressure

The key to the physiology of the pericardium is to understand the critical importance of transmural pressure. The LV, like any elastic chamber, distends in proportion to its transmural pressure, not in proportion to its intracavity pressure *per se*. Although physicists and engineers understand the distinction, it is frequently overlooked in medicine. Whether we are aware of it or not, pressure is always measured in relation to another pressure. Electrical potential (voltage) is always measured in relation to another voltage and, strictly speaking, voltage is a *potential difference*. Analogously, effective distending pressure[2] is a *pressure difference* across the chamber wall, i.e. transmural pressure. Although this principle is only rarely important with respect to systolic pressures[3], it may be critical in particular with respect to LV end-diastolic pressure (LVEDP)[4]. If we report that LVEDP is 12 mm Hg, we mean that LVEDP is 12 mm Hg higher than atmospheric pressure, because we measured LVEDP with a transducer that mechanically compared it to atmospheric pressure. However, if pericardial pressure happens to be 4 mm Hg, the actual transmural LVEDP is only 8 mm Hg. Furthermore, if LVEDP increases to 15 mm Hg but pericardial pressure also increases to 7 mm Hg, transmural LVEDP remains unchanged and so does LV end-diastolic volume (LVEDV).

The truth of these statements is persuasively demonstrated by an observation that is commonplace to a cardiac physiologist or a surgeon. Assuming that normal values of right ventricular end-diastolic

pressure (RVEDP) and LVEDP are 4 and 12 mm Hg, respectively, consider what happens when the pericardium is opened widely and held back from the heart and when both those pressures are maintained constant, by an infusion of volume. The LV expands somewhat, but the more thin-walled RV and the right atrium (RA) expand substantially, to an extent that could never be accommodated within the normal pericardium. The chambers of the heart expand because their transmural pressures increase. Because the intracavity pressures remained constant, pericardial pressures could not have been zero when the pericardium was closed. When the pericardium was closed, RVEDP was 4 mm Hg, and pericardial pressure was approximately 4 mm Hg, giving a transmural RVEDP of ~ 0 mm Hg. When the pericardium was opened, RVEDP was still 4 mm Hg, but, as pericardial pressure was then zero, transmural RVEDP now equalled 4 mm Hg. RV volume increased according to the increase in transmural RVEDP. Such observations underscore the importance of the pericardium in preventing excessive dilation of the RV, with its attendant increased irritability[5,6], an example of MEC[7].

Figure 39.1 illustrates these relationships[8]. Pressures are represented semi-quantitatively by opposing arrows of different lengths and, if unit surface areas are considered, are equivalent to force balances across the LV free wall, the interventricular septum and the RV free wall. Inertial and viscous effects can be ignored when the heart is approximately stationary at end diastole, so this constitutes a static-equilibrium analysis. At each wall, intracavity pressure is equal to the opposing transmural pressure plus the pressure on the opposite side. As suggested above, if the pericardium is removed and held back from the heart, pericardial pressure becomes zero (i.e. atmospheric pressure) and intracavity pressure must then be exactly equal to the transmural pressure, which is the rationale for our measurement of pericardial pressure (see below). Except under conditions in which the RV is hypertrophied[9], RVEDP is approximately equal to pericardial pressure[10,11] and, except when the RV or the LV are selectively afterloaded by arterial constriction, right and left pericardial pressures are equal[12]. Thus, LV pericardial pressure approximately equals RVEDP, and RVEDP approximately equals RV pericardial pressure. This implies that

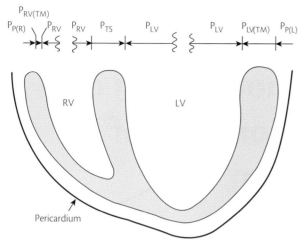

Fig. 39.1 A schematic diagram representing an end-diastolic, static-equilibrium analysis of the heart and pericardium. Arrows indicate direction and approximate magnitude of opposing end-diastolic pressures (P), equivalent to opposing forces if the pressures are applied over unit area. At each wall, intracavity pressure is equal to transmural (TM) pressure plus the pressure outside the wall. For the left and right ventricular free walls, intracavity pressure is equal to transmural pressure when the pericardium is removed. PP(R) and PP(L), right and left pericardial pressure; PTS, transseptal pressure. [Reproduced, with permission, from Tyberg JV (1985) Ventricular interaction and the pericardium. In: *The Ventricle: Basic and Clinical Aspects* (eds HJ Levine, WH Gaasch). Martinus Nijhoff, Boston, pp. 171–184.]

transmural RVEDP approaches zero, a contentious conclusion for a time[13,14], but one that was ultimately verified[15,16] and supported by other investigators[17].

How can pericardial pressure be measured?

It was long thought that the relationship between LVEDP and LVEDV, so-called diastolic compliance[18], was practically invariant. Indeed, this assumption was the basis for Sarnoff and Berglund's ventricular function curve analysis in which they used LV filling pressure rather than LVEDV as the measure of LV preload[19]. However, investigators in the 1970s demonstrated that diastolic compliance could change substantially and rapidly, for example, by giving nitroglycerin to a patient with heart failure[20]. We then suggested that such changes were due to unappreciated decreases in pericardial pressure[21], but many thought this hypothesis unlikely, because pericardial pressure had been shown to be negative and unchanging, even as RVEDP had been raised to very high values by pulmonary artery obstruction[22].

This prompted a re-examination of what was meant by pericardial pressure and how it should be measured[23,24]. We compared pericardial pressure measured using a flat, liquid-containing balloon transducer[25] to that measured using an open catheter[22] and compared both pressure measurements to 'true' pericardial pressure, which we suggested should be the difference between LVEDP measured with the pericardium closed and that measured with the pericardium open and held back, at the same LVEDV. As explained above, this rationale was based on our understanding of transmural pressure, such that LVEDP = transmural LVEDP +

pericardial pressure. The study demonstrated that the balloon-measured pressure was always correct, but that the open catheter seriously underestimated pericardial pressure unless substantial volumes of liquid (~ 30 ml) were added to the pericardium. We then measured pericardial pressure in patients during surgery who were transiently volume-loaded until mean right atrial pressure increased up to as much as 20 mm Hg and compared this to mean RA pressure; both pressures increased in parallel and, in most cases, were effectively identical[11] (see Fig. 39.2). Thus, we concluded that pericardial pressure is changeable acutely and that it is approximately equal to RV filling pressure under most circumstances[9]. In a normal pericardium without an excess of liquid[23], pericardial pressure is fundamentally a compressive contact stress[24] and is equal to measured hydrostatic pressure only when special care is taken to eliminate the artifacts due to the presence of a large catheter[26]. These conclusions have been supported by experimental[17] and clinical[9,27] studies.

Ventricular interaction

Ventricular interaction is the reciprocal, complementary change in the volumes of the RV and LV such that, when RVEDV increases, LVEDV decreases and *vice versa*[28]. Ventricular interaction involves the septum moving toward the LV or the RV, and it is profoundly diminished when the heart is not constrained by the pericardium[28,29] or other mediastinal structures[30]. The stretched pericardium is relatively stiff compared to the RV or LV myocardium so, as viewed with respect to an 'equatorial' cross-sectional plane, the heart is surrounded by an effectively unyielding band or belt. (Changes in shape translate into alterations, such as in the long axis of the LV, but these will be ignored in this discussion of steady-state diastolic volumes.) Thus, for the most part, RVEDV can increase only at the 'expense' of LVEDV. These changes in volume occur because the septum is elastic and moves leftward or rightward with small decreases or increases in the difference between LVEDP and RVEDP [i.e. the transseptal 'gradient' (TSG) = LVEDP – RVEDP][31,32]. Ventricular interaction is diminished when pericardial pressure is very low and, effectively, it does not occur when the pericardium is open[28].

Ventricular interaction was first illustrated clearly by a series of studies of the effects of acute pulmonary artery embolization and volume loading, with and without the pericardium[29,33,34]. With the pericardium intact, pulmonary embolization and volume loading appeared to decrease LV diastolic compliance and LV contractility, as evaluated conventionally by plots of LVEDP vs LVEDV (upper-left panel, Fig. 39.3) and LV stroke work vs LVEDP (lower-left panel), respectively[33]. However, when diastolic compliance and contractility were evaluated using transmural LVEDP to reflect the effective distending pressure, there was no change in LV compliance (upper-right panel) or contractility (lower-right panel)[35]. These concepts are re-capitulated in the left-hand panels of Fig. 39.4. When the same experiment was repeated after opening the pericardium (see right-hand panels), ventricular interaction was absent[29].

Ventricular interaction and its effects on apparent contractility were also illustrated in the newborn lamb[36]. Before the lamb had taken its first breath, pressures and LV performance (stroke work) were measured while blood volume was momentarily increased and decreased by transfusion and withdrawal. These measurements

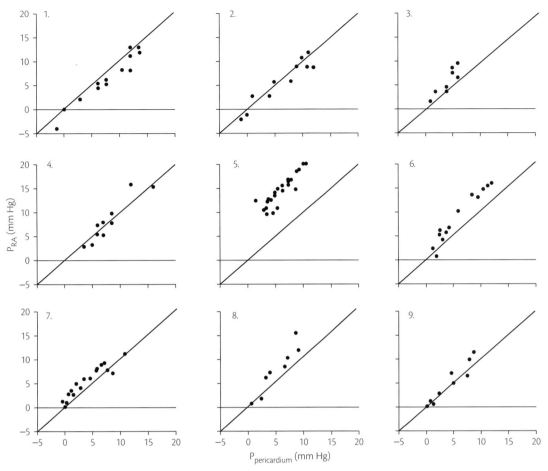

Fig. 39.2 Simultaneously measured mean right atrial pressure (y axes) and pericardial pressure (x axes; measured over the LV free wall) in nine patients during volume loading before initiation of cardiopulmonary bypass. Note that right atrial pressure increased in proportion to the increase in pericardial pressure in each patient. Note also that, except for one patient (#5), the absolute value of right atrial pressure was equal to pericardial pressure. Thus, pericardial pressure is highly variable and is usually equal to right atrial pressure. [Reproduced, with permission, from Tyberg JV, Taichman GC, Smith ER, Douglas NWS, Smiseth OA, Keon WJ (1986) The relation between pericardial pressure and right atrial pressure: an intraoperative study. *Circulation* **73**:428–432.]

were repeated after ventilation had been initiated and then, again, after the pericardium was opened and the lungs had been pulled away from the heart. Ventilation increased LV compliance and apparent contractility (i.e. greater stroke work was performed at the same level of LVEDP), and complete removal of pericardial and pleural constraints to LV filling appeared to increase compliance and contractility further. However, under all these conditions, LV stroke work was predicted by LVEDV or by transmural LVEDP, which is directly proportional to LVEDV.

As suggested, the constraining effect of the lungs and associated thoracic structures produces measurable effects on LV filling[37,38]. When the chest is closed, pericardial pressure is the sum of pleural pressure and transpericardial pressure (i.e. pericardial pressure – pleural pressure). Pleural pressure (i.e. cardiac fossa pressure) naturally increases with positive end-expiratory pressure, but it is measurable (~ 5 mm Hg) after volume loading even in the absence of positive end-expiratory pressures[39]. Transpericardial pressure is a measure of the effective distending pressure of the pericardium and, thus, reflects total cardiac volume[39,40]. Recent work suggests that substantial mediastinal and pleural constraint remains, even after surgical pericardiotomy[30].

Recently, we demonstrated how the pericardium modulates LV and RV stroke volumes to compensate for sudden changes in atrial volume[28]. In anaesthetized dogs, we suddenly infused or removed ~ 25 ml of blood into or from the left or right atrium. With infusions, ipsilateral ventricular end-diastolic transmural pressure, diameter and stroke volume all increased. With the pericardium closed, there were compensatory decreases in contralateral transmural end-diastolic pressure, diameter and stroke volume. The sum of the ipsilateral increases and the contralateral decreases in stroke volume approximated the infused volume. Corresponding and opposite changes were seen with blood withdrawals. Changes in LV septum-to-free-wall diameter were inversely related to changes in RV septum-to-free-wall diameter, a relation we called 'complementarity' and feel to be a hallmark of ventricular interaction. All these manifestations of direct ventricular interaction were diminished when pericardial pressure was less than 5 mm Hg and were absent when the pericardium was opened. Thus, constraint by a taut pericardium (in this experiment, pericardial pressure was equal to a transpericardial pressure, as the lungs were held back) appears essential for immediate biventricular compensatory responses to acute atrial volume changes. This not only demonstrates new

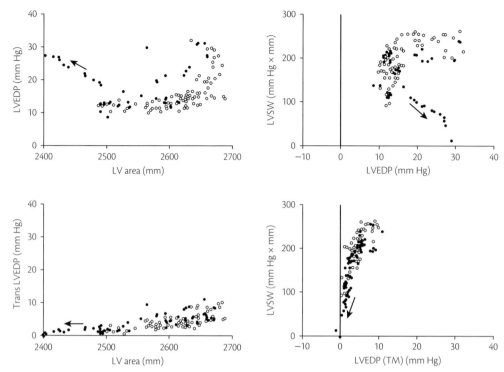

Fig. 39.3 The effect of pericardial pressure on apparent LV compliance and ventricular function curves in dogs after acute pulmonary embolization and volume loading by rapid intravenous infusion of Ringer's lactate solution. In each panel, arrows indicate direction of beat-by-beat changes during a pre-terminal infusion of saline. Upper panels represent conventional measures of compliance (left) and contractility (right) based on LVEDP measurement relative to atmospheric pressure; lower panels utilize transmural LVEDP. The upper left panel shows an apparent decrease in LV diastolic compliance, as LVEDP increased while LV area (LVEDV) decreased. However, the properties of the ventricular wall did not really change as, in the lower left panel, the transmural LVEDP–LV area relationship was unchanged and all the data fell on a single curve. In the upper right panel, a conventional ventricular function curve indicates that contractility has decreased, as LV stroke work (LVSW) decreased while LVEDP increased. However, as shown in the lower right panel, there was no real change in contractility because there was no shift in the LVSW–transmural LVEDP relationship. [Reproduced, with permission, from Tyberg JV, Smith ER (1990) Ventricular diastole and the role of the pericardium. *Herz* **15**:354–361. Data from Belenkie et al.[33].]

dynamic aspects of ventricular interaction, but also highlights a mechanism whereby pulmonary blood volume is stabilized. The pericardium acts as a mechanical servo-control system whereby one ventricle can immediately respond to changes in the volume of the other ventricle, adjusting its output to compensate.

Further, we suggested that this mechanism might normally be a first line of defence against orthostatic hypotension (i.e. the drop in arterial blood pressure that results from assuming a standing position). When a person stands up, venous return to the RA is momentarily decreased as blood pools in the lower body. This reduces RVEDV which, by the mechanism outlined above, increases LVEDV and LV stroke volume, tending to minimize the hypotension. If pericardial pressure is reduced for any reason, this mechanism might be impaired and the individual might be more prone to develop orthostatic hypotension (e.g. in both the endurance athlete at rest and the over-diuresed or excessively vasodilated heart-failure patient, the pericardium might be 'too big' for the heart). This hypothesis is supported by data from a study by Esch *et al.* in endurance-trained athletes[41]. Although all eight of the normally active men completed the orthostatic tolerance test, seven of the eight athletes were unable to do so, because of light-headedness or syncope. The LVEDP–LVEDV relation was shifted substantially to the right in athletes and, in response to lower-body negative

pressure (−80 mm Hg), LVEDV and stroke volume decreased more in endurance-trained athletes than in normally active men.

Because the complementary changes in RV and LV volumes (i.e. ventricular interaction) occur largely through the displacement of the septum, and because the driving force for septal displacement is the TSG[31,42], changes in the TSG become a convenient indicator of ventricular interaction. Such considerations led Mirsky and Rankin to observe that the LV is surrounded by the pericardium only over approximately two-thirds of its circumference, the remaining one-third being surrounded by the RV[43]. Therefore, because we hold that LVEDV is the most fundamental chamber parameter of LV preload and the best predictor of systolic performance according to the Frank–Starling law, it is sometimes useful to modify the definition of transmural pressure accordingly to better account for the contribution of a changing RVEDP and predict LVEDV[44].

Physiological implications

When LV filling pressure is used as the parameter of preload in a ventricular function curve analysis[19], a change in compliance[18] can lead erroneously to the conclusion that LV contractility has changed, as Glantz and Parmley pointed out[35] (see Fig. 39.5).

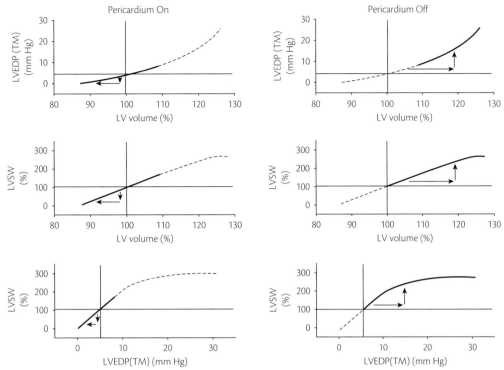

Fig. 39.4 A schematic diagram illustrating ventricular interaction (left panel) and showing how the effects of intravenous volume loading after pulmonary embolism differ qualitatively, depending on whether the pericardium is present. In order to compare the results of two investigations[33,34], data were normalized such that LVEDV and LVSW were set equal to 100% when transmural LVEDP (i.e. in the left panel, LVEDP minus pericardial pressure; in the right panel, LVEDP) was equal to 5 mmHg. The top panels shows diastolic compliance (transmural LVEDP vs end-diastolic volume); the middle panels show LV function (LV stroke work) in terms of LV end-diastolic volume; the bottom panels show LV function in terms of transmural LVEDP. The left and right paired relations are identical; the thickened lines indicate the operating regions of the relations, with or without the pericardium. In both the left and right panels, the paired arrows (representing the sides of a triangle) describe the typical effects of volume loading. In the right panel, volume loading increases end-diastolic volume and transmural LVEDP (top panel), and the increases in LV stroke work are predicted by both the increases in end-diastolic volume (middle panel) and transmural LVEDP (bottom panel). In the left panel, because of pericardial constraint volume loading paradoxically *decreases* end-diastolic volume and transmural LVEDP (top panel). The magnitudes of the decreases in LV stroke work are predicted by both the decreases in end-diastolic volume and transmural LVEDP. [Reproduced, with permission, from Tyberg JV, Belenkie I (2000) Mechanical interactions between the respiratory and circulatory systems. In: *Sleep Apnea: Implications in Cardiovascular and Cerebrovascular Disease* (eds TD Bradley, JS Floras). Marcel Dekker, New York, pp. 99–112.]

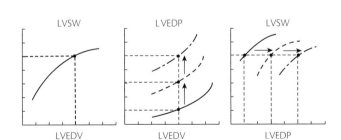

Fig. 39.5 Schematic diagram illustrating the relation of diastolic compliance to contractility. At any given LV stroke work (LVSW) (left panel), a decrease in diastolic compliance (middle panel) might be mistakenly interpreted as a decrease in contractility, if assessed as a function of LVEDP (right panel). [Modified, with permission, from Tyberg JV, Grant DA, Kingma I, Mitchell JR, Sun Y-H, Belenkie I (2001) Effects of positive intrathoracic pressure on the evaluation of cardiac performance. In: *Proceedings of the 2nd Dresden Postgraduate Course on Mechanical Ventilation* (eds MG de Abreu, T Koch). Drager Medical, Lubeck. Data from Glantz and Parmley[35].]

If compliance decreases (see middle panel), LVEDP increases at a given value of LVEDV. That being so, when ventricular systolic performance (i.e. LV stroke work) is evaluated in terms of LVEDP (right-hand panel), the ventricular function curve is shifted to the right. This indicates that the same value of LV stroke work is accomplished at increasing values of LVEDP, and this may erroneously suggest that contractility is decreased. LVEDP increases but LVEDV, the ultimate measure of LV preload, does not, consistent with the unchanged value of stroke work. Thus, the Frank–Starling law is accurate and useful when LVEDV (or transmural LVEDP, as shown elsewhere) is used as a measure of LV preload, but may be seriously misleading when LVEDP is assumed to be a reliable measure of LV preload.

The paramount importance of transmural pressure has crucial physiological implications. By recording from single cervical vagal afferent fibres, we demonstrated that the activity of ventricular mechano-receptors is dependent on LV transmural pressure and consequent distension, not on intracavity pressure[45]. Similarly, serum atriopeptin (atrial natriuretic peptide, ANP) concentrations are dependent on atrial transmural pressure and distension[46].

These interpretations of pericardial physiology might also have the effect of focusing relatively more attention on changes in LV preload and less on LV contractility, when attempting to understand the basis for short-term changes in systolic performance. As shown above[29,33,34,36], profound changes in systolic performance can be explained when preload is understood as transmural LVEDP. In normal, instrumented, conscious dogs, volume loading has negligible effects on stroke volume, although cardiac output increases because of the increased heart rate[47]. However, LVEDV fails to increase further when LVEDP is raised above 10–15 mm Hg[48], which, based on our cumulative experience, could well be due to pericardial constraint. Similarly, volume loading beyond an LVEDP of 10–15 mm Hg fails to increase systolic performance in human subjects[49], which also could be due to pericardial constraint.

Clinical implications

Perhaps one of the detrimental effects of an inappropriate P–R interval relates to the pericardium. In dogs with atrio-ventricular block that were paced independently from the RA and RV, we assessed LV diastolic compliance and systolic function when P–R intervals were normal and when the atrium and ventricle were stimulated simultaneously (P–R interval = 0). In the latter situation, as conventionally assessed, diastolic compliance and systolic performance were decreased, because of atrio-ventricular interaction. The unemptied atria compromised the pericardial volume, increasing pericardial pressure and decreasing transmural LVEDP and LVEDV for a given value of intracavitary LVEDP[50].

A similar mechanism seems to provide a partial explanation for the effectiveness of cardiac resynchronization therapy[51]. Recently, Williams et al. reported that it is also effective in patients with a narrow QRS[52,53]. In 30 heart-failure patients in sinus rhythm (QRS duration < 120 ms; ejection fraction ≤ 35%), biventricular or LV pacing increased cardiac output and stroke work by 25%. The authors suggested that pacing allowed the LV to fill earlier and, in so doing, was less impeded by pericardial constraint because the RV was smaller[52].

Because pacemaker activity[54] and other heart rate disturbances depend on myocardial stretch[7] and, thus chamber volume, the effects of performing the Valsalva manoeuvre may be difficult to predict[55–57]. Ventricular volumes decrease during the strain phase of the Valsalva manoeuvre in normal subjects (presumably due to combined effect of reduced venous return, arterial blood drainage from the chest and a decrease in transmural pressure, even during the initial increase in intracavity pressure), but not in failing ventricles affected by severe cardiomyopathy[58].

Using isolated, Langendorff-perfused rabbit hearts, Ravelli and Allessie demonstrated an increased vulnerability to atrial fibrillation with atrial distension, an increased vulnerability that was closely correlated with the decrease in the atrial effective refractory period[59]. This is believed to be related to stretch-activation of ion channels, as blocking them using the tarantula venom peptide GsMTx-4 prevented the atrial-distension-induced increase in AF vulnerability[60]. Because the pericardium had been removed in both studies, atrial pressures of up to 20 or 30 cm H$_2$O corresponded to substantial transmural pressures. Ninio and Saint extended these findings to document the effect of the pericardium[6]. At an atrial pressure of 16 cm H$_2$O, the atrial

refractory period was reduced to ~55 from ~105 ms in the absence of the pericardium; no change in the refractory period was observed at that pressure when the pericardium was intact. These decreases in refractory period were accompanied by increased vulnerability and prolonged duration of atrial fibrillation[6]. These findings are supported by interesting case reports[61,62].

Perhaps the most important clinical implication of these aspects of pericardial physiology is the role of the pericardium in heart failure. In 1946, Howarth et al. reported the effects of venesection in patients with low-output heart failure[63]. They described a patient with very high venous pressure and low cardiac output in whom the removal of 800 ml of venous blood almost doubled cardiac output, as venous pressure fell precipitously. As shown in Fig. 39.6, this long-puzzling observation might be explained by the action of the pericardium. As blood was withdrawn from a dog in pacing-induced heart failure[64], LVEDP decreased as expected. However, because pericardial pressure actually decreased more than LVEDP, transmural LVEDP increased. The increase in transmural LVEDP was accompanied by an increase in LVEDV and LV systolic performance (i.e. stroke work)[64,65].

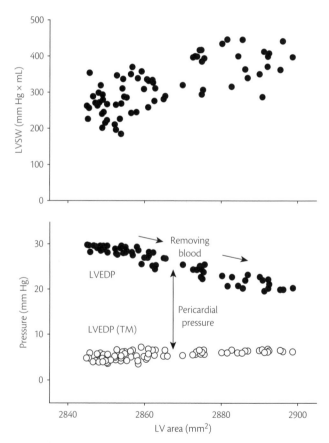

Fig. 39.6 Effect of removing blood volume in a dog in whom heart failure was produced by pacing[64]. Removing venous blood decreased LVEDP. However, because pericardial pressure (vertical arrow) decreased more than LVEDP, transmural LVEDP increased, consistent with the increase in LVEDV (i.e. Area). In turn, LV stroke work increased, consistent with the increase in transmural LVEDP and LVEDV.]

These observations bring to mind the classical therapy of blood letting – whether effected by venesection or the application of leeches – and raise the question of whether the benefits of nitrate therapy in heart failure are at least partly related to the mechanisms described above (in addition to decreased mitral regurgitation, if present). Nitrates increase venous capacitance and decrease central venous pressure; therefore they decrease pericardial pressure[66], which shifts the LV diastolic pressure–volume relationship downward[20,21,67]. LVEDV may increase or decrease slightly but, if so, much less than would have been expected from the profound decrease in LVEDP. Both nitrates and reduction of blood volume reduce central venous pressure, which decreases pericardial pressure *pari passu*[11], thus effectively increasing the compliance of the LV.

As shown in Fig. 39.7[68], a reduction in LV afterload and a modest increase in heart rate typically help to maintain cardiac output after the administration of nitrates[69]. However, the role of pericardium-mediated ventricular interaction is critical. There would be no possibility of reducing LVEDP so much (thereby effectively treating pulmonary oedema) and reducing LVEDV so little (thereby tending to maintain LV preload), except for the downward shift in the diastolic pressure–volume relationship, a downward shift that all the evidence now suggests is due to a reduction in pericardial pressure.

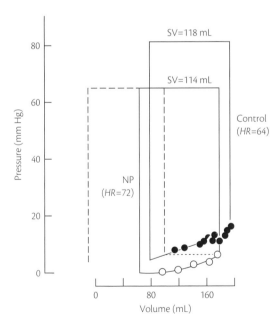

Fig. 39.7 The importance of the shift in the LV diastolic pressure-volume relationship for the maintenance of stroke volume (SV) after administration of sodium nitroprusside (NP). Because of the shift in the relationship, stroke volume was maintained despite large reductions in LVEDP. Had the control pressure–volume relationship been followed, this reduction in LVEDP would have corresponded to such a small LVEDV that stroke volume would have decreased greatly. HR, heart rate. [Reproduced, with permission, from Tyberg JV, Misbach GA, Parmley WW, Glantz SA (1980) Effects of the pericardium on ventricular performance. In: *Cardiac Dynamics* (eds J Baan, EL Yellin, AC Arntzenius). Martinus Nijhoff, The Hague, Boston, pp. 159–168. Data from Alderman and Glantz[69].]

Conclusions and outlook

This overview of recent developments in pericardial physiology was incisively anticipated by L.N. Katz in 1955[4]:

> "Even the use of end-diastolic pressure as an index of end-diastolic volume is not justified…. Furthermore, if the expansion of the heart is limited, for example by the pericardium, changes in end-diastolic pressure lose much of their meaning in terms of changes in end-diastolic volume."

With the benefit of this past insight and of the results of more recent experimental work, it is hoped that future generations of clinicians will not assume that interventions that increase LVEDP will necessarily also increase stroke volume and cardiac output; the opposite may occur in some circumstances. **Transmural** LV end-diastolic pressure predicts end-diastolic volume and end-diastolic volume predicts systolic performance; thus, the Frank–Starling law continues to be useful. The implications of the pericardium for research into MEC need to be addressed better. The physical constraint offered by the pericardium should be taken into account when comparing data across biological model systems. This may require a conceptual reorientation, and could be helped by the rapidly developing techniques for whole organ computational modelling of cardiac mechano-electrical behaviour.

References

1. Shabetai R. (1981) *The Pericardium*. Grune and Stratton, New York.
2. Henderson Y, Barringer TBJ. The relation of venous pressure to cardiac efficiency. *Am J Physiol* 1913;**13**:352–369.
3. Haykowsky M, Taylor D, Teo K, Quinney A, Humen D. Left ventricular wall stress during leg-press exercise performed with a brief Valsalva maneuver. *Chest* 2001;**119**:150–154.
4. Katz LN. Analysis of the several factors regulating the performance of the heart. *Physiol Rev* 1955;**35**:91–106.
5. Levine JH, Guarnieri T, Kadish AH, White RI, Calkins H, Kan JS. Changes in myocardial repolarization in patients undergoing balloon valvuloplasty for congenital pulmonary stenosis: evidence for contraction-excitation feedback in humans. *Circulation* 1988;**77**: 70–77.
6. Ninio DM, Saint DA. Passive pericardial constraint protects against stretch-induced vulnerability to atrial fibrillation in rabbits. *Am J Physiol* 2006;**291**:H2547–H2549.
7. Kohl P, Ravens U. Cardiac mechano-electric feedback: past, present, and prospect. *Prog Biophys Mol Biol* 2003;**82**:3–9.
8. Tyberg JV. Ventricular interaction and the pericardium. In: *The Ventricle: Basic and Clinical Aspects* (eds. HJ Levine, WH Gaasch), Boston: Martinus Nijhoff Publishing; 1985, pp. 171–184.
9. Boltwood CM, Skulsky A, Drinkwater DC, Lang S, Mulder DG, Shah PM. Intraoperative measurement of pericardial constraint: role in ventricular diastolic mechanics. *J Am Coll Cardiol* 1986;**8**: 1289–1297.
10. Smiseth OA, Refsum H, Tyberg JV. Pericardial pressure assessed by right atrial pressure: a basis for calculation of left ventricular transmural pressure. *Am Heart J* 1983;**108**:603–605.
11. Tyberg JV, Taichman GC, Smith ER, Douglas NWS, Smiseth OA, Keon WJ. The relation between pericardial pressure and right atrial pressure: an intraoperative study. *Circulation* 1986;**73**:428–432.
12. Smiseth OA, Scott-Douglas NW, Thompson CR, Smith ER, Tyberg JV. Nonuniformity of pericardial surface pressure in dogs. *Circulation* 1987;**75**:1229–1236.
13. Assanelli D, Lew WYW, Shabetai R, LeWinter MM. Influence of the pericardium on right and left ventricular filling in the dog. *J Appl Physiol* 1987;**63**:1025–1032.

14. Slinker BK, Ditchey RV, Bell SP, LeWinter MM. Right heart pressure does not equal pericardial pressuure in the potassium chloride arrested in situ dog heart. *Circulation* 1987;**76**:357–362.

15. Traboulsi M, Scott-Douglas NW, Smith ER, Tyberg JV. The right and left ventricular intracavitary and transmural pressure-strain relationships. *Am Heart J* 1992;**123**:1279–1287.

16. Hamilton DR, Dani RS, Semlacher RA, Smith ER, Kieser TM, Tyberg JV. Right atrial and right ventricular transmural pressures in dogs and humans. Effects of the pericardium. *Circulation* 1994;**90**:2492–2500.

17. Applegate RJ, Johnston WE, Vinten-Johansen J, Klopfenstein HS, Little WC. Restraining effect of intact pericardium during acute volume loading. *Am J Physiol* 1992;**262**:H1725–H1733.

18. Braunwald E, Ross J, Jr. The ventricular end-diastolic pressure (editorial). *Am J Med* 1963;**34**:147–150.

19. Sarnoff SJ, Berglund E. Ventricular function. 1. Starling's law of the heart studied by means of simultaneous right and left ventricular function curves in the dog. *Circulation* 1954;**9**:706–718.

20. Ludbrook PA, Byrne JD, Kurnik PB, McKnight RC. Influence of reduction of preload and afterload by nitroglycerin on left ventricular diastolic pressure-volume relations and relaxation in man. *Circulation* 1977;**56**:937–943.

21. Tyberg JV, Misbach GA, Glantz SA, Moores WY, Parmley WW. A mechanism for the shifts in the diastolic, left ventricular, pressure-volume curve: the role of the pericardium. *Europ J Cardiol* 1978;**7**(Suppl.):163–175.

22. Kenner HM, Wood EH. Intrapericardial, intrapleural, and intracardiac pressures during acute heart failure in dogs studied without thoracotomy. *Circ Res* 1966;**19**:1071–1079.

23. Smiseth OA, Frais MA, Kingma I, Smith ER, Tyberg JV. Assessment of pericardial constraint in dogs. *Circulation* 1985;**71**:158–164.

24. Hamilton DR, deVries G, Tyberg JV. Static and dynamic operating characteristics of a pericardial balloon. *J Appl Physiol* 2001;**90**:1481–1488.

25. Holt JP, Rhode EA, Kines H. Pericardial and ventricular pressure. *Circ Res* 1960;**8**:1171–1180.

26. deVries G, Hamilton DR, ter Keurs HE, Beyar R, Tyberg JV. A novel technique for measurement of pericardial pressure. *Am J Physiol* 2001;**280**:H2815–H2822.

27. Dauterman K, Pak PH, Maughan WL, *et al.* Contribution of external forces to left ventricular diastolic pressure. Implications for the clinical use of the Starling law. *Ann Intern Med* 1995;**122**:737–742.

28. Gibbons Kroeker CA, Shrive NG, Belenkie I, Tyberg JV. The pericardium modulates LV and RV stroke volumes to compensate for sudden changes in atrial volume. *Am J Physiol* 2003;**284**:H2247–H2254.

29. Belenkie I, Dani R, Smith ER, Tyberg JV. The importance of pericardial constraint in experimental pulmonary embolism and volume loading. *Am Heart J* 1992;**123**:733–742.

30. Belenkie I, Kieser TM, Sas R, Smith ER, Tyberg JV. Evidence for left ventricular constraint during open heart surgery. *Canad J Cardiol* 2002;**18**:951–959.

31. Kingma I, Tyberg JV, Smith ER. Effects of diastolic transseptal pressure gradient on ventricular septal position and motion. *Circulation* 1983;**68**:1304–1314.

32. Dong S-J, Beyar R, Zhou Z-N, Fick GH, Smith ER, Tyberg JV. Determinants of midwall circumferential segmental length of the canine ventricular septum at end diastole. *Am J Physiol* 1993;**265**:H2057–H2065.

33. Belenkie I, Dani R, Smith ER, Tyberg JV. Ventricular interaction during experimental acute pulmonary embolism. *Circulation* 1988;**78**:761–768.

34. Belenkie I, Dani R, Smith ER, Tyberg JV. Effects of volume loading during experimental acute pulmonary embolism. *Circulation* 1989;**80**:178–188.

35. Glantz SA, Parmley WW. Factors which affect the diastolic pressure-volume curve. *Circ Res* 1978;**42**:171–180.

36. Grant DA, Kondo CS, Maloney JE, Walker AM, Tyberg JV. Changes in pericardial pressure during the perinatal period. *Circulation* 1992;**86**:1615–1621.

37. Marini JJ, Culver BH, Butler J. Mechanical effect of lung distension with positive pressure on cardiac function. *Am Rev Respir Dis* 1980;**124**:382–386.

38. Butler J. The heart is in good hands. *Circulation* 1983;**67**:1163–1168.

39. Kingma I, Smiseth OA, Frais MA, Smith ER, Tyberg JV. Left ventricular external constraint: Relationship between pericardial, pleural and esophageal pressures during positive end-expiratory pressure and volume loading in dogs. *Ann Biomed Eng* 1987;**15**:331–346.

40. Grant DA, Kondo CS, Maloney JE, Tyberg JV. Pulmonary and pericardial limitations to diastolic filling of the left ventricle of the lamb. *Am J Physiol* 1994;**266**:H2327–H2333.

41. Esch BT, Scott JM, Haykowsky MJ, McKenzie DC, Warburton DE. Diastolic ventricular interactions in endurance-trained athletes during orthostatic stress. *Am J Physiol* 2007;**293**:H409–H415.

42. Dong S-J, Smith ER, Tyberg JV. Changes in the radius of curvature of the ventricular septum at end diastole during pulmonary arterial and aortic constrictions in the dog. *Circulation* 1992;**86**:1280–1290.

43. Mirsky I, Rankin JS. The effects of geometry, elasticity, and external pressures on the diastolic pressure-volume and stiffness-stress relations. How important is the pericardium? *Circ Res* 1979;**44**:601–611.

44. Baker AE, Belenkie I, Dani R, Smith ER, Tyberg JV. Quantitative assessment of the independent contributions of the pericardium and septum to direct ventricular interaction. *Am J Physiol* 1998;**275**:H476–H483.

45. Wang SY, Sheldon RS, Bergman DW, Tyberg JV. Effects of pericardial constraint on left ventricular mechanoreceptor activity in cats. *Circulation* 1995;**92**:3331–3336.

46. Stone JA, Wilkes PRH, Keane PM, Smith ER, Tyberg JV. Pericardial pressure attenuates release of atriopeptin in volume-expanded dogs. *Am J Physiol* 1989;**256**:H648–H654.

47. Vatner SF, Boettcher DH. Regulation of cardiac output by stroke volume and heart rate in conscious dogs. *Circ Res* 1978;**42**:557–561.

48. Boettcher DH, Vatner SF, Heyndrickx GR, Braunwald E. Extent of utilization of the Frank-Starling mechanism in conscious dogs. *Am J Physiol* 1978;**234**:H338–H345.

49. Parker JO, Case RB. Normal left ventricular function. *Circulation* 1979;**60**:4–12.

50. Linderer T, Chatterjee K, Parmley WW, Sievers RE, Glantz SA, Tyberg JV. Influence of atrial systole on the Frank-Starling relation and the end-diastolic pressure-diameter relation of the left ventricle. *Circulation* 1983;**67**:1045–1053.

51. Bleasdale RA, Turner MS, Mumford CE, *et al.* Left ventricular pacing minimizes diastolic ventricular interaction, allowing improved preload-dependent systolic performance. *Circulation* 2004;**110**:2395–2400.

52. Williams LK, Ellery S, Patel K, *et al.* Short-term hemodynamic effects of cardiac resynchronization therapy in patients with heart failure, a narrow QRS duration, and no dyssynchrony. *Circulation* 2009;**120**:1687–1694.

53. Smiseth OA, Russell K, Remme EW. Pacing in heart failure patients with narrow QRS: is there more to gain than resynchronization? *Circulation* 2009;**120**:1651–1653.

54. Cooper PJ, Lei M, Cheng LX, Kohl P. Axial stretch increases spontaneous pacemaker activity in rabbit isolated sinoatrial node cells. *J Appl Physiol* 2000;**89**:2099–2104.

55. Waxman MB, Cameron DA, Wald RW. Role of ventricular vagal afferents in the vasovagal reaction. *J Am Coll Cardiol* 1993;**21**:1138–1141.

56. Kohl P, Hunter P, Noble D. Stretch-induced changes in heart rate and rhythm: clinical observations, experiments and mathematical models. *Prog Biophys Mol Biol* 1999;**71**:91–138.

57. Ambrosi P, Habib G, Kreitmann B, Faugere G, Metras D. Valsalva manoeuvre for supraventricular tachycardia in transplanted heart recipient. *Lancet* 1995;**346**:713.

58. Little WC, Barr WK, Crawford MH. Altered effect of the Valsalva maneuver on left ventricular volume in patients with cardiomyopathy. *Circulation* 1985;**71**:227–233.

59. Ravelli F, Allessie M. Effects of atrial dilatation on refractory period and vulnerability to atrial fibrillation in the isolated Langendorff-perfused rabbit heart. *Circulation* 1997;**96**:1686–1695.

60. Bode F, Sachs F, Franz MR. Tarantula peptide inhibits atrial fibrillation. *Nature* 2001;**409**:35–36.

61. Renner U, Busch UW, Sebening H, et al. [Slow increase in the size of the left atrium with atrial fibrillation–a congenital pericardial defect or aneurysm of the left atrium?]. *Z Kardiol* 1987;**76**: 581–584.

62. Misthos P, Neofotistos K, Drosos P, Kokotsakis J, Lioulias A. Paroxysmal atrial fibrillation due to left atrial appendage herniation and review of the literature. *Int J Cardiol* 2009;**133**:e122–e124.

63. Howarth S, McMichael J, Sharpey-Schafer EP. Effects of venesection in low output heart failure. *Clin Sci* 1946;**6**:41–50.

64. Moore TD, Frenneaux MP, Sas R, et al. Ventricular interaction and external constraint account for decreased stroke work during volume loading in CHF. *Am J Physiol* 2001;**281**:H2385–H2391.

65. Atherton JJ, Moore TD, Lele SS, et al. Diastolic ventricular interaction in chronic heart failure. *Lancet* 1997;**349**:1720–1724.

66. Smiseth OA, Manyari DE, Lima JA, et al. Modulation of vascular capacitance by angiotensin and nitroprusside: a mechanism of changes in pericardial pressure. *Circulation* 1987;**76**:875–883.

67. Kingma I, Smiseth OA, Belenkie I, et al. A mechanism for the nitroglycerin-induced downward shift of the left ventricular diastolic pressure-diameter relationship of patients. *Am J Cardiol* 1986;**57**: 673–677.

68. Tyberg JV, Misbach GA, Parmley WW, Glantz SA. Effects of the pericardium on ventricular performance. In: *Cardiac Dynamics* (eds J Paan, EL Yellin, AC Arntzenius), The Hague, Boston: Martinus Nijhoff; 1980, pp. 159–168.

69. Alderman EL, Glantz SA. Acute hemodynamic interventions shift the diastolic pressure- volume curve in man. *Circulation* 1976;**54**:662–671.

70. Tyberg JV, Smith ER. Ventricular diastole and the role of the pericardium. *Herz* 1990;**15**:354–631.

71. Tyberg JV, Belenkie I. Mechanical interactions between the respiratory and circulatory systems. In: *Sleep Disorders and Cardiovascular and Cerebrovascular Disease* (eds. TD Bradley, JS Floras), New York: Marcel Dekker, Inc.; 2000, pp. 99–112.

72. Tyberg JV, Grant DA, Kingma I, Mitchell JR, Sun Y-H, Belenkie I. Effects of positive intrathoracic pressure on the evaluation of cardiac performance. In: *Proceedings of the Second Dresden Postgraduate Course on Mechanical Ventilation* (eds. MG de Abreu, T Koch), Lubeck: Drager Medical; 2001.

73. Tyberg JV. Mechanical modulation of cardiac function: role of the pericardium. In: *Cardiac Mechano-Electric Feedback & Arrhythmias: From Pipette to Patient* (eds. P Kohl, F Sachs, MR Franz), Elsevier (Saunders), Philadelphia, 2005, pp. 208–214.

Mechanically induced electrical remodelling in human atrium

Geoffrey Lee, Prashanthan Sanders, Joseph B. Morton and Jonathan M. Kalman

Background

In humans, both paroxysmal and chronic atrial fibrillation (AF) are frequently associated with structural heart disease. Common to many of the conditions associated with a high incidence of AF is the presence of atrial stretch or atrial dilatation. Such conditions include congestive heart failure, mitral valve disease and congenital heart diseases such as atrial septal defect. Despite this well-recognized clinical association, until recently little was known of the type of electrical remodelling associated with chronic atrial stretch in these conditions and the mechanism that leads to the development of AF.

Wijffels et al. initially described the concept that the atria remodel due to AF in a landmark study in conscious chronically instrumented goats[1]. These investigators observed that while induced AF was initially short lived, the artificial maintenance of AF resulted in progressive increase of its propensity to become sustained with time providing the seminal observation that 'AF begets AF'. This persistence of AF has been demonstrated to be associated with an abbreviation of the fibrillatory interval (FI) and the atrial effective refractory period (ERP), loss of rate adaptation, increased ERP heterogeneity and regional conduction slowing[2–5].

Remarkably similar and consistent observations have also been made in humans following the termination of chronic AF and flutter[6–9].

While the initial focus of atrial electrical remodelling was on the role of the atrial ERP, emerging data suggest that the development of structural changes of atrial fibrosis accompanied by conduction slowing is more important for the pathogenesis of chronic AF[10]. These chronic remodelling changes may occur as a result either of sustained atrial arrhythmias or of underlying processes such as those mediated by stretch.

As our understanding of the mechanisms underlying AF has grown over recent years, so has our appreciation of its heterogeneity. This is reflected by the diversity of pathophysiological processes and underlying conditions that create the substrate for the development of AF. While recent studies of atrial remodelling have emphasized the importance of rapid atrial rates, attention has also been directed toward the role of stretch and mechano-electric coupling. Atrial stretch appears to play a role in the development of AF in a wide spectrum of clinical conditions, ranging from the acute effects of supraventricular tachycardia (SVT) and myocardial infarction, to chronic conditions such as heart failure, mitral regurgitation, atrial septal defects and on-demand pacing with a single sensing and stimulating electrode in the right ventricle (VVI) pacing.

This chapter focuses on changes in atrial electrophysiology occurring as a result of atrial stretch and the importance of these changes in providing the electrophysiological substrate for AF.

Effects of acute atrial stretch on atrial electrophysiology

Studies in humans of the effects of acute atrial stretch have provided differing and sometimes confusing results. These differences may relate to the different methods of achieving atrial stretch in these studies, and the confounding effects of the population under study and the atrial rate. One method of achieving atrial stretch utilized simultaneous atrial and ventricular pacing. Calkins et al. reported that simultaneous atrioventricular pacing produced no change in atrial ERP at a drive cycle length of 400 ms in patients without structural heart disease, and they observed no increase in the frequency of AF induction[11]. However, the same group found a decrease in atrial ERP in response to acute changes in atrial pressure brought about by pacing just the final two beats of the drive train at an atrioventricular interval of 0 ms[12]. Tse et al. studied patients without structural heart disease and observed that simultaneous atrioventricular pacing caused atrial stretch and was associated with a decrease in right atrial (RA) ERP accompanied by an increased propensity to develop AF[13]. In contrast, Klein et al. demonstrated an increase in atrial ERP during pacing at a cycle length of 400 ms associated with an increase in atrial pressure occurring when the atrioventricular interval was decreased from 160 ms to 0 ms[14].

Other studies have also observed a non-uniform increase in atrial ERP in patients without structural heart disease due to an increase in atrial pressure associated with simultaneous atrio-ventricular pacing[15]. There was a significant increase in the atrial ERP measured at the distal coronary sinus and the posterior lateral RA but not at the RA appendage. As a result they observed an increase in the dispersion of ERP.

Antoniou *et al.* studied the effects of acute atrial stretch on the inducibility of AF in patients with a history of paroxysmal AF[16]. In these patients atrial stretch was induced by volume loading with 0.9% saline to double the RA pressure. While at low atrial pressure AF of >3 minutes was inducible in 3 of 16 patients, an increase of atrial pressure resulted in persistent AF in 10 patients.

Further studies have examined the impact of atrial stretch, brought about by rapid SVT with near simultaneous atrioventricular activation. While these studies may be confounded by the impact of a rapid rate, they mimic a real clinical situation where there is an increased risk of AF. Klein *et al.* observed an increase in RA ERP associated with an increase in RA pressure during SVT[14]. Similarly Chen *et al.* observed an increase in atrial ERP and dispersion of ERP with an increase in atrial pressure during supraventricular tachycardia[17]. Interestingly, these investigators observed a greater dispersion of ERP with acute atrial stretch in patients with a history of AF.

The reasons for the variable results in these studies on acute atrial stretch may relate to the different populations studied, the wide variation in atrial rates, failure to control for secondary autonomic effects, and the heterogeneous effects of stretch on regional atrial ERP. Indeed, an increase in ERP heterogeneity may be one factor in the pro-arrhythmic effect of atrial stretch.

At the cellular level, variable effects of acute mechanical stimulation on action potential duration (APD), for example by calcium handling-related APD shortening or stretch-activated ion channel-induced APD lengthening, may also contribute to apparently opposite effects of acute stretch on ERP. Acute stretch-induced AP repolarization crossover, where early APD is reduced and late APD is prolonged, is discussed in more detail in Chapters 14 and 22.

It is certainly striking that despite the variation in reported effects on ERP, all studies have demonstrated that acute atrial stretch results in an acute increase in AF inducibility.

Effects of chronic atrial stretch on atrial electrophysiology

In order to obtain information regarding the impact of chronic atrial stretch on atrial electrophysiology in humans it is necessary to study the effects of a variety of pathophysiological conditions, or situations that have in common the development of chronic atrial enlargement.

Asynchronous (VVI) pacing

An association between asynchronous ventricular pacing and an increased incidence of AF has been well established. In order to better understand the mechanism underlying this relationship, Sparks *et al.* studied the impact of long-term asynchronous ventricular pacing on the electrical properties and mechanical function of the atria[18,19]. This study was a prospective randomized comparison between 18 patients paced in the VVI mode and 12 patients paced in the DDD (synchronous atrioventricular pacing) mode for 3 months. After chronic VVI pacing, atrial ERP increased significantly in a non-uniform fashion at all sites evaluated (lateral RA, RA appendage, RA septum and distal coronary sinus). This was associated with prolongation of the P wave duration and sinus node remodelling. In a parallel study these authors demonstrated significant enlargement of the atria associated with

impairment of atrial mechanical function as evidenced by a decrease in emptying velocities and fractional area change in the left atrial (LA) appendage[19]. Importantly, these studies also documented that these changes associated with 3 months of VVI pacing could be reversed by 3 months of physiological (DDD) pacing.

Electrophysiological properties of the atria have been studied in a range of clinical conditions associated with atrial enlargement that provide further information on the substrate for AF.

Mitral stenosis

Mitral stenosis (MS) due to rheumatic heart disease is frequently complicated by the development of AF. While the incidence of this condition has diminished significantly in Western communities, it remains a significant illness in many countries worldwide. Fan *et al.* studied electrophysiological parameters in the RA of 31 patients with mitral valve stenosis at the time of percutaneous mitral commissurotomy[20]. Of these, 19 were in chronic AF and 12 in sinus rhythm at the time of the procedure. Following cardioversion of AF, these patients demonstrated significantly shortened atrial ERP, sinus node remodelling and no significant difference in atrial conduction delay to extra-stimuli compared to patients in sinus rhythm. At repeat study 3 months following mitral commissurotomy the atrial ERP had increased significantly from baseline to be comparable to patients who were in sinus rhythm. While this increase in ERP may be attributed to reversal of AF-induced remodelling, the study also observed an increase in ERP in the sinus rhythm group immediately following balloon valvuloplasty. This latter observation suggested that under circumstances of MS, atrial stretch might reversibly shorten the atrial ERP. There was no change in conduction delay in the AF group following valvuloplasty, but, interestingly, a significant decrease in delay was seen immediately after valvuloplasty in the sinus rhythm group, consistent with the hypothesis that atrial stretch may induce conduction delay. Whether additional, and irreversible, changes in conduction persist in the long term could not be evaluated in this study.

John and colleagues compared the bi-atrial electrophysiological properties of 24 patients with severe MS presenting for percutaneous balloon mitral commissurotomy with 24 control patients without MS[21]. Twelve patients in each group underwent multi-electrode studies with catheters placed in both atria to characterize atrial electrophysiology and AF inducibility. In a further 12 patients in each group, biatrial eletro-anatomical maps were created to determine conduction velocity and to identify regions of low voltage and scar. They found that compared to controls, patients with severe MS had prolonged P-wave duration and prolonged ERP in both the LA and RA. They also observed a reduction in conduction velocities in both atria and pronounced conduction delay along the *Crista terminalis*. AF was also more easily inducible in patients with severe MS. Electroanatomical mapping revealed LA dilatation with more frequent evidence of electrical scar in the MS group than normal control patients. Areas of low voltage and electrical silence suggest that severe MS is a process associated with a loss of atrial myocardium (Fig. 40.1).

In patients with rheumatic heart disease it would be expected that the disease itself might lead to regional fibrosis, causing conduction delay in addition to the effects of chronic stretch. The study by John *et al.* is consistent with this hypothesis, as MS disease progression is associated with conduction abnormalities such as

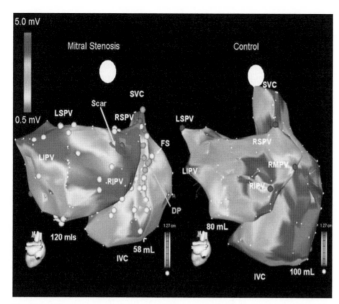

Fig. 40.1 Electroanatomical map of a patient with mitral stenosis (MS; left) and a representative control (right) (for voltage colour coding see scale bar in color plate section). The MS patient has an enlarged left atrium with extended regions of low voltage, inexcitable scar tissue and evidence of conduction abnormalities such as fractionated signals (FS) and double potentials (DP). [Reproduced, with permission, from John B, Stiles MK, Kuklik P, *et al.* (2008) Electrical remodelling of the left and right atria due to rheumatic mitral stenosis. *Eur Heart J* **29**:2234–2243] (See color plate section.)

regions of double potentials (DP), fractionated electograms, prolonged conduction times and P wave duration, and site-specific conduction delay, which parallel the progressive atrial structural changes. Although these abnormalities were seen in both atria, the extent was greater in the LA, suggesting that the substrate for AF in MS patients is related to both structural abnormalities and associated local conduction abnormalities.

Mitral regurgitation

Chronic mitral regurgitation (mR) is one of the most potent risk factors for the development of AF. In recent years a number of studies have provided an emerging picture of the substrate for AF in chronic AF. In a chronic canine model of AF, Verheule *et al* observed a homogeneous increase in LA and RA ERP[22]. Despite this, there was an increase in inducibility of sustained AF in the presence of areas of pathologically increased interstitial fibrosis and chronic inflammation.

Tieleman *et al.* measured atrial ERP in a heterogenous group of patients undergoing cardiac surgery: 15 with chronic AF, 16 with paroxysmal AF and 15 with no history of AF[23]. Of these, 22 had a history of mR. They report that mR was associated with prolongation of the atrial ERP irrespective of the underlying atrial rhythm compared to the patients without mR.

These data are consistent with preliminary data from our institution. We studied the electrophysiological characteristics of ten patients with severe mR due to mitral valve prolapse without prior AF, and compared these with ten age-matched controls. Patients with mR had significantly increased LA and RA volumes. These patients demonstrated an increase in atrial ERP at the RA septum

and in the distal coronary sinus (Fig. 40.2). However, there was an increase in the dispersion of ERP. In addition, patients with mR showed electrophysiological evidence of both significant regional conduction delay and prolongation of P wave duration.

In an attempt to further define the mechanism by which chronic stretch leads to AF, Roberts-Thomson *et al.* performed detailed epicardial mapping of the posterior LA in 23 patients at the time of cardiac surgery[24]. Patients investigated were divided into three groups: group A included those in sinus rhythm with normal left ventricular function undergoing coronary artery bypass surgery; group B consisted of patients in sinus rhythm with mR undergoing mitral valve surgery; group C patients were in persistent AF with mR undergoing mitral valve surgery.

Patients in each of the three groups demonstrated at least one line of functional delay in a constant anatomic location, which typically ran vertically in the posterior LA between the pulmonary veins. Patients with mR and AF (group C) demonstrated a greater number of lines of conduction delay compared to those with mR and no AF (group B) and those without mR (group A) (see Fig. 40.3). The greater number of lines of functional block resulted in markedly circuitous activation patterns in this region, which may promote the development of AF. However, it is unclear whether the increase in lines of functional block is a cause or a consequence of AF.

It is now widely recognized that rapid atrial rates produce shortening of the atrial ERP, contributing to the maintenance of AF[1]. In contrast, studies that examine conditions associated with chronic atrial dilation have usually observed prolonged refractoriness[19,22,25,26]. Consistent with these observations, this study demonstrated prolongation of atrial ERP on the posterior LA. This effect was abolished by superimposition of AF, suggesting that in patients with chronic atrial stretch, structural and conduction abnormalities are greater determinants of the predisposition to AF than alterations in ERP.

This study demonstrated that patients with both chronic stretch and AF have a greater degree of slow conduction and conduction heterogeneity in the posterior LA. There were no significant difference between groups B (mR) and C (AF-mR) in terms of severity of mR or in terms of LA or ventricular size, which indicates that at least some of the chronic remodelling occurred as a result of AF itself.

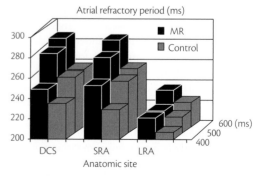

Fig. 40.2 Patients with chronic mitral regurgitation (MR) demonstrated increased ERP compared with control patients at the distal coronary sinus (DCS) and the septal right atrium (SRA) at all cycle lengths tested (400, 500 and 600 ms). LRA, low right atrium.

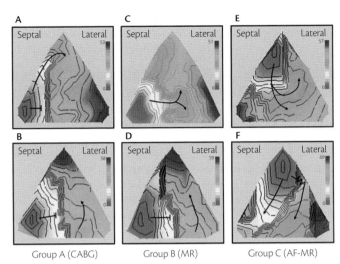

Group A (CABG)   Group B (MR)   Group C (AF-MR)

Fig. 40.3 Activation patterns on the posterior left atrium (LA) in patients from three different groups. Activation proceeds from *red* to *blue* (see color plate) with pacing from a corner of the plaque. Patients in group A (sinus rhythm, undergoing coronary artery bypass grafting, CABG) and group B (mitral regurgitation, MR) had one line of slow conduction, running vertically down the posterior LA between the pulmonary veins (**A–D**). Activation proceeded either around the line of conduction delay (**B, D**), through a gap in the line (**C**), or slowly across the line. Patients in group C (MR plus atrial fibrillation, AF) showed two (**E**) or more (**F**) lines of conduction delay with more complex patterns of activation across the LA. [Reproduced, with permission, from Roberts-Thomson K, Sanders P, Kalman J (2009) The role of chronic atrial stretch and atrial fibrillation on posterior left atrial wall conduction. *Heart Rhythm* **6**:1109–1117.] (See color plate section.)

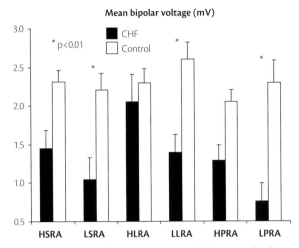

Fig. 40.4 Patients with CHF demonstrate lower atrial voltage amplitude in each of the six atrial regions mapped, when compared to control patients. HSRA, high septal right atrium; LSRA, low septal RA; HLRA, high lateral RA; LLRA, low lateral RA; HPRA, high posterior RA; LPRA, low posterior RA.

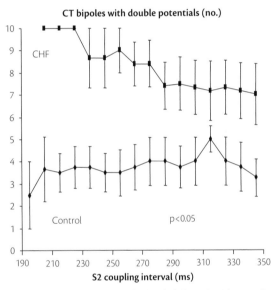

Fig. 40.5 A 20 pole mapping catheter (10 bipoles) along the *Crista terminalis* (CT) demonstrated that CHF patients had more bipoles showing double potentials (DP) than control patients, and that the number of bipoles with DP changed in inverse relationship to the S2 coupling interval.

Congestive heart failure

Congestive heart failure (CHF) is one of the most common conditions to be complicated by the development of AF, which occurs in up to 30% of patients during the course of the disease. Sanders *et al.* described the nature of atrial electrical remodelling in patients with advanced CHF. Twenty-one patients with CHF due to idiopathic or chronic ischaemic cardiomyopathy underwent electrophysiological and electroanatomical evaluation and were compared with 21 age-matched controls[25]. Patients with CHF had extensive electrophysiological abnormalities. They demonstrated structural and anatomic abnormalities as well, with extensive atrial regions of low voltage amplitude (Fig. 40.4) and areas of spontaneous electrical silence (scarring).

Together with, and possibly as a result of, these structural changes there was evidence of significantly impaired atrial conduction. Abnormalities of conduction were observed throughout the RA using both conventional and electroanatomical mapping techniques. There was also anatomically determined regional conduction delay at the *Crista terminalis* (Fig. 40.5). Furthermore, in contrast to the type of atrial remodelling seen in response to rapid atrial rates, patients with CHF did not demonstrate an abbreviation of the atrial ERP. Indeed in these patients there was an increase in ERP at all sites compared with the control group. There was no change in dispersion or the rate adaptation of ERP. These patients also demonstrated impairment of sinus node function. Perhaps as a consequence of the demonstrated electrophysiological abnormalities, these patients had an increased

propensity for AF and a significantly increased duration of induced AF.

This study suggests that the substrate for AF in patients with CHF may be predominantly due to the development of structural abnormalities and conduction delay, rather than changes in atrial ERP as occurs in remodelling due to rapid atrial rates.

Congenital heart disease, atrial septal defects, atrial stretch and atrial remodelling

The natural history of adults with an atrial septal defect (ASD) and chronic atrial volume overload is characterized by an increased risk for the development of atrial arrhythmias, which appears minimally affected by ASD closure. While surgical lines of block may form the substrate for 'scar-related' atrial macro-re-entry post-surgical ASD repair, the impact of chronic atrial stretch and volume overload on atrial electrophysiology in ASD patients has been the subject of study. Morton *et al.* studied the RA electrophysiological properties of 13 patients with haemodynamically significant ASD[26]. These patients demonstrated significant prolongation of the atrial ERP at the low lateral RA, high lateral RA and high septal RA. These changes in ERP were not associated with changes in the heterogeneity of ERP. Additionally, these patients demonstrated evidence of anatomically determined functional conduction delay at the *Crista terminalis*. Compared with age-matched controls, ASD patients had extensive and widely split double potentials recorded along the *Crista terminalis*. Conduction delay at this site increased with increasing pre-maturity during S_2 extra-stimulus testing. Importantly, when a proportion of the patients were restudied more than 6 months after ASD closure, these regional abnormalities of conduction persisted. The role of anisotropy and functional conduction delay at the *Crista terminalis* in a range of atrial arrhythmias has been extensively detailed. It has previously been shown that this structure plays an important role in the development of typical atrial flutter[27], atypical forms of flutter [such as lower loop re-entry[28]] and in AF[29,30].

Patients with an ASD had evidence of sinus node remodelling with significant prolongation of the corrected sinus node recovery time. The authors hypothesized that regional conduction delay formed the substrate for re-entry in patients with an ASD and had an important pro-arrhythmic effect despite modest increases in atrial ERP.

Importantly, this study also suggested that these regional conduction abnormalities, presumably a result of chronic atrial stretch and central to the development of an arrhythmia substrate, might not reverse when the underlying defect is corrected. Chen *et al.* studied ten patients with atrial dilatation and no history of atrial arrhythmias and found significantly longer atrial ERP compared to 20 control patients with normal atrial size[31].

Roberts-Thomson *et al.* extended the observations made by Morton by characterizing LA remodelling of patients with haemodynamically significant ASD[32]. LA electrical remodelling of 11 patients undergoing percutaneous closure of an ASD were compared with 12 control patients. Multipolar catheters were used to evaluate effective ERP at seven sites, P-wave duration, conduction time and inducibility of AF. In addition, electroanatomical maps were created to determine atrial activation and regional conduction voltage abnormalities from within the LA.

ERP at different LA sites were the same or prolonged in patients with ASD compared to control subjects. However, there was no difference in the heterogeneity of ERP (Fig. 40.6). Conduction time was significantly prolonged in patients with ASD, and in keeping with this finding the P-wave duration was significantly prolonged compared to controls.

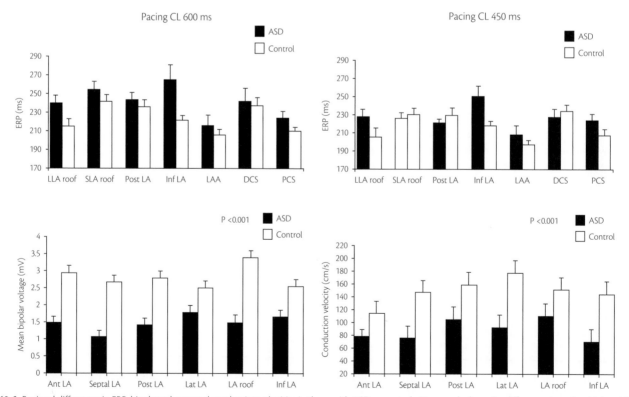

Fig. 40.6 Regional differences in ERP, bipolar voltages and conduction velocities in those with ASD vs controls. Top panels show the differences in regional left atrial (LA) refractoriness (effective refractory period, ERP) at a pacing cycle length (CL) of 600 ms (left) and 450 ms (right). Bottom panels show the differences in regional bipolar voltage (left) and regional conduction velocity (right). DCS, distal coronary sinus; Inf, inferior; LAA, LA appendage; LLA, lateral LA roof; PCS, proximal coronary sinus; SLA, septal LA roof; Ant, anterior; Post, posterior; Lat, lateral. [Reproduced, with permission, from Roberts-Thomson K, Sanders P, Kalman J (2009) Left atrial remodeling in patients with atrial septal defects. *Heart Rhythm* **6**:1000–1006.]

Structural and voltage mapping revealed that patients with ASD had significantly greater LA volumes compared to controls. Mean LA bipolar voltages were significantly reduced (Fig. 40.7), as was the relative surface area of the LA that showed low voltage (≤ 0.5 mV) in patients with ASD compared with controls (15.7% vs 3.9%). This was associated with a greater degree of voltage heterogeneity. Mapped potentials were significantly lower at all LA sites in ASD patients (Fig. 40.6). In addition, scar areas (defined as bipolar voltage < 0.05 mV) were only seen in ASD (6 of 11 patients), preferentially in the posterior wall of the LA. These changes were accompanied by an increased inducibilty of sustained AF. Patients with ASD developed sustained episodes of AF (> 5 min) more frequently than control patients with single extra stimuli (4 of 11 ASD patients vs 0 of 12 control patients). In addition AF persisted and required electrical cardioversion to revert back to sinus rhythm.

This study shows that patients with haemodynamically significant ASD show evidence of pronounced LA remodelling, characterized by atrial enlargement, regions of low voltage and areas of electrical scarring, with associated widespread conduction abnormalities but with either no change or increased atrial refractoriness.

Structural remodelling, AF and the coexistence of sinus node dysfunction

The above studies have shed new light on the nature of structural remodelling associated with chronic atrial enlargement, whether it was due to volume overload, cardiac failure or related to valvular pathology.

The extensive atrial pathology observed in these patients suggests that there may be a mechanism that couples AF and sinus node dysfunction (SND). That is, the primary pathological process leads to diffuse structural and functional abnormalities. These then cause loss of functioning atrial myocardium and slowed conduc-tion. This process thus not only creates the substrate for AF, but also may contribute to sinus node pacemaker dysfunction.

Sanders et al. hypothesized that given the widely distributed nature of the functional sinus pacemaker complex[33] and the frequent association of SND and AF, patients with SND would necessarily have widespread atrial abnormalities[34]. They compared electrophysiological and electroanatomical properties of atria in 16 patients with symptomatic SND with 16 age-matched controls. Patients with SND demonstrated very similar atrial remodelling to that seen in patients with conditions of chronic atrial stretch. The SND patients showed a significant increase in atrial ERP without changes in the heterogeneity of ERP; a slowing of atrial conduction, and evidence of anatomically determined conduction delay at the *Crista terminalis*. Electroanatomical mapping demonstrated the sinus node complex in SND patients was a localized structure, frequently in the region of the low *Crista terminalis*, which corresponds to the site of the largest residual voltage amplitude on voltage mapping. Elsewhere in the atrium, and particularly along the long axis of the original pacemaker complex, there were significant areas of low voltage and electrical silence (or scarring). Induced AF persisted for longer, or became sustained, in patients with SND. These electrophysiological abnormalities resemble those seen in conditions of chronic atrial stretch. Why these patients developed such changes in the absence of chronic stretch is unknown, but it is worthwhile to briefly examine the nature of atrial remodelling that occurs with ageing.

Age and atrial remodelling

Advancing age is one of the most significant predictors for the development of AF. It is detected in 3–4% of the population over age 60 years and has a prevalence of almost 9% in octogenarians. Kistler et al. described the electrophysiological and electroanatomical remodelling that occurs with age[35]. Patients without atrial arrhythmias underwent RA mapping and data were stratified according to age group (< 30 years, 30–60 years and > 60 years). Aging was associated with an increase in atrial refractoriness and both generalized and anatomically determined conduction slowing. Electroanatomical mapping revealed diffuse areas of low voltage which were associated with regional conduction slowing. There was a significant age-related increase in sites showing fractionation and double potentials, particularly in the region of the *Crista terminalis*. These changes also resembled those seen with chronic stretch, although they were less severe and consistent with the development of atrial fibrosis, which has been found in pathological studies of aging.

Stretch-related triggers

While this chapter has discussed the role of stretch in development of the atrial substrate required to sustain multiple wavelet re-entry, the triggers that initiate the process may also have a relationship to stretch. The most common anatomic location for these triggers are the pulmonary veins[36]. However, while clinical impression suggests that sudden changes in venous return may stimulate these triggers, by producing pulmonary venous stretch, definitive data are lacking (see also Chapters 15 and 29).

There have been a number of recent studies describing the electrophysiological features of pulmonary vein musculature, and showing how these sleeves of tissue may contribute to the development of AF. Hocini et al. using canine pulmonary veins found

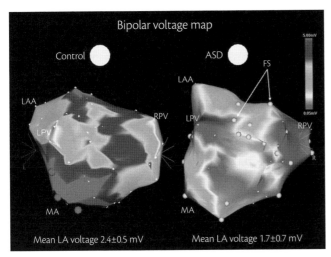

Fig. 40.7 Bipolar voltage maps of the left atrium (LA) projected in the posterior–anterior view. On the right is a representative map of a patient with ASD, and on the left a control patient. The ASD patient shows significantly lower voltages, particularly on the posterior LA, associated with fractionated signals (FS). [Reproduced, with permission, from Roberts-Thomson K, Sanders P, Kalman J (2009) Left atrial remodeling in patients with atrial septal defects. *Heart Rhythm* **6**:1000–1006.] (See color plate section.)

significant conduction delay within the pulmonary veins. This was correlated with myocardial fibre orientation, producing non-uniform anisotropy and fractionated electrograms[37]. Clinically, this is also apparent in patients with paroxysmal AF. They demonstrate decremented conduction to and from the atrium, with documentation of long fractionated electrograms in close juxtaposition to sharp spikes within the pulmonary veins[38,39]. Chen *et al.* have demonstrated delayed and early after-depolarizations following rapid atrial pacing of isolated myocytes from canine pulmonary veins, and hypothesized that triggered automaticity may be the mechanism underlying these rapidly firing foci[40,41].

However, while these studies have advanced our understanding of pulmonary vein electrophysiology, a link between the above observations and the role of *in vivo* atrial stretch remains to be further elucidated. Clinical studies have suggested that patients with pulmonary vein ectopy initiating AF have significantly dilated pulmonary veins compared to controls. This suggests a possible contribution of anatomic remodelling and stretch in predisposing the pulmonary vein to become arrhythmogenic[42,43]. By altering pulmonary vein diameter, chronic atrial stretch may change the wavelength and facilitate the development of re-entry within pulmonary venous muscle bundles. Acute stretch may have similar effects, but might also result in stretch-induced calcium-mediated after-depolarizations.

It is quite possible that atrial stretch contributes to the development of AF, not only by modifying substrate but also by initiating the triggers.

Conclusions and outlook

Studies in humans of chronic atrial stretch have consistently demonstrated an unchanged or prolonged atrial ERP, which is likely to prolong the atrial wavelength and, theoretically, should protect against the development of AF. As such, these studies have alluded to the important contribution of other factors to the substrate for AF. These factors include structural abnormalities, such as interstitial fibrosis and an apparently progressive loss of functioning atrial myocardium. Associated with these abnormalities is significant generalized conduction slowing, which may also be focused in certain anatomic regions. These changes, which may be stretch related or reflect the primary pathophysiological processes, do not appear to be reversible once significant structural change has developed.

Although we have discussed the important electrophysiological changes that result from chronic atrial stretch and left atrial remodelling in the pathogenesis of AF, the underlying molecular mechanism by which these changes occur is not fully understood. Recent studies have suggested a molecular link between atrial fibrosis, structural remodelling and electrical remodelling. Adam *et al.* found that the LA of patients with AF was characterized by an increased tissue concentration of angiotensin II and increased expression of collagen and connective tissue growth factor (CTGF)[44]. The activation of CTGF via the small G protein Rac-1 led to increased production of adherens junctional protein, N-cadherin and gap junction protein connexion 43. Both are considered to be important mediators of signal transduction within the LA. Further characterization of the molecular signalling pathways involved in atrial fibrosis and resultant left atrial remodelling is needed. Future research in this area may potentially lead to the development of novel pharmacological drugs for the prevention and treatment of AF.

References

1. Wijffels MC, Kirchhof CJ, Dorland R, Allessie MA. Atrial fibrillation begets atrial fibrillation. A study in awake chronically instrumented goats. *Circulation* 1995;**92**:1954–1968.

2. Fareh S, Villemaire C, Nattel S. Importance of refractoriness heterogeneity in the enhanced vulnerability to atrial fibrillation induction caused by tachycardia- induced atrial electrical remodeling. *Circulation* 1998;**98**:2202–2209.

3. Gaspo R, Bosch RF, Talajic M, Nattel S. Functional mechanisms underlying tachycardia-induced sustained atrial fibrillation in a chronic dog model. *Circulation* 1997;**96**:4027–4035.

4. Morillo CA, Klein GJ, Jones DL, Guiraudon CM. Chronic rapid atrial pacing. Structural, functional, and electrophysiological characteristics of a new model of sustained atrial fibrillation. *Circulation* 1995;**91**: 1588–1595.

5. Morton JB, Byrne MJ, Power JM, Raman J, Kalman JM. Electrical remodeling of the atrium in an anatomic model of atrial flutter: relationship between substrate and triggers for conversion to atrial fibrillation. *Circulation* 2002;**105**:258–264.

6. Kamalvand K, Tan K, Lloyd G, Gill J. Alterations in atrial lectrophysiology associated with chronic atrial fibrillation in man. *Eur Heart J* 1999;**20**:888–895.

7. Kumagai K, Akimitsu S, Kawahira K, Kawanami F, Yamanouchi Y, Hiroki T, Arakawa K. Electrophysiological properties in chronic lone atrial fibrillation. *Circulation* 1991;**84**:1662–1668.

8. Sparks PB, Jayaprakash S, Vohra JK, Kalman JM. Electrical remodeling of the atria associated with paroxysmal and chronic atrial flutter. *Circulation* 2000;**102**:1807–1813.

9. Yu WC, Lee SH, Tai CT, *et al.* Reversal of atrial electrical remodeling following cardioversion of long-standing atrial fibrillation in man. *Cardiovasc Res* 1999;**42**:470–476.

10. Allessie M, Ausma J, Schotten U. Electrical, contractile and structural remodeling during atrial fibrillation. *Cardiovasc Res* 2002;**54**:230–246.

11. Calkins H, el-Atassi R, Leon A, Kalbfleisch S, Borganelli M, Langberg J, Morady F. Effect of the atrioventricular relationship on atrial refractoriness in humans. *Pacing Clin Electrophysiol* 1992;**15**:771–778.

12. Calkins H, el-Atassi R, Kalbfleisch S, Langberg J, Morady F. Effects of an acute increase in atrial pressure on atrial refractoriness in humans. *Pacing Clin Electrophysiol* 1992;**15**:1674–1680.

13. Tse HF, Pelosi F, Oral H, Knight BP, Strickberger SA, Morady F. Effects of simultaneous atrioventricular pacing on atrial refractoriness and atrial fibrillation inducibility: role of atrial mechano-electric feedback. *J Cardiovasc Electrophysiol* 2001;**12**:43–50.

14. Klein LS, Miles WM, Zipes DP. Effect of atrioventricular interval during pacing or reciprocating tachycardia on atrial size, pressure, and refractory period. Contraction–excitation feedback in human atrium. *Circulation* 1990;**82**:60–68.

15. Chen YJ, Tai CT, Chiou CW, Wen ZC, Chan P, Lee SH, Chen SA. Inducibility of atrial fibrillation during atrioventricular pacing with varying intervals: role of atrial electrophysiology and the autonomic nervous system. *J Cardiovasc Electrophysiol* 1999;**10**:1578–1585.

16. Antoniou A, Milonas D, Kanakakis J, Rokas S, Sideris DA. Contraction–excitation feedback in human atrial fibrillation. *Clin Cardiol* 1997;**20**:473–476.

17. Chen YJ, Chen SA, Tai CT, Wen ZC, Feng AN, Ding YA, Chang MS. Role of atrial electrophysiology and autonomic nervous system in patients with supraventricular tachycardia and paroxysmal atrial fibrillation. *J Am Coll Cardiol* 1998;**32**:732–738.

18. Sparks PB, Mond HG, Vohra JK, Jayaprakash S, Kalman JM. Electrical remodeling of the atria following loss of atrioventricular synchrony: a long-term study in humans. *Circulation* 1999;**100**:1894–1900.

19. Sparks PB, Mond HG, Vohra JK, Yapanis AG, Grigg LE, Kalman JM. Mechanical remodeling of the left atrium after loss of atrioventricular synchrony. A long-term study in humans. *Circulation* 1999;**100**: 1714–1721.

20. Fan K, Lee KL, Chow WH, Chau E, Lau CP. Internal cardioversion of chronic atrial fibrillation during percutaneous mitral commissurotomy: insight into reversal of chronic stretch-induced atrial remodeling. *Circulation* 2002;**105**:2746–2752.

21. John B, Stiles MK, Kuklik P, *et al.* Electrical remodelling of the left and right atria due to rheumatic mitral stenosis. *Eur Heart J* 2008; **29**:2234–2243.

22. Verheule S, Wilson EE, Everett T 4th, Shanbhag S, Golden C, Olgin J. Alterations in atrial electrophysiology and tissue structure in a canine model of chronic atrial dilatation due to mitral regurgitation. *Circulation* 2003;**107**:2615–2622.

23. Tieleman RG, Van Gelder IC, Brundel BJJM, *et al.* Mitral regurgitation is associated with prolongation of the atrial refractory period. *Circulation* 2002;**106**:II–370.

24. Roberts-Thomson K, Sanders P, Kalman J. The role of chronic atrial stretch and atrial fibrillation on posterior left atrial wall conduction. *Heart Rhythm* 2009;**6**:1109–1117.

25. Sanders P, Morton JB, Davidson NC, Spence SJ, Vohra JK, Sparks PB, Kalman JM. Electrical remodeling of the atria in congestive heart failure: electrophysiologic and electroanatomic mapping in humans. *Circulation* 2003;**108**:1461–1468.

26. Morton JB, Sanders P, Vohra JK, *et al.* The effect of chronic atrial stretch on atrial electrical remodeling in patients with an atrial septal defect. *Circulation* 2003;**107**:1775–1782.

27. Olgin JE, Kalman JM, Fitzpatrick AP, Lesh MD. Role of right atrial endocardial structures as barriers to conduction during human type I atrial flutter. Activation and entrainment mapping guided by intracardiac echocardiography. *Circulation* 1995;**92**:1839–1848.

28. Cheng J, Cabeen WR, Jr., Scheinman MM. Right atrial flutter due to lower loop reentry: mechanism and anatomic substrates. *Circulation* 1999;**99**:1700–1705.

29. Cox JL, Canavan TE, Schuessler RB, *et al.* The surgical treatment of atrial fibrillation. II. Intraoperative electrophysiologic mapping and description of the electrophysiologic basis of atrial flutter and atrial fibrillation. *J Thorac Cardiovasc Surg* 1991;**101**:406–426.

30. Liu TY, Tai CT, Chen SA. Treatment of atrial fibrillation by catheter ablation of conduction gaps in the Crista terminalis and cavotricuspid isthmus of the right atrium. *J Cardiovasc Electrophysiol* 2002;**13**: 1044–1046.

31. Chen YJ, Chen SA, Tai CT, Yu WC, Feng AN, Ding YA, Chang MS. Electrophysiologic characteristics of a dilated atrium in patients with paroxysmal atrial fibrillation and atrial flutter. *J Interv Card Electrophysiol* 1998;**2**:181–186.

32. Roberts-Thomson K, Sanders P, Kalman J. Left atrial remodeling in patients with atrial septal defects. *Heart Rhythm* 2009;**6**:1000–1006.

33. Boineau JP, Canavan TE, Schuessler RB, Cain ME, Corr PB, Cox JL. Demonstration of a widely distributed atrial pacemaker complex in the human heart. *Circulation* 1988;**77**:1221–1237.

34. Sanders P, Morton JB, Spence SJ, *et al.* Electrophysiologic and electroanatomic characterization of the atria in sinus node disease: Evidence of diffuse atrial remodeling. *Circulation* 2004;**109**:1514–1522.

35. Kistler P, Sanders P, Fynn SP, *et al.* Electrophysiologic and electroanatomic changes in the atrium associated with age. *J Am Coll Cardiol* 2004;**44**:109–116.

36. Haissaguerre M, Jais P, Shah DC, *et al.* Spontaneous initiation of atrial fibrillation by ectopic beats originating in the pulmonary veins. *N Engl J Med.* 1998;**339**:659–666.

37. Hocini M, Ho SY, Kawara T, *et al.* Electrical conduction in canine pulmonary veins: electrophysiological and anatomic correlation. *Circulation* 2002;**105**:2442–2448.

38. Tada H, Oral H, Ozaydin M, *et al.* Response of pulmonary vein potentials to premature stimulation. *J Cardiovasc Electrophysiol* 2002;**13**:33–37.

39. Jais P, Hocini M, Macle L, *et al.* Distinctive Electrophysiological Properties of Pulmonary Veins in Patients With Atrial Fibrillation. *Circulation* 2002;**106**:2479–2485.

40. Chen YJ, Chen SA, Chen YC, Yeh HI, Chan P, Chang MS, Lin CI. Effects of rapid atrial pacing on the arrhythmogenic activity of single cardiomyocytes from pulmonary veins: implication in initiation of atrial fibrillation. *Circulation* 2001;**104**:2849–2854.

41. Chen YJ, Chen SA, Chang MS, Lin CI. Arrhythmogenic activity of cardiac muscle in pulmonary veins of the dog: implication for the genesis of atrial fibrillation. *Cardiovasc Res* 2000;**48**:265–273.

42. Lin WS, Prakash VS, Tai CT, *et al.* Pulmonary vein morphology in patients with paroxysmal atrial fibrillation initiated by ectopic beats originating from the pulmonary veins: implications for catheter ablation. *Circulation* 2000;**101**:1274–1281.

43. Tsao HM, Yu WC, Cheng HC, *et al.* Pulmonary vein dilation in patients with atrial fibrillation: detection by magnetic resonance imaging. *J Cardiovasc Electrophysiol* 2001;**12**:809–813.

44. Adam O, Lavall D, Laufs U, *et al.* Rac-1 induced connective tissue growth factor regulates connexin 43 and N-cadherin expression in atrial fibrillation. *J Am Coll Cardiol* 2010;**55**:469–480.

Drug effects and atrial fibrillation: potential and limitations

Jurren M. van Opstal, Yuri Blaauw and Harry J.G.M. Crijns

Background

Atrial fibrillation (AF) is the most common sustained arrhythmia and occurs in the setting of specific structural and electrophysiological changes in the atria that contribute to the perpetuation of the arrhythmia. These alterations are termed 'atrial remodelling'[1].

Atrial remodelling can involve changes in the function and distribution of cardiac ion channels (electrical remodelling) or changes in atrial tissue architecture, particularly interstitial fibrosis and atrial dilatation (structural remodelling). Most often, structural and electrical remodelling co-exist.

While remodelling provides a substrate to maintain AF, triggers that initiate the arrhythmia may originate from the pulmonary veins[2], or relate to Ca^{2+} handling abnormalities associated with the arrhythmia[3] or with underlying AF-promoting conditions such as systemic hypertension and chronic heart failure[4]. In addition to remodelling, related to underlying cardiac conditions, AF itself causes changes that play a significant role in AF pathophysiology (AF begets AF; see also Chapter 28)[5].

Despite advances in ablation therapy, antiarrhythmic drug therapy will remain a cornerstone in the treatment and prevention of AF.

This chapter discusses the different remodelling and electromechanical coupling processes in AF and the various potentials of antiarrhythmic and upstream therapies related to these processes.

Electrical remodelling

In a landmark study in conscious chronically instrumented goats, Wijffels et al.[5] were the first to propose the concept that the atria remodel as a result of AF. These investigators observed that after artificial maintenance of AF the propensity of the arrhythmia to become sustained increased markedly. This persistence of AF has been demonstrated to be associated with an abbreviation of the fibrillatory interval and the atrial effective refractory period (AERP), loss of rate adaptation, increased ERP heterogeneity and regional conduction slowing. These phenomena are the main constituents of electrical remodelling.

The AF-induced fast atrial rate may cause a large increase in intracellular Na^+ relative to Ca^{2+} and switch the Na^+/Ca^{2+} exchanger (NCX) into the reverse mode and shorten the action potential[6]. Furthermore, increased intracellular Ca^{2+} concentrations and abnormalities in Ca^{2+} handling have been linked to initiation of AF by promoting delayed and late phase III early after-depolarizations sufficient to initiate ectopic activation[7,8]. These changes usually occur (sub)acutely and are mostly reversible. Apart from high atrial rate, also stretch at normal atrial rate is associated with short-term electrical remodelling (see section on 'Electromechanical coupling' below).

The sustained shortening of atrial action potential duration (APD) was found to be due to downregulation of L-type Ca^{2+} current[9,10], and an increase in inward rectifier K^+ currents such as the background current (I_{K1}) and the constitutively activated acetylcholine-regulated current ($I_{K,ACh}$)[11]. The transient outward current (I_{to}) and ultra-rapid-delayed rectifier (I_{Kur}) are also decreased in atrial myocytes isolated from patients with permanent AF[12–14]. However, the rapid and slow components of the delayed rectifier K^+ currents, I_{Kr} and I_{Ks}, were not altered in dog myocytes subjected to atrial tachycardia[10].

A recent study showed that in patients with lone AF and a polymorphism in the angiotensin-converting enzyme (ACE) gene who may be exposed to higher angiotensin II levels, electrical remodelling, specifically a prolonged PR interval and heart block, was present. The authors, however, could not exclude that underlying structural remodelling formed the basis for these findings[15].

Structural remodelling

Several studies have shown that atrial fibrosis plays an important role in the induction and continuation of AF. Atrial fibrosis causes intra- and interatrial inhomogeneity in conduction, thus creating a substrate for local re-entry[16–19]. Atrial stretch associated with AF increases local synthesis of angiotensin II and initiates a cascade of phosphorylation processes that activate mitogen-activated protein kinases. Mitogen-activated protein kinases promote atrial myocyte hypertrophy, fibroblast proliferation and accumulation of collagen.

Atrial interstitial fibrosis can lead to non-uniform anisotropy in conduction[20]. In addition, angiotensin II modifies atrial electrophysiology by indirect effects on ion channels, increases Ca^{2+} influx, promotes inflammation and may also impair cell-to-cell coupling associated with gap junctional remodelling[21]. There is evidence that links an absence of connexin 40 (Cx40) to enhanced atrial vulnerability and increased risk of AF attributable to increased dispersion of refractoriness[22].

Other factors likely to be involved in structural remodelling are oxidative stress and inflammation. Mihm et al.[23] investigated oxidative stress and energetic impairment in myofibrils in right atrial appendage biopsies of patients with chronic AF. The formation of peroxynitrite was used as a parameter of oxidative stress. During periods of high oxidative stress, loss of nitric oxide control occurs and peroxynitrite is formed. This may result in selective nitration of protein tyrosine residues and disruption of cellular energetic control resulting in contractile dysfunction[24].

Electromechanical coupling

A unifying feature of many conditions which lead to the development of AF has been that of atrial stretch. Atrial dilatation may produce electrophysiological effects on the atria by mechano-electrical coupling which involves stretch-activated channels[25]. These include non-specific channels[26] and channels that are selective to potassium or chloride ions. Such mechanical gradients caused by stretch can induce electrical gradients, resulting in increased automaticity. Additionally, atrial stretch causes the AERP to shorten and conduction to slow, which provides a substrate for functional re-entry. Stretch, when applied continuously, is also involved in structural remodelling by inducing fibrosis and thereby producing anisotropic conduction[27].

The importance of triggers for the development of AF is well recognized. The pulmonary veins have consistently been observed to be the dominant source of these triggers. Although many studies have explored the consequences of stretch in the atria, the effects of stretch on the pulmonary veins is largely unknown. In clinical studies it has been suggested that patients with AF have significantly dilated pulmonary veins compared with control subjects[28]. Chronic atrial stretch by altering pulmonary vein diameter may change the wavelength and facilitate the development of re-entry within pulmonary venous muscle bundles. Acute stretch may have similar effects but might also result in stretch-induced, Ca^{2+}-mediated after-depolarizations[8].

Upstream therapy

Because of the adverse effects and limited efficacy of conventional antiarrhythmic agents, research has focused not only on new antiarrhythmic agents, but also on efforts to prevent development of the AF substrate[29].

Angiotensin receptor antagonists and ACE inhibitors

Drugs interfering with the renin–angiotensin system were among the first non-antiarrhythmic compounds tested with respect to their potential efficacy for AF prevention. Experimental studies have shown that inhibition of angiotensin-related signalling pathways ameliorates the AF substrate[30]. These effects are associated with suppression of the conduction abnormalities caused by atrial fibrosis. The potential mechanisms include haemodynamic, antiproliferative, anti-inflammatory and antioxidant effects that may prevent the development of atrial stretch and enlargement, thereby reducing the development of interstitial fibrosis and adverse atrial electrical remodelling. Clinically, retrospective analyses of classical trials[31,32] that evaluated ACE inhibitors for indications such as hypertension, heart failure and coronary artery disease post-MI indicate protective effects of ACE-inhibitor treatment with respect to AF development[33]. Data from the LIFE (Losartan Intervention For End point reduction in hypertension) trial demonstrated reductions in AF occurrence for losartan- versus atenolol-treated patients[34]. Retrospective analysis of rhythm-control patients within AFFIRM (Atrial Fibrillation Follow-up Investigation of Rhythm Management) indicated fewer AF relapses in ACE-inhibitor treated patients with heart failure[35]. This has been prospectively addressed by adding irbesartan to amiodarone treatment after electrical cardioversion, leading to reduced AF recurrences in irbesartan-treated patients[36]. This effect happened in the first month after electrical cardioversion suggesting that the protection against AF occurs in the short phase of reversed remodelling after conversion, a period known for its high arrhythmogenicity. However, the recently completed GISSI-AF (Gruppo Italiano per lo Studio della Sopravvivenza nell'Infarto Miocardico) trial failed to confirm benefit in AF of the addition of the angiotensin-II receptor blocker valsartan to conventional management, including amiodarone and ACE inhibitors[37]. It should be noted, however, that this trial was a study of secondary prevention of AF (i.e. prevention of recurrent AF). It is possible that irbesartan failed to provide protective effects in this group of patients because these drugs might prevent but not reverse the development of the substrate for AF. Another possible explanation could be that genetic variations [e.g. ACE inhibitor polymorphism[15]] may modulate the response to ACE inhibitors and angiotensin receptor blockers (ARB). This may account for the fact that some patients respond favourably to these agents for prevention of AF and others do not[38].

Preclinical studies suggest that aldosterone antagonists may prevent AF[39]. However, at present, trials of aldosterone antagonists in patients susceptible to AF and impaired left ventricular function are not yet available.

3-Hydroxy-3-methylglutaryl coenzyme A reductase inhibitors (statins)

Atrial tissue fibrosis is particularly important in the pathophysiology of AF associated with heart failure. Experimental data indicate effective reduction in CHF-related structural remodelling and AF promotion by simvastatin. In addition, simvastatin improved haemodynamic function and inhibited atrial fibroblast activation[40]. Clear evidence of corresponding clinical benefit is lacking, but the inherent anti-inflammatory properties of statin therapy may confer protection against AF in some subgroups, particularly patients undergoing cardiothoracic surgery[41]. The recent subanalysis of GISSI-HF showed a minor benefit of statins for the—mainly primary—prevention of AF in heart failure patients[42]. Currently, several ongoing prospective randomized controlled trials have been designed to assess the antiarrhythmic value of statins. The contradicting results of clinical data, however, do not allow recommending statins for prevention of AF at this point in time.

Antifibrotic therapy

Pirfenidone is a newly developed antifibrotic agent which inhibits collagen synthesis, downregulates production of profibrotic cytokines and blocks cytokine-induced fibroblast proliferation. The antiarrhythmic potential of pirfenidone has recently been shown in a canine model of heart failure induced by rapid ventricular pacing[43]. Pirfenidone reduced the amount of mitogen-activated protein kinases which mediate the effects of angiotensin II at the tissue level and also modified the expression of matrix degrading enzymes [matrix metalloproteinases (MMP)] and their endogenous inhibitors.

An imbalance between expression of MMP and their natural tissue inhibitors plays an important role in extracellular matrix remodelling associated with AF. As such, an increase in MMP activity can induce matrix degradation and lead to dilatation, whereas a decrease can reduce the extracellular matrix breakdown and lead to fibrosis[44,45].

Stretch receptor antagonists

The non-selective stretch-activated channel blocker gadolinium prevented burst-pacing-mediated induction of AF and suppressed the occurrence of spontaneous AF during increased atrial pressures in isolated rabbit hearts, whereas in the absence of gadolinium, AF could be induced[46]. GsMTx-4, a 35-amino acid peptide toxin, which was isolated from the venom of the Chilean Rose tarantula *Grammostola spatulata* in 2000, is a selective and potent blocker of cationic stretch-activated channels. GsMTx-4 has been shown to prevent inducibility of AF in the rabbit atria without any measurable effect on the duration and shape of the atrial action potential[47]. In the presence of GsMTx-4, induction of AF was possible only at significantly higher atrial pressures compared with control preparations.

Gap junction modulators

Gap junction organization is a critical component of cell-to-cell coupling and rapid myocardial conduction. Alteration of gap junction kinetics or cellular distribution slows conduction velocity and is arrhythmogenic[48-50]. Drugs that enhance gap junction conduction may prove to be a novel tool for treating atrial arrhythmias. For example, during atrial ischaemia and acidosis, alteration in gap junction kinetics slows conduction velocity and thereby promotes AF[48]. Rotigaptide is a stable peptide analogue that maintains myocardial conduction velocity during metabolic stress such as ischaemia and acidosis[51]. In models of AF, rotigaptide improves conduction and suppresses AF in the setting of acute ischaemia. In contrast, rotigaptide does not appear to play a role in AF suppression in CHF or atrial tachypacing remodelling[52]. Despite the potential niche in treating arrhythmias, e.g. in patients with mutations in the connexion gene(s), rotigaptide and other peptide analogues have a significant practical limitation: poor oral bioavailability due to presystemic enzymatic degradation and inadequate mucosal penetration[53].

Conventional antiarrhythmic drug therapy

When considering a rhythm control strategy it is important to realize that there is no evidence that maintenance of sinus rhythm is associated with improved survival[54,55]. Therefore the main goal of antiarrhythmic drug treatment is to alleviate symptomatic AF episodes. Antiarrhythmic drugs are classified according to the Vaughan Williams classification. Based on their electrophysiological action on normal myocardium these agents can be divided into four different categories. For cardioversion of AF both class I and class III drugs have been shown to be effective.

Class IC drugs (e.g. flecainide, propafenone) exert their antiarrhythmic effect by slowing of conduction by blockade of the fast Na^+ channels. The mechanism underlying AF termination is incompletely understood, but it has been suggested that as a result of Na^+ channel blockade, myocardial excitability is reduced which causes preferential depression of conduction of fibrillation wavelets with a strong curvature[56]. The arrhythmia will then become more organized, the number of circulating wavelets decreases and eventually the arrhythmia extinguishes.

A second mechanism of the efficacy of Na^+ channel blockers could be the counteraction of the transient rise in Na^+ entry into atrial myocytes during the fast atrial rate. Cytosolic Na^+ accumulation is believed to worsen myocardial injury mainly as a result of increased Ca^{2+} entry through sarcolemmal NCX[57]. Cytosolic Ca^{2+} overload, which also induces increased Ca^{2+} entry through L-type Ca^{2+} channels, leads to mitochondrial Ca^{2+} overload, which can worsen cell injury by disrupting mitochondrial function[58,59]. Cytosolic Ca^{2+} overload can also favour reperfusion arrhythmias through delayed after-depolarizations[60,61]. Interestingly, Iwai et al.[62] reported that cytosolic Na^+ overload may directly alter mitochondrial function by depolarizing its inner membrane and reducing the rate of oxidative phosphorylation.

Currently available class III drugs (e.g. sotalol, dofetilide) prolong the atrial refractory period by predominantly blocking the I_{Kr}. During fibrillation, this prolongs the atrial wavelength, and multiple wavelets are now unable to co-exist simultaneously. The success rate of cardioversion of recent onset AF with currently available class IC drugs is approximately 60–80%[63]. Amiodarone also terminates AF, but its slow onset of action is an important disadvantage[64]. The 'pill-in-the-pocket' approach using class IC agents may be a feasible and safe alternative to cardiovert AF in the outpatient setting[65].

Of all available drugs, amiodarone appears to be most effective in preventing AF recurrences. The Canadian Trial of AF (CTAF) showed that after 1 year of treatment with amiodarone approximately 75% of patients were in sinus rhythm versus 45% of patients using sotalol or propafenone[66]. Similar efficacy rates were observed in the AFFIRM trial and the recent Sotalol Amiodarone Atrial Fibrillation Efficacy Trial (SAFE-T)[67,68]. Although amiodarone is most effective, it should be reserved for second-line treatment because of the serious side effects[69].

Additionally, blockade of $I_{K,Ach}$ may potentially be antiarrhythmic and, because $I_{K,Ach}$ is absent in the ventricles, its antiarrhythmic effect will be specific to the atria. Some antiarrhythmic agents, such as amiodarone, flecainide and ibutilide, exhibit $I_{K,Ach}$-blocking properties[70].

It should be noted that all these drugs possess potential serious proarrhythmic side effects [QRS widening, ventricular arrhythmias and Torsade de Pointes (TdP)] which limits their general use.

Novel antiarrhythmic drug strategies

Newer and investigational class III compounds

Numerous class III or repolarization-delaying compounds have been partly developed and then abandoned, largely because of the risk of TdP brought about by the effect of ventricular repolarization. This is why amiodarone derivatives have been developed as it is the only class III drug which does not increase the propensity for TdP tachycardia[71].

Amiodarone derivatives

Dronedarone is an agent with multiple electrophysiological effects, similar to amiodarone, and is believed to have a better side effect profile because it is devoid of iodine. In experimental studies dronedarone inhibited trans-membrane potassium currents: I_{Kur}, I_{Ks}, I_{Kr}, I_{to} and I_{K1}[72]. The antiarrhythmic potential of dronedarone has been extensively studied. EURIDIS (EURopean trial In atrial fibrillation or flutter patients receiving Dronedarone for the maIntenance of Sinus rhythm) and ADONIS (American–Australian–African trial with DronedarONe In atrial fibrillation/flutter patients for the maintenance of Sinus rhythm) have shown that dronedarone 400 mg twice daily was superior to placebo in prevention of recurrent AF and was also effective in controlling ventricular rates during ongoing AF[73]. In EURIDIS, the median time to the recurrence of arrhythmia (the primary endpoint) was 41 days in the placebo group and 96 days in the dronedarone group. Dronedarone did not significantly prolong the QT interval and probably has a low potential for causing TdP. However, as with amiodarone, there may be some risk of pulmonary fibrosis, ocular side effects and skin photosensitivity, although very substantially less than with amiodarone. In EURIDIS and ADONIS, the ventricular rates during the recurrence of AF were on average 12–15 bpm lower in the dronedarone arm than in the placebo arm.

EURIDIS and ADONIS were not designed to assess mortality and excluded patients with significant left ventricular dysfunction. The ANDROMEDA (ANtiarrhythmic trial with DROnedarone in Moderate to severe heart failure Evaluating morbidity DecreAse) study was initiated to explore the effects of dronedarone on all-cause death and hospitalizations for heart failure in patients with New York Heart Association function class III or IV heart failure. The trial was, however, stopped prematurely after 627 patients out of the 1000 planned were enrolled, because an interim safety analysis revealed a potential excess risk of death in patients on active treatment: 25/310 (8%) vs 12/317 (3.8%) on placebo[74]. The adverse outcome of ANDROMEDA is thought to be due to an increase in creatinin in the dronedarone arm, which prompted inappropriate discontinuation of potentially life-saving therapy with ACE inhibitors. Dronedarone inhibits tubular absorption of creatinin and therefore has the potential to increase plasma creatinin, which may be an issue of concern in some patients.

The ATHENA (A placebo-controlled, double-blind, parallel arm Trial to assess the efficacy of dronedarone 400 mg bid for the prevention of cardiovascular Hospitalization or death from any cause in patieNts with AF/atrial flutter) study enrolled 4,628 high risk patients[75]. Mean follow-up was 21 ± 5 months. Dronedarone prolonged time to first cardiovascular hospitalization or death from any cause (the composite primary endpoint) by 24% ($p < 0.001$) compared with placebo. This effect was driven by the reduction in cardiovascular hospitalizations (25%), particularly hospitalizations for AF (37%). All-cause mortality was similar in the dronedarone and placebo groups (5% and 6%, respectively; hazard ratio 0.84, 95% CI, 0.66–1.08, $p < 0.176$); however, dronedarone significantly reduced deaths from cardiovascular causes[75]. Thus, the development portfolio of this drug is practically complete and the approval for several indications concerning AF may soon be assessed in the real world.

Budiodarone is another compound that structurally resembles amiodarone and retains two iodine atoms in its molecular structure. Only limited clinical data are available. Two phase 2 trials demonstrated a reduction of up to 75% of paroxysmal AF in patients with implanted pacemakers[76,77]. Some patients manifested a rise in thyroid stimulating hormone (TSH), but clinical symptoms did not appear. However, the potential for chronic toxicity is not known.

Celivarone is a non-iodinated benzofuran derivative with electrophysiological effects similar to amiodarone. A preliminary eport from the dose-ranging study showed the lowest rate of AF recurrence at the 50 mg dose, with no enhanced efficacy at higher doses[78].

Ranolazine

Ranolazine is a unique drug with both antianginal and electrophysiological properties. In tissue and wedge preparations, ranolazine has ion channel effects similar to those of amiodarone (reduced I_{Kr}, I_{Ks}, late I_{Na}, I_{Ca})[79]. The clinical effects appear to be principally mediated by the drug's inhibition of late I_{Na}, which subsequently reduces intracellular Na^+ and Ca^{2+} overload A large randomized controlled trial, MERLIN-TIMI (Metabolic Efficiency with Ranolazine for Less Ischaemia in Non-ST-elevation acute coronary syndrome Thrombolysis In Myocardial Infarction), demonstrated a significant decrease in occurrence of new-onset AF, supraventricular tachycardia and ventricular tachycardia in patients admitted with acute coronary syndrome[80]. In addition, animal models show that use-dependent blockade of Na^+ channels is highly atrium selective and is effective in terminating persistent AF[81].

Atrial repolarization-delaying agents

The mechanism of action of currently used class III antiarrhythmic agents such as sotalol and dofetilide is mediated by prolongation of APD, principally by targeting I_{Kr}[82]. This translates to an increase in refractoriness with a resultant increase in atrial wavelength, which may be important in suppressing the functional re-entry underlying AF substrates. However, I_{Kr} is present in both atrial and ventricular tissue, which increases the risk of ventricular early after-depolarizations, phase 2 re-entry and TdP[83]. Newer drugs exploit atrium-specific expression of certain potassium channel subunits that may be important for modulating repolarization in the electrically remodelled atrium. The I_{Kur} is an attractive target because it is carried by the Kv1.5 subunit, which is not expressed in ventricular myocardium. I_{Kur} blockers are expected to demonstrate atrial selectivity without affecting the electrophysiological properties of the ventricles. These investigational agents are also known as atrial repolarization- delaying agents (ARDA). Presently, there are several potential antiarrhythmic drugs with an ARDA mode of action which are currently in clinical development, of which vernakalant is furthest in development.

Intravenous vernakalant rapidly and effectively terminated recent-onset AF in a dose-finding study[84]. In this study, 56 patients with AF of 3–72 h duration were randomized to one of two vernakalant dose groups or to placebo. The vernakalant groups received either 0.5 mg/kg of the agent followed by 1 mg/kg or 2 mg/kg followed by 3 mg/kg via intravenous infusion over 10 min. Patients treated with the higher dose of vernakalant had a greater rate of AF termination compared with placebo. There were more patients in sinus rhythm at 30 min and at 1 h and median time to AF conversion was shorter. There were no serious adverse events related to vernakalant administration, indicating safety as well as efficacy of drug treatment.

In a phase III clinical trial, patients with short-lasting (3–7 days, $n = 220$) or long-lasting (8–45 days, $n = 116$) AF were randomized to receive either vernakalant 3 mg/kg or placebo[85]. In the short-duration group, 51.7% of patients converted rapidly to sinus rhythm compared with only 4.0% of patients receiving placebo. Median time to conversion with vernakalant was 11 min. Vernakalant was ineffective for conversion of longstanding AF and effects were not statistically different from placebo.

There were no incidences of TdP arrhythmia within the 24-h period following cardioversion despite mild but statistically significant QT interval prolongation. One episode of TdP was observed 32 h after drug administration.

Other promising therapies

Atrial $I_{K,Ach}$ inhibition[70], agents targeting abnormal Ca^{2+} handling, NCX inhibitors and agents targeting ischaemia-related channels and proteins (e.g. $I_{K,ATP}$ channel blockers and Na^+/H^+ exchanger inhibitors) are potentially promising but are still in an early phase of development[86].

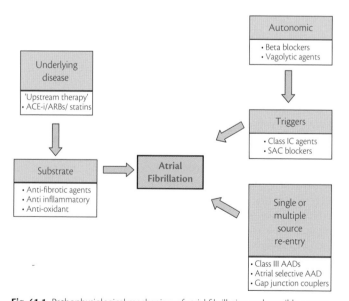

Fig. 41.1 Pathophysiological mechanism of atrial fibrillation and possible targets for intervention. ACE-i, angiotensin-converting enzyme inhibitor; ARB, angiotensin receptor blockers; SAC, stretch-activated channel; AAD, antiarrhythmic drug. [Reproduced, with permission, from Savelieva I, Kourliouros A, Camm J (2010) Primary and secondary prevention of atrial fibrillation with statins and polyunsaturated fatty acids: review of evidence and clinical relevance. *Naunyn-Schmiedeberg Arch Pharmacol* **381**:1–13.]

Conclusions and outlook

During the last decade important progress has been made in understanding the mechanisms of AF. It can be hypothesized that a better characterization of the substrate or type of AF in an individual patient may guide the choice of treatment. With an expanding pharmacological treatment arsenal we may be able to individualize or tailor our drug treatment (Fig. 41.1). For example, a patient with frequent short-lasting episodes of AF is likely to have a focal trigger and may be best treated with drugs that suppress automaticity. On the other hand, a patient with infrequent episodes but immediate persistent AF may have more structural remodelling and may benefit from upstream therapies such as gap junction modulators, stretch receptor antagonists and anti-inflammatory and anti-fibrotic therapy.

Unfortunately the risk–benefit ratio of old and currently available antiarrhythmic drugs has been troublesome. Since no survival benefit of maintenance of sinus rhythm has been demonstrated so far, the safety aspect of novel drugs is crucial. In this respect, the development of atrial-specific drugs may be an important step forward.

References

1. Nattel S, Maguy A, Le Bouter S, Yeh YH. Arrhythmogenic ion-channel remodeling in the heart: heart failure, myocardial infarction, and atrial fibrillation. *Physiol Rev* 2007;**87**:425–456.
2. Haïssaguerre M, Jaïs P, Shah DC, *et al.* Spontaneous initiation of atrial fibrillation by ectopic beats originating in the pulmonary veins. *N Engl J Med* 1998;**339**:659–666.
3. Vest JA, Wehrens XH, Reiken SR, *et al.* Defective cardiac ryanodine receptor regulation during atrial fibrillation. *Circulation* 2005;**111**: 2025–2032.
4. Yung-Hsin Yeh, Reza Wakili, Xiao-Yan Qi, *et al.* Calcium-handling abnormalities underlying atrial arrhythmogenesis and contractile dysfunction in dogs with congestive heart failure. *Circ Arrhythm Electrophysiol* 2008;**1**:93–102.
5. Wijffels MC, Kirchhof CJ, Dorland R, Allessie MA. Atrial fibrillation begets atrial fibrillation. A study in awake chronically instrumented goats. *Circulation* 1995;**92**:1954–1968.
6. Dobrev D. Atrial Ca^{2+} signaling in atrial fibrillation as an antiarrhythmic drug target. *Naunyn-Schmiedeberg Arch Pharmacol* 2010;**381**:195–206.
7. Schlotthauer K, Bers DM. Sarcoplasmic reticulum Ca^{2+} release causes myocyte depolarization. Underlying mechanism and threshold for triggered action potentials. *Circ Res* 2000;**87**: 774–780.
8. Chen YJ, Chen SA, Chen YC, *et al.* Effects of rapid atrial pacing on the arrhythmogenic activity of single cardiomyocytes from pulmonary veins: implication in initiation of atrial fibrillation. *Circulation* 2001;**104**:2849–2854.
9. Nattel S. New ideas about atrial fibrillation 50 years on. *Nature* 2002;**415**:219–226.
10. Yue L, Feng J, Gaspo R, Li GR, Wang Z, Nattel S. Ionic remodeling underlying action potential changes in a canine model of atrial fibrillation. *Circ Res* 1997;**81**:512–525.
11. Cha TJ, Ehrlich JR, Chartier D, Qi XY, Xiao L, Nattel S. Kir3-based inward rectifier potassium current: potential role in atrial tachycardia remodeling effects on atrial repolarization and arrhythmias. *Circulation* 2006;**113**:1730–1737.
12. Van Wagoner DR, Pond AL, Lamorgese M, Rossie SS, McCarthy PM, Nerbonne JM. Atrial L-type Ca^{2+} currents and human atrial fibrillation. *Circ Res* 1999;**85**:428–436.

13. Van Wagoner DR, Pond AL, McCarthy PM, Trimmer JS, Nerbonne JM. Outward K$^+$ current densities and Kv1.5 expression are reduced in chronic human atrial fibrillation. *Circ Res* 1997;**80**: 772–781.

14. Brandt MC, Priebe L, Böhle T, Südkamp M, Beuckelmann DJ. The ultrarapid and the transient outward K$^+$ current in human atrial fibrillation. Their possible role in postoperative atrial fibrillation. *J Mol Cell Cardiol* 2000;**32**:1885–1896.

15. Watanabe H, Kaiser DW, Makino S, et al. ACE I/D polymorphism associated with abnormal atrial and atrioventricular conduction in lone atrial fibrillation and structural heart disease: implications for electrical remodeling. *Heart Rhythm.* 2009;**6**:1327–1332.

16. Li D, Fareh S, Leung TK, Nattel S. Promotion of atrial fibrillation by heart failure in dogs: atrial remodeling of a different sort. *Circulation* 1999;**100**:87–95.

17. Verheule S, Sato T, Everett T 4th, et al. Increased vulnerability to atrial fibrillation in transgenic mice with selective atrial fibrosis caused by overexpression of TGF-beta1. *Circ Res* 2004;**94**: 1458–1465.

18. Kostin S, Klein G, Szalay Z, Hein S, Bauer EP, Schaper J. Structural correlate of atrial fibrillation in human patients. *Cardiovasc Res* 2002;**54**:361–379.

19. Frustaci A, Chimenti C, Bellocci F, Morgante E, Russo MA, Maseri A. Histological substrate of atrial biopsies in patients with lone atrial fibrillation. *Circulation* 1997;**96**:1180–1184.

20. Eckstein J, Verheule S, de Groot NM, Allessie M, Schotten U. Mechanisms of perpetuation of atrial fibrillation in chronically dilated atria. *Prog Biophys Mol Biol* 2008;**97**:435–451.

21. Dhein S. Role of connexins in atrial fibrillation. *Adv Cardiol* 2006;**42**:161–174.

22. Firouzi M, Ramanna H, Kok B, et al. Association of human connexin40 gene polymorphisms with atrial vulnerability as a risk factor for idiopathic atrial fibrillation. *Circ Res* 2004;**95**:e29–e33.

23. Mihm MJ, Yu F, Carnes CA, Reiser PJ, McCarthy PM, Van Wagoner DR, Bauer JA. Impaired myofibrillar energetics and oxidative injury during human atrial fibrillation. *Circulation* 2001;**104**:174–180.

24. Beckman JS, Koppenol WH. Nitric oxide, superoxide, and peroxynitrite: the good, the bad, and ugly. *Am J Physiol* 1996;**271**:C1424–C1437.

25. Nazir SA, Lab MJ. Mechanoelectric feedback and atrial arrhythmias. *Cardiovasc Res* 1996;**32**:52–61.

26. Cooper PJ, Lei M, Cheng LX, Kohl P. Selected contribution: axial stretch increases spontaneous pacemaker activity in rabbit isolated sinoatrial node cells. *J Appl Physiol* 2000;**89**:2099–2104.

27. Thijssen VL, Ausma J, Borgers M. Structural remodelling during chronic atrial fibrillation: act of programmed cell survival. *Cardiovasc Res* 2001;**52**:14–24.

28. Tsao HM, Yu WC, Cheng HC, et al. Pulmonary vein dilation in patients with atrial fibrillation: detection by magnetic resonance imaging. *J Cardiovasc Electrophysiol* 2001;**12**:809–813.

29. Ehrlich JR, Nattel S. Novel approaches for pharmacological management of atrial fibrillation. *Drugs* 2009;**69**:757–774.

30. Burstein B, Nattel S. Atrial fibrosis: mechanisms and clinical relevance in atrial fibrillation. *J Am Coll Cardiol* 2008;**51**:802–809.

31. Pedersen OD, Bagger H, Kober L, Torp-Pedersen C. Trandolapril reduces the incidence of atrial fibrillation after acute myocardial infarction in patients with left ventricular dysfunction. *Circulation* 1999;**100**:376–380.

32. Vermes E, Tardif JC, Bourassa MG, et al. Enalapril decreases the incidence of atrial fibrillation in patients with left ventricular dysfunction: insight from the Studies Of Left Ventricular Dysfunction (SOLVD) trials. *Circulation* 2003;**107**:2926–2931.

33. Ehrlich JR, Nattel S, Hohnloser SH. Atrial fibrillation and congestive heart failure: specific considerations at the intersection of two common and important cardiac disease sets. *J Cardiovasc Electrophysiol* 2002;**13**:399–405.

34. Wachtell K, Hornestam B, Lehto M, et al. Cardiovascular morbidity and mortality in hypertensive patients with a history of atrial fibrillation: The Losartan Intervention For End Point Reduction in Hypertension (LIFE) study. *J Am Coll Cardiol* 2005;**45**:705–711.

35. Murray KT, Rottman JN, Arbogast PG, et al. AFFIRM Investigators. Inhibition of angiotensin II signaling and recurrence of atrial fibrillation in AFFIRM. *Heart Rhythm* 2004;**1**:669–675.

36. Madrid AH, Bueno MG, Rebollo JM, et al. Use of irbesartan to maintain sinus rhythm in patients with long-lasting persistent atrial fibrillation: a prospective and randomized study. *Circulation* 2002;**106**:331–336.

37. GISSI-AF Investigators, Disertori M, Latini R, Barlera S, et al. Valsartan for prevention of recurrent atrial fibrillation. *N Engl J Med* 2009; **360**:1606–1617.

38. van den Berg MP, Van Gelder IC. New insight into the association among atrial fibrillation, electrophysiological remodeling, and the ACE insertion/deletion polymorphism–toward a more patient-tailored therapy? *Heart Rhythm* 2009;**6**:1333–1334.

39. Milliez P, Deangelis N, Rucker-Martin C, et al. Spironolactone reduces fibrosis of dilated atria during heart failure in rats with myocardial infarction. *Eur Heart J* 2005;**26**:2193–2199.

40. Shiroshita-Takeshita A, Brundel BJ, Burstein B, Leung TK, Mitamura H, Ogawa S, Nattel S. Effects of simvastatin on the development of the atrial fibrillation substrate in dogs with congestive heart failure. *Cardiovasc Res* 2007;**74**:75–84.

41. Bachmann JM, Majmudar M, Tompkins C, Blumenthal RS, Marine JE. Lipid-altering therapy and atrial fibrillation. *Cardiol Rev* 2008;**16**: 197–204.

42. Maggioni AP, Fabbri G, Lucci D, et al. GISSI-HF Investigators. Effects of rosuvastatin on atrial fibrillation occurrence: ancillary results of the GISSI-HF trial. *Eur Heart J* 2009;**30**:2327–2336.

43. Lee KW, Everett TH 4th, Rahmutula D, Guerra JM, Wilson E, Ding C, et al. Pirfenidone prevents the development of a vulnerable substrate for atrial fibrillation in a canine model of heart failure. *Circulation* 2006;**114**:1703–1712.

44. Savelieva I, Camm J. Statins and polyunsaturated fatty acids for treatment of atrial fibrillation. *Nat Clin Pract Cardiovasc Med* 2008;**5**:30–41.

45. Saygili E, Rana OR, Meyer C, et al. The angiotensin-calcineurin-NFAT pathway mediates stretch-induced up-regulation of matrix metalloproteinases-2/-9 in atrial myocytes. *Basic Res Cardiol* 2009;**104**:435–448.

46. Bode F, Katchman A, Woosley RL, Franz MR. Gadolinium decreases stretch-induced vulnerability to atrial fibrillation. *Circulation* 2000;**101**:2200–2205.

47. Bode F, Sachs F, Franz MR. Tarantula peptide inhibits atrial fibrillation. *Nature* 2001;**409**:35–36.

48. Kanno S, Saffitz JE. The role of myocardial gap junctions in electrical conduction and arrhythmogenesis. *Cardiovasc Pathol* 2001;**10**: 169–177.

49. Gutstein DE, Morley GE, Tamaddon H, et al. Conduction slowing and sudden arrhythmic death in mice with cardiac-restricted inactivation of connexin43.*Circ Res* 2001;**88**:333–339.

50. Leaf DE, Feig JE, Vasquez C, et al. Connexin40 imparts conduction heterogeneity to atrial tissue. *Circ Res* 2008;**103**:1001–1008.

51. Eloff BC, Gilat E, Wan X, Rosenbaum DS. Pharmacological modulation of cardiac gap junctions to enhance cardiac conduction: evidence supporting a novel target for antiarrhythmic therapy. *Circulation* 2003;**108**:3157–3163.

52. Shiroshita-Takeshita A, Sakabe M, Haugan K, Hennan JK, Nattel S. Model-dependent effects of the gap junction conduction-enhancing antiarrhythmic peptide rotigaptide (ZP123) on experimental atrial fibrillation in dogs. *Circulation* 2007;**115**:310–318.

53. Hamman JH, Enslin GM, Kotzé AF, Awie F. Oral delivery of peptide drugs: barriers and developments. *BioDrugs* 2005;**19**: 165–177.

54. Wyse DG, Waldo AL, DiMarco JP, *et al.* Atrial Fibrillation Follow-up Investigation of Rhythm Management (AFFIRM) Investigators. A comparison of rate control and rhythm control in patients with atrial fibrillation. *N Engl J Med* 2002;**347**:1825–1833.

55. Van Gelder IC, Hagens VE, Bosker HA, *et al.* Rate Control versus Electrical Cardioversion for Persistent Atrial Fibrillation Study Group. A comparison of rate control and rhythm control in patients with recurrent persistent atrial fibrillation. *N Engl J Med* 2002;**347**: 1834–1840.

56. Wijffels MC, Dorland R, Mast F, Allessie MA. Widening of the excitable gap during pharmacological cardioversion of atrial fibrillation in the goat: effects of cibenzoline, hydroquinidine, flecainide, and d-sotalol. *Circulation* 2000;**102**:260–267.

57. Wang S, Radhakrishnan J, Ayoub IM, Kolarova JD, Taglieri DM, Gazmuri RJ. Limiting sarcolemmal Na$^+$ entry during resuscitation from ventricular fibrillation prevents excess mitochondrial Ca^{2+} accumulation and attenuates myocardial injury. *J Appl Physiol* 2007;**103**:55–65.

58. Bukowska A, Schild L, Keilhoff G, *et al.* Mitochondrial dysfunction and redox signaling in atrial tachyarrhythmia. *Exp Biol Med (Maywood)* 2008;**233**:558–574.

59. Yamamoto S, Matsui K, Ohashi N. Protective effect of Na$^+$/H$^+$ exchange inhibitor, SM-20550, on impaired mitochondrial respiratory function and mitochondrial Ca^{2+} overload in ischemic/reperfused rat hearts. *J Cardiovasc Pharmacol* 2002;**39**:569–575.

60. Fozzard HA. Afterdepolarizations and triggered activity. *Basic Res Cardiol* 1992;**87**:S105–S113.

61. Anderson ME, Braun AP, Wu Y, Lu T, Wu Y, Schulman H, Sung RJ. KN-93, an inhibitor of multifunctional Ca^{2+}/calmodulin-dependent protein kinase, decreases early afterdepolarizations in rabbit heart. *J Pharmacol Exp Ther* 1998;**287**:996–1006.

62. Iwai T, Tanonaka K, Inoue R, Kasahara S, Kamo N, Takeo S. Mitochondrial damage during ischemia determines post-ischemic contractile dysfunction in perfused rat heart. *J Mol Cell Cardiol* 2002;**34**:725–738.

63. McNamara RL, Tamariz LJ, Segal JB, Bass EB. Management of atrial fibrillation: review of the evidence for the role of pharmacologic therapy, electrical cardioversion, and echocardiography. *Ann Intern Med* 2003;**139**:1018–1033.

64. Joseph AP, Ward MR. A prospective, randomized controlled trial comparing the efficacy and safety of sotalol, amiodarone, and digoxin for the reversion of new-onset atrial fibrillation. *Ann Emerg Med* 2000;**36**:1–9.

65. Alboni P, Botto GL, Baldi N, *et al.* Outpatient treatment of recent-onset atrial fibrillation with the "pill-in-the-pocket" approach. *N Engl J Med* 2004;**351**:2384–2391.

66. Roy D, Talajic M, Dorian P, *et al.* Amiodarone to prevent recurrence of atrial fibrillation. Canadian Trial of Atrial Fibrillation Investigators. *N Engl J Med* 2000;**342**:913–920.

67. AFFIRM First Antiarrhythmic Drug Substudy Investigators. Maintenance of sinus rhythm in patients with atrial fibrillation: an AFFIRM substudy of the first antiarrhythmic drug. *J Am Coll Cardiol* 2003;**42**:20–29.

68. Singh BN, Singh SN, Reda DJ, *et al.* Sotalol Amiodarone Atrial Fibrillation Efficacy Trial (SAFE-T) Investigators. Amiodarone versus sotalol for atrial fibrillation. *N Engl J Med* 2005;**352**:1861–1872.

69. Goldschlager N, Epstein AE, Naccarelli GV, Olshansky B, Singh B, Collard HR, Murphy E; Practice Guidelines Sub-committee, North American Society of Pacing and Electrophysiology (HRS). A practical guide for clinicians who treat patients with amiodarone: 2007. *Heart Rhythm* 2007;**4**:1250–1259.

70. Voigt N, Rozmaritsa N, Trausch A, Zimniak T, Christ T, Wettwer E, *et al.* Inhibition of I$_{(K,ACh)}$ current may contribute to clinical efficacy of class I and class III antiarrhythmic drugs in patients with atrial fibrillation. *Naunyn-Schmiedebergs Arch Pharmacol* 2010;**381**:251–259.

71. Singh BN. Amiodarone as paradigm for developing new drugs for atrial fibrillation. *J Cardiovasc Pharmacol* 2008;**52**:300–305.

72. Wegener FT, Ehrlich JR, Hohnloser SH. Dronedarone: an emerging agent with rhythm- and rate-controlling effects. *J Cardiovasc Electrophysiol* 2006;**17**:S17–S20.

73. Singh BN, Connolly SJ, Crijns HJ, *et al.* EURIDIS and ADONIS Investigators. Dronedarone for maintenance of sinus rhythm in atrial fibrillation or flutter. *N Engl J Med* 2007;**357**:987–999.

74. Køber L, Torp-Pedersen C, McMurray JJ, *et al.* Dronedarone Study Group. Increased mortality after dronedarone therapy for severe heart failure. *N Engl J Med* 2008;**358**:2678–2687.

75. Hohnloser SH, Crijns HJ, van Eickels M, Gaudin C, Page RL, Torp-Pedersen C, Connolly SJ; ATHENA Investigators. Effect of dronedarone on cardiovascular events in atrial fibrillation. *N Engl J Med* 2009;**360**:668–678.

76. Arya A, Silberbauer J, Teichman SL, Milner P, Sulke N, Camm AJ. A preliminary assessment of the effects of ATI-2042 in subjects with paroxysmal atrial fibrillation using implanted pacemaker methodology. *Europace* 2009;**11**:458–464.

77. Ezekowitz, Hohnloser SH, Lubunski A, Bandman O, Canafax D, Ellis DJ, *et al.* A randomized double-blind, placebo-controlled study of budiodarone in patients with paroxysmal atrial fibrillation and pacemakers with atrial fibrillation data logging capabilities. *Abstract presented at Heart Rhythm Society Boston* 2009.

78. Kowey PR, Aliot EM, Cappucci A, *et al.* Placebo-controlled double-blind dose-ranging study of the efficacy and safety of SSR149744C in patient with recent atrial fibrillation/flutter (abstract). *Heart Rhythm* 2007;**5**:S72.

79. Antzelevitch C, Belardinelli L, Zygmunt AC, *et al.* Electrophysiological effects of ranolazine, a novel antianginal agent with antiarrhythmic properties. *Circulation* 2004;**110**:904–910.

80. Scirica BM, Morrow DA, Hod H, *et al.* Effect of ranolazine, an antianginal agent with novel electrophysiological properties, on the incidence of arrhythmias in patients with non ST-segment elevation acute coronary syndrome: results from the Metabolic Efficiency With Ranolazine for Less Ischemia in Non ST-Elevation Acute Coronary Syndrome Thrombolysis in Myocardial Infarction 36 (MERLIN-TIMI 36) randomized controlled trial. *Circulation* 2007;**116**:1647–1652.

81. Burashnikov A, Di Diego JM, Zygmunt AC, Belardinelli L, Antzelevitch C. Atrium-selective sodium channel block as a strategy for suppression of atrial fibrillation: differences in sodium channel inactivation between atria and ventricles and the role of ranolazine. *Circulation* 2007; **116**:1449–1457.

82. Mazzini MJ, Monahan KM. Pharmacotherapy for atrial arrhythmias: present and future. *Heart Rhythm* 2008;**5**:S26–S31.

83. Yan GX, Wu Y, Liu T, Wang J, Marinchak RA, Kowey PR. Phase 2 early afterdepolarization as a trigger of polymorphic ventricular tachycardia in acquired long-QT syndrome: direct evidence from intracellular recordings in the intact left ventricular wall. *Circulation* 2001;**103**:2851–2856.

84. Roy D, Rowe BH, Stiell IG, *et al.* CRAFT Investigators. A randomized, controlled trial of RSD1235, a novel anti-arrhythmic agent, in the treatment of recent onset atrial fibrillation. *J Am Coll Cardiol* 2004; **44**:2355–2361.

85. Roy D, Pratt CM, Torp-Pedersen C, *et al.* Atrial Arrhythmia Conversion Trial Investigators. Vernakalant hydrochloride for rapid conversion of atrial fibrillation: a phase 3, randomized, placebo-controlled trial. *Circulation* 2008;**117**:1518–1525.

86. Savelieva I, Camm J. Anti-arrhythmic drug therapy for atrial fibrillation: current anti-arrhythmic drugs, investigational agents, and innovative approaches. *Europace* 2008;**10**:647–665.

87. Savelieva I, Kourliouros A, Camm J. Primary and secondary prevention of atrial fibrillation with statins and polyunsaturated fatty acids: review of evidence and clinical relevance. *Naunyn-Schmiedeberg Arch Pharmacol* 2010;**381**:1–13.

Stretch as a mechanism linking short- and long-term electrical remodelling in the ventricles

Eugene A. Sosunov, Evgeny P. Anyukhovsky and Michael R. Rosen

Background

The aim of this chapter is to explore stretch as a unifying factor in the causality of the electrophysiological changes characterizing ventricular electrical remodelling of brief and of long duration. To achieve this goal we use the T-wave changes induced by ventricular pacing as an example of remodelling, follow their transduction through brief and long periods of pacing, and consider the role of altered stretch on the myocardium.

'Electrical remodelling' refers to an alteration in myocardial electrophysiological properties in response to a variety of physiological interventions or pathological conditions. These can range from changes in heart rate or activation sequence unassociated with structural change through pathologies that cause structural change at the macroscopic or microscopic level. A useful example of ventricular electrical remodelling induced by an altered ventricular activation sequence is referred to as cardiac memory (CM)[1]. The clinical markers of CM are T-wave morphology changes that persist for considerable intervals after cessation of altered ventricular activation (e.g. induced by ventricular pacing or intraventricular conduction delay) and resumption of normal supraventricular activation[1,2].

Origin of the T-wave

In selecting the T-wave as a marker of remodelling it is useful to understand the origin of the T-wave: there is a history of disagreement here. At the simplest level, it is understood that the T-wave reflects the occurrence of repolarization in all cells in the ventricular myocardium[3–5]. Beyond this are three areas of contention: (1) the extent to which transmural (epicardial–endocardial) gradients contribute to the T-wave and to what extent the mid-myocardium plays a role; (2) the importance of apico-basal versus transmural gradients as aetiologies of T-waves and T-wave changes; (3) the roles of the septum and the right ventricle in complementing the dominant electrical forces generated by the left ventricle.

Given the consensus that the T-wave reflects epicardial potential gradients during ventricular repolarization that result from the spatial heterogeneity in repolarization time of normal hearts[3–5], the altered T-wave morphology in CM would imply that ventricular pacing induces spatially heterogeneous changes in ventricular repolarization. In other words, because no consistent QT interval changes have been demonstrated in CM[1,5–7], this form of ventricular electrical remodelling likely reflects a shortening of repolarization in some ventricular regions and prolongation of repolarization in other regions. The ventricular electrical remodelling of CM demonstrates 'accumulation' that is dependent on site of initiation of activation and on duration of altered ventricular activation[1,6,7]. Consequently, the T-wave changes may be of short (minutes to hours) or long (weeks to months) duration[2,6,7]. Evolving knowledge suggests a difference in signalling pathways and molecular mechanisms of short-term and long-term ventricular electrical remodelling and a transition from one mechanism to another during periods of sustained ectopic ventricular activation [see[8] for review].

Initiation of pacing-induced electrical remodelling

Changing the pacemaker site from atrium to ventricle or moving it from one to another ventricular site alters the sequence of ventricular electrical activation. This in turn affects spatial stress–strain relationships and contractile patterns of the ventricular wall[9,10]. It was initially suggested that altered spatial electrotonic interactions occurring during ventricular pacing create the stimulus for ventricular electrical remodelling[1,11]. In short-term CM, Costard-Jackle et al.[12] observed action potential duration (APD) prolongation in rabbit ventricle close to the site of altered activation, and progressive APD shortening in regions distal to the site of pacing. The authors suggested that altered electrotonic interactions among myocytes during ventricular pacing account for these APD changes.

An alternative proposal has been that a pacing-induced altered ventricular activation pattern modifies the spatial stress–strain relationships of the myocardial wall to initiate memory. Close association of alterations in ventricular activation with regional changes in myocardial stretch has been demonstrated[13].

Short-term remodelling

A number of studies have demonstrated that (1) changing the pacemaker site from atrium to ventricle alters ventricular activation and the mechanical pattern of ventricular contraction, and (2) ventricular pacing induces spatial changes in ventricular repolarization that alter T-wave morphology[5–13]. These studies have been performed in intact animals using invasive methods requiring sonomicrometry crystals or other implanted markers of motion or non-invasive techniques such as echocardiography or magnetic resonance imaging (MRI). The key to understanding all of them resides in comprehension of the changes in strain that occur with pacing.

Strain was initially defined as 'a dimensionless quantity [representing] the percent change in dimension from a resting state to one achieved following application of a force,' in this case stress[14,15]. Strain may be negative, indicating compression or shortening, or positive, reflecting the lengthening of a segment or region. Key questions in relating pacing and its effect on repolarization to strain would be (1) whether changes in ventricular activation modify repolarization in the absence of altered strain, (2) whether altered strain can affect repolarization when activation remains constant, and (3) whether the effects of pacing to alter strain at a specific site mirror the outcome of altering strain at that site directly.

We explored these questions in an isolated rabbit heart model[12] modified to permit the recording of a pseudo-electrocardiogram (ECG) and to allow alteration of activation and of contractile pattern in concert or independently of one another[16]. Figure 42.1 illustrates an experiment in which three-dimensional vector images were reconstructed, and the T-wave vector was defined as a line from the origin of the T-wave loop to its most remote point (Fig. 42.1C). Hearts were paced at a constant rate from either the right atrial appendage or left ventricular (LV) lateral wall. Panel B shows the prominent alteration of the QRS complex during ventricular pacing (as compared to right atrial pacing) reflecting a change of the ventricular activation pattern. Ten seconds after resuming atrial pacing, T-wave shapes differ in all leads in comparison to those before ventricular pacing, leading to altered T-wave vector angles and amplitudes (Fig. 42.1C) and in a prominent T-wave vector displacement (Fig. 42.1D). Fifteen minutes after resuming atrial pacing all three ECG leads and T-wave vectors have returned to their respective controls. Pressure measured in the right ventricle remained unchanged throughout the course of the experiment. The results demonstrate ventricular pacing-induced short-term ventricular electrical remodelling in isolated rabbit hearts.

In the experiment in Fig. 42.1, both ventricles contracted isovolumetrically and developed normal intraventricular pressures. We then used interventions that decrease either ventricular load (shunting both ventricles to the bath) or contractility [using the excitation–contraction uncoupler blebbistatin[17]] to explore the role of altered mechanical pattern in inducing ventricular electrical remodelling. Both interventions resulted in a marked fall of ventricular developed pressure and eliminated T-wave vector displacement

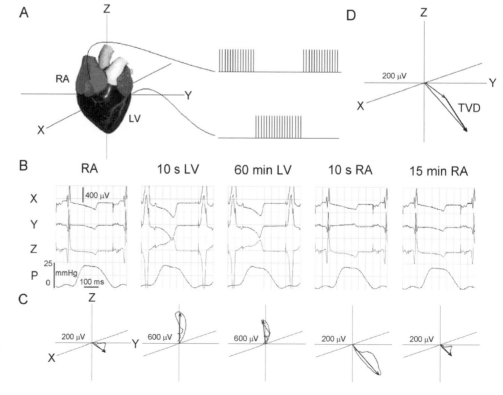

Fig. 42.1 A Schematic of isolated heart, ECG leads and pacing protocol for inducing short-term memory. **B** Memory induced by 60 min of left ventricular (LV) pacing at the same rate. Representative recordings of three orthogonal ECG leads and right ventricular pressure (P) are shown. Shown from left to right are: steady-state at right atrial (RA) pacing, 10 s of LV pacing, 60 min of LV pacing, 10 s after resumption of RA pacing and 15 min after resumption of RA pacing. **C** Corresponding T-wave loops and vectors (arrows). **D** T-wave vector displacement (TVD, measured in microvolts) is the distance between T-wave vector peaks before LV pacing (RA) and 10 s after resumption of atrial pacing (10 s RA). [Reproduced, with permission, from Sosunov EA, Anyukhovsky EP, Rosen MR (2008) Altered ventricular stretch contributes to initiation of cardiac memory. *Heart Rhythm* **5**:106–113.]

while not altering the QRS complex during ventricular pacing, suggesting that the pattern of stretch might be the primary trigger of the remodelling.

To assess the quantitative relationship between ventricular load and expression of CM, ventricular pressure was decreased or increased by changing volume in a fluid-filled latex balloon inserted into the LV (Fig. 42.2). Note that 5-min ventricular pacing performed at a high LV-developed pressure led to prominent T-wave changes in leads X and Y [Fig. 42.2A – compare control trace (C) with the trace recorded 10 s after the end of LV pacing (to assess CM)]. After the ECG had completely recovered, the extent of balloon inflation was decreased and the ventricular pacing protocol repeated (Fig. 42.2B). T-wave changes were seen again, but they were less prominent than at higher developed pressure (compare Figs 42.2A and B). Further decreases in balloon inflation resulted in progressive reductions of ventricular-developed pressure and T-wave changes (Figs 42.2C, D), whereas partial restoration of

balloon inflation led to an increase of developed pressure and T-wave changes (Fig. 42.2E). T-wave vector displacement was calculated for all these experimental conditions and plotted against LV-developed pressure (Fig. 42.2F). Note the direct relationship between these values.

The experiment in Fig. 42.2 demonstrates a direct role for pressure change in the evolution of T-wave changes, which is a long-known physiological phenomenon. Direct evidence for the role of stretch in initiating memory was demonstrated in separate experiments in which CM was induced by mechanically stretching the ventricle in the absence of altered activation and while not altering intracavitary pressure. To apply local stretch to the LV myocardium, small plastic pads sliding along steel shafts were sutured to two epicardial sites. Calibrated mechanical manipulators allowed us to change the distance between the pads. Figure 42.3 shows typical results from an experiment in which ~15% stretch was applied locally to the LV while the heart was continuously paced from the right atrium at a constant cycle length. Local stretch applied for 5 min produced changes in T-wave morphology in all ECG leads (Fig. 42.3B), and release of stretch led to a gradual recovery of T-wave morphology. On complete recovery, 5-min ventricular pacing produced T-wave vector displacement comparable to that of stretch (Figs 42.3C and D, respectively). The time course of dissipation of the vector change after resumption of atrial pacing in the ventricular pacing protocol was similar to that after release of stretch. Because stretch is a final common pathway for load, contraction or pressure changes, we concluded that stretch is the ultimate determinant of short-term ventricular electrical remodelling.

How are these short-term changes transduced?

Studies in cultured myocytes have shown that increasing stretch increases tissue angiotensin II synthesis and release[18,19]. Moreover, the ventricular electrical remodelling resulting from pacing the heart for brief periods (up to 1–2 h) can be attenuated by pretreating with angiotensin-converting enzyme (ACE) inhibitors, angiotensin II receptor type 1 (AT-I), blockers or L-type Ca^{2+} current ($I_{Ca,L}$) channel blockers[20]. In other words, the pacing/stretch-induced initiation of remodelling appears to be an angiotensin II/Ca^{2+}-determined mechanism. The question of how this comes about has two components: (1) if repolarization is changing, what are the ion channel determinants of repolarization that contribute? and (2) how does angiotensin II influence the ion channels? A schematic of the pathways involved is provided in Fig. 42.4.

There is a long understanding of the role of angiotensin II in increasing $I_{Ca,L}$[21]. More recently it was discovered that angiotensin II modulates the transient outward K^+ current (I_{to})[22]. The effect on I_{to} is site-dependent within the ventricle in the following sense: I_{to} is large in epicardial myocytes and far smaller in endocardial myocytes. When epicardial myocytes are disaggregated from the ventricle and incubated with AT-I blockers, the magnitude of the current decreases; in contrast, when disaggregated endocardial myocytes are incubated with angiotensin II, I_{to} magnitude increases[22]. There is general agreement that there is a transmural distribution of I_{to} with epicardium > endocardium and that by providing a 'set-point' for the onset of repolarization, the magnitude of I_{to} influences the transmural dispersion of repolarization[23–25]. However, none of these observations explains the mechanism whereby angiotensin II decreases epicardial I_{to} to alter repolarization.

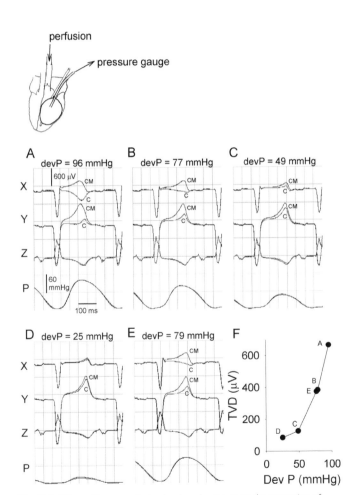

Fig. 42.2 Effects of intraventricular developed pressure on the expression of T-wave memory. ECG leads during right atrial pacing before (trace C) and 10 s after 5 min of left ventricular (LV) pacing (trace CM) are superimposed. **A–E** Pacing protocol was performed at different degrees of balloon inflation resulting in different LV developed pressure (devP). **F** Dependence of T-wave vector displacement (TVD) on LV developed pressure. [Reproduced, with permission, from Sosunov EA, Anyukhovsky EP, Rosen MR (2008) Altered ventricular stretch contributes to initiation of cardiac memory. *Heart Rhythm* **5:**106–113.]

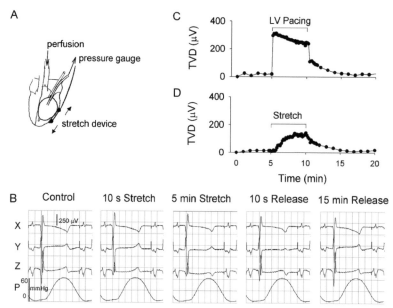

Fig. 42.3 Effects of local ventricular stretch on T-wave morphology and T-wave vector displacement (TVD). **A** Schematic showing application of stretching device on left ventricular (LV) surface. LV balloon is in place. **B** Representative recordings show ECG leads and LV pressure at various times during the stretching protocol. The heart was continuously paced from the right atrium. Shown from left to right are: steady-state before stretch, 10 s of local LV stretch, 5 min of local LV stretch, 10 s after release of stretch and 15 min after release of stretch. **C** and **D** Time course of TVD induced by 5 min ventricular pacing or 5 min local ventricular stretch, respectively. [Reproduced, with permission, from Sosunov EA, Anyukhovsky EP, Rosen MR (2008) Altered ventricular stretch contributes to initiation of cardiac memory. *Heart Rhythm* **5**:106–113.]

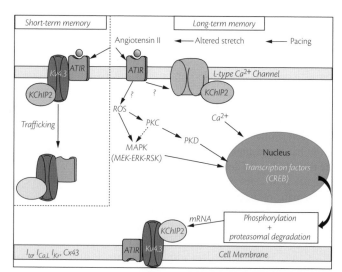

Fig. 42.4 Pathways in short- and long-term cardiac memory. Initiation is via ventricular pacing to alter stretch resulting in increased angiotensin II synthesis and release. Short-term memory results from angiotensin II-induced internalization of AT-I (AT1R)/Kv4.3/KChIP2 macromolecular complex leading to I_{to} reduction. Long-term memory is initiated by angiotensin II binding to its receptor resulting in reduction of the transcription factor CREB. Production of reactive oxygen species (ROS) results in mitogen-activated protein kinase (MAPK)- and protein kinase C (PKC)/protein kinase D (PKD)-determined pathways currently under investigation. CREB is phosphorylated and then proteasomally degraded. Other ion currents involved are $I_{Ca,L}$ and I_{Kr}. Connexin 43 is reduced as well and translocated to the lateral margins of myocytes. [Reproduced, with permission, from Ozgen N, Rosen MR (2009) Cardiac memory: a work in progress. *Heart Rhythm* **6**:564–570.]

Understanding of the mechanism came about with a pivotal experiment by Doronin *et al.*[26] performed first in a cell line and then in myocytes. In brief, they transfected human embryo kidney cell line (HEK) cells with Kv4.3 and KChIP2 (respectively the alpha and accessory subunits that contribute to I_{to}) as well as with AT-I. Experiments in the cell line and in myocytes demonstrated that the Kv4.3/KChIP2 complex forms a macromolecular entity with AT-I; the three components reside closely in the cell membrane as demonstrated in co-immunoprecipitation experiments and using fluorescence resonance energy transfer. When the complex resides in the membrane, there is a large I_{to}. However, when the cell is exposed to angiotensin II, there is internalization of the complex. Preliminary data demonstrate block of the process by colchicine, suggesting that the tubulin component of the cytoskeleton is involved in the trafficking. The fate of the components of the complex beyond this step is not yet known.

Short-term pacing and the resultant ventricular electrical remodelling have also been studied in the intact heart[5]. Epicardial and transmural mapping of the ventricles during atrial pacing showed a minimal epicardial–endocardial gradient and the expected apico-basal gradient. The apicobasal gradient changed markedly during brief periods of ventricular pacing, resulting in an altered T-wave characteristic of CM. In contrast, the epicardial–endocardial gradient remained unchanged.

Long-term remodelling

It is important to note that long-term ventricular electrical remodelling can occur in the absence of structural remodelling. Three weeks of ventricular pacing in dogs induced no changes in myocardial blood flow to the ventricles and no sign of heart failure or ischaemia[7]. The pacing protocol did not affect the capacitance of ventricular myocytes, indicating that myocyte size had not changed[27]. Histological analysis performed by Jeyaraj *et al.*[28] revealed no myocyte hypertrophy, fibrosis or necrosis after 4 weeks of ventricular pacing. This is important because extension of pacing beyond 4 weeks can lead to hypertrophy[29] and the structural remodelling of hypertrophy has been associated with APD prolongation[30]. Hence, ventricular electrical remodelling appears before the development of structural remodelling.

The relative roles of altered activation and mechanical stretch in triggering long-term ventricular electrical remodelling have received limited study. To test the hypothesis that mechanoelectric coupling triggered by regional strain is the mechanism for long-term ventricular electrical remodelling, Jeyaraj *et al.*[28] studied the relationship between regional changes in repolarization and local circumferential strain in long-term ventricular pacing experiments. Canine hearts were paced either from the anterior or from the posterior LV wall for 4 weeks, and after successful induction of memory the hearts were harvested and the LV was divided into anterior, lateral and posterior segments. Myocardial wedges

dissected from these segments were arterially perfused and action potentials (AP) were recorded using a multisegment transmural optical system. In a separate group of dogs, tagged MRI was performed *in vivo* to measure the effect of pacing direction on mechanical strain in different segments of the LV. Figure 42.5 illustrates the relationship found between regional AP remodelling and myocardial strain. During sinus activation (control), AP waveforms recorded from both anterior and posterior LV segments were essentially identical. Similarly, the timing and amplitude of peak strain were almost identical in both segments, consistent with temporally synchronized LV contraction. The absence of segmental differences in strain (Δstrain) and APD (ΔAPD) was observed consistently across all experiments (Fig. 42.5A, lower panel). In contrast to sinus activation, after anterior LV pacing (Fig. 42.5B), marked APD prolongation was observed in posterior (blue) compared with anterior (red) myocytes. This was paralleled by a substantial increase in circumferential strain in the late (blue point) relative to the early (red point) activated myocardial segments. After reversing the direction of propagation by pacing the posterior LV wall (Fig. 42.5C), essentially the identical but inverted

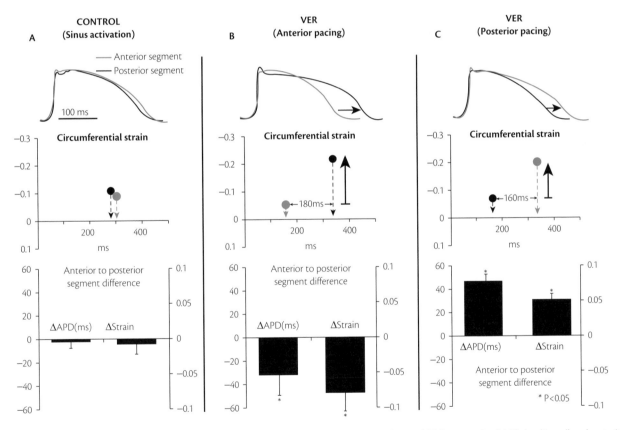

Fig. 42.5 Circumferential strain as a mechanism triggering ventricular electrical remodelling. Top: superimposed AP from anterior (highlighted in red) and posterior LV segments. Middle: temporal occurrence of peak systolic circumferential strain during the cardiac cycle in the anterior (red) and posterior LV segments measured with tagged MRI. Bottom: calculated difference in anterior–posterior APD (ΔAPD) and anterior–posterior strain (Δstrain). In control (**A**), AP and temporal occurrence of peak circumferential strain in both anterior and posterior LV segments are identical. Therefore, an almost indistinguishable ΔAPD and Δstrain is noted. In ventricular electrical remodelling induced by anterior LV pacing (**B**), a selective prolongation of APD is noted in the late-activated anterior segment (arrow). Interestingly, there is not only a temporal dyssynchrony in occurrence of peak-systolic strain, but also a significant increase in circumferential strain in the late-activated posterior segment (arrow). Therefore, anterior–posterior ΔAPD and Δstrain are shifted in the same direction. In ventricular electrical remodelling induced by posterior LV pacing (**C**), selective prolongation of APD is noted in the late-activated anterior segment, and this is paralleled by a selective increase in strain in the late-activated anterior segment. Again, the anterior–posterior ΔAPD and Δstrain are shifted in the same direction. [Reproduced, with permission, from Jeyaraj D, Wilson LD, Zhong J, *et al.* (2007) Mechanoelectrical feedback as novel mechanism of cardiac electrical remodeling. *Circulation* **115**:3145–3155.]

pattern of circumferential strain and ventricular electrical remodelling was produced. Thus, under each of the three circumstances tested, localized ventricular electrical remodelling was closely paralleled by regional circumferential strain. These data suggest the locally enhanced circumferential strain as the mechanism responsible for triggering remodelling of ion channel function in settings of long-term ventricular pacing.

In the study by Jeyaraj et al.[28] the effects of long-term ventricular pacing on mechanical strain in different LV segments were determined in vivo and local repolarization was measured in vitro in arterially perfused LV segments. Coronel et al. used a similar pacing protocol to induce long-term CM in dogs and measured local ventricular repolarization in situ by recording multiple unipolar electrograms[31]. No measure of contractile indices was obtained. While in the study by Jeyaraj et al.[28] CM was associated with a significant increase in segmental dispersion of repolarization and not with changes in transmural dispersion of repolarization, Coronel et al. found that long-term T-wave changes were associated with evolution of transmural repolarization gradients[31]. To resolve this discrepancy and test a link between local alterations in strain and repolarization in long-term ventricular electrical remodelling, both variables likely should be recorded in heart in situ.

Molecular mechanisms for long-term ventricular electrical remodelling

There is a continuum of repolarization change between short- and long-term ventricular electrical remodelling as pacing periods are prolonged. However, the mechanisms for the short-term change and for the long-term change differ markedly[8]. Whereas the ion channel changes in short-term memory are largely seen in the components of I_{to}, there is in long-term memory the additional involvement of $I_{Ca,L}$[32] and of rapid component of the delayed rectifier K$^+$ current (I_{Kr})[33]. Moreover, there are changes in the connexins that regulate cell–cell current flow and transfer of small molecules [See [34]; also Chapter 18]. A schematic is provided in Fig. 42.4.

With regard to the connexins, a reduction of connexin 43 protein and lateralization of this connexin has been demonstrated in myocytes near the ventricular pacing site[34]. However, the mechanisms responsible for these connexin changes have not been detailed. In contrast, there is a good deal of information concerning ion channels, especially I_{to} which has served as a bellwether for memory studies. What is remarkable in the segue from short- to long-term memory is that channel internalization no longer seems to be a major factor; instead, gene transcription comes to the fore. The transcriptional changes do not take long to commence. In an early study by Meghji et al., stretch was altered on pig ventricular epicardium in the absence of any change in activation[35]. Within 30 min upregulation was noted in immediate early gene expression.

A major focus in studies of transcription in long-term pacing has been the cyclic adenosine monophosphate (cAMP) response element binding protein (CREB)[36,37]. We studied CREB, initially because review of the literature on memory revealed that several minutes of electrical shock in aplysia increase CREB levels which in turn contribute to the evolution of long-term potentiation[38]. At first we thought that the association of shock (or pacing) with a stereotypical behaviour like long-term potentiation (or T-wave change) might provide an entrée into our understanding of the

transcriptional changes associated with altered activation and stretch. In fact we hypothesized that CM might be a variant on long-term potentiation.

While it turned out that CREB is important to the transcription of CM (with the onset of change in minutes to hours) the association is antithetical to that in long-term potentiation. The following factors are involved: (1) there is a cAMP response element in the promoter region of KChIP2, the accessory protein for I_{to}[36]. However, pacing (or myocardial stretch in the absence of altered activation) does not increase CREB protein: rather there is a decrease in CREB[36]. In other words, a basal CREB level appears to be required for appropriate KChIP2 gene transcription and as levels of CREB fall, so does the amount of the KChIP2 protein. To test whether the change in CREB and that in KChIP2 and I_{to} might be epiphenomena we injected CREB antisense into canine ventricle in the absence of ventricular pacing or altered stretch. The result was reduced CREB protein, a smaller AP notch and a reduced I_{to}[37]. These results strengthened our appreciation of the importance of CREB to maintenance of KChIP2 and I_{to}.

During long-term LV epicardial pacing, not only does the epicardial AP notch diminish (likely reflecting the decreased I_{to}) but also the plateau is higher, consistent with a change in $I_{Ca,L}$, and AP duration is longer, consistent with a reduction of I_{Kr}[39]. In keeping with this observation, studies of $I_{Ca,L}$ have shown an alteration in activation and inactivation kinetics that would be associated with an increased plateau height[32], while those of I_{Kr} have shown a decrease in current density that would be associated with a prolongation of AP duration[33]. Moreover, the change in I_{Kr} occurs in a gradient across the myocardial wall (in controls, epicardial I_{Kr} exceeds endocardial; in memory, epicardial I_{Kr} is not different from endocardial) in a fashion that may contribute to the transmural changes in repolarization in long-term memory in situ (see above).

Whereas we are still in the early stages of studying I_{Kr} transcription, we have recent data concerning the control of $I_{Ca,L}$[40]. It appears that KChIP2 is an accessory subunit of the $I_{Ca,L}$, such that in KChIP2 knockout mice, current density is reduced. This appears to result from a direct interaction between KChIP2 and the CaV1.2 alpha-1C subunit N terminus. KChIP2 binding to the N-terminal inhibitory module of alpha-1C augments $I_{Ca,L}$ density without increasing CaV1.2 protein expression or changing trafficking to the cell membrane. It is therefore proposed that 'KChIP2 impedes the N-terminal inhibitory module of CaV1.2, to increase $I_{Ca,L}$'[40]. Hence it is likely that the role CREB plays with regard to regulation of I_{to} in long-term ventricular electrical remodelling is complemented by its action on $I_{Ca,L}$.

How are these long-term changes transduced?

Paralleling our consideration of short-term memory, we must ask how stretch and altered activation intrude on the transcriptional pathways involved to alter the levels and function of the relevant ion channel subunits. Certainly in the initial stages, angiotensin II and Ca^{2+} are critical. We noted that the reduction of CREB so readily induced by 2 h of pacing could be blocked completely by exposure to the angiotensin II receptor blocker saralasin or the dihydropyridine receptor blocker nifedipine[36]. However, long-term exposure to similar blocking agents did not prevent the long-term ventricular electrical remodelling from occurring, they simply attenuated the process[7,32].

So the question 'why' comes to the fore. We know that ventricular pacing reduces CREB protein levels[36]. We also know that AT-I blockade and $I_{Ca,L}$ blockade prevent the reduction of CREB in short-term pacing experiments, resulting in prevention of ventricular electrical remodelling[20]. Now under investigation is the role of oxidative stress in this process. Although we have not measured tissue H_2O_2 levels, our preliminary data show that ventricular pacing does increase malondialdehyde levels, providing evidence for oxidative stress[41]. Experiments in cell culture have shown that downstream to reactive oxygen species (ROS) production, CREB reduction appears to derive from a pathway regulated by protein kinase C and protein kinase D[42]. The end-point is the proteasomal degradation of CREB[43]. Interestingly, in the intact animal, proteasomal inhibiton prevents the reduction of CREB levels that otherwise would result from pacing[43].

Conclusions and outlook

The results discussed point to altered stretch as a trigger for ventricular electrical remodelling, with altered ventricular activation being important primarily because it initiates the new contractile pattern. While we are confident in the role of stretch in these processes, we recognize as well that much regarding the pathways and their transduction remains to be discovered. Because of the multiplicity of channels involved in the remodelling processes discussed, it is likely that the final road map will be far more complex than the already complicated map we have at present.

References

1. Rosenbaum MB, Blanco HH, Elizari MV, Lazzari JO, Davidenko JM. Electrotonic modulation of the T-wave and cardiac memory. *Am J Cardiol* 1982;**50**:213–222.

2. Libbus I, Rosenbaum DS. Remodeling of cardiac repolarization: mechanisms and implications of memory. *Card Electrophysiol Rev* 2002;**6**:302–310.

3. Spach MS, Barr RC, Lanning CF, Tucek PC. Origin of body surface QRS and T-wave potentials from epicardial potential distributions in the intact chimpanzee. *Circulation* 1977;**55**:268–278.

4. Ghanem RN, Jia P, Ramanathan C, Ryu K, Markowitz A, Rudy Y. Noninvasive electrocardiographic imaging (ECGI): Comparison to intraoperative mapping in patients. *Heart Rhythm* 2005;**2**: 339–354.

5. Janse MJ, Sosunov EA, Coronel R, *et al.* Repolarization gradients in the canine left ventricle before and after induction of short-term cardiac memory. *Circulation* 2005;**112**:1711–1718.

6. del Balzo U, Rosen MR. T-wave changes persisting after ventricular pacing in canine heart are altered by 4-aminopyridine but not by lidocaine. Implications with respect to phenomenon of cardiac 'memory'. *Circulation* 1992;**85**:1464–1472.

7. Shvilkin A, Danilo P, Jr., Wang J, *et al.* Evolution and resolution of long-term cardiac memory. *Circulation* 1998;**97**:1810–1817.

8. Ozgen N, Rosen MR. Cardiac memory: a work in progress. *Heart Rhythm* 2009;**6**:564–570.

9. Prinzen FW, Peshar M. Relation between the pacing induced sequence of activation and left ventricular pump function in animals. *Pacing Clin Electrophysiol* 2002;**25**:484–498.

10. Wyman BT, Hunter WC, Prinzen FW, Faris OP, McVeigh ER. Effects of single- and biventricular pacing on temporal and spatial dynamics of ventricular contraction. *Am J Physiol* 2002;**282**:H373–H379.

11. Franz MR, Bargheer K, Costard-Jackle A, Miller DC, Lichtlen P. Human ventricular repolarization and T-wave genesis. *Prog Cardiovasc Dis* 1991;**33**:369–384.

12. Costard-Jackle A, Goetsch B, Antz M, Franz MR. Slow and long-lasting modulation of myocardial repolarization produced by ectopic activation in isolated rabbit hearts. Evidence for cardiac "memory". *Circulation* 1989;**80**:1412–1420.

13. Prinzen FW, Hunter WC, Wyman BT, McVeigh ER. Mapping of regional myocardial strain and work during ventricular pacing: experimental study using magnetic resonance imaging tagging. *J Am Coll Cardiol* 1999;**33**:1735–1742.

14. Mirsky I, Parmley WW. Assessment of passive elastic stiffness for isolated heart muscle and the intact heart. *Circ Res* 1973;**33**:233–243.

15. Abraham TP, Nishimura RA. Myocardial Strain: Can we finally measure contractility? *JACC* 2001;**37**:731–734.

16. Sosunov EA, Anyukhovsky EP, Rosen MR. Altered ventricular stretch contributes to initiation of cardiac memory. *Heart Rhythm* 2008;**5**: 106–113.

17. Fedorov VV, Lozinsky IT, Sosunov EA, *et al.* Application of blebbistatin as an excitation-contraction uncoupler for electrophysiologic study of rat and rabbit hearts. *Heart Rhythm* 2007;**4**:619–626.

18. Sadoshima J, Izumo S. Mechanical stretch rapidly activates multiple signal transduction pathways in cardiac myocytes: potential involvement of an autocrine/paracrine mechanism. *EMBO J* 1993;**12**:1681–1692.

19. Sadoshima J, Xu Y, Slayter HS, *et al.* Autocrine release of angiotensin II mediates stretch-induced hypertrophy of cardiac myocytes in vitro. *Cell* 1993;**75**:977–984.

20. Ricard P, Danilo P, Jr., Cohen IS, Burkhoff D, Rosen MR. A role for the renin–angiotensin system in the evolution of cardiac memory. *J Cardiovasc Electrophysiol* 1999;**10**:545–551.

21. Kass RS, Blair ML. Effects of angiotensin II on membrane current in cardiac Purkinje fibers. *J Mol Cell Cardiol* 1981;**13**:797–809.

22. Yu H, Gao J, Wang H, *et al.* Effects of the renin-angiotensin system on the current Ito in epicardial and endocardial ventricular myocytes from the canine heart. *Circ Res* 2000;**86**:1062–1068.

23. Litovsky SH, Antzelevitch C. Transient outward current prominent in canine ventricular epicardium but not endocardium. *Circ Res* 1988;**62**:116–126.

24. Rosati B, Grau F, Rodriguez S, Li H, Nerbonne JM, McKinnon D. Concordant expression of KChIP2 mRNA, protein and transient outward current throughout the canine ventricle. *J Physiol* 2003;**548**:815–822.

25. Rosati B, Pan Z, Lypen S, *et al.* Regulation of KChIP2 potassium channel beta subunit gene expression underlies the gradient of transient outward current in canine and human ventricle. *J Physiol* 2001;**533**:119–125.

26. Doronin SV, Potapova IA, Lu Z, Cohen IS. Angiotensin receptor type 1 forms a complex with the transient outward potassium channel Kv4.3 and regulates its gating properties and intracellular localization. *J Biol Chem* 2004;**279**:48231–48237.

27. Gao J, Yu J, Wymore RR, Rosen MR, Danilo P Jr. Long-standing cardiac memory in dogs is attributable to an altered activation threshold for I_{to}. *Circulation* 1995;**92**:I-428 (abstract).

28. Jeyaraj D, Wilson LD, Zhong J, *et al.* Mechanoelectrical feedback as novel mechanism of cardiac electrical remodeling. *Circulation* 2007;**115**:3145–3155.

29. Van Oosterhout MFM, Prinzen FW, *et al.* Asynchronous electrical activation induces asymmetrical hypertrophy of the left ventricular wall. *Circulation* 1998;**98**:588–595.

30. Volders PGA, Sipido KR, Vos MA, *et al.* Downregulation of delayed rectifier K+ currents in dogs with chronic complete atrioventricular block and acquired torsades de pointes. *Circulation* 1999;**100**: 2455–2461.

31. Coronel R, Opthof T, Plotnikov AN, *et al.* Long-term cardiac memory in canine heart is associated with the evolution of a transmural repolarization gradient. *Cardiovasc Res* 2007;**74**:416–425.

32. Plotnikov AN, Yu H, Geller JC, *et al*. Role of L-type calcium channels in pacing-induced short-term and long-term cardiac memory in canine heart. *Circulation* 2003;**107**:2844–2849.

33. Obreztchikova MN, Patberg KW, Plotnikov AN, *et al*. I$_{Kr}$ contributes to the altered ventricular repolarization that determines long-term cardiac memory. *Cardiovasc Res* 2006;**71**:88–96.

34. Patel PM, Plotnikov A, Kanagaratnam P, *et al*. Altering ventricular activation remodels gap junction distribution in canine heart. *J Cardiovasc Electrophysiol* 2001;**12**:570–577.

35. Meghji P, Nazir SA, Dick DJ, Bailey MES, Johnson KJ, Lab MJ. Regional workload induced changes in electrophysiology and immediate early gene expression in intact in situ porcine heart. *J Mol Cell Cardiol* 1997;**29**:3147–3155.

36. Patberg KW, Plotnikov AN, Quamina A, *et al*. Cardiac memory is associated with decreased levels of the transcriptional factor CREB modulated by angiotensin II and calcium. *Circ Res* 2003;**93**:472–478.

37. Patberg KW, Obreztchikova MN, Giardina SF, *et al*. The cAMP response element binding protein modulates expression of the transient outward current: implications for cardiac memory. *Cardiovasc Res* 2005;**68**:259–267.

38. Kandel ER. The molecular biology of memory storage: a dialogue between genes and synapses. *Science* 2001;**294**:1030–1038.

39. Yu H, McKinnon D, Dixon JE, *et al*. Transient outward current, Ito1, is altered in cardiac memory. *Circulation* 1999;**99**:1898–1905.

40. Thomsen MB, Wang C, Ozgen N, Wang HG, Rosen MR, Pitt GS. Accessory subunit KChIP2 modulates the cardiac L-type calcium current. *Circ Res* 2009;**104**:1382–1389.

41. Özgen N, Plotnikov AN, Shlapakova IN, *et al*. A reactive oxygen species-mediated PKC-ERK-RSK pathway decreases the cyclic AMP response element binding protein and may initiate transcriptional changes in cardiac memory. *Circulation* 2007;**116**:88.

42. Ozgen N, Guo J, Gertsberg Z, Danilo P, Rosen MR, Steinberg SF. Reactive oxygen species decrease cAMP response element binding protein expression in cardiomyocytes via a protein kinase D1-dependent mechanism that does not require Ser133 phosphorylation. *Mol Pharmacol* 2009;**76**:896–902.

43. Ozgen N, Lau DH, Shlapakova IN, Sherman W, Danilo P Jr, Rosen MR. The decreased CREB level determining K channel transcription in cardiac memory results from its ubiquitination and subsequent proteosomal degradation. *Heart Rhythm* 2008;**5**:S358.

Volume and pressure overload and ventricular arrhythmogenesis

Michiel J. Janse and Ruben Coronel

Background

Congestive heart failure (HF) is a major public health problem. Its incidence and prevalence has increased in the past decades, mainly because of the aging of the general population and the increased survival rate following acute myocardial infarction. In the United States, 1.5% of the adult population is affected[1]. HF carries a poor prognosis: the 5 year survival rate varies between 25% and 38%[2]. Half of the deaths are classified as sudden[3], and of these about half are due to ventricular tachycardia or fibrillation, the other half to bradyarrhythmias and electromechanical dissociation[4–6].

In about half of patients with congestive HF, complex ventricular arrhythmias, including non-sustained ventricular tachycardia, are present and sudden death is common. It is not clear whether there is a relationship between presence of arrhythmias and the subsequent occurrence of sudden death, since there are studies that both support such a relationship[7–9] and deny it[10,11]. There is also controversy regarding the question whether sudden death is related to the severity of HF. Kjekshus reported that in patients with New York Heart Association class I and II, 50–60% of all deaths were sudden, whereas in patients with more severe HF (class III and IV) this was only 20–30%[12]. In patients with end-stage HF, awaiting cardiac transplantation, sudden death was due to ventricular tachyarrhythmias in about 50%, and due to bradycardia, asystole or electromechanical dissociation in the other 50%[5,6]. These findings contrast with those of recent randomized trials on the prevention of sudden death by implantable cardioverter defibrillator therapy, in which the device was most effective in patients with the lowest ejection fraction[13–15]. It is difficult to see how a defibrillator shock would be effective in electromechanical dissociation. In other words, there is still much to learn about arrhythmias and sudden death in HF.

There is an extraordinary variety of animal models of HF, including cow, baboon, dog, pig, sheep, cat, rabbit, turkey, ferret, guinea pig, Syrian hamster, rat and mouse, as well as genetically determined HF models, for example in Syrian hamsters, Doberman Pinscher dogs and transgenic mice. Techniques to induce HF include coronary artery occlusion, volume overload (aorta-caval fistulae, mitral regurgitation, aortic regurgitation, tricuspid regurgitation), pressure overload (aortic or pulmonary banding, salt-sensitive or spontaneous hypertension), combined volume and pressure overload, toxic cardiomyopathy (by, for example, doxorubicin or monocrotaline administration), rapid pacing and hyperthyroidism [for details see the excellent reviews of Hasenfuss[16] and Doggrell and Brown[17].

For electrophysiological studies, rat and mouse models have the disadvantage that the ventricular action potential (AP) lacks a plateau and that Ca^{2+} removal from the cytosol is predominantly via the activity of the sarcoplasmic reticulum (SR) Ca^{2+} pump, whereas activity of the Na^+/Ca^{2+} exchanger (NCX) is less relevant[16]. The species that, as far as AP characteristics are concerned, resemble humans most appear to be rabbits and dogs.

The rabbit model in which HF is induced by a combination of volume and pressure overload has been used by many investigators to study electrophysiologic changes and mechanisms of arrhythmias[18–25], and this chapter is limited mainly to a discussion of findings obtained in this model. Briefly, the rabbits undergo two operations. Initially aortic insufficiency is induced under sterile conditions by rupturing the aortic valves with a catheter tip introduced via the carotid artery, resulting in an increase in pulse pressure of 70% or more. Three weeks after the first operation, the rabbits are again anaesthetized. The abdomen is opened, a stainless-steel rod (external diameter 2.3 mm) is positioned next to the abdominal aorta and a ligature is firmly tied around the aorta and the rod. The rod is removed, resulting in a reduction of the aortic diameter by approximately 50%.

Figure 43.1 shows M-mode echocardiographic recordings of the left ventricle in a rabbit before HF induction and 40 days thereafter. Dilation of the left ventricular cavity is evident, while left ventricular wall diameter has not increased. This rabbit showed ventricular premature beats and non-sustained ventricular tachycardias on the Holter recordings of the electrocardiogram (ECG) (not shown).

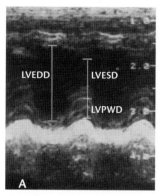
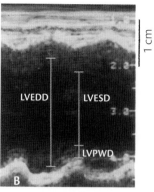

Fig. 43.1 Echographic M-mode recordings (parasternal long axis view) of the left ventricle of a rabbit before induction of heart failure (HF) (**A**) and 40 days after induction of combined volume and pressure overload (**B**). Numbers indicate centimetres. LVEDD, left ventricular end diastolic diameter; LVESD, left ventricular end systolic diameter; LVPWD, left ventricular posterior wall diameter. [Reproduced, with permission, from Rademaker H (1997) Arrhythmogenesis during the development of heart failure in rabbits. PhD Thesis, University of Amsterdam, ISBN 90-9011009-7.]

Electrophysiological changes and arrhythmogenesis

Several review articles on the mechanisms of arrhythmias in HF have appeared in the last decade[26–34]. We limit ourselves to the findings in the rabbit model subjected to combined volume and pressure overload. Hypertrophy in the absence of HF can cause changes in the ventricular AP, and it is often difficult, if not impossible, to separate changes due to HF *per se* and those due to hypertrophy and dilatation. Vermeulen *et al.*[19] used a 'heart failure index', based on measurements of relative heart weight, relative lung weight, left ventricular end diastolic pressure, presence of a third heart sound and ascites. HF was considered to be present if at least three of the five parameters were abnormal.

Changes in sinus node function

It is interesting that combined volume and pressure overload causes changes not only at the level of the left ventricle but also in sinus node function. In nine rabbits, implanted transmitters for Holter recording documented changes in sinus cycle length and occurrence of arrhythmias during the development of HF for periods up to 490 days[24,25]. Three rabbits died suddenly and two had to be euthanized because of development of serious dyspnoea. In these five rabbits, the RR intervals prior to death were significantly shorter than those in the surviving four animals (257 ± 29 vs 304 ± 12 ms, $p < 0.05$, t-test). In the surviving rabbits, sinus cycle length increased above the control levels. Eight of the nine rabbits developed ventricular arrhythmias. Figure 43.2 shows consecutive ECG recordings of a rabbit during the final 10 min before sudden death. Three hours before the terminal events the animal had a supraventricular tachycardia of 1.5 h duration with a cycle length of 170 ms (not shown). Ten minutes before the onset of ventricular fibrillation, sinus rhythm (cycle length 200 ms) was present, followed by sinus bradycardia (cycle length 410 ms) and sinus arrest with a ventricular escape rhythm. Total atrio-ventricular (AV) block developed and ST segment changes occurred. Finally, following extreme bradycardia, ventricular fibrillation ensued. It is difficult

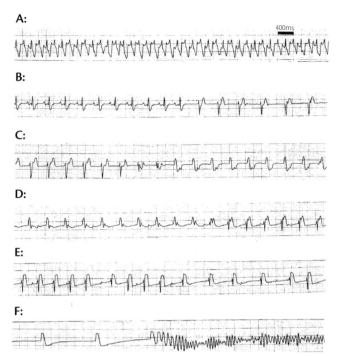

Fig. 43.2 Consecutive recordings of the ECG of a rabbit during the final 10 min before sudden death. **A** –10 min: sinus rhythm, cycle length 200 ms; **B** –9 min 30 s: sinus bradycardia, cycle length 410 ms followed by a ventricular escape rhythm (cycle length 610 ms); **C** –7 min: widening of the QRS complex; **D** –3 min: ST segment elevation; **E** –2 min: total AV block; **F** ventricular fibrillation. [Reproduced, with permission, from Rademaker H (1997) Arrhythmogenesis during the development of heart failure in rabbits. PhD Thesis, University of Amsterdam, ISBN 90-9011009-7.]

to say whether the animal was already dead at the time of the extreme bradycardia or died because of ventricular fibrillation.

In isolated preparations from the failing rabbits, the intrinsic cycle length was significantly longer than in preparations from control rabbits [406 ± 13 vs 353 ± 9 ms[24]]. Also, the response to acetylcholine was enhanced, while the response to norepinephrine was unchanged compared to control preparations. Verkerk *et al.*[35], using the same model, found that in isolated sinus node cells intrinsic cycle length was decreased by 15% and diastolic depolarization rate by 30%, whereas other AP parameters were unchanged. These effects were caused by a reduction of the hyperpolarization-activated inward (pacemaker) current (I_f) by 40%.

It would appear, therefore, that in HF sinus rate can be both increased and decreased. A rapid sinus rate is a harbinger of sudden death and is most likely caused by an excess of sympathetic activity that overrides the intrinsic decrease of sinus cycle length caused by downregulation of I_f. In survivors, the decrease in sinus rate may be a protective mechanism since at rapid rates the likelihood of the occurrence of triggered activity is enhanced[19]. Also, because the force–frequency relation is reversed in HF[36], a lowering of the heart rate leads to improved 'pumping' efficiency.

The fact that combined volume and pressure overload affects sinus node function indicates that the effects of stretch of the left ventricle are not confined to the heart itself, but cause systemic effects as well, in this case a change in the balance of the two arms of the autonomic nervous system.

Changes in action potential duration and ionic currents

A consistent finding in various models of HF is the prolongation of the ventricular AP [for the most recent details, see[33] and[34]]. In most studies this was documented at unphysiologically long cycle lengths, ranging from 1–5 s, and most often it was measured in isolated myocytes. Since AP prolongation promotes the occurrence of early after-depolarizations (EAD), which may produce Torsade de Pointes (TdP) types of arrhythmias, it has been suggested that this may be one of the arrhythmogenic mechanisms in HF. A caveat must be given here: AP duration is very much longer in isolated myocytes than in intact hearts or multicellular preparations. Thus, at a cycle length of 1,000 ms, AP duration in isolated myocytes from humans with end-stage HF was around 600 ms[37], whereas at the same cycle length in isolated trabeculae from humans with end-stage HF it was only about 350 ms[19]. In the presence of norepinephrine, EAD were elicited in the isolated myocytes[37], but in view of the extreme prolongation of the AP in these conditions, it is doubtful whether these results can be extrapolated to the intact heart.

Figure 43.3 shows the relation between steady-state AP duration and cycle length from 25 ventricular trabeculae from control rabbit hearts and from 26 trabeculae from failing hearts subjected to volume and pressure overload. With decreasing cycle lengths, the difference in AP duration between normal and failing myocardium decreases. Differences were statistically significant at cycle lengths longer than 350 ms[19].

Although not all results of the various studies are in agreement, the most consistent findings are that the AP prolongation is due to a reduction in the transient outward K^+ current (I_{to}) and the slowly activating component of delayed rectifier K^+ current (I_{Ks}) and an upregulation of the late Na^+ current $I_{Na,L}$[33,34].

Delayed after-depolarizations

In the study of Vermeulen et al.[19], delayed after-depolarizations (DAD) could not be induced when the trabeculae were superfused with normal Tyrode's solution. However, in modified Tyrode's solution (K^+ 3 mmol/L and noradrenaline 1 µmol/L) DAD and triggered activity were frequently observed and occurred reproducibly. In other studies on the same rabbit model, DAD have been recorded as well[21,22,38,39].

The basis for DAD is the Ca^{2+} after-transients resulting from spontaneous Ca^{2+} release from the SR (see Fig. 43.4). The after-transient-related Ca^{2+} is removed from the cell by the electrogenic NCX or by a Ca^{2+}-activated Cl^- current, providing the transient inward current that causes the delayed after-depolarization [[39,40]; NCX is electrogenic because it removes one Ca^{2+} for every three Na^+ ions entering, thus causing a net flow of positive ions to enter and depolarize the cell]. Pogwizd et al.[38] concluded that three factors combine to enhance the propensity for the occurrence of DAD: (1) increased activity of the NCX, providing more transient inward current for any given SR Ca^{2+} release; (2) a reduced inward rectifier K^+ current (I_{K1}), allowing more depolarization for any given transient inward current; and (3) residual beta-adrenergic responsiveness, required to raise the low SR Ca^{2+} content ($[Ca^{2+}]_{SR}$) to the point at which more spontaneous Ca^{2+} release occurs. They[38,39] noted the paradox that normally a high $[Ca^{2+}]_{SR}$ is required for spontaneous Ca^{2+} release, whereas in HF $[Ca^{2+}]_{SR}$ is reduced[22,41]. They[38,39] resolved this paradox by the preserved beta-adrenergic responsiveness which allows, in the presence of adrenergic drive, the $[Ca^{2+}]_{SR}$ to reach the threshold for spontaneous Ca^{2+} release. As already noted, DAD and Ca^{2+}-after transients only occur in the presence of noradrenaline[19,22]. Another factor facilitating Ca^{2+} release is the increased open probability of the ryanodine receptor[22].

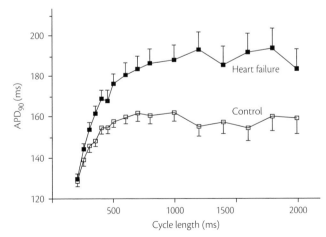

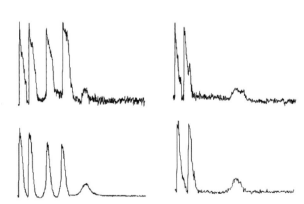

Fig. 43.4 Ca^{2+} after-transients (lower panels) and trans-membrane potentials (upper panels) recorded by optical methods (fluorescence from myocytes loaded with the voltage-sensitive dye di-4-ANEPPS) from myocytes of rabbits with HF due to combined volume and pressure overload. After-transients, DAD and triggered activity were induced by cessation of a 10 s burst stimulation (3 Hz) in the presence of 100 nmol/L noradrenaline. Arrows mark the last two stimulated beats. The dotted lines are included to show that the Ca^{2+} after-transients precede the triggered AP and the DAD. [Reproduced, with permission, from Baartscheer A, Schumacher CA, Belterman CNW, Coronel R, Fiolet JWT (2003) SR calcium handling and calcium after-transients in a rabbit model of heart failure. *Cardiovasc Res* **58**:99–108.]

Fig. 43.3 Steady-state AP duration at 90% repolarization (APD_{90}) of pooled ventricular trabeculae as a function of cycle length. Empty squares indicate data from normal rabbit hearts, filled squares data from hearts subjected to volume and pressure overload. APD_{90} of failing myocardium was significantly longer at cycle lengths longer than 350 ms. [Reproduced, with permission, from Vermeulen JT, McGuire MA, Opthof T, *et al.* (1994) Triggered activity and automaticity in ventricular trabeculae of failing human and rabbit hearts. *Cardiovasc Res* **28**: 1547–1554.]

An important mechanism leading to Ca^{2+} overload is the increased activity of the Na^+/H^+ exchanger-1 (NHE-1), which results in elevated intracellular Na^+ concentration and consequently leads to Ca^{2+} overload via NCX[42,43]. Recently it was shown that chronic inhibition of the NHE-1 by treatment with dietary cariporide in the rabbit volume and pressure overload model, initiated at the time when HF had already developed, reduced the electrophysiological and ionic remodelling to almost normal values. The propensity to develop Ca^{2+} after-transients, which underlie the development of triggered arrhythmias, was reduced to normal[44].

Conduction velocity

DAD can induce triggered activity leading to sustained arrhythmias. However, the salvos of triggered activity in *in vitro* preparations have longer cycle lengths than the ventricular tachycardias in the intact animal. It is likely that triggered activity due to DAD may induce re-entrant rhythms. One of the factors that promotes the occurrence of re-entry is slow conduction. Patients with HF often have an increased QRS interval, and those with a QRS duration of > 150 ms have a higher mortality than patients with shorter QRS duration[45,46]. Increased QRS duration is usually interpreted as slowing of ventricular conduction. Actual measurements of conduction velocity revealed that in the subepicardium both longitudinal and transverse conduction velocity were increased, while transmural conduction was unchanged[47]. The increase in conduction velocity was attributed to the increase in cell size by about 30%. The increased conduction velocity could not compensate for the increased strand size of longitudinally coupled cells and, consequently, total activation time, and thus QRS duration was longer. It is possible that the antiarrhythmic effect of the increase in conduction velocity is offset by the increase in muscle mass, which in itself predisposes to re-entry.

Changes in cell-to-cell coupling

In the rabbit model of volume and pressure overload, the expression of connexin 43 (Cx43) was heterogeneously reduced in the left ventricular mid-myocardium by about 50%, whereas in the subepicardium it was unchanged[48]. Despite the reduction in cellular coupling in the mid-myocardial regions, transmural conduction velocity was unchanged compared to control rabbits. It could be that the reduction in Cx43 expression is compensated by the increase in myocyte dimensions, thus rescuing conduction velocity to control values[47,48]. The decrease in cellular coupling was responsible for an increased dispersion in transmural refractory periods and heterogeneous transmural conduction. Both factors may have been responsible for the observation that in the failing rabbits, ventricular arrhythmias were more easily induced than in control rabbits[48]. Attempts to improve cellular coupling in explanted human hearts (of patients with end-stage HF) by pharmacological means led to a paradoxical increase of lines of activation block in some of the hearts, secondary to an increase in longitudinal but a decrease in transversal conduction[49]. This increased anisotropy is a potentially proarrhythmic condition.

Conclusions and outlook

Rabbits subjected to combined volume and pressure overload develop spontaneous non-sustained ventricular tachycardias and often die suddenly. It is not clear whether sudden death is only due to ventricular tachyarrhythmias. Extreme bradycardia and electromechanical dissociation may also be involved. In rabbits dying suddenly, heart rate prior to the fatal event was rapid, probably caused by extreme sympathetic activation. In surviving rabbits sinus rhythm is slower than in control rabbits. This is due to a reduction in the pacemaker current (I_f).

Ventricular AP duration is prolonged, especially at cycle lengths longer than 350 ms. In isolated ventricular trabeculae of failing hearts, DAD and salvos of triggered activity occur, but only in the presence of noradrenaline. Cycle lengths of triggered activity are longer than cycle lengths of ventricular tachycardias *in vivo*, suggesting that re-entrant mechanisms may also occur.

The basis for DAD is abnormal cellular Ca^{2+} handling. Ca^{2+} after-transients *may* give rise to after-contractions, which would appear to precede after-depolarizations that can trigger TdP[50]. Spontaneous release of Ca^{2+} from the SR causes a transient inward current via NCX which removes one Ca^{2+} from the cell in exchange for three Na^+ ions entering the cell. Several factors are involved in spontaneous Ca^{2+} release, such as adrenergic drive, increased open probability of the ryanodine receptor and increased activity of the NHE.

QRS duration in the ECG is increased, and this is usually interpreted as due to a slowing of conduction in the ventricles. However, conduction velocity is actually increased due to the increase in cell size by about 30%. Because of a reduction in the expression of Cx43, transmural conduction is heterogeneous and dispersion in transmural refractory periods is increased. These factors, as well as the increase in muscle mass, may predispose to re-entry.

HF is primarily a loss of haemodynamic function and, as demonstrated in this chapter, is related to severe electrophysiological alterations that may eventually lead to sudden death. Although mechano-electrical coupling is a potential contributor to many of the mechanisms listed here, HF is a complex process and it is difficult, if not impossible, to assign causality to a single mechanism.

Most studies on mechano-electrical coupling have addressed the effects of acute stretch. In the model described here, stretch is chronic and the electrophysiological changes occur over periods of weeks or months. It might be possible to study the effects of chronic stretch *per se* in a tissue culture model[51].

References

1. Garg R, Packer M, Pitt B, Yusuf S. Heart failure in the 1990s: evolution of a major public health problem in cardiovascular medicine. *J Am Coll Cardiol* 1993;**22**(Suppl A):3A–5A.
2. Kannel WB, Ho K, Thom T. Changing epidemiological features of cardiac failure. *Br Heart J* 1994;**72**(Suppl):S3–S9.
3. Tomaselli GF, Zipes DP. What causes sudden death in heart failure? *Circ Res* 2004;**95**:754–763.
4. Kempf FC, Josephson ME. Cardiac arrest recorded on ambulatory electrocardiograms. *Am J Cardiol* 1984;**427**:241–251.
5. Luu M, Stevenson WG, Stevenson LW, Baron K, Walden J. Diverse mechanisms of unexpected cardiac arrest in advanced heart failure. *Circulation* 1989;**80**:1675–1680.
6. Stevenson WG, Stevenson LW, Middlekauff HR, Saxon LA. Sudden death prevention in patients with advanced ventricular dysfunction. *Circulation* 1993;**88**:2953–2961.
7. De Maria R, Gavazzi A, Caroli A, *et al*. Ventricular arrhythmia in dilated cardiomyopathy as an independent prognostic hallmark. *Am J Cardiol* 1992;**69**:1451–1457.
8. Romeo F, Pellicia F, Cianfrocca C, *et al*. Predictors of sudden death in idiopathic dilated cardiomyopathy. *Am J Cardiol* 1996;**63**:138–140.

9. Doval HC, Nul DR, Grancelli HO, *et al.* Non sustained ventricular tachycardia in severe heart failure: independent marker of increased mortality due to sudden death. *Circulation* 1996;**94**:3189–3203.

10. Packer M. Lack of relation between ventricular arrhythmias and sudden death in patients with chronic heart failure. *Circulation* 1992;**85**:I-50–6.

11. Teerlink JR, Jaladuddin M, Anderson S, *et al.* Ambulatory ventricular arrhythmias in patients with heart failure do not specifically predict an increased risk of sudden death. *Circulation* 2000;**101**:40–46.

12. Kjekshus J. Arrhythmias and mortality in congestive heart failure. *Am J Cardiol* 1990;**65**:421–481.

13. Moss AJ. Implantable cardioverter defibrillator therapy. *The sickest patients benefit most. Circulation* 2000;**101**:1638–1640.

14. The Antiarrhythmics Versus Implantable Defibrillators (AVID) Investigators. A comparison of antiarrhythmic drug therapy with implantable defibrillators in patients resuscitated from near-fatal ventricular arrhythmias *N Engl J Med* 1997;**337**:1576–1583.

15. Moss AJ, Zareba W, Hall W, *et al.* Prophylactic implantation of a defibrillator in patients with myocardial infarction and reduced ejection fraction. *N Engl J Med* 2002;**346**:877–883

16. Hasenfuss G. Animal models of human cardiovascular disease, heart failure and hypertrophy. *Cardiovasc Res* 1998;**39**:60–76.

17. Doggrell SA, Brown L. Rat models of hypertension, cardiac hypertrophy and heart failure. *Cardiovasc Res* 1998;**39**:89–105.

18. Bril A, Forrest M, Gout B. Ischemia and reperfusion-induced arrhythmias in rabbits with chronic heart failure. *Am J Physiol* 1991;**261**:H301–H307.

19. Vermeulen JT, McGuire MA, Opthof T, *et al.* Triggered activity and automaticity in ventricular trabeculae of failing human and rabbit hearts. *Cardiovasc Res* 1994;**28**:1547–1554.

20. Vermeulen JT, Tan HL, Rademaker H, *et al.* Electrophysiologic and extracellular ionic changes during acute ischemia in failing and normal rabbit myocardium. *J Mol Cell Cardiol* 1996;**28**:123–131.

21. Pogwizd. Nonreentrant mechanisms underlying spontaneous ventricular arrhythmias in a model of nonischemic heart failure. *Circulation* 1995;**92**:1034–1084.

22. Baartscheer A, Schumacher CA, Belterman CNW, Coronel R, Fiolet JWT. SR calcium handling and calcium after-transients in a rabbit model of heart failure. *Cardiovasc Res* 2003;**58**:99–108.

23. Baartscheer A Schumacher CA, van Borren MMGJ, *et al.* Increased Na/H-exchange activity is the cause of increased $[Na^+]_i$ and underlies disturbed calcium handling in the rabbit pressure and volume overload heart failure model. *Cardiovasc Res* 2003;**57**:1015–1024.

24. Opthof T, Coronel R, Rademaker JME, Vermeulen JT, Wilms-Schopman FJG, Janse MJ. Changes in sinus node function in a rabbit model of heart failure with ventricular arrhythmias and sudden death. *Circulation* 2000;**101**:2975–2980.

25. Rademaker H (1997). Arrhythmogenesis during the development of heart failure in rabbits. PhD Thesis, University of Amsterdam, ISBN 90-9011009-7.

26. Vermeulen JT. Mechanisms of arrhythmias in heart failure. *J Cardiovasc Electrophysiol* 1998;**9**:208–221.

27. Marban E. Heart failure: the electrophysiologic connection. *J Cardiovasc Electrophysiol* 1999;**10**:1425–1428.

28. Tomaselli GF, Marban E. Electrophysiological remodelling in hypertrophy and heart failure. *Cardiovasc Res* 1999;**47**:270–283.

29. Eckardt L, Haverkamp W, Johna R, *et al.* Arrhythmias in heart failure: current concepts of mechanisms and therapy. *J Cardiovasc Electrophysiol* 2000;**11**:106–117.

30. Janse MJ, Vermeulen JT, Opthof T, *et al.* Arrhythmogenesis in heart failure. *J Cardiovasc Electrophysiol* 2001;**12**:496–499.

31. Amoundas AA, Wu R, Juang G, *et al.* Electrical and structural remodelling of the failing ventricle. *Pharmacol Ther* 2001;**92**: 213–230.

32. Janse MJ. Electrophysiological changes in heart failure and their relationship to arrhythmogenesis. *Cardiovasc Res* 2004;**61**:208–217.

33. Nattel S, Maguey A, Le Bouter S, Yeh Y-H. Arrhythmogenic ion-channel remodelling in the heart: heart failure, myocardial infarction, and atrial fibrillation. *Physiol Rev* 2007;**87**:425–456.

34. Michael G, Xiao L, Qi X-Y, Dobrev D, Nattel S. Remodelling of cardiac repolarization: how homeostatic responses can lead to arrhythmogenesis. *Cardiovasc Res* 2009;**81**:491–499.

35. Verkerk AO, Wilders R, Coronel R, *et al.* Ionic remodeling of sinoatrial cells by heart failure. *Circulation* 2003;**108**:760–767.

36. Hasenfuss G, Reinecke H, Studer R, *et al.* Calcium cycle proteins and force-frequency relationship in heart failure. *Basic Res Cardiol* 1996;**91**(Suppl 2):17–22.

37. Veldkamp MW, Verkerk AO, Van Ginneken ACG, *et al.* Norepinephrine induces action potential prolongation and early afterdepolarizations in ventricular myocytes isolated from human end-stage failing hearts. *Eur Heart J* 2001;**22**:055–963.

38. Pogwizd SM, Schlotthauer K, Li L, Yuan W, Bers DM. Arrhythmogenesis and contractile dysfunction in heart failure. Roles of sodium-calcium exchange, inward rectifier potassium current, and residual beta-adrenergic responsiveness. *Circ Res* 2001;**88**:1159–1167.

39. Pogwizd SM, Sipido KR, Verdonck F, Bers DM. Intracellular Na in animal models of hypertrophy and heart failure: contractile function and arrhythmogenesis. *Cardiovasc Res* 2003;**57**:887–896.

40. Verkerk AO, Veldkamp MW, Bouman LN, *et al.* Calcium-activated Cl⁻ current contributes to delayed afterdepolarizations in single Purkinje and ventricular myocytes. *Circulation* 2000;**101**:2639–2644.

41. Pogwizd SM, Qi M, Yuan W, Samarel AM, Bers DM. Upregulation of Na/Ca exchanger expression and function in an arrhythmogenic model of heart failure. *Circ Res* 1999;**85**:1015–1025.

42. Baartscheer A, Schumacher CA, Belterman CNW, Coronel R, Fiolet JWT. Na^+_i and the driving force of the Na/Ca exchanger in heart failure. *Cardiovasc Res* 2003;**57**:986–995.

43. Cingolani HE, Ennis IL. Sodium-hydrogen exchanger, cardiac overload and myocardial hypertrophy. *Circulation* 2007;**115**:1090–1100.

44. Baartscheer A, Hardziyenka M, Schumacher CA, *et al.* Chronic inhibition of the Na^+/H^+-exchanger causes regression of hypertrophy, heart failure, and ionic and electrophysiological remodelling. *Br J Pharmacol* 2009;**154**:1266–1275.

45. Bode-Schnurbus L, Bocker D, Block M, *et al.* QRS duration: a simple marker for predicting cardiac mortality in ICD patients with heart failure. *Heart* 2003;**89**:1157–1162.

46. Kearney MT, Zaman A, Eckberg, *et al.* Cardiac size, autonomic function, and 5-year follow-up of chronic heart failure patients with severe prolongation of ventricular activation. *J Card Fail* 2003;**9**:93–99.

47. Wiegerinck RF, Verkerk AO, Belterman CN, *et al.* Larger cell size in rabbits with heart failure increases myocardial conduction velocity and QRS duration. *Circulation* 2006;**113**:806–813.

48. Wiegerinck RF, van Veen TAB, Belterman CN, *et al.* Transmural dispersion of refractoriness and conduction velocity is associated with heterogeneously reduced connexin43 in a rabbit model of heart failure. *Heart Rhythm* 2008;**5**:1178–1185.

49. Wiegerinck RF, de Bakker JM, Opthof T, de Jonge N, Kirkels H, Wilms-Schopman FJ, Coronel R. The effect of enhanced gap junctional conductance on ventricular conduction in explanted hearts from patients with heart failure. *Basic Res Cardiol* 2009;**104**:321–332.

50. Gallacher DJ, Van de Water A, van der Linde H, Hermans AN, Lu HR, Towart R, Volders PGA. In vivo mechanisms precipitating torsades de pointes in a canine model of drug-induced long-QT1 syndrome. *Cardiovascular Research* 2007;**76**:247–256.

51. Zhuang J, Yamada KA, Saffitz JE, Kleber AG. Pulsatile stretch remodels cell-to-cell communication in cultured myocytes. *Circ Res* 2000; **87**:316–322.

Stretch effects on fibrillation dynamics

Masatoshi Yamazaki and Jérôme Kalifa

Background

In the last decades, the exploration of the mechanisms linking myocardial stretch to atrial and ventricular fibrillation[1,2] has benefited from advances in high-resolution electrical and/or optical mapping[3,4]. In comparison with initial reports – mostly electrocardiographic – these approaches have enabled us to describe with an improved accuracy the general organization of fibrillation (also called fibrillation dynamic)[5,6]. In particular, a relatively higher spatiotemporal resolution has eased the examination of the fibrillatory activity in specific myocardial regions such as the pulmonary veins (PV) and at changing levels of intra-atrial and intraventricular pressure. Thus, it has been feasible to monitor parameters such as local frequency, wave patterns and wavebreak formation during prolonged episodes of fibrillation and in the presence of controlled myocardial stretch. In this chapter we present examples that illustrate how myocardial stretch reproducibly modulates fibrillation dynamics.

Effect of acute myocardial stretch on atrial fibrillation dynamics

Effect of stretch on frequency

Among the parameters of atrial fibrillation (AF) dynamics, the frequency of activation has been reported to vary substantially upon acute and/or chronic atrial stretch in several stretch-related AF experimental models. For instance, in a dog model of chronic mitral regurgitation obtained after mitral avulsion, an increase in the highest dominant frequency (DF), in the number of DF domains and in the frequency gradient were observed during AF in comparison with control[7]. It was also shown that the maximal DF located in the left atrium (LA) posterior wall increased during acute atrial dilatation (7.1 ± 0.8 vs 8.8 ± 2.1, $p = 0.02$)[8]. Recently our laboratory adapted a well-characterized model of stretch-related AF using sheep[3,4] to test the hypothesis that atrial dilation associates with arrhythmogenic sources at the PV. As initially reported in a rabbit model[9], an intra-atrial pressure of 10 cm H_2O was found to be the lower level above which sustained AF episodes were inducible. In comparison, below 10 cm H_2O, AF usually terminated after 10–20 min and stretch-activated ion channels blockade using GsMTx-4 caused a significant decrease in AF inducibility for comparable pressure values[10]. In sheep, we evaluated the frequency of activation with fast-Fourier transformation of both optical and electrical signals and determined the organization of the activity during AF at various levels of intra-atrial pressure (IAP) (for a detailed technical description please refer to references[3,4,11–14]). In Fig. 44.1, panels A and B are representative DF maps obtained simultaneously from the LA free wall (LAFW) and the LA superior pulmonary vein junction (JPV) in one isolated sheep heart at IAP of 5 and 18 cm H_2O, respectively. These maps clearly illustrate the dependence of frequency on IAP. Below 10 cm H_2O, the difference between the maximum dominant frequency (DF_{Max}) in the JPV and LAFW was not significant (10.8 ± 0.3 vs 10.2 ± 0.3; $p = 0.6$; Fig. 44.1C). However, at pressures > 10 cm H_2O, DF_{Max} in the JPV was significantly higher than that in LAFW [12.0 ± 0.2 and 10.5 ± 0.2 Hz, respectively (mean ± SEM); $n = 9$; $p < 0.001$; see also representative single-pixel recordings in Fig. 44.1D]. Importantly at all pressures, DF_{Max} in both JPV and LAFW was significantly higher than the largest frequency recorded in the right atrial free wall (7.8 ± 0.3 Hz; $p < 0.001$). Altogether, the above results from three laboratories point toward a correlation between the frequency of excitation during AF and the level of myocardial stretch. Specifically, they indicate that the fibrillation dynamics of regions harbouring the fastest frequency of activation are reproducibly sensitive to a change in atrial mechano-electric feedback.

Effects of stretch on AF wave directionality

As described in several works, propagation of waves in AF may be highly periodic, both spatially and temporally[11,15]. Such spatiotemporal periodicities (STP) may take various forms, including periodic waves emerging from the edge of the recording field, breakthroughs occurring at constant frequencies or rotors[15]. We found similar STP waves in high IAP-associated AF. In Fig.44.1E,F we present evidence of the correlation of STP of electrical activation with IAP values. Clearly, the direction of propagation from left superior pulmonary vein (LSPV) to LAFW (grey symbols) was very consistent in that the local direction of excitation at the JPV correlated strongly with IAP ($r = 0.79$, $p = 0.02$; Fig. 44.1E). In contrast, the wave directionality LAFW-to-LSPV had a negative and statistically non-significant correlation with pressure ($r = 0.54$, $p = 0.09$). Further, we show in Fig. 44.1F that the number of STP wavefronts (normalized to the maximum number of STP

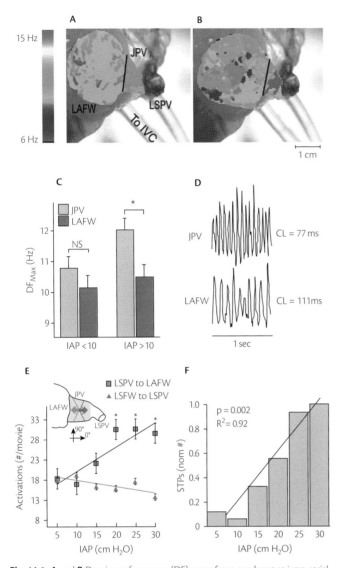

Fig. 44.1 **A** and **B** Dominant frequency (DF) maps from one heart at intra-atrial pressures of 5 and 18 cm H$_2$O, respectively. DF maps are superimposed on colour picture of a heart for illustrative purposes. **C** Bar graph showing DF$_{max}$ (mean ± SEM) in the JPV (blue) and LAFW (red) at IAp < 10 and > 10 cm H$_2$O (*p < 0.001). **D** Single-pixel recordings from JPV and LAFW at 30 cm H$_2$O. IVC, inferior *vena cava*; CL, cycle length. **E** Number of activations (mean ± SEM) moving from LSPV to LAFW and from LAFW to LSPV (*p < 0.01 compared with LAFW to LSPV). Left inset: directionality of activity from the PV to LAFW (grey arrow) and from the LAFW to LSPV (red arrow) assessed at the JPV region. **F** Relation between the normalized number of STP wavefronts by episode and the level of pressure. [Reproduced, with permission, from Kalifa J, Jalife J, Zaitsev AV, *et al.* (2003) Intra-atrial pressure increases rate and organization of waves emanating from the superior pulmonary veins during atrial fibrillation. *Circulation* **108**:668–671.] (See color plate section.)

Previous works have indicated that STP and breakthrough waves are indications of spontaneous focal discharges, re-entrant activities or both. Thus, we further explored the mechanisms – **re-entry** and/or **focal discharges** – maintaining atrial fibrillation under conditions of atrial stretch.

Effect of acute stretch on the interplay rotors – spontaneous focal discharges

To examine which of the re-entrant or focal discharge mechanisms is preponderant during stretch-related atrial fibrillation (SRAF), we utilized optical mapping techniques as described above, and perfused ryanodine (RyR) 10–40 µM. Our rationale was to abolish calcium overload-related-triggered activity during SRAF in order to examine the changes in fibrillatory dynamics. Besides, we also observed SRAF dynamics in the presence of a vago-sympathetic input – mimicked by the simultaneous perfusion of acetylcholine 1 µM plus isoproterenol 0.03 µM (adrenocholinergic stimulation, ACS)[4] – and thereafter abolished focal discharges with RyR.

Stretch-related AF mechanism

During SRAF alone, the perfusion of RyR yielded contrasting results. In five out of eight animals AF terminated and in three out of eight it did not. Figure 44.2 shows representative examples of electrograms with DF time course at three atrial locations in a case of AF termination and in a case of absence of AF termination. In the former, DF significantly decreased at all atrial locations before AF termination (right), while DF at the LA roof did not change significantly in the animal in which AF did not terminate (left). As also presented in the left panel, we gradually increased RyR concentration to 40 µM during the AF episode that did not terminate, without additional frequency changes or AF termination.

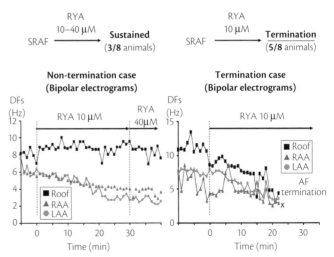

Fig. 44.2 Representative examples of a termination case and a non-termination case of stretch-related AF (SRAF) during perfusion of ryanodine 10–40 µM (RYA). While DF significantly decreased at all atrial locations before AF termination (right), DF at the LA roof did not change significantly in an animal in which AF did not terminate (left). [Reproduced, with permission, from Yamazaki M, Vaquero LM, Hou L, *et al.* (2009) Mechanisms of stretch-induced atrial fibrillation in the presence and the absence of adrenocholinergic stimulation: interplay between rotors and focal discharges. *Heart Rhythm* **6**: 1009–1017.]

wavefronts by level of pressure) in the JPV was also strongly linked to IAP values ($r = 0.92$, $p = 0.002$). These data relate well to patients with paroxysmal AF in whom it was suggested that the superior PV were the most arrhythmogenic and markedly dilated in comparison with the inferior PV[16,17]. However, the nature of the electrophysiological mechanism(s) causing STP remained to be evaluated.

These results suggest that in some animals fibrillation was insensitive to the suppression of calcium-dependent focal discharges, while in others fibrillation rapidly terminated. In total, it seemed that in the presence of atrial stretch both re-entry and spontaneous focal discharges had the ability to maintain AF.

Stretch-related AF mechanism in the presence of a vago-sympathetic input

We then examined AF dynamics under a pharmacologically induced vago-sympathetic input (ACS) to further promote re-entrant and focal discharge mechanisms. Figure 44.3A, B is a

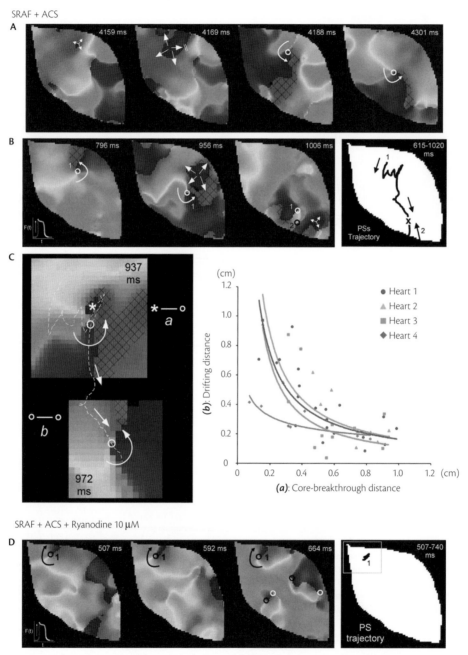

Fig. 44.3 Interaction between rotors and spontaneous breakthroughs in the setting of adrenocholinergic stimulation (ACS). **A** Representative phase maps during ACS; repeated breakthroughs gave rise to rotor formation after wavebreak. **B** Left: a breakthrough induced substantial rotor drift. Right: the corresponding PS trajectory is shown for rotor 1, which was forced to drift inferiorly and terminate after collision with counter-rotating rotor 2; both rotors mutually annihilated. **C** Quantification of breakthrough-induced-rotor drift. Left: example of measurements between PS and breakthrough centre (distance a: asterisk to open circle) and breakthrough-induced rotor drifting (distance b: between open circles) in the presence of ACS. Right: relationship between (a) and (b). We added a trend line to fit a line according to a power function $y = x^n$. A black shaded area depicts the excitable gap for the rotors presented. **D** Representative example of phase maps and corresponding rotor PS trajectory in the setting of ACS in the presence of RYA. A long-lasting and stable rotor (left) with a stationary PS trajectory (right) was visualized. Notably, a decrease in the number of breakthroughs was also noted. This re-entry showed the fastest atrial frequency of activation (12.2 Hz). SRAF stretch-related AF; PS, phase singularity. [Reproduced, with permission, from Yamazaki M, Vaquero LM, Hou L, et al. (2009) Mechanisms of stretch-induced atrial fibrillation in the presence and the absence of adrenocholinergic stimulation: interplay between rotors and focal discharges. *Heart Rhythm* **6**:1009–1017.] (See color plate section.)

representative example of the two opposite situations that were visualized during SRAF in the presence of ACS. First, as shown in Fig. 44.3A, breakthroughs resulted in wavebreak and rotor formation. In this example, at 4,188 ms the breakthrough that emerged on the upper LA appendage underwent wavebreak, leading to the formation of a counterclockwise rotor with a cycle length (72 ms) equal to the inverse of the maximum DF (1/DF$_{Max}$). Second, although several rotors could be observed during a given AF episode, most were forced to drift and eventually terminate after three to four rotations by their interaction with the repetitively emerging breakthroughs. In Fig. 44.3B the breakthrough that appeared near the centre of the optical field at frame 956 ms (location 1) forced the nearby rotor 1 to drift over a long distance toward the LA roof (location 2). Then, collision of this rotor with a second rotor (2) led to its annihilation. These results indicate that SRAF mechanisms in the presence of ACS resulted from a constant interplay between rotors and spontaneous focal discharges. In Fig. 44.3C, we quantified the substantial drift that rotors underwent during SRAF in the presence of ACS. We followed the trajectory of the phase singularities (PS) at the rotor tip and quantified the spatiotemporal relationship between PS and breakthrough site as follows: first, as depicted on the left of Fig. 44.3C, the PS-to-centre of breakthrough distance at the onset of the breakthrough was noted as distance a; i.e. from the asterisk to the white circle in the top frame of Fig. 44.3C. Distance a was then plotted against the PS-to-centre of breakthrough distance after the rotor had undergone a half rotation; the latter was noted as distance b and measured between the white circles in the top and bottom frames of Fig. 44.3C. As plotted in Fig. 44.3C rightmost panel ($n = 4$), there was a non-linear inverse relationship between rotor drifting and PS-breakthrough distance. Breakthroughs caused the most drifting when they occurred in the immediate vicinity of the PS, and the drifting effect tended to fade as the PS-breakthrough distance increased above 6 mm. Interestingly, when spontaneous focal discharges were abolished the rotors were long-lasting and no longer drifted. Figure 44.3D shows a long-lasting and stable rotor with a stationary PS trajectory after perfusion of RYA in the presence of ACS. Altogether these results indicate that in the presence of a vago-sympathetic input, SRAF is governed by **an evolving interplay between re-entries and spontaneous focal discharges.**

Effect of acute myocardial stretch on ventricular fibrillation dynamics

Although the pathophysiological factors at play are profoundly different, two elegant studies have examined how acute ventricular myocardial stretch modulates VF dynamics and have presented results consistent with the atrial studies. In isolated rabbit hearts, Chorro et al.[18] indicated that a mechanically induced stretch – obtained with an L-shaped tube-connected platform device – induced a significant DF increase blunted in the presence of an Na$^+$/Ca^{2+} (NCX) exchange-blocking pharmacological agent (KBR7943) or propranolol (see Fig. 44.4). It should be mentioned, however, that in this work NCX might not have been the main mechano-sensitive component as it is likely to have been activated in both the forward and the reverse mode, leading to both calcium extrusion and loading. Also, Moreno et al.[19] showed that acute ventricular stretch slightly modulated DF in control and failing

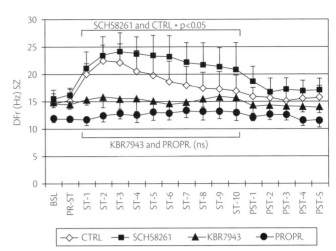

Fig. 44.4 Mean values ± SD of the ventricular fibrillation dominant frequency in the stretched zones (SZ) obtained at baseline, before stretch, each minute during stretch and after stretch suppression. BSL, baseline; CTRL, control; DFr, dominant frequency; KBR7943, NCX blocker; SCH5826, adenosine A2 receptor antagonist; PROPR, propranolol; PR-ST pre-stretch; PST 1–5 post-stretch; ST1–10, stretch; differences with respect to pre-stretch: *$p < 0.05$; ns, non-significant. [Reproduced, with permission, from Chorro FJ, Trapero I, Such-Miquel L, et al. (2009) Pharmacological modifications of the stretch-induced effects on ventricular fibrillation in perfused rabbit hearts. *Am J Physiol* **297**:H1860–H1869.]

hearts but altered significantly PS density and rotor numbers. As depicted in Fig. 44.5, an elevation of the intraventricular pressure from 0–5 to 25–30 mmHg significantly increased PS density, from 15.5 ± 2.0 to 17.9 ± 1.9 PS/cm^2/s in failing hearts and from 21.3 ± 1.5 to 23.9 ± 1.1 PS/cm^2/s in controls. Besides, stretch induced a significant rise in rotor density, from 0.24 ± 0.06 to 0.41 ± 0.1 rotors/cm^2/s in heart failure (HF) animals and from 0.81 ± 0.2 to 1.0 ± 0.2 rotors/cm^2/s in controls ($p < 0.002$). Thus, these works indicate that myocardial stretch tends to increase the complexity of ventricular fibrillation dynamics. Such a stretch-dependent modulation in fibrillation organization could be relevant to patients with congestive heart failure, which are known to be at risk of ventricular arrhythmias (see also Chapters 43 and 47).

Conclusions and outlook

Various reports presented here clearly show that acute and/or chronic myocardial stretch directly modulates fibrillation dynamics. The most striking effect observed by several investigators, at both atrial and ventricular levels, is a steady increase in fibrillation frequency in the stretched areas. Besides, the increased complexity of fibrillatory waves after stretch may well result from an interplay between spontaneous activity and rotors. It is unclear, however, how such observations relate to the electrophysiological effects of stretch at the cellular level. In future investigations, the use of specific stretch-activated channel blockers together with advanced mapping methodologies will certainly help elucidate the mechanisms of these changes.

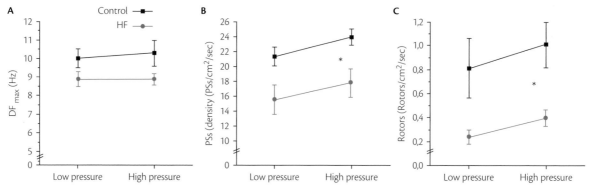

Fig. 44.5 Effects of increased intraventricular pressure on DF$_{max}$, PS and rotor density in control and HF groups (**A**, **B** and **C**, respectively). Values are mean ± SEM. Applying stretch did not modify frequencies but significantly increased PS and rotors density in both groups. *$p < 0.004$; †$p < 0.02$. PS, singularity point. [Reproduced, with permission, from Moreno J, Zaitsev AV, Warren M, *et al.* (2005) Effect of remodelling, stretch and ischaemia on ventricular fibrillation frequency and dynamics in a heart failure model. *Cardiovasc Res* **65**:158–166.]

References

1. Vaziri SM, Larson MG, Benjamin EJ, Levy D. Echocardiographic predictors of nonrheumatic atrial fibrillation. The Framingham Heart Study. *Circulation* 1994;**89**:724–730.

2. Manyari DE, Patterson C, Johnson D, Melendez L, Kostuk WJ, Cape RD. Atrial and ventricular arrhythmias in asymptomatic active elderly subjects: correlation with left atrial size and left ventricular mass. *Am Heart J* 1990;**119**:1069–1076.

3. Kalifa J, Jalife J, Zaitsev AV, *et al.* Intra-atrial pressure increases rate and organization of waves emanating from the superior pulmonary veins during atrial fibrillation. *Circulation* 2003;**108**:668–671.

4. Yamazaki M, Vaquero LM, Hou L, *et al.* Mechanisms of stretch-induced atrial fibrillation in the presence and the absence of adrenocholinergic stimulation: interplay between rotors and focal discharges. *Heart Rhythm* 2009;**6**:1009–1017.

5. Eijsbouts SC, Majidi M, van Zandvoort M, Allessie MA. Effects of acute atrial dilation on heterogeneity in conduction in the isolated rabbit heart. *J Cardiovasc Electrophysiol* 2003;**14**:269–278.

6. Eckstein J, Verheule S, de Groot NM, Allessie M, Schotten U. Mechanisms of perpetuation of atrial fibrillation in chronically dilated atria. *Prog Biophys Mol Biol* 2008;**97**:435–451.

7. Everett THt, Verheule S, Wilson EE, Foreman S, Olgin JE. Left atrial dilatation resulting from chronic mitral regurgitation decreases spatiotemporal organization of atrial fibrillation in left atrium *Am J Physiol* 2004;**286**:H2452–H2460.

8. Huang JL, Tai CT, Lin YJ, *et al.* The mechanisms of an increased dominant frequency in the left atrial posterior wall during atrial fibrillation in acute atrial dilatation. *J Cardiovasc Electrophysiol* 2006;**17**:178–188.

9. Ravelli F, Allessie M. Effects of atrial dilatation on refractory period and vulnerability to atrial fibrillation in the isolated Langendorff-perfused rabbit heart. *Circulation* 1997;**96**:1686–1695.

10. Bode F, Katchman A, Woosley RL, Franz MR. Gadolinium decreases stretch-induced vulnerability to atrial fibrillation. *Circulation* 2000;**101**:2200–2205.

11. Mandapati R, Skanes A, Chen J, Berenfeld O, Jalife J. Stable microreentrant sources as a mechanism of atrial fibrillation in the isolated sheep heart. *Circulation* 2000;**101**:194–199.

12. Sanders P, Berenfeld O, Hocini M, *et al.* Spectral analysis identifies sites of high-frequency activity maintaining atrial fibrillation in humans. *Circulation* 2005;**112**:789–797.

13. Berenfeld O, Zaitsev AV, Mironov SF, Pertsov AM, Jalife J. Frequency-dependent breakdown of wave propagation into fibrillatory conduction across the pectinate muscle network in the isolated sheep right atrium. *Circ Res* 2002;**90**:1173–1180.

14. Mansour M, Mandapati R, Berenfeld O, Chen J, Samie FH, Jalife J. Left-to-right gradient of atrial frequencies during acute atrial fibrillation in the isolated sheep heart. *Circulation* 2001;**103**:2631–2636.

15. Skanes AC, Mandapati R, Berenfeld O, Davidenko JM, Jalife J. Spatiotemporal periodicity during atrial fibrillation in the isolated sheep heart. *Circulation* 1998;**98**:1236–1248.

16. Lin WS, Prakash VS, Tai CT, *et al.* Pulmonary vein morphology in patients with paroxysmal atrial fibrillation initiated by ectopic beats originating from the pulmonary veins: implications for catheter ablation. *Circulation* 2000;**101**:1274–1281.

17. Yamane T, Shah DC, Jais P, *et al.* Dilatation as a marker of pulmonary veins initiating atrial fibrillation. *J Interv Card Electrophysiol* 2002;**6**:245–249.

18. Chorro FJ, Trapero I, Such-Miquel L, *et al.* Pharmacological modifications of the stretch-induced effects on ventricular fibrillation in perfused rabbit hearts. *Am J Physiol* 2009;**297**:H1860–H1869.

19. Moreno J, Zaitsev AV, Warren M, *et al.* Effect of remodelling, stretch and ischaemia on ventricular fibrillation frequency and dynamics in a heart failure model. *Cardiovasc Res* 2005;**65**:158–166.

SECTION 6

Pathophysiology of cardiac mechano-electric coupling: specific cases

45. *Commotio cordis*: sudden death from blows to the chest wall   325
Mark S. Link

46. Repolarization changes in the synchronously and dyssynchronously contracting failing heart   330
Takeshi Aiba and Gordon F. Tomaselli

47. Ventricular arrhythmias in heart failure: link to haemodynamic load   340
Steven N. Singh and Pamela Karasik

48. Mechanical heterogeneity and after contractions as trigger for Torsades de Pointes   345
Annerie M.E. Moers and Paul G.A. Volders

49. Stretch-induced arrhythmias in ischaemia   352
Ruben Coronel, Natalia A. Trayanova, Xiao Jie and Michael J. Janse

Commotio cordis: sudden death from blows to the chest wall

Mark S. Link

Background

Commotio cordis (CC) is defined as sudden cardiac death or aborted sudden cardiac death resulting from blunt and often innocent-appearing chest wall blows. CC is not associated with structural heart disease, and is primarily an electrical event, with the instantaneous induction of ventricular fibrillation (VF) resulting from non-penetrating chest wall impacts that do not cause structural damage to the ribs, sternum or heart itself[1–3]. The lack of structural damage distinguishes CC from *Contusio cordis*, in which high-impact blows result in myocardial and thoracic damage. Many instances of CC occur as a result of chest impact with projectiles used in sports, particularly baseball, hockey and lacrosse[4]. In the United States, CC has now been recognized as the second most common cause of sudden death in youth athletes and is being reported with increasing frequency[5]. Over the last decade, CC has achieved broad visibility through a series of detailed reports describing its epidemiology[2,4]. At the same time, the development of an experimental animal and Langendorff models have led to a greater understanding of its mechanism[1,6–10].

Epidemiology: patient characteristics

Since being initiated in 1996, the United States *Commotio cordis* Registry (US CCR; Minneapolis, Minnesota) now includes more than 190 cases[2,4]. As awareness of this phenomenon grows, CC is being reported with increasing frequency, with most cases in the registry (75%) clustered from 1988 to the present[11]. However, the actual prevalence may be even greater as many cases go unreported. Young males (median age 14 years) appear to be most at risk[4]. This susceptibility may be the result of the compliant chest walls of children that allow for greater transmission of impact energy to the myocardium. Only 28% of the cases in the US CCR were aged over 18 years.

Sport characteristics

Most victims are struck in the chest by projectiles used in sports and they generally have a dense solid core, such as a baseball, hockey puck or lacrosse ball. Projectiles with a soft core tend to collapse on contact and probably absorb much of the impact energy. Only one event has been attributed to chest impact with an air-filled ball, which was a soccer ball. In almost all cases, chest impacts that resulted in CC occurred to the left of the sternum, directly over the cardiac silhouette. Estimated velocities of baseballs were 13–22 m $\times$ s^{-1} (30–50 mph). Interestingly, 38% of the individuals competing in organized sports were wearing standard chest wall protection[12]. However, in 25 of these 32 cases, the chest wall protector did not adequately cover the left chest or precordium at the time of impact. In sports such as football and hockey, raising the arms lifts the protector, thereby exposing the chest. In lacrosse and baseball, the projectiles struck the chest protector directly over the heart and still caused CC. Although commonly associated with sports, CC has now been reported in a diverse spectrum of non-sports activity[13] with unintentional and innocuous-appearing chest blows.

Arrhythmias

Initial electrocardiogram (ECG) data (recorded in the emergency room or by emergency medical technicians in the field) are available for 82 patients in the US CCR. There are 33 cases of VF, three with ventricular tachycardia, three with bradyarrhythmias, two with idioventricular rhythm and one with complete heart block[4]. Forty of the cases had asystole, which was unlikely to be the initial rhythm after impact, but is more likely the result of prolonged time elapsed from event to rhythm documentation.

Resuscitation

The survival rate in the US CCR is only about 15%, probably due to a lack of early recognition and the failure to initiate timely aggressive resuscitation and defibrillation. Survival is most likely to occur with cardiopulmonary resuscitation and defibrillation, applied within 3 min of the incident event[4,14]. Not unexpectedly, application of early resuscitation and defibrillation appears to be the most important determinant of survival, as with other causes of VF. Cardiopulmonary resuscitation is known to have been performed in 106 of the individuals in the US CCR. Of 68 cases in which early resuscitation was instituted (estimated < 3 min), 17 survived (25%). In the cases where resuscitation was substantially delayed (estimate > 3 min) only 1 out of 38 survived (3%). However, not even early resuscitation and defibrillation guarantees a good outcome[14].

Prevention

Strategies to protect young athletes include chest protectors and softer-than-normal baseballs. Using data from the US CCR, we found that almost 40% of the competitive athletes in the Registry who died of CC had in fact worn chest barriers under the assumption that this equipment would protect the chest from effects of a blow or trauma[12]. These unsuccessful chest barriers were all similar in design. They utilized closed or open-cell polymer foam covered by fabric and/or a hard plastic shell. These protectors were not designed or specifically promoted to protect from CC, but more likely to protect against structural injury to the chest wall. Indeed, seven events in the Registry included baseball catchers and hockey or lacrosse goalies, for whom precordial blows are common and therefore chest protection is mandatory.

In the United States, the use of softer balls for youth sports has been recommended[15,16]. However, in the Registry, deaths have been noted even with safety balls. Nonetheless, given not only the reduction in CC but also the reduction in eye and other bodily injury, the US Consumer Product Safety Commission has called for the use of these age-appropriate safety baseballs in youth sport[15,16].

Animal models and pathological mechanisms

Porcine model

Early experimental efforts to replicate CC were limited by the considerable chest wall trauma inflicted causing severe cardiac and thoracic injuries[17-19]. Over the last decade an animal model of low energy chest impact replicated the clinical scenario of CC and, more recently, Langendorff models have been developed[6,20]. In the juvenile male swine model, first described in 1998, an anaesthetized swine is placed prone in a sling to approximate physiological cardiac and vascular haemodynamics[1]. This animal is struck by a baseball or lacrosse ball propelled at 5.5–20 m × s^{-1} (20–70 mph). Impacts over the cardiac silhouette, timed relative to the cardiac cycle, can cause VF (Fig. 45.1)[9]. The VF is immediate and not preceded by ischaemic changes, premature ventricular contractions, ventricular tachycardia or heart block.

Timing

Timing of the chest blow is perhaps the single most important determinant of VF (Fig. 45.2a)[1]. The vulnerable window appears to be narrower than that observed with experimental induced VF from electrical shock application during the T-wave. Only impacts occurring 0–40 ms prior to the peak of the T-wave cause VF, and the impacts that are most effective in inducing VF occur during the 10–30 ms window. Impacts at other phases of the cardiac cycle may cause transient heart block, left bundle branch block (BBB) or ST elevation, but these abnormalities are self-terminating. Of these three, BBB and ST elevation appear independent of the timing of the strike, but transient heart block is more common during QRS impacts.

Site of impact

The location of the blow over the cardiac silhouette affects sensitivity, with the most arrhythmogenic site being the centre of the heart[9]. In the animal model, only those impacts directly over the heart triggered VF (12 of 78: 15% vs 0 of 100 for non-cardiac sites: $p < 0.0001$). Blows over the centre of the heart (7 of 23; 30%) more

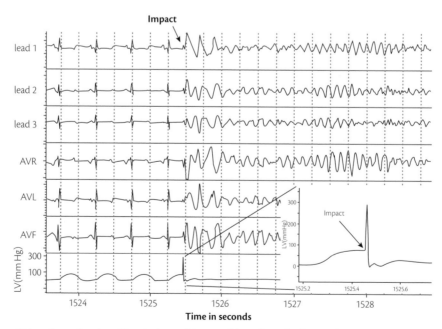

Fig. 45.1 Six-lead ECG from an 11-kg swine undergoing a 30-mph chest wall impact with an object the shape and weight of a standard baseball. VF is produced immediately on impact within the vulnerable zone of repolarization (10–30 ms prior to the peak of the T-wave). Lead 1-3 and AVR, AVL and AVF are ECG recording configurations. [Reproduced, with permission, from Link MS, Maron BJ, VanderBrink BA, *et al.* (2001) Impact directly over the cardiac silhouette is necessary to produce VF in an experimental model of *Commotio cordis. J Am Coll Cardiol* **37**:649–654.]

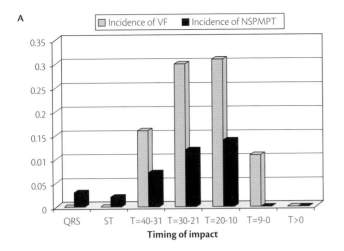

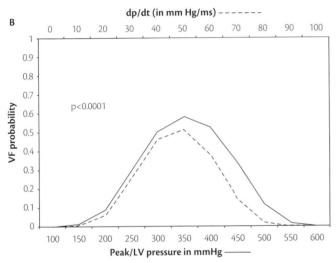

Fig. 45.2 A The incidence of VF and non-sustained polymorphic ventricular tachycardia (NSPMVT) in our animal model of CC. Note the narrow window of vulnerability for VF and a slightly wider window for NSPMVT. [Reproduced, with permission, from Link MS, Estes NA, 3rd (2007) Mechanically induced ventricular fibrillation (*Commotio cordis*). *Heart Rhythm* **4**:529–532.] **B** The probability of VF relative to the peak LV pressure (solid line) and change in LV pressure over time (dp/dt) (dotted line) in 8–12 kg swine undergoing 30 mph chest wall impacts with a baseball. The data exhibit a Gaussian distribution (*p* < 0.0001 by logistic regression). VF began to occur at a threshold peak pressure of around 250 mmHg in all experimental protocols including variations of sites of impact, energy of impact, stretch-activated channel inhibitors and colchicine application. The highest incidence of VF was evident with peak LV pressures between 250 and 450 mmHg. [Reproduced , with permission, from Link MS, Maron BJ, Wang PJ, VanderBrink BA, Zhu W, Estes NA, 3rd (2003) Upper and lower limits of vulnerability to sudden arrhythmic death with chest-wall impact (*Commotio cordis*). *J Am Coll Cardiol* **41**:99–104.]

likely initiated VF than impacts at other precordial sites (5 of 55; 9%: *p* = 0.02). Peak left ventricular (LV) pressures generated by the chest impact were directly related to the risk of VF (*p* < 0.0006; Fig. 45.2b). Impacts that did not lie directly over the heart produced neither VF nor other arrhythmias, nor wall motion abnormalities identified by echocardiography. Peak LV pressures became markedly elevated as an immediate consequence of impacts directly over the centre (280 ± 36 mmHg), base (258 ± 60 mmHg) and apex

(224 ± 48 mmHg) of the LV, but not with impacts at sites outside of the cardiac silhouette.

Stiffness of the impact object

Increased stiffness of the impact object correlated with the probability of VF[1,21]. The susceptibility of VF initiation with four different hardnesses [reduced injury factor (RIF) Worth® levels 1, 5 and 10] and a wood sphere propelled at ~8 m × s⁻¹ (30 mph) revealed significant differences in the occurrence of VF[1]. With baseballs at ~11 m × s⁻¹ (40 mph)[21], the risk of VF linearly correlated with hardness of the projectile. Differences in the incidence of VF between the standard baseball and the safety balls were statistically significant.

Velocity of impact

The velocity of impact object is a key variable[22]. With baseballs propelled at 5.5 to 20 m × s⁻¹ (20 to 70 mph), the incidence of VF relative to the velocity of chest impact was Gaussian, with the peak incidence of VF at ~11 m × s⁻¹ (40 mph; *p* < 0.0001). There was no VF at 5.5 m × s⁻¹ (20 mph). Chest impacts at ~7 m × s⁻¹ (25 mph) caused VF in 7% of the animals, while ~8 m × s⁻¹ (30 mph) impacts produced VF in 27%. VF incidence increased to a maximum of 68% at ~11 m × s⁻¹ (40 mph), and then decreased to 53%, 37% and 38% at ~14, 17 and 20 m × s⁻¹ (50, 60 and 70 mph), respectively. However, with increasing velocity impacts, cardiac rupture and contusion were more frequently observed, arguing that the model at these velocities was more of *Contusio cordis* than CC.

Langendorff model

In a Langendorff rabbit model of CC, an increase in LV pressure resulted in VF only when it occurred at or near the peak of the T-wave[6,23,24], where the mechanical stimulus significantly increased the dispersion of repolarization. Ventricular pressure pulse amplitudes that exceeded 138 ± 29 mmHg were able to trigger action potentials during diastole by mechano-electric coupling and if the action potentials fell within the vulnerable period, VF could be initiated (for more detail see Chapter 31).

Cellular and subcellular mechanisms

In vivo and experimental data from the porcine[1] and Langendorff models show instantaneous induction of arrhythmias by mechanical impact or pressure changes. These observations do not support a VF genesis secondary to myocardial ischaemia, haemorrhage or conduction system block[25–27], but suggest a primary electrical event due to mechanically induced changes in the myocardium. Mechanical stimuli have been recognized to produce electrical effects in the myocardium, including arrhythmias[28]. The phenomenon of mechano-electric coupling has been attributed to the existence of specific stretch-activated channels (SAC)[29–32] and/or other ion channels that exhibit mechano-sensitivity[33]. Non-selective cationic stretch-activated channels (SAC$_{NS}$) might lead to depolarization by generation of inward cation currents. Block of SAC$_{NS}$ suppresses stretch-induced depolarization[34] and arrhythmias[35,36] in isolated hearts[10]. Suppression of VF with 200μM streptomycin, a non-selective inhibitor of SAC$_{NS}$, suggested their involvement. However, in the porcine CC model, animals received either 2 g streptomycin intravenously (mean serum concentration 115 + 18 μM) or sterile water, but neither prevented VF[37]. The differences between the rabbit and the porcine results may have resulted from differences in the free streptomycin concentration, or possibly differences in the channels. Thus, the role of mechano-sensitive channels in *CC* remains to be further elucidated.

In vivo experiments in the porcine model indicate a role of the mechano-sensitive adenosine triphosphate (ATP)-sensitive K$^+$ channel (K$_{ATP}$) for arrhythmia generation[10]. Glibenclamide, a blocker of K$_{ATP}$, significantly decreased the occurrence of VF and the magnitude of ST segment elevation produced by chest blows. With T-wave impacts, animals that received glibenclamide had significantly fewer occurrences of VF (one episode in 27 impacts; 4%) compared to controls (six episodes in 18 impacts; 33%; $p = 0.01$). With QRS impacts, the maximal ST elevation was significantly less in animals given glibenclamide (0.16 + 0.10 mV) compared to controls (0.35 + 0.20 mV; $p = 0.004$).

Mechano-sensitive ion channels may be activated by stress in membranes produced by pressure changes in the ventricle. Dissolution of microtubules with colchicine increased VF incidence with no change in intracardiac pressure in the porcine model[8]. Unfortunately this experiment does not give us information on whether strain, stretch or deformation of the cell membrane is the critical event.

Putting it all together

The necessary ingredients for chest blow-induced VF include a mechanically induced change in the myocardial substrate (amplified dispersion of repolarization) and an appropriately timed trigger. The mechanical force generated by the precordial blow during repolarization causes an abrupt and marked rise in peak intracavity LV systolic pressure (by 250 mmHg to 500 mmHg), which stretches the cells and initiates a cascade of cellular events. This deformation presumably activates ion channels, whose increased current flow prolongs repolarization and amplifies dispersion of repolarization, creating the substrate for VF. The trigger is an appropriately timed ventricular depolarization, caused by direct stimulation at the point of impact, highlighting the relevance of a local stimulus (Fig. 45.3)[38]. The ectopic action potential propagates inhomogeneously through the ventricular myocardium, establishing a spiral wave that degenerates into VF.[38,39] This scenario of altered repolarization and amplified dispersion of repolarization, combined with a depolarization trigger, is common to other cardiac conditions characterized by primary VF[40–46], such as acquired and congenital long QT[41–43], Brugada[41,44–46], short QT syndromes and catecholaminergic polymorphic ventricular tachycardia (82), which share similar abnormalities of repolarization and the need for an electrophysiological trigger. Thus, the mechanism by which VF occurs in CC shares a common theme with other pathophysiological states in which abnormal repolarization constitutes the electrophysiological substrate, but an independent trigger is required to initiate VF.

Conclusions and outlook

CC is being reported with increasing frequency, with young athletes at greatest risk. Sudden cardiac death results from the instantaneous induction of VF following a precordial blow. A narrow time window of vulnerability exists just prior to the peak

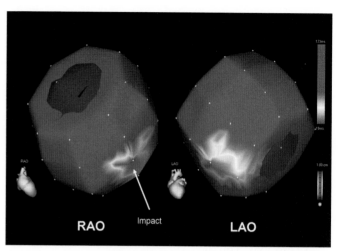

Fig. 45.3 A three-dimensional electrical activation map of the LV in a swine. The earliest ventricular depolarization occurs at the site of impact on the myocardium. This depolarization initiates a continuing re-entry circuit which then anchors in the septum. RAO, right anterior oblique view; LAO, left anterior oblique view. [Reproduced, with permission from Alsheikh-Ali AA, Akelman C, Madias C, Link MS (2008) Endocardial mapping of ventricular fibrillation in *Commotio cordis*. *Heart Rhythm* **5**:1355–1356] (See color plate section.)

of the T-wave. In addition, several other variables, including impact location over the heart and the hardness and velocity of the projectile, are key determinants of arrhythmogenicity. The rapid rise in LV pressure following chest impact results in myocardial stretch and activation of ion channels, including K$_{ATP}$ channels, via mechano-electric coupling. Current flow, presumably through SAC$_{NS}$, may trigger focal excitation, while the interplay of all involved factors increases the spatial dispersion of repolarization, resulting in VF induction and sustenance. By inference, mechanisms of reducing or eliminating stretch-related currents may ultimately be agents to prevent or treat ventricular arrhythmias, important not for CC but for ventricular arrhythmias in other conditions.

References

1. Link MS, Wang PJ, Pandian NG, *et al.* An experimental model of sudden death due to low-energy chest-wall impact (*Commotio cordis*). *N Engl J Med* 1998;**338**:1805–1811.
2. Madias C, Maron BJ, Weinstock J, Estes NA, 3rd, Link MS. *Commotio cordis*– sudden cardiac death with chest wall impact. *J Cardiovasc Electrophysiol* 2007;**18**:115–122.
3. Maron BJ, Poliac LC, Kaplan JA, Mueller FO. Blunt impact to the chest leading to sudden death from cardiac arrest during sports activities. *N Engl J Med* 1995;**333**:337–342.
4. Maron BJ, Gohman TE, Kyle SB, Estes NA, 3rd, Link MS. Clinical profile and spectrum of *Commotio cordis*. *JAMA* 2002; **287**:1142–1146.
5. Maron BJ. Sudden death in young athletes. *N Engl J Med* 2003;**349**:1064–1075.
6. Bode F, Franz MR, Wilke I, Bonnemeier H, Schunkert H, Wiegand UK. Ventricular fibrillation induced by stretch pulse: implications for sudden death due to *Commotio cordis*. *J Cardiovasc Electrophysiol* 2006;**17**:1011–1017.
7. Link MS, Estes NA, 3rd. Mechanically induced ventricular fibrillation (*Commotio cordis*). *Heart Rhythm* 2007; **4**:529–532.

8. Madias C, Maron BJ, Supron S, Estes NA, 3rd, Link MS. Cell membrane stretch and chest blow-induced ventricular fibrillation: *Commotio cordis*. *J Cardiovasc Electrophysiol* 2008;**19**:1304–1309.

9. Link MS, Maron BJ, VanderBrink BA, *et al*. Impact directly over the cardiac silhouette is necessary to produce ventricular fibrillation in an experimental model of *Commotio cordis*. *J Am Coll Cardiol* 2001;**37**:649–654.

10. Link MS, Wang PJ, VanderBrink BA, *et al*. Selective activation of the K^+_{ATP} channel is a mechanism by which sudden death is produced by low-energy chest-wall impact (*Commotio cordis*). *Circulation* 1999;**100**:413–418.

11. Maron BJ, Doerer JJ, Haas TS, Estes NA, 3rd, Link MS. Historical observation on *Commotio cordis*. *Heart Rhythm* 2006;**3**:605–606.

12. Doerer JJ, Haas TS, Estes NA, 3rd, Link MS, Maron BJ. Evaluation of chest barriers for protection against sudden death due to *Commotio cordis*. *Am J Cardiol* 2007;**99**:857–859.

13. Maron BJ. Hypertrophic cardiomyopathy; A systemic review. *J Am Med Assoc* 2002;**287**:1308–1320.

14. Maron BJ, Wentzel DC, Zenovich AG, Estes NA, 3rd, Link MS. Death in a young athlete due to *Commotio cordis* despite prompt external defibrillation. *Heart Rhythm* 2005;**2**:991–993.

15. Adler P, Monticone RCJ. *Injuries and deaths related to baseball*. In: Kyle SB, ed. *Youth Baseball Protective Equipment Project Final Report*. Washington, D. C.: United States Consumer Product Safety Commission, 1996:1–43.

16. Kyle SB. *Youth baseball protective equipment project final report*. Washington, D. C.: United States Consumer Product Safety Commission, 1996.

17. Liedtke AJ, Gault JH, Demuth WE. Electrocardiographic and hemodynamic changes following nonpenetrating chest trauma in the experimental animal. *Am J Physiol* 1974;**226**:377–382.

18. Cooper GJ, Pearce BP, Stainer MC, Maynard RL. The biomechanical response of the thorax to nonpenetrating impact with particular reference to cardiac injuries. *J Trauma* 1982;**22**:994–1008.

19. Viano DC, Andrzejak DV, Polley TZ, King AI. Mechanism of fatal chest injury by baseball impact: development of an experimental model. *Clin J Sports Med* 1992;**2**:166–171.

20. Cooper PJ, Epstein A, Macleod IA, et a.. Soft tissue impact characterisation kit (STICK) for ex situ investigation of heart rhythm responses to acute mechanical stimulation. *Prog Biophys Mol Biol* 2006;**90**:444–468.

21. Link MS, Maron BJ, Wang PJ, Pandian NG, VanderBrink BA, Estes NA, 3rd. Reduced risk of sudden death from chest wall blows (*Commotio cordis*) with safety baseballs. *Pediatrics* 2002;**109**:873–877.

22. Link MS, Maron BJ, Wang PJ, VanderBrink BA, Zhu W, Estes NA, 3rd. Upper and lower limits of vulnerability to sudden arrhythmic death with chest-wall impact (*Commotio cordis*). *J Am Coll Cardiol* 2003;**41**:99–104.

23. Franz MR, Bargheer K, Rafflenbeul W, Haverich A, Lichtlen PR. Monophasic action potential mapping in human subjects with normal electrocardiograms: direct evidence for the genesis of the T-wave. *Circulation* 1987;**75**:379–386.

24. Yue AM, Paisey JR, Robinson S, Betts TR, Roberts PR, Morgan JM. Determination of human ventricular repolarization by noncontact mapping: validation with monophasic action potential recordings. *Circulation* 2004;**110**:1343–1350.

25. Louhimo I. Heart injury after blunt thoracic trauma: an experimental study on rabbits. *Acta Chir Scand Suppl* 1968; **380**:1–60.

26. Pringle SD, Davidson KG. Myocardial infarction caused by coronary artery damage from blunt chest injury. *Br Heart J* 1987;**57**:375–376.

27. Schlomka G. *Commotio cordis* und ihre Folgen. Die Einwirkung stumpfer Brustwandtraumen auf das Herz. *Ergebn Inn Med Kinderheilk* 1934;**47**:1–91.

28. Zabel M, Portnoy S, Franz MR. Electrocardiographic indexes of dispersion of ventricular repolarization: an isolated heart validation study. *J Am Coll Cardiol* 1995;**25**:746–752.

29. Hu H, Sachs F. Mechanically activated currents in chick heart cells. *J Membr Biol* 1996;**154**:205–216.

30. Hu H, Sachs F. Stretch-activated ion channels in the heart. *J Mol Cell Cardiol* 1997; **29**:1511–1523.

31. Kohl P, Nesbitt AD, Cooper PJ, Lei M. Sudden cardiac death by *Commotio cordis*: role of mechanico-electrical feedback. *Cardiovasc Res* 2001;**50**:280–289.

32. Kohl P, Ravens U. Cardiac mechano-electric feedback: past, present, and prospect. *Prog Biophys Mol Biol* 2003; **82**:3–9.

33. Van Wagoner DR. Mechanosensitive gating of atrial ATP-sensitive potassium channels. *Circ Res* 1993;**72**:973–983.

34. Hansen DE, Borganelli M, Stacey GP, Taylor LK. Dose-dependent inhibition of stretch-induced arrhythmias by gadolinium in isolated canine ventricles; evidence for a unique mode of antiarrhythmic action. *Circ Res* 1991;**69**:820–831.

35. Bode F, Sachs F, Franz MR. Tarantula peptide inhibits atrial fibrillation. *Nature* 2001; **409**:35–36.

36. Bode F, Katchman A, Woosley RL, Franz MR. Gadolinium decreases stretch-induced vulnerability to atrial fibrillation. *Circulation* 2000;**101**:2200–2205.

37. Garan AR, Maron BJ, Wang PJ, Estes NA, 3rd, Link MS. Role of streptomycin-sensitive stretch-activated channel in chest wall impact induced sudden death (*Commotio cordis*). *J Cardiovasc Electrophysiol* 2005;**16**:433–438.

38. Alsheikh-Ali AA, Akelman C, Madias C, Link MS. Endocardial mapping of ventricular fibrillation in *Commotio cordis*. *Heart Rhythm* 2008;**5**:1355–1356.

39. Gelzer AR, Koller ML, Otani NF, *et al*. Dynamic mechanism for initiation of ventricular fibrillation in vivo. *Circulation* 2008;**118**: 1123–1129.

40. Turitto G, Dini P, Prati PL. The R on T phenomenon during transient myocardial ischemia. *Am J Cardiol* 1989;**63**:1520–1522.

41. Haissaguerre M, Extramiana F, Hocini M, *et al*. Mapping and ablation of ventricular fibrillation associated with long-QT and Brugada syndromes. *Circulation* 2003;**108**:925–928.

42. Shimizu W, Antzelevitch C. Cellular basis for the ECG features of the LQT1 form of the long-QT syndrome: effects of beta-adrenergic agonists and antagonists and sodium channel blockers on transmural dispersion of repolarization and torsade de pointes. *Circulation* 1998;**98**:2314–2322.

43. Viswanathan PC, Rudy Y. Cellular arrhythmogenic effects of congenital and acquired long-QT syndrome in the heterogeneous myocardium. *Circulation* 2000;**101**:1192–1198.

44. Gussak I, Antzelevitch C, Bjerregaard P, Towbin JA, Chaitman BR. The Brugada syndrome: clinical, electrophysiologic and genetic aspects. *J Am Coll Cardiol* 1999;**33**:5–15.

45. Yan GX, Antzelevitch C. Cellular basis for the Brugada syndrome and other mechanisms of arrhythmogenesis associated with ST-segment elevation. *Circulation* 1999;**100**:1660–1666.

46. Antzelevitch C, Oliva A. Amplification of spatial dispersion of repolarization underlies sudden cardiac death associated with catecholaminergic polymorphic VT, long QT, short QT and Brugada syndromes. *J Intern Med* 2006;**259**:48–58.

Repolarization changes in the synchronously and dyssynchronously contracting failing heart

Takeshi Aiba and Gordon F. Tomaselli

Background

Over 5 million Americans suffer from heart failure (HF) and more than 250,000 die annually. The incidence and prevalence has continued to increase with the aging of the US population, with approximately 600,000 new diagnoses made annually, at a cost of nearly 30 billion dollars annually[1].

Dilated cardiomyopathy is common in patients with HF, and among these many develop dyssynchronous left ventricular (LV) contraction associated with intraventricular conduction delays. The presence of dyssynchrony markedly worsens HF morbidity and mortality independent of traditional prognostic factors[2]. Dyssynchronous contraction generates marked regional heterogeneity of both mechanical function and loading, effectively dividing the heart into early and late contracting zones. The early-activated territory (anterior and septal LV) becomes relatively unloaded, but its work is largely wasted first by pre-stretching the quiescent lateral wall. The delayed contracting lateral wall reciprocally stretches the anterior territory but later in systole, creating regional disparities in wall stress[3], associated with diminished net chamber function and efficiency.

In response to therapeutic gaps in the pharmacological management of ventricular dysfunction, device-based therapies have secured a firm place in the treatment of advanced HF. A number of studies have shown that biventricular pacing in patients with HF and intraventricular conduction delays producing discoordinate ventricular contraction acutely increases LV ejection fraction[4] with a reduction in myocardial oxygen consumption[5]. The remarkable improvement in the efficiency of myocardial energy utilization helped to fast-track implementation of cardiac resynchronization therapy (CRT) and a number of clinical trials have been performed that demonstrate the efficacy of this therapy in reducing symptoms, HF hospitalizations and overall mortality[6] in HF patients with left bundle branch block (LBBB).

Despite the clear demonstration of the effectiveness of CRT, a number of studies have raised several key questions regarding the use of this invasive and expensive therapy. The trials serve to emphasize the shortcomings of CRT including the limited utility of prospective predictors of a therapeutic response, variable effects on arrhythmic mortality and the role of defibrillation capacity of CRT devices. Interestingly the foundation of the clinical benefit of CRT remains incompletely understood. The notion that mechanical resynchronization of contraction is the *sine qua non* of the beneficial effects of CRT has been challenged by several clinical studies. Prominently, patients with mechanical dyssynchrony and a narrow QRS complex did not benefit from CRT[7].

In patients with cardiomyopathy and LBBB, positron emission tomography studies have revealed regionally heterogeneous myocardial oxygen consumption, glucose metabolism and blood flow[8]. In most but not all studies, CRT acutely[5] and chronically[9] improves myocardial energetics, efficiency and reserve. Several studies have demonstrated improvement in the exaggerated regional heterogeneity of oxidative metabolism associated with dyssynchronous HF by CRT[9]. The links between reactive oxygen species, cellular electrophysiology, Ca^{2+} handling and HF have been well established[10]. The role of CRT in correcting regional heterogeneities in cardiac electrophysiology and signalling is the subject of this chapter.

The molecular and cellular basis of electrical remodelling in dyssynchronous HF and CRT

Myocytes have a characteristically long action potential (AP) depolarizing currents, primarily Na^+ and Ca^{2+}, and are responsible for the AP upstroke and maintenance of the AP plateau, while repolarizing currents, primarily K^+, in concert with a reduction in depolarizing currents, are responsible for restoration of the resting membrane potential. A number of electrogenic transporters contribute to the AP profile, and the magnitude and direction of the current depends upon the trans-membrane voltage and concentration gradient of the ions being transported.

Remodelling of myocyte electrophysiology in HF is well described[11]. Indeed, abnormalities of atrial[12] and ventricular[13] electrophysiology in diseased human hearts have been recognized for over four decades. The hallmark signature of cells and tissues isolated from failing hearts independent of the aetiology is AP prolongation[14]. The AP prolongation is heterogeneous particularly across the ventricular wall, resulting in exaggeration of the physiological inhomogeneity of electrical properties in the failing heart[15] (Fig. 46.1). In addition to transmural heterogeneity, in the dyssynchronously contracting failing heart, there is significant variation in the APD within the LV. The AP are longest with a steep rate dependence in the lateral, late-activated region of the LV, with less pronounced prolongation in cells isolated from the anterior wall when compared to non-failing controls. AP prolongation in HF is arrhythmogenic with frequent early after-depolarizations (EAD) that are typically not observed in myocytes isolated from the non-failing hearts. Remarkably, CRT has the unique effect of regional shortening of the action potential duration (APD), reducing heterogeneity of repolarization and frequency of EAD in dyssynchronous HF[16] (Fig. 46.2).

K$^+$ channel remodelling in HF

Downregulation of K$^+$ currents is the most consistent ionic current change in animal models and human HF[17,18]. K$^+$ current downregulation may promote ventricular tachycardia/fibrillation (VT/VF) either by direct prolongation of AP in the voltage range at which L-type Ca^{2+} current ($I_{Ca,L}$) reactivation occurs predisposing to the development of EAD or by heterogeneously reducing repolarization reserve and promoting functional re-entry.

Transient outward K$^+$ current (I_{to})

Although expressed cardiac K$^+$ channels vary in different species, I_{to} downregulation is the most consistent ionic current change in failing mammalian hearts[14,19]. However, the effect on ventricular repolarization is complex and species-dependent[20].

I_{to} activates shortly following the onset of the AP and is responsible for the early phase of repolarization (phase 1 notch of the AP) and setting the membrane potential at which the $I_{Ca,L}$ reactivates. Since I_{to} is an early transient current, it may not directly affect the ventricular APD in large mammalian hearts[20] as it does in

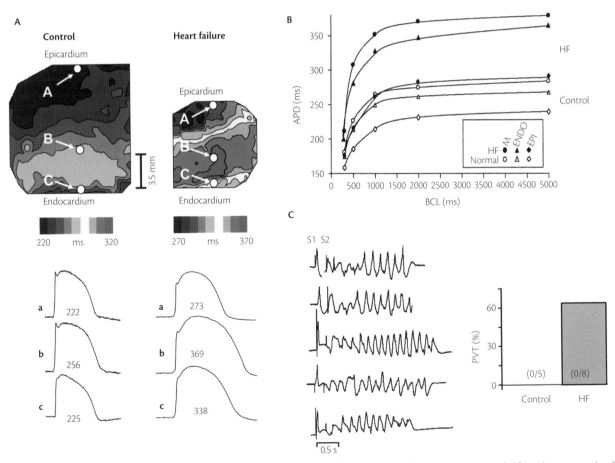

Fig. 46.1 Heart failure (HF) induced transmural dispersion of repolarization. **A** Upper panel: representative APD contour maps recorded from the transmural surfaces of a control (left) and canine tachypacing HF wedge (right). APD was heterogeneously prolonged across all layers in HF. Lower panel: representative action potentials from sub-epicardial (EPI; a), mid-myocardial (M; b) and sub-endocardial (ENDO; c) layers of the control (left) and HF wedges (right). **B** HF wedges exhibited a significant prolongation of APD, which was associated with a marked increase in arrhythmia inducibility (**C**) with a single premature stimulus. PVT, polymorphic ventricular arrhythmia; BCL, basic cycle length. [Modified, with permission, from Akar FG, Rosenbaum DS (2003) Transmural electrophysiological heterogeneities underlying arrhythmogenesis in heart failure. *Circ Res* **93**:638–645.] (See color plate section.).

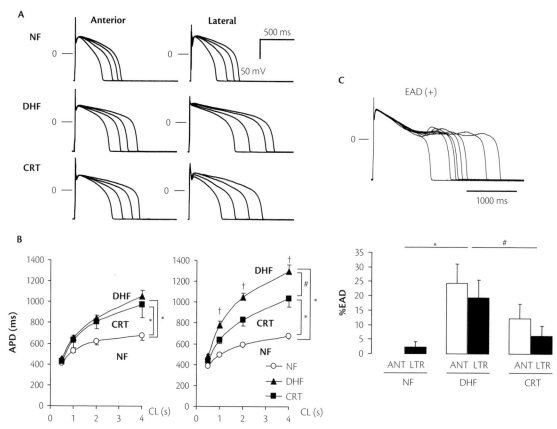

Fig. 46.2 Regional APD differences and development of EAD in dyssynchronous heart failure and CRT. **A** APD were significantly prolonged in dyssynchronous heart failure (DHF) especially in lateral (LTR) cells, and CRT abbreviated APD in LTR cells but not in anterior (ANT) cells (**B**) over a range of pacing cycle lengths. **C** Early after-depolarizations (EAD) as the percentage of AP with one or more EAD were more frequent in DHF and significantly reduced in CRT. NF, non-failing hearts; CL, cycle length. [Modified, with permission, from Aiba T, Hesketh GG, Barth AS, et al. (2009) Electrophysiological consequences of dyssynchronous heart failure and its restoration by resynchronization therapy. *Circulation* **119**:1220–1230.]

rodent ventricle[21]. Interestingly, downregulation of I_{to} in cells isolated from terminally failing human hearts is not associated with a change in the voltage dependence or kinetics of the current[14].

Kv4.3 is the gene that encodes the α subunit of cardiac I_{to} in large mammals[19]. Other accessory subunits may also participate in the formation of native I_{to} channels. For example, Kv4 subunits may form heteromeric complexes with a class of Kv-channel interacting proteins (KChIP)[22]. In the heart, KChIP2 along with several splice variants is expressed[23]. Although KChIP2 significantly modulates Kv4.3 function when expressed in heterologous systems and may impart Ca^{2+} sensitivity to the gating of Kv4.3[24], it remains uncertain whether KChIP2 or other accessory subunits, such as the potassium channel accessory protein (KChAP) or the voltage-activated potassium channel beta subunit (Kvβ), merely act to increase the sarcolemmal expression of Kv4.3 or in fact directly participate in the formation and active phenotypic expression and modulation of native ventricular I_{to}.

The molecular mechanism of I_{to} downregulation in HF is likely to be multifactorial. For one, I_{to} is tightly regulated by neurohumoral factors, which are significantly altered in HF. In addition, there is compelling evidence for a component of transcriptional regulation of I_{to} in HF. For example, reduced steady-state levels of Kv4 messenger RNA (mRNA) are highly correlated with functional

downregulation of I_{to} in both humans[25] and canines[19]. In a canine pacing model of HF, tachycardia downregulates I_{to} expression, with the Ca^{2+}/calmodulin-dependent protein kinase II (CaMKII) and calcineurin/nuclear factor of activated T-cells (NFAT) systems playing key Ca^{2+}-sensing and signal-transducing roles in rate-dependent I_{to} control[26].

The downregulation of I_{to} is regionally uniform in the LV and is unique among regulated K^+ currents in HF in that it is *not* reversed by CRT (Fig. 46.3A). In parallel, Kv4.3 and KChIP2 mRNA and protein expression are downregulated in dyssynchronous HF without restoration by CRT (Fig. 46.3D)[16].

Inward rectifier K^+ current (I_{K1})

Changes in other K^+ currents have also been reported in HF, but not with the consistency of I_{to} downregulation. The inward rectifier K^+ current (Kir2 family of genes, I_{K1}) maintains the resting membrane potential and contributes to terminal repolarization (phase 3). Reduced inward I_{K1} density in HF[19,27] may contribute to prolongation of APD and enhanced susceptibility to spontaneous membrane depolarizations including delayed after-depolarizations (DAD)[27,28].

Reported changes in I_{K1} functional expression are more variable than I_{to}. Even within the same experimental model of HF induction

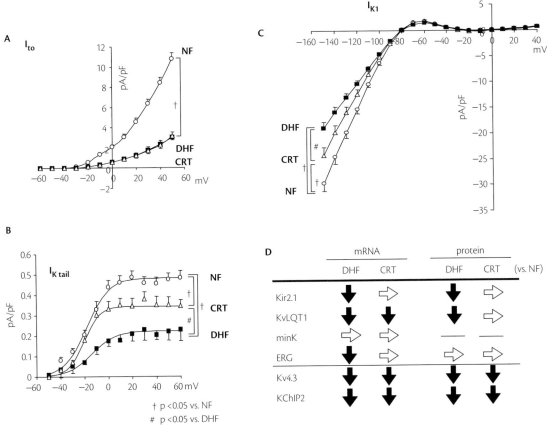

Fig. 46.3 CRT partially reverses DHF-induced downregulation of I_{K1} and I_K but not I_{to}. **A–C** DHF significantly reduces the inward rectifier (I_{K1}), delayed rectifier (I_K) and transient outward K+ currents (I_{to}) in both anterior (ANT) and lateral (LTR) cells. CRT partially restores the DHF-induced reduction of I_{K1} and I_K but not I_{to} in both ANT and LTR cells (**D**) consistent with changes in steady-state K+ channel mRNA subunit and protein expression. NF, non-failing hearts. [Modified, with permission, from Aiba T, Hesketh GG, Barth AS, *et al.* (2009) Electrophysiological consequences of dyssynchronous heart failure and its restoration by resynchronization therapy. *Circulation* **119**:1220–1230.]

(e.g. pacing-tachycardia), inconsistencies have been observed across species: reduced I_{K1} density in canine[19,29] but no change in rabbit[30]. In terminal human HF, I_{K1} is significantly reduced at negative voltages[14], but the underlying basis for such downregulation appears to be post-transcriptional in light of the absence of changes in the steady-state level of Kir2.1 mRNA[25]. Interestingly, a differential reduction in I_{K1} was noted between cells isolated from failing hearts with dilated versus ischaemic cardiomyopathy, with the former group exhibiting a lower whole-cell slope conductance at the reversal potential for K+ than the latter[31].

The underlying molecular basis of I_{K1} downregulation in HF remains controversial in the absence of consistent changes in the expression of the Kir2 family of genes. The specific subunit(s) that underlie I_{K1} vary as a function of species and cardiac chamber, although Kir2.1 and 2.2 knockout[32] and Kir2.1 dominant negative overexpressing mice[33] exhibit prolonged APD.

CRT even in the setting of continued HF partially restores I_{K1} density (Fig. 46.3B)[16] and decreases membrane resistance and in the setting of improved Ca2+ handling in CRT (see below) may reduce the frequency of arrhythmogenic DAD generation. Kir2.1 mRNA and protein levels are partially restored by CRT in the canine model (Fig. 46.3D)[16], suggesting that different mechanisms of regulation of the current are operative in some animal models and human HF.

Delayed rectifier K+ currents (I_{Kr} and I_{Ks})

The delayed rectifier K+ currents play a prominent role in the late phase of repolarization, and therefore changes in either the slow (I_{Ks}) or fast (I_{Kr}) activating components of this current could contribute significantly to AP prolongation in HF. Reduced I_K density, slower activation and faster deactivation kinetics have been observed in hypertrophied feline ventricles[34]. In addition, downregulation of both I_{Kr} and I_{Ks} has been reported in a rabbit model of rapid ventricular pacing HF[35], whereas I_{Ks} but not I_{Kr} was downregulated in all layers of the LV myocardium in a canine model of tachypacing HF[29].

The molecular basis for I_K downregulation in HF remains controversial. We recently measured messenger ribonucleic acid (mRNA) levels of the genes encoding the α subunits for the rapidly (ERG) and slowly (KvLQT1) activating components of I_K in normal and dyssynchronously contracting failing canine hearts and found a modest but significant reduction in steady-state mRNA levels[16].

CRT partially restores dyssynchronous HF-induced downregulation of I_K density in both anterior and lateral LV myocytes (Fig. 46.3C,D) without a significant change in mRNA or protein levels of KvLQT1 or minK compared with dyssynchronous HF, whereas ERG mRNA levels were partially restored by CRT in either the anterior or lateral LV wall[16].

Ca²⁺ handling and arrhythmic risk

Altered Ca^{2+} homeostasis underlies abnormalities in excitation–contraction (EC) coupling and arrhythmic risk in HF. Intracellular Ca^{2+} conecentration ($[Ca^{2+}]_i$) and the AP are intricately linked by a variety of Ca^{2+}-mediated cell surface channels and transporters such as $I_{Ca,L}$, I_K, Ca^{2+}-activated Cl^- current ($I_{Ca,Cl}$) and the Na^+/Ca^{2+} exchanger current (I_{NCX}).

L-type Ca²⁺ current (I_Ca,L)

$I_{Ca,L}$ density is unchanged or reduced in HF, the latter typically occurring in more advanced disease[17,18,36]. Remarkably in human HF baseline $I_{Ca,L}$ density is consistently unchanged[37] although single channel studies suggest a reduction in channel number with an increase in open probability perhaps due to altered phosphorylation or subunit composition[38,39]. The molecular bases of changes in the density of $I_{Ca,L}$ are incompletely understood and subunit mRNA expression in HF is variable. The complexity of the molecular basis of channel remodelling is highlighted by reports of isoform switching of both $\alpha 1C$[40,41] and β subunits[42] in the failing heart.

In canine dyssynchronous HF models, there are intraventricular regional changes in $I_{Ca,L}$ that are partially restored by CRT. Dyssynchronous HF produced a reduction in peak $I_{Ca,L}$ density and slowed current decay in myocytes isolated from the lateral LV wall. In contrast, the peak $I_{Ca,L}$ density in anterior myocytes was increased compared with non-failing controls; thus dyssynchronous HF produced regional heterogeneity of current density and kinetics. CRT restored the peak current density but did not alter the $I_{Ca,L}$ decay in the lateral cells, eliminating the anterior–lateral current density gradient[16] (Fig. 46.4A).

Sarcoplasmic reticulum function

HF is associated with major changes in intracellular and SR Ca^{2+} homeostasis[43]. The amplitude of the calcium transient (CaT) and its rate of decay are reduced in intact preparations and cells isolated from failing ventricles. The sarcoplasmic/endoplasmatic reticulum Ca^{2+} ATPase (SERCA2a), its inhibitor phospholamban (PLB) and NCX are primary mediators of Ca^{2+} removal from the cytoplasm. In HF, ventricular myocytes exhibit a greater reliance on NCX for removal of Ca^{2+} from the cytosol and an increase in NCX function[44], which leads to defective SR Ca^{2+} loading. The enhanced NCX function in the failing heart, particularly in the setting of changes in intracellular Na^+ concentration ($[Na^+]_i$),

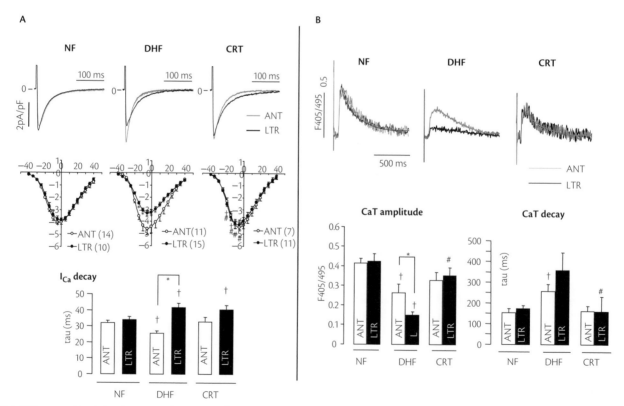

Fig. 46.4 CRT restores DHF-induced regional differences in Ca^{2+} currents ($I_{Ca,L}$) and transients (CaT). **A** In DHF, the peak $I_{Ca,L}$ density was smaller and the decay was slower in LTR myocytes, whereas the peak current density was larger and decay is faster in the ANT myocytes. The reduced current density is observed over a wide range of activation voltages. CRT restored the peak $I_{Ca,L}$ density in LTR cells, but the decay remained slow. **B** Compared with the control, DHF significantly reduced the CaT amplitude and slowed the rate of decay of the transient prominently in the LTR myocytes. CRT partially restored the CaT amplitude of LTR cells but did not significantly change the amplitude of ANT myocytes, but did hasten the decay to nearly that of normal ANT control cells. F405/F495, ratiometric fluorescence wavelengths; NF, non-failing hearts.

contribute to the augmented transient inward current (I_{ti}) that underlies arrhythmogenic DAD induction[27].

HF-associated changes in the function of the key Ca^{2+} release channel in the SR, the cardiac-specific ryanodine receptor (RyR2), also contribute to defective SR loading and EC coupling. In failing hearts, the stoichiometry and function of the RyR2 macromolecular complex is altered[45]. Decreased levels of protein phosphatases (PP1 and PP2A) and hyperphosphorylation by protein kinase A (PKA) result in dissociation of the regulatory protein FKBP12.6 from RyR2 with increased Ca^{2+} sensitivity, resulting in an increase in open probability that produces a Ca^{2+} leak from the SR (Fig. 46.5)[46]. The enhanced Ca^{2+} sensitivity that causes the leak also increases the fractional release of Ca^{2+} during EC coupling, so the effect on systolic function and the role of phosphorylation of RyR2 continues to be hotly debated[43]. However, it is likely that defects in RyR2 function contribute to the development of triggered arrhythmias in failing heart and as such they remain an attractive therapeutic target. Beta-adrenergic receptor blockers reverse PKA hyperphosphorylation of RyR2, restore the stoichiometry of the RyR2 macromolecular complex and normalize single-channel function in a canine model and human HF[47].

A number of studies have demonstrated reductions in SERCA2a and PLB mRNA, but fewer have shown a reduction in immunoreactive protein; however, reductions in PLB phosphorylation may result in enhanced inhibition of SERCA in HF. Increases in NCX mRNA and protein have been regularly observed in failing hearts[17,18]. Levels of RyR mRNA and protein in HF are variable.

Abnormal SR Ca^{2+} handling in dyssynchronous HF is also functionally restored by CRT[16,48]. CRT dramatically increases the amplitude and hastens the decay kinetics of the CaT particularly in cells isolated from the lateral LV wall (Fig. 46.4B). The reversal in SR function by CRT occurs without a change in mRNA or protein levels of PLB, SERCA2a, NCX or RyR2[16] and thus is likely to be the result of altered post-translational modifications.

Intracellular Na^+ concentration in HF

The mechanisms governing $[Na^+]_i$ and Ca^{2+} handling are intimately linked and $[Na^+]_i$ is increased in failing ventricular myocytes. Increases in $[Na^+]_i$ may be the result of diminished efflux by reduced Na^+/K^+ ATPase activity or an increase in Na^+ influx via I_{Na}, Na^+/H^+ exchanger, NCX or other Na^+ co-transporters. Below we briefly address changes in Na^+ current and Na^+/K^+ ATPase.

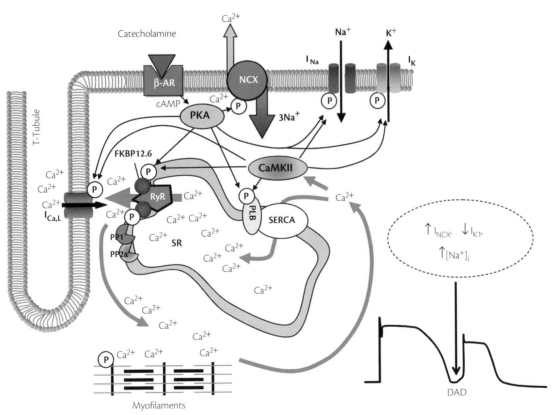

Fig. 46.5 Summary of intracellular Ca^{2+} cycling and associated signalling pathways in cardiomyocytes. On a beat-by-beat basis, a CaT is elicited by the influx of a small amount of Ca^{2+} through the $I_{Ca,L}$ and the subsequent large-scale Ca^{2+} release from the SR through the ryanodine receptor (RyR). During diastole, cytosolic Ca^{2+} is taken up into the SR by the PLB-regulated SERCA2a pump. β-Adrenergic receptor (β -AR)-mediated PKA stimulation regulates this Ca^{2+} cycling by phosphorylating $I_{Ca,L}$, RyR and PLB. In normal hearts, sympathetic stimulation activates the β1-adrenergic receptor, which in turn stimulates the production of cAMP by adenylyl cyclase and thereby activates PKA. PKA phosphorylates PLB and RyR, both of which contribute to an increased intracellular CaT and enhanced cellular contractility. PP1 and PP2A regulate the dephosphorylation process of these Ca^{2+} regulatory proteins (RyR, PLB and $I_{Ca,L}$). The PLB hypophosphorylation inhibits SERCA2a activity, thereby decreasing SR Ca^{2+} uptake. The increased Ca^{2+} level in the cytosol activates CaMKII, which affects the functions of RyR and PLB. Activation or deactivation of these molecules at a node in the signalling cascade affects beat-by-beat Ca^{2+} cycling, and such manoeuvres have recently been highlighted as potential new therapeutic strategies against HF. Increased I_{NCX}, reduced I_{K1} and residual coupling to β-AR signalling may predispose to arrhythmogenic DAD formation[27].

Cardiac I_{Na} in HF

A prominent increase in late Na^+ current ($I_{Na,L}$) and slowing of I_{Na} decay has been described in several models of HF[49]. The mechanism(s) of the increase in $I_{Na,L}$ in HF are uncertain, but block of the late current inhibits oxidant-induced EAD and contractile dysfunction[50] and alterations in calmodulin kinase (CaMK) signalling influence I_{Na} decay and the magnitude of $I_{Na,L}$[51–53], suggesting post-translational modifications of the Na^+ current. There are no consistent changes in cardiac Na^+ channel subunit expression in HF; however, aberrant splicing of $Na_V1.5$ transcripts has been reported in failing human ventricular myocardium[54]. HF increases $I_{Na,L}$ and slows I_{Na} decay, whereas CRT partially restores dyssynchronous HF-induced altered I_{Na} gating kinetics. I_{Na} blockers have an infamous history in the treatment of cardiac arrhythmias with substantial proarrhythmic liability; however, new strategies that target the late current may have more promise.

Na^+/K^+ ATPase

The Na^+/K^+ ATPase, or Na^+ pump, is responsible for the establishment and maintenance of the major ionic gradients across the cell membrane and belongs to the widely distributed class of P-type ATPases that are responsible for transporting a number of cations. The Na^+/K^+ ATPase hydrolyzes a molecule of ATP to transport K^+ into the cell and Na^+ out with a stoichiometry of 2:3, thereby generating a time-independent outward current.

The consensus of experimental data reveal that the expression and function of the Na^+/K^+ ATPase are reduced in HF compared with control hearts. The density as assessed by $[^3H]$-ouabain binding of the Na^+/K^+ ATPase is decreased in HF. The decrease occurs without a significant impact on the inotropic effect of digitalis glycosides in human ventricular myocardium[55]. Decreased Na^+ pump function in HF has several consequences that might be relevant to production of arrhythmias. First, the reduction in the outward repolarizing current could prolong APD. Second, reduced pump function reduces Na^+ efflux and may increase $[Na^+]_i$. Finally, cells with less Na^+/K^+ ATPase activity have greater difficulty handling changes in extracellular K^+ concentration ($[K^+]_o$). Low $[K^+]_o$ itself tends to inhibit the ATPase, while increases in $[K^+]_o$ would tend to be cleared less rapidly in the setting of relative pump inhibition.

The consequences of increased Na^+ influx or decreased efflux in HF, particularly in the setting of regionally variable lengthening of the APD, are heterogenous cytosolic Na^+ loading and subsequent activation of 'reverse mode' NCX. NCX functioning in the reverse mode in response to increased $[Na^+]_i$ may be adaptive, promoting an increased influx in activator Ca^{2+} (Fig. 46.5). However, the slowed I_{Na} decay and increased $I_{Na,L}$ may contribute to the regional AP prolongation and more frequent EAD occurrence in dyssynchronous HF (Fig. 46.2).

Gap junctions and connexins

Gap junction channels are intercellular channel proteins that permit electrical and chemical communication between cells. These channels are major mediators of conduction in the heart. Mammalian gap junction channels or connexons are built by the oligomerization of a family of closely related genes encoding connexins (Cx)[56]. Three different Cx have been identified in the mammalian heart, Cx40, Cx43 and Cx45, named for their respective molecular masses.

Slowed intraventricular conduction is a prominent feature of HF and is associated with a reduction in the density, altered distribution and post-translational modification of the major cardiac gap junction protein (Cx43)[57]. Similar findings have been observed in hypertrophied and ischaemic human ventricular myocardium. Cx43 is downregulated and redistributed from the intercalated disk to the entire cell border (lateralization)[58], a pattern observed in early cardiac development. Downregulation and lateralization of Cx43 in tachypacing-induced HF is progressive[59] and associated with conduction slowing. The mechanism of Cx43 downregulation is not completely understood but may involve altered renin-angiotensin-aldosterone system signalling changes in binding partners or defective trafficking. In the pacing tachycardia HF, Cx43 downregulation is associated with a reduction in Cx43 mRNA and may be regulated by a microRNA (miR-1)[60].

Purkinje fibres – link to synchronous activation of the ventricle

Synchronous activation of the ventricles requires conduction over the His-Purkinje network. Ionic current remodelling is distinct in different regions of the failing heart. In HF, changes in Purkinje cell ionic currents include a reduction of I_{to} and I_{K1} density with slowing of $I_{Ca,L}$ decay. There were no significant changes in I_{Kr} or I_{Ks} but Purkinje cells exhibit a reduction in repolarizing reserve in HF manifest by APD prolongation and exaggerated prolongation of the duration in the presence of class III antiarrhythmic drugs. In Purkinje fibres downregulation of $K_V4.3$, $K_V3.4$, Kir2.1 mRNA and protein was observed consistent with the K current changes[61]. Pacing-induced HF in the canine model slowed conduction in Purkinje fibres false tendons with an associated reduction in $Na_V1.5$, Cx40, Cx43 and phospho-Cx43 protein levels. Immunohistochemistry revealed reduced Cx40, Cx43 and phospho-Cx43 protein at the intercalated disk[61]. The changes in electrophysiological properties of Purkinje fibres may serve as a substrate for ventricular arrhythmia; moreover, reduction in conduction in the Purkinje network may result in dyssynchronous activation of the ventricle and progression of the HF phenotype.

Autonomic signalling

Changes in adrenergic signalling in the failing heart have been well characterized[62–64]. The β_1, β_2 and α_1 adrenergic receptors mediate the effects of increased catecholamines, both circulating epinephrine and norepinephrine, released from cardiac nerve terminals, in the heart. These receptor subtypes are coupled to different signalling systems.

Chronic β-adrenergic receptor (β-AR) stimulation can be cardiotoxic, and multiple regulatory adjustments produce desensitization of downstream effector responses in the failing heart, such as functional upregulation of inhibitory G proteins ($G\alpha_i$) and inhibitory regulators of G protein signalling (RGS). In human and animal models of HF the cardiac response to β-adrenergic stimulation is blunted and there is a positive correlation between increased plasma catecholamine levels and the degree of the diminution of the β-AR response. In most studies of end-stage human HF and some failing animal models, the β_1-AR undergoes subtype-selective downregulation such that the proportion of β_1-AR:β_2-AR is nearly equal in abundance[65,66] compared to the dominance of the

β_1-subtype in normal hearts. In addition, the remaining β-AR are significantly desensitized due to uncoupling of the receptors from their respective signalling pathways[67,68]. HF in both humans and animal models has been associated with a marked increase in $G\alpha_i$ mRNA levels. Studies in rat and guinea pig have shown that chronic infusion of catecholamines increases the expression of $G\alpha_i$[69,70]; in parallel, overexpression of the human β_2-AR in transgenic mice was associated with increased $G\alpha_i$ protein abundance[71].

Protein phosphorylation mediated by β-adrenergic activation is decreased in the failing human heart. The PKA signalling pathway appears to be downregulated at several levels beyond the β-receptor, with the functional implication of limiting PKA targeting to important subcellular locations such as the sarcolemma and the SR in failing cardiac myocytes[72]. There is increasing evidence for local regulation of PKA activity by binding of PKA to A-kinase anchoring proteins (AKAP). Such compartmentalization of PKA in the human heart may be disrupted in HF as yet another mechanism of abnormal autonomic signalling in the failing heart[72].

Adrenergic signalling pathways affect the function of a number of ion channels and transporters. The net effect of β-adrenergic stimulation is to shorten the ventricular APD due to an increase of I_K current density[73], despite β_1 receptor stimulation of depolarizing current through the L-type Ca^{2+} channel. α_1-Adrenergic receptor stimulation inhibits several K^+ currents in the mammalian heart, including I_{to}, I_{K1} and I_K in rat ventricle, with the net effect of prolonging APD. In a rat HF model, the inotropic responses to β-stimulation and to direct stimulation of adenylyl cyclase, but not to Ca^{2+}, were diminished due to desensitization of the stimulatory side of the adenylyl cyclase signal transduction system. In parallel, the responses to inhibitory receptors were augmented, leading to a pronounced G_i-mediated negative inotropic effect on failing heart muscle cells[74].

Interestingly, CRT produces a striking improvement in β-AR reserve in cells and tissues isolated from dyssynchronous HF. The effects were particularly prominent in myocytes isolated from the high-stress lateral wall of dyssynchronous HF hearts where isoproterenol augmentation of $I_{Ca,L}$ density and CaT amplitude were nearly completely restored in myocytes from CRT hearts. The profoundly slowed CaT decay in dyssynchronous HF myocytes was dramatically hastened by CRT. This restoration is the result of augmentation of $\beta 1$ receptor abundance and a reduction in $G\alpha_i$ (presumably via $\beta 2$-AR) signalling mediated by an increase in the inhibitory regulator of G protein signalling, RGS3, in CRT[75].

Calmodulin kinase

Calmodulin (CaM) is the most ubiquitous Ca^{2+}-binding protein in mammalian cells. CaM is a vital signalling molecule that regulates the function of many proteins critical to cellular metabolism, Ca^{2+} transport, contraction, electrophysiology, gene expression and cell proliferation[76]. CaMKII is the main target of CaM binding in the heart and is a multifunctional enzyme capable of phosphorylating several substrates, including K channels, RyR and PLB[77,78]. CaMKII activity is increased, possibly as a compensatory mechanism for altered Ca^{2+} homeostasis in both human[77] and animal[79] models of HF. However, the regional differences in Ca^{2+} homeostasis and associated regulatory proteins in dyssynchronous HF and their restoration by CRT have not been studied.

Conclusions and outlook

Structural remodelling and HF-induced regional changes in ionic currents and transporters and Ca^{2+} handling in the ventricle create a highly susceptible substrate for both triggered and re-entrant and potentially lethal ventricular arrhythmias. Understanding electrical remodelling of the diseased heart creates opportunities for interventions to reduce structural changes and arrhythmic risk. Remarkably, CRT produces both global and regional improvement in cardiac performance, Ca^{2+} handling and reversal of many aspects of electrophysiological remodelling. Biventricular pacing that is the basis of CRT restores mechanical synchronization of contraction but also alters the electrical activation of the ventricles. The extent to which changes in the pattern of contraction and electrical activation contribute to the salutary effects of CRT remain to be determined. What is remarkable is that even in the setting of ongoing systolic dysfunction, biventricular pacing dramatically alters the molecular electrophysiology and Ca^{2+} handling of the failing heart.

References

1. Rosamond W, Flegal K, Furie K, *et al.* Heart disease and stroke statistics – 2008 update: a report from the American Heart Association Statistics Committee and Stroke Statistics Subcommittee. *Circulation* 2008;**117**:e25–e146.
2. Iuliano S, Fisher SG, Karasik PE, Fletcher RD, Singh SN. QRS duration and mortality in patients with congestive heart failure. *Am Heart J* 2002;**143**:1085–1091.
3. Prinzen FW, Hunter WC, Wyman BT, McVeigh ER. Mapping of regional myocardial strain and work during ventricular pacing: experimental study using magnetic resonance imaging tagging. *J Am Coll Cardiol* 1999;**33**:1735–1742.
4. Blanc JJ, Etienne Y, Gilard M, *et al.* Evaluation of different ventricular pacing sites in patients with severe heart failure: results of an acute hemodynamic study. *Circulation* 1997;**96**:3273–3277.
5. Nelson GS, Berger RD, Fetics BJ, *et al.* Left ventricular or biventricular pacing improves cardiac function at diminished energy cost in patients with dilated cardiomyopathy and left bundle-branch block. *Circulation* 2000;**102**:3053–3059.
6. McAlister FA, Ezekowitz J, Hooton N, *et al.* Cardiac resynchronization therapy for patients with left ventricular systolic dysfunction: a systematic review. *JAMA* 2007;**297**:2502–2514.
7. Beshai JF, Grimm RA, Nagueh SF, *et al.* Cardiac-resynchronization therapy in heart failure with narrow QRS complexes. *N Engl J Med* 2007;**357**:2461–2471.
8. Thompson K, Saab G, Birnie D, *et al.* Is septal glucose metabolism altered in patients with left bundle branch block and ischemic cardiomyopathy? *J Nucl Med* 2006;**47**:1763–1768.
9. Ukkonen H, Beanlands RS, Burwash IG, *et al.* Effect of cardiac resynchronization on myocardial efficiency and regional oxidative metabolism. *Circulation* 2003;**107**:28–31.
10. Heymes C, Bendall JK, Ratajczak P, *et al.* Increased myocardial NADPH oxidase activity in human heart failure. *J Am Coll Cardiol* 2003;**41**:2164–2171.
11. Nass RD, Aiba T, Tomaselli GF, Akar FG. Mechanisms of disease: ion channel remodeling in the failing ventricle. *Nat Clin Pract Cardiovasc Med* 2008;**5**:196–207.
12. van Dam RT, Durrer D. Excitability and electrical activity of human myocardial strips from the left atrial appendage in cases of rheumatic mitral stenosis. *Circ Res* 1961;**9**:509–514.
13. Trautwein W, Kassebaum DG, Nelsol RM, Hecht HH. Electrophysiological study of human heart muscle. *Circ Res* 1962;**10**:306–312.

14. Beuckelmann DJ, Nabauer M, Erdmann E. Alterations of K$^+$ currents in isolated human ventricular myocytes from patients with terminal heart failure. *Circ Res* 1993;**73**:379–385.

15. Akar FG, Rosenbaum DS. Transmural electrophysiological heterogeneities underlying arrhythmogenesis in heart failure. *Circ Res* 2003;**93**:638–645.

16. Aiba T, Hesketh GG, Barth AS, *et al.* Electrophysiological consequences of dyssynchronous heart failure and its restoration by resynchronization therapy. *Circulation* 2009;**119**:1220–1230.

17. Nattel S, Maguy A, Le Bouter S, Yeh YH. Arrhythmogenic ion-channel remodeling in the heart: heart failure, myocardial infarction, and atrial fibrillation. *Physiol Rev* 2007;**87**:425–456.

18. Tomaselli GF, Marban E. Electrophysiological remodeling in hypertrophy and heart failure. *Cardiovasc Res* 1999;**42**:270–283.

19. Kaab S, Nuss HB, Chiamvimonvat N, *et al.* Ionic mechanism of action potential prolongation in ventricular myocytes from dogs with pacing-induced heart failure. *Circ Res* 1996;**78**:262–273.

20. Greenstein JL, Wu R, Po S, Tomaselli GF, Winslow RL. Role of the calcium-independent transient outward current i(to1) in shaping action potential morphology and duration. *Circ Res* 2000;**87**: 1026–1033.

21. Nerbonne JM. Molecular basis of functional voltage-gated K$^+$ channel diversity in the mammalian myocardium. *J Physiol* 2000;**525**: 285–298.

22. An WF, Bowlby MR, Betty M, *et al.* Modulation of A-type potassium channels by a family of calcium sensors. *Nature* 2000;**403**:553–556.

23. Deschenes I, DiSilvestre D, Juang GJ, Wu RC, An WF, Tomaselli GF. Regulation of Kv4.3 current by KChIP2 splice variants: a component of native cardiac I$_{to}$? *Circulation* 2002;**106**:423–429.

24. Patel SP, Parai R, Campbell DL. Regulation of Kv4.3 voltage-dependent gating kinetics by KChIP2 isoforms. *J Physiol* 2004; **557**:19–41.

25. Kaab S, Dixon J, Duc J, *et al.* Molecular basis of transient outward potassium current downregulation in human heart failure: a decrease in Kv4.3 mRNA correlates with a reduction in current density. *Circulation* 1998;**98**:1383–1393.

26. Xiao L, Coutu P, Villeneuve LR, *et al.* Mechanisms underlying rate-dependent remodeling of transient outward potassium current in canine ventricular myocytes. *Circ Res* 2008;**103**:733–742.

27. Pogwizd SM, Schlotthauer K, Li L, Yuan W, Bers DM. Arrhythmogenesis and contractile dysfunction in heart failure: Roles of sodium-calcium exchange, inward rectifier potassium current, and residual beta-adrenergic responsiveness. *Circ Res* 2001;**88**: 1159–1167.

28. Nuss HB, Kaab S, Kass DA, Tomaselli GF, Marban E. Cellular basis of ventricular arrhythmias and abnormal automaticity in heart failure. *Am J Physiol* 1999;**277**:H80–H91.

29. Li GR, Lau CP, Ducharme A, Tardif JC, Nattel S. Transmural action potential and ionic current remodeling in ventricles of failing canine hearts. *Am J Physiol* 2002;**283**:H1031–H1041.

30. Rozanski GJ, Xu Z, Whitney RT, Murakami H, Zucker IH. Electrophysiology of rabbit ventricular myocytes following sustained rapid ventricular pacing. *J Mol Cell Cardiol* 1997;**29**:721–732.

31. Koumi S, Backer CL, Arentzen CE. Characterization of inwardly rectifying K$^+$ channel in human cardiac myocytes. Alterations in channel behavior in myocytes isolated from patients with idiopathic dilated cardiomyopathy. *Circulation* 1995;**92**:164–174.

32. Zaritsky JJ, Eckman DM, Wellman GC, Nelson MT, Schwarz TL. Targeted disruption of Kir2.1 and Kir2.2 genes reveals the essential role of the inwardly rectifying K$^+$ current in K$^+$-mediated vasodilation. *Circ Res* 2000;**87**:160–166.

33. McLerie M, Lopatin AN. Dominant-negative suppression of I$_{K1}$ in the mouse heart leads to altered cardiac excitability. *J Mol Cell Cardiol* 2003;**35**:367–378.

34. Furukawa T, Bassett AL, Furukawa N, Kimura S, Myerburg RJ. The ionic mechanism of reperfusion-induced early afterdepolarizations in feline left ventricular hypertrophy. *J Clin Invest* 1993;**91**:1521–1531.

35. Tsuji Y, Opthof T, Kamiya K, *et al.* Pacing-induced heart failure causes a reduction of delayed rectifier potassium currents along with decreases in calcium and transient outward currents in rabbit ventricle. *Cardiovasc Res* 2000;**48**:300–309.

36. Pitt GS, Dun W, Boyden PA. Remodeled cardiac calcium channels. *J Mol Cell Cardiol* 2006;**41**:373–388.

37. Beuckelmann DJ, Erdmann E. Ca^{2+}-currents and intracellular [Ca^{2+}]i-transients in single ventricular myocytes isolated from terminally failing human myocardium. *Basic Res Cardiol* 1992; **87**:235–243.

38. Handrock R, Schroder F, Hirt S, Haverich A, Mittmann C, Herzig S. Single-channel properties of L-type calcium channels from failing human ventricle. *Cardiovasc Res* 1998;**37**:445–455.

39. Schroeder F, Handrock R, Beuckelmann DJ, *et al.* Increased availability and open probability of single L-type calcium channels from failing compared with nonfailing human ventricle. *Circulation* 1998;**98**: 969–976.

40. Gidh-Jain M, Huang B, Jain P, Battula V, el-Sherif N. Reemergence of the fetal pattern of L-type calcium channel gene expression in non infarcted myocardium during left ventricular remodeling. *Biochem Biophys Res Comm* 1995;**216**:892–897.

41. Yang Y, Chen X, Margulies K, *et al.* L-type Ca^{2+} channel alpha 1c subunit isoform switching in failing human ventricular myocardium. *J Mol Cell Cardiol* 2000;**32**:973–984.

42. Hullin R, Khan IF, Wirtz S, *et al.* Cardiac L-type calcium channel beta-subunits expressed in human heart have differential effects on single channel characteristics. *J Biol Chem* 2003;**278**:21623–21630.

43. Bers DM. Altered cardiac myocyte Ca regulation in heart failure. *Physiology* 2006;**21**:380–387.

44. O'Rourke B, Kass DA, Tomaselli GF, Kaab S, Tunin R, Marban E. Mechanisms of altered excitation-contraction coupling in canine tachycardia-induced heart failure, I: experimental studies. *Circ Res* 1999;**84**:562–570.

45. Yano M, Ikeda Y, Matsuzaki M. Altered intracellular Ca^{2+} handling in heart failure. *J Clin Invest* 2005;**115**:556–564.

46. Marx SO, Reiken S, Hisamatsu Y, *et al.* PKA phosphorylation dissociates FKBP12.6 from the calcium release channel (ryanodine receptor): defective regulation in failing hearts. *Cell* 2000;**101**: 365–376.

47. Reiken S, Wehrens XH, Vest JA, *et al.* Beta-blockers restore calcium release channel function and improve cardiac muscle performance in human heart failure. *Circulation* 2003;**107**:2459–2466.

48. Nishijima Y, Sridhar A, Viatchenko-Karpinski S, *et al.* Chronic cardiac resynchronization therapy and reverse ventricular remodeling in a model of nonischemic cardiomyopathy. *Life Sci* 2007;**81**:1152–1159.

49. Undrovinas AI, Maltsev VA, Sabbah HN. Repolarization abnormalities in cardiomyocytes of dogs with chronic heart failure: role of sustained inward current. *Cell Mol Life Sci* 1999;**55**:494–505.

50. Song Y, Shryock JC, Wagner S, Maier LS, Belardinelli L. Blocking late sodium current reduces hydrogen peroxide-induced arrhythmogenic activity and contractile dysfunction. *J Pharmacol Exp Ther* 2006;**318**:214–222.

51. Aiba T, Hesketh GG, Liu T, *et al.* Na$^+$ channel regulation by Ca^{2+}/calmodulin and Ca^{2+}/calmodulin-dependent protein kinase II in guinea-pig ventricular myocytes. *Cardiovasc Res* 2009;**85**:454–463.

52. Deschenes I, Neyroud N, DiSilvestre D, Marban E, Yue DT, Tomaselli GF. Isoform-specific modulation of voltage-gated Na$^+$ channels by calmodulin. *Circ Res* 2002;**90**:E49–E57.

53. Wagner S, Dybkova N, Rasenack EC, *et al.* Ca^{2+}/calmodulin-dependent protein kinase II regulates cardiac Na$^+$ channels. *J Clin Invest* 2006;**116**:3127–3138.

54. Shang LL, Pfahnl AE, Sanyal S, *et al*. Human heart failure is associated with abnormal C-terminal splicing variants in the cardiac sodium channel. *Circ Res* 2007;**101**:1146–1154.

55. Erdmann E, Schwinger R, Bohm M. Beta-blocking agents and positive inotropic agents in the therapy of chronic heart failure. *J Cardiovasc Pharmacol* 1990;**16**:S138–S144.

56. Saffitz JE, Schuessler RB, Yamada KA. Mechanisms of remodeling of gap junction distributions and the development of anatomic substrates of arrhythmias. *Cardiovasc Res* 1999;**42**:309–317.

57. Akar FG, Spragg DD, Tunin RS, Kass DA, Tomaselli GF. Mechanisms underlying conduction slowing and arrhythmogenesis in nonischemic dilated cardiomyopathy. *Circ Res* 2004;**95**:717–725.

58. Peters NS, Green CR, Poole-Wilson PA, Severs NJ. Reduced content of connexin43 gap junctions in ventricular myocardium from hypertrophied and ischemic human hearts. *Circulation* 1993;**88**: 864–875.

59. Akar FG, Nass RD, Hahn S, *et al*. Dynamic changes in conduction velocity and gap junction properties during development of pacing-induced heart failure. *Am J Physiol* 2007;**293**: H1223–H1230.

60. Yang B, Lin H, Xiao J, *et al*. The muscle-specific microRNA miR-1 regulates cardiac arrhythmogenic potential by targeting GJA1 and KCNJ2. *Nat Med* 2007;**13**: 486–491.

61. Maguy A, Le Bouter S, Comtois P, *et al*. Ion channel subunit expression changes in cardiac Purkinje fibers: a potential role in conduction abnormalities associated with congestive heart failure. *Circ Res* 2009;**104**:1113–1122.

62. Bristow MR, Minobe WA, Raynolds MV, *et al*. Reduced beta 1 receptor messenger RNA abundance in the failing human heart. *J Clin Invest* 1993;**92**:2737–2745.

63. Bristow MR, Ginsburg R, Minobe W, *et al*. Decreased catecholamine sensitivity and beta-adrenergic-receptor density in failing human hearts. *N Engl J Med* 1982;**307**:205–211.

64. Bohm M, Flesch M, Schnabel P. Beta-adrenergic signal transduction in the failing and hypertrophied myocardium. *J Mol Med* 1997;**75**: 842–848.

65. Bristow MR, Ginsburg R, Umans V, *et al*. Beta 1- and beta 2-adrenergic-receptor subpopulations in nonfailing and failing human ventricular myocardium: coupling of both receptor subtypes to muscle contraction and selective beta 1-receptor down-regulation in heart failure. *Circ Res* 1986;**59**:297–309.

66. Brodde OE. Beta-adrenergic receptors in failing human myocardium. *Basic Res Cardiol* 1996;**91**:35–40.

67. Bristow MR, Anderson FL, Port JD, *et al*. Differences in beta-adrenergic neuroeffector mechanisms in ischemic versus idiopathic dilated cardiomyopathy. *Circulation* 1991;**84**:1024–1039.

68. Brodde OE, Vogelsang M, Broede A, *et al*. Diminished responsiveness of Gs-coupled receptors in severely failing human hearts: no difference in dilated versus ischemic cardiomyopathy. *J Cardiovasc Pharmacol* 1998;**31**:585–594.

69. Mende U, Eschenhagen T, Geertz B, *et al*. Isoprenaline-induced increase in the 40/41 kDa pertussis toxin substrates and functional consequences on contractile response in rat heart. *Naunyn Schmiedebergs Arch Pharmacol* 1992;**345**:44–50.

70. Eschenhagen T, Mende U, Nose M, *et al*. Increased messenger RNA level of the inhibitory G protein alpha subunit Gi alpha-2 in human end-stage heart failure. *Circ Res* 1992;**70**:688–696.

71. Xiao RP, Avdonin P, Zhou YY, *et al*. Coupling of beta2-adrenoceptor to Gi proteins and its physiological relevance in murine cardiac myocytes. *Circ Res* 1999;**84**:43–52.

72. Zakhary DR, Moravec CS, Bond M. Regulation of PKA binding to AKAPs in the heart: alterations in human heart failure. *Circulation* 2000;**101**:1459–1464.

73. Hartzell HC, Duchatelle-Gourdon I. Regulation of the cardiac delayed rectifier K current by neurotransmitters and magnesium. *Cardiovasc Drugs Ther* 1993;**7**:547–554.

74. Borst MM, Szalai P, Herzog N, Kubler W, Strasser RH. Transregulation of adenylyl-cyclase-coupled inhibitory receptors in heart failure enhances anti-adrenergic effects on adult rat cardiomyocytes. *Cardiovasc Res* 1999;**44**:113–120.

75. Chakir K, Daya SK, Tunin RS, *et al*. Mechanisms of Enhanced Beta-adrenergic Reserve From Cardiac Resynchronization Therapy. *Circulation* 2009;**119**:1231–1240.

76. Zhang T, Brown JH. Role of Ca^{2+}/calmodulin-dependent protein kinase II in cardiac hypertrophy and heart failure. *Cardiovasc Res* 2004;**63**:476–486.

77. Kirchhefer U, Schmitz W, Scholz H, Neumann J. Activity of cAMP-dependent protein kinase and Ca^{2+}/calmodulin-dependent protein kinase in failing and nonfailing human hearts. *Cardiovasc Res* 1999; **42**:254–261.

78. Maier LS, Bers DM. Role of Ca^{2+}/calmodulin-dependent protein kinase (CaMK) in excitation-contraction coupling in the heart. *Cardiovasc Res* 2007;**73**:631–640.

79. Netticadan T, Temsah RM, Kawabata K, Dhalla NS. Sarcoplasmic reticulum Ca^{2+}/Calmodulin-dependent protein kinase is altered in heart failure. *Circ Res* 2000;**86**:596–605.

Ventricular arrhythmias in heart failure: link to haemodynamic load

Steven N. Singh and Pamela Karasik

Background

Heart failure (HF) is characterized by an inadequate volume of blood to meet the metabolic demands of the body. It is usually classified as either systolic HF, where there is depressed ejection fraction, or diastolic HF, an abnormality in ventricular relaxation. This chapter deals with ventricular arrhythmias in systolic HF with links to haemodynamic load. The aetiologies of HF include coronary artery disease especially in those with prior myocardial infarction, valve pathology as in aortic stenosis or mitral regurgitation, and chronic hypertension. Other reasons include a primary cardiomyopathy associated with toxin or infection. Finally a sustained tachyarrhythmia may eventually lead to HF.

Ventricular arrhythmias in heart failure

Ventricular arrhythmias are quite common in systolic HF and these include premature ventricular contractions (PVC), non-sustained ventricular tachycardia (NSVT), sustained ventricular tachycardia (VT), Torsades de Pointes (TdP) and ventricular fibrillation (VF).

PVC as measured by Holter recordings are very common in HF patients[1]. They convey excess mortality in those with > 10/h[2]. However, suppression of such arrhythmias does not appear to provide a survival benefit[1]. NSVT is frequently seen in HF patients and exceeds an incidence of 90% if the PVC count is greater than 10/h. However, the presence of NSVT may not worsen prognosis[3]. In patients with depressed ejection fraction and NSVT, electrophysiological inducible sustained VT will benefit from an implantable cardioverter-defibrillator (ICD)[4]. Sustained VT is not uncommon in patients with or without ischaemic cardiomyopathy. While inducibility of this arrhythmia is possible in those with coronary artery disease, it is uncommon to reproduce the arrhythmia in a non-ischaemic cardiomyopathy patient.

TdP is not often seen in HF patients except with the concomitant use of antiarrhythmic drugs that prolong repolarization. This is most likely due to increased dispersion of refractoriness between the epicardium and endocardium[5].

VF may follow sustained VT and may account for 50% of all deaths in HF patients. Bradyarrhythmias and electromechanical dissociation are also common, especially in those with end-stage cardiomyopathy (Fig. 47.1).

Arrhythmia mechanisms in heart failure

The mechanisms for arrhythmogenesis include re-entry, abnormal automaticity, triggered activity and altered stretch. Re-entry requires two pathways, unidirectional block and conduction-slowing of sufficient magnitude to allow recovery of excitability in part of the tissue before it is reached by re-entrant excitation. In HF, fibrosis, scarring and downregulation of the gap junction protein connexin 43 (Cx43), leading to cell–cell uncoupling, present a perfect milieu for re-entrant arrhythmia[6]. These arrhythmias are easily reproduced and terminated with electrophysiological testing, and also respond to antiarrhythmic drugs that either slow conduction or prolong repolarization.

Microvolt T-wave alternans (TWA) has been identified in HF patients when submitted to heart rate increases above 110 beats/minute and has been found predictive of sudden cardiac arrest or

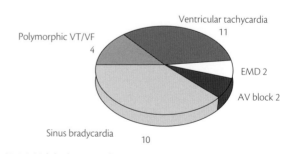

Fig. 47.1 Initial rhythm at cardiac arrests in patients with advanced heart failure (HF).EMD, electromechanical dissociation; AV, atrio-ventricular. [Data reproduced, with permission, from Luu M, Stevenson WG, Stevenson LW, Baron K, Walden J (1989) Diverse mechanisms of unexpected cardiac arrest in advanced heart failure. *Circulation* **80**:1675–1680.]

ICD discharge[7,8]. Newer investigations using monophasic action potential (AP) recordings have shown that in patients with HF there is alternans of AP amplitudes in the presence of increased heart rate. Based on experimental and modelling studies, this alternans is considered to be due to abnormal calcium cycling and has been shown to predict the risk for VT or VF[7].

Stretch-activated channels (SAC) play an important role in arrhythmogenesis. Stretch affects both conduction and refractoriness, and any alteration in such may predispose to arrhythmia generation in HF patients[9]. Electromechanical coupling may lead to electrical remodelling, with changes in conduction and repolarization creating a situation of increased electrophysiological heterogeneity, known to predispose to ventricular arrhythmias.

Micro-electrode studies of single myocytes isolated from animal hearts with experimentally induced severe HF or patients with end-stage HF have shown a significant prolongation of AP duration, a greater heterogeneity of AP duration and early after-depolarizations (EAD) compared to control myocytes[10]. Such changes, attributed to functional downregulation of potassium and altered calcium currents, clearly have arrhythmogenic potential. One would expect that such AP prolongation would cause an increase in the QT interval, or more specifically in the JT interval. However, in the absence of left bundle branch block, QT interval prolongation has rarely been reported even in patients with stage IV HF. In one recent study of patients admitted to the emergency department with acute decompensated HF, QRS duration but not QT interval duration was associated with mortality during long-term follow up[11].

Therapies

Pharmacological

The Class I (Vaughn-Williams) antiarrhythmic agents are contraindicated in HF patients because of the excess risk of proarrhythmia. This may be related to the worsening of the slower conduction seen in the failing heart, creating a lower threshold for re-entrant arrhythmias.

Use of beta-blockers (class II) has consistently been shown to reduce sudden cardiac deaths (SCD) presumably related to malignant arrhythmias[12–14]. This effect is independent of

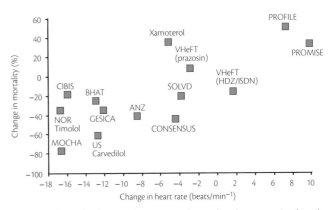

Fig. 47.2 Relationship between heart rate and mortality, documents in a broad range of published clinical studies. [Reproduced, with permission, from Kjekshus J, Gullestad L (1999) Heart rate as a therapeutic target in heart failure. *Eur Heart J* **1**(Suppl):H64–H69.]

PVC suppression[15]. The exact mechanism by which beta-blockers prevent SCD is unclear but may be related to multiple factors such as sympathetic blockade, reduced ischaemia and improved ejection fraction. Of note, in HF there is an inverse relationship between heart rate and mortality: the slower the heart rate, the lower the mortality (Fig. 47.2)[16]. Interestingly, with beta-blockers the improvement in survival is seen in the patient with HF and left ventricular dysfunction and not in the patient with normal ventricle. This could all be explained by the higher event rates in the sicker patients.

Class III drugs such as sotalol and dofetilide can suppress ventricular arrhythmias but without beneficial effects on outcome[17–19]. The risk of proarrhythmia is high in HF patients, and if used extreme caution is advised. Amiodarone is a very complex antiarrhythmic agent. It blocks multiple channels (Na^+, K^+, Ca^{2+}) and has indirect activities on alpha and beta receptors. It is very effective in suppression of PVC and NSVT but has no benefit on mortality in patients with HF (Fig. 47.3). Proarrhythmia is seldom seen with this compound. There are many cardiac and non-cardiac side effects, limiting its use.

Class IV drugs include the calcium channel blockers. These drugs may be harmful in HF patients and are of limited use[20–22].

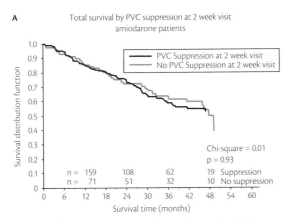
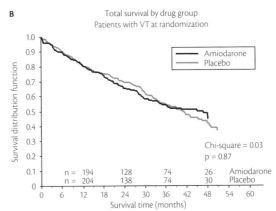

Fig. 47.3 A Total survival by PVC suppression at 2 week after hospital discharge – amiodarone patients. **B** Total survival by drug group – patients with VT at randomization. [Reproduced, with permission, from Singh SN, Fletcher RD, Fisher SG, *et al.* (1995) The Survival Trial of Antiarrhythmic Therapy in Congestive Heart Failure: amiodarone in patients with congestive heart failure and asymptomatic ventricular arrhythmia. *N Eng J Med* **333**:77–82, © Massachusetts Medical Society.]

Blockade of the renin–angiotensin system with either the converting enzyme or the angiotensin II receptor type 1(AT-I) has been shown to reduce ventricular arrhythmias. Perhaps they accomplish this indirect antiarrhythmic effect by preventing the reversal of structural, functional and electrical remodelling[23].

The aldosterone receptor blockers, spironolactone and eplerenone, have been shown to decrease mortality in patients with HF[24,25]. Both drugs reduce SCD. This may be related to a reduction of fibrosis and scarring which promote arrhythmogenesis.

In the effect of n-3 polyunsaturated fatty acids in patients with chronic HF trial (GISSI-HF) trial, polyunsaturated fatty acids (PUFA) have been shown to reduce all causes of mortality and cardiovascular admissions[26]. In addition, in the GISSI-Prevenzione Trial, in patients after myocardial infarction (MI), PUFA reduced all causes of mortality and SCD[27]. The mechanisms may possibly be related to the suppression of malignant arrhythmias by inhibition of Na^+, Ca^{2+} and K^+current, or even inflammation[28]. Of course, this is highly speculative.

Non-pharmacological

Coronary artery bypass grafting has been shown to reduce the incidence of SCD[29,30]. This effect may be upstream prevention of ischaemia, thereby suppressing ischaemia-related arrhythmias. However, there are no data on revascularization and arrhythmia suppression in HF patients. ICD therapies have consistently shown beneficial effects on survival in HF patients[31,32]. Clearly this is related to the arrhythmia-aborting effects of the device, suggesting perhaps that an ideal antiarrhythmic drug is still possible.

Cardiac resynchronization therapy (CRT) has also been shown to reduce HF hospitalizations and mortality[33,34]. Of note, responders to CRT have shown a significant reduction in ventricular arrhythmias and ICD shocks compared to non-responders[35]. This reduction in arrhythmia density could be related to reverse remodelling.

Ablation of frequent PVC foci and/or recurrent VT, both of which may contribute to left ventricular dysfunction, may provide improvement of the cardiomyopathy. However, the 1-year mortality rate is still high[36,37].

Links to haemodynamic load

The link between mechanical and electrical activities of the heart has been termed mechano-electric coupling (MEC). This interaction is real and has been validated in multiple experiments[38]. An increase in preload or afterload may induce electrophysiological changes, and via stretch may shorten or lengthen the AP duration which may provide a milieu for arrhythmogenesis[39]. Moreover, sudden increases in left ventricular pressure with aortic occlusion resulted in triggered arrhythmias and premature beats. In addition, in the rabbit isolated heart model critical volume pulses create diastolic depolarization. In patients with hypertension and left ventricular hypertrophy, development of new electrocardiogram (ECG) strain pattern is an independent risk factor for increased cardiovascular deaths[40]. In HF patients, while bradycardia may predispose to excessive stretch through greater diastolic filling and provoke malignant arrhythmias, the greater the heart rate reduction with beta-blockers, the greater the reduction in mortality. Interestingly, in patients with aortic insufficiency who have a predisposition for excess diastolic volume load with potential for arrhythmias, the use of beta-blockers once thought to be contraindicated has recently been shown to be beneficial[41].

The aforementioned trials and therapies point to a link between HF and ventricular arrhythmias, thereby supporting the presence of MEC in the chronic disease setting. However, the effect of acute ventricular loading and unloading, while shown to influence PVC and VT occurrence in experimental interventions, has not been convincingly demonstrated in the clinical setting. Clinicians are aware of amelioration of ventricular arrhythmias in intensive care patients when acute volume overload has been corrected by diuretic drugs or haemofiltration, but these 'anecdotal' observations have not been tested or confirmed in clinical trials.

Conclusions and outlook

The failing heart is compromised in a chronic overload situation. As the left ventricle dilates, the wall tension increases. An adaptive response is development of left ventricular hypertrophy. Electrical, structural and functional remodelling occur. There is increased expression of angiotension II and enhanced activities of the sympathetic and renin–angiotension–aldosterone systems. With scarring, fibrosis, downregulation of currents and gap junction abnormalities, ventricular arrhythmias frequently occur. Mechano-electrical coupling from SAC may further enhance arrhythmogenesis. Pardoxically, while beta-blockers in theory may provoke stretch and arrhythmogenesis from bradycardia and aortic insufficiency, their uses have been associated with better outcome. Perhaps the stretch may not have reached a critical threshold to provoke lethal arrhythmias.

It would be of interest to study the antiarrhythmic effects of a selective SAC blocker, such as GsMTx-4, in patients with HF. If this was found to be positive with respect to activity and safety, then clinical outcomes could be determined. Volume reduction may decrease stretch. However, results of volume reduction with use of diuretics in HF patients have been inconsistent in that the potassium sparing diuretics appear to be safer than loop diuretics. Of note, spironolactone has beneficial effects on outcome without a diuretic effect. The true anti-stretch effects of diuretics are 'contaminated' by other effects, such as electrolyte imbalances, and thus cannot be measured. Perhaps a good model to study the effects of volume (and perhaps stretch) is to measure arrhythmia density before and after dialysis. Of note and as a general rule, dialysis patients are vulnerable to SCD, which seldom occurs during dialysis with volume depletion.

Such future trials may improve our understanding of the relationship between stretch and arrhythmias, with the hope of specific treatments that may effect beneficial outcomes.

References

1. Singh SN, Fletcher RD, Fisher SG, *et al*. The Survival Trial of Antiarrhythmic Therapy in Congestive Heart Failure: amiodarone in patients with congestive heart failure and asymptomatic ventricular arrhythmia. *N Eng J Med* 1995;**333**:77–82.

2. Maggioni AP, Zuanetti G, Franzosi MG, *et al*. Prevalence and prognostic significance of ventricular arrhythmias after acute myocardial infarction in the fibrinolytic era. GISSI-2 results. *Circulation* 1993;**87**:312–322.

3. Singh SN, Fisher SG, Carson PE, Fletcher RD. Prevalence and significance of nonsustained ventricular tachycardia in patients

with premature ventricular contractions and heart failure treated with vasodilator therapy. *J Am Coll Cardiol* 1998;**32**:942–947.

4. Buxton AE, Lee KL, DiCarlo L, *et al.* Electrophysiologic testing to identify patients with coronary artery disease who are at risk for sudden death Multicenter Unsustained Tachycardia Trial Investigators. *N Engl J Med* 2000;**342**:1937–1945.

5. Antzelevitch C. Cardiac repolarization. The long and short of it. *Europace* 2005;**7**(Suppl 2):2:S3–S9.

6. Wiegerinck RF, vanVeen TAB, Belterman CH, Schumacher CA, Noorman M, deBakker JMT. Transmural dispersion of refractoriness and conduction velocity is associated with heterogeneously reduced connexin43 in a rabbit model of heart failure. *Heart Rhythm* 2008; **5**:1178–1185.

7. Narayan SM, Bayer JD, Lalan G, Trayanova NA. Action potential dynamics explain arrhythmic vulneratiblity in human heart failure. *J Am Coll Cardiol* 2008;**52**:1782–1792.

8. Culter MJ, Rosenbaum DS. Risk stratification for sudden cardiac death: is there a clinical role for T-wave alternans? *Heart Rhythm* 2009;**6** (Suppl 8):S56–S61.

9. Tomaselli GF, Beuckemann DF, Calkins HG, *et al.* Sudden cardiac death in heart failure: The role of abnormal repolarization. *Circulation* 1994;**90**:2534–2539.

10. Jin H, Lyon AR, Akar FG. Arrhythmia mechanisms in the failing heart. *PACE* 2008;**31**:1048–1056.

11. Kirchhof P, Eckardt L, Arslan O, *et al.* Prolonged QRS duration increases QT dispersion but does not relate to arrhythmias in survivors of acute myocardial infarction. *Pacing Clin Electrophysiol* 2001;**24**: 789–795.

12. CIBIS-II Investigators and Committees. The cardiac insufficiency bisoprolol study-II (CIBIS=II): a randomized trial. *Lancet* 1999;**353**: 9–13.

13. MERIT-HF Study Group. Effect of metoprolol CR/XL in chronic heart failure: metoprolol CR/XL randomized intervention trial in congestive heart failure. *Lancet* 1999;**353**:2001–2007.

14. Poole-Wilson PA, Swedberg K, Cleland JGF, *et al.*; for the COMET Investigators. Comparison of carvedilol and metoprolol on clinical outcomes in patients with chronic heart failure. Results of the Carvedilol or Metoprolol European Trial. *Lancet* 2003;**362**:7–13.

15. Ryden L, Ariniego R, Ainman K, *et al.* A double-blind trial of metoprolol in acute myocardial infarction: effects on ventricular tachyarrhythmia. *N Eng J Med* 1983;**308**:614–618.

16. Kjekshus J, Gullestad L Heart rate as a therapeutic target in heart failure. *Eur Heart J* 1999;**1**(Suppl):H64–H69.

17. Julian DG, Presccott RJ, Jackson FS, Szekely P. Controlled trial of sotalol for one year after myocardial infarction. *Lancet* 1982;**319**: 1142–1147.

18. Torp-Pedersen C, Moller M, Block-Thomsen PE, *et al.* Dofetilide in patients with converstive heart failure and left ventricular dysfunction. Danish Investigations of Arrhythmia and Mortality on Dofetilide Study Drug. *N Engl J Med* 1999;**341**:857–865.

19. Kober L. Bloch Thomsen PE, *et al.* Danish Investigations of Arrhythmia and Mortality on Dofetilide (DIAMOND) Study Group. Effect of dofetilide in patients with recent infarction and left-ventricular dysfunction: a randomized trial. *Lancet* 2000;**356**: 2052–2058.

20. Gibson RS, Boden WE, Theroux P, *et al.* Diltiazem and reinfarction in patients with non-Q-wave myocardial infarction. Results of a double-blind, randomized, multicenter trial. *N Eng J Med* 1986;**315**:423–429.

21. The Danish Study Group on Verapamil in Myocardial Infarction. Effect of varapamil on mortality and major events after acute myocardial infarction (the Danish Varapamil Tiral II-DAVIT II). *Am J Cardiol* 1990;**66**:779–785.

22. Packer M, O'Connor CM, Ghali JK, *et al.*; for the Prospective Randomized Amlodipine Survival Evaluation Study Group. Effect of Amlodipine on Morbidity and Mortality in Severe Chronic Heart Failure. *N Eng J Med* 1996;**335**:1107–1114.

23. Makkar KM, Sanoski CA, Spinler SA. Role of angiotensin-converting enzyme inhibitors, angiotensin II receptor blockers and aldosterone antagonists in the prevention of atrial and ventricular arrhythmias. *Phamacotherapy* 2009;**29**:31–48.

24. Pitt B, Zannad F, Remme WJ, *et al.*; for the Randomized Aldactone Evaluation Study Investigators. The effect of spironolactone on morbidity and mortality in patients with severe heart failure. *N Eng J Med* 1999;**341**:709–717.

25. Pitt B, Remme W, Zannad F, *et al.*; for the Eplerenone Post-Acute Myocardial Infarction Heart Failure Efficacy and Survival Study Investigators. *N Eng J Med* 2003;**348**:1309–1321.

26. GISSI-HF Investigators. Effect of n-3 polyunsaturated fatty acids in patients with chronic heart failure (The GISSI-HF trial): a randomised double-blind, placebo-controlled trial. *Lancet* 2008; **372**:1223–1230.

27. Marchioli R, Barzi F, Bomba E, *et al.*; on behalf of the GISSI-Prevenzione Investigators. Early protection against sudden death by n-3 polyunsaturated fatty acids after myocardial infarction time-course analysis of the results of the gruppo intialiano per lo studio della ssopravvivenza nell'infarto miocardico (GISSI)-prevenzione. *Circulation* 2002;**105**:1897–1903.

28. Calo L, Bianconi L, Colivicchi F, *et al.* N-3 fatty acids for the prevention of atrial fibrillation after coronary artery bypass surgery. *J Am Coll Cardiol* 2005;**45**:1723–1728.

29. Holmes DR Jr, Davis KB, Mock MB, *et al.* Risk factor profiles of patients with sudden cardiac death and death from other cardiac causes: A report from the Coronary Artery Surgery Study. *J Am Coll Cardiol* 1989;**13**:524–530.

30. Bigger JT Jr. Prophylactic use of implanted cardiac defibrillators in patients at high risk for ventricular arrhythmias after coronary-artery bypass graft surgery. Coronary Artery Bypass Graft (CABG) Patch Trial Investigators. *N Engl J Med* 1997;**337**:1569–1575.

31. Moss AJ, Zareba W, Hall WJ, *et al.*; for the Multicenter Automatic Defibrillator Implantation Trial II Investigators. Prophylactic implantation of a defibrillator in patients with myocardial infarction and reduced ejection fraction. *N Eng J Med* 2002;**346**:877–883.

32. Bardy GH, Lee KL, Mark DB, *et al.*; for the Sudden Cardiac Death in Heart Failure Trial (SCD-HeFT) Investigators. *N Engl J Med* 2005;**352**:21–46.

33. Bristow MR, Saxon LA, Boehmer J, *et al.*; for the Comparison of Medical Therapy, Pacing, and Defibrillation in Heart Failure (COMPANION) Investigators. Cardiac-Resynchronization therapy with or without an implantable defibrillator in advanced chronic heart failure. *N Engl J Med* 2004;**350**:2140–2150.

34. Cleland JG, Daubert JC, Erdmann E, *et al.*; on behalf of the CARE-HF Investigators. Longer-term effects of cardiac resynchronization therapy on mortality in heart failure [The CArdiac REsynchroniztion-Heart Failure (CARE-HF) trial extension phase]. *Eur Heart J* 2006;**27**: 1928–1932.

35. DiBiase L, Gasparini M, Lunati M, *et al.* Antiarrhythmic effect of reverse ventricular remodeling induced by cardiac resynchronization therapy. *J Am Coll Cardiol* 2008;**52**:1442–1449.

36. Chugh SS, Shen WK, Luria DM, Smith HC. First evidence of premature ventricular complex-induced cardiomyopathy: a potentially reversible cause of heart failure. *J Cardiovasc Electrophysiol* 2000;**11**:328–329.

37. Kottkamp H, Hindricks G, Chen X, *et al.* Radiofrequency catheter ablation of sustained ventricular tachycardia in idiopathic dilated cardiomyopathy. *Circulation* 1995;**92**:1159–1168.

38. Kohl P, Sachs F, Franz MR (2005) Stretch-activated channels in the heart. In: *Cardiac Mechano-Electric Feedback and Arrhythmias: from Pipette to Patient* (eds P Kohl, F Sachs, MR Franz). Elsevier Saunders, Philadelphia, pp.2–9.

39. Zabel M, Franz M (2005) Mechanical triggers and facilitators of cardiac excitation and arrhythmias. In: *Cardiac Mechano-Electric Feedback and Arrhythmias: from Pipette to Patient* (eds P Kohl, F Sachs, MR Franz). Elsevier Saunders, Philadelphia, pp.119–115.

40. Okin PM, Oikarinen L, Viitasalo M, *et al.* Devereux RB for the LIFE Study Investigators. Prognsostic value of changes in the electrocardiographic strain pattern during antihypertensive treatment. The Lorsartan Intervention of End-point Reduction in Hypertension Study (LIFE). *Circulation* 2009;**119**:1883–1891.

41. Sampat U, Varadarajan P, Turk R, Kamath A, Khandhar S, Pai RG. Effect of beta-blocker therapy on survival in patients with severe aortic regurgitation. *J Am Coll Cardiol* 2009;**54**:452–457.

42. Luu M, Stevenson WG, Stevenson LW, Baron K, Walden J. Diverse mechanisms of unexpected cardiac arrest in advanced heart failure. *Circulation* 1989;**80**:1675–1680.

Mechanical heterogeneity and after contractions as trigger for Torsades de Pointes

Annerie M.E. Moers and Paul G.A. Volders

Background

Intrinsic mechanical heterogeneity of the beating heart optimizes overall cardiac function during physiological conditions. However, via mechano-electrical coupling (MEC), it can contribute to the occurrence of polymorphic ventricular tachycardia, including Torsades de Pointes (TdP), in the structurally normal heart. A major role of altered myocardial Ca^{2+} handling is suspected here. In the human congenital long-QT syndrome, considered a primary electrical cardiomyopathy, mechanical wall abnormalities are found in some patients, which may precipitate arrhythmias under provocative conditions. This chapter focuses on mechano-electrical heterogeneity and the mechanisms by which this can trigger ventricular arrhythmia.

Intrinsic basal mechanical heterogeneity

Cardiac mechanical load is the integrated sum of distinct elementary quantities and can be quantified in terms of stress and strain. These terms are derived from physics, where *stress* is defined as the force acting on the surface of an object and *strain* as the resultant deformation of this object. Strain is dimensionless and expressed as the length of the object after the deformation relative to its unstressed baseline length. In the heart, this is closely related to sarcomere length (when describing behaviour in the tissue plane) and cavity volume (when considering whole heart; note that these two representations of the heart's mechanical environment are not linearly related). By definition, positive strain represents lengthening or expansion of an object, and negative strain indicates shortening or compression.

Intrinsic mechanical heterogeneity of the normal ventricles is characterized by gradients of non-uniform responses to stimuli between (1) the endo- and epicardium, (2) the apex and base, (3) the left and right ventricle (LV and RV, respectively), and (4) at the circumferential diameter[1]. In disease, these are altered and often further complicated by step-discontinuities (e.g. near scar tissue). Under physiological conditions, mechanical heterogeneity plays a key role in the optimization of global excitation–contraction (EC) coupling (see also Chapter 21).

Electrical heterogeneity of the ventricular myocardium roughly follows similar patterns. Ashikaga *et al.*[2] investigated the relationship between three-dimensional transmural myofibre mechanics and electrical properties in the anterior LV of anaesthetized adult mongrel dogs. While finding transmural differences in myofibre shortening and relaxation, they did not find significant gradients of repolarization *in vivo*. The latter corroborates earlier *in vivo* results by Anyukhovsky *et al.*[3] Figure 48.1 shows the temporal relation between electrical depolarization and myofibre shortening (left panel), and electrical repolarization and myofibre relaxation (right panel). Transmural electrical conduction (slope of 0.49 m/s) occurs faster than mechanical activation (0.25 m/s) and relaxation (0.10 m/s). Both electrical and mechanical activation originate at the endocardium, proceeding towards the epicardium. For relaxation, this pattern is reversed. Electrical repolarization is almost synchronous at sub-endocardial, mid-wall and sub-epicardial levels. Interestingly, Ashikaga *et al.* reported a second peak of myofibre shortening at several LV transmural layers in 8 out of 14 animals during diastolic filling, which was smaller in magnitude than the initial peak shortening[2]. The potential importance of this second peak under pathological conditions will become apparent in later sections of this chapter.

In humans, sub-epicardial relaxation may precede sub-endocardial relaxation, which is consistent with the *in vivo* animal studies by Ashikaga *et al.*[2,4] In healthy humans undergoing magnetic resonance imaging, wall thickness and strain are larger at the base than at the apex of the LV. Strain decreases from the sub-endocardium to the sub-epicardium[4,5]. In patients with LV hypertrophy due to aortic stenosis, this transmural gradient in strain is often reversed, while transmural relaxation orientation remains unchanged[4]. Abnormal repolarization is not necessarily the consequence of abnormal wall thickness and may be independent of ventricular dimensions and systolic function. However, it is consistently associated with abnormal diastolic function. Abnormal pressure wave forms, consisting of continuous LV pressure decay throughout diastole and/or a secondary pressure rise in mid-diastole, have been reported for patients with aortic stenosis and hypertrophic cardiomyopathy[6]. Post-extrasystolic potentiation causes further

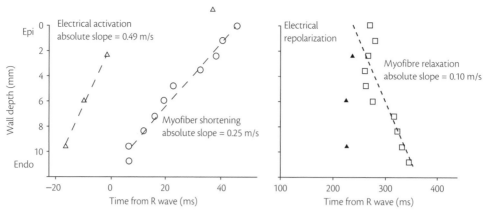

Fig. 48.1 Left panel: temporal relation between electrical activation and myofibre shortening in the normal canine left ventricle. The open triangles represent the onset of electrical activation and open circles the onset of myofibre shortening, both measured from the onset of the R-wave on the ECG. Electrical activation starts earlier and proceeds faster than myofibre shortening. In either case, patterns proceed from the endocardium towards the epicardium. Right panel: temporal relation between electrical repolarization (closed triangles) and myofibre relaxation (open squares). Relaxation occurs at a slope of 0.10 m/s, starting from the epicardium. Electrical repolarization at sub-endocardial, mid-wall and sub-epicardial levels was almost synchronous, and overall delay between electrical and mechanical recovery was small, compared to the activation delay shown in the left panel. (Reproduced, with permission, from Ashikaga H, Coppola BA, Hopenfeld B, Leifer ES, McVeigh ER, Omens JH (2007) Transmural dispersion of myofiber mechanics. Implications for electrical heterogeneity in vivo. *J Am Coll Cardiol* **49**:909–916.]

accentuation of this abnormal diastolic pressure pattern. During simultaneous recording of LV monophasic action potentials (MAP), dyssynchronous LV relaxation and diastolic after-contractions are accompanied by delayed after-depolarizations (DAD)[6], suggesting abnormal myocardial Ca^{2+} handling as the underlying mechanism.

The molecular basis for physiological mechano-electrical non-uniformity is determined, at least partly, by the differential expression of ion channels (both subunits and channel density may be affected) and proteins involved in myocyte Ca^{2+} handling. Na^+ channels function differently across the canine LV transmural wall. At similar Na^+-current density, epicardial cells have a more negative half-inactivation voltage than endocardial cells[7]. Along with this, Nav1.5 messenger ribonucleic acid (mRNA) and protein expressions are lowest in epicardium compared to mid- and endocardium, both in canine and human[8,9]. Transmural molecular and functional expressions of L-type Ca^{2+} channels appear similar in these species[8,9]. In the LV free wall, Kv4.3 and KChIP2 expressions encode for a gradient of transient outward K^+ current (I_{to})[10], with highest amplitudes measured at the epicardium. Transmural expressions of KCNQ1 and the slowly activating delayed-rectifier K^+ current (I_{Ks}) are consistently found to be lowest in the mid-myocardium[8,11,12], whereas in this same layer KCNE1 mRNA and protein are expressed more abundantly than in epi- or endocardium[8,9,12]. No transmural differences are reported for the rapidly activating delayed-rectifier K^+ current (I_{Kr}), a finding that is corroborated by similar expressions of KCNH2 and KCNE2 across the wall, at least in the canine[8,11]. The same applies for the inward rectifier K^+ current (I_{K1}) and its channel subunit encoded by Kir2.1. Na^+/K^+-pump current is larger in canine epicardial than in endocardial myocytes, and concentrations of intracellular Na^+ show the opposite gradient, both in quiescent and in paced cells[13]; see[9] for transmural mRNA expression of Na^+/K^+ ATPase (ATP1A1) in non-failing human hearts. For the Na^+/Ca^{2+} exchanger (NCX),

current densities are found to be larger in epi- and mid-myocardial layers than in the endocardium[14,15], paralleling mRNA and protein levels[15]. See[9] for transmural expressions of NCX1 in non-failing human hearts. For the cardiac ryanodine receptor (RyR2), protein density and message are greater in the canine sub-endo-than sub-epicardial myocardium[16]. In human hearts, RyR2 mRNA is found most abundantly in the mid-myocardium[9]. By contrast, the sarcoplasmic reticulum Ca^{2+} ATPase (SERCA2a) is expressed significantly less in the sub-endo- and mid-myocardium than in the sub-epicardium, and this may explain a slower decay of the intracellular Ca^{2+} transient at the endocardium, as depicted in Fig. 48.2[17].

The functional and molecular differences described above are reflected prominently in the distinct morphologies of action potentials, cell shortening and intracellular Ca^{2+} transients across the ventricular wall, at least in cellular and tissue experiments. Figure 48.2 shows typical examples for canine epi-, mid-myo- and endocardium[17,18]. Epicardial action potentials have the most pronounced spike-and-dome morphology. The hallmark of mid-myocardial action potentials is their ability to prolong with slowing of the pacing rate with much more accentuation than at the epi- and endocardium, although the extent to which this will happen *in situ* is a matter of ongoing debate[19]. Epi- and mid-myocardial cells express a shorter latency in the onset and time to peak of cell shortening than endocardial myocytes. The relaxation of cell shortening and Ca^{2+} transient lasts significantly longer in endo- than epicardial myocytes (Fig. 48.2). As a possible consequence, Ca^{2+} transient alternans and increased diastolic levels of intracellular Ca^{2+} may occur preferentially closer to the endocardial surface. In line with this, pharmacological studies have shown that Ca^{2+}-dependent DAD and early after-depolarizations (EAD), as well as triggered activity, develop much more readily in tissues from the sub-endocardial/mid-myocardial region than at the epicardium.

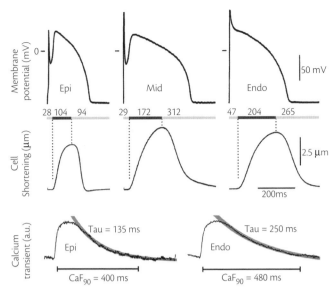

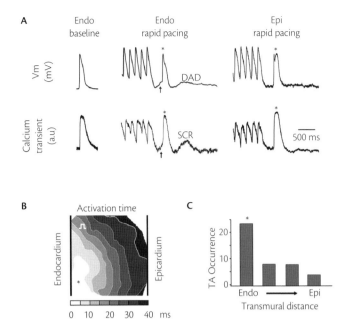

Fig. 48.2 Transmural differences in action potentials, cell shortening and Ca²⁺ transients in the canine left ventricle. Representative action potentials (top) and corresponding unloaded cell shortening (middle) recorded from epi-, mid- and endocardial myocytes paced at a cycle length of 2000 ms. Bottom panel: Ca²⁺ transients simultaneously recorded from epi- and endocardium in a canine left-ventricular wedge preparation at an endocardial pacing cycle length of 600 ms. Return of intracellular Ca²⁺ transients to diastolic levels is slower for endo- than for epicardium as indicated by the exponential fit (thick grey line), the time constant of decay (Tau) and the duration of the Ca²⁺ transient (CaF₉₀). (Reproduced, with permission, from Cordeiro JM, Greene L, Heilmann C, Antzelevitch D, Antzelevitch C (2004) Transmural heterogeneity of calcium activity and mechanical function in the canine left ventricle. *Am J Physiol* **286**:H1471–H1479, and from Laurita KR, Katra RP, Wible B, Wan X, Koo MH (2003) Transmural heterogeneity of calcium handling in canine. *Circ Res* **92**:668–675.]

Fig. 48.3 Triggered activity under conditions of increased myocardial Ca²⁺ entry caused by the simultaneous administration of the I_{Ks} blocker HMR1556 and the β-adrenergic agonist isoproterenol in canine LV wedge preparations. **A** Representative action potentials (Vm) and Ca²⁺ transients recorded during baseline pacing (600 ms) from the endocardium (left) and during rapid pacing (180 ms) followed by an abrupt halt in pacing from the same endocardial site (middle) and an epicardial site (right). After cessation of rapid pacing, an ectopic excitation is evident (askerisk). At the endocardium, a DAD and spontaneous Ca²⁺ release (SCR) occurred after the ectopic excitation. **B** shows an activation map with the origin of the ectopic excitation (askerisk). **C** Based on experiments in 12 LV wedges from 12 dogs, triggered activity (TA) occurred more frequently at the endocardium than in other transmural layers. (Reproduced, with permission, from Katra RP, Laurita KR (2005) Cellular mechanism of calcium-mediated triggered activity in the heart. *Circ Res* **96**:535–542.]

Ca²⁺ after-transients and after-contractions as triggers for Torsades de Pointes

Katra and Laurita[20] reported a study in which canine LV-wedge preparations were exposed to the I_{Ks} inhibitor HMR1556 and the β-adrenergic agonist isoproterenol, effectively leading to enhanced myocardial Ca²⁺ entry[20]. This model mimics the clinical condition of long-QT syndrome type 1. The aim was to examine the relationship between elevated intracellular Ca²⁺ levels and triggered activity originating from specific transmural locations. The wedge preparations were electro-mechanically uncoupled by Cytochalasin-D to avoid motion artefacts during optical mapping (of course, motion is no 'artifact' for cardiac tissue, but immobilization is a currently necessary, if undesirable, limitation of our experimental abilities). Figure 48.3A shows representative action potentials and Ca²⁺ transients at baseline and during rapid pacing from the endocardium in the presence of HMR1556 and isoproterenol. Triggered ectopic excitations occurred, both at the endo- and epicardium, after sudden termination of the rapid pacing. However, spontaneous Ca²⁺ release from the sarcoplasmic reticulum, and concomitant DAD, were only visible at the endocardium (not at the epicardium) *after* the ectopic beat. Nonetheless, Ca²⁺-induced DAD were also considered the mechanism *of* the ectopic excitation

at that site (arrows in Fig. 48.3A; also note local Ca²⁺ transient alternans during pacing). Triggered activity originated most frequently at the endocardium, with resultant ectopic beats propagating to other transmural regions (Fig. 48.3B,C). From a mechanistic standpoint, the absence of mechanical influences (by Cytochalasin-D) in these preparations strongly indicates that Ca²⁺-overload-dependent, and not mechano-sensitive, membrane currents are involved in abnormal impulse formation.

Gallacher *et al.*[21] administered HMR1556 to anaesthetized beagle dogs, thus creating an *in vivo* model of drug-induced long-QT 1 syndrome. The anaesthetics lofentanil and etomidate were purposefully chosen in this study to minimize influences on autonomic (particularly β-adrenergic) sensitivity. Bolus injections of 2.5 μg/kg isoproterenol provoked TdP in 17 out of 18 animals. Figure 48.4 illustrates the primary events leading to arrhythmia, based on simultaneous recordings of the ECG, MAP from the LV endocardium and epicardium, and LV pressure. Isoproterenol, in the presence of HMR1556, led to paradoxical prolongation and beat-to-beat instability of repolarization during heart-rate acceleration, particularly at the LV endocardium (but not at the epicardium or in the RV). Along with these electrophysiological changes, after-contractions emerged in the LV before TdP ensued. These after-contractions commenced well before the completion of LV

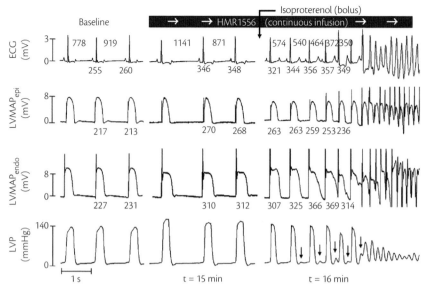

Fig. 48.4 Beat-to-beat repolarization prolongation and instability by isoproterenol occur predominantly at the left-ventricular (LV) endocardium in a canine model of drug-induced long-QT 1 syndrome. Simultaneous ECG (mV), LVMAP (mV) from epicardium (epi) and endocardium (endo), and LV pressure (LVP) (mm Hg) recorded from an anaesthetized open-chest beagle dog at baseline, during 0.05 mg/kg/min HMR 1556 (t = 15 min) and upon a bolus of 2.5 μg/kg isoproterenol (t = 16 min). Numbers at ECG trace indicate RR intervals (above) and QT times (below) in milliseconds. Numbers below MAP recordings indicate MAP duration at 90% repolarization in milliseconds. Arrows at LVP trace indicate after-contractions. (Reproduced, with permission, from Gallacher DJ, Van de Water A, van der Linde H, *et al.* (2007) In vivo mechanisms precipitating torsades de pointes in a canine model of drug-induced long-QT1 syndrome. *Cardiovasc Res* **76**:247–256.]

repolarization (so before the end of electrical systole) and equally *before* the onset of concomitant late EADs. After-contraction amplitudes grew beat-by-beat, reaching averaged peak pressures of 25 ± 6 mm Hg (17% of primary 'normal' contractions) just prior to arrhythmia induction, and they coincided with delayed activity in the nadir of the T-wave on the ECG (more so than did EAD). Prevention of TdP with esmolol, verapamil or mexiletine was only achieved if after-contractions (more than other proarrhythmic precursors) remained absent.

These *in vivo* results correlate with the data of Katra and Laurita[20,22], forming a bridge from mechanistic studies at the ventricular tissue level to catheter-based clinical investigations during adrenergic-provocation testing in selected patients (see below).

With regard to the *in vivo* origins of arrhythmogenic after-contractions, various explanations are offered. First, after-contractions could be initiated by stretch-evoked membrane depolarizations during a state of ß-adrenergic increased inotropy. This would implicate trans-membrane Na^+ or Ca^{2+} influx via non-selective stretch-activated ion channels and subsequent Ca^{2+}-induced Ca^{2+} release from the sarcoplasmic reticulum (perhaps secondary to effects on NCX activity) as their probable cause. Previous work by Franz *et al.*[23] has demonstrated that increases in LV volume and pressure in the intact beating canine heart (e.g. by transient clamping of the aorta or intraventricular balloon inflation) led to the development of after-depolarizations and a reduction in the maximum diastolic potential of LV epicardial MAP. The timing of stretch at end-diastole is critical here, as after-depolarizations are often associated with ventricular ectopic beats[23], including in human heart[24].

As an alternative mechanism, EAD carried by ß-adrenergic-enhanced window L-type Ca^{2+} current could be the generators of after-contractions via Ca^{2+}-induced Ca^{2+} release from the sarcoplasmic reticulum during repolarization[25]. This explanation presumes that EAD in MAP signals are truly representative of trans-membrane EAD. However, the finding of Gallacher *et al.*[21] that most after-contractions started *earlier* than the onset of late EAD, at least in their model, raises doubt about the relevance of this mechanism *in vivo*.

Finally, after-contractions and after-depolarizations (via NCX) can share the same underlying mechanism of spontaneous Ca^{2+} release from the sarcoplasmic reticulum in the setting of Ca^{2+} overload. The latter has been demonstrated for isoproterenol-induced Ca^{2+} overload in canine ventricular myocytes[26,27], while sarcoplasmic reticulum Ca^{2+} release has recently been demonstrated to be enhanced (in isolated ventricular myocytes) by mechanical stretch[28]. Given the strong connection of these data[26,27], and those of Katra and Laurita[20] and Gallacher *et al.*[21], a central role of spontaneous Ca^{2+} release for *in vivo* after-contractions, triggered activity and initiation of TdP is likely, although the precise pathway needs further investigation.

Ventricular mechanical wall abnormalities in the long-QT syndrome

Ever since its first description by Jervell and Lange-Nielsen in 1957 and by Romano *et al.* and Ward in 1963 and 1964, the congenital long-QT syndrome has been considered a purely electrical disorder. Long-QT patients can have variable symptoms, ranging from mild palpitations to syncope and sudden death due to TdP and ventricular fibrillation. Mutations leading to this syndrome have been identified in at least 12 different genes. Loss-of-function mutations of the KCNQ1 gene affect I_{Ks} and account for long-QT 1 syndrome, the most common form (up to 55% of all cases).

In 1991, Nador *et al.*[29] reported unexpected ventricular mechanical abnormalities in this 'purely electrical' disorder. In a group of 42 patients, 23 exhibited a shortened time to half systolic contraction and a prolonged late contraction phase on M-mode long-axis parasternal views. Examples are illustrated in Fig. 48.5. Moreover, a peculiar double-peak pattern of late thickening was observed in 11 of the 23 patients. The finding of these mechanical abnormalities was associated with a history of syncope and cardiac arrest. Treatment with the Ca^{2+}-channel blocker verapamil normalized the contraction pattern[30].

Similar ventricular mechanical abnormalities were observed by other investigators using tissue Doppler imaging[31,32]. However, genotype-specific patterns were not recognized. In 73 long-QT mutation carriers (mixed genotypes), Haugaa *et al.*[32] identified significantly increased mechanical dispersion of the LV, assessed as the standard deviation of contraction duration of basal LV segments from apical four-chamber, two-chamber and long-axis views. Prolonged contraction duration was superior to heart-rate corrected QT interval (QTc) for the risk assessment of cardiac events. It is tempting to speculate that the prolonged contraction duration, increased mechanical dispersion and double-peak pattern of late thickening are consequences of (locally) prolonged

repolarization, abnormal myocardial Ca^{2+} handling and after-contractions.

Clinical data based on isoproterenol or epinephrine provocation testing indicate differential responses of the QT interval and the T_{peak}–T_{end} interval in long-QT 1, long-QT 2 (KCNH2; loss-of-function I_{Kr} channel) and long-QT 3 (SCN5A; gain-of-function Na^+ channel) patients. In long-QT 1 patients, isoproterenol or epinephrine infusion prolongs the QTc with a peak effect at maximal heart-rate increase. QTc remains prolonged for a considerable time thereafter. EAD in MAP recordings are frequently observed under these conditions[33,34]. By contrast, QTc prolongation is (much) less pronounced in long-QT 2 and 3 patients. In long-QT 1 patients with a non-diagnostic QT interval at baseline ('concealed long-QT'), adrenergic provocation testing can unmask the typical phenotype with high accuracy[35]. For similar diagnostic purposes, provocation testing is sometimes performed in genotype-negative patients with long-QT intervals at baseline and ventricular tachyarrhythmias and/or unexplained syncope.

Figure 48.6 illustrates such a case from our own centre. The patient is a 51-year-old male who was admitted because of unexplained syncope while standing in a crowd. Note his abnormal T-wave morphology at baseline and a prolonged QT time > 600 ms. During invasive cardiac electrophysiological testing, he exhibited normal conduction times. No ventricular tachycardia could be induced by standard programmed electrical stimulation. Isoproterenol provocation testing was performed after the

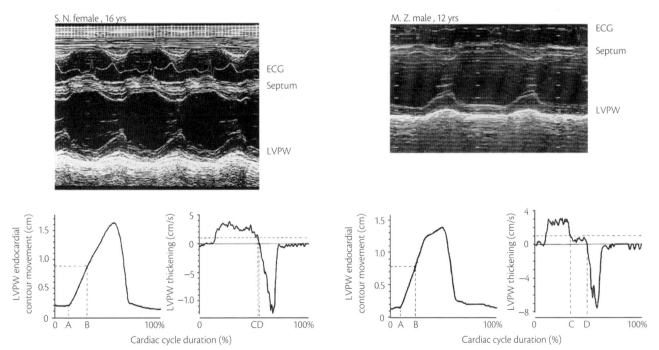

Fig. 48.5 Ventricular wall-motion abnormalities in patients with idiopathic long-QT syndrome. Representative M-mode echocardiograms of a control subject (left panel) and a long-QT patient (right panel) during sinus rhythm. Long-axis parasternal view, 100 mm/s. In the lower panel, the first and third trace represent the endocardial contour movement of the left-ventricular posterior wall (LVPW). Segment A–B indicates the time to half systolic contraction as a percentage of cardiac cycle (Th1/2). Second and fourth trace, first derivative of LVPW wall thickening. Segment C–D indicates the time spent during the late thickening phase, before rapid relaxation, at a rate smaller than 1 cm/s (TSTh). In the right lower panel, note the abnormal movement of the LVPW caused by a shorter early systolic thickening (segment A–B) and a longer late thickening phase (segment C–D) resulting in a plateau morphology. (Reproduced, with permission, from Nador F, Beria G, De Ferrari GM, Stramba-Badiale M, Lotto LEH, Schwartz PJ (1991) Unsuspected echocardiographic abnormality in the long QT syndrome. Diagnostic, prognostic, and pathogenetic implications. *Circulation* **84**:1530–1542.]

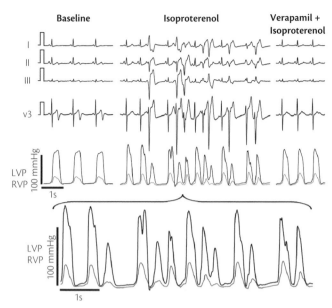

Fig. 48.6 Arrhythmogenic mechano-electrical instability during isoproterenol-provocation testing in a 51-year-old male patient with unexplained syncope. Shown are ECG leads I, II, III and V3, simultaneously recorded with left- (LVP) and right- (RVP) ventricular pressure. Recordings are taken at baseline, after bolus i.v. infusion of 40 µg/min isoproterenol, and subsequent administration of 10 mg verapamil. In this patient, the baseline echocardiogram and cardiac magnetic resonance imaging showed no significant abnormalities. He had a normal coronary angiogram. ECG calibration bars indicate 1 mV. [Courtesy of Laurent Pison, MD, and Jurren M. van Opstal, MD, PhD, Department of Cardiology, Maastricht University Medical Centre, The Netherlands.]

positioning of LV- and RV- pressure catheters. As a first ECG change, leads with T-wave negativity or bipolarity showed a reversal to positivity. The QT interval shortened. Dramatic alterations occurred in the LV pressure signals (but not in the RV), mainly characterized by significant relaxation delays and systolic after-contractions. The latter were often followed by ventricular premature complexes or bursts of non-sustained ventricular tachycardias. Infusion of esmolol and verapamil normalized all of these derangements. This case illustrates the clinical importance of arrhythmogenic mechano-electrical instability in the human heart with particular vulnerability to adrenergic stress. To date, genotyping in this patient has revealed a normal expression of the major 'long-QT' genes, as well as calsequestin and the RyR.

Conclusions and outlook

Physiological mechano-electrical heterogeneity of the myocardium optimizes overall cardiac function. At the molecular level, it is characterized by the differential expression of ion channels and proteins involved in myocyte Ca^{2+} handling. In normal canine and human hearts, electrical and mechanical activation originate at the endocardium, proceeding towards the epicardium, and myofibre strain gradually declines from the endocardium towards the epicardium. For relaxation, the electro-mechanical wave pattern is reversed. In patients with cardiac hypertrophy, transmural gradients of myofibre strain decline from the epicardium towards

the endocardium. Simultaneous recordings of LV MAP, dyssynchronous LV relaxation, diastolic after-contractions and DAD strongly suggest abnormal myocardial Ca^{2+} handling as the underlying mechanism.

The long-QT syndrome has long been considered a 'pure' electrical disorder. However, late contraction phase is prolonged at least in some patients with arrhythmia vulnerability. Dispersion of contraction is increased, consistent with electrical abnormalities. Mechanical wall abnormalities normalize after verapamil, suggesting abnormal myocardial Ca^{2+} handling as an underlying mechanism. It has been demonstrated that intracellular diastolic Ca^{2+} levels are higher and Ca^{2+} transient alternans is more prevalent at the endocardium than in other transmural layers. *In vitro* and *in vivo* studies mimicking long-QT 1 syndrome demonstrated ectopic, electrical and mechanical activity preferentially at the endocardium. *In vivo*, after-contractions preceded EAD if TdP ensued. Adrenergic provocation testing in some patients with phenotypic long-QT syndrome, whether or not based on demonstrable genetic mutations, reveals major mechano-electrical instability and after-contractions, associated with ventricular premature complexes or bursts of non-sustained ventricular tachycardias. While interesting as a mechanistic observation, future studies should reveal whether these combined recordings of ECG and ventricular pressure during provocation testing enhance assessment of arrhythmia risk.

Acknowledgements

Dr Volders was supported by a Vidi grant from The Netherlands Organization for Scientific Research (ZonMw 91710365). Roel L.H.M.G. Spätjens, BSc, Department of Cardiology, Cardiovascular Research Institute Maastricht, The Netherlands, assisted in the making of the figures.

References

1. Brutsaert DL. Nonuniformity: a physiologic modulator of contraction and relaxation of the normal heart. *J Am Coll Cardiol* 1987;**9**: 341–348.
2. Ashikaga H, Coppola BA, Hopenfeld B, Leifer ES, McVeigh ER, Omens JH. Transmural dispersion of myofiber mechanics: implications for electrical heterogeneity in vivo. *J Am Coll Cardiol* 2007;**49**:909–916.
3. Anyukhovsky EP, Sosunov EA, Rosen MR. Regional differences in electrophysiological properties of epicardium, midmyocardium, and endocardium. In vitro and in vivo correlations. *Circulation* 1996;**94**:1981–1988.
4. Hasegawa T, Nakatani S, Kanzaki H, Abe H, Kitakaze M. Heterogeneous onset of myocardial relaxation in subendocardial and subepicardial layers assessed with tissue strain imaging: comparison of normal and hypertrophied myocardium. *JACC Cardiovasc Imaging* 2009;**2**:701–708.
5. Bogaert J, Rademakers FE. Regional nonuniformity of normal adult human left ventricle. *Am J Physiol* 2001;**280**:H610–H620.
6. Paulus WJ, Goethals MA, Sys SU. Failure of myocardial inactivation: a clinical assessment in the hypertrophied heart. *Basic Res Cardiol* 1992;**87** Suppl 2:145–161.
7. Cordeiro JM, Mazza M, Goodrow R, Ulahannan N, Antzelevitch C, Di Diego JM. Functionally distinct sodium channels in ventricular epicardial and endocardial cells contribute to a greater sensitivity of the epicardium to electrical depression. *Am J Physiol* 2008;**295**: H154–H162.

8. Szabó G, Szentandrássy N, Bíró T, *et al.* Asymmetrical distribution of ion channels in canine and human left-ventricular wall: epicardium versus midmyocardium. *Pflugers Arch* 2005;**450**:307–316.

9. Soltysinska E, Olesen S-P, Christ T, *et al.* Transmural expression of ion channels and transporters in human nondiseased and end-stage failing hearts. *Pflugers Arch* 2009;**459**:11–23.

10. Zicha S, Xiao L, Stafford S, *et al.* Transmural expression of transient outward potassium current subunits in normal and failing canine and human hearts. *J Physiol* 2004;**561**:735–748.

11. Liu DW, Antzelevitch C. Characteristics of the delayed rectifier current (IKr and IKs) in canine ventricular epicardial, midmyocardial, and endocardial myocytes. A weaker IKs contributes to the longer action potential of the M cell. *Circ Res* 1995;**76**:351–365.

12. Luo X, Xiao J, Lin H, *et al.* Transcriptional activation by stimulating protein 1 and post-transcriptional repression by muscle-specific microRNAs of I_{Ks}-encoding genes and potential implications in regional heterogeneity of their expressions. *J Cell Physiol* 2007; **212**:358–367.

13. Gao J, Wang W, Cohen IS, Mathias RT. Transmural gradients in Na/K pump activity and $[Na^+]_i$ in canine ventricle. *Biophys J* 2005;**89**: 1700–1709.

14. Zygmunt AC, Goodrow RJ, Antzelevitch C. I_{NaCa} contributes to electrical heterogeneity within the canine ventricle. *Am J Physiol* 2000;**278**:H1671–H1678.

15. Xiong W, Tian Y, DiSilvestre D, Tomaselli GF. Transmural heterogeneity of Na^+-Ca^{2+} exchange: evidence for differential expression in normal and failing hearts. *Circ Res* 2005;**97**:207–209.

16. Hittinger L, Ghaleh B, Chen J, *et al.* Reduced subendocardial ryanodine receptors and consequent effects on cardiac function in conscious dogs with left ventricular hypertrophy. *Circ Res* 1999;**84**:999–1006.

17. Laurita KR, Katra R, Wible B, Wan X, Koo MH. Transmural heterogeneity of calcium handling in canine. *Circ Res* 2003;**92**: 668–675.

18. Cordeiro JM, Greene L, Heilmann C, Antzelevitch D, Antzelevitch C. Transmural heterogeneity of calcium activity and mechanical function in the canine left ventricle. *Am J Physiol* 2004;**286**:H1471–H1479.

19. Taggart P, Sutton P, Opthof T, Coronel R, Kallis P. Electrotonic cancellation of transmural electrical gradients in the left ventricle in man. *Prog Biophys Mol Biol* 2003;**82**:243–254.

20. Katra RP, Laurita KR. Cellular mechanism of calcium-mediated triggered activity in the heart. *Circ Res* 2005;**96**:535–542.

21. Gallacher DJ, Van de Water A, van der Linde H, *et al.* In vivo mechanisms precipitating torsades de pointes in a canine model of drug-induced long-QT1 syndrome. *Cardiovasc Res* 2007;**76**:247–256.

22. Laurita KR, Katra RP. Delayed afterdepolarization-mediated triggered activity associated with slow calcium sequestration near the endocardium. *J Cardiovasc Electrophysiol* 2005;**16**:418–424.

23. Franz MR, Burkhoff D, Yue DT, Sagawa K. Mechanically induced action potential changes and arrhythmia in isolated and in situ canine hearts. *Cardiovasc Res* 1989;**23**:213–223.

24. Levine JH, Guarnieri T, Kadish AH, White RI, Calkins H, Kan JS. Changes in myocardial repolarization in patients undergoing balloon valvuloplasty for congenital pulmonary stenosis: evidence for contraction–excitation feedback in humans. *Circulation* 1988;**77**:70–77.

25. De Ferrari GM, Viola MC, D'Amato E, Antolini R, Forti S. Distinct patterns of calcium transients during early and delayed afterdepolarizations induced by isoproterenol in ventricular myocytes. *Circulation* 1995;**91**:2510–2515.

26. Volders PG, Kulcsár A, Vos MA, *et al.* Similarities between early and delayed afterdepolarizations induced by isoproterenol in canine ventricular myocytes. *Cardiovasc Res* 1997;**34**:348–359.

27. Volders PG, Vos MA, Szabo B, *et al.* Progress in the understanding of cardiac early afterdepolarizations and torsades de pointes: time to revise current concepts. *Cardiovasc Res* 2000;**46**:376–392.

28. Iribe G, Ward CW, Camelliti P, *et al.* Axial stretch of rat single ventricular cardiomyocytes causes an acute and transient increase in Ca^{2+} spark rate. *Circ Res* 2009;**104**:787–795.

29. Nador F, Beria G, De Ferrari GM, *et al.* Unsuspected echocardiographic abnormality in the long QT syndrome. Diagnostic, prognostic, and pathogenetic implications. *Circulation* 1991;**84**: 1530–1542.

30. De Ferrari GM, Nador F, Beria G, Sala S, Lotto A, Schwartz PJ. Effect of calcium channel block on the wall motion abnormality of the idiopathic long QT syndrome. *Circulation* 1994;**89**:2126–2132.

31. Savoye C, Klug D, Denjoy I, *et al.* Tissue Doppler echocardiography in patients with long QT syndrome. *Eur J Echocardiogr* 2003;**4**:209–213.

32. Haugaa KH, Edvardsen T, Leren TP, Gran JM, Smiseth OA, Amlie JP. Left ventricular mechanical dispersion by tissue Doppler imaging: a novel approach for identifying high-risk individuals with long QT syndrome. *Eur Heart J* 2009;**30**:330–337.

33. Shimizu W, Kurita T, Matsuo K, *et al.* Improvement of repolarization abnormalities by a K^+ channel opener in the LQT1 form of congenital long-QT syndrome. *Circulation* 1998;**97**:1581–1588.

34. Shimizu W, Ohe T, Kurita T, *et al.* Early afterdepolarizations induced by isoproterenol in patients with congenital long QT syndrome. *Circulation* 1991;**84**:1915–1923.

35. Vyas H, Hejlik J, Ackerman MJ. Epinephrine QT stress testing in the evaluation of congenital long-QT syndrome: diagnostic accuracy of the paradoxical QT response. *Circulation* 2006;**113**:1385–1392.

Stretch-induced arrhythmias in ischaemia

Ruben Coronel, Natalia A. Trayanova, Xiao Jie and Michiel J. Janse

Background

It has been well established experimentally that a sudden increase in cardiac wall stress or a sudden direct impact on the chest may induce cardiac arrhythmias and even may lead to sudden death[1–5]. 'Commotio cordis', however, is a relatively rare phenomenon and direct evidence that mechanical effects may lead to life-threatening arrhythmias in other clinical conditions is sporadic[6]. One of the reasons for this lack of evidence is the impossibility of directly and non-invasively measuring myocardial wall stress.

Ventricular arrhythmias resulting from acute myocardial ischaemia are a major cause of sudden – arrhythmic – cardiac death[7]. Because the ischaemic tissue ceases to contract[8] in the early phase of acute myocardial ischaemia[9,10] or contractions become dyssynchronous, mechano-electrical coupling (MEC) potentially plays a role in arrhythmogenesis during ischaemia. In particular when part of the myocardium becomes rigid ('stone heart') after about 30 min of ischaemia, the remaining healthy myocardium is expected to exert strong forces on the interface between healthy and ischaemic myocardium. This is in contrast to the early phase of ischaemia when the ischaemic myocardium is flaccid.

Ischaemia-induced arrhythmias occur in two distinct phases. These phases were first defined by Kaplinsky et al.[11] in dogs subjected to coronary ligation. Kaplinsky surmised that the mechanisms of arrhythmogenesis were different between these two phases of ischaemia based on the morphology of local electrograms. The authors concluded that re-entry was not the probable mechanism of the delayed (1b) ventricular arrhythmias[11]. The idea of different mechanisms in the two phases of arrhythmogenesis was substantiated by the work of Smith et al.[12] who related the second phase of arrhythmias (now commonly named 1b arrhythmias) to a rise in tissue resistivity in pig hearts. In their key figure the authors show the cumulative number of arrhythmia events as a function of duration of ischaemia with a superimposed plot of tissue resistivity (Rt). The two phases of arrhythmias are clearly seen, as well as the coincidence of the second, 1b, phase with the rising phase of Rt[12]. It is of interest that they demonstrate that the second (1b) phase of arrhythmias is much more often associated with ventricular fibrillation (VF) than the first (1a) phase.

The rise in tissue resistivity is caused by the closure of gap junctions which, in turn, is initiated by an increase in cytoplasmatic free Ca^{2+}-concentration and acidification of the intracellular milieu[13–16].

Preconditioning the myocardium with several short episodes of ischaemia and reperfusion may postpone the rise in Rt[17] and, indeed, delays the second phase of arrhythmias as well[18]. Thus, there is circumstantial evidence that the second (1b) phase of arrhythmias may be causally related to mechanical effects and cellular uncoupling.

For the generation of arrhythmias, the co-incidence of a pre-existing condition ('the substrate') and a sudden 'discharging' event ('the trigger') is required[19]. Both trigger and substrate may be modulated by, for example, the presence of drugs, mutations and the effects of the autonomic nervous system[19]. Identification of both the trigger and the substrate is needed to define the arrhythmogenic mechanism of 1b-arrhythmias. MEC appears to play a role in the genesis of the trigger, and uncoupling in the formation of the substrate.

Phase 1b-arrhythmias *in vivo* and in isolated hearts

The involvement of MEC in the spontaneous 1b-arrhythmia during ischaemia was demonstrated by our own group[20]. Figure 49.1 is derived from our paper and demonstrates the occurrence of spontaneous arrhythmias in 5 min episodes after the occlusion of the left anterior descending artery in pig hearts. In the isolated blood-perfused hearts arrhythmias are rare and only one of eight hearts developed VF (Fig. 49.1B). This is in contrast to the arrhythmias encountered *in vivo* (Fig. 49.1A) where arrhythmias are more common and more lethal. *In vivo* the heart performs work and is under the influence of the autonomic nervous system. When a fluid-filled balloon was inserted through the mitral orifice of the Langendorff-perfused heart and the left ventricle (LV) was allowed to perform work arrhythmias were again more abundant (Fig. 49.1C)[20]. This demonstrates that MEC is an important modifier of arrhythmogenesis during ischaemia, although it is not possible to identify whether the modification is at the level of the trigger of the substrate. Barrabes et al. counted spontaneous premature beats in the presence of a blocker of stretch-activated channels – gadolinium – in *in vivo* pig hearts, but failed to demonstrate a reduction of arrhythmias with gadolinium[21]. It is not clear how to reconcile these contradictory observations although it is possible that gadolinium was only injected into the ischaemic

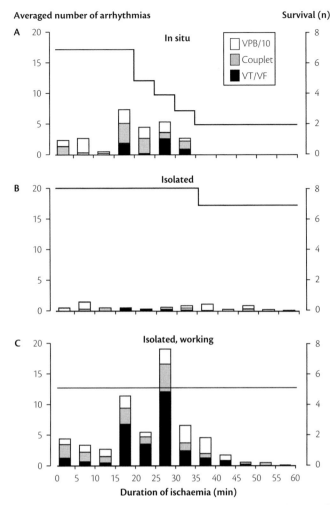

Fig. 49.1 Distribution of ventricular arrhythmias during the course of 60 min of regional ischaemia in pigs. **A** *In situ*. **B** Isolated unloaded perfused hearts. **C** Isolated perfused working hearts. VPB, ventricular premature beat. [Modified, with permission, from Coronel R, Wilms-Schopman FJG, de Groot JR (2002) Origin of ischemia-induced phase 1b ventricular arrhythmias in pig hearts. *J Am Coll Cardiol* **39**:166–167.]

zone. Alternatively, gadolinium may not act very well in the presence of bicarbonate[22].

By providing one or more premature beats ('the trigger') and by subsequently observing whether VF (re-entry) occurs, one may study the development of an arrhythmic substrate. De Groot *et al.* did this in unloaded isolated perfused pig hearts[23]. Figure 49.2 shows an example of one experiment. Premature beats were applied to the ischaemic zone (coupling intervals were adjusted to the refractory period, the stimulus artefacts are indicated by arrows) at various times during ischaemia. If VF was not induced by a single premature beat, progressively more premature beats were given (up to a maximum of three). Prior to ischaemia three premature beats did not result in VF. In the 1b-phase, however, a single (see tracing D) premature beat was sufficient to induce VF, pointing to the maximum availability of the arrhythmic substrate. Later on (after about 50 min of ischaemia) three premature beats were required to induce VF. These experiments show that during ischaemia an arrhythmogenic substrate waxes and wanes. Figure 49.2B shows

the relation between the relative rise in tissue impedance (recorded with the four-electrode technique). The maximum substrate (at arrow D) is present when uncoupling is only moderate.

Although the evidence so far indicates that MEC has a potential role in the induction of the triggering premature beat, we need to go into some detail to describe the arrhythmogenic substrate of 1b-arrhythmias.

Phase 1b: arrhythmogenic mechanisms: substrate

De Groot *et al.* demonstrated that epicardial re-entry is the predominant mechanism of 1b-arrhythmias[23]. Figure 49.3 shows an example of epicardial activation maps of two subsequent activation waves during VF, from the ischaemic tissue. A complete re-entrant wave is seen. Slow conduction, a short refractory period and heterogeneity in action potential (AP) duration are required for the initiation and maintenance of re-entry[24]. Indeed, simulation studies have indicated that with the electrophysiological conditions occurring during the second phase of arrhythmogenesis it is possible to induce re-entry by providing a premature beat[25].

The closure of gap junctions is associated with an increase in intracellular $[Ca^{2+}]$[26,27] and/or a decrease in intracellular pH[28] and leads to slowing of conduction and conduction block[29,30]. De Groot *et al.* demonstrated that arrhythmogenesis in the 1b phase occurred when uncoupling was moderate (up to about 40% of maximal) and terminated when uncoupling was complete (see Fig. 49.2)[23]. Because a larger degree of intercellular uncoupling is needed to result in conduction slowing than was encountered at the moment of 1b-arrhythmias[30], alternative mechanisms for the arrhythmogenic substrate have to be considered.

One possibility is that uncoupling may unmask pre-existing differences in AP duration, a mechanism that has been demonstrated in heart failure[31]. In normal myocardium, heterogeneity in AP duration is minimized through the high degree of electrotonic coupling between cells. When the coupling is diminished, AP heterogeneity may become apparent[32]. In computer simulations of Jie *et al.* epicardial re-entry was demonstrated but only in the presence of heterogeneities in AP duration (see below)[25].

Another potential mechanism is related to the interaction between surviving subendocardial or subepicardial myocardium and severely depressed intramural myocardium during the 1b-phase of acute ischaemia. For this mechanism, the inexcitable – intramural – myocardium may act as a passive load for surviving and relatively normal tissue, if intercellular coupling is (residually) intact. The surviving and intrinsically normal layers are then depolarized by being coupled to the severely depolarized midmyocardial tissue[23,33]. This may result in epicardial conduction slowing and unmasking of AP heterogeneities[25]. A similar mechanism has been demonstrated in cell pairs[34] and in a simulation study[35]. When the uncoupling is total, the electrotonic interaction between the two layers ceases, the arrhythmogenic substrate disappears and the 1b phase is terminated. Jie *et al.* executed a computer modelling study in which a surviving and a depolarized sheet of myocardium were coupled. The normal 'epicardial' sheet contained heterogeneities. Indeed, epicardial re-entry could be induced by moderate uncoupling of the two layers alone[25].

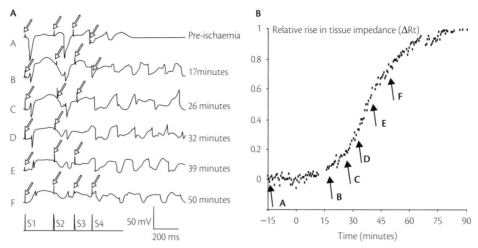

Fig. 49.2 A Local electrograms from the ischaemic tissue at times A–F from the start of ischaemia. Open arrows point to stimulus artefacts (stimulus protocol indicated at bottom). **B** Rise of tissue resistance (ΔRt) recorded in the same animal. The minimum number of premature beats necessary to induce ventricular fibrillation concurs with a moderate rise of tissue resistance. S1, basic stimulus; S2/S3/S4, premature stimuli. [Reproduced, with permission, from de Groot JR, Wilms-Schopman FJG, Opthof T, Remme CA, Coronel R (2001) Late ventricular arrhythmias during acute regional ischemia in the isolated blood perfused pig heart. Role of electrical cellular coupling. *Cardiovasc Res* **50**:362–372.]

Phase 1b: arrhythmogenic mechanisms: trigger

In the presence of the arrhythmogenic substrate a single premature beat is sufficient to induce re-entry and VF. This is demonstrated during the 1b-phase of ischaemia-induced arrhythmias [Fig. 49.2[23]], where a single premature beat initiates re-entry. The mechanism of this initiating beat is not clear. Although triggered activity emanating from Purkinje fibres during cellular uncoupling and the local release of catecholamines have been suggested to play a role[36–39], mechanical stretch exerted by the normally contracting myocardium on the rigid ischaemic tissue is involved. A clear indication for MEC is provided by potentiated contractions provoked in the isolated working pig heart [Fig. 49.4[20]]. A stimulation protocol with a long interval after eight basic cycles (see Fig. 49.4, lower tracing) during the 1b-phase of regional ischaemia incites a spontaneous premature beat following the potentiated beat originating from the LV myocardium (see the bipolar electrograms from the left and right ventricular myocardium). This stimulus protocol also led to the induction of VF (not shown)[40]. One may argue that the stimulus protocol leads to triggered activity based on early after-depolarizations. However, the activation-recovery intervals of the beats before and following the pause were the same. Also, the QT-times of the bipolar electrograms in Fig. 49.4 were not prolonged after the pause. Indeed, the pig lacks the transient outward current that is responsible for the AP duration changes induced by a long interval[41]. Therefore, early after-depolarizations cannot explain the genesis of the premature beats in phase 1b.

Origin of the triggering premature beat

We argued that the forces exerted by the healthy, contracting myocardium on the ischaemic tissue would cause MEC effects preferentially at the interface between the two domains. We therefore performed mapping studies *in vivo* and in Langendorff-perfused pig hearts. Figures 49.5 and 49.6 [from ref[20]] show some

examples of the mapping of the site of origin of a premature beat: one that did and another that did not lead to VF. The tracings in both figures are unipolar electrograms recorded from the sites indicated by a star in the maps. Figure 49.5 shows how the rectangular electrode matrix was positioned over the ischaemic area. In Fig. 49.5A the activation pattern of the last stimulated beat is shown, and in Fig. 49.5B the initiating beat of VF. At 310 ms after the last stimulus artefact a spontaneous activation is generated at the border between the ischaemic and the normal tissue (star), which is blocked towards the ischaemic zone (see the crowding of isochrones). The absence of an R-wave in the electrogram recorded at that site also indicates that this area is the origin of the premature beat. A similar case is shown in Fig. 49.6. Here, no VF was induced, but a remarkable double origin of the premature beat was recorded, both located at the border between the ischaemic and non-ischaemic tissue. Again, the electrograms recorded at both sites showed the absence of R-waves.

Thus, strong evidence exists that MEC is a principal cause for arrhythmogenesis in myocardial ischaemia. Ischaemia, however, is a complicated process, and it is difficult to attribute causality to a single factor by experimental means. In simulation studies, however, it is possible to address these issues more systematically.

Simulation studies

Unravelling the exact mechanisms underlying mechanically induced spontaneous arrhythmias is hampered by the lack of adequate experimental protocols to measure the three-dimensional (3D) electromechanical activity, with high spatiotemporal resolution, in the beating heart with ischaemic injury. Also, the electrophysiological changes in acute ischaemia are very rapid, rendering the assessment of mechanically induced arrhythmogenic mechanisms technically difficult. Jie *et al.* used a novel anatomically realistic dynamic 3D electromechanical model of the rabbit ventricles to gain insight into the role of electromechanical dysfunction on arrhythmogenesis during acute ischaemia[42]. The model contained

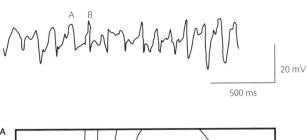

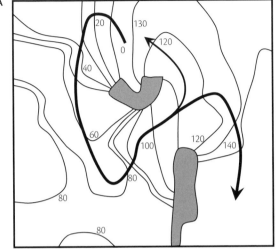

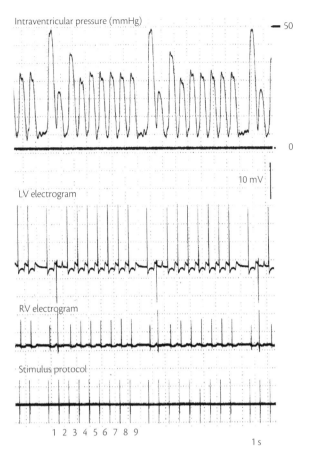

Fig. 49.4 Simultaneous recording of intraventricular pressure (top panel), a left and right ventricular bipolar electrogram (middle panels) and the stimulus protocol (bottom panel) during the second phase of arrhythmogenesis. A pause in the stimulation protocol was followed by a potentiated beat. Following the potentiated beat a spontaneous left ventricular premature beat occurred. [Modified, with permission, from Coronel R, Wilms-Schopman FJG, de Groot JR (2002) Origin of ischemia-induced phase 1b ventricular arrhythmias in pig hearts. *J Am Coll Cardiol* **39**:166–167.]

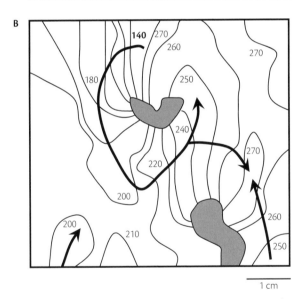

Fig. 49.3 Subsequent activation maps showing re-entrant activation between the two beats marked A and B in the top unipolar tracing. Lines are isochrones (numbers indicate time in milliseconds from an arbitrary reference time). [Modified, with permission, from Coronel R, Wilms-Schopman FJG, de Groot JR (2002) Origin of ischemia-induced phase 1b ventricular arrhythmias in pig hearts. *J Am Coll Cardiol* **39**:166–167.]

stretch-activated channels and demonstrated that large myofibre strain developed in the ischaemic region, increasing from the border zone (BZ) towards the central ischaemic zone (CIZ). The maximum distribution of maximum strain rate occurred endocardially in the LV within the CIZ.

Figure 49.7B shows that local depolarization and even triggered activity occurred following the AP during ischaemia. These

'after-depolarization-like events' (named because they are not dependent on intracellular calcium concentration) were absent if the stretch-activated channels were omitted from the model.

Figure 49.7 depicts the activation sequence of the last paced beat and the spontaneous induced beat during ischaemia (in the presence of stretch-activated channels). The cross-sectional views show that a premature beat originated from two locations in the LV endocardial BZ (arrows in the 191-ms inset) and led to epicardial breakthrough at 198 ms (ellipse in the 198-ms inset). Note that in this view the ventricles were tilted for better visualization of the epicardial activation pattern. Another epicardial breakthrough is shown in the rectangle in the 200-ms inset. Both sites of epicardial breakthrough were located close to the anterior ischaemic border in close resemblance to the experimentally obtained data mentioned earlier.

Figure 49.7B also presents the AP recorded at sites 1 (in BZ) and 2 (in CIZ) marked in the bottom 191-ms inset. At site 1, the mechanically induced membrane depolarization (black arrow) evoked spontaneous firing with a takeoff potential of −56.2 mV. At site 2, despite the fact that the peak magnitude of

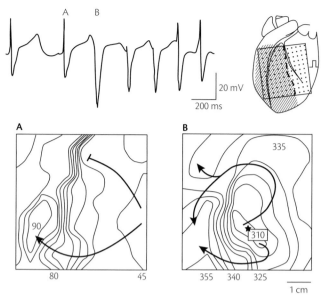

Fig. 49.5 Spontaneous occurrence of a premature beat during the 1b-phase followed by ventricular fibrillation. Top panel: local unipolar electrogram recorded from a site at the border between the ischaemic and non-ischaemic myocardium (star). **A** and **B** Activation maps of the last stimulated beat and the premature beat. Note the focal origin of the premature beat and the absence of an R-wave at the site of origin. [Modified, with permission, from Coronel R, Wilms-Schopman FJG, de Groot JR (2002) Origin of ischemia-induced phase 1b ventricular arrhythmias in pig hearts. *J Am Coll Cardiol* **39**:166–167.]

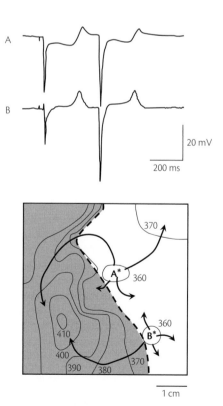

Fig. 49.6 Spontaneous occurrence of a premature beat during the 1b-phase. Note the double origin of the premature beat (stars). [Modified, with permission, from Coronel R, Wilms-Schopman FJG, de Groot JR (2002) Origin of ischemia-induced phase 1b ventricular arrhythmias in pig hearts. *J Am Coll Cardiol* **39**: 166–167.]

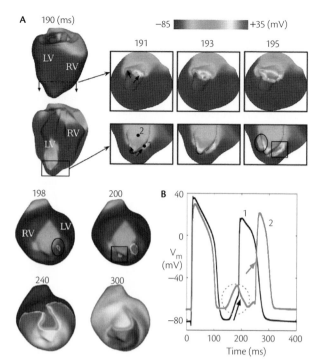

Fig. 49.7 A Evolution of the mechanically induced ventricular premature beat (VPB) for regional ischaemia stage I. The 191- to 195-ms insets present both short and long axis views of the apical region. The 198- to 300-ms insets present a tilted anterior view of the ventricles for better observation of epicardial activation. Arrows in the 191-ms inset indicate locations of earliest spontaneous firing. Ellipse and rectangle in the bottom 195-ms inset indicate the parts of the wavefront that make the earliest epicardial breakthrough at the locations encircled with an ellipse in the 198-ms inset and a rectangle in the 200-ms inset, respectively. **B** Traces of trans-membrane potential (V_m) recorded at site 1 [black, border zone (BZ)] and 2 [red, central ischaemic zone (CIZ)] marked in the bottom 191-ms inset in **A**. Black arrow and red dashed circle denote mechanically induced depolarization at sites 1 and 2, respectively. Red arrow indicates activation at site 2 by the propagation of the mechanically induced VPB. [Reproduced, with permission, from Jie X, Gurev V, Trayanova N (2010) Mechanisms of mechanically-induced spontaneous arrhythmias in acute regional ischemia. *Circ Res* **106**:185–192.] (See color plate section)

subthreshold depolarization (dashed circle) was 8.5 mV larger, no AP was triggered, probably caused by the decreased resting membrane potential in the more ischaemic CIZ myocardium. The site was subsequently activated in the course of the propagating wave.

In addition to the role of MEC in the genesis of the triggering premature beat, Jie *et al.* also describe how the arrhythmogenic substrate characteristic for acute ischaemia is modified by wall stress. Its modifying action can make the difference between the successful induction of VF by the premature beat or not, or between life and death.

The paper by Jie *et al.* shows the unique application of simulation studies to scientific questions that cannot be addressed otherwise[42].

Conclusions and outlook

There is a strong case for the arrhythmogenic potential of MEC, especially in acute ischaemia. MEC appears to be causal to the genesis of premature beats, and likely is a strong modulator of the arrhythmogenic substrate. Pharmacological interventions aimed at reducing the impact of MEC on ischaemia-induced arrhythmogenesis are hampered by low specificity of blockers of the stretch-activated channels, and by scant insight on the exact pathophysiological mechanism of MEC in ischaemia. Because wall stress can only be calculated and not directly measured, studies combining an experimental and a mathematical approach, like the one by Jie et al.[42], are most likely to contribute to progress in this field, especially if they incorporate the intricate architecture of the intact heart.

References

1. Kamkin A, Kiseleva I, Isenberg G. Stretch-activated currents in ventricular myocytes: amplitude and arrhythmogenic effects increase with hypertrophy. *Cardiovasc Res* 2000;**48**:402–408.

2. Franz MR, Cima R, Wang D, Profitt D, Kurz R. Electrophysiological effects of myocardial stretch and mechanical determinants of stretch-activated arrhythmias. *Circulation* 1992;**86**:968–978.

3. Hansen DE, Craig CS, Hondeghem LM. Stretch-induced arrhythmias in the isolated canine ventricle. Evidence for the importance of mechanoelectrical feedback. *Circulation* 1990;**81**:1094–1105.

4. Babuty D, Lab MJ. Mechanoelectric contributions to sudden cardiac death. *Cardiovasc Res* 2001;**50**:270–279.

5. Lerman BB, Burkoff D, Yue DT, Franz MR, Sagawa K. Mechanoelectrical feedback: independent role of preload and contractility in modulation of canine ventricular excitability. *J Clin Invest* 1985;**76**:1843–1850.

6. Maron BJ, Doerer JJ, Haas TS, Tierney DM, Mueller FO. Sudden deaths in young competitive athletes: analysis of 1866 deaths in the United States, 1980–2006. *Circulation* 2009;**119**:1085–1092.

7. Janse MJ, Wit AL. Electrophysiological mechanisms of ventricular arrhythmias resulting from myocardial ischemia and infarction. *Physiol Rev* 1989;**69**:1049–1169.

8. Silverman HS, Stern MD. Ionic basis of ischaemic cardiac injury: Insights from cellular studies. *Cardiovasc Res* 1994;**28**:581–597.

9. Jennings RB, Reimer KA, Steenbergen C, Schaper J. Total ischemia III: effect of inhibition of anaerobic glycolysis. *J Mol Cell Cardiol* 1989;**21**:37–54.

10. Fiolet JWT, Baartscheer A, Schumacher CA, Coronel R, ter Welle HF. The change of the free energy of ATP hydrolysis during global ischemia and anoxia in the rat heart. *J Mol Cell Cardiol* 1984;**26**:1023–1036.

11. Kaplinsky E, Ogawa S, Blake CW, Dreifus LS. Two periods of early ventricular arrhythmias in the canine acute myocardial infarction model. *Circulation* 1979;**60**:397–403.

12. Smith IV WT, Fleet WF, Johnson TA, Engle CL, Cascio WE. The 1B phase of ventricular arrhythmias in ischemic in situ porcine heart is related to changes in cell-to-cell coupling. *Circulation* 1995;**92**:3051–3060.

13. Beardslee MA, Lerner DL, Tadros PN, et al. Dephosphorylation and intracellular redistribution of ventricular Connexin-43 during electrical uncoupling induced by ischemia. *Circ Res* 2000;**87**:656–662.

14. Dekker LR, Rademaker H, Vermeulen JT, et al. Cellular uncoupling during ischemia in hypertrophied and failing rabbit ventricular myocardium: effects of preconditioning. *Circulation* 1998;**97**:1724–1730.

15. Kléber AG, Riegger CB, Janse MJ. Electrical uncoupling and increase of extracellular resistance after induction of ischemia in isolated, arterially perfused rabbit papillary muscle. *Circ Res* 1987;**61**:271–279.

16. Kléber G. The potential role of Ca^{2+} for electrical cell-to-cell uncoupling and conduction block in myocardial tissue. *Basic Res Cardiol* 1992;**87**(Suppl 2):131–143.

17. Tan HL, Mazon P, Verberne HJ, Sleeswijk ME, Coronel R, Opthof T, Janse MJ. Ischaemic preconditioning delays ischaemia induced cellular electrical uncoupling in rabbit myocardium by activation of ATP sensitive potassium channels. *Cardiovasc Res* 1993;**27**:664–651.

18. Cinca J, Warren M, Carreno A, Tresanchez M, Armadans L, Gomez P, Soler-Soler J. Changes in myocardial electrical impedance induced by coronary artery occlusion in pigs with and without preconditioning. Correlation with local ST segment potential and ventricular arrhytmias. *Circulation* 1997;**96**:3079–3086.

19. Coumel P. The management of clinical arrhythmias. An overview on invasive versus non-invasive electrophysiology. *Eur Heart J* 1987;**8**:92–99.

20. Coronel R, Wilms-Schopman FJG, de Groot JR. Origin of ischemia-induced phase 1b ventricular arrhythmias in pig hearts. *J Am Coll Cardiol* 2002;**39**:166–167.

21. Barrabes JA, Garcia-Dorado D, Agullo L, et al. Intracoronary infusion of Gd^{3+} into ischemic region does not suppress phase Ib ventricular arrhythmias after coronary occlusion in swine. *Am J Physiol* 2006;**290**:H2344–H2350.

22. Caldwell RA, Clemo HF, Baumgarten CM. Using gadolinium to identify stretch-activated channels: technical considerations. *Am J Physiol* 1998;**275**:C619–C621.

23. de Groot JR, Wilms-Schopman FJG, Opthof T, Remme CA, Coronel R. Late ventricular arrhythmias during acute regional ischemia in the isolated blood perfused pig heart. Role of electrical cellular coupling. *Cardiovasc Res* 2001;**50**:362–372.

24. Mines GR. On circulating excitations in heart muscles and their possible relation to tachycardia and fibrillation. *Trans R Soc Canada* 1914;**IV**:43–53.

25. Jie X, Rodriguez B, de Groot JR, Coronel R, Trayanova N. Reentry in survived subepicardium coupled to depolarized and inexcitable midmyocardium: Insights into arrhythmogenesis in ischemia phase 1B. *Heart Rhythm* 2008;**5**:1036–1044.

26. De Mello WC. Effect of intracellular injection of calcium and strontium on cell communication in heart. *J Physiol* 1975;**250**:231–245.

27. Dekker LRC, Fiolet JWT, VanBavel E, et al. Intracellular Ca^{2+}, intercellular electrical coupling and mechanical activity in ischemic rabbit papillary muscle. Effects of preconditioning and metabolic blockade. *Circ Res* 1996;**79**:237–246.

28. Yan GX, Kleber AG. Changes in extracellular and intracellular pH in ischemic rabbit papillary muscle. *Circ Res* 1992;**71**:460–470.

29. Weingart R, Maurer P. Action potential transfer in cell pairs isolated from adult rat and guinea pig ventricles. *Circ Res* 1988;**63**:72–80.

30. Jongsma HJ, Wilders R. Gap junctions in cardiovascular disease. *Circ Res* 2000;**86**:1193–1197.

31. Wiegerinck RF, van Veen AA, Belterman CN, et al. Transmural dispersion of refractoriness and conduction velocity is associated with heterogeneously reduced connexin43 in a rabbit model of heart failure. *Heart Rhythm* 2008;**5**:1178–1185.

32. Lesh MD, Pring M, Spear JF. Cellular uncoupling can unmask dispersion of action potential duration in ventricular myocardium. A computer modeling study. *Circ Res* 1989;**65**:1426–1440.

33. de Groot JR, Coronel R. Acute ischemia-induced gap junctional uncoupling and arrhythmogenesis. *Cardiovasc Res* 2004;**62**:323–334.

34. Tan RC, Joyner RW. Electrotonic influences on action potentials from isolated ventricular cells. *Circ Res* 1990;**67**:1071–1081.

35. Pollard AE, Cascio WE, Fast VG, Knisley SB. Modulation of triggered activity by uncoupling in the ischemic border: A model study with phase 1b-like conditions. *Cardiovasc Res* 2002;**56**:381–392.

36. Verkerk AO, Veldkamp MW, Coronel R, Wilders R, van Ginneken ACG. Effects of cell-to-cell uncoupling and catecholamines on Purkinje and ventricular action potentials: implications for phase-1b arrhythmias. *Cardiovasc Res* 2001;**51**:30–40.

37. Dart AM, Schömig A, Dietz R, Mayer E, Kubler W. Release of endogenous catecholamines in the ischemic myocardium of the rat. Part B: Effect of sympathetic nerve stimulation. *Circ Res* 1984;**55**:702–706.

38. Opthof T, Ramdat Misier AR, Coronel R, *et al.* Dispersion of refractoriness in canine ventricular myocardium: Effects of sympathetic stimulation. *Circ Res* 1991;**68**:1204–1215.

39. Remme CA, Schumacher CA, de Jong JW, Fiolet JW, Coronel R, Wilde AA. K_{ATP} channel opening during ischemia: effects on myocardial noradrenaline release and ventricular arrhythmias. *J Cardiovasc Pharmacol* 2001;**38**:406–416.

40. Janse MJ, Coronel R, Wilms-Schopman FJG, De Groot JR. Mechanical effects on arrhythmogenesis: from pipette to patient. *Prog Biophys Mol Biol* 2003;**82**:187–195.

41. Verkerk AO, van Ginneken AC, Berecki G, *et al.* Incorporated sarcolemmal fish oil fatty acids shorten pig ventricular action potentials. *Cardiovasc Res* 2006;**70**:509–520.

42. Jie X, Gurev V, Trayanova N. Mechanisms of mechanically-induced spontaneous arrhythmias in acute regional ischemia. *Circ Res* 2010;**106**:185–192.

SECTION 7

Mechano-electric coupling as a mechanism involved in therapeutic interventions

50. **Anti-arrhythmic effects of acute mechanical stimulation** *361*
Tommaso Pellis and Peter Kohl

51. **Termination of arrhythmias by haemodynamic unloading** *369*
Peter Taggart and Peter Sutton

52. **Mechanical modulation of defibrillation and resuscitation efficacy** *374*
Derek J. Dosdall, Harish Doppalapudi and Raymond E. Ideker

53. **Anti- and proarrhythmic effects of cardiac assist device implantation** *381*
Paul J. Joudrey, Roger J. Hajjar and Fadi G. Akar

54. **Anti- and proarrhythmic effects of cardiac resynchronisation therapy** *387*
Nico H.L. Kuijpers and Frits W. Prinzen

Anti-arrhythmic effects of acute mechanical stimulation

Tommaso Pellis and Peter Kohl

(With special thanks to Angie M. King and Christian Boulin for contributions to this chapter in the first edition)

Background

"No procedure in modern medicine has aroused more controversial thought than the attempt to revive the dead."

This statement by Albert Hyman[1] introduced his 1930 paper on the mechanical component of 'intracardiac therapy' – the injection of drugs into arrested hearts. Hyman noted that, while epinephrine seemed to be the drug of choice, injection of atropine, caffeine and even dextrose produced similarly favourable results. This apparent drug-independence of the intervention led him to propose that the mechanical stimulation, afforded by needle insertion into the myocardium, was sufficient to restart asystolic hearts – a hypothesis that he went on to illustrate in several patients. In line with the opening statement, Hyman's paper initiated one of the most controversial debates in medicine of his time.

The use of mechanical interventions to reset disturbed heart rhythms is still a subject of contention. As anticipated by Hyman, the controversy in the field of resuscitation is a general one, at times including widely accepted interventions such as the utility of pharmacological agents *during* cardiac arrest, which has equally become a matter of debate[2]. This chapter summarizes the means and anti-arrhythmic utility of cardiac mechanical stimulation, recapitulates regulatory aspects and addresses the mechanisms and potential utility of this intervention.

Means of cardiac mechanical stimulation

Direct manual stimulation

Direct mechanical stimulation of cardiac muscle by 'finger tap' is a well-established method used by surgeons to prompt rhythmic contractile activity in hearts after induced arrest during open heart surgery. While this may be one of the most regularly used mechanical interventions to restore the heart beat, it is equally one of the least well characterized, in terms of mechanics and mechanisms.

Trans-thoracic needle insertion

Hyman found that the mechanical interaction of a trans-thoracically inserted needle with the myocardium may resuscitate arrested hearts[1].

He used both straight needles (for ventricular stimulation) and curved needles (to reach the right atrial appendage) to trigger ectopic beats, followed in about 25% of cases by temporary or full restoration of sinus rhythm. While his observations are largely of historical interest, the mechanical component is worth consideration.

Intracardiac catheter tip prodding

Cardiac catheterization is often associated with induction of premature ventricular contractions (PVC). Interestingly, catheter tip interactions with the cardiac wall can also lead to cardioversion from tachyarrhythmia. This was systematically studied by Befeler in 68 patients undergoing diagnostic catheterization[3]. Catheter tip stimulation of atrial and ventricular muscle was found to be effective in reverting atrial tachycardia in 24% of cases, junctional tachycardia in 60% and ventricular tachycardia (VT) in 14% [another 27% of VT patients in this study were treated by precordial thump (PT), discussed below]. Catheter tip-induced conversion of fibrillation was not attempted in this study. There is, however, a case report on successful and maintained cardioversion of chronic atrial fibrillation by catheter prodding[4]. In terms of 'practical utility', while the regularly observed PVC induction can be used to judge the final approach of a catheter to the heart, reports of anti-arrhythmic effects of intracardiac mechanical stimulation have remained anecdotal. Nonetheless, the concept has given rise to device development ideas, such as a piezo-driven endocardial stimulator developed by Pacesetter AB (US Patent 5433731; 1995).

Intrathoracic pressure increase

Several reports have highlighted the link between an abrupt increase in intrathoracic pressure and *termination* of tachyarrhythmias. This type of mechanical cardioversion can be self-administered[5], for example by coughing[6], or via the Valsalva manoeuvre[7], which has been found to also work in heart transplant recipients[8]. The distinction between direct mechano-electrical coupling (MEC) effects of intrathoracic pressure increase on cardiac electrophysiology and those mediated haemodynamically (via 'respiratory pump' action) has remained incomplete.

Extra-corporal impact

The best-known form of acute cardiac mechanical stimulation is probably PT, a forceful fist thump, usually applied to the sternum (although cases of successful spinal impact have been reported[9]). First described as a trigger of competent ventricular contraction in asystolic patients[10], PT has been used to pace hearts[11] and to terminate tachycardia[12] and fibrillation[13]. This procedure has also been proposed for patient self-administration[14], although not without serious objection[15], and it has inspired the design of external mechanical pacemakers, pioneered by Paul Zoll (US Patent 4265228; 1981).

Serial application of precordial impacts (so-called precordial percussion) may be used to pace the asystolic heart. Pre-cordial percussion differs from PT in that lower energy impacts (passive fall of the fist from 20–30 cm height), delivered at a rate of approximately 50–70 min^{-1}, are used to target the left sternal edge[16].

Anti-arrhythmic effects: case studies and experiments

Asystole

In 1920, Schott reported that a single blow to the chest could restore a palpable pulse in a patient with ventricular standstill, caused by a Stokes-Adams attack[10]. Building on Schott's observations, it was subsequently shown that rhythmic thumps, applied to the pre-cordium (precordial percussion) of patients in ventricular standstill, can trigger ventricular contractions[17]. These mechanically induced beats have a greater haemodynamic effect than external chest compression[18] and may be used to maintain consciousness in patients during extended periods of ventricular standstill (up to 2h 45min of successful fist-pacing has been reported[11,19]).

While of historical and mechanistic interest, asystole caused by Stokes-Adams attacks plays a less prominent role in modern-day 'Western' medicine (where such patients will normally carry an implanted electronic pacemaker). Nonetheless, acute asystole can occur as a rhythm secondary to electrical defibrillation, and manual mechanical pacing has a place as a bridge to instrumentation-based approaches, in particular in out-of-hospital and emergency settings (Fig. 50.1A).

This finds a reflection in reports on PT-effects in asystole, derived from single case reports[10,23–26] and case series[27,28]. Given the low case numbers involved in these studies, and the limited information on patient backgrounds and interventions, one must be careful not to over-interpret apparent success rates. Still, PT was effective in restoring normal sinus rhythm (NSR) in acutely asystolic patients in 14 out of 15 cases reported above (93%). Similarly, recent experimental evidence from anaesthetized pigs supports the view that PT may be particularly efficient in asystole[29].

Tachycardia

Following reports on successful application of PT as a means of re-starting asystolic hearts, it was found that PT may also be used to revert VT to NSR (see Fig. 50.1B)[12,21]. The success rate of optimally performed PT in VT may exceed 40%[3,30], and best results are seen if impacts coincide with the electrocardiogram (ECG) R-wave[31] (i.e. occur at a time when at least some of the ventricular tissue is already excited).

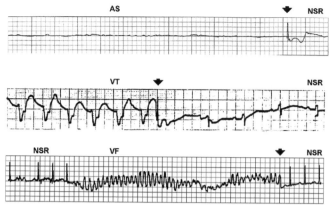

Fig. 50.1 ECG recordings from arrhythmic patients in whom normal sinus rhythm (NSR) was restored by single precordial thump. Presenting rhythm was (**A**) asystole (AS; reproduced, with permission, from Pellis T, Kette F, Lovisa D, *et al.* (2009) Utility of precordial thump for treatment of out of hospital cardiac arrest: a prospective study. *Resuscitation* **80**:17–23); (**B**) ventricular tachycardia (VT; reproduced, with permission, from Pennington JE, Taylor J, Lown B (1970) Chest thump for reverting ventricular tachycardia. *N Engl J Med* **283**:1192–1195, © Massachusetts Medical Society, all rights reserved.); and (**C**) early ventricular fibrillation (VF; reproduced, with permission, from Barrett JS (1971) Chest thumps and the heart beat. *N Engl J Med* **284**:392–393, © Massachusetts Medical Society, all rights reserved.)

Since the timing, relative to the cardiac cycle, of manually applied PT cannot be controlled reliably, there is concern about mechanical stimulation during the vulnerable period (T-wave), which could have detrimental effects on heart rhythm (see Chapter 45).

The expectation, however, that ill-timed PT would readily convert VT to ventricular fibrillation (VF) has largely not been confirmed[30], except in patients[32] and experiments[33] involving severe pre-existing hypoxia. This highlights that PT is more efficient if applied early into the development of VT, where it appears to pose little risk for rhythm deterioration[30].

To control impact timing, mechanical stimulators have been developed (Fig. 50.2), which can be triggered via cardiac rhythm monitors[34,35].

In a study by Zoll, ventricular excitation was reliably evoked in eight out of ten patients (nine were suffering from different cardiac rhythm disturbances including atrial fibrillation and one was in NSR undergoing a haemodynamic study) with not a single observation of repetitive responses, tachycardia or fibrillation[34].

It was furthermore found that the threshold for mechanical stimulation of PVC in adults is as low as 0.04–1.5 J[34]. This is a fraction only of the energy required for external electrical stimulation (usually ~150 J for biphasic defibrillatory stimuli, 200 J or more for monophasic).

Interestingly, this is also several orders of magnitude less than the mechanical energy levels involved in *Commotio cordis* in adults during competitive sports. By way of illustration, a standard regulation baseball (weight 0.142 kg) at a speed of 45 m × s^{-1} (common value for batted balls in major league games) has a kinetic energy of 144 J.

This discrepancy in a key parameter of the mechanical intervention may help to explain the rarity of negative side-effects of precordial impacts. In fact, controlled chest impacts, applied at energies ten

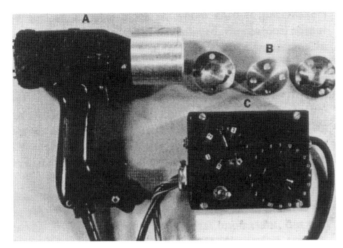

Fig. 50.2 Modified industrial stapling gun (A), projectiles with varying impact area (B) and control box for ECG synchronization (C), used by Paul Zoll for precordial thump studies. [Reproduced, with permission, from Zoll PM, Belgard AH, Weintraub MJ, Frank HA (1976) External mechanical cardiac stimulation. *N Engl J Med* **294**:1274–1276, © Massachusetts Medical Society, all rights reserved.]

times the threshold level for mechanical action potential (AP) stimulation, did not trigger VT or VF – even if applied during the T-wave[34]. Thus, there would appear to be a minimum 'permissive' energy level (tens of Joules in the adult), which has to be exceeded before impact timing becomes the decisive factor in determining impact arrhythmogeneity.

Fibrillation

In contrast to the relatively optimistic reports on PT effectiveness in patients with asystole or VT, successful treatment of VF by mechanical interventions has only occasionally been achieved (success rates near 2%, but often lower, have been observed[27,36]). In all documented successful cases, PT was applied very early during the development of VF, either at the verge of deterioration from VT[37] or within the first few seconds of VF (Fig. 50.1C), as verified by ECG and, occasionally, arterial pressure recordings[3,22,38].

Clinical utility: prospective data

The use of mechanical stimulation as a means of cardioversion in the hospital setting shows a large variation among societies, hospitals and even within single healthcare organizations. Medical personnel in China and Japan, for example, will use PT as a matter of course for patients developing life-threatening dysrhythmias. Personnel of specialized cardiac catheter laboratories, on the other hand, will usually opt for attaching defibrillator pads to patients before any intervention is conducted and, thus, do not normally consider application of PT, except for research purposes.

Tachycardia

Motivated by the previous lack of prospective studies, two recent catheter laboratory-based studies analyzed the effects of PT in over 200 patients with freshly induced VT (~20 s duration). Both demonstrated a low overall success rate of 1.3%,[39,40] even though earlier application of PT is unlikely to be possible in 'real life'

scenarios. In the rather different setting of out-of-hospital cardiac arrest, the only study to prospectively investigate PT using data from 144 'real life' victims of cardiac arrest, arrived at similar conclusions[20].

Compared to prior expectations that were largely driven by individual case reports, the exceedingly low success rates observed upon PT application to tachycardic patients are possibly a reflection of 'positive result selection bias' associated with many case reports. On the other hand, it is worth noting that PT had an excellent safety profile record (as already anticipated from the majority of non-prospective reports), with no episodes of rhythm deterioration or other adverse events in the catheter laboratory and only one deterioration of VT into pulseless electrical activity in the out-of-hospital setting (in a patient with prolonged cardiac arrest).

Asystole

The use of extracorporally applied mechanical stimulation for asystole deserves special consideration, since asystole may develop in several completely different situations. These can be split roughly into: (1) terminal agonal rhythm, when cardiac arrest (mainly from VF) is not promptly treated with chest compressions, reflecting late electrophysiological changes after prolonged collapse; and (2) complete atrio-ventricular (AV) block, as a result of conduction disturbances, which in the absence of adequate escape foci determines ventricular standstill. While the first type of asystole is, almost by definition, non-witnessed (i.e. it is not an acute event detected be first-aiders), the second type can be witnessed, either because of the recurrent nature of AV block (i.e. previous collapse) or because other symptoms may have given rise to attendance by emergency medical service (EMS) personnel before the onset of complete ventricular standstill. Interestingly, this is precisely the context in which PT was initially described by Schott[10].

In line with this reasoning the only prospective study reporting out-of-hospital cardiac arrest victims presenting in asystole observed return of spontaneous circulation after application of PT, but only in EMS-witnessed asystole (Fig. 50.1A)[20]. Of six patients in witnessed asystole who were treated by PT, three were resuscitated with prompt neurological recovery. However, current international resuscitation guidelines do not specifically recommend PT application in the asystolic patient.

In summary, methodologically robust and numerically adequate data on PT efficacy in asystole patients are still lacking. However, the currently available evidence suggests that for *witnessed* onset of asystole, a single PT might be a suitable strategy to successfully restore sinus rhythm. Automated mechanical stimulator technology could overcome concerns about impact timing, location and energy, as well as ethical issues ('hitting a conscious patient'), and – if used as a preventive means (for example during patient evacuation or transport) – reduce the time-delay between onset of an arrhythmia and the attempted mechanical termination.

Special case study: clinical utility of PT in the US versus the UK

As mentioned above, there are marked international differences in the approach to mechanical cardioversion. As it is only since 2000 that the UK and the US have shared a common set of advanced life support (ALS) recommendations (see next section), a questionnaire-based investigation tried to compare PT use and utility in the

US and UK. Particulars of PT application were assessed from verbal descriptions and subsequent biomechanical measurements in a subgroup of participants[41].

Out of 567 healthcare professionals approached (UK: 279, US: 288), 95 replied (UK: 52, US: 43), reporting a total of 1,740 PT applications (UK: 813, US: 927). While non-representative, some of the insight of this study may be of broader interest.

'Speed of delivery' was ranked by 92.5% of the participants as the most important reason for using PT, while 'perceived inefficiency' (60.2%), 'other established procedures' (45.9%) and 'unawareness of technique' (37.8%) precluded more frequent use. Of note, only 54.3% of professionals were taught PT as part of their curriculum, and no established tools for training or assessment were identified.

There was a pronounced difference in opinions on appropriateness of PT application in various dysrhythmias. Tachyarrhythmias were regarded as the key targets for thump-version, where UK participants ranked onset of VF (89.5%) as a prime indication for PT, followed by established VF (54.4%) and VT (35.1%). In the US, VT was the prime target (62.8%), leading over onset of VF (58.1%) and established VF (25.6%). PT in asystole was, in both populations, regarded as a distant fourth, considered appropriate only by 2.9% (US) to 10.4% (UK) of healthcare professionals.

Self-reported success rate was significantly higher among US participants, who stated 'at least temporary cardioversion to NSR' in 27.7% of PT cases, compared to only 13.3% in the UK. Adverse side effects were rare (0.5% of cases; UK: 0.8%, US: 0.2%) and largely of structural nature (broken ribs).

To determine whether PT application mechanics might contribute to the differences observed, pre-impact fist speed was measured in a subgroup of participants. Healthcare professionals in both countries (UK: 22, US: 22) performed three PT-like impacts each on a custom-build thump-o-meter[41]. Biomechanical recordings were then correlated to individual reported success rates in the application of PT. Inter-individual differences in pre-impact fist speed ranged from 0.42–8.14 $m \times s^{-1}$ (Fig. 50.3). Participants with fist speeds of < 2.25 $m \times s^{-1}$ reported successful cardioversion in 18 ± 3% of PT cases, compared to 36 ± 2% for those who performed faster impacts ($p < 0.01$).

The national distribution of pre-impact fist speeds showed a significantly higher average among US participants (UK: 1.55 ± 0.68 $m \times s^{-1}$, US: 4.17 ± 1.68 $m \times s^{-1}$; $p < 0.01$).

Thus, PT success rates, assessed in a small and non-representative selection of healthcare professionals, were more than two times higher in the US, compared to the UK. This may be related to differences in arrhythmia targeted and/or mechanics of PT application (as a minimum severity of impact may be required to achieve optimal mechanical cardioversion rates). The majority of participants regard tachycardias, rather than asystole, as indications for PT, and roughly half of those who use PT have never been formally trained in the procedure. Both the possibility of a minimum energy requirement and the lack of training highlight the need for clear procedural instructions and training aids.

Legislation

History

Formal guidelines for ALS were first issued by the American Heart Association (AHA) in 1974, and have been regularly revised since. The UK Resuscitation Council started publishing ALS guidelines in 1984. Since 2000, the International Liaison Committee on Resuscitation (ILCOR), an association of key international resuscitation organizations, publishes a 'Consensus on Science and Treatment Recommendations' in 5-yearly intervals. This now lays foundation to ALS guidelines worldwide (adopted, among others, by both the AHA and the European Resuscitation Council).

Recommendations

In the 1970s and 1980s, ALS guidelines tended to recommend PT for treatment of asystole, VT and VF. It was felt that – even though success rates of PT differed widely between investigators – the swiftness of delivery and the overall low incidence of negative side-effects warranted regular PT application. This applied, in particular, to the clinical setting, where other treatment modalities (such as electrical defibrillators) are available as back-up (even though with some delay). Out-of-hospital, PT was considered appropriate for any pulseless rhythm disturbance.

Since the 1990s, the utility of PT has been progressively de-emphasized. In 1992, the AHA removed asystole as an indication. In the 2000 ILCOR consensus statement, PT was listed as the first ALS procedure after witnessed or monitored cardiac arrest, and it is highlighted that PT is unlikely to succeed after more than 30 s of cardiac arrest. In the 2005 consensus statement PT is further de-emphasized: it is no longer regarded as an integral part of the general ALS algorithm, although PT is mentioned as a possible intervention (in part III of the statement on 'defibrillation'), stating that *one immediate precordial thump may be considered after a monitored cardiac arrest, if an electrical defibrillator is not immediately available*;[42] see 'Note added in print'.

Procedural instructions

Written descriptions in previous editions of the guidelines and explanatory notes described PT as a sharp impact to the lower half of the sternum, usually delivered from a height of 20–40 cm, using the ulnar edge of the tightly clenched fist (see Fig. 50.4 for one of the rare graphic representations[43]). This might suitably be extended by the suggestion to actively retract the fist after full impact, to emphasize the impulse-like nature of the optimal stimulus.

Of note, the therapeutically efficient PT speeds depicted in Fig. 50.3 were associated with a pre-impact kinetic energy of 2–8 J. These were in most cases close to the maximum impact energy that the individual healthcare professional was able to apply from a pre-impact height of about 20 cm.

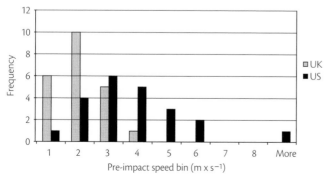

Fig. 50.3 Pre-impact fist speed distribution of PT recordings reveal higher average speeds for US participants (black columns) compared to UK (grey).

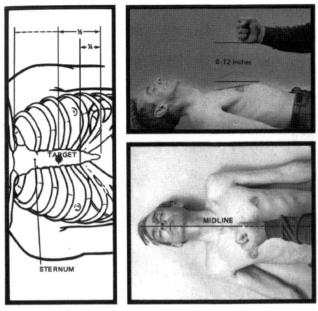

Fig. 50.4 One of the few 'how-to' illustrations on PT application, from the early 1980s. [Reproduced from Huszar RJ (1982) *Emergency Cardiac Care*, 2nd edn. Robert J. Brady Co., Bowie, Maryland.]

Of course it is beyond the scope of this chapter to offer treatment recommendations (instead, the reader is advised to consult the 2010 revision of the ILCOR 'Consensus on Science and Treatment Recommendation'; see 'Note added in print'). With this premise, and taking into account the limitations imposed by the quantity and quality of published reports, the available evidence suggests that PT is not effective in treating VF and of limited use for VT. However, low success rates in reverting ventricular tachyarrhythmias are contrasted by the fact that PT is the fastest resuscitation manoeuvre possible, with a very good safety profile. The effectiveness of extracorporeal mechanical stimulation (PT and/or precordial percussion) appears to be highest in witnessed asystolic arrest, for example secondary to AV conduction block. This indication, as stated in the 2010 ILCOR consensus, poses a target for further research (also because energy levels required for triggering extra beats in quiescent tissue appear to be even lower than those used in thump-version of tachyarrhythmias).

Mechanisms

General considerations

The theory underlying PT, developed in the 1970s, assumes that the mechanical stimulation causes, via MEC, a change in myocardial electrical properties[13,35]. This has been proposed, in particular, to depolarize excitable ventricular tissue. If this depolarization is large enough, it will trigger ectopic excitation in quiescent tissue, obliterating the excitable gap required for re-entrant excitation[12,38].

Experimental findings

Experimental studies have overwhelmingly confirmed that stretch of resting myocardium does indeed cause depolarization (for review see[44] and Chapter 22). If the mechanically induced depolarizations reach the threshold for AP generation (supra-threshold mechanical stimulus), they give rise to ectopic beats in ventricular tissue preparations[45]. In the quiescent heart, rhythmic application of supra-threshold mechanical stimuli can be used to mechanically pace ventricles in isolated perfused hearts[46], mimicking the effects of PT or precordial percussion during asystole in man.

At the cellular levels, mechanically induced depolarizations may be explained by activation of cation non-selective stretch-activated channels (SAC_{NS}), chiefly in ventricular cardiomyocytes[47], but possibly also in electrically connected[48] mechano-sensitive[49] fibroblasts. Most SAC_{NS} have a reversal potential between 0 mV and –15 mV, and their activation is capable of triggering AP in isolated cardiomyocytes[50]. Fittingly, pharmacological inhibition of SAC_{NS} prevents mechanical induction of PVC in asystolic isolated hearts[51].

Another group of SAC is K^+ selective (SAC_K), with a reversal potential near –95 mV[52,53]. These channels will only have a moderate effect on resting cardiomyocytes, whose intrinsic trans-membrane voltage is near the K^+ reversal potential during diastole (for review see[54]).

In contrast to mechanical effects on the asystolic heart, experimental insight into mechanical cardioversion of VT and VF is still scarce. The few studies reporting successful mechanical termination of VT and VF did not quantify mechanical interventions and could not exclude structural tissue damage, which complicates their interpretation[55]. Nonetheless, the *instantaneous* conversion from VT and VF to NSR, observed in patients and experimental models, suggests that stretch-activation of ion channels is likely to play a role here as well. The dynamic interaction of SAC effects with ectopic foci or re-entrant excitation is complex, however, and has not been experimentally elucidated in detail for their potential to terminate tachycardias.

In VT or VF, some cells will be at resting potential levels, and their response to a mechanical stimulus would be similar to that detailed above for diastolic cells. Other cells will be at various stages of the AP, and the effect of a mechanical stimulus will be affected by the difference between the actual trans-membrane potential of a cell and the reversal potential of SAC_{NS} and/or SAC_K. This is a highly dynamic setting, in space and time, whose interpretation benefits from quantitative modelling[54].

Quantitative modelling

Biophysically detailed computer models of the heart have seen an impressive improvement in recent years[56]. It is now possible to represent cardiac anatomy, locally prevailing cell orientation, cell properties, coupling and regional gradients in mechano-electrical factors in simulations of the cardiac electro-mechanical cycle. These quantitative models have started to possess predictive power, and can aid data interpretation and hypothesis formation[54,57].

We have studied the potential anti-arrhythmic effects of a mechanical stimulus in a comparatively simple VT model (figure-of-eight re-entry), using a two-dimensional grid of ventricular cardiomyocytes (Fig. 50.5A). Mechanical impact is simulated via brief (5 ms), impulse-like activation of SAC_{NS} and/or SAC_K (stretch-activated conductance 25 nS).

Mechanical activation of SAC_{NS} (reversal potential –10 mV) reliably terminates re-entry in the ventricular tissue model, exactly via the mechanism proposed three decades ago: depolarization of the tissue forming the excitable gap (Fig. 50.5B).

Addition of increasing amounts of SAC_K to the population of ion channels activated by the mechanical stimulus moves the reversal potential of the 'net stretch-activated current' towards more negative potentials. This reduces the ability to depolarize cells in the excitable gap and shortens AP duration. At an $SAC_{NS}:SAC_K$ ratio of about 1:0.4 [corresponding to a net stretch-activated reversal potential of −35 mV (Fig. 50.5C)], this results in failure to instantaneously terminate VT in the model.

This is of interest in the context of the reported reduction in PT efficacy during pre-existing hypoxia. Hypoxia reduces tissue adenosine triphosphate (ATP) levels and thereby reduces inhibition of ATP-dependent K^+ channel (K_{ATP}). These channels show combined ATP- and mechano-sensitivity in atrial[53] and ventricular[54] cardiomyocytes. As a consequence, ischaemia has been shown to potentiate K_{ATP} channel mechano-sensitivity[60]. Pre-existing hypoxia may therefore 'sensitize' K_{ATP} channels to respond more readily to a mechanical stimulus, thereby potentially rendering PT less effective, or even detrimental. Similar conclusions have been drawn from three-dimensional simulation studies employing an anatomically representative rabbit heart model[61].

These modelling-derived predictions, while in keeping with clinical insight into PT limitations, require thorough experimental validation. They illustrate, though, how clinical motivation, theoretical simulation, and experimental validation may facilitate new insight and targeted research.

Conclusions and outlook

Mechanical stimulation affects cardiac electrophysiology via MEC. Like externally applied electrical current discharges, this may either cause or terminate arrhythmias. A potentially important advantage of mechanical energy delivery for cardioversion is that the necessary electrical currents are 'generated' on-site, i.e. in the heart. The mechanical stimulus is passed on from precordium to cardiac tissue in a relatively direct fashion, without massive 'loss' to other regions of the body (during trans-thoracic defibrillation in humans, only 4% of the applied current actually traverses the heart[62]). PT therefore allows application of much lower energy levels (reducing trauma), and it can be tolerated by the conscious patient.

Insight into mechanisms underlying mechanical cardioversion is still patchy. Given the swift response to mechanical stimulation, it is highly probable that stretch-activation of ion channels plays a role in this process. Quantitative computational modelling suggests that the relative contribution of SAC_{NS} and SAC_K may be a determinant of the success or failure of interventions such as PT. This ratio may be affected by regional differences in myocardial properties, impact characteristics, or disease states such as myocardial ischaemia. Future progress in our understanding of the utility and limitations of mechanical termination of heart rhythm disturbances requires suitable multicellular experimental (and matching computational) models.

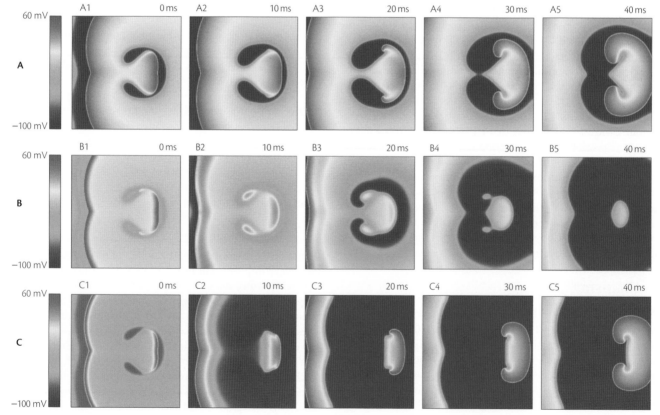

Fig. 50.5 Two-dimensional model (2.5 × 2.5 cm) of ventricular myocardium, consisting of 251 × 251 Noble'98[58] single cell models (trans-membrane voltage is colour coded; for mesh implementation see[59]). **A** Control figure-of-eight re-entry activity. **B** Mechanical stimulation, modelled by activation for 5 ms of SAC_{NS} (reversal potential −10 mV), causes depolarization of tissue in the excitable gap and terminates re-entry. **C** Mechanical stimulation of tissue after simulated ischaemic sensitization of SAC_K to stretch shifts net mechanically induced reversal potential to more negative levels (here −35 mV), which (1) prevents depolarization of resting tissue and (2) shortens action potential duration, rendering mechanical stimulation incapable of instantaneously terminating re-entry. [Figure courtesy of Dr Alan Garny, University of Oxford.] (See color plate section.)

Acknowledgements

We thank Patricia Cooper and Alan Garny from the Oxford Cardiac Mechano-Electric Feedback Laboratory for important contributions to this research and colleagues at the following Hospitals for participation in the fist thump measurements: University of Miami School of Medicine, Florida Hospital Orlando Campus; Royal Brompton Hospital, London; Hammersmith Hospital, London; John Radcliffe Hospital, Oxford. This work is supported by the British Heart Foundation and the UK Medical Research Council.

References

1. Hyman AS. Resuscitation of the stopped heart by intracardiac therapy. *Arch Intern Med* 1930;**46**:553–568.

2. Olasveengen TM, Sunde K, Brunborg C, Thowsen J, Steen PA, Wik L. Intravenous drug administration during out-of-hospital cardiac arrest: a randomized trial. *JAMA*. 2009;**302**:2222–2229.

3. Befeler B. Mechanical stimulation of the heart: its therapeutic value in tachyarrhythmias. *Chest* 1978;**73**:832–838.

4. Lee HT, Cozine K. Incidental conversion to sinus rhythm from atrial fibrillation during external jugular venous catheterization. *J Clin Anesth* 1997;**9**:664–667.

5. Criley JM, Blaufuss AH, Kissel GL. Cough-induced cardiac compression: self-administered from of cardiopulmonary resuscitation. *JAMA* 1976;**236**:1246–1250.

6. Wei JY, Greene HL, Weisfeldt ML. Cough-facilitated conversion of ventricular tachycardia. *Am J Cardiol* 1980;**45**:174–176.

7. Waxman MB, Wald RW, Sharma AD, Huerta F, Cameron DA. Vagal techniques for termination of paroxysmal supraventricular tachycardia. *Am J Cardiol* 1980;**46**:655–664.

8. Ambrosi P, Habib G, Kreitmann B, Faugere G, Metras D. Valsalva manoeuvre for supraventricular tachycardia in transplanted heart recipient [letter]. *Lancet* 1995;**346**:713.

9. Moore EW, Davies MW. A slap on the back. *Anaesthesia* 1999; **54**:308.

10. Schott E. Über Ventrikelstillstand (Adam-Stokes'sche Anfälle) nebst Bemerkungen über andersartige Arrhythmien passagerer Natur. ["On Ventricular Standstill (Adam-Stokes Attacks) together with other Arrhythmias of Temporary Nature."] *Dtsch Arch klin Med* 1920; **131**:211–229.

11. Don Michael TA, Lond MB, Stanford RL. Precordial percussion in cardiac asystole. *Lancet* 1963;**1**:699.

12. Befeler B, Juan M. Termination of ventricular tachycardia by a chest thump over the area of paradoxical pulsation. *Am Heart J* 1977;**94**: 773–775.

13. Lown B, Taylor J. "Thump-version". *N Engl J Med* 1970;**283**: 1223–1224.

14. Conner D, Shander D, Deegan C, Craddock D, Wolf PS, Baum RS. Self-administered chest thump for cardioversion of recurrent ventricular tachycardia. *Chest* 1978;**73**:877.

15. Rozanski JJ. Ventricular tachycardia and the chest thump. *Chest* 1978;**74**:694–695.

16. Eich C, Bleckmann A, Schwarz SK. Percussion pacing – an almost forgotten procedure for haemodynamically unstable bradycardias? A report of three case studies and review of the literature. *Br J Anaesth* 2007;**98**:429–433.

17. Scherf D, Bornemann C. Thumping of the precordium in ventricular standstill. *American Journal of Cardiology* 1960;**5**:30–40.

18. Phillips JH, Burch GE. Management of cardiac arrest. *Am Heart J* 1964;**67**:265–277.

19. Albano A, Di Comite A, Tursi F. La percussione ritmica a pugno chiuso del precordio come primo intervento nella terapia dell'arresto cardiaco. *Minerva Medica* 1967;**58**:2659–2665.

20. Pellis T, Kette F, Lovisa D, *et al.* Utility of pre-cordial thump for treatment of out of hospital cardiac arrest: a prospective study. *Resuscitation* 2009;**80**:17–23.

21. Pennington JE, Taylor J, Lown B. Chest thump for reverting ventricular tachycardia. *N Engl J Med* 1970; **283**:1192–1195.

22. Barrett JS. Chest thumps and the heart beat. *N Engl J Med* 1971;**284**: 392–393.

23. Antonelli D, Barzilay J. Complete atrioventricular block after sublingual isosorbide dinitrate. *Int J Cardiol* 1986;**10**:71–73.

24. Patros RJ, Goren CC. The precordial thump: an adjunct to emergency medicine. *Heart Lung* 1983;**12**:61–64.

25. Brandenburg JT. Successful treatment by a chest blow of cardiac arrest during myocardial infarction. *JAMA* 1959;**170**:1307–1308.

26. Marmor BM, Black MM. Unusual manifestations of severe sick sinus syndrome. *Am Heart J* 1980;**100**:95–98.

27. Caldwell G, Millar G, Quinn E. Simple mechanical methods for cardioversion: Defence of the precordial thump and cough version. *BMJ* 1985;**291**:627–630.

28. Cotol S, Moldovan D, Carasca E. Precordial thump in the treatment of cardiac arrhythmias (electrophysiologic considerations). *Physiologie* 1980;**17**:285–288.

29. Madias C, Maron BJ, Alsheikh-Ali AA, M. R, Estees III NAM, Link MS. Precordial thump for cardiac arrest is effective for asystole but not for ventricular fibrillation. *Heart Rhythm* 2009;**6**:1495-1500.

30. Goldberg E. Mechanical factors and the electrocardiogram. *Am Heart J* 1977;**93**:629–644.

31. Rajagopalan RS, Appu KS, Sultan SK, Jagannadhan TG, Nityanandan K, Sethuraman S. Precordial thump in ventricular tachycardia. *J Assoc Physicians India* 1971;**19**:725–729.

32. Miller J, Tresch D, Horwitz L, Thompson BM, Aprahamian C, Darin JC. The precordial thump. *Ann Emerg Med* 1984;**13**:791–794.

33. Yakaitis RW, Redding JS. Precordial thumping during cardiac resuscitation. *Crit Care Med* 1973;**1**:22–26.

34. Zoll PM, Belgard AH, Weintraub MJ, Frank HA. External mechanical cardiac stimulation. *N Engl J Med* 1976;**294**:1274–1276.

35. Wirtzfeld A, Himmler FC, Forßmann B, *et al.* External mechanical cardiac stimulation - Methods and possible applications. *Z Kardiol* 1979;**68**:583–589.

36. Haman L, Parizek P, Vojacek J. Precordial thump efficacy in termination of induced ventricular arrhythmias. *Resuscitation* 2009;**80**:14–16.

37. Baderman H, Robertson NR. Thumping the precordium. *Lancet* 1965;**2**:1293.

38. Bierfeld JL, Rodriguez-Viera V, Aranda JM, Castellanos A, Jr., Lazzara R, Befeler B. Terminating ventricular fibrillation by chest thump. *Angiology* 1979;**30**:703–707.

39. Haman L, Parizek P, Vojacek J. Precordial thump efficacy in termination of induced ventricular arrhythmias. *Resuscitation* 2008; **80**:14–16.

40. Amir O, Schliamser JE, Nemer S, Arie M. Ineffectiveness of precordial thump for cardioversion of malignant ventricular tachyarrhythmias. *Pacing Clin Electrophysiol* 2007;**30**:153–156.

41. Kohl P, King AM, Boulin C. Anti-arrhythmic effects of acute mechanical stimulation. In: *Cardiac Mechano-Electric Feedback and Arrhythmias: from Pipette to Patient* (eds P Kohl, F Sachs, MR Franz), Philadelphia: Saunders (Elsevier); 2005:304–314.

42. Deakin CD, Nolan JP. European Resuscitation Council guidelines for resuscitation 2005. Section 3. Electrical therapies: automated external defibrillators, defibrillation, cardioversion and pacing. *Resuscitation* 2005;**67** Suppl 1:S25–S37.

43. Huszar RJ (1982) *Emergency Cardiac Care*, 2nd edn. Robert J. Brady Co., Bowie, Maryland.

44. Kohl P, Hunter P, Noble D. Stretch-induced changes in heart rate and rhythm: clinical observations, experiments and mathematical models. *Prog Biophys Mol Biol* 1999;**71**:91–138.

45. Kaufmann R, Theophile U. Automatie-fördernde Dehnungseffekte an Purkinje-Fäden, Papillarmuskeln und Vorhoftrabekeln von Rhesus-Affen. *Pflügers Archiv* 1967;**297**:174–189.

46. Franz MR, Cima R, Wang D, Profitt D, Kurz R. Electrophysiological effects of myocardial stretch and mechanical determinants of stretch-activated arrhythmias. *Circulation* 1992;**86**:968–978.

47. Craelius W, Chen V, el-Sherif N. Stretch activated ion channels in ventricular myocytes. *Biosci Rep* 1988;**8**:407–414.

48. Camelliti P, Green CR, LeGrice I, Kohl P. Fibroblast network in rabbit sinoatrial node: structural and functional identification of homogeneous and heterogeneous cell coupling. *Circ Res* 2004;**94**:828–835.

49. Kohl P, Kamkin AG, Kiseleva IS, Noble D. Mechanosensitive fibroblasts in the sino-atrial node region of rat heart: interaction with cardiomyocytes and possible role. *Exp Physiol* 1994;**79**:943–956.

50. Craelius W. Stretch-activation of rat cardiac myocytes. *Exp Physiol* 1993;**78**:411–423.

51. Hansen DE, Borganelli M, Stacy GP, Jr., Taylor LK. Dose-dependent inhibition of stretch-induced arrhythmias by gadolinium in isolated canine ventricles. Evidence for a unique mode of antiarrhythmic action. *Circ Res* 1991;**69**:820–831.

52. Niu W, Sachs F. Dynamic properties of stretch-activated K$^+$ channels in adult rat atrial myocytes. *Prog Biophys Mol Biol* 2003;**82**:121–135.

53. Van Wagoner DR. Mechanosensitive gating of atrial ATP-sensitive potassium channels. *Circ Res* 1993;**72**:973–983.

54. Kohl P, Bollensdorff C, Garny A. Effects of mechanosensitive ion channels on ventricular electrophysiology: experimental and theoretical models. *Exp Physiol* 2006;**91**:307–321.

55. Kawakami T, Lowbeer C, Valen G, Vaage J. Mechanical conversion of post-ischaemic ventricular fibrillation: Effects on function and myocyte injury in isolated rat hearts. *Scand J Clin Lab Invest* 1999;**59**:9–16.

56. Plank G, Burton RA, Hales P, *et al.* Generation of histo-anatomically representative models of the individual heart: tools and application. *Phil Trans R Soc (Lond) A* 2009;**367**:2257–2292.

57. Kohl P, Nesbitt AD, Cooper PJ, Lei M. Sudden cardiac death by *Commotio cordis*: role of mechano-electric feedback. *Cardiovasc Res* 2001;**50**:280–289.

58. Noble D, Varghese A, Kohl P, Noble P. Improved guinea-pig ventricular cell model incorporating a diadic space, I_{Kr} and I_{Ks}, and length- and tension-dependent processes. *Can J Cardiol* 1998;**14**:123–134.

59. Garny A, Kohl P. Mechanical induction of arrhythmias during ventricular repolarization: modeling cellular mechanisms and their interaction in two dimensions. *Ann N Y Acad Sci* 2004;**1015**:133–143.

60. Van Wagoner DR, Lamorgese M. Ischemia potentiates the mechanosensitive modulation of atrial ATP-sensitive potassium channels. *Ann N Y Acad Sci* 1994;**723**:392–395.

61. Li W, Kohl P, Trayanova N. Myocardial ischemia lowers precordial thump efficacy: an inquiry into mechanisms using three-dimensional simulations. *Heart Rhythm* 2006;**3**:179–186.

62. Lerman BB, Deale OC. Relation between transcardiac and transthoracic current during defibrillation in humans. *Circ Res* 1990;**67**:1420–1426.

63. Sayre MR, Koster RW, Botha M, Cave DM, Cudnik MT, Handley AJ, *et al.* (on behalf of the Adult Basic Life Support Chapter Collaborators). 2010 international consensus on cardiopulmonary resuscitation and emergency cardiovascular care science with treatment recommendations. Part 5: adult basic life support. *Circulation* 2010;**122**:S298–S324.

Note added in print

The latest ILCOR Consensus on Science and Treatment Recommendation[63], published in October 2010, summarise the utility of PT as follows: *"The PT should not be used for unwitnessed out-of-hospital cardiac arrest. The PT may be considered for patients with monitored, unstable ventricular tachycardia if a defibrillator is not immediately available. There is insufficient evidence to recommend for or against the use of the PT for witnessed onset of asystole."*

Termination of arrhythmias by haemodynamic unloading

Peter Taggart and Peter Sutton

Background

Experimental evidence from animal models indicates that increased loading may enhance the inducibility of arrhythmias and unloading may suppress stretch- or loading-induced arrhythmias. However, clinical evidence that reducing the volume within the heart, i.e. reducing stretch, is antiarrhythmic is at present incomplete. Although a number of clinical scenarios incorporating unloading are associated with suppression or termination of arrhythmias, the acquisition of hard evidence for a cause and effect relationship has so far not been possible. These issues are discussed in this chapter.

Haemodynamic unloading should be antiarrhythmic

Two main mechanisms of arrhythmia are re-entry and triggered activity[1]. Re-entry is facilitated by shortening of the refractory period, inhomogeneity of refractoriness and local conduction slowing. Under normal conditions the refractory period is mainly voltage dependent and approximates to the action potential duration (APD). Increased volume loading, or stretch, has been shown to shorten APD and refractoriness in *in vitro* and *in vivo* animal studies and in humans[2–10]. In addition these effects on APD and refractoriness have been shown to be inhomogeneous[4,11,12]. T-wave alternans has also been shown to be modulated by volume loading. In a canine model of volume overload T-wave alternans was induced by incremental pacing. Under conditions of increased load T-wave alternans increased in magnitude and developed at lower heart rates compared to control conditions[13]. However, as pointed out by the authors, extrapolation of volume loading from animal models to humans is not straightforward and this effect needs to be examined in humans, and in particular in humans with myocardial disease.

Physiological levels of stretch appear to exert relatively little, if any, effect on conduction [[4,12,14,15]; but see also Chapter 25]. Increased loading therefore would be expected to influence predominantly two of the three main requirements for re-entrant arrhythmias in a proarrhythmic manner.

Arrhythmias due to triggered activity arise from depolarization occurring either during the repolarization phase of the action potential (AP) as early after-depolpolarizations (EAD) or after AP repolarization is complete as delayed after-depolpolarizations (DAD). If these after-depolarizations reach sufficient amplitude they may trigger an AP and generate a premature ventricular contraction (PVC) or trigger a series of AP and generate a focal tachycardia. Increased ventricular loading, or acute stretch, has been shown to induce depolarizations resembling both EAD and DAD[2,5,8,10,16–18]. There is also evidence that stretch alters APD and refractoriness in the atrium[19–24], including in humans[21,23]. However, the effect in the atrium is less clear than in the ventricle, with some studies reporting a lengthening and some a shortening in response to stretch. On this basis, ventricular or atrial unloading should tend to be protective against focal tachycardias due to triggered activity.

These foregoing theoretical predictions are supported by several studies in different animal models in which arrhythmias were induced during increased stretch or volume loading.

Experimental evidence that haemodynamic unloading is antiarrhythmic

The majority of experimental work has been directed towards the demonstration of arrhythmia induction by increased haemodynamic loading, rather than arrhythmia termination by decreased loading. Evidence that haemodynamic unloading is antiarrhythmic is therefore to a large extent derived by inference rather than by direct proof.

An abrupt increase in ventricular volume in rabbit and canine ventricles during diastole has been shown to induce depolarizations resembling DAD and PVC, and in some instances couplets and non-sustained ventricular tachycardia (VT)[5,17,18]. The probability of inducing PVC by an abrupt stretch was greater in the presence of ventricular dilatation[17]. The likelihood of inducing arrhythmia was shown to depend on both the amount of stretch and rate of increase of the stretch. However, these arrhythmias do not arise from perturbations during the repolarization phase of the AP and so are not strictly within the remit of this chapter. Several studies have shown that acute stretch or volume loading may either result in depolarization during the terminal phase of the AP resembling EAD, or shorten APD and hence refractoriness which, in both cases, may be associated with arrhythmias[5,15,17,25,26] (see Figs 51.1 and 51.2).

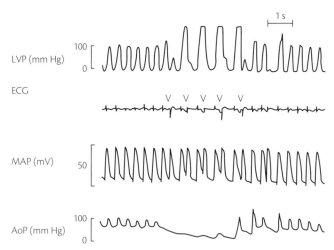

Fig. 51.1 Transient aortic occlusion of *in situ* canine hearts induced after-depolpolarizations and arrhythmia. LVP, left ventricular pressure; ECG, electrocardiogram; MAP, monophasic action potential; AoP, aortic pressure; V, ventricular ectopic beat. [Reproduced, with permission, from Franz MR, Burkhoff D, Yue DT, Sagawa K (1989) Mechanically induced action potential changes and arrhythmia in isolated and in situ canine hearts. *Cardiovasc Res* **23**:213–223.]

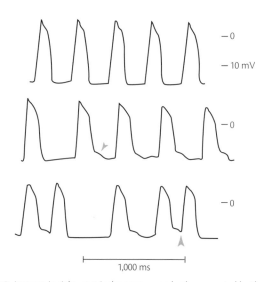

Fig. 51.2 Increase in right ventricular pressure and volume created by the insertion of a balloon catheter into the pulmonary valve orifice prior to dilating the narrowed valve in patients induced deflections during repolarization (slanted arrow). These resembled EAD and were associated with spontaneous ectopic beats (upward arrow). Top panel: Background activity; middle and bottom panel: recordings during balloon inflation. [Reproduced, with permission, from Levine JH, Guarnieri T, Kadish AH, White RI, Calkins H, Khan JS (1988) Changes in myocardial repolarisation in patients undergoing balloon valvuloplasty for congenital pulmonary stenosis: evidence for contraction excitation feedback in humans. *Circulation* **77**:70–77.]

In a study in isolated rabbit hearts the inducibility of arrhythmias was increased substantially when the ventricle was already dilated. The increase in arrhythmia inducibility was accompanied by an increased heterogeneity of refractoriness attributed to the dilatation[4]. In the isolated canine ventricle the probability of arrhythmia initiation by stretch was shown to be increased as a function of the volume of diastolic increments[17] (Fig. 51.3).

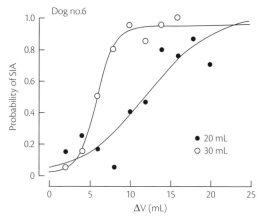

Fig. 51.3 In an isolated canine ventricle preparation the probability of inducing arrhythmia increased as a function of the volume of diastolic increments (filled circles). This effect was enhanced when the baseline volume was increased from 20 to 30 mL (open circles). [Reproduced, with permission, from Lab MJ (1989) Contribution of mechano-electric coupling to ventricular arrhythmias during reduced perfusion. *Int J Microcirc Clin Exp* **8**:433–442.]

Increased loading decreases the ventricular fibrillation (VF) threshold, i.e. facilitates the induction of VF, and decreased loading increases the threshold, i.e. reduces the ease of induction of VF[27].

Similarly increased loading in isolated rabbit hearts has been shown to increase the defibrillation threshold, i.e. to increase the voltage requirement necessary to achieve electrical conversion of VF to regular rhythm[28] (Fig. 51.4; see also Chapter 52). Increased loading in atria increased inducibility of atrial fibrillation (AF) in rabbit hearts[22] and guinea pig[24]. In a Langendorff guinea pig heart model the number of stretch-induced atrial premature beats increased with increased atrial volume loading[24] (Fig. 51.5).

The mechanisms by which changes in loading and stretch influence membrane currents, i.e. mechano-electric transduction, probably involve both non-selective cation stretch-activated channels and calcium transients and are discussed in other chapters.

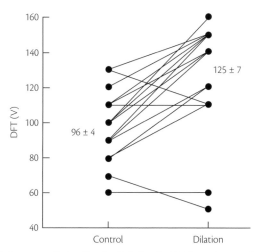

Fig. 51.4 Acute ventricular dilatation in isolated rabbit hearts increased the defibrillation threshold from 96 ± 4 to125 ± 7 V. DFT, defibrillation threshold. [Reproduced, with permission, from Jalal S, Williams GR, Mann DE, Reiter MJ (1992) Effect of ventricular dilatation on fibrillation thresholds in the isolated rabbit heart. *Am J Physiol* **263**:H1306–H1310.]

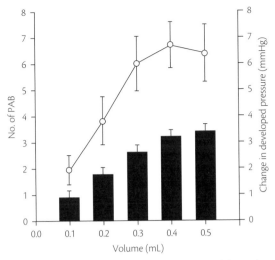

Fig. 51.5 Relationship between left atrial balloon volume and the incidence of stretch-induced premature atrial beats (PAB) in isolated Langendorff guinea pig hearts. The number of atrial premature beats (solid bars) increased with elevated atrial volume loading and atrial pressure (open circles).[Reproduced, with permission, from Klein LS, Miles WM, Zipes DP (1990) Effect of atrioventricular interval during pacing or reciprocating tachycardia on atrial size, pressure and refractory period: contraction–excitation feedback in human atrium. *Circulation* **82**:60–68.]

Gadolinium, which is a non-selective stretch-activated channel, blocker has been shown to block stretch-induced depolarizations and PVC[29] (Fig. 51.6). Both gadolinium and GsMTx-4 (tarantula peptide) have been shown to reduce the susceptibility to the induction of AF by burst pacing in an animal model[30,31]. In Langendorff rabbit hearts with a perforated atrial septum to equalize pressures, the atria were pressure and volume loaded by increasing the pulmonary outflow fluid column. The vulnerability to AF induced by

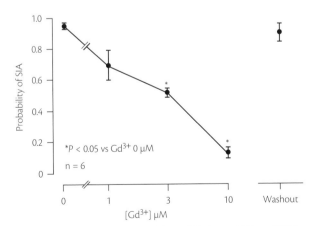

Fig. 51.6 Effect of the stretch-activated channel blocker gadolinium (Gd^{3+}) on ventricular arrhythmia inducibility studied in an isolated canine preparation. The probability of the initiation of stretch-induced arrhythmias was reduced by gadolinium in a dose-dependent manner. After washout of the drug the probability returned to control values. [Reproduced, with permission, from Ou P, Reiter MJ (1997) Effect of ventricular dilation on defibrillation threshold in isolated perfused rabbit heart. *J Cardiovasc Electrophysiol* **8**:1013–1019.]

burst pacing was increased with increasing loading conditions. gadolinium and GsMTx-4 both reduced the vulnerability to AF under increased load. Atrial refractory period shortened with increased load but gadolinium had no effect on refractory period. Both agents appeared to work without suppressing the stretch dependence of the refractory period. A suggestion made by the authors[31] is that K$^+$ selective stretch-activated channels which are resistant to gadolinium and perhaps GsMTx-4 as well act to shorten APD under stretch.

Clinical evidence that haemodynamic unloading is antiarrhythmic

Despite a wealth of experimental evidence for a potential role of mechano-electric coupling (MEC) in the initiation and termination of arrhythmias, evidence that this is the case in humans is remarkably limited. Still, there are several clinical scenarios in which MEC may play a role (see also Chapters 53 and 59 on rhythm effects of cardiac assist devices).

Cardiopulmonary bypass

Many cardiac surgical operations incorporate cardiopulmonary bypass to achieve a bloodless operating field. Deoxygenated blood returning to the heart is diverted through a canula placed in the right atrium to a pump oxygenator, and reoxygenated blood is then returned to the circulation through a canula in the ascending aorta. The circulation thereby bypasses the heart and lungs while maintaining systemic perfusion and coronary flow. During the time the patient is on bypass the heart has reduced volume and is flaccid and non-working. At the end of the surgical procedure the normal circulation is restored and the heart is refilled and takes over the work of maintaining the circulation. Arrhythmias developing at this time may, on occasions, prove difficult to manage. It is well known amongst anaesthetists and cardiac surgeons that reverting to the on-bypass situation, i.e. unloading the heart, may terminate the arrhythmia. A likely explanation for both the development of arrhythmia during discontinuing cardiopulmonary bypass, i.e. loading the heart, and the termination of the arrhythmia on reinstating bypass, i.e. unloading the heart, is MEC. In keeping with this suggestion, it has been shown that the process of discontinuing cardiopulmonary bypass, i.e. restoring ventricular loading, shortens APD[9]. The consequent shortening of refractory periods would be expected to facilitate re-entrant arrhythmias, such as VT and VF. However, proof of a central role of MEC is lacking, and it is clearly not practical to conduct a formal study. Nevertheless, the anecdotal evidence is sufficiently compelling to warrant inclusion as a probable example of termination of arrhythmias by mechanical unloading in this clinical scenario.

Valsalva manoeuvre

The Valsalva manoeuvre is frequently effective in terminating supraventricular and right ventricular outflow tract arrhythmias. To perform the Valsalva manoeuvre the subject takes a deep breath in, occludes the nostrils by pinching the nose, and attempts to exhale hard against a closed glottis for 15 s. During the forced isovolumic expiration 'strain' phase the raised intrathoracic pressure impedes venous return and reduces cardiac filling and cardiac output. Upon release, venous return, cardiac filling and cardiac output increase rapidly. Heart rate increases during the ventricular unloading phase and decreases during ventricular reloading, due to reflex-based enhancement of sympathetic and parasympathetic nerve activity, respectively. In a study on patients undergoing cardiac catheterization, monophasic AP were recorded from the right ventricular septum during the performance of the Valsalva manoeuvre resulting in changes in APD during the strain and release phases[32]. Particular note is that whereas in patients with normal ventricular wall motion the effect on APD was similar between patients and repeatable, in patients with regional wall motion abnormality the changes in APD were markedly heterogeneous. These results were attributed mainly to the effects of heterogeneous stretch and suggest that regional wall motion abnormality may enhance dispersion of repolarization. The Valsalva manoeuvre is also accompanied by changes in autonomic sympathetic and parasympathetic activity, which may have influenced the results. However, it is noteworthy that one of the patients studied had received an orthotopic heart transplant just a few months previously and showed similar changes in APD during the Valsalva manoeuvre. Ambrosi et al.[33] described a case report of an orthotopic heart transplant patient who was able to suppress a supraventricular arrhythmia by the Valsalva manoeuvre, although the possibility of autonomic nerve reinnervation in this patient cannot be excluded. Nanthakumar and colleagues studied patients with a stimulus to T-wave pacemaker-given autonomic blockade (atropine and propranolol) to minimize any autonomic influence[34]. The majority of patients had coronary artery disease. The Valsalva manoeuvre altered the surrogate measure of APD in a manner similar to the patients with heart disease described above[32]. It has been shown in patients with ventricular wall motion abnormality that dispersion of repolarization is sensitive to small changes in volume loading in studies where ventricular load was manipulated by an abrupt alteration in the presence or absence of the atrial component of ventricular filling[35]. Since increased dispersion of repolarization is well known to provide a major substrate for arrhythmogenesis, these observations suggest a mechanistic link for the high incidence of arrhythmias in patients with ventricular wall motion abnormality.

Intra-aortic balloon assist

Several reports have described the benefit of intra-aortic balloon counter pulsation (IABCP) in the control of ventricular arrhythmias after myocardial infarction and for refractory ventricular arrhythmias[36–40]. One study reported 21 patients with ventricular arrhythmias and severe left ventricular impairment. Ten patients had monomorphic VT and 11 had paroxysmal VT and/or VF. The use of the IABCP resulted in termination of the arrhythmia in 14 patients and significant reduction in the frequency of episodes of sustained VT in four patients. The ten patients with incessant monomorphic VT terminated within 30–85 min of commencing IABCP. Nineteen patients were subsequently discharged from hospital. The authors discussed the possible mechanisms. Ventricular unloading with the increase in mean aortic diastolic pressure and the decrease in peak systolic pressure that they observed would be expected to increase coronary blood flow and myocardial oxygen delivery. Ventricular unloading also reduces wall tension and oxygen requirement. These possibilities were considered less likely since patients with normal coronary arteries benefited equally to those with significant coronary artery disease, and reversible ischaemia was seen in one patient only. Another possibility suggested was reduction in adrenergic drive due to improved haemodynamic status and general well-being. However, the very nature of the intervention suggests a possible mechanical explanation such as via MEC. These various alternatives are by no means mutually exclusive. For example, experiments in canines have shown that ventricular ectopy and VT induced by increasing afterload occur more readily in the presence of induced coronary disease[17].

Pharmacological load reduction

Angiotensin-converting enzyme (ACE) inhibitors incorporate load reduction and have been shown to reduce mortality in patients with congestive heart failure[41,42]. However, this is thought to be due to mainly a reduction in overall mortality rather than a decrease in arrhythmic deaths[41], although there is evidence for a reduction in VT in these patients[42].

Conclusions and outlook

There is ample experimental evidence to suggest that ventricular unloading might be an effective antiarrhythmic strategy in humans. For example, MEC has been shown to influence several of the key electrophysiological parameters involved in arrhythmogenesis, such as APD and refractoriness which are key components of re-entrant arrhythmias, as well as inducing depolarizations resembling EAD and DAD which may generate triggered activity. Increased haemodynamic loading not only influences these electrophysiological parameters in a pro-arrhythmic manner but also may induce or facilitate the induction of arrhythmias. A cautionary note, however, is necessary in the interpretation of these experimental findings in that the majority of research work has focused on the effects of increased loading rather than the effects of unloading. Therefore much of the evidence on the effects of unloading is derived by inference rather than direct proof. Evidence that haemodynamic unloading in humans is antiarrhythmic is difficult to acquire due to the multiplicity of variables that accompany load manipulation, the lack of feasibility for clinical trials and the absence of clinically useful blockers of the electrophysiological effects of load alteration. Hopefully in the not too distant future the development of suitable blocking agents will enable the potential of MEC as a therapeutic target to be realized.

References

1. Janse MJ, Wit AL. Electrophysiological mechanisms of ventricular arrhythmias resulting from myocardial ischaemia and infarction. *Physiol Rev* 1989;**69**:1049–1089.
2. Lab MJ. Contraction excitation feedback in myocardium: physiological basis and clinical relevance. *Circ Res* 1982;**50**:757–766.
3. Lerman BB, Burkhoff D, Yue DT, Sagawa K. Mechanoelectrical feedback: independent role of preload and contractility in modulation of canine ventricular excitability. *J Clin Invest* 1985;**76**:1843–1850.
4. Reiter MJ, Synhorst DP, Mann DE. Electrophysiologic effects of acute ventricular dilatation in the isolated rabbit heart. *Circ Res* 1988;**62**:554–562.
5. Franz MR, Burkhoff D, Yue DT, Sagawa K. Mechanically induced action potential changes and arrhythmia in isolated and in situ canine hearts. *Cardiovasc Res* 1989;**22**:213–223.
6. Franz MR, Cima R, Wang D, Profitt D, Kurz R. Electrophysiologic effects of myocardial stretch and mechanical determinants of stretch-activated arrhythmias. *Circulation* 1992;**86**:968–978.

7. Hansen DE. Mechanoelectrical feedback effects of altering preload, afterload, and ventricular shortening. *Am J Physiol* 1993;**264**: H423–H432.

8. Levine JH, Guarnieri T, Kadish AH, White RI, Calkins H, Khan JS. Changes in myocardial repolarisation in patients undergoing balloon valvuloplasty for congenital pulmonary stenosis: evidence for contraction excitation feedback in humans. *Circulation* 1988;**77**:70–77.

9. Taggart P, Sutton PMI, Treasure T, *et al*. Monophasic action potentials at discontinuation of cardiopulmonary bypass: Evidence for contraction-excitation feedback in man. *Circulation* 1988;**77**:1266–1275.

10. Taggart P, Sutton P, Lab M, Runnalls ME, O'Brien W, Treasure T. Effect of abrupt changes in ventricular loading on repolarisation induced by transient aortic occlusion in man. *Am J Physiol* 1992;**636**:H816–H823.

11. Dean JW, Lab MJ. Regional changes in ventricular excitability during load manipulation of the in situ pig heart. *J Physiol* 1990;**429**:387–400.

12. Zabel M, Portnoy S, Franz MR. Effect of sustained load on dispersion of ventricular repolarisation and conduction time in the isolated rabbit heart. *J Cardiovasc Electrophysiol* 1996;**7**:9–16.

13. Narayan SM, Drinan DD, Lackey RP, Edman CF. Acute volume overload elevates T-wave alternans magnitude. *J Appl Physiol* 2007;**102**:1462–1468.

14. Reiter MJ, Zetelakiz, Kirchof CJH, Boersma L, Allessie MA. Interaction of acute ventricular dilatation and d-sotalol during sustained ventricular tachycardia around a fixed obstacle. *Circulation* 1994;**89**:423–431.

15. Reiter MJ, Landers M, Zetelaki Z, Kirchhof CJ, Allessie MA. Electrophysiologic effects of acute dilatation in the isolated rabbit heart: Cycle length-dependent effects on epicardial refractoriness and conduction velocity. *Circulation* 1997;**96**:4050–4056.

16. Lab MJ. Contribution of mechano-electric coupling to ventricular arrhythmias during reduced perfusion. *Int J Microcirc Clin Exp* 1989;**8**:433–442.

17. Hansen DE, Craig CS, Hondeghem LM. Stretch-induced arrhythmias in the isolated canine ventricle: Evidence for the importance of mechanoelactrical feedback. *Circulation* 1990;**81**:1094–1105.

18. Stacy GP, Jobe RL, Taylor LK, Hansen DE. Stretch-induced depolarisations as a trigger of arrhythmias in isolated canine left ventricles. *Am J Physiol* 1992;**263**:H613–H621.

19. Kaseda S, Zipes DP. Contraction-excitation feedback in the atria: A cause of changes in refractoriness. *J Am Coll Cardiol* 1988;**11**: 1327–1336.

20. Solti F, Veesey T, KekesiV, Juhasz-Nagy A. The effect of atrial dilatation on atrial arrhythmias. *Cardiovasc Res* 1989;**23**:882–886.

21. Ravelli F, Disertori M, Cozzi F, Antolini R, Allessie MA. Ventricular beats induce variations in cycle length of rapid (type 11) atrial flutter in humans: Evidence of leading circle reentry. *Circulation* 1994;**89**:2107–2116.

22. Ravelli F, Allessie MA. Effects of atrial dilation on refractory period and vulnerability to atrial fibrillation in the isolated Langendorff-perfused rabbit heart. *Circulation* 1997;**96**:1686–1695.

23. Klein LS, Miles WM, Zipes DP. Effect of atrioventricular interval during pacing or reciprocating tachycardia on atrial size, pressure and refractory period: contraction–excitation feedback in human atrium. *Circulation* 1990;**82**:60–68.

24. Nazir SA, Lab MJ. Mechanoelectric feedback in the atrium of the isolated guinea-pig heart. *Cardiovasc Res* 1996;**32**:112–119.

25. Calkins H, Maughan L, Weisman HF, Sugiura S, Sagawa K, Levine JH. Effects of acute volume load on refractoriness and arrhythmia development in isolated chronically infarcted canine hearts. *Circulation* **1989**;79:687–697.

26. Calkins H, Maughan WL, Kass DA, Sagawa K, Levine JH. Electrophysiological effect of volume load in isolated canine hearts. *Am J Physiol* 1989;**256**:H1697–H1706.

27. Jalal S, Williams GR, Mann DE, Reiter MJ. Effect of ventricular dilatation on fibrillation thresholds in the isolated rabbit heart. *Am J Physiol* 1992;**263**:H1306–H1310.

28. Ou P, Reiter MJ. Effect of ventricular dilation on defibrillation threshold in isolated perfused rabbit heart. *J Cardiovasc Electrophysiol* 1997;**8**:1013–1019.

29. Hansen DE, Borganelli M, Stacey GP, Taylor LK. Dose-dependent inhibition of stretch-induced arrhythmias by gadolinium in isolated canine ventricles: Evidence for a unique mode of antiarrhythmic action. *Circ Res* 1991;**69**:820–831.

30. Bode F, Katchman A, Woolsley RL, Franz MR. Gadolinium decreases stretch induced vulnerability to atrial fibrillation. *Circulation* 2000;**101**:2200–2205.

31. Bode F, Sachs F, Franz MR. Tarantula peptide inhibits atrial fibrillation. *Nature* 2001;**409**:35–36.

32. Taggart P, Sutton P, John R, Lab M, Swanton H. Monophasic action potential recordings during acute changes in ventricular loading induced by the valsalva manoeuvre. *Br Heart J* 1992;**67**:221–229.

33. Ambrosi P, Habib G, Kreitmann B, Faugere G, Metras D. Valsalva manoeuvre for supraventricular tachycardia in transplant heart recipient. *Lancet* 1995;**346**:713.

34. Nanthakumar K, Dorian P, Paquette M, Hutchison S, Andrews J, Newman D. Effect of physiological mechanical perturbations on intact human myocardial repolarization. *Cardiovasc Res* 2000;**45**: 303–309.

35. James PR, Hardman SM, Taggart P. Physiological changes in ventricular filling alter cardiac electrophysiology in patients with abnormal ventricular function. *Heart* 2002;**88**:149–152.

36. Willerson JT, Curry GC, Watson JT, *et al*. Intra-aortic balloon counterpulsation in patients in cardiogenic shock, medically refractory left ventricular failure and/or recurrent ventricular tachycardia. *Am J Med* 1975;**58**:183–191.

37. Hanson EC, Levine FH, Kay HR, *et al*. Control of post infarction ventricular irritability with the intra aortic balloon pump. *Circulation* 1980;**62**:1130–1137.

38. Culliford AY, Madden MR, Isom OW, Glassman E. Intra-aortic balloon counterpulsation: refractory ventricular tachycardia. *JAMA* 1978;**239**:431–432.

39. Fotopoulos GD, Mason MJ, Walker S, *et al*. Stabilisation of medically refractory arrhythmia by intra-aortic balloon counterpulsation. *Heart* 1999;**82**:96–100.

40. Kurose K, Okamoto K, Sato T, *et al*. Successful treatment of life threatening ventricular tachycardia with high dose propranolol under extracorporeal life support and intraaortic balloon pumping. *Jpn Circ J* 1993;**57**:1106–1110.

41. The CONSENSUS Trial Study Group. Effects of enalapril on mortality in severe congestive heart failure. *N Engl J Med* 1987;**316**: 1429–1435.

42. Fletcher RD, Cintron GB, Johnson G, *et al*.; for the V-HeFT 11 VA Cooperative Studies Group: Enalapril decreases prevalence of ventricular tachycardia in patients with chronic congestive heart failure. *Circulation* 1993;**87**:V149–V155.

Mechanical modulation of defibrillation and resuscitation efficacy

Derek J. Dosdall, Harish Doppalapudi and Raymond E. Ideker

Background

Changes in cardiac size and volume may influence the efficacy of defibrillation by altering the current distribution of the shock through the heart, or by changing the electrophysiological properties of the myocardium. The former mechanism involves a change in the electric field produced by the shock without requiring a change in the electrophysiological properties of the myocardium and may be termed 'extrinsic' mechano-electric coupling (MEC), whereas the latter mechanism involves the traditional concept of MEC and may be termed 'intrinsic'. This chapter reviews experimental insight from animal and human studies into the effect of changes in cardiac size and volume on defibrillation, and then discusses the likely mechanisms responsible for these findings. Finally, this chapter discusses some clinical implications of mechanical modulation of defibrillation and resuscitation efficacy.

Evidence

Animal studies

A decrease in the size and volume of the ventricles by cardiac compression or by a decrease in cardiac preload has been shown to improve defibrillation efficacy. Idriss and colleagues[1] showed that delivery of a shock during external cardiac compression decreased the 50% effective dose (ED50) required for ventricular defibrillation by 37% in voltage, 49% in current and 63% in energy in pigs (Fig. 52.1). In this study, cardiac compression was achieved by direct mechanical ventricular compression, and defibrillation was performed using a biphasic waveform shock delivered between a left ventricular (LV) apex patch and a superior *Vena cava* (SVC) catheter electrode. In another study, Strobel and colleagues[2] inflated a balloon catheter in the inferior *vena cava* of pigs to decrease cardiac preload. Although the reduced preload significantly decreased the ED50 of voltage (6%), current (12%) and energy (13%) for defibrillation, this decrease was less than that in

the previous study. A biphasic waveform shock was used for defibrillation, but, in contrast to the first study, the shock was delivered between an endocardial right ventricular (RV) lead and an SVC catheter.

Other studies have shown that defibrillation threshold (DFT) increases with LV dilation and an increase in preload. Using a fluid-filled latex balloon in the LV of isolated Langendorff-perfused rabbit hearts, Ott and Reiter[3] demonstrated a 30% increase in DFT voltage (which would correspond approximately to a 70% increase in DFT energy) with acute LV dilation. They used a monophasic waveform shock between a patch electrode positioned over the posterior LV and a metallic aortic cannula. This study not only increased LV size, but also replaced the highly conductive blood or perfusate in the LV cavity by an insulated balloon, which altered the shock current distribution through the heart. Vigh and colleagues[4] investigated DFT in dogs under three conditions: at baseline, after inducing LV dysfunction with norepinephrine infusion (to achieve an LV ejection fraction < 0.35) and, finally, after volume overload with normal saline (to achieve a pulmonary capillary wedge pressure > 19 mm Hg) in the setting of norepinephrine-induced LV dysfunction. A biphasic waveform was used for defibrillation delivered between a subcutaneous patch and an intravenous RV apex lead. DFT energy was not significantly different between baseline (3.3 ± 2.0 J) and after norepinephrine infusion (4.8 ± 2.2 J), but was nearly double baseline after volume overload in the presence of LV dysfunction (6.4 ± 2.5 J, $p < 0.02$).

Human studies

Brooks and colleagues[5] studied 101 consecutive patients requiring an implantable cardioverter-defibrillator (ICD), of whom 72 underwent successful non-thoracotomy implantation and 29 required thoracotomy for placement of epicardial patches because of a high DFT. A smaller cardiac size on chest radiographs and a smaller echocardiographic LV size in diastole were found to be predictors of successful non-thoracotomy implantation.

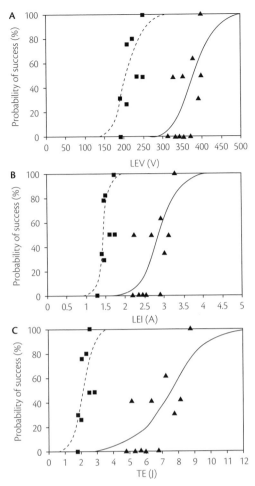

Fig. 52.1 Plots of defibrillation shock strength versus probability of success for (**A**) leading edge voltage (LEV), (**B**) leading edge current (LEI) and (**C**) total energy (TE) for a single pig. In each panel, the fitted curves for the normal heart state (solid line) and the compressed heart state (dashed line) are plotted. For each heart state, the binned raw data points are shown as solid squares for compression and solid triangles for normal control. The data for the normal heart state are positioned to the right of the data for the compressed heart state for each shock parameter. This indicates that shock delivery during cardiac compression improved defibrillation efficacy. [Modified and reproduced, with permission, from Idriss SF, Anstadt MP, Anstadt GL, Ideker RE (1995) The effect of cardiac compression on defibrillation efficacy and the upper limit of vulnerability. *J Cardiovasc Electrophysiol* **6**:368–378.]

Likewise, in a study of 101 patients who underwent placement of a transvenous defibrillation system, Raitt and colleagues[6] reported that radiographic cardiac size and echocardiographic LV end-diastolic diameter showed a significant positive correlation with the DFT ($r = 0.36$, $p < 0.0003$; and $r = 0.40$, $p < 0.0001$, respectively).

In 114 patients undergoing transvenous ICD insertion, Gold *et al.* measured 38 parameters involving demographic, electrocardiographic, echocardiographic and radiographic measurements[7]. Multivariable analysis revealed that LV dilatation (odds ratio = 0.16, $p = 0.003$) and body size (odds ratio = 0.36, $p = 0.005$) were independent predictors of a high DFT (> 20 J). In a subsequent study of 119 patients by the same investigators, LV dilation (odds ratio = 0.47, $p \leq 0.005$), body size (odds ratio = 0.51, $p \leq 0.006$) and

amiodarone use (odds ratio = 5.8, $p \leq 0.002$) were independent predictors of a high DFT (> 20 J)[8].

Mechanisms

To understand how changes in preload can affect defibrillation, the basic mechanism of defibrillation must be understood[9]. To defibrillate, a shock must not only halt the fibrillation wavefronts, but also not create new wavefronts that reinduce fibrillation. A small shock fails to defibrillate because it does not halt all ventricular fibrillation (VF) activation fronts. A stronger shock, still well below the DFT, fails to defibrillate because of re-entry induced by virtual electrodes or by shock-induced prolongation of refractoriness and block. A still stronger shock of near DFT strength may fail to defibrillate because of the induction of several rapidly activating post-shock cycles arising from a focus where the shock field is weak. To defibrillate, a shock must be sufficiently strong that any post-shock ectopic cycles of activation are too few or too slow to induce re-entry that degenerates into VF. Thus, the concept of an initiator and a substrate, as has been previously applied to understanding the initiation of arrhythmias, also applies to defibrillation, with several rapidly activating focal post-shock cycles serving as the initiator, and the region of the myocardium where re-entry later develops serving as the substrate.

The ability of a given shock to defibrillate depends on the potential gradient field generated within the myocardium by the shock. There appears to be a minimum potential gradient that must be created throughout the ventricles by the shock to defibrillate consistently[10]. Alteration in current distribution changes the potential gradient field produced by the shock. For a given potential gradient field that is generated, the electrophysiological properties of the myocardium may determine whether a greater minimum potential gradient is required in the low-gradient areas, and may thus influence the defibrillation efficacy. Changes in preload can influence defibrillation efficacy at both these levels – that is, by alteration of the potential gradient field that is generated by the shock because of alteration in current distribution, and by alteration of the minimum potential gradient field that is required because of changes in the electrophysiological properties of the myocardium.

Extrinsic

The first level involves alteration of the potential gradient field generated in the myocardium by a change in the current distribution because of a variation in ventricular volume or dimensions. Because this mechanism does not involve a direct change in the electrophysiological properties of the myocardium, it may be termed extrinsic.

Compression of the heart decreases the ventricular blood pool by mechanically forcing blood out of the ventricles. For a given shock strength, decreasing the low-impedance ventricular blood pool results in a greater proportion of the shock current being passed through the high-impedance myocardial tissue[11]. This, in turn, increases the potential gradient in the myocardium. In support of this view, the impedance during defibrillation has been shown to increase with cardiac compression[1,2], suggesting that less current is shunted through the blood and more current is passed through the myocardium when the volume of blood within the ventricles is decreased by cardiac compression (see also Chapter 64). In the study by Ott and Reiter[3], however, acute LV dilation increased the impedance. Notably, though, in this study, LV dilation was achieved by an inflated, insulated balloon in the LV cavity that offered more resistance to current flow than free blood would.

Compression also decreases the cross-sectional area of the heart. Decreasing chamber dimensions, and hence the distance between shock electrodes, also decreases the distance from the electrodes to the portion of the ventricles most remote from them. Because the potential gradient field in any portion of the myocardium decreases exponentially with increasing distance from the shock electrodes, decreasing the distance of the myocardial region that is situated farthest from the shock electrodes could result in a significantly greater minimum potential gradient field within the myocardium.

These effects of compression lead to more efficient current distribution, resulting in improvement in defibrillation efficacy[12]. Volume overload of the heart causes the opposite effects and thus decreases defibrillation efficacy. Indeed, as shown in Fig. 52.2, a

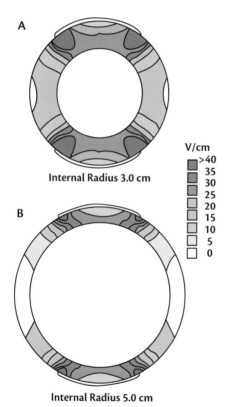

Fig. 52.2 Computer simulation of effect of cardiac dilatation on the electrical potential gradient field produced by a 200 V shock. Each circle represents a cross section of the LV. The defibrillation electrodes are curved discs applied to the top and bottom portions of the heart and have the same surface area in **A** and **B**. The volume of myocardium is the same for both. In **A** the internal radius of the LV is 3.0 cm, while in **B** it is 5.0 cm. The central portion of each panel represents the blood-filled chamber. The conductivity of the myocardium is assumed to be 0.003 S /cm and the conductivity of the blood 0.0065 S /cm. The key depicts the resulting potential gradients, with light regions corresponding to regions of lowest potential gradient and dark representing areas of highest potential gradient. The low gradient area is considerably larger for the dilated heart (**B**). [Reproduced, with permission, from Hillsley RE, Wharton JM, Cates AW, Wolf PD, Ideker RE (1994) Why do some patients have high defibrillation thresholds at defibrillator implantation? Answers from basic research. *Pacing Clin Electrophysiol* **17**: 222–239.]

computer simulation of a defibrillation shock delivered to a ventricle (electrode locations above and below the modelled tissue) with the same volume of myocardium but an increased diameter and cavity size, simulating a dilated ventricle, demonstrates a larger volume of ventricle exposed to a low-potential gradient[12].

Defibrillation during compression also has been shown to decrease the animal-to-animal variation in the ED50 estimate compared with defibrillation without compression[1]. This suggests that geometric differences among animals, either before or after initiation of VF, may account for a proportion of the inter-animal variability in defibrillation requirements. Because static cardiac compression creates a more similar cardiac geometry among animals, the potential gradient field for a given defibrillation lead configuration becomes more similar across animals.

Intrinsic

For a given potential gradient, mechanical changes can influence the defibrillation efficacy by altering the electrical properties of the myocardium. This may be termed intrinsic MEC. The electrophysiological changes, in turn, can be direct, or they may be mediated through the autonomic nervous system (indirect).

Direct

An increase in preload stretches the ventricle. Various studies in isolated tissue, intact hearts, patients and simulations have shown that stretch of the ventricular muscle may decrease conduction velocity, action potential duration (APD) and refractory period, increasing the dispersion of refractoriness, and induce depolarizations[13–17].

Preload alterations can consist of a static, baseline volume overload or of a rapid, dynamic volume change. Similarly, stretch can be acute (caused by a rapid, dynamic volume change) or chronic (caused by a gradually developing, static volume overload). Stretch-induced depolarizations are predominantly caused by acute stretch and are probably mediated through non-selective, stretch-activated ion channels (SAC)[13,18]. SAC activity is increased by oxidative stress, which occurs during prolonged VF[19], and metabolically gated channels (such as the ATP-dependent K+ channel; K_{ATP}) are sensitive to mechanical modulation in atrial[20] and ventricular cells[21]. Changes in APD and refractory period can be caused both by acute stretch, through SAC, and by chronic stretch, possibly through changes in the expression of Ca^{2+} handling proteins[13,18]. Chronic stretch also causes structural remodelling including changes in connexin expression that can increase anisotropy and cause slowing of conduction[16,22,23]. Hypertrophy also increases the risk of stretch-induced arrhythmias[24]. All these changes, caused by acute or chronic stretch, can influence the ability of a shock to defibrillate, either by increasing the likelihood of post-shock activation (initiator) or by altering the substrate for re-entry (substrate).

Effect on substrate

A successful defibrillation shock can be classified as type A if earliest post-shock activation appears more than 130 ms after the shock, or as type B if it appears less than or equal to 130 ms after the shock[25]. For shocks of near DFT strength, unsuccessful shocks have a similar post-shock activation pattern as type B successful shocks of the same shock strength for the first cycle after the shock[25,26]. However, in the former, the rapid cycles of post-shock activation continue until refibrillation occurs through re-entry, whereas in the latter, the ectopic activation cycles terminate, usually in a few cycles in healthy hearts, before re-entry is induced (Fig. 52.3). Thus, altering the substrate may increase DFT by causing a shock to fail because the few rapid post-shock cycles induce re-entry in this altered substrate, whereas they would not have induced re-entry in a healthy heart, so that a type B success would have occurred instead. Ventricular dilation (both acute and chronic) decreases the refractory period and increases the dispersion of refractoriness. Chronic volume overload induces structural changes that increase non-uniform anisotropy and cause slowing of conduction, thus facilitating conduction block. Both these effects may facilitate re-entry and cause a shock to fail that would have been a type B success in a heart with a normal substrate.

Effect on initiator

Acute volume overload (acute stretch) increases the excitability of the myocardium and causes stretch-induced depolarizations[13,18]. Increased baseline ventricular volume increases the sensitivity to acute stretch-induced depolarizations. Based on our previous discussion that shocks of near-DFT strength fail because of induction of rapidly activating post-shock cycles arising from a focus where the shock field is weak, we can conceptualize that volume overload increases the threshold shock field required to prevent the focal post-shock activations, thus increasing the strength of current required for defibrillation.

Trayanova and others developed shock-sensitive models of pressure- or volume-overloaded cardiac tissue including SAC

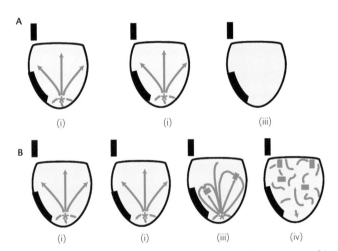

Fig. 52.3 Diagram illustrating the differences in responses following a successful type B shock (**A**) and a failed shock (**B**) delivered from electrodes in the right ventricular apex and the superior *vena cava* during VF (black bars). **A** Successful type B shock. Following the shock, two cycles of activation arise from a region of the ventricles where the shock field is weak (asterisk) and spread over the entire ventricular epicardium (red arrows), as shown in (i) and (ii). After the two cycles, spontaneous activations terminate, leaving the ventricles electrically quiescent, as shown in (iii). An organized recovery rhythm is then established. **B** Failed shock. Three post-shock foci of activation arise from a region where the shock field is weak, as shown in (i), (ii) and (iii). The third activation encounters refractory tissue so that conduction block occurs (red bars), as shown in (iii), setting up re-entry, which ultimately leads to refibrillation (iv). Focal activations act as initiators and the myocardium where conduction block occurs as the substrate in the genesis of refibrillation following a failed shock.

[17,27,28]; see also Chapter 36]. They demonstrated that inclusion of cationic SAC in the model caused a decrease in post-shock conduction velocity and an increase in trans-membrane voltage following repolarization, which facilitated post-shock re-entry and elevated DFT by 31%[17]. When SAC were incorporated into their anatomically realistic model of geometric deformation and fibre architecture, heterogeneous activation of the SAC led to increased dispersion of electrophysiological properties, and created a substrate that facilitated unidirectional block and re-entry[27].

Indirect

Changes in preload can cause baroreceptor-mediated alteration of parasympathetic and sympathetic tone. Changes in autonomic tone have been reported to affect ventricular vulnerability and the VF threshold[29]. Augmented preload has been shown by Lerman and colleagues to decrease ventricular APD and refractoriness through activation of β-adrenergic receptors[30]. This may occur by catecholamine release from intramyocardial nerve endings[30]. These effects were abolished by β-blockers and by catecholamine depletion. A shortening of APD was reported with dobutamine infusion in another study[31]. As discussed previously, a decrease in APD and refractoriness can increase DFT. Epinephrine has been shown by Sousa and colleagues to increase DFT[32]. Thus, augmentation of preload can increase DFT by activating the sympathetic system. However, other studies have shown either a decrease[33,34] or no change[35] in DFT with adrenergic stimulation.

Clinical implications

Heart failure

Heart failure (HF) is a complex pathophysiological condition in which several different factors, including haemodynamic changes, morphological alterations and neurohormonal activation, may influence DFT. Preload changes can explain the failure of internal defibrillation devices in patients with decompensated HF. As discussed previously, ventricular volume has been shown to positively correlate with DFT[5–8]. Canines with rapid pacing-induced heart failure have a larger baseline LV volume than control dogs and tend to have higher DFT[36,37]. More importantly, acute ventricular dilation (e.g. acute haemodynamic decompensation and acute myocardial ischaemia) may result in a significant increase in defibrillation energy requirements. This is because, in addition to the extrinsic effects of increased volume, chronic stretch from baseline elevated ventricular volume increases the sensitivity to acute, stretch-induced, electrophysiological changes[38]. This may result in defibrillation failure in these situations, even if the DFT obtained at the time of implantation was below the programmed or maximum energy delivered by the device.

Volume changes may also have indirect effects on the defibrillation energy requirements in HF. HF usually is associated with cardiac hypertrophy and an increase in LV mass. Chapman and colleagues[39] found a significant positive correlation between LV mass and DFT in humans and dogs. Finite element modelling of pulmonary oedema has shown that increased current flow through the lungs increases DFT[40]. Several studies in animals[2,37,41] and humans[6,42] showed a similar correlation, but other studies did not[3,43–45]. Volume overload (chronic stretch) likely does play a role by affecting expression of connexins that affect hypertrophy, fibrosis and other structural changes in HF[22,23].

Interestingly, several studies found no correlation between ejection fraction and defibrillation efficacy[5,41–43,46], whereas two small studies[6,45] showed a negative correlation. This may be because ejection fraction is a poor surrogate of HF (and of volume overload), or because of the different aetiological factors of HF in different patients.

The DFT in HF may be affected by LV dilation[3,7,8], hypertrophy[47], wall thinning[41] and other chronic structural alterations. Although most of these changes tend to increase DFT, some changes (particularly wall thinning) tend to decrease it[41]. Hence, it is difficult to predict DFT in HF. In a canine model of rapid pacing-induced HF, Lucy and colleagues[37] showed a fourfold increase in DFT energy compared with control subjects, which was significantly correlated with ventricular weight (the ventricular weight being significantly greater in the rapidly paced group). Even when expressed as DFT per gram of ventricular tissue, the authors found a significant increase in DFT in the rapidly paced group compared with control subjects, thus suggesting that both myocardial hypertrophy and LV dysfunction independently affect DFT. They used two sequential monophasic shocks for defibrillation, with the first shock delivered between an anterior RV mesh electrode and a mesh electrode on the left lateral free wall, and the second shock delivered between a posterior RV mesh electrode and the left lateral free wall mesh electrode. Likewise, Huang and colleagues[36] showed that HF, induced by rapid pacing, increased DFT energy by 180% in dogs when a biphasic defibrillation waveform was delivered between an RV apical electrode and an SVC electrode. They also showed that an auxiliary shock to the LV through an electrode in the great cardiac vein decreased DFT in HF. However, in a similar dog model, Friedman and colleagues[41] found no difference in the ED50 or DFT between failing and non-failing hearts when a biphasic waveform was delivered between a rectangular cutaneous patch on the left lateral chest wall and an endovenous RV coil. In their study, rapid pacing produced no change in LV mass. However, it induced ventricular cavity dilation and wall thinning, which may have had opposing effects on defibrillation energy requirements, resulting in no net change in the ED50 in HF.

Prolonged VF

Blood is pooled in the venous circulation during VF, so that the right heart becomes progressively distended and the left heart progressively empty over about 3 min of VF[48,49]. Some studies report that defibrillation energy requirements increase with time during VF, whereas other studies report no change in DFT[1]. Interestingly, those studies showing no change in DFT over time used subcutaneous or epicardial patches combined with an endocardial electrode. In the former studies, the increase in DFT may be attributed to increased shunting of current from the endocardial electrode through the increased blood pool of the RV cavity.

Electrophysiological effects of chest compressions during resuscitation

Osorio *et al.* demonstrated that chest compressions can electrically stimulate the heart and induce refibrillation in pigs after defibrillation following approximately 3 min of VF[50], possibly by a mechanism similar to that which causes *Commotio cordis*[51–53]. In 11 pigs, chest compressions were required in 46 episodes to achieve return of spontaneous circulation. In 12 of these episodes, refibrillation occurred due to a long–short sequence of activation within 2 s of initiating chest compressions (Fig. 52.4). The first chest compression caused an activation, and then an escape beat often followed 700–900 ms later. The second chest compression was delivered 1 s after the first, which stimulated a second activation superimposed on the T-wave of the escape beat. This often led to immediate refibrillation. Chest compressions following defibrillation have been associated with early recurrence of VF[54]. Cardiac excitation by mechanical chest compressions during resuscitation has also been demonstrated in humans[55]. Computational modelling suggests that this kind of mechanically induced refibrillation may be linked to an increased contribution of metabolically activated mechano-sensitive K_{ATP} channels[21,56]. This would be expected to become more prominent with increased duration of the preceding cardiac arrest period. Another study tested DFT in six pigs at various times during cardiac compression[57]. Shocks were

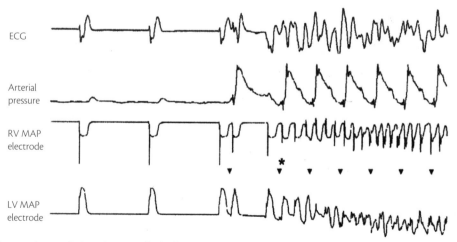

Fig. 52.4 Chest compressions causing ventricular activation and refibrillation. Following approximately 2.5 min of VF, successful defibrillation was followed by pulseless electrical activity. Chest compressions (marked with triangles) were delivered. Ventricular capture is seen for the first two compressions with an interposed spontaneous depolarization associated with long and short intervals that is immediately followed by VF (asterisk). On the horizontal axis, 8 s of data are shown. LV, left ventricle; RV, right ventricle; MAP, monophasic action potential. [Reproduced, with permission, from Osorio J, Dosdall DJ, Robichaux RP Jr, Tabereaux PB, Ideker RE (2008) In a swine model, chest compressions cause ventricular capture, and by means of a long-short sequence, ventricular fibrillation. *Circ Arrhythmia Electrophysiol* **1**:282–289.]

delivered (1) at the beginning of compression, (2) at the end of compression, (3) at the beginning of decompression, (4) at the end of decompression, (5) randomly throughout chest compressions or (6) following a 2–3 s pause in chest compressions. The DFT was significantly higher when shocks were delivered at the beginning of chest compressions, but none of the other groups showed significant differences. A separate study conducted in pigs determined that the DFT was significantly lower when shocks were delivered during the upstroke of the chest compressions.[58] A combination of extrinsic effects (modified current paths due to compression of the heart) and direct intrinsic effects (stretch activation during the vulnerable period) may have been responsible for the observed changes in DFT.

Conclusions and outlook

Cardiac volume changes affect the efficacy of defibrillation by altering the current distribution (extrinsic MEC) or by changing the electrophysiological properties of the myocardium (intrinsic MEC), or both. Cardiac compression and a decrease in preload decrease DFT, whereas cardiac dilation and an increase in preload increase DFT. Although patients with heart failure have a larger baseline ventricular volume than the normal level, which tends to increase DFT, the baseline DFT is difficult to predict because hypertrophy, wall thinning and other chronic alterations also affect DFT in HF. Clinical situations causing an increase in ventricular volume, such as acute haemodynamic compensation in patients with heart failure and prolonged VF, tend to increase DFT. Cardiac compression during resuscitation may stimulate the heart and initiate VF.

Additional work is needed to determine whether there are pharmacological interventions that may reverse the effects of chronic and acute stretch on defibrillation efficacy. This may be important for patients prone to arrhythmias with abnormally high DFT, such as those with HF. Further work is also needed to determine the effects of stretch activation during chest compressions and the incidence of refibrillation due to chest compressions.

Acknowledgments

This chapter was supported in part by National Institutes of Health grants HL085370 and HL091138.

References

1. Idriss SF, Anstadt MP, Anstadt GL, Ideker RE. The effect of cardiac compression on defibrillation efficacy and the upper limit of vulnerability. *J Cardiovasc Electrophysiol* 1995;**6**:368–378.

2. Strobel JS, Kay GN, Walcott GP, Smith WM, Ideker RE. Defibrillation efficacy with endocardial electrodes is influenced by reductions in cardiac preload. *J Interv Card Electrophysiol* 1997;**1**:95–102.

3. Ott P, Reiter MJ. Effect of ventricular dilatation on defibrillation threshold in the isolated perfused rabbit heart. *J Cardiovasc Electrophysiol* 1997;**8**:1013–1019.

4. Vigh AG, Lowder J, Deantonio HJ. Does acute volume overloading in the setting of left ventricular dysfunction and pulmonary hypertension affect the defibrillation threshold? *Pacing Clin Electrophysiol* 1999;**22**:759–764.

5. Brooks R, Garan H, Torchiana D, *et al*. Determinants of successful nonthoracotomy cardioverter-defibrillator implantation: experience in 101 patients using two different lead systems. *J Am Coll Cardiol* 1993;**22**:1835–1842.

6. Raitt MH, Johnson G, Dolack GL, Poole JE, Kudenchuk PJ, Bardy GH. Clinical predictors of the defibrillation threshold with the unipolar implantable defibrillation system. *J Am Coll Cardiol* 1995;**25**:1576–1583.

7. Gold MR, Khalighi K, Kavesh NG, Daly B, Peters RW, Shorofsky SR. Clinical predictors of transvenous biphasic defibrillation thresholds. *Am J Cardiol* 1997;**79**:1623–1627.

8. Khalighi K, Daly B, Leino EV, *et al*. Clinical predictors of transvenous defibrillation energy requirements. *Am J Cardiol* 1997;**79**:150–153.

9. Dosdall DJ, Fast V, Ideker RE. Mechanisms of defibrillation. In: Cardiac electrophysiology: from cell to bedside. (eds Zipes DP, Jalife J) 5th ed. Philadelphia: Saunders; 2009.

10. Wharton JM, Wolf PD, Smith WM, *et al*. Cardiac potential and potential gradient fields generated by single, combined, and sequential shocks during ventricular defibrillation. *Circulation* 1992;**85**:1510–1523.

11. Sepulveda NG, Wikswo JP, Jr., Echt DS. Finite element analysis of cardiac defibrillation current distributions. *IEEE Trans Biomed Eng* 1990;**37**:354–365.

12. Hillsley RE, Wharton JM, Cates AW, Wolf PD, Ideker RE. Why do some patients have high defibrillation thresholds at defibrillator implantation? Answers from basic research. *Pacing Clin Electrophysiol* 1994;**17**:222–239.

13. Ravens U. Mechano-electric feedback and arrhythmias. *Prog Biophys Mol Biol* 2003;**82**:255–266.

14. Taggart P, Sutton PM. Cardiac mechano-electric feedback in man: clinical relevance. *Prog Biophys Mol Biol* 1999;**71**:139–154.

15. Riemer TL, Sobie EA, Tung L. Stretch-induced changes in arrhythmogenesis and excitability in experimentally based heart cell models. *Am J Physiol* 1998;**275**:H431–H442.

16. Taggart P, Lab M. Cardiac mechano-electric feedback and electrical restitution in humans. *Prog Biophys Mol Biol* 2008;**97**:452–460.

17. Trayanova N, Li W, Eason J, Kohl P. Effect of stretch-activated channels on defibrillation efficacy. *Heart Rhythm* 2004;**1**:67–77.

18. Janse MJ, Coronel R, Wilms-Schopman FJ, de Groot JR. Mechanical effects on arrhythmogenesis: from pipette to patient. *Prog Biophys Mol Biol* 2003;**82**:187–195.

19. Wang Y, Joyner RW, Wagner MB, Cheng J, Lai D, Crawford BH. Stretch-activated channel activation promotes early afterdepolarizations in rat ventricular myocytes under oxidative stress. *Am J Physiol* 2009;**296**:H1227–H1235.

20. Van Wagoner DR. Mechanosensitive gating of atrial ATP-sensitive potassium channels. *Circ Res* 1993;**72**:973–983.

21. Kohl P, Bollensdorff C, Garny A. Effects of mechanosensitive ion channels on ventricular electrophysiology: experimental and theoretical models. *Exp Physiol* 2006;**91**:307–321.

22. Kanno S, Saffitz JE. The role of myocardial gap junctions in electrical conduction and arrhythmogenesis. *Cardiovasc Pathol* 2001;**10**:169–177.

23. Severs NJ. Gap junction remodeling in heart failure. *J Card Fail* 2002;**8**:S293–S299.

24. Kamkin A, Kiseleva I, Isenberg G. Stretch-activated currents in ventricular myocytes: amplitude and arrhythmogenic effects increase with hypertrophy. *Cardiovasc Res* 2000;**48**:409–420.

25. Chen PS, Shibata N, Dixon EG, *et al*. Activation during ventricular defibrillation in open-chest dogs. Evidence of complete cessation and regeneration of ventricular fibrillation after unsuccessful shocks. *J Clin Invest* 1986;**77**:810–823.

26. Chattipakorn N, Fotuhi PC, Chattipakorn SC, Ideker RE. Three-dimensional mapping of earliest activation after near-threshold ventricular defibrillation shocks. *J Cardiovasc Electrophysiol* 2003;**14**:65–69.

27. Li W, Gurev V, McCulloch AD, Trayanova NA. The role of mechanoelectric feedback in vulnerability to electric shock. *Prog Biophys Mol Biol* 2008;**97**:461–478.

28. Gurev V, Maleckar MM, Trayanova NA. Cardiac defibrillation and the role of mechanoelectric feedback in postshock arrhythmogenesis. *Ann N Y Acad Sci* 2006;**1080**:320–333.

29. Ng GA, Brack KE, Patel VH, Coote JH. Autonomic modulation of electrical restitution, alternans and ventricular fibrillation initiation in the isolated heart. *Cardiovasc Res* 2007;**73**:750–760.

30. Lerman BB, Engelstein ED, Burkhoff D. Mechanoelectrical feedback: role of beta-adrenergic receptor activation in mediating load-dependent shortening of ventricular action potential and refractoriness. *Circulation* 2001;**104**:486–490.

31. Horner SM, Murphy CF, Coen B, Dick DJ, Lab MJ. Sympathomimetic modulation of load-dependent changes in the action potential duration in the in situ porcine heart. *Cardiovasc Res* 1996;**32**:148–157.

32. Sousa J, Kou W, Calkins H, Rosenheck S, Kadish A, Morady F. Effect of epinephrine on the efficacy of the internal cardioverter-defibrillator. *Am J Cardiol* 1992;**69**:509–512.

33. Ruffy R, Schechtman K, Monje E. Beta-adrenergic modulation of direct defibrillation energy in anesthetized dog heart. *Am J Physiol* 1985;**248**:H674–H677.

34. Ruffy R, Schechtman K, Monje E, Sandza J. Adrenergically mediated variations in the energy required to defibrillate the heart: observations in closed-chest, nonanesthetized dogs. *Circulation* 1986;**73**:374–380.

35. Kalus JS, White CM, Caron MF, Guertin D, McBride BF, Kluger J. The impact of catecholamines on defibrillation threshold in patients with implanted cardioverter defibrillators. *Pacing Clin Electrophysiol* 2005;**28**:1147–1156.

36. Huang J, Rogers JM, Killingsworth CR, *et al.* Improvement of defibrillation efficacy and quantification of activation patterns during ventricular fibrillation in a canine heart failure model. *Circulation* 2001;**103**:1473–1478.

37. Lucy SD, Jones DL, Klein GJ. Pronounced increase in defibrillation threshold associated with pacing-induced cardiomyopathy in the dog. *Am Heart J* 1994;**127**:366–376.

38. Hansen DE, Craig CS, Hondeghem LM. Stretch-induced arrhythmias in the isolated canine ventricle. Evidence for the importance of mechanoelectrical feedback. *Circulation* 1990;**81**:1094–1105.

39. Chapman PD, Sagar KB, Wetherbee JN, Troup PJ. Relationship of left ventricular mass to defibrillation threshold for the implantable defibrillator: a combined clinical and animal study. *Am Heart J* 1987;**114**:274–278.

40. Yang F, Patterson RP. Effect of cardiogenic pulmonary edema on defibrillation efficacy. *Int J Cardiol* 2010;**114**:76–79.

41. Friedman PA, Foley DA, Christian TF, Stanton MS. Stability of the defibrillation probability curve with the development of ventricular dysfunction in the canine rapid paced model. *Pacing Clin Electrophysiol* 1998;**21**:339–351.

42. Kopp DE, Blakeman BP, Kall JG, Olshansky B, Kinder CA, Wilber DJ. Predictors of defibrillation energy requirements with nonepicardial lead systems. *Pacing Clin Electrophysiol* 1995;**18**:253–260.

43. Engelstein ED, Hahn RT, Stein KM, Lerman BB. Noninvasive predictors of successful implantation of transvenous defibrillator lead systems. *J Am Coll Cardiol* 1995;**25**:110A–111A.

44. Haberman RJ, Mower MM, Veltri EP. LV mass and defibrillation threshold. *Am Heart J* 1988;**115**:1340–1341.

45. O'Donoghue S, Platia EV, Mispireta L, Goldstein S, Waclawski S. Relationships between left ventricular mass and ejection fraction, and defibrillation threshold. *J Am Coll Cardiol* 1990;**15**:51A.

46. Strickberger SA, Brownstein SL, Wilkoff BL, Zinner AJ. Clinical predictors of defibrillation energy requirements in patients treated with a nonthoracotomy defibrillator system. The ResQ Investigators. *Am Heart J* 1996;**131**:257–260.

47. Almquist AK, Montgomery JV, Haas TS, Maron BJ. Cardioverter-defibrillator implantation in high-risk patients with hypertrophic cardiomyopathy. *Heart Rhythm* 2005;**2**:814–819.

48. Steen S, Liao Q, Pierre L, Paskevicius A, Sjoberg T. The critical importance of minimal delay between chest compressions and subsequent defibrillation: a haemodynamic explanation. *Resuscitation* 2003;**58**:249–258.

49. Mashiro I, Cohn JN, Heckel R, Nelson RR, Franciosa JA. Left and right ventricular dimensions during ventricular fibrillation in the dog. *Am J Physiol* 1978;**235**:H231–H236.

50. Osorio J, Dosdall DJ, Robichaux R.P Jr., Tabereaux PB, Ideker RE. In a swine model, chest compressions cause ventricular capture, and by means of a long-short sequence, ventricular fibrillation. *Circ Arrhythmia Electrophysiol* 2008;**1**:282–289.

51. Link MS, Estes NA, 3rd. Mechanically induced ventricular fibrillation (*Commotio cordis*). *Heart Rhythm* 2007;**4**:529–532.

52. Madias C, Maron BJ, Weinstock J, Estes NA, 3rd, Link MS. *Commotio cordis*–sudden cardiac death with chest wall impact. *J Cardiovasc Electrophysiol* 2007;**18**:115–122.

53. Kohl P, Nesbitt AD, Cooper PJ, Lei M. Sudden cardiac death by *Commotio cordis*: role of mechano-electric feedback. *Cardiovasc Res* 2001;**50**:280–289.

54. Berdowski J, Tijssen JG, Koster RW. Chest compressions cause recurrence of ventricular fibrillation after the first successful conversion by defibrillation in out-of-hospital cardiac arrest. *Circ Arrhythm Electrophysiol* 2010;**3**:72–78.

55. Osorio J, Dosdall DJ, Tabereaux P, *et al.* Mechanoelectrical coupling during cardiopulmonary resuscitation: chest compressions can cause ventriular activation in humans (abstract). *Heart Rhythm* 2009;**6**:S465.

56. Li W, Kohl P, Trayanova N. Myocardial ischemia lowers precordial thump efficacy: an inquiry into mechanisms using three-dimensional simulations. *Heart Rhythm* 2006;**3**:179–186.

57. Walcott GP, Melnick SB, Banville I, Chapman FW, Killingsworth CK, Ideker RE. Pauses for defibrillation not necessary during mechanical chest compressions during pre-hospital cardiac arrest (abstract). *Circulation* 2007;**116**:II_386.

58. Li Y, Wang H, Cho JH, *et al.* Defibrillation delivered during the upstroke phase of manual chest compression improves shock success. *Crit Care Med* 2010;**38**:910–915.

Anti- and proarrhythmic effects of cardiac assist device implantation

Paul J. Joudrey, Roger J. Hajjar and Fadi G. Akar

Background

Less than 2,500 donor hearts are available yearly for the over 100,000 Americans with advanced heart failure (HF) who would benefit from transplantation[1]. This extreme mismatch between supply and demand has mandated the development of alternative strategies for the acute management of high risk patients with end-stage HF. The surgically implanted left ventricular (LV) assist device (LVAD) was originally created to provide short-term mechanical circulatory support to the failing heart until a suitable donor organ became available. The LVAD, which actively unloads the decompensated failing ventricle through a cannula inserted through the LV apex, efficiently routes blood in a controlled manner to the aorta by an electrically driven pump. Although early LVAD use was severely hampered by inflammatory complications and high device failure rates, second generation LVAD have, to a large extent, circumvented these limitations, improving 1-year survival rates among patients from ~55 to 75%[2]. Indeed, these marked improvements in survival have fundamentally transformed the role of the LVAD, from a primitive device used merely as a temporary bridge to organ transplantation, to a more sophisticated device that can act as a destination therapy for HF patients[2,3]. With the widespread expansion of LVAD use, however, previously unrecognized benefits and complications associated with short- and long-term LVAD therapy are becoming increasingly recognized. In this chapter, we discuss pro- and antiarrhythmic effects associated with LVAD use in end-stage HF. We provide an overview of potential mechanisms by which LVAD-mediated alterations in cardiac loading and stretch may alter the electrophysiological substrate of the failing heart in multiple ways that can promote the incidence of arrhythmias in the short term, while offering long-term antiarrhythmic benefits.

Incidence of ventricular arrhythmias in LVAD patients

One of the major consequences of LVAD-mediated unloading of the failing ventricle is the incidence of arrhythmic events.

The prevalence and nature of ventricular arrhythmias in LVAD patients have been investigated in recent years. Specifically, Refaat et al. examined the occurrence of ventricular arrhythmias and the risk factors that gave rise to them in 42 LVAD recipients over a 2-year period[4]. While 35% of LVAD patients exhibited ventricular arrhythmias, the vast majority of rhythm disturbances occurred very early (within 25 days) following device implantation. Interestingly, these arrhythmias appeared to be mechanistically dependent on LVAD use, since pre-LVAD arrhythmic events were not a significant predictor of post-LVAD arrhythmias in the same patients[4]. This highlights the notion that acute mechanical unloading by LVAD therapy, and consequent alterations in ventricular stretch, may form a unique mechano-electrical coupling mechanism that underlies complex remodelling and arrhythmias in these patients.

In another study, Bedi et al.[5] retrospectively investigated the incidence of pre- and post-LVAD arrhythmias in 116 patients over a 14-year period (1987–2001). About 22% of patients developed ventricular arrhythmias after LVAD implantation, and those patients had a higher mortality rate than their arrhythmia-free counterparts. Although the mean duration of LVAD support in these patients was 14 weeks, over 50% of arrhythmic events occurred during the first 7 days after surgery. These events, which were unrelated to the relatively rare surgical complications associated with the LVAD implantation procedure, were likely caused by the acute activation of a mechano-sensitive signalling cascade and the opening of non-selective stretch-activated ion channels (Fig. 53.1). Importantly, the subset of patients exhibiting early onset ventricular arrhythmias following LVAD use was at higher risk for sudden death than patients who developed late-onset arrhythmias[5]. Again, the clear predominance of arrhythmias following LVAD support suggests an active role for acute ventricular unloading and associated changes in ventricular stretch levels in the genesis of arrhythmic triggers. These findings also suggest a potential role for chronic LVAD-mediated enhancement of cardiac function in the suppression of ventricular arrhythmias in the long term. Finally, while arrhythmic events were observed in patients with HF caused by ischaemic and non-ischaemic aetiologies,

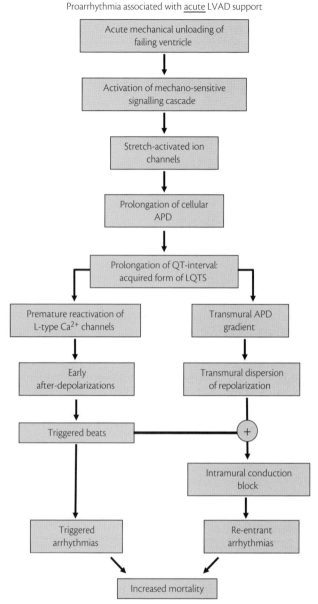

Fig. 53.1 Schematic illustration of signalling cascade associated with increased arrhythmic risk following acute LVAD support of the failing ventricle.

sustained ventricular arrhythmias were more common in the ischaemic cardiomyopathy group[5]. These clinical findings underscored the importance of investigating the potential pathophysiological effects of LVAD therapy on electrical remodelling in an aetiology-specific manner.

Electrophysiological alterations during mechanical support of the failing ventricle

As mentioned above, abrupt mechanical unloading of the failing ventricles by LVAD may increase short-term abnormalities in electrophysiological properties that lead to the incidence of malignant arrhythmias. In sharp contrast, long-term improvement of cardiac function by LVAD use is thought to suppress the incidence of

arrhythmias, potentially by causing a complex programme of reverse remodelling that counters, at least in part, some of the key pathophysiological alterations associated with LV dysfunction in HF (Fig. 53.2).

To better understand the mechanisms by which LVAD-mediated changes in mechanical load of the failing ventricle can predispose to or prevent arrhythmias, it is important to first consider the major electrophysiological abnormalities that are associated with HF, independent of LVAD use. Cells and tissues isolated from hypertrophied and failing hearts are electrophysiologically distinguished by a prolonged action potential (AP) duration (APD), reflecting delayed terminal repolarization of cardiac myocytes. This fundamental change in myocyte biology underlies QT-interval prolongation of the surface electrocardiogram (ECG) in patients with HF. Underlying these changes in repolarization properties of the failing heart are fundamental alterations in key ion channels and Ca^{2+} cycling proteins (Fig. 53.2).

Akar and Rosenbaum investigated the nature of APD prolongation in HF and its mechanistic relationship to arrhythmias in a canine model of LV dysfunction caused by rapid pacing[6]. Specifically, they found that APD prolongation in HF was heterogeneous across the ventricular wall, giving rise to a twofold enhancement in transmural repolarization heterogeneity. They also found that differential sensitivity of mid-myocardial cells to HF-related electrical remodelling increased transmural dispersion of repolarization across the failing ventricle. This created an electrophysiological substrate that was amenable to intramural conduction block and the genesis of transmural re-entrant circuits. Rapid activation circuits supported the early maintenance of polymorphic ventricular tachyarrhythmias. Other studies have also demonstrated a proarrhythmic tendency of class III antiarrhythmic agents because of their excessive APD and QT-prolonging effects specifically in the setting of reduced repolarization reserve, which is a hallmark of the failing heart[7]. These findings strongly suggest that therapeutic interventions known to further delay the already prolonged repolarization of the failing heart (such as acute LVAD use; see below) may be highly proarrhythmic.

Acute and chronic effects of LVAD therapy on global cardiac repolarization have been characterized in two consecutive studies by Harding et al.[7,8]. They investigated the effects of mechanical unloading of the ventricle on the electrophysiological properties of LVAD patients with and without ventricular arrhythmias. The first study addressed the effects of acute mechanical unloading by comparing LVAD patients with those who underwent cardiac surgery without mechanical support. The retrospective analysis of 12-lead ECG recordings taken shortly before, immediately following and more than 1 week after surgery revealed dynamic changes in global repolarization of LVAD-treated patients that were not present in patients undergoing cardiac surgery without LVAD support. Specifically, an immediate prolongation of the QT interval upon LVAD implantation was followed by a gradual decease after 1 week of LVAD therapy. The decrease in QT interval in response to extended LVAD support had a cellular basis as it coincided with an observed decrease in APD in isolated myocytes from LVAD patients[8]. In the second study, changes in 12-lead ECG recordings were monitored in 17 consecutive patients receiving LVAD support. ECG measurements were acquired 4 days prior to surgery, less than 12 h after surgery and weekly thereafter. Among these patients, 59% developed ventricular arrhythmias. QT interval

Reverse remodelling cascade associated with <u>chronic</u> LVAD support

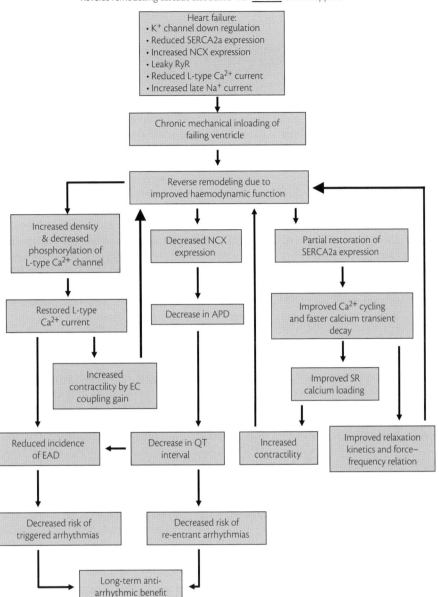

Fig. 53.2 Schematic illustration of the signalling cascade associated with reverse remodelling and protection against arrhythmias following term LVAD therapy.

changes during the first day after surgery were the only variable that significantly correlated with arrhythmic events[9].

These clinical investigations highlight the notion that mechanical unloading of the failing ventricle by LVAD alters repolarization globally (QT interval) and locally (APD), thereby modulating cardiac electrical function of these high-risk patients. Abrupt unloading of the failing ventricle appears to immediately worsen the electrophysiological substrate by prolonging APD and potentially predisposing cells to the incidence of early after-depolarization-induced triggered beats (Fig. 53.1). As such, acute LVAD use may predispose to a previously unrecognized form of the acquired long QT syndrome (LQTS). The exact nature and distribution of APD prolongation caused by acute LVAD therapy has not been investigated to date. Chronic mechanical support by LVAD therapy appears to reverse key pathophysiological properties, leading to

improved electrophysiological function and the suppression of arrhythmic triggers (Fig. 53.2).

LVAD-mediated form of the acquired long QT syndrome

As mentioned above, one of the major electrophysiological consequences of short-term unloading of the failing ventricle is a significant prolongation in the QT interval of the surface ECG, which gives rise to an acquired form of LQTS (Fig. 53.1). Therefore, the proarrhythmic nature of short-term LVAD use may be understood in light of recent advances in our understanding of mechanisms by which defective spatio-temporal repolarization kinetics across a host of congenital and acquired cardiac disorders can predispose to malignant arrhythmias. Of particular importance is LQTS, in which either a deficit in the magnitude of K^+ currents or an abnormality in the inactivation properties of Ca^{2+} or late Na^+ currents can lead to a pathophysiological prolongation of the AP at the cellular-tissue levels and corresponding QT interval prolongation at the organ-system levels. A long line of evidence highlights the importance of repolarization lability in the genesis of arrhythmic triggers in acquired and congenital forms of the LQTS. It is well known that excessive prolongation of the AP by disease or pharmacological agents predisposes to the incidence of arrhythmic triggers in the form of early after-depolarizations that can be caused by the premature reactivation of the L-type Ca^{2+} current ($I_{Ca,L}$) prior to terminal repolarization. These triggers are thought to give rise to the initial beats of Torsade de Pointes arrhythmias in LQTS.

We and others have elucidated the role of transmural heterogeneities of repolarization under conditions of prolonged QT interval, such as in LQTS and HF, in the maintenance of polymorphic ventricular tachyarrhythmias[6,10]. Using a novel technique of transmural AP mapping, Akar, Rosenbaum and colleagues assessed the electrophysiological substrate under conditions of prolonged QT interval in the arterially perfused canine wedge preparation. They found that mid-myocardial cells were more sensitive to AP prolongation relative to their epicardial and endocardial neighbours. Selective delays in mid-myocardial repolarization created discrete refractory borders across the transmural myocardium. The functional significance of this dispersion of repolarization was unmasked by the application of single premature stimuli, which resulted in intramural conduction block and transmural re-entrant circuits underlying polymorphic ventricular tachyarrhythmias[10]. We further characterized the transmural electrophysiological substrate of the failing heart, which also exhibited QT interval prolongation, and were able to identify qualitatively similar transmural repolarization heterogeneities that again appeared to underlie the early maintenance of arrhythmias in HF[6]. These findings demonstrate that the disease process associated with HF induces pathophysiological changes that preferentially target mid-myocardial cells in a manner that increases transmural repolarization heterogeneity and predisposes to intramural conduction block and re-entrant arrhythmias. Since abrupt mechanical unloading of the failing ventricle is known to further prolong the QT-interval of the failing heart, it is likely that similar mechanisms underlie the genesis of arrhythmic triggers and the formation of an electrically heterogeneous substrate in LVAD-treated patients (Fig. 53.1). Whether acute alterations in myocardial stretch levels by LVAD-induced mechanical unloading of the failing ventricle lead to selective enhancement of APD within certain cell types remains unknown. Future studies designed to investigate the cellular, ionic and molecular bases of LVAD-mediated arrhythmogensis are required to elucidate underlying mechanisms.

Calcium cycling in LVAD patients

LVAD-mediated changes in Ca^{2+} cycling and their functional consequences in terms of excitation–contraction (EC) coupling may play an important role in the long-term electrophysiological benefits associated with mechanical circulatory support. EC coupling is the vital process linking electrical stimuli to mechanical contraction. The process is initiated by Ca^{2+} entry through $I_{Ca,L}$ channels in response to depolarization of the cellular membrane.

Only a limited amount of Ca^{2+} enters the cell during each beat because of the time-dependent inactivation of these channels. This limited Ca^{2+} entry, while not sufficient to initiate myofilament contraction, activates the positive feedback process of Ca^{2+}-induced Ca^{2+} release from the sarcoplasmic reticulum (SR) through Ca^{2+} release channels, known as the ryanodine receptors (RyR). The tenfold rise in cytosolic Ca^{2+} levels initiates actin–myosin interaction and myofilament contraction. Cytosolic Ca^{2+} levels are subsequently restored by rapid reuptake into the SR by the cardiac sarco- /endoplasmatic reticulum Ca^{2+} ATPase (SERCA2a) and extrusion by the electrogenic Na^+/Ca^{2+} exchanger (NCX), which generates a net depolarizing transient inward current. All key players of the cellular Ca^{2+} handling machinery have been found to be mechano-sensitive, in terms of both acute modulation and chronic remodelling (for detail see Chapter 10).

HF modifies the expression and function of several EC coupling proteins, resulting in mechanical and electrical dysfunction. Failing hearts typically display, in addition to a prolonged APD, slower Ca^{2+} transient decay, revealing a deficit in the restoration of diastolic Ca^{2+} levels following each heart beat. Functionally, these Ca^{2+} abnormalities result in slowed rates of relaxation, a negative force frequency relationship and diminished contractile reserve. Such deviations from normal Ca^{2+} cycling and EC coupling can render the heart vulnerable to ventricular arrhythmias by a number of mechanisms. Prolonged LVAD support may reverse some of these modifications and protect against the development of arrhythmic triggers (Fig. 53.2). Several studies have examined changes in EC coupling resulting from LVAD support of failing ventricles. Dipla et al.[11] characterized the contractile properties of isolated myocytes from HF patients with and without LVAD support. The LVAD group represented failing hearts following prolonged mechanical support and significantly improved contractile performance compared to unsupported failing hearts. Isolated myocytes from the LVAD group displayed a greater magnitude of contraction, a reduction in time to peak contraction, a shortening in time to 50% relaxation and an improvement in the force–frequency relationship[11]. The evidence for mechanically induced improvement in EC coupling was further related to Ca^{2+} cycling by Chaudhary et al., who compared the kinetics of intercellular Ca^{2+} decay in cells from non-failing versus failing hearts, with and without LVAD therapy[12]. Changes in Ca^{2+} transient decay could be explained by alterations in the expression and function of key Ca^{2+} handling proteins. Abnormal Ca^{2+} cycling in these cells also accounted for changes in the force–frequency relationship among the three groups. As expected, cells from failing hearts exhibited a blunted Ca^{2+} transient decay rate relative to those from non-failing hearts. Remarkably, LVAD support normalized the Ca^{2+} transient decay rate to non-failing levels. The improvement in Ca^{2+} transient kinetics in the LVAD group correlated with improvement in relaxation kinetics and force–frequency properties. Failing and non-failing hearts exhibited negative and positive force–frequency relationships, respectively. While not completely corrected, the force–frequency relationship of the LVAD group was significantly improved compared to unsupported failing hearts. As expected, failing hearts exhibited decreased SERCA2a and increased NCX protein levels. Surprisingly, SERCA2a levels were not restored in LVAD-supported hearts despite the improved Ca^{2+} transient decay. In contrast, NCX levels decreased significantly by mechanical unloading[12], highlighting its importance in the mechanism of LVAD-mediated improvement in EC coupling.

Alterations in L-type Ca^{2+} current

As previously described, $I_{Ca,L}$ facilitates the entry of Ca^{2+} into the cytosol, thereby triggering further Ca^{2+} release from the SR and subsequent myocyte contraction. HF alters $I_{Ca,L}$ density and regulation, typically resulting in decreased function and responsiveness to β-adrenergic stimulation. Recent evidence suggests that mechanical unloading of the failing ventricle with LVAD can modulate EC coupling, in large part, by restoring $I_{Ca,L}$ function.

Chen *et al.* investigated changes in $I_{Ca,L}$ channel density and regulation in response to mechanical unloading[13]. They compared $I_{Ca,L}$ in myocytes from failing hearts with and without LVAD support with non-failing myocytes. As expected, myocytes from failing hearts exhibited decreased $I_{Ca,L}$ density, which was associated with increased phosphorylation of Cav1.2, and reduced responsiveness by β-adrenergic stimulation relative to cells from non-failing hearts. Mechanical unloading of the failing heart by chronic LVAD therapy caused a reversal of these defects, as Cav1.2 expression was increased to non-failing levels and current responsiveness to beta-stimulation was restored[13]. In a subsequent study, Chen *et al.* examined the relationship between the phosphorylation state of $I_{Ca,L}$ channels and the decreased response of $I_{Ca,L}$ to β-adrenergic stimulation. Mechanical support appears to at least partially reverse the pathological regulation of $I_{Ca,L}$ by HF. In LVAD-supported failing hearts phosphorylation levels decline and channel density improves, implicating a central role for mechanical unloading in the normalization of $I_{Ca,L}$ function and associated improvement in Ca^{2+} cycling[14]. Further investigation is needed to dissect the signalling cascade underlying these fundamental changes that occur during disease progression and in response to acute and chronic LVAD-mediated mechanical support.

Conclusions and outlook

Patients receiving LVAD therapy typically have advanced HF and therefore are at increased risk for developing ventricular and atrial arrhythmias. With the progression of HF, pathophysiological remodelling occurs at multiple levels, spanning the spectrum from molecular and subcellular changes to those occurring at the organ system level. Highly complex, interactive and dynamic changes in mechanical, structural, neurohumoral, metabolic and electrophysiological properties collectively predispose the failing heart to electrical disturbances. As such, the vast majority of pharmaco-therapies for HF patients are highly problematic because of their risk for lethal arrhythmias.

Mechanical support by LVAD therapy has proven to be a highly useful clinical tool in the combat against HF. Of key importance was the surprising finding of progressively increased cardiac function in LVAD patients even when their devices were temporarily turned off. This clearly signalled that complex physiological (reverse) remodelling processes were being activated as a consequence of mechanical unloading by the LVAD. Subsequent experiments have characterized this unique reversal of key structural, mechanical and molecular changes associated with heart failure by chronic LVAD therapy. The onset, rate and extent of these improvements remain unclear, but mechanical unloading does modify the electrophysiological substrate and key Ca^{2+} handling properties of the failing heart (see also chapter 59).

Unfortunately, LVAD therapy may give rise to a transient increase in the susceptibility of the failing ventricle to arrhythmic triggers. The underlying complex and multifactorial mechanisms that involve multiple proteins and signalling cascades are as yet incompletely identified. Several studies show that LVAD patients are indeed at increased risk of arrhythmias immediately after implantation, presumably before beneficial remodelling can take place. This risk appears to decline substantially after prolonged mechanical support, further implicating an important role for LVAD-mediated reverse remodelling in the mechanism of protection against arrhythmias in the long run.

The complex and dynamic electrophysiological changes associated with LVAD therapy provide a unique opportunity to further our understanding of mechanisms by which acute and chronic alterations in cardiac workload and stretch–strain relationships predispose to arrhythmias. Despite the clear advancement in our understanding of the molecular, mechanical and structural remodelling that occur in the failing heart and upon LVAD therapy, detailed descriptions of the mechanisms underlying the generation of arrhythmias remain elusive.

References

1. Rosamond W, Flegal K, Furie K, *et al.* Heart disease and stroke statistics – 2008 update: a report from the American Heart Association Statistics Committee and Stroke Statistics Subcommittee. *Circulation* 2008;**117**:e25–e146.

2. Badiwala MV, Rao V. Left ventricular device as destination therapy: are we there yet? *Curr Opin Cardiol* 2009;**24**:184–189.

3. Maybaum S, Kamalakannan G, Murthy S. Cardiac recovery during mechanical assist device support. *Semin Thorac Cardiovasc Surg* 2008;**20**:234–246.

4. Refaat M, Chemaly E, Lebeche D, Gwathmey JK, Hajjar RJ. Ventricular arrhythmias after left ventricular assist device implantation. *Pacing Clin Electrophysiol* 2008;**31**:1246–1252.

5. Bedi M, Kormos, R, Winowich S, McNamara DM, Mathier MA, Murali S. Ventricular arrhythmias during left ventricular assist device support. *Am J Cardiol* 2007;**99**:1151–1153.

6. Akar FG, Rosenbaum DS. Transmural electrophysiological heterogeneities underlying arrhythmogenesis in heart failure. *Circ Res* 2003;**93**:638–645.

7. Chugh SS, Johnson SB, Packer DL. Amplified effects of d,l-sotalol in canine dilated cardiomyopathy. *Pacing Clin Electrophysiol* 2001;**24**:1783–1788.

8. Harding JD, Piacentino V, 3rd, Gaughan JP, Houser SR, Margulies KB. Electrophysiological alterations after mechanical circulatory support in patients with advanced cardiac failure. *Circulation* 2001;**104**:1241–1247.

9. Harding JD, Piacentino V, 3rd, Rothman S, Chambers S, Jessup M, Margulies KB. Prolonged repolarization after ventricular assist device support is associated with arrhythmias in humans with congestive heart failure. *J Card Fail* 2005;**11**: 227–232.

10. Akar FG, Yan GX, Antzelevitch C, Rosenbaum DS. Unique topographical distribution of M cells underlies reentrant mechanism of torsade de pointes in the long-QT syndrome. *Circulation* 2002;**105**:1247–1253.

11. Dipla K, Mattiello JA, Jeevanandam V, Houser SR, Margulies KB. Myocyte recovery after mechanical circulatory support in humans with end-stage heart failure. *Circulation* 1998;**97**: 2316–2322.

12. Chaudhary KW, Rossman EI, Piacentino V, 3rd, Kenessey A, Weber C, Gaughan JP, *et al.* Altered myocardial Ca^{2+} cycling after left ventricular assist device support in the failing human heart. *J Am Coll Cardiol* 2004;**44**:837–845.

13. Chen X, Piacentino V, 3rd, Furukawa S, Goldman B, Margulies KB, Houser SRL-type Ca^{2+} channel density and regulation are altered in failing human ventricular myocytes and recover after support with mechanical assist devices. *Circ Res* 2002;**91**:517–524.

14. Chen X, Zhang X, Harris DM, Piacentino V, 3rd, Berretta RM, Margulies KB, Houser SR. Reduced effects of BAY K 8644 on L-type Ca^{2+} current in failing human cardiac myocytes are related to abnormal adrenergic regulation. *Am J Physiol* 2008;**294**:H2257–H2267.

Anti- and proarrhythmic effects of cardiac resynchronization therapy

Nico H.L. Kuijpers and Frits W. Prinzen

Background

Asynchronous electrical activation, as caused by left bundle branch block (LBBB), hampers cardiac function[1]. To restore electrical synchrony, cardiac resynchronization therapy (CRT) is often applied in patients with a severe stage of heart failure. CRT involves implantation of a pacemaker with multiple leads to enable biventricular pacing. To reduce the risk of sudden cardiac death (SCD), CRT is often combined with an implantable cardioverter-defibrillator (ICD). In animal experiments, it was found that CRT restores both electrical and haemodynamic malfunctioning of the heart[1]. From several large randomized clinical trials, it was concluded that CRT improves cardiac function and quality of life and decreases all-cause mortality as well as cardiovascular mortality[2,3].

Heart failure is associated with SCD. An unsettled debate is, however, whether CRT is pro- or antiarrhythmic. On the one hand, CRT improves cardiac function and decreases asynchrony, thus reducing the risk of SCD[4]. On the other hand, it has been suggested that altered electrical activation during biventricular pacing increases (transmural) dispersion of repolarization, which may lead to serious arrhythmia[5].

A topic not yet considered in this discussion, is the potential role of electrical remodelling as a consequence of abnormal electrical activation. Electrical remodelling is mainly studied in the context of 'cardiac memory'[6], but also appears to be present in hearts with LBBB[7]. Evidence is increasing that 'cardiac memory' is triggered by changes in mechanical load[8]. In this chapter, we discuss the potential role of mechano-electric coupling (MEC) on pro- and antiarrhythmic effects of CRT, using information primarily from animal experiments and computer simulations.

Data from clinical studies

Medina-Ravell et al.[5] showed that, in CRT patients, JTc time is longer during epicardial left ventricular (LV) pacing than during right ventricular (RV) pacing, while QRS duration was equal. From these observations the investigators concluded that the specific (epicardial to endocardial) sequence of electrical activation during epicardial LV pacing elicits prolongation of transmural dispersion

of repolarization. Subsequently, these investigators showed that in rabbit hearts, switching from endocardial to epicardial pacing produced a net increase in QT interval and transmural dispersion of repolarization. The potential proarrhythmic effects of CRT have been supported by a number of case reports[9,10] and small clinical studies[11]. Ermis et al. studied the effect of CRT upgrade on ventricular arrhythmias in 18 patients with pre-existing ICD and found a reduction in the rate of appropriate therapy after biventricular ICD placement[12]. More insight into the issue of proarrhythmia remains unclear, partly because of a non-systematic investigation of arrhythmia. An example of the latter is seen in the InSync ICD trial[13]. While no proarrhythmia was reported, upon close review one patient developed 'incessant ventricular tachycardia (VT)' after receiving CRT with ICD (CRT-D). In reports from other randomized trials, information about the patients who experienced VT after biventricular pacing is typically lacking. However, closely studying results from these studies shows that a proarrhythmic effect of CRT cannot be excluded.

In the Comparison Medical Therapy, Pacing and Defibrillation in Chronic Heart Failure (COMPANION) study[2], CRT reduced the composite of all-cause mortality and all-cause hospital admission by 20%. In the case of CRT-P (CRT without ICD), the risk of death from any cause was reduced by 24%. However, when CRT was combined with an ICD (CRT-D), all-cause mortality was significantly more reduced, by 36%[2]. In the outcome study on class IV heart failure patients within the COMPANION trial, Lindenfeld et al. showed a moderate increase in sudden death compared with patients medically treated as well as compared with the CRT-D group during the first year[14]. Moreover, after > 300 days, the lines for CRT-P and CRT-D are parallel, suggesting that risk of sudden death due to CRT is only increased during the first year.

Similarly, in the Cardiac Resynchronization in Heart Failure (CARE-HF) extension study[15] the Kaplan Meier curves for death by heart failure of the medical treatment versus CRT group seem to diverge immediately after onset of CRT, whereas the curves for SCD do not separate within 400 days (Fig. 54.1). These studies support the idea that, in the long run, improvement of cardiac function and presumably reverse myocardial and electrical remodelling

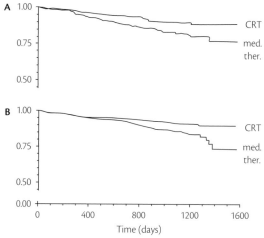

Fig. 54.1 Time to death from worsening heart failure (**A**) and SCD (**B**) over an average follow-up time of 900 days in the CARE-HF extension trial. CRT, resynchronization group (CRT pacemakers); med. ther., medical therapy (control group). [Modified, with permission, from Cleland JGF, Daubert JC, Erdmann E, Freemantle N, Gras D, Kappenberger L, Tavazzi L, on behalf of the CARE-HF Study Investigators (2006) Longer-term effects of cardiac resynchronization therapy on mortality in heart failure [the Cardiac REsynchronization-Heart Failure (CARE-HF) trial extension phase]. *Eur Heart J* **27**:1928–1932.]

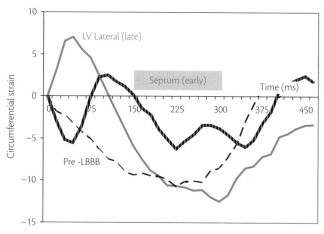

Fig. 54.2 Circumferential strain (strain units × 100; negative values represent shortening) in a canine heart before LBBB (pre-LBBB) as well as after LBBB in the LV lateral wall and septum. Note that in the early activated septum, early systolic shortening is quickly followed by rebound stretch and that net systolic shortening is decreased. In contrast, in the LV lateral wall, early systolic stretch occurs, followed by pronounced systolic shortening. Example from studies as described in reference[18].

reduce SCD, but that during the first year of CRT this beneficial effect is counteracted by a proarrhythmic effect.

Mechanical and electrical consequences of asynchronous activation

The ideal animal model for studying effects of CRT is the canine heart, where LBBB is induced by radiofrequency ablation. Changes due to LBBB as well as effects of CRT are well in the range of those observed in human patients[16]. In this model, as well as in models of ventricular pacing, it was demonstrated that early-activated regions are mechanically unloaded, whereas late-activated regions undergo early systolic stretch followed by supra-normal systolic shortening[17,18] (Fig. 54.2).

Changes in regional mechanics (stretch, systolic shortening, mechanical work) seem to have an important impact on regional growth. This was initially demonstrated in dogs with chronic LV pacing[19,18]. Within 2 months of experimental LBBB, hypertrophy is observed specifically in the late-activated LV lateral wall, the region where mechanical work is increased. There, local wall mass increases by 30%, whereas mass of the septum hardly changes. Similar to the normalization of regional workload after initiation of biventricular pacing, regional differences in hypertrophy also disappear within 2 months[1].

Mechano-electric coupling

For decades it was known that asynchronous electrical activation also leads to electrical remodelling. It is well known that after stopping asynchronous activation (e.g. ending ventricular pacing or ablation of the accessory pathway in Wolf–Parkinson–White (WPW) syndrome) the T-wave of the surface electrocardiogram (ECG) remains abnormal, a phenomenon called cardiac (or T-wave) memory. Costard-Jäckle *et al.*[20] were the first to show that this cardiac memory is due to prolongation of the action

potential (AP) at the site of pacing and AP shortening in the late-activated region. This was later confirmed in the LBBB model, both after 4 weeks of isolated LBBB and during LBBB in combination with heart failure[7,12].

Electrical remodelling could be of benefit due to minimization of dispersion of repolarization, which reduces the risk for development of arrhythmia. It has indeed been shown in the canine heart that dispersion of repolarization increases with acute LBBB, but subsequently becomes smaller with longer duration of LBBB[16].

Evidence is increasing that abnormal and regionally different mechanics during asynchronous activation is a major determinant of electrical remodelling. Jeyaraj *et al.*[22] showed the association of changes in AP duration with myocardial strains. Even more elegantly, Sosunov *et al.* demonstrated that ventricular pacing did not lead to electrical remodelling when the left ventricle was mechanically unloaded in the isolated heart preparation. In addition, they showed that electrical remodelling may be induced by stretching the ventricular wall without changing activation sequence[8].

Therefore, the intriguing paradigm emerges that abnormal electromechanical activation leads to mechano-electric coupling (MEC), a mechanism that does not seem to reduce asynchrony of activation but primarily dispersion of repolarization. The question is therefore how cardiac function benefits from this long-term form of MEC.

Computer simulations

In order to better understand the effect of long-term MEC in CRT, others[23] as well as ourselves have used computer simulations. We hypothesized that electrical remodelling, as observed during chronic asynchrony, should be placed in a broader perspective: a (negative) feedback system aiming at equalizing differences in workload, as occurs after changing the sequence of electrical activation. Since cardiac cell contraction is triggered by the calcium transient, a logical place for a feedback mechanism would be calcium release from the sarcoplasmic reticulum (SR), which is triggered by the inflow of calcium ions through L-type calcium channels. These channels play a pivotal role in both excitation–contraction coupling and action potential duration (APD)[24] and are known to adapt to changes in activation sequence[25].

The computer model employs a cardiac fibre strand, allowing the simulation of the effects of changes in mechanical workload on ion channel behaviour, leading to adaptation of the calcium transient, contractile force and APD[26,27]. The fibre strand can be regarded as mimicking half the circumference of the left ventricular short axis, while transmural differences are neglected for this first-order approximation. This approach was chosen because in electrical remodelling the segmental dispersion was shown to be more important than the transmural dispersion[22]. In our model, the unloaded fibre strand is 3 cm long and is represented by a string of 300 segments that are electrically and mechanically coupled[27]. Cardiac excitation–contraction coupling is modelled by integrating the model of Courtemanche et al.[28], representing ionic membrane currents and intracellular calcium handling, with the model of Rice et al.[29] to compute contractile forces. Local differences between ionic membrane behaviour and calcium handling are accounted for by changes in the L-type calcium current ($l_{Ca,L}$)[27]. Since the calcium transient is affected by these differences, also contractile forces generated by the sarcomeres are affected as well as the distribution of mechanical workload over the fibre.

To simulate the cardiac cycle, a constant load was applied during filling, ejection and isotonic relaxation, whereas during isovolumic contraction and isovolumic relaxation fibre length was kept constant. The amount of workload (W_{tot}) during the cardiac cycle was determined for each individual fibre segment by computing the stress–strain area from the stress–strain excursion of that segment[30]. To initiate cardiac contraction, either the segment at 0.0 cm (representing activation mimicking RV pacing and LBBB) or the segments at 0.0 and 3.0 cm (representing biventricular pacing) were electrically stimulated. MEC was simulated by adapting the dynamical behaviour of $l_{Ca,L}$ for each segment such that a more homogeneous distribution of W_{tot} was obtained. Workload of the centre segment was used as reference, i.e., $l_{Ca,L}$ was not changed for that segment. Adaptation of $l_{Ca,L}$ was performed iteratively until steady-state was reached, which was always the case after 150 cardiac cycles[27].

With this model, we investigated the effects of MEC during LBBB (normal activation) and subsequent CRT (biventricular pacing), assuming that after acute change of the activation sequence a negative feedback occurs aiming at equalizing the total mechanical work of all fibres through modulation of the L-type calcium channel. Since all fibres in the strand were assumed to be equal, perfectly synchronous electrical activation also results in perfectly uniform contraction and APD. Four simulations were performed: acute (A) and chronic (B) LBBB and, following chronic LBBB, acute (C) and chronic (D) CRT. During LBBB, electrical activation started at one end of the strand (indicated with an asterisk in Fig. 54.4 later in this chapter) and was assumed to be conducted cell-to-cell to the other side. Total activation of the fibre took 98 ms, representing slow conduction during LBBB. CRT reduced total activation time to 48 ms.

Figure 54.3 shows that acute LBBB caused significant redistribution of W_{tot}, with a figure-of-eight-shaped work loop in the early-activated region (0.5 cm) and increased W_{tot} in the late-activated region.

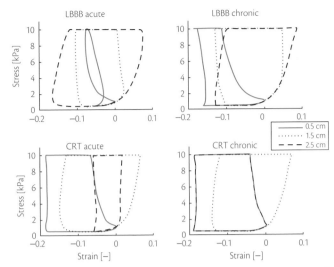

Fig. 54.3 Stress–strain loops in the simulations of acute and chronic LBBB as well as acute and chronic CRT.

Due to the assumed effect of MEC on $l_{Ca,L}$ the difference in W_{tot} decreased, but the assumed feedback system is clearly not capable of creating uniform workload during asynchronous electrical activation. Acute CRT reduced the regional differences in W_{tot}, which further decreased during chronic CRT. These changes are also illustrated in the upper row of Fig. 54.4.

MEC was able to reduce the dispersion of repolarization from 77 to 39 ms (Fig. 54.4, lower left panel), especially by increasing APD in early-activated segments (middle left panel).

After onset of CRT, dispersion of repolarization increased because regions with shortest APD now became early activated

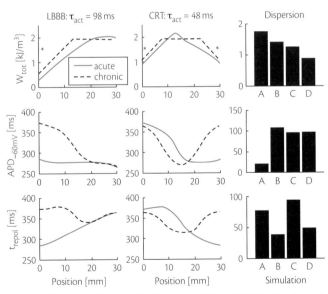

Fig. 54.4 The effect of (long-term) MEC during LBBB and CRT. Total stroke work density (W_{tot}), action potential duration (APD$_{-60mV}$) and time of repolarization (t_{repol}) of all segments along the fibre during acute and chronic LBBB and CRT (see text for details). During LBBB the fibre strand is activated from position 0 mm (left), while during CRT activation occurs from positions 0 and 30 mm (asterisks).

(the rightmost region along the X-axis). Since early-activated regions (near both pacing sites) now performed the lowest amount of work, MEC lead to an increase in APD in these regions (center panel of Fig. 54.4) and a reduction of the dispersion of repolarization from 94 to 49 ms (lower middle panel).

Figure 54.5 further substantiates these data by presenting traces of the AP, Ca²⁺ transient and shortening signal during chronic LBBB and during acute and chronic CRT. During chronic LBBB, the AP and Ca²⁺ transient of the early-activated segment envelop the AP and Ca²⁺ transients of the other two segments, so that their end is almost simultaneous. The middle panels illustrate that acute CRT results in increased dispersion in repolarization as well as in end of the Ca²⁺ transient. During chronic LBBB, systolic shortening is lower in early-activated regions (0.5 cm from pacing site), despite MEC. Acute CRT reduced the non-uniformity of strain and this was further reduced during chronic CRT.

The observed APD differences and reversible changes in dispersion of repolarization compare well, both qualitatively and quantitatively, with data from animal experiments, as discussed in the first paragraph of this chapter. Therefore, the computer simulations support the idea that MEC in asynchronous hearts may also affect mechanical loading and calcium handling, a hypothesis which needs to be tested. More important probably, our model predicts a sudden increase in dispersion of repolarization in the early phase of CRT. Such dispersion could fade away over time, again due to long-term MEC.

Conclusions and outlook

These computer simulations indicate that long-term MEC in asynchronous hearts may be a coin with two sides: it may help to reduce dispersion during long-term asynchrony, but it also leads to, temporarily, increased dispersion when activation is resynchronized. Clearly, there is a large difference between this highly simplified computer model and a patient's heart. Also, various predictions by

the model require experimental validation. Nevertheless, these computer simulations may stimulate further research into the effects of MEC in asynchronous and resynchronized hearts. Such research seems important, because it may aid the decision whether a patient should receive a CRT device with or without an implantable defibrillator. In the extended CARE-HF study, 7.8% of patients with New York Heart Association (NYHA) class III/IV heart failure and a CRT pacemaker died from sudden death within 30 months. On the other hand, costs of a CRT defibrillator are at least three times higher than that of a CRT pacemaker.

References

1. Vernooy K, Comelussen RNM, Verbeek XAAM, *et al.* Cardiac resynchronization therapy cures dyssynchronopathy in canine left bundle-branch block hearts. *Eur Heart J* 2007;**28**:2148–2155.
2. Bristow MR, Saxon LA, Boehmer J, et al. On behalf of the Comparison of Medical Therapy, Pacing, and Defibrillation in Heart Failure (COMPANION) Investigators. Cardiac-resynchronization therapy with or without an implantable defibrillator in advanced chronic heart failure. *N Engl J Med* 2004;**350**:2140–2150.
3. Cleland JG, Daubert JC, Erdmann E, et al. On behalf of the Cardiac Resynchronization-Heart Failure (CARE-HF) Study Investigators. The effect of cardiac resynchronization on morbidity and mortality in heart failure. *N Engl J Med* 2005;**352**:1539–1549.
4. Lepillier A, Piot O, Gerritse B, et al. Relationship between New York Heart Association class change and ventricular tachyarrhythmia occurrence in patients treated with cardiac resynchronization plus defibrillator. *Europace* 2009;**11**:80–85.
5. Medina-Ravell VA, Lankipalli RS, Yan GX, et al. Effect of epicardial or biventricular pacing to prolong QT interval and increase transmural dispersion of repolarization: does resynchronization therapy pose a risk for patients predisposed to long QT or torsade de pointes? *Circulation* 2003;**107**:740–746.
6. Rosen MR. The heart remembers: clinical implications. *Lancet* 2001;**357**:468–471.
7. Spragg DD, Akar FG, Helm RH, Tunin RS, Tomaselli GF, Kass DA. Abnormal conduction and repolarization in late-activated myocardium of dyssynchronously contracting hearts. *Cardiovasc Res* 2005; **67**:77–86.
8. Sosunov EA, Anyukhovsky EP, Rosen MR Altered ventricular stretch contributes to initiation of cardiac memory. *Heart Rhythm* 2008; **5**:106–113.
9. Myktsey A, Maheshwari P, Dhar G, Razminia M, Zheutlin T, Wang T, Kehoe R. Ventricular tachycardia induced by biventricular pacing in patient with severe ischemic cardiomyopathy. *J Cardiovasc Electrophysiol* 2005;**16**:655–658.
10. Guerra JM, Wu J, Miller JM, Groh WJ. Increase in ventricular tachycardia frequency after biventricular implantable cardioverter defibrillator upgrade. *J Cardiovasc Electrophysiol* 2003;**14**:1245–1247.
11. Nayak HM, Verdino RJ, Russo AM, et al. Ventricular tachycardia storm after initiation of biventricular pacing: incidence, clinical characteristics, management, and outcome. *J Cardiovasc Electrophysiol* 2008;**19**:708–715.
12. Ermis C, Seutter R, Zhu AX, et al. Impact of upgrade to cardiac resynchronization therapy on ventricular arrhythmia frequency in patients with implantable cardioverter-defibrillators. *J Am Coll Cardiol* 2005;**46**:2258–2263.
13. Kuhlkamp V, InSync World Wide Investigators. Initial experience with an implantable cardioverter defibrillator incorporating cardiac resynchronization therapy. *J Am Coll Cardiol* 2002;**39**:790–797.
14. Lindenfeld J, Feldman AM, Saxon L, et al. Effects of cardiac resynchronization therapy with or without a defibrillator on survival and hospitalizations in patients with New York Heart Association class IV heart failure. *Circulation* 2007;**115**:204–212.

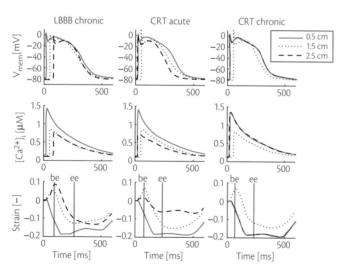

Figure 54.5 Membrane potential (V_{mem}), intracellular Ca²⁺ concentration ($[Ca^{2+}]_i$) and strain for segments located at 0.5, 1.5 and 2.5 cm. Beginning and end of ejection are indicated with be and ee, respectively. Note that the electromechanical behaviour of the segments at 0.5 and 2.5 cm is exactly the same in the case of chronic CRT (right column).

15. Cleland JGF, Daubert JC, Erdmann E, *et al.*; on behalf of the CARE-HF Study Investigators. Longer-term effects of cardiac resynchronization therapy on mortality in heart failure [the CArdiac REsynchronization-Heart Failure (CARE-HF) trial extension phase]. *Eur Heart J* 2006;**27**:1928–1932.

16. Kerckhoffs RCP, Lumens J, Vemooy K, *et al.* Cardiac resynchronization: insight from experimental and computational models. *Progr Biophys Mol Biol* 2008;**97**:543–561.

17. Prinzen FW, Hunter WC, Wyman BT, McVeigh ER. Mapping of regional myocardial strain and work during ventricular pacing: experimental study using magnetic resonance imaging tagging. *J Am Coll Cardiol* 1999;**33**:1735–1742.

18. Vernooy K, Verbeek XAAM, Peschar M, Crijns HJ, Arts T, Cornelussen RN, Prinzen FW. Left bundle branch block induces ventricular remodeling and functional septal hypoperfusion. *Eur Heart J* 2005;**26**:91–98.

19. Van Oosterhout MFM, Prinzen FW, Arts T, Schreuder JJ, Vanagt WY, Cleutjens JP, Reneman RS. Asynchronous electrical activation induces inhomogeneous hypertrophy of the left ventricular wall. *Circulation* 1998;**98**:588–595.

20. Costard-Jäckle A, Franz MR. Slow and long-lasting modulation of myocardial repolarization produced by ectopic activation in isolated rabbit hearts: evidence for cardiac "memory". *Circulation* 1989;**80**:1412–1420.

21. Spragg DD, Leclercq C, Loghmani M, *et al.* Regional alterations in protein expression in the dyssynchronous failing heart. *Circulation* 2003;**108**:929–932.

22. Jeyaraj D, Wilson LD, Zhong J, *et al.* Mechanoelectrical feedback as novel mechanism of cardiac electrical remodeling. *Circulation* 2007;**115**:3145–3155.

23. Solovyova O, Katsnelson L, Konovalov P, Lookin O, Moskvin A, Protsenko Yu, *et al.* Activation sequence as a key factor in spatio-temporal optimization of myocardial function. *Phil Trans Roy Soc Lond (A)* 2006;**364**:1367–1383.

24. Brette F, Leroy J, Le Guennec JY, Sallé L. Ca^{2+} currents in cardiac myocytes: old story, new insights. *Prog Biophys Mol Biol* 2006;**91**:1–82.

25. Plotnikov AN, Yu H, Geller JC, *et al.* Role of L-type calcium channels in pacing-induced short-term and long-term cardiac memory in canine heart. *Circulation* 2003;**107**:2844–2849.

26. Kuijpers NHL, ten Eikelder HMM, Bovendeerd PHM, Verheule S, Arts T, Hilbers PAJ. Mechano-electric feedback leads to conduction slowing and block in acutely dilated atria: a modeling study of cardiac electromechanics. *Am J Physiol* 2007;**292**:H2832–H2853.

27. Kuijpers NH, Ten Eikelder HM, Bovendeerd PH, Verheule S, Arts T, Hilbers PA. Mechanoelectric feedback as a trigger mechanism for cardiac electrical remodeling: a model study. *Ann Biomed Eng* 2008;**36**:1816–1835.

28. Courtemanche M, Ramirez RJ, Nattel S. Ionic mechanisms underlying human atrial action potential properties: insights from a mathematical model. *Am J Physiol* 1998;**275**:H301–H321.

29. Rice JJ, Winslow RL, Hunter WC. Comparison of putative cooperative mechanisms in cardiac muscle: length dependence and dynamic responses. *Am J Physiol* 1999;**276**:1734–1754.

30. Delhaas T, Arts T, Prinzen FW, Reneman RS. Regional fibre stress–fibre strain area as estimate of regional oxygen demand in the canine heart. *J Physiol* 1994;**477**:481–496.

SECTION 8

Evidence for mechano-electric coupling from clinical trials

55. **Evidence for mechano-electric coupling from clinical trials on AF** 395
Matthias Hammwöhner and Andreas Goette

56. **Evidence for mechano-electric coupling from clinical trials on heart failure** 402
Paulus Kirchhof and Günter Breithardt

57. **Mechano-electrical coupling and the pathogenesis of arryhthmogenic right ventricular cardiomyopathy** 407
Hayden Huang, Angeliki Asimaki, Frank Marcus and Jeffrey E. Saffitz

58. **Evidence for mechano-electric coupling from clinical trials on cardiac resynchronization therapy** 412
Nico R.L. Van de Veire and Jeroen J. Bax

59. **Mechano-electric coupling in patients treated with ventricular assist devices: insights from individual cases and clinical trials** 420
Cesare M. Terracciano, Michael Ibrahim, Manoraj Navaratnarajah and Magdi H. Yacoub

Evidence for mechano-electric coupling from clinical trials on AF

Matthias Hammwöhner and Andreas Goette

Background

Atrial fibrillation (AF) is the most common not immediately life-threatening cardiac arrhythmia, with a prevalence of 0.5–2% in the general population[1–3]. Cardiac diseases like hypertensive heart disease, congestive heart failure (HF) and valve diseases are present in about 90% of patients with AF[4]. The impact of these diseases on atrial pathophysiology is commonly considered to be due to pressure and/or volume overload of the atria. Pure pharmacological antiarrhythmic therapy of patients with AF is often ineffective, if concomitant diseases like hypertension, HF and valvular deficiency are not well treated or corrected[5–8]. Acute pressure overload can cause changes in atrial action potential duration (APD) and may increase the rate of focal ectopy. Furthermore, chronic atrial pressure and volume overload cause atrial dilation, hypertrophy of atrial myocytes and interstitial fibrosis, all of which may provide a 'morphologic substrate' for AF (see also Chapter 28). Some of these molecular and structural changes may also be relevant for atrial thrombus formation[3,9–11]. This chapter summarizes the present evidence concerning effects of atrial pressure and volume overload on development of AF, derived from clinical trials.

Acute profibrillatory atrial changes due to atrial pressure overload in patients

Recent studies in humans have improved our understanding of electrophysiological remodelling of the atrial myocardium. Changes encompass shortening of the effective refractory period (ERP), loss of rate adaptation, increase in ERP dispersion and regional slowing of conduction after a prolonged period of AF[12,13]. Although the electrophysiological effects of atrial pressure and volume overload are still incompletely understood, it is clear that mechano-electrical coupling (MEC) caused by atrial dilatation plays an important role in the development of AF (Fig. 55.1). Few studies have assessed the role of MEC on the vulnerability for AF in human atrial tissue[14]. The study by Fan et al.[15] systematically assessed the effect of a reduction of left atrial (LA) stretch on the electrophysiological changes in patients with rheumatic mitral stenosis undergoing percutaneous balloon mitral commissurotomy (Fig. 55.2). The study showed that a reduction of LA pressure in patients with sinus rhythm was associated with rapid restitution (homogenous increase) of regional atrial ERP. Interestingly, in patients with AF, an inhomogeneous distribution of regional ERP occurred. The heterogeneity index of ERP improved significantly after LA stretch reduction. Both AF vulnerability and the index of heterogeneity of conduction delay showed a significant correlation with changes in LA pressures.

In contrast, Calkins et al.[16] assessed the acute effects of increased atrial pressure on atrial ERP in patients without valvular diseases. The objective of their study was to investigate the effect of acute alterations in atrial pressure, induced by varying the atrio-ventricular (AV) interval, on atrial refractoriness. Peak right atrial pressure was increased from 7 ± 3 to 15 ± 5 mmHg. The increase in atrial pressure resulted in shortening of the atrial ERP and absolute refractory period (ARP) by 7.3 ± 5.2 and 6.2 ± 3.5 ms, respectively. Similar results were obtained during autonomic blockade.

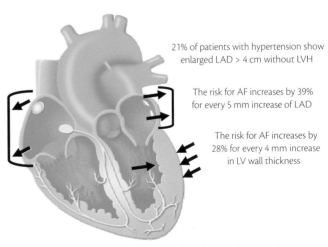

21% of patients with hypertension show enlarged LAD > 4 cm without LVH

The risk for AF increases by 39% for every 5 mm increase of LAD

The risk for AF increases by 28% for every 4 mm increase in LV wall thickness

Fig. 55.1 Impact of arterial hypertension and cardiac chamber morphology on the occurrence of atrial fibrillation (AF). LAD, left atrial diameter; LVH, left ventricular hypertrophy; LV, left ventricular.

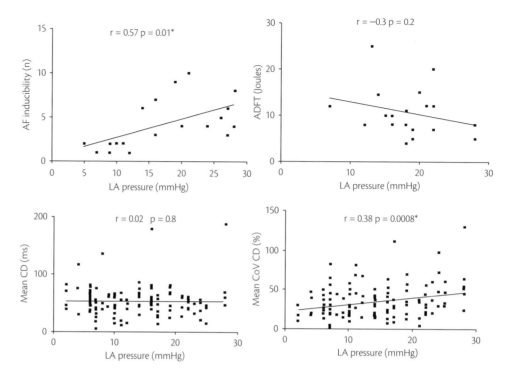

Fig. 55.2 Top left: correlation between left atrial (LA) pressure and atrial fibrillation (AF) inducibility. Top right: atrial defibrillation threshold (ADFT). Bottom left: correlation between LA pressure and conduction delay (CD). Bottom right: index of heterogeneity of conduction delay (CoV-CD). * $p < 0.05$. [Reproduced, with permission, from Fan K, Lee KL, Chow WH, Chau E, Lau CP (2002) Internal cardioversion of chronic atrial fibrillation during percutaneous mitral commissurotomy: insight into reversal of chronic stretch-induced atrial remodeling. *Circulation* **105**: 2746–2752.]

Thus, acute effects of pressure overload appear to depend on the underlying pathophysiological substrate contributing to various alterations in atrial refractory periods. Despite different conditions, all findings confirm the presence of MEC in human atria.

AF due to chronic atrial pressure overload in hypertensive patients

Long-term follow-up in patients with arterial hypertension has shown a positive correlation between blood pressure and occurrence of AF[17,18]. Katritsis *et al.*[19] reported that 44% of 292 patients with lone AF had borderline increased blood pressure. Furthermore, therapy-refractory lone AF led to a 46 times higher risk for arterial hypertension within the following 3 years. An increase in arterial blood pressure corresponds to LA enlargement[20–22]. Atrial dilatation can be both a cause and a consequence of AF[23]. In patients, atrial enlargement correlates with the incidence of AF, and LA size is a strong independent predictor for the development of AF. On the other hand, several studies imply that AF itself causes atrial enlargement[22,24]. Furthermore, cardioversion of AF leads to a decrease in atrial dimensions. In animal models of chronic hypertension, LA surface area increased by 20% due to pressure overload and by an estimated 80% due to volume overload in a canine chronic HF model. The surface electrocardiogram (ECG) P-wave duration is clearly prolonged in patients with hypertension and paroxysmal AF[25]. AV dyssynchrony due to VVI pacing (on-demand pacing with a single sensing and stimulating electrode in the right ventricle) causes biatrial dilatation associated with a non-uniform increase in atrial ERP in humans. Lengthening of the atrial ERP was accompanied by a prolongation of P-wave duration. These electrophysiological phenomena, occurring as a consequence of long-term VVI pacing, were reversible. After the

re-establishment of AV synchrony with DDD pacing (on demand and atrially triggered ventricular pacing with sensing and stimulating electrodes in the right atrium and ventricle) for 3 months, all parameters returned to values comparable to baseline[26].

The association between blood pressure and atrial size was reported in humans by Vaziri *et al.*[22]. The study consisted of 1,849 male and 2,152 female participants of the Framingham Heart Study and Framingham Offspring Study. In correlation analyses, systolic and pulse pressures were identified as statistically significant determinants of LA size after adjustment for age and body mass index, although the magnitudes of these relations were modest. In logistic analyses, increasing levels of the pressure variables were significantly predictive of LA enlargement. Subjects with 8-year average systolic pressure of 140 mmHg or higher were twice as likely to have LA enlargement as those with values of 110 mmHg or lower. However, concerning prediction of LA size, multivariable linear regression models showed relative contributions of pressure variables to be substantially less than those of age and, in particular, body mass index (BMI). Importantly, inclusion of left ventricular mass in these multivariable models eliminated or attenuated the associations of the pressure variables with LA size. Overall, this population-based study demonstrated that increased levels of systolic and pulse pressures (but not diastolic or mean arterial pressures) were significantly associated with increased LA size, although the magnitude of these associations was modest.

Gottdiener *et al.*[27] reported that antihypertensive drugs differ in their effects on LA size. Hydrochlorothiazide was associated with greater overall reduction of LA size than other drugs effective for the treatment of hypertension (Fig. 55.3). Reduction of LA size with therapy is in part independent of other factors known to influence LA size, including LV mass and reduction of LV mass with treatment. Milan *et al.*[28] assessed the association between blood

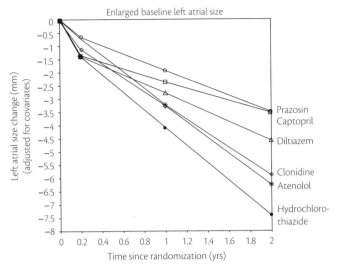

Fig. 55.3 Impact of antihypertensive drugs on atrial size. [Reproduced, with permission, from Gottdiener JS, Reda DJ, Williams DW, Materson BJ, Cushman W, Anderson RJ (1998) Effect of single-drug therapy on reduction of left atrial size in mild to moderate hypertension: comparison of six antihypertensive agents. *Circulation* **98**:140–148.]

pressure levels, left ventricular mass and function with LA volume (LAV) in mild to moderate hypertensive patients. They demonstrated that the LAV index is significantly increased in patients with essential hypertension. Furthermore, the LAV index significantly depended on blood pressure levels and BMI. Of note, the LV mass index was the most important variable associated with LAV in mild to moderate essential hypertensive adult patients. The measurement of LAV might be a better parameter than atrial size in predicting the occurrence of AF.

So far, several studies have shown that arterial hypertension is an independent risk factor for AF[11,29], but 'optimal' blood pressure levels for AF prevention have not been established. Few studies have assessed in more detail the association between different blood pressure components or their change over time and subsequent risk of AF. Given the non-linear relationship between age and diastolic blood pressure, but not systolic blood pressure[30], alterations in systolic or diastolic blood pressure may also differentially affect the risk of AF. Along these lines, a recent study suggested that pulse pressure may be more predictive of AF than either systolic or diastolic blood pressure alone. However, these relationships may differ in younger individuals or women, in whom the prevalence, outcome and underlying comorbidities associated with AF are different[4,5,11].

The relationship between systolic and diastolic blood pressure levels and the risk of AF was recently assessed in a large cohort of middle-aged women, who were free of cardiovascular disease at baseline[18]. A total of 34,221 women participating in the Women's Health Study were prospectively followed up for AF incidence. The risk of AF across categories of systolic and diastolic blood pressure was compared by use of Cox proportional hazard models[31]. During 12.4 years of follow-up, 644 AF events occurred. Using blood pressure measurements at baseline, the study showed that the long-term risk of AF was significantly increased across categories of systolic and diastolic blood pressure. Of note, systolic blood pressure was a better predictor than diastolic blood pressure. Systolic blood pressure levels within the non-hypertensive range were independently associated with AF incidence even after blood pressure changes over time were taken into account. This interesting finding points toward a direct MEC interaction of pressure and AF.

Other factors: aortic stiffness

Another study indicated that pulse pressure is an important risk factor for AF. One factor that might help to explain the association between AF and aortic pressure is aortic stiffness. Interestingly, the exponential rise in AF incidence with age parallels a rapid age-related increase in aortic stiffness. The concomitant increase in pulse pressure adds to pulsatile load on the heart[32], thereby promoting ventricular hypertrophy[33], impaired ventricular relaxation[34–36] and increased LA size[22]. Elevated LA size and pressure, and impaired ventricular diastolic function may lead to fibrosis and electrical remodelling in the atria, providing a substrate for the development of AF. Consistently, echocardiographic measures of abnormal left ventricular diastolic function are associated with increased risk for developing AF[37]. Thus, age-associated increased pulsatile load (as measured with pulse pressure) may be a key determinant for the increasing incidence of AF in the elderly.

The study by Mitchell *et al.*[17] tested prospectively the hypothesis that pulse pressure may represent an easily measured and potentially modifiable risk factor for the development of AF in the Framingham Study sample. In that study, pulse pressure was associated with increased risk for AF (adjusted hazard ratio 1.26 per 20 mmHg increment; 95% confidence interval, 1.12–1.43; $p < 0.001$). In contrast, mean arterial pressure was unrelated to incident AF. Systolic pressure was also related to AF; however, if diastolic pressure was added, model fit improved and the diastolic relation was inverse, consistent with a pulse pressure effect. The authors speculated that, pathophysiologically, episodic increases in systolic and pulse pressure in individuals with a stiff aorta contribute to relations between pulse pressure and AF incidence, independently of effects on LA size or left ventricular mass. Importantly, interventions known to reduce pulse pressure, such as blockade of the renin–angiotensin II system, have been shown to reduce the incidence of new or recurrent AF[17,38–41].

Interestingly, a recent statistical model indicates that women with a diastolic blood pressure below 65 mmHg have the highest risk of developing AF, further supporting the concept that elevated pulse pressure and aortic stiffness play a role[18]. Thus, the very close association between blood pressure, AF incidence and subsequent cardiovascular events suggests that treatment of hypertension should take the risk for AF into account[5,6,11,42]. Given the tight correlation between blood pressure and occurrence of AF, it was suggested that individuals with AF may benefit from a lower blood pressure treatment threshold of < 140/90 mmHg, which is the usually recommended blood pressure threshold for AF-free patients. The analysis from Conen *et al.*[18] further supports the concept that a substantial risk reduction may be obtained if systolic blood pressure levels were maintained at, or lowered to, levels less than 120 mmHg. Importantly, a reduction in atrial pressure also reduces the incidence of atrial ectopy, which serves as a trigger for AF episodes[43,44]. Further, the impact of atrial pressure on the occurrence of ectopic beats originating from the pulmonary veins has been well documented[45] (see also Chapter 15).

Results from clinical hypertension trials

Clementy et al.[46] performed a multicentre trial including 251 untreated patients with mild to moderate hypertension. Atrial arrhythmias such as premature beats, fibrillation, flutter and paroxysmal atrial tachycardia were detected in 16% of patients. Monomorphic premature ventricular contractions (PVC) were detected in 41% of patients and polymorphic PVC or couplets/ triplets in 14%. A correlation was present between the level of hypertensive cardiomyopathy, age of patients and severity of arrhythmias. Sotalol treatment was effective on blood pressure and arrhythmias (82% improvement of severe PVC).

More recently, the Losartan Intervention for Endpoint Reduction in Hypertension (LIFE) study clearly showed that the risk for AF increases by 6% for every 10 mmHg increase in systolic blood pressure[41]. Secondary analyses of clinical trial data suggest that, compared with other agents, angiotensin-converting enzyme (ACE) inhibitors and angiotensin receptor blockers (ARB) are associated with lower risk of AF incidence in patients with hypertension. Heckbert et al.[47] conducted a population-based case-control study to determine whether antihypertensive treatment with ACE inhibitors/ARB or beta-blockers, compared with diuretics, was associated with the risk of AF incidence in a community practice setting. All patients (810 AF cases, 1,512 control subjects) were members of Group Health (GH), an integrated healthcare delivery system. All patients were pharmacologically treated for hypertension and none had HF. Single-drug users of an ACE inhibitor/ARB had a lower risk of AF compared with single-drug users of a diuretic (adjusted odds ratio 0.63, 95% confidence interval 0.44–0.91). Single-drug use of beta-blockers was not significantly associated with lower AF risk and also none of the most commonly used two-drug regimens (usually a diuretic or Ca^{2+} antagonist with any other antihypertensive drug) were significantly associated with AF risk when compared to single-drug use of a diuretic. Thus, this study showed that in a general hypertensive population without HF, single-drug use of ACE inhibitors/ARB is associated with lower AF risk.

The importance of angiotensin II blocking drugs is further supported by several studies[40,41,47]. Although adequate treatment of arterial hypertension has significant effects on atrial size and occurrence of AF, studies point towards specific effects of ACE inhibitors and ARB to prevent AF[47,48]. Antihypertensive studies have shown that ACE inhibitors/ARB are more beneficial in preventing AF occurrence compared to Ca^{2+} antagonists or beta-blockers. Nevertheless, clinical data showed that reduction of systolic blood pressure by 30 mmHg or more has the same effect that ARB therapy has[41]. This may also, at least partially, explain the negative results from some hypertension trials. The Swedish Trial in Old Patients with Hypertension (STOP H2) found that the rate of new-onset AF was significantly increased by 43% on ACE inhibitors compared with 'conventional' therapy[49].

Nevertheless, among hypertensive patients with electrocardiographic left ventricular hypertrophy (LVH) in the LIFE randomized trial, ARB therapy with losartan reduced the incidence of AF by 33% and resulted in significant reduction in the incidence of subsequent stroke compared with an atenolol-based therapy[41].

Baseline severity of LVH has been demonstrated to be an additional predictor of AF in many studies[4,11,41,50–53]. In the LIFE trial, baseline severity LVH (Cornell product[54]) was a significant predictor of the development of new-onset AF[41]. The presence of LVH might be a much stronger parameter for increased intracardiac pressure and cardiac remodelling compared to systemic arterial hypertension. Okin et al.[55] tested the hypothesis that LVH regression during treatment, or continued absence of electrocardiographic LVH during antihypertensive therapy, is associated with a decreased incidence of AF. After a mean follow-up of 4.7 years, new-onset AF occurred in patients with in-treatment regression or continued absence of Cornell product LVH at a rate of 14.9 per 1,000 patient-years. In contrast, AF occurred in patients with in-treatment persistence or development of LVH at a rate of 19.0 per 1,000 patient-years. Thus, the study demonstrated that lower Cornell product electrocardiographic LVH during antihypertensive therapy is associated with a lower likelihood of new-onset AF, independent of blood pressure lowering and treatment modality in essential hypertension. The authors speculated that antihypertensive therapy targeted at regression or prevention of electrocardiographic LVH may reduce the incidence of new-onset AF. Nevertheless, the LIFE study also demonstrated that the absolute reduction of systolic blood pressure is the most important factor to reduce the incidence of AF[41].

Aggressive treatment of hypertension is particularly beneficial in patients with concomitant diabetes mellitus. Interestingly, AF is commonly observed in diabetic patients, with prevalence rates estimated to be twice that among people without diabetes[56], and up to three times higher in patients with coexistent hypertension[57]. The Action in Diabetes and Vascular disease: preterAx and diamicroN-MR Controlled Evaluation (ADVANCE) study investigated the routine administration of a fixed combination of perindopril (an ACE inhibitor) and indapamide (a diuretic) on major vascular outcomes in patients with type 2 diabetes at elevated cardiovascular risks[58]. The trial showed that AF is a strong, independent marker of overall mortality and cardiovascular events in diabetics. The study emphasizes the greater absolute benefit that would be expected from routine blood pressure-lowering treatment for patients with type 2 diabetes and coexisting AF. These findings are of direct relevance for the routine clinical management of diabetic patients and indicate that detection of AF in a patient with diabetes should prompt more aggressive treatment of all cardiovascular risk factors[59]. Ueng et al. demonstrated that the most important variable to predict the recurrence of AF after successful electrical cardioversion is LA size > 40 mm prior to cardioversion. They showed that use of enalapril (an ACE inhibitor) to prevent AF recurrence was most effective in this subgroup of patients[44].

Results from clinical CHF trials

Chronic atrial dilatation due to systolic HF has been shown to lead to increased AF vulnerability, both in experimental animal models[60,61] and in patients. Thirty to forty percent of HF patients will develop AF during the course of the disease[62]. When AF develops, it is associated with increased morbidity and mortality[42]. Sanders et al.[63] demonstrated that patients with chronic HF and no prior atrial arrhythmias have significant atrial remodelling, characterized by anatomic and structural changes. These include atrial enlargement, regions of low voltage and scarring, abnormalities of conduction with widespread conduction slowing and anatomically determined conduction delay or block, increased refractoriness and sinus node dysfunction. These abnormalities were associated with an increased inducibility and sustainability of AF.

Treatment of HF has been shown to reduce the incidence of AF in experimental models and clinical studies. Interestingly, in this setting, the renin–angiotensin II system appears to play a substantial role in reducing AF. Experimental studies revealed that the antiarrhythmic effects of ACE inhibitors and ARB related to their effect on atrial morphology and structure[40,64]. The findings are clearly supported by retrospective analyses of several clinical trials [Valsartan Heart Failure Trial (Val-HeFT), Studies of Left Ventricular Dysfunction (SOLVD), Candesartan in Heart Failure – Assessment of Reduction in Mortality and Morbidity (CHARM)][65].

Furthermore, the Randomized Aldactone Evaluation Study (RALES) trial clearly showed that spironolactone (an aldosterone antagonist) reduces circulating pro-collagen I and III levels in patients with HF, which was associated with an improved survival[66].

Conclusions and outlook

The results of many clinical studies support the relevance of MEC in atrial tissue. Although not all mechanisms of the underlying processes are yet fully understood, comorbidities causing volume and/or pressure overload have a strong impact on electrophysiological and morphological properties of human atria, which may facilitate the occurrence of AF.

Acute atrial volume and pressure changes have been demonstrated to affect electrophysiological properties, with (at least initially) reversible changes in conduction and refractoriness. Long-term volumetric and pressure load changes, however, also lead to morphological changes (interstitial matrix alterations leading to atrial dilatation, hypertrophy of myocytes, fibrosis, etc.) fostering AF habituation. Hypertension is the most common concomitant disease in patients with AF. Experimental and clinical data imply that inhibition of the renin–angiotensin II system has several positive effects in reducing blood pressure and attenuating pressure-induced ultrastructural atrial changes. These effects appear to be of particular importance for primary prevention of AF. Nevertheless, the 'true' effect of ACE inhibitors and ARB for secondary prevention of AF has not been well defined. Further studies are warranted to delineate the true benefit of 'upstream therapy' in AF. These studies should provide more facts on cellular mechanisms and the time course of upstream therapy influencing MEC in AF. One study currently underway is CREATIVE-AF (Impact of Irbesartan on Oxidative Stress and C-Reactive Protein Levels in Patients with Persistent Atrial Fibrillation), testing the effects of angiotensin receptor blockade on adhesion molecules and inflammatory markers in AF[67]. If results are promising, further prospective studies should evaluate upstream therapy effects in patients at risk for developing AF in the future. In addition, novel ion channel and non-ion channel drug targets need further investigational evaluation in upstream and downstream AF treatment[68].

References

1. Go AS, Hylek EM, Phillips KA, *et al.* Prevalence of diagnosed atrial fibrillation in adults: national implications for rhythm management and stroke prevention: the AnTicoagulation and Risk Factors in Atrial Fibrillation (ATRIA) Study. *JAMA* 2001;**285**:2370–2375.
2. Miyasaka Y, Barnes ME, Gersh BJ, *et al.* Secular trends in incidence of atrial fibrillation in Olmsted County, Minnesota, 1980 to 2000, and implications on the projections for future prevalence. *Circulation* 2006;**114**:119–125.
3. Wolf PA, Benjamin EJ, Belanger AJ, Kannel WB, Levy D, D'Agostino RB. Secular trends in the prevalence of atrial fibrillation: The Framingham Study. *Am Heart J* 1996;**131**:790–795.
4. Benjamin EJ, Wolf PA, D'Agostino RB, Silbershatz H, Kannel WB, Levy D. Impact of atrial fibrillation on the risk of death: the Framingham Heart Study. *Circulation* 1998;**98**:946–952.
5. Stewart S, Hart CL, Hole DJ, McMurray JJ. A population-based study of the long-term risks associated with atrial fibrillation: 20-year follow-up of the Renfrew/Paisley study. *Am J Med* 2002;**113**:359–364.
6. Wolf PA, Abbott RD, Kannel WB. Atrial fibrillation as an independent risk factor for stroke: the Framingham Study. *Stroke* 1991;**22**:983–988.
7. Wang TJ, Larson MG, Levy D, *et al.* Temporal relations of atrial fibrillation and congestive heart failure and their joint influence on mortality: the Framingham Heart Study. *Circulation* 2003;**107**:2920–2925.
8. Ott A, Breteler MM, de Bruyne MC, van HF, Grobbee DE, Hofman A. Atrial fibrillation and dementia in a population-based study. The Rotterdam Study. *Stroke* 1997;**28**:316–321.
9. Cappato R, Calkins H, Chen SA, *et al.* Worldwide survey on the methods, efficacy, and safety of catheter ablation for human atrial fibrillation. *Circulation* 2005;**111**:1100–1105.
10. Waldo AL. A perspective on antiarrhythmic drug therapy to treat atrial fibrillation: there remains an unmet need. *Am Heart J* 2006;**151**:771–778.
11. Benjamin EJ, Levy D, Vaziri SM, D'Agostino RB, Belanger AJ, Wolf PA. Independent risk factors for atrial fibrillation in a population-based cohort. The Framingham Heart Study. *JAMA* 1994;**271**:840–844.
12. Hobbs WJ, Fynn S, Todd DM, Wolfson P, Galloway M, Garratt CJ. Reversal of atrial electrical remodeling after cardioversion of persistent atrial fibrillation in humans. *Circulation* 2000;**101**:1145–1151.
13. Franz MR, Karasik PL, Li C, Moubarak J, Chavez M. Electrical remodeling of the human atrium: similar effects in patients with chronic atrial fibrillation and atrial flutter. *J Am Coll Cardiol* 1997;**30**:1785–1792.
14. Klein LS, Miles WM, Zipes DP. Effect of atrioventricular interval during pacing or reciprocating tachycardia on atrial size, pressure, and refractory period. Contraction-excitation feedback in human atrium. *Circulation* 1990;**82**:60–68.
15. Fan K, Lee KL, Chow WH, Chau E, Lau CP. Internal cardioversion of chronic atrial fibrillation during percutaneous mitral commissuro-tomy: insight into reversal of chronic stretch-induced atrial remodeling. *Circulation* 2002;**105**:2746–2752.
16. Calkins H, el-Atassi R, Kalbfleisch S, Langberg J, Morady F. Effects of an acute increase in atrial pressure on atrial refractoriness in humans. *Pacing Clin Electrophysiol* 1992;**15**:1674–1680.
17. Mitchell GF, Vasan RS, Keyes MJ, *et al.* Pulse pressure and risk of new-onset atrial fibrillation. *JAMA* 2007;**297**:709–715.
18. Conen D, Tedrow UB, Koplan BA, Glynn RJ, Buring JE, Albert CM. Influence of systolic and diastolic blood pressure on the risk of incident atrial fibrillation in women. *Circulation* 2009;**119**:2146–2152.
19. Katritsis DG, Toumpoulis IK, Giazitzoglou E, *et al.* Latent arterial hypertension in apparently lone atrial fibrillation. *J Interv Card Electrophysiol* 2005;**13**:203–207.
20. Mureddu GF, Cioffi G, Stefenelli C, Boccanelli A. Relationships of the appropriateness of left ventricular mass to left atrial size and function in arterial hypertension. *J Cardiovasc Med (Hagerstown)* 2007;**8**:445–452.
21. Triantafyllidi H, Ikonomidis I, Lekakis J, *et al.* Pulse pressure determines left atrial enlargement in non-dipper patients with never-treated essential hypertension. *J Hum Hypertens* 2007;**21**:897–899.
22. Vaziri SM, Larson MG, Lauer MS, Benjamin EJ, Levy D. Influence of blood pressure on left atrial size. The Framingham Heart Study. *Hypertension* 1995;**25**:1155–1160.
23. Schotten U, Neuberger HR, Allessie MA. The role of atrial dilatation in the domestication of atrial fibrillation. *Prog Biophys Mol Biol* 2003;**82**:151–162.

24. Kannel WB, Wolf PA, Benjamin EJ, Levy D. Prevalence, incidence, prognosis, and predisposing conditions for atrial fibrillation: population-based estimates. *Am J Cardiol* 1998;**82**:2N–9N.

25. Aytemir K, Amasyali B, Abali G, *et al*. The signal-averaged P-wave duration is longer in hypertensive patients with history of paroxysmal atrial fibrillation as compared to those without. *Int J Cardiol* 2005;**103**:37–40.

26. Sparks PB, Mond HG, Vohra JK, Jayaprakash S, Kalman JM. Electrical remodeling of the atria following loss of atrioventricular synchrony: a long-term study in humans. *Circulation* 1999;**100**:1894–1900.

27. Gottdiener JS, Reda DJ, Williams DW, Materson BJ, Cushman W, Anderson RJ. Effect of single-drug therapy on reduction of left atrial size in mild to moderate hypertension: comparison of six antihypertensive agents. *Circulation* 1998;**98**:140–148.

28. Milan A, Caserta MA, Dematteis A, *et al*. Blood pressure levels, left ventricular mass and function are correlated with left atrial volume in mild to moderate hypertensive patients. *J Hum Hypertens* 2009;**23**: 743–750.

29. Krahn AD, Manfreda J, Tate RB, Mathewson FA, Cuddy TE. The natural history of atrial fibrillation: incidence, risk factors, and prognosis in the Manitoba Follow-Up Study. *Am J Med* 1995;**98**: 476–484.

30. Burt VL, Whelton P, Roccella EJ, *et al*. Prevalence of hypertension in the US adult population. Results from the Third National Health and Nutrition Examination Survey, 1988-1991. *Hypertension* 1995;**25**: 305–313.

31. Cox DR. Regression Models and Life Tables. *Journal of the Royal Statistical Society Series B* 1972;**34**:187–220.

32. Mitchell GF, Parise H, Benjamin EJ, *et al*. Changes in arterial stiffness and wave reflection with advancing age in healthy men and women: the Framingham Heart Study. *Hypertension* 2004;**43**:1239–1245.

33. Gardin JM, Arnold A, Gottdiener JS, *et al*. Left ventricular mass in the elderly. The Cardiovascular Health Study. *Hypertension* 1997;**29**: 1095–1103.

34. Hundley WG, Kitzman DW, Morgan TM, *et al*. Cardiac cycle-dependent changes in aortic area and distensibility are reduced in older patients with isolated diastolic heart failure and correlate with exercise intolerance. *J Am Coll Cardiol*, 2001;**38**:796–802.

35. Zile MR, Gaasch WH. Mechanical loads and the isovolumic and filling indices of left ventricular relaxation. *Prog Cardiovasc Dis* 1990;**32**: 333–346.

36. Leite-Moreira AF, Correia-Pinto J, Gillebert TC. Afterload induced changes in myocardial relaxation: a mechanism for diastolic dysfunction. *Cardiovasc Res* 1999;**43**:344–353.

37. Tsang TS, Gersh BJ, Appleton CP, *et al*. Left ventricular diastolic dysfunction as a predictor of the first diagnosed nonvalvular atrial fibrillation in 840 elderly men and women. *J Am Coll Cardiol* 2002;**40**:1636–1644.

38. Goette A, Staack T, Rocken C, *et al*. Increased expression of extracellular signal-regulated kinase and angiotensin-converting enzyme in human atria during atrial fibrillation. *J Am Coll Cardiol* 2000;**35**:1669–1677.

39. Goette A, Arndt M, Rocken C, *et al*. Regulation of angiotensin II receptor subtypes during atrial fibrillation in humans. *Circulation* 2000;**101**:2678–2681.

40. Healey JS, Baranchuk A, Crystal E, *et al*. Prevention of atrial fibrillation with angiotensin-converting enzyme inhibitors and angiotensin receptor blockers: a meta-analysis. *J Am Coll Cardiol* 2005;**45**:1832–1839.

41. Wachtell K, Lehto M, Gerdts E, *et al*. Angiotensin II receptor blockade reduces new-onset atrial fibrillation and subsequent stroke compared to atenolol: the Losartan Intervention For End Point Reduction in Hypertension (LIFE) study. *J Am Coll Cardiol* 2005;**45**:712–719.

42. Wang TJ, Larson MG, Levy D, *et al*. Temporal relations of atrial fibrillation and congestive heart failure and their joint influence on mortality: the Framingham Heart Study. *Circulation* 2003;**107**: 2920–2925.

43. Webster MW, Fitzpatrick MA, Nicholls MG, Ikram H, Wells JE. Effect of enalapril on ventricular arrhythmias in congestive heart failure. *Am J Cardiol* 1985;**56**:566–569.

44. Ueng KC, Tsai TP, Yu WC, *et al*. Use of enalapril to facilitate sinus rhythm maintenance after external cardioversion of long-standing persistent atrial fibrillation. Results of a prospective and controlled study. *Eur Heart J* 2003;**24**:2090–2098.

45. Kalifa J, Jalife J, Zaitsev AV, *et al*. Intra-atrial pressure increases rate and organization of waves emanating from the superior pulmonary veins during atrial fibrillation. *Circulation* 2003;**108**:668–671.

46. Clementy J, Safar M, Vrancea F. [Cardiac arrhythmia in moderate arterial hypertension. Epidemiologic survey of 251 cases. Effect of sotalol]. *Ann Cardiol Angeiol (Paris)* 1989;**38**:47–51.

47. Heckbert SR, Wiggins KL, Glazer NL, *et al*. Antihypertensive treatment with ACE inhibitors or beta-blockers and risk of incident atrial fibrillation in a general hypertensive population. *Am J Hypertens* 2009;**22**:538–544.

48. Dagres N, Karatasakis G, Panou F, *et al*. Pre-treatment with Irbesartan attenuates left atrial stunning after electrical cardioversion of atrial fibrillation. *Eur Heart J* 2006;**27**:2062–2068.

49. Ekbom T, Linjer E, Hedner T, *et al*. Cardiovascular events in elderly patients with isolated systolic hypertension. A subgroup analysis of treatment strategies in STOP-Hypertension-2. *Blood Press* 2004;**13**:137–141.

50. Vaziri SM, Larson MG, Benjamin EJ, Levy D. Echocardiographic predictors of nonrheumatic atrial fibrillation. The Framingham Heart Study. *Circulation* 1994;**89**:724–730.

51. Verdecchia P, Reboldi G, Gattobigio R, *et al*. Atrial fibrillation in hypertension: predictors and outcome. *Hypertension* 2003;**41**:218–223.

52. Okin PM, Devereux RB, Jern S, *et al*. Regression of electrocardiographic left ventricular hypertrophy by losartan versus atenolol: The Losartan Intervention for Endpoint reduction in Hypertension (LIFE) Study. *Circulation* 2003;**108**:684–690.

53. Okin PM, Devereux RB, Jern S, *et al*. Regression of electrocardiographic left ventricular hypertrophy during antihypertensive treatment and the prediction of major cardiovascular events. *JAMA* 2004;**292**:2343–2349.

54. Molloy TJ, Okin PM, Devereux RB, Kligfield P. Electrocardiographic detection of left ventricular hypertrophy by the simple QRS voltage-duration product. *J Am Coll Cardiol* 1992;**20**:1180–1186.

55. Okin PM, Wachtell K, Devereux RB, *et al*. Regression of electrocardiographic left ventricular hypertrophy and decreased incidence of new-onset atrial fibrillation in patients with hypertension. *JAMA* 2006;**296**:1242–1248.

56. Movahed MR, Hashemzadeh M, Jamal MM. Diabetes mellitus is a strong, independent risk for atrial fibrillation and flutter in addition to other cardiovascular disease. *Int J Cardiol* 2005;**105**:315–318.

57. Ostgren CJ, Merlo J, Rastam L, Lindblad U. Atrial fibrillation and its association with type 2 diabetes and hypertension in a Swedish community. *Diabetes Obes Metab* 2004;**6**:367–374.

58. Institute for International Health. Study rationale and design of ADVANCE: action in diabetes and vascular disease – preterax and diamicron MR controlled evaluation. *Diabetologia* 2001;**44**: 1118–1120.

59. Du X, Ninomiya T, de Galan B, *et al*.; on behalf of the ADVANCE Collaborative Group. Risks of cardiovascular events and effects of routine blood pressure lowering among patients with type 2 diabetes and atrial fibrillation: results of the ADVANCE study. *Eur Heart J* 2009;**30**:1128–1135.

60. Shinagawa K, Shi YF, Tardif JC, Leung TK, Nattel S. Dynamic nature of atrial fibrillation substrate during development and reversal of heart failure in dogs. *Circulation* 2002;**105**:2672–2678.

61. Nattel S, Shiroshita-Takeshita A, Brundel BJ, Rivard L. Mechanisms of atrial fibrillation: lessons from animal models. *Prog Cardiovasc Dis* 2005;**48**:9–28.

62. Stevenson WG, Stevenson LW. Atrial fibrillation in heart failure. *N Engl J Med* 1999;**341**:910–911.

63. Sanders P, Morton JB, Kistler PM, Vohra JK, Kalman JM, Sparks PB. Reversal of atrial mechanical dysfunction after cardioversion of atrial fibrillation: implications for the mechanisms of tachycardia-mediated atrial cardiomyopathy. *Circulation* 2003;**108**:1976–1984.

64. Hammwöhner M, D'Alessandro A, Dobrev D, Kirchhof P, Goette A. New antiarrhythmic drugs for therapy of atrial fibrillation: II. Non-ion channel blockers. *Herzschr Elektrophys* 2006;**17**:73–80.

65. Ehrlich JR, Hohnloser SH, Nattel S. Role of angiotensin system and effects of its inhibition in atrial fibrillation: clinical and experimental evidence. *Eur Heart J* 2006;**27**:512–518.

66. Zannad F, Alla F, Dousset B, Perez A, Pitt B. Limitation of excessive extracellular matrix turnover may contribute to survival benefit of spironolactone therapy in patients with congestive heart failure: insights from the randomized aldactone evaluation study (RALES). Rales Investigators. *Circulation* 2000;**102**:2700–2706.

67. Goette A, D'Alessandro A, Bukowska A, *et al.* Rationale for and design of the CREATIVE-AF trial: randomized, double-blind, placebo-controlled, crossover study of the effect of irbesartan on oxidative stress and adhesion molecules in patients with persistent atrial fibrillation. *Clin Drug Investig* 2008;**28**:565–572.

68. Hammwöhner M, Smid J, Lendeckel U, Goette A. New drugs for atrial fibrillation. *J Interv Card Electrophysiol* 2008;**23**:15–21.

Evidence for mechano-electric coupling from clinical trials on heart failure

Paulus Kirchhof and Günter Breithardt

Background

Heart failure (HF) is a major cause of death, hospitalizations and reduced quality of life in developed countries[1]. Usually, HF is a consequence of left ventricular dysfunction (systolic or diastolic). The initial damage to the heart may have different aetiologies such as myocardial infarction and chronic ischaemic heart disease[2], an inherited contractile cardiac dysfunction[3], tachycardiomyopathy and extra-cardiac diseases such as arterial hypertension. Independent of the initial damaging factor, the increased work load of the (remaining) myocardium can intensify the damage conferred to the heart and aggravate HF. Increased intracellular calcium accumulation, shifts of calcium between different cellular compartments and increased death rates (apoptosis) of the 'overworked' cardiomyocytes probably mediate this process, which has been summarized as 'ventricular remodelling'. Many aspects of this complex adaptive process relate to 'chronic' mechano-electric coupling (MEC). Their pathophysiology is discussed in earlier chapters of this book. Unfortunately, a maladaptive vicious cycle based on these processes may develop which maintains and intensifies left ventricular dysfunction as a consequence of chronically increased work load of the left ventricle.

Patients with heart failure often die from arrhythmic mechanisms

Approximately every second HF patient dies suddenly[1]. Although a documentation of the heart rhythm during the clinical event that leads to death is usually not available, it is reasonable to assume that the majority of these deaths are arrhythmic and usually caused by ventricular fibrillation or rapid ventricular tachycardia[4]. Especially in patients in whom sudden arrhythmia occurs as a consequence of deteriorating left ventricular function, sudden cardiac death (SCD) in HF is a sign of MEC 'gone wrong'.

Reduced left ventricular ejection fraction identifies patients at risk for sudden arrhythmic death

The implantable cardioverter defibrillator (ICD)[5,6] protects patients from SCD due to ventricular fibrillation as an 'implanted emergency system'. Implantation of a ICD improves survival in patients at high risk for SCD[7]. The possibility to protect patients at risk for SCD by an ICD spurred a long search for clinical parameters that could identify patients at risk for sudden death: while a physician usually waits for a disease to occur, prevention of sudden death requires identification of subjects at risk before the first manifestation of those ventricular arrhythmias that are often lethal.

Many invasive and non-invasive markers have been proposed and tested to identify patients at risk for sudden death, but, to date, this diagnostic need is still partially unmet. The single most powerful predictor of SCD in patients with heart disease is the presence of a markedly reduced left ventricular contractile function, usually assessed by reduced left ventricular ejection fraction. In such patients, implantation of a ICD improves survival by preventing ventricular arrhythmic death[7–10].

Left ventricular volume may relate better to outcome than ejection fraction

The major multicentre clinical trials that demonstrated a survival benefit of ICD implantation often used left ventricular ejection fraction as the clinical measure to quantify the degree of left ventricular HF. This measure is adequate for clinical trials because its ratiometric nature allows comparison of values almost independent of the measurement technique. Such a ratio, on the other hand, reduces the amount of information markedly. Interestingly, left ventricular volume – a non-ratiometric measurement that is therefore less well applicable in large-scale clinical trials – appears to be a better predictor of outcome in HF, suggesting that chronic dilation (and its implicit mechano-electric feedback mechanisms) may be more relevant to outcome than contractile function alone.

A landmark study that related excessive ventricular dilatation to an increased mortality after myocardial infarction came from White and co-workers[11]. They showed that left ventricular end-systolic volume (ESV) was a major determinant of survival and had a greater predictive value than end-diastolic volume (EDV) or ejection fraction (EF). Stepwise analysis showed that once the relationship between survival and end-systolic volume had been fitted, there was no additional significant predictive information in either end-diastolic volume or ejection fraction. When EF and ESV were compared in individual patients, addition of ESV clearly added prognostic power to stratification of mortality risk by EF alone[11].

Their conclusion that treatment of infarction should be aimed at limitation of infarct size and prevention of ventricular dilatation is even more a goal as it was in 1987.

Infarct expansion occurs between 3 days and 2 weeks after infarction, and patients showing expansion by 10–21 days after transmural infarction may continue to have expansion over a period of 3–30 months[12]. Infarct expansion would increase left ventricular systolic and diastolic volumes, with a resultant increase in wall stress, which in turn may act as a stimulus to cardiac hypertrophy.

Drugs that prevent ventricular remodelling reduce sudden death rates

Ventricular remodelling is, at least in part, mediated by chronic activation of myocardial signalling pathways that were designed to allow acute adaptation of cardiac function to increased demands. These signalling pathways are chronically activated in failing hearts (Fig. 56.1).

Prognosis in HF patients can be improved by a cocktail of drugs that interrupt myocardial signalling pathways, which was evolutionarily helpful in allowing an acute, rapid increase in cardiac performance. These drugs, ß-adrenoreceptor blockers, angiotensin converting enzyme (ACE) inhibitors and aldosterone antagonists,

prevent the process of left ventricular remodelling, i.e. progressive dilation of the left ventricle, and thereby improve survival in patients with severe HF. Interestingly, many of these substances not only prevent deterioration of haemodynamic left ventricular function – usually the main motivation for therapy and the main outcome in controlled trials – but also reduce sudden death rates (Table 56.1). It is very likely that the antiarrhythmic effects of these therapies are in part attributable to preventing a proarrhythmic milieu in the failing left ventricle that is most likely related to cardiomyocyte hypertrophy (see Chapter 32) and to increased interstitial fibrosis and subsequent conduction disturbances (Fig. 56.2).

Inhibition of the angiotensin receptor (or of the conversion of angiotensin I to angiotensin II) reduces activation of profibrotic signalling in the heart, prevents formation of extracellular matrix and may even have direct effects on cardiac repolarization, although the latter effect is rather small. This 'antifibrotic' effect of ACE inhibitors or angiotensin receptor inhibitors therefore likely improves electrical contacts between cardiomyocytes and may thereby prevent both formation of re-entrant arrhythmias and triggered activity. These effects are likely candidates to explain the effects of ACE inhibitors on sudden death rates in HF patients[13,14].

Pharmacological inhibition of ß-adrenoreceptors prevents excessive sympathetic stimulation in the heart and can thereby prevent intracellular calcium overload, increased pre- and afterload of

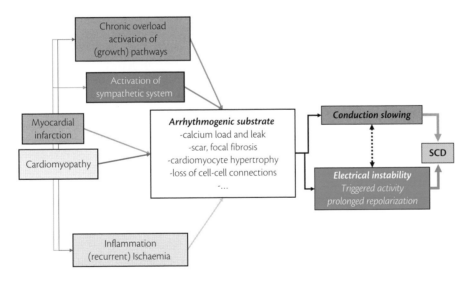

Fig. 56.1 Myocardial damage pathways in heart failure (HF) that may lead to sudden cardiac death (SCD). An initial damage to the heart, often a myocardial infarction, but also as a consequence of other external damaging factors or of an inherited cardiomyopathy, damages a portion of or the whole left ventricle. The remaining myocardium attempts to maintain contractile function by activation of several acutely force-conserving signalling pathways which help to increase cardiac function acutely. Unfortunately, these signalling pathways persevere chronic damage to the heart, thereby creating a vicious circle of 'left ventricular remodelling'.

Table 56.1 Recommended drug therapies in HF with known prognostic benefit and their effects on SCD. While the main therapeutic effect, and the main outcome tested in clinical trials, is usually stabilization of contractile and haemodynamic function and improvement in overall survival, some therapies have antiarrhythmic effects and prevent SCD.

Class of drugs	Effect on sudden (presumably arrhythmic) death in HF populations
Beta-blockers	Reduce sudden death rates in meta-analyses, especially in survivors of a myocardial infarction[15,16]
Aldosterone-antagonists (spironolactone and eplerenone)	Reduce sudden death rates as secondary outcome in controlled trials[17,18]
Angiotensin converting enzyme (ACE) inhibitors and angiotensin-receptor inhibitors (ART)	Reduce sudden death rates in meta-analysis (demonstrated for ACE inhibitors; likely but not shown for ART)[13,14]

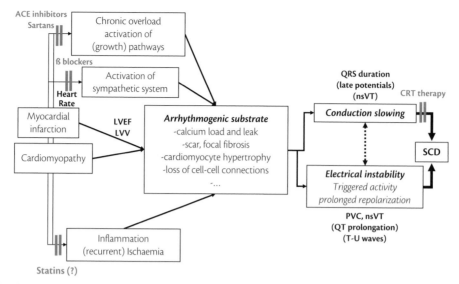

Fig. 56.2 Diagnostic markers for SCD in HF (black) and therapeutic modalities known to affect SCD in HF (red). The markers and therapeutic options are placed in their putative position within the vicious circles that convey myocardial damage and death in HF. The best markers for SCD in HF directly relate to left ventricular function or volume, and many of the interventions that disrupt deleterious myocardial signalling in HF prevent SCD. Most of the diagnostic markers and most of the drug interventions relate to mechano-electric coupling, while QRS duration and CRT therapy relate to 'reverse' mechano-electric coupling. LVEF, left ventricular ejection fraction; LVV, left ventricular volume; CRT, cardiac resynchronization; PVC, premature ventricular contractions; nsVT, non-sustained ventricular tachycardia; SCD, sudden cardiac death.

the left ventricle, cellular mechanisms of triggered activity, abnormal cardiomyocyte growth and cardiac hypertrophy. A combination of these effects is likely to convey the effects of β-blockers on prevention of SCD in clinical trials[15,16].

Inhibition of aldosterone-mediated gene expression reduces mortality when added to ß-blocker and ACE inhibitor therapy, at least in patients with severe HF[17,18]. In the context of this chapter, it is remarkable that eplerenone reduced the risk for sudden death numerically more than the total death rate[18].

Furthermore, HF also activates pro-inflammatory signalling cascades in the heart[19–22]. While there is no direct evidence for this hypothesis, it is conceivable that statins reduce sudden death rate not only through prevention of acute coronary syndromes, but also through modulation of abnormally increased myocardial inflammation[23].

Electromechanics reversed: improving electrical activation of the left ventricle improves outcome in heart failure

Prolongation of the QRS complex is associated with death in heart failure patients

Abnormal electrical activation of the ventricles can result in inefficient contraction of the left ventricle, resulting in an impaired stroke volume. This is probably one of the reasons why patients with prolonged QRS interval on the surface electrocardiogram (ECG) suffer from a poorer prognosis than persons with a narrow QRS complex[24–26]. While most analyses of QRS duration and outcome included a majority of patients who survived a myocardial infarction, prolongation of the QRS complex may also be associated with outcome in dilative cardiomyopathy[27].

Electrical 'resynchronization' by biventricular stimulation improves survival in heart failure patients with prolonged QRS duration

In the past 5 years, several large trials have shown that an electrical therapy aimed at reversing asynchronous electrical activation, termed 'cardiac resynchronization therapy' (CRT), can improve outcomes in patients with left bundle branch block, reduced left ventricular ejection fraction and clinically overt HF[28–32]. In patients with a prolonged QRS complex and reduced left ventricular ejection fraction, resynchronization therapy improves survival on top of ICD therapy, suggesting that resynchronization therapy improves HF and prevents deaths related to haemodynamic compromise[33]. Thereby, this electrical therapy improves contractile function, representing clinical evidence for 'reverse MEC' or 'electro-mechanic coupling' (EMC).

CRT aims at synchronizing left contraction through optimally timed electrical activation of the lateral and septal left ventricular wall. This is done in clinical practice through 'biventricular' pacing that allows electrical stimulation from the (right ventricular) apical septum and the lateral left ventricular wall. The timing between these two stimuli is optimized to achieve synchronous contraction of the septal and lateral left ventricular wall. When such 'biventricular stimulation' therapy is applied in patients with evidence of asynchronous electrical activation – identified by a long QRS complex duration – biventricular stimulation improves survival[30]. In fact, a pooled analysis of data from several resynchronization trials suggests that the degree of QRS prolongation prior to implantation of a CRT device and the degree of QRS shortening on therapy are among the best predictors of those patients who will benefit from this therapy[32]. Applying such therapy aimed at improving electrical activation of the left ventricle to patients with narrow QRS complexes, in contrast, does not improve outcome[34–36].

The survival benefit of CRT in HF patients with a broad QRS complex is conveyed by improved contractile function and prevention of haemodynamic failure as well as by prevention of SCD – both in trials that implanted a biventricular pacemaker 'only'[29] and in trials that implanted a biventricular pacemaker with the capacity to defibrillate the heart as well[30]. The recently published Multicenter Automatic Defibrillator Implantation Trial with Cardiac Resynchronization Therapy (MADIT-CRT) trial in early stages of HF [partly New York Heart Association (NYHA) class I and mostly class II patients] with markedly reduced left ventricular ejection fraction strongly suggests that a main effect of resynchronization therapy is prevention of haemodynamic deterioration and 'HF events'[33]. It is worthy of note that resynchronization therapy in MADIT-CRT did not prevent deaths ($p = 0.99$) in a population where mortality was low anyway, but markedly reduced HF hospitalizations. Furthermore, the effect on HF events was very similar in patients with low or high left ventricular volumes[33]. At present, it is not clear to what extent the prevention of SCD by CRT is conveyed by the ICD function of most devices or by an indirect effect of 'reverse MEC'.

Conclusions and outlook

Data from clinical trials in HF can only convey indirect information on the clinical impact of MEC. Detailed pathophysiological, mechanistic studies are difficult to conduct. Within this limitation, there is ample indirect evidence for MEC and EMC:

♦ MEC 1: Reduced left ventricular function and – probably related better to outcome – increased left ventricular systole volume strongly associates with lethal ventricular arrhythmias.

♦ MEC 2: Drugs that preserve left ventricular function in HF patients also prevent SCD to a certain degree. This effect is mediated via disruption of chronically activated myocardial signalling pathways.

♦ EMC: Electrical resynchronization of left ventricular activation prevents deterioration of left ventricular function in patients with HF and abnormal left ventricular electrical activation, most likely by improving cardiac mechanical function.

References

1. Dickstein K, Cohen-Solal A, Filippatos G, *et al*. ESC Guidelines for the diagnosis and treatment of acute and chronic heart failure 2008: the Task Force for the Diagnosis and Treatment of Acute and Chronic Heart Failure 2008 of the European Society of Cardiology. Developed in collaboration with the Heart Failure Association of the ESC (HFA) and endorsed by the European Society of Intensive Care Medicine (ESICM). *Eur Heart J* 2008;**29**:2388–2442.

2. Gheorghiade M, Bonow RO. Chronic heart failure in the United States: a manifestation of coronary artery disease. *Circulation* 1998;**97**:282–289.

3. Maron BJ, Towbin JA, Thiene G, *et al*. Contemporary definitions and classification of the cardiomyopathies: an American Heart Association Scientific Statement from the Council on Clinical Cardiology, Heart Failure and Transplantation Committee; Quality of Care and Outcomes Research and Functional Genomics and Translational Biology Interdisciplinary Working Groups; and Council on Epidemiology and Prevention. *Circulation* 2006;**113**:1807–1816.

4. Hinkle LE, Jr., Thaler HT. Clinical classification of cardiac deaths. *Circulation* 1982;**65**:457–464.

5. Mirowski M, Mower MM, Staeven WS, Tabatznik B, Mendeloff AI. Standby automatic defibrillator: an approach to prevention of sudden coronary death. *Arch Intern Med* 1970;**126**:158–161.

6. Mirowski M, Reid PR, Mower MM, *et al*. Clinical experience with the automatic implantable defibrillator. *Arch Mal Coeur Vaiss* 1985;**78**:39–42.

7. Zipes DP, Camm AJ, Borggrefe M, *et al*. ACC/AHA/ESC 2006 guidelines for management of patients with ventricular arrhythmias and the prevention of sudden cardiac death – executive summary: a report of the American College of Cardiology/American Heart Association Task Force and the European Society of Cardiology Committee for Practice Guidelines (Writing Committee to Develop Guidelines for Management of Patients with Ventricular Arrhythmias and the Prevention of Sudden Cardiac Death) Developed in collaboration with the European Heart Rhythm Association and the Heart Rhythm Society. *Eur Heart J* 2006;**27**:2099–2140.

8. Moss AJ, Hall WJ, Cannom DS, *et al*. Improved survival with an implanted defibrillator in patients with coronary disease at high risk for ventricular arrhythmia. Multicenter Automatic Defibrillator Implantation Trial Investigators. *N Engl J Med* 1996;**335**:1933–1940.

9. Moss AJ, Zareba W, Hall WJ, *et al*. Prophylactic implantation of a defibrillator in patients with myocardial infarction and reduced ejection fraction. *N Engl J Med* 2002;**346**:877–883.

10. Nanthakumar K, Epstein AE, Kay GN, Plumb VJ, Lee DS. Prophylactic implantable cardioverter-defibrillator therapy in patients with left ventricular systolic dysfunction: a pooled analysis of 10 primary prevention trials. *J Am Coll Cardiol* 2004;**44**:2166–2172.

11. White HD, Norris RM, Brown MA, Brandt PW, Whitlock RM, Wild CJ. Left ventricular end-systolic volume as the major determinant of survival after recovery from myocardial infarction. *Circulation* 1987;**76**:44–51.

12. Erlebacher JA, Weiss JL, Eaton LW, Kallman C, Weisfeldt ML, Bulkley BH. Late effects of acute infarct dilation on heart size: a two dimensional echocardiographic study. *Am J Cardiol* 1982;**49**:1120–1126.

13. Domanski MJ, Exner DV, Borkowf CB, Geller NL, Rosenberg Y, Pfeffer MA. Effect of angiotensin converting enzyme inhibition on sudden cardiac death in patients following acute myocardial infarction. A meta-analysis of randomized clinical trials. *J Am Coll Cardiol* 1999;**33**:598–604.

14. Granger CB, McMurray JJ, Yusuf S, *et al*. Effects of candesartan in patients with chronic heart failure and reduced left-ventricular systolic function intolerant to angiotensin-converting-enzyme inhibitors: the CHARM-Alternative trial. *Lancet* 2003;**362**:772–776.

15. Huikuri HV, Castellanos A, Myerburg RJ. Sudden death due to cardiac arrhythmias. *N Engl J Med* 2001;**345**:1473–1482.

16. Effect of metoprolol CR/XL in chronic heart failure: Metoprolol CR/XL Randomised Intervention Trial in Congestive Heart Failure (MERIT-HF). *Lancet* 1999;**353**:2001–2007.

17. Pitt B, Zannad F, Remme WJ, *et al*. The effect of spironolactone on morbidity and mortality in patients with severe heart failure. Randomized Aldactone Evaluation Study Investigators. *N Engl J Med* 1999;**341**:709–717.

18. Pitt B, Remme W, Zannad F, *et al*. Eplerenone, a selective aldosterone blocker, in patients with left ventricular dysfunction after myocardial infarction. *N Engl J Med* 2003;**348**:1309–1321.

19. Rohde LE, Ducharme A, Arroyo LH, *et al*. Matrix metalloproteinase inhibition attenuates early left ventricular enlargement after experimental myocardial infarction in mice. *Circulation* 1999;**99**:3063–3070.

20. Nian M, Lee P, Khaper N, Liu P. Inflammatory cytokines and postmyocardial infarction remodeling. *Circ Res* 2004;**94**:1543–1553.

21. Lee KL, Pryor DB, Pieper KS, *et al*. Prognostic value of radionuclide angiography in medically treated patients with coronary artery disease.

A comparison with clinical and catheterization variables. *Circulation* 1990;**82**:1705–1717.

22. Pfeffer MA, Braunwald E. Ventricular remodeling after myocardial infarction. Experimental observations and clinical implications. *Circulation* 1990;**81**:1161–1172.

23. Priori SG, Aliot E, Blomstrom-Lundqvist C, Bossaert L, Breithardt G, Brugada P. Update of the guidelines on sudden cardiac death of the European Society of Cardiology. *Eur Heart J* 2003;**24**:13–15.

24. Bunch TJ, White RD, Bruce GK, *et al.* Prediction of short- and long-term outcomes by electrocardiography in survivors of out-of-hospital cardiac arrest. *Resuscitation* 2004;**63**:137–143.

25. Bode-Schnurbus L, Bocker D, Block M, Gradaus R, Heinecke A, Breithardt G, Borggrefe M. QRS duration: a simple marker for predicting cardiac mortality in ICD patients with heart failure. *Heart* 2003;**89**:1157–1162.

26. Yerra L, Anavekar N, Skali H, *et al.* Association of QRS duration and outcomes after myocardial infarction: the VALIANT trial. *Heart Rhythm* 2006;**3**:313–316.

27. Akar FG, Spragg DD, Tunin RS, Kass DA, Tomaselli GF. Mechanisms underlying conduction slowing and arrhythmogenesis in nonischemic dilated cardiomyopathy. *Circ Res* 2004;**95**:717–725.

28. Young J, Abraham W, Smith A, *et al.* on behalf of the Multicenter InSync ICD Randomized Clinical Evaluation (MIRACLE ICD) Trial Investigators. Combined cardiac resynchronization and implantable cardioversion defibrillation in advanced chronic heart failure: the MIRACLE ICD Trial. *JAMA* 2003;**289**:2685–2694.

29. Cleland JG, Daubert JC, Erdmann E, Freemantle N, Gras D, Kappenberger L, Tavazzi L. The effect of cardiac resynchronization on morbidity and mortality in heart failure. *N Engl J Med* 2005;**352**:1539–1549.

30. Bristow MR, Saxon LA, Boehmer J, *et al.* Cardiac-resynchronization therapy with or without an implantable defibrillator in advanced chronic heart failure. *N Engl J Med* 2004;**350**: 2140–2150.

31. Cleland JG, Daubert JC, Erdmann E, Freemantle N, Gras D, Kappenberger L, Tavazzi L. Longer-term effects of cardiac resynchronization therapy on mortality in heart failure [the CArdiac REsynchronization-Heart Failure (CARE-HF) trial extension phase]. *Eur Heart J* 2006;**27**:1928–1932.

32. McAlister FA, Ezekowitz J, Hooton N, *et al.* Cardiac resynchronization therapy for patients with left ventricular systolic dysfunction: a systematic review. *JAMA* 2007;**297**:2502–2514.

33. Moss A, Hall WJ, Cannom D, *et al.* Cardiac-resynchronization therapy for the prevention of heart-failure events. *N Engl J Med* 2009;**361**: 1329–1338.

34. Beshai JF, Grimm RA, Nagueh SF, *et al.* Cardiac-resynchronization therapy in heart failure with narrow QRS complexes. *N Engl J Med* 2007;**357**:2461–2571.

35. Yu CM, Abraham WT, Bax J, *et al.* Predictors of response to cardiac resynchronization therapy (PROSPECT) – study design. *Am Heart J* 2005;**149**:600–605.

36. van Bommel RJ, Bax JJ, Abraham WT, *et al.* Characteristics of heart failure patients associated with good and poor response to cardiac resynchronization therapy: a PROSPECT (Predictors of Response to CRT) sub-analysis. *Eur Heart J* 2009;**30**:2470–2477.

Mechano-electric coupling and the pathogenesis of arrhythmogenic right ventricular cardiomyopathy

Hayden Huang, Angeliki Asimaki, Frank Marcus and Jeffrey E. Saffitz

Background

Arrhythmogenic right ventricular cardiomyopathy (ARVC) is a primary disease of heart muscle associated with ventricular arrhythmias and/or sudden death which may occur early in the disease before significant structural remodelling and contractile dysfunction develop[1]. It typically affects the right ventricular free wall, although left-dominant and biventricular forms are being increasingly recognized[2]. The characteristic pathological features are degeneration of cardiac myocytes and replacement of healthy heart muscle by fat and fibrous tissue, but the extent of this change can be quite variable and it is not always conspicuous in patients who die suddenly[1].

ARVC is a familial disease, which may affect 1 in 5,000 individuals, although the true incidence may be higher due to reduced penetrance, age-related progression and marked phenotypic variations which are characteristic of this condition. Mutations in genes encoding desmosomal proteins have been identified in ~40% of ARVC patients[3]. Desmosomes are intercellular junction structures that anchor intermediate filaments to membrane-associated plaques to reinforce cell–cell adhesion. Mutations in every known desmosomal gene have been identified in ARVC, including those encoding desmosomal adhesion molecules (desmoglein-2 and desmocollin-2) and intracellular linker proteins of the plakin and catenin families (plakoglobin, plakophilin-2 and desmoplakin)[3,4]. Mutations in non-desmosomal genes have also been implicated in ARVC pathogenesis, including genes encoding the cardiac ryanodine receptor (RyR2)[5], transforming growth factor-β3 (TGF-β3)[6] and trans-membrane protein 43 (TMEM43)[7]. However, in more than half of the cases, no pathogenic mutation has been identified.

Although there has been significant progress in identifying mutations that lead to ARVC, much less is known about how genetic defects in desmosomal proteins cause disease. One hypothesis is that disruption of mechanical linkage between cells under mechanical stress conditions leads to injury and eventual degeneration of cardiac myocytes with subsequent replacement by fat and fibrous tissue. Remodelling of gap junctions has also been reported in ARVC, suggesting that abnormalities of cell–cell adhesion may prevent normal assembly and/or maintenance of gap junctions, which, in turn, could alter conduction and act synergistically with the structural defects of ARVC to promote ventricular arrhythmias[8,9]. If these hypotheses are correct, then ARVC would be an important example of a disease in which altered mechano-electric (MEC) coupling plays a major pathogenic role. However, the data supporting these hypotheses are limited. This chapter reviews current information about disease mechanisms in ARVC. First, we review some recent work implicating dislocation of plakoglobin (also known as γ-catenin) from intercalated disks in ventricular myocardium in patients with ARVC. Then we review observations on potential alterations in cell biomechanics caused by expression of mutant forms of plakoglobin implicated in causing ARVC. We discuss MEC in ARVC as a potential link between the desmosome and remodelling of gap junctions.

Altered distribution of plakoglobin occurs in ARVC

Initial studies implicating abnormal sub-cellular localization of desmosomal proteins in ARVC were focused on Naxos disease[8] and Carvajal syndrome[9], rare cardiocutaneous syndromes caused by recessive mutations resulting in truncation of the C-terminal portions of plakoglobin and desmoplakin, respectively. The clinical phenotypes of these severe, highly penetrant syndromes include cardiomyopathies that are similar to autosomal dominant ARVC. Analysis of myocardial tissues revealed that immunoreactive signal for the intracellular desmosomal linker protein plakoglobin failed to localize properly at cell–cell junctions in both Naxos disease[8] and Carvajal syndrome[9].

More recent studies have involved analysis of tissues from patients with more common forms of ARVC inherited in a dominant pattern[10]. To determine whether altered distribution of plakoglobin is a consistent feature of ARVC, we performed immunohistochemical analysis on cardiac tissue samples from 11 subjects with ARVC but no skin or hair abnormalities. Eight subjects had a documented desmosomal gene mutation, whereas the remaining three had no identifiable desmosomal gene mutation despite careful analysis of candidate genes. In every case, immunoreactive signal for plakoglobin was reduced at intercalated disks, while strong signal was present in myocardium obtained from ten control subjects with no clinical or pathological evidence of heart disease (Fig. 57.1)[10]. Signal levels for other desmosomal proteins such as plakophilin-2 and desmoplakin were reduced at intercalated disks in some patients with ARVC but appeared normal in others. However, all 11 samples showed a clear reduction in the amount of immunoreactive signal for the major ventricular gap junction protein, connexin43 (Cx43) (Fig. 57.1). Junctional plakoglobin and Cx43 signal levels were reduced in right ventricular regions showing typical pathological changes of fibrofatty replacement but also in normal-appearing left ventricle and interventricular septum, including the sub-endocardium in these areas[10].

To determine whether a reduced junctional signal level for plakoglobin is specific for ARVC or merely a marker of heart disease, tissue samples from 15 subjects with end-stage hypertrophic, dilated or ischaemic cardiomyopathies were analyzed. In every case, plakoglobin signal at intercalated disks was strong and indistinguishable from controls. These observations suggest that loss of normal levels of plakoglobin and Cx43 at cell–cell junctions occurs commonly in ARVC[10]. Because plakoglobin can participate in signalling functions regulated by Wnt pathways, these results also raise the possibility that dislocation of plakoglobin from desmosomes may be an important component of a disease pathogenesis pathway involving aberrant signalling[11]. However, the extent to which this interesting 'molecular pathology' reflects altered biomechanical properties of the myocardium and/or contributes to disease expression cannot be determined from simple immunohistochemical studies. Additional studies are required to address these important questions.

ARVC mutations in plakoglobin alter cellular responses to mechanical load

Two different mutations in plakoglobin have been linked to the development of ARVC. The first to be identified was the recessive mutation that causes Naxos disease. This 2-bp deletion (2157del2) introduces a premature stop codon resulting in truncation of 56 amino acids from the C-terminus of the plakoglobin protein[12]. The second is a 3-bp insertion (S39_K40insS) which is predicted to cause insertion of an additional serine residue within the N-terminal domain of the plakoglobin protein. This mutation has been linked to dominant inheritance of ARVC without cutaneous abnormalities[13]. To assess the effects of these two distinct disease-causing plakoglobin mutations on a broad range of cell mechanical behaviour, we characterized a model system consisting of stably transfected human embryonic kidney cell-line 293 (HEK293) cells which are well suited for analyses of cell migration, adhesion and other aspects of cell biomechanics[14].

First, we grew confluent monolayers of HEK cells expressing wild-type plakoglobin or the mutant forms of plakoglobin known to cause Naxos disease (Naxos) or dominant ARVC (insS) on deformable silicone membranes and subjected them to uniaxial, pulsatile stretch (110% of resting length, frequency of 3 Hz) for 1 or 4 h. Under these culture conditions, cells form numerous intercellular junctions which can be readily visualized by immunohistochemical staining of adhesion junction or gap junction proteins and quantified by confocal microscopy and digital image processing. In response to either 1 or 4 h of pulsatile stretch, cells

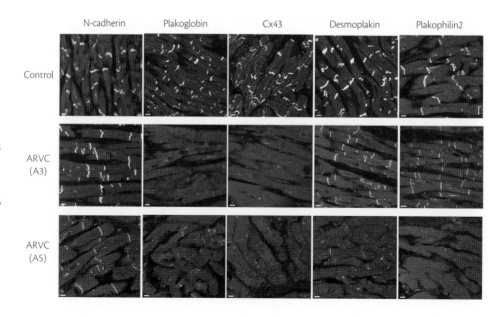

Fig. 57.1 Representative images showing that immunoreactive signal for plakoglobin at intercalated disks is reduced in subjects with ARVC compared with normal control subjects. [Reproduced, with permission, from Asimaki A, Tandri H, Huang H, *et al.* (2009) A new diagnostic test for arrhythmogenic right ventricular cardiomyopathy. *New Engl J Med* **360**:1075–1084, © Massachusetts Medical Society, all rights reserved.] (See color plate section.)

expressing wildtype plakoglobin showed a marked increase in the amount of immunoreactive signals for N-cadherin, plakoglobin and Cx43 at points of cell–cell apposition (Fig. 57.2). These results suggest that the normal cellular response to an external mechanical load is enhanced assembly of cell–cell adhesion proteins at both fascia adherens junctions (N-cadherin) and desmosomes (plakoglobin). Enhanced cell–cell communication also appears to be part of the normal response to mechanical load, based on the increased accumulation of Cx43 at cell–cell junctions. These responses were significantly blunted, however, in cells that expressed either the Naxos mutation or the serine-insertion mutation

implicated in ARVC (Fig. 57.2). Interestingly, even baseline expression levels of Cx43 were reduced in cells expressing either mutant form of plakoglobin, as shown by confocal microscopy and protein assays. This observation is in agreement with the reduced Cx43 at intercalated disks seen in patients with ARVC[8–10]. It suggests, however, that blunted upregulation of Cx43 cells cannot be attributed solely to abnormal responses to stretch. It is possible that the mutation has a direct effect on Cx43 expression independent of effects on cellular biomechanical behaviour. This possibility is supported by evidence suggesting that Cx43 gene expression can be regulated by Wnt signalling pathways[15].

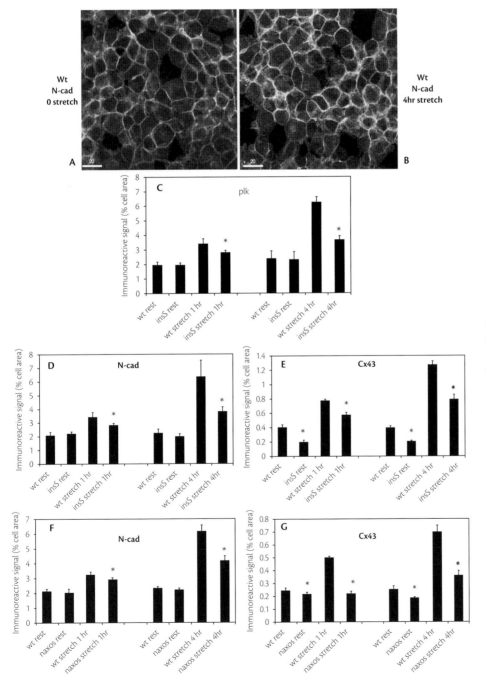

Fig. 57.2 **A** and **B** Application of stretch to normal HEK cells leads to accumulation of proteins at cell–cell junctions. Signals for plakoglobin (plk) (**C**), N-cadherin (N-cad) (**D**) and connexin 43 (Cx43) (**E**) were increased at cell–cell junctions after 1 and 4 h of stretch in cells expressing wild-type (wt) plakoglobin, but these responses were blunted in cells expressing the serine insertion (insS) mutant form of plakoglobin. A blunted response to stretch was also observed for N-cadherin (**F**) and Cx43 (**G**) in cells expressing the Naxos mutant form of plakoglobin. Cx43 levels were reduced at baseline in cells expressing either mutant form of plakoglobin. Asterisks indicate statistically significant difference compared to wild-type (WT) response. [Reproduced, with permission, from Huang H, Asimaki A, Lo D, McKenna W, Saffitz J (2008) Disparate effects of different mutations in plakoglobin on cell mechanical behavior. *Cell Motil Cytoskeleton* **65**:964–978.]

ARVC mutations in plakoglobin have complex effects on cellular biomechanical properties

Expression of wild-type plakoglobin and two distinct disease-causing forms of plakoglobin in separate lines of HEK cells provides an opportunity to determine how mutant plakoglobin might alter cell biomechanical behaviour and to define the specific effects of different mutations in the same protein. First, to determine whether expression of mutant plakoglobin affects cell stiffness, magnetic beads (4.5 μm diameter) coated with antibodies against β1-integrins were added to cultures of confluent cells in a limiting dilution such that a typical cell would have one bead attached to its surface. Then, a magnetic micromanipulator was used to apply graded magnetic force and the extent of bead displacement was quantified as a measure of cell stiffness (expression of integrins was the same in all cell lines and the extent to which beads became detached was not statistically different)[16,17]. Expression of plakoglobin with the serine insertion mutation resulted in a significant increase in bead displacement, reflecting reduced cell stiffness when compared to cells expressing wild-type plakoglobin. However, no change in cell stiffness was observed in cells expressing Naxos plakoglobin[14].

Next, we measured the effects of mutant plakoglobin expression on the strength of cell–cell adhesion. Two different techniques were employed. The first involved dispase dissociation assays which have been used previously as a qualitative measure of cell–cell adhesiveness in cultured keratinocytes[18]. Briefly, this method uses the matrix-lysing enzyme dispase to separate a confluent cell monolayer from a culture dish without significantly affecting cell–cell connections. Once removed as an intact monolayer, the cell sheet is subjected to shear forces with a mixing protocol and the extent to which the monolayer becomes fragmented is determined. In this assay, cell sheets composed of cells with stronger cell–cell adhesion dissociate into fewer, larger fragments[18]. Application of this assay to the HEK cell models of ARVC demonstrated a dramatic decrease in cell–cell adhesion in the cells expressing Naxos plakoglobin, but not for those expressing the serine insertion mutant form of plakoglobin (Fig. 57.3)[14].

A second assay was used to assess cell–cell adhesion while the cells were still attached to a matrix. This method, called the 'deform-drag assay', involves the use of a glass rod to shear cells off the substratum. As cells in the path of the glass rod are removed, adjacent cells to which they are attached are pulled along. The extent to which these connected cells are displaced when the rod is dragged across the dish is a function of the strength of intercellular adhesion. The lateral excursion of adjacent cells can be measured by imaging the shearing as a function of time, resulting in a more quantitative measure compared to the dispase assay. When frames from all time-points are merged, cells that move during the imaging interval are smeared in the final composite image. The lateral distance of this smearing can then be used as a measure of cell–cell adhesion strength relative to cell–substrate adhesion. Deform-drag assays showed a dramatic reduction in the strength of cell–cell adhesion in HEK cells expressing the Naxos mutation when compared to cells expressing wild-type plakoglobin (Fig. 57.4). In contrast, no apparent effect on intercellular adhesion was seen in cells expressing the serine insertion mutant form of plakoglobin (Fig. 57.4)[14].

These results provide clear evidence that mutations in desmosomal proteins known to cause ARVC can alter the biomechanical properties of cells, but the effects can vary dramatically even when different mutations in the same protein are being compared. In this analysis, two different mutations in plakoglobin, both known to cause disease, were compared. One mutation (serine insertion) caused a marked reduction in the stiffness of cells, perhaps reflecting a change in interactions between desmosomes and intermediate filaments of the cytoskeleton. However, this mutation had no apparent effect on the strength of cell–cell adhesion. In marked contrast, a different mutation in the same protein (Naxos mutation) had no effect on cell stiffness but caused a dramatic decrease in cell–cell adhesion[14]. Thus, while is seems likely that altered biomechanical properties play a fundamental role in ARVC pathogenesis, these results suggest that the range of potential alterations

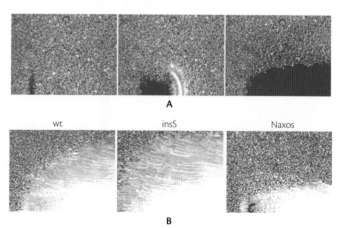

A

wt insS Naxos

B

Fig. 57.4 Deform-drag assays can be used to assess cell–cell adhesiveness on cells that remain adhered on a substrate. **A** The assay uses a glass rod that is dragged from left to right, shearing off cells in its path. Cells immediately adjacent to the cells being sheared are pulled along. **B** The extent of lateral excursion can be visualized by combining all frames acquired during the assay into a single image; cells that move are blurred. Cells expressing Naxos plakoglobin (Naxos) exhibited the lowest amount of movement, suggesting that cell–cell adhesive strength is significantly diminished compared with cells expressing either wild-type (wt) or serine insertion (insS) forms of plakoglobin. [Reproduced, with permission, from Huang H, Asimaki A, Lo D, McKenna W, Saffitz J (2008) Disparate effects of different mutations in plakoglobin on cell mechanical behavior. *Cell Motil Cytoskeleton* **65**:964–978.]

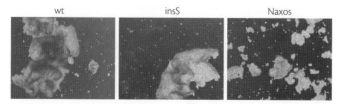

wt insS Naxos

Fig. 57.3 A dispase dissociation assay revealed smaller, more numerous fragments in cells expressing Naxos plakoglobin (Naxos), indicating that the presence of the Naxos mutation significantly reduces the strength of cell–cell adhesion. wt, wild-type plakoglobin; insS, serine insertion form of plakoglobin. [Reproduced, with permission, from Huang H, Asimaki A, Lo D, McKenna W, Saffitz J (2008) Disparate effects of different mutations in plakoglobin on cell mechanical behavior. *Cell Motil Cytoskeleton* **65**:964–978.]

is large, and that different disease-causing mutations may have disparate effects. It will be of interest in future studies to characterize the effects of these mutations on the biomechanical properties of cardiac myocytes and to link altered cellular biomechanics to altered cell signalling.

Conclusions and outlook

Mutations in genes encoding all five of the known desmosomal proteins have been identified in ARVC patients, supporting the idea that ARVC is, at least in part, a disease of abnormal cell–cell adhesion. It is now widely believed that genetic defects in desmosomal proteins reduce cell–cell coupling under conditions of mechanical stress, ultimately causing cellular degeneration and subsequent replacement by fibro-fatty scar tissue. At the same time, there is increasing evidence that ARVC mutations activate signalling pathways that can modulate gene expression, promote cardiac myocyte apoptosis and mediate expression of fibrogenic and/or adipogenic phenotypes[13,19]. Considerable work remains to be done to elucidate the roles of MEC disruption and identify pathological alterations in specific signalling pathways in the development of ARVC.

Identification of ARVC-causing mutations in genes encoding non-desmosomal proteins such as TMEM43[7] raises questions about whether these mutations can affect MEC. Furthermore, it must be emphasized that more than half of all ARVC patients have no identifiable mutation[4]. Many other aspects of this disease remain unexplained. Myocardial loss and fibro-fatty replacement occur preferentially in specific regions, including the inferior tricuspid annulus, the outflow tract and apical areas of the right ventricle[1]. Perhaps these areas are subjected to specific mechanical forces which promote myocyte injury, but this remains unexplored. Indeed, the reasons for the right ventricular free wall predominance in classical ARVC and the determinants of biventricular and left-dominant forms of the disease are entirely unknown. It is also not understood why the disease is generally not manifest until adolescence. Various environmental factors, chief among them vigorous exercise and athletic activities, are known to exacerbate disease progression[1]. While this suggests a link between increased mechanical stress and myocardial injury, the underlying mechanisms are not known. It does appear, however, that ARVC is a human heart disease in which altered mechano-electric coupling plays an especially prominent role in disease pathogenesis. Insights gained from future studies will undoubtedly advance this understanding and could potentially be applicable to other forms of heart muscle disease such as valvular and hypertensive heart disease in which an increased mechanical burden plays a role.

Acknowledgements

Angeliki Asimaki was supported by the Kenneth M. Rosen Fellowship in Pacing and Electrophysiology from the Heart Rhythm Society. Hayden Huang was supported by the Lerner Fund.

References

1. Sen-Chowdhry S, Lowe MD, Sporton SC, McKenna WJ. Arrhythmogenic right ventricular cardiomyopathy: clinical presentation, diagnosis and management. *Am J Med* 2004;**117**:685–695.

2. Sen-Chowdhry S, Syrris P, Prasad SK, *et al.* Left-dominant arrhythmogenic cardiomyopathy: an under-recognized clinical entity. *J Am Coll Cardiol* 2008;**52**:2175–2187.

3. Thiene G, Corrado D, Basso C. Arrhythmogenic right ventricular cardiomyopathy/dysplasia. *Orphanet J Rare Dis* 2007;**2**:45.

4. Sen-Chowdhry S, Syrris P, McKenna WJ. Role of genetic analysis in the management of patients with arrhythmogenic right ventricular dysplasia/cardiomyopathy. *J Am Coll Cardiol* 2007;**50**:1813–1821.

5. Tiso N, Stephan DA, Nava A, *et al.* Identification of mutations in the cardiac ryanodine receptor gene in families affected with arrhythmogenic right ventricular cardiomyopathy type 2 (ARVD2). *Hum Mol Genet* 2001;**10**:189–194.

6. Beffagna G, Occhi G, Nava A, *et al.* Regulatory mutations in transforming growth factor beta3 gene cause arrhythmogenic right ventricular cardiomyopathy type 1. *Cardiovasc Res* 2005;**65**: 366–373.

7. Merner ND, Hodgkinson KA, Haywood AF, *et al.* Arrhythmogenic right ventricular cardiomyopathy type 5 is a fully penetrant, lethal, arrhythmic disorder caused by a missense mutation in the TMEM43 gene. *Am J Hum Genet* 2008;**82**:809–821.

8. Kaplan SR, Gard JJ, Protonotarios N, *et al.* Remodeling of myocyte gap junctions in arrhythmogenic right ventricular cardiomyopathy due to a deletion in plakoglobin (Naxos disease). *Heart Rhythm* 2004; **1**:3–11.

9. Kaplan SR, Gard JJ, Carvajal-Huerta L, Ruiz-Cabezas JC, Thiene G, Saffitz JE. Structural and molecular pathology of the heart in Carvajal syndrome. *Cardiovasc Pathol* 2004;**13**:26–32.

10. Asimaki A, Tandri H, Huang H, *et al.* A new diagnostic test for arrhythmogenic right ventricular cardiomyopathy. *New Engl J Med* 2009;**360**:1075–1084.

11. Zhurinsky J, Shtutman M, Ben-Ze'ev A. Plakoglobin and β-catenin: protein interactions, regulation and biological roles, *J Cell Sci* 2000;**113**:3127–3139.

12. McKoy G, Protonotarios N, Crosby A, *et al.* Identification of a deletion in plakoglobin in arrhythmogenic right ventricular cardiomyopathy with palmoplantar keratoderma and woolly hair (Naxos disease). *Lancet* 2000;**355**:2119–2124.

13. Asimaki A, Syrris P, Wichter T, Matthias P, Saffitz JE, McKenna WJ. A novel mutation in plakoglobin causes arrhythmogenic right ventricular cardiomyopathy. *Am J Hum Genet* 2007;**81**:964–973.

14. Huang H, Asimaki A, Lo D, McKenna W, Saffitz J. Disparate effects of different mutations in plakoglobin on cell mechanical behavior. *Cell Motil Cytoskeleton* 2008;**65**:964–978.

15. Ai Z, Fischer A, Spray DC, Brown AM, Fishman GI. Wnt-1 regulation of connexin43 in cardiac myocytes. *J Clin Invest* 2000;**105**: 161–171.

16. Huang H, Kamm RD, So PT, Lee RT. Receptor-based differences in human aortic smooth muscle cell membrane stiffness. *Hypertension* 2001;**38**:1158–1161.

17. Huang H, Sylvan J, Jonas M, Barresi R, So PT, Campbell KP, Lee RT. Cell stiffness and receptors: Evidence for cytoskeletal subnet works. *Am J Physiol* 2005;**288**:C72–C80.

18. Yin T, Getsios S, Caldelari R, Kowalczyk AP, Muller EJ, Jones JC, Green KJ. Plakoglobin suppresses keratinocyte motility through both cell–cell adhesion-dependent and –independent mechanisms. *Proc Natl Acad Sci USA* 2005;**102**:5420–5425.

19. Garcia-Gras E, Lombardi R, Giocondo MJ, Willerson JT, Schneider MD, Khoury DS, Marian AJ. Suppression of canonical Wnt/beta catenin signaling by nuclear plakoglobin recapitulates phenotype of arrhythmogenic right ventricular cardiomyopathy. *J Clin Invest* 2006;**116**:2012–2021.

Evidence for mechano-electric coupling from clinical trials on cardiac resynchronization therapy

Nico R.L. Van de Veire and Jeroen J. Bax

Background

Heart failure (HF) is an important cardiovascular disorder in developed countries[1]. Due to the improved survival of other cardiovascular conditions such as myocardial infarction, the prevalence and burden of HF is likely to increase further[1]. Despite advances in diagnosis and medical treatment, the morbidity and mortality of HF patients remain high. Cardiac resynchronization therapy (CRT) has shown to be an effective strategy to improve prognosis and left ventricular (LV) systolic function of patients with end-stage, drug-refractory HF[1].

Patients with depressed LV systolic function and HF symptoms may show impaired electromechanical coupling, which may further impair LV function[2]. This impaired electromechanical coupling is translated into a disparity in regional contraction timing called mechanical dyssynchrony[3]. There are three levels of dyssynchrony: atrio-ventricular (AV) dyssynchrony, interventricular dyssynchrony (conduction delay between the right and left ventricle) and intraventricular dyssynchrony. Particularly prolonged ventricular conduction causing regional mechanical delay within the LV (intraventricular dyssynchrony) reduces LV systolic function and causes mitral regurgitation and LV dilatation, with further impairment of LV performance[4]. CRT devices have been designed to improve LV performance by restoring synchronicity at all three levels. To achieve resynchronization, three different pacing leads are implanted: one lead in the right atrium, one in the right ventricle (RV) and the third one placed via the coronary sinus close to the LV wall[5]. These leads are connected to a device that controls all pacing outputs with programmable timing. Intraventricular resynchronization can be achieved by simultaneously stimulating the interventricular septum and the LV lateral wall, resulting in coordinated septal and free wall contraction and thus improved LV pumping efficiency. In addition, AV resynchronization allows for optimization of the AV delay between atrial and LV pacing leads. By modulating preload this can result in an effective LV filling period. Interventricular resynchronization can be achieved via either simultaneous or sequential LV and RV pacing to improve the dyssynchronous contraction between the ventricles.

Clinical evidence for efficacy and safety of CRT

The efficacy and safety of CRT in drug refractory HF patients have been widely investigated. Table 58.1 summarizes the findings of ten landmark, randomized, multicentre trials. Most trials included highly symptomatic HF patients [New York Heart Association (NYHA) class III/IV] with poor LV ejection fraction (< 35–40%) and wide QRS complex (> 120–130 ms). The Resynchronization Reverses Remodelling in Systolic Left Ventricular Dysfunction (REVERSE) and Multicenter Automatic Defibrillator Implantation Trial with Cardiac Resynchronization Therapy (MADIT-CRT) trials focused on patients with mild HF (NYHA class I/II).

Data from the ten landmark trials listed in Table 58.1, including over 6,200 patients, demonstrate that CRT improves functional status (reducing NYHA class, improving quality-of-life scores and increasing 6-min walking distance) and reduces all-cause mortality and HF hospitalizations. Moreover, echocardiographic data of these trials demonstrated that CRT induces a significant reduction in LV volumes (reverse remodelling), improvement in LV systolic function and reduction in mitral regurgitation. These favourable results have been confirmed in two recent meta-analyses[1,16]. Rivero-Ayerza et al. pooled five randomized controlled studies including 1,028 controls and 1,343 CRT-treated patients[16]. The analysis demonstrated that CRT alone, as compared with optimal medical therapy, significantly reduced all-cause mortality by 29% and mortality due to progressive HF by 38%. McAlister et al. pooled the data from the five randomized trials, including 1,411 subjects, that reported on HF hospitalizations[1]. CRT markedly reduced the proportion of patients hospitalized with HF compared with medical therapy alone (relative risk 0.51; 95% CI 0.41–0.64).

Table 58.1 Outcome of CRT in randomized clinical trials

Trial reference	No. of subjects	Clinical improvement	Functional improvement
MUSTIC-SR[6]	58	NYHA class QOL, 6MWT Peak VO$_2$ Less hospitalizations	LV volumes MR
PATCH-CHF[7]	41	NYHA class QOL, 6MWT Less hospitalizations	
MIRACLE[8]	453	NYHA class QOL, 6MWT	LVEF LVEDD MR
MIRACLE-ICD[9]	362	NYHA class QOL	
PATCH-CHF II[10]	86	QOL, 6MWT Peak VO$_2$	
CONTAK-CD[11]	490	NYHA class QOL, 6MWT	LVEF LV volumes
COMPANION[12]	1,520	Reduced all-cause mortality/ hospitalization	
CARE-HF[13]	813	NYHA class QOL Reduced morbidity/mortality	LVEF LVESV
REVERSE[14]	610	HF clinical composite response	LVESV index
MADIT-CRT[15]	1,820	Reduced all-cause mortality/ HF events	LVEF LV volumes

CARE-HF, Cardiac Resynchronization-Heart Failure; COMPANION, Comparison of Medical Therapy, Pacing and Defibrillation in Heart Failure; CONTAK-CD, CONTAK-Cardiac Defibrillator; CRT, cardiac resynchronization therapy; EDD, end-diastolic diameter; EF, ejection fraction; ESV, end-systolic volume; LV, left ventricular; MADIT-CRT, Multicenter Automatic Defibrillator Implantation Trial with Cardiac Resynchronization Therapy; MIRACLE, Multicenter InSync Randomized Clinical Evaluation; MIRACLE-ICD, Multicenter InSync Implantable Cardioverter Defibrillator; MR, mitral regurgitation; MUSTIC, Multisite Stimulation in Cardiomyopathies; NYHA, New York Heart Association; PATCH-CHF, Pacing Therapies in Congestive Heart Failure; QOL, quality-of-life score; REVERSE, Resynchronization Reverses Remodeling in Systolic Left Ventricular Dysfunction; VO$_2$, oxygen uptake; 6MWT, 6-min walking test.

dyssynchrony, extent and location of scar and position of the LV lead[18]. This section focuses on the most controversial factor, dyssynchrony.

Current guidelines define dyssynchrony by QRS duration. However, several studies have demonstrated the limited value of the QRS width to predict response to CRT[19,20]. There is a poor relation between LV dyssynchrony and QRS width, as one third of patients with a QRS > 150 ms do not show dyssynchrony, whereas patients with a narrow QRS often show dyssynchrony[19,20]. Subsequently, echocardiographic parameters have been proposed to define **mechanical** dyssynchrony. Several studies have suggested that both the magnitude of basal dyssynchrony and its reduction by CRT predicted chronic chamber functional improvement and enhanced exercise capacity and clinical status[18]. Dyssynchrony was also found to be an independent predictor of clinical events and poor survival in HF patients[18].

Various echocardiographic techniques have been proposed to quantify LV dyssynchrony, including simple methods such as Doppler and M-mode echocardiography and more complex methods such as pulsed wave and colour tissue Doppler imaging (TDI), deformation imaging and more recently three-dimensional echocardiography.

Simple methods

Pulsed wave Doppler echocardiography

Pulsed wave Doppler echocardiography is the method of choice for assessment of interventricular dyssynchrony. For this purpose pulsed wave recordings across the aortic and pulmonary valves are obtained, and aortic and pulmonary pre-ejection times are defined as the intervals between the onset of the QRS complex and the onset of aortic and pulmonary flow, respectively (Fig. 58.1). An aortic pre-ejection time > 140 ms is considered indicative of intraventricular dyssynchrony[13]. The difference between the aortic and pulmonary pre-ejection times is considered a measure of interventricular dyssynchrony[13]. Ghio *et al.* (using a cut-off value of 40 ms) reported that 72% of patients with QRS duration > 150 ms exhibited interventricular dyssynchrony[20]. The Cardiac Resynchronization-Heart Failure (CARE-HF) trial assessed aortic pre-ejection time and interventricular dyssynchrony as selection

Based on these findings, the European Society of Cardiology guidelines consider CRT a class I indication in HF patients who remain symptomatic in NYHA classes III–IV despite optimal medical treatment, with LV ejection fraction ≤ 35%, LV dilatation, normal sinus rhythm and wide QRS complex (> 120 ms).[17]

Echocardiographic assessment of mechanical dyssynchrony

Despite careful selection of CRT candidates, up to 30% of the patients do not show clinical improvement (clinical non-responder). If echocardiographic criteria are applied to define response (e.g. reduction in LV end-systolic volume > 10–15% or LV ejection fraction improvement > 5%), the percentage of non-responders increases up to 40%[4]. Therefore several additional issues need to be addressed in potential CRT candidates, including

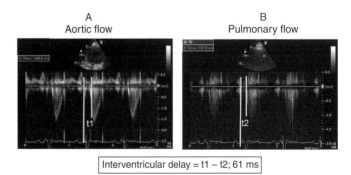

Interventricular delay = t1 – t2; 61 ms

Fig. 58.1 The aortic (**A**) and pulmonary (**B**) pre-ejection times are measured as the time differences between the onset of the QRS complex and the onset of aortic flow (t1) and pulmonary flow (t2) as obtained with pulsed wave Doppler imaging. The difference between the aortic (189 ms) and pulmonary pre-ejection times (128 ms) is a measure of interventricular dyssynchrony: 61 ms (> 40 ms) indicates significant interventricular dyssynchrony.

criteria in order to include HF patients with a QRS duration between 120 and 149 ms[13]. Available evidence on the predictive value of these dyssynchrony parameters is still limited. Bordachar *et al.* evaluated 41 HF patients; despite a significant reduction of interventricular dyssynchrony after CRT initiation, no relation was found between interventricular dyssynchrony and haemodynamic improvement acutely after CRT[21].

M-mode echocardiography

M-mode echocardiography is a relatively simple technique to assess LV dyssynchrony. Using the parasternal short-axis view of the LV at the level of the papillary muscles, the time interval between peak systolic contraction of the septum and the peak inward contraction of the posterior wall can be obtained [septal-to-posterior wall motion delay (SPWMD)] (Fig. 58.2A). Pitzalis evaluated SPWMD in 20 HF patients scheduled for CRT[22]. A SPWMD > 130 ms appeared to be predictive of a 15% reduction in LV end-systolic volume after 1 month of CRT. However, in a retrospective analysis of 79 patients from the CONTAK-CD trial, SPWMD had only modest value in predicting response to CRT (sensitivity 24%, specificity 66%)[23]. In almost half of the study population, the SPWMD could not be measured reliably. According to another analysis involving 98 HF patients the poor feasibility of SPWMD was confirmed. Possible reasons are the absence of clear systolic deflection on M-mode echocardiography in the case of scar in the antero-septal and posterior wall or poor acoustic windows[24].

Complex methods

Several studies have elucidated the role of TDI to quantify mechanical dyssynchrony. TDI includes assessment of myocardial velocities in different LV segments and relating the timing of these myocardial velocities to electrical activity (QRS complex), providing mechano-electrical delays.

Pulsed-wave TDI

Initially the widespread modality, pulsed-wave TDI offering high spatial resolution was used to quantify dyssynchrony. A sample volume can be positioned on-line in any LV segment, allowing measurement of time to onset of systolic ejection phase. Penicka *et al.* measured time intervals in the four basal LV segments and in the basal segment of the free wall of the RV[25]. The authors reported a cut-off value of 102 ms (sum of intra- and interventricular dyssynchrony) for the prediction of improved LV function after CRT yielding 96% sensitivity and 77% specificity. However, sampling is restricted to a single position during each cardiac cycle, precluding post-hoc repositioning and analysis. Comparison of multiple segments requires separate acquisitions in different cycles and is limited by differences in heart rate and respiration[26].

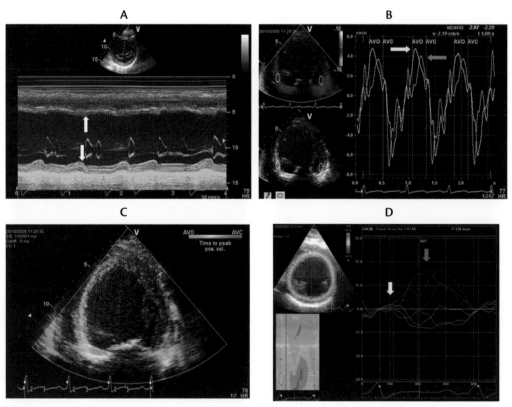

Fig. 58.2 Echocardiographic parameters of intraventricular dyssynchrony. **A** The septal to posterior wall motion delay (SPWMD) measurement by M-mode echocardiography obtained from the short-axis view. A delay of 150 ms between the maximal systolic excursion of the septum and posterior walls (arrows) indicates significant intraventricular dyssynchrony. **B** Dyssynchrony assessment by measuring the time difference between the peak myocardial systolic velocities of the septal and lateral wall on tissue Doppler images; aortic valve opening (AVO) and closure (AVC) are indicated to facilitate identification of systolic peak velocities (arrows). **C** Automated measurement of time to peak myocardial systolic velocities by tissue synchronization imaging (TSI). Timings are translated in a colour scheme (see color plate section for detail) **D** Short-axis slice of the left ventricle at the level of the papillary muscles, with reconstruction of six LV segments. Separate 2D strain time curves for each individual segment are depicted. In this example severe baseline intraventricular dyssynchrony was present as expressed by the delay in time to peak systolic radial 2D strain > 130 ms between the anterior and posterior wall peak strain. (See color plate section.)

Colour-coded TDI

Colour-coded TDI stores myocardial velocities superimposed on two-dimensional cine loops, allowing off-line analysis of various segments during the same cardiac cycle[26]. In the early colour-coded TDI studies, samples were placed in the basal septal and lateral segments[27] (Fig. 58.2B). The time difference was calculated by measuring the time to peak systolic velocity of the individual segments with reference to the QRS complex. A delay exceeding 60 ms appeared predictive of an immediate response after CRT[27]. Subsequently a four-segment model was proposed including the septal, lateral, inferior and anterior basal segments[28]. A delay ≥ 65 ms was predictive of both clinical (sensitivity/specificity 80%) and echocardiographic (sensitivity/specificity 92%) improvement after 6 months of CRT[28]. Yu *et al.* proposed a 12-segment model including six basal and six mid LV segments to quantify dyssynchrony. Intraventricular dyssynchrony was quantified by using the standard deviation of all 12 time intervals. In an initial study involving 30 patients, a standard deviation ≥ 32.6 ms was predictive of reverse LV remodelling after CRT[29]. In a more recent study involving 256 CRT patients, a standard deviation exceeding 33 ms predicted reverse LV remodelling with 93% sensitivity and 78% specificity[30]. Multisegment analysis of TDI velocity curves is time consuming and automated analysis may be preferred.

Tissue synchronization imaging

Tissue synchronization imaging (TSI) is a TDI-based modality that automatically calculates time to peak myocardial systolic velocities of each LV segment within a pre-specified time frame (usually the systolic ejection phase)[31]. The resultant colour-coded images permit quick visualization of the earliest activated segments (displayed in green) and the latest activated segments (displayed in orange) (Fig. 58.2C). Moreover automated quantitative calculation of various TDI-derived dyssynchrony parameters is available. In a validation study involving 60 subjects, LV dyssynchrony was measured manually (time difference between the basal septum and the lateral wall) and automatically by the TSI software[32]. An excellent correlation was found between manually and automatically derived intraventricular dyssynchrony ($r = 0.95$, $p < 0.0001$). In addition, similar to TDI, TSI was able to predict LV reverse remodelling after 6 months of CRT (sensitivity 81%, specificity 89%) using a cut-off value of 65 ms[32].

TDI-derived strain

TDI myocardial velocities are inherently inaccurate due to incorporation of translational cardiac motion, rotation and tethering by adjacent segments. In contrast, strain measures myocardial deformation, differentiating between passive displacement and active systolic contraction[26]. Strain imaging can be performed by off-line analysis of colour-coded TDI images. Initial studies applied strain imaging on the apical views, thereby measuring longitudinal strain, and reported low reproducibility due to the relatively high operator and angle dependence[33]. Yu *et al.* evaluated the value of TDI-derived strain as compared to TDI in 256 CRT patients[30]. The standard deviation of 12 LV segments of time to peak systolic velocity was significantly higher in responders compared to non-responders [46 ± 13 ms vs 29 ± 11 ms, p = non-significant (NS)]. Consequently, longitudinal strain was not able to predict response to CRT in this study. Applying TDI-derived strain to short axis views, measuring radial strain, showed more promising results[34].

Intraventricular dyssynchrony, defined as the time difference of peak radial strain in the septum versus the posterior wall, was significantly larger in patients with an acute haemodynamic response to CRT[34]. Patients with ≥ 130 ms dyssynchrony experienced an immediate improvement in stroke volume (sensitivity 95%, specificity 88%). High signal noise, artefacts, angle dependence, respiratory drift and complex data processing all overshadow the theoretical merits. The resulting high intraobserver and interobserver variability limit the reproducibility of TDI-derived strain[26].

Speckle tracking or two-dimensional strain

A new echocardiographic technique, speckle tracking, can calculate myocardial strain from conventional two-dimensional echocardiography. The most important advantage of two-dimensional strain over TDI-derived strain is its lack of angle dependency. Suffoletto *et al.* applied speckle tracking in 48 patients undergoing CRT[35]. Strain curves were derived from routine two-dimensional short axis images and time to peak radial strain was measured from six LV segments (Fig. 58.2D). A time difference in peak anteroseptal wall to posterior wall strain ≥ 130 ms yielded a sensitivity of 91% and a specificity of 75% to predict an immediate increase ≥ 15% in stroke volume. Delgado *et al.* used speckle tracking in 161 HF patients undergoing CRT to evaluate radial, circumferential and longitudinal strain[36]. Only radial strain predicted response to CRT; a cut-off value of 130 ms intraventricular dyssynchrony was able to predict reverse LV remodelling after 6 months of CRT.

Three-dimensional echocardiography: tri-plane imaging

Colour-coded TDI only compares opposing walls within one plane. Interrogation of all segments requires three separate acquisitions in orthogonal planes, with unavoidable heart rate variability. Recently, it has become possible to acquire a tri-plane dataset and colour-coded TDI of the LV simultaneously. Combined with TSI, this technique presents the timing of the peak systolic velocities in a colour-map in the apical two-, three- and four-chamber views. Furthermore, a three-dimensional volume can be generated semi-automatically by tracing the endocardial borders manually, allowing for a quick identification of the latest activated area. Tri-plane TSI was applied in 60 patients and intraventricular dyssynchrony was calculated as the standard deviation of time to peak systolic velocity of 12 LV segments[37]. Patients showing reverse LV remodelling after 6 months of CRT had higher baseline dyssynchrony values (42 ± 14 ms vs 22 ± 12 ms, $p < 0.05$). As a result, a cut-off value of 33 ms was able to predict response with a sensitivity of 90% and a specificity of 83%.

Three-dimensional echocardiography: full-volume acquisition

Dyssynchrony may be characterized without TDI using a three-dimensional model of the LV. During acquisition, four consecutive cardiac cycles are combined to form a larger pyramidal volume (Fig. 58.3). Regional time–volume curves allow measurement of time to minimum systolic volume. The standard deviation of 16 segments creates a systolic dyssynchrony index, expressed as percentage of the cardiac cycle. This method can rapidly quantify LV dyssynchrony, as demonstrated by Kapetanakis *et al.* who evaluated 174 unselected patients referred for routine echocardiography[38]. Ajmone *et al.* found that a systolic dyssynchrony index of 5.6% was predictive for an immediate decrease in LV end-systolic volume of 15% with 88% sensitivity and 86% specificity[39]. In a

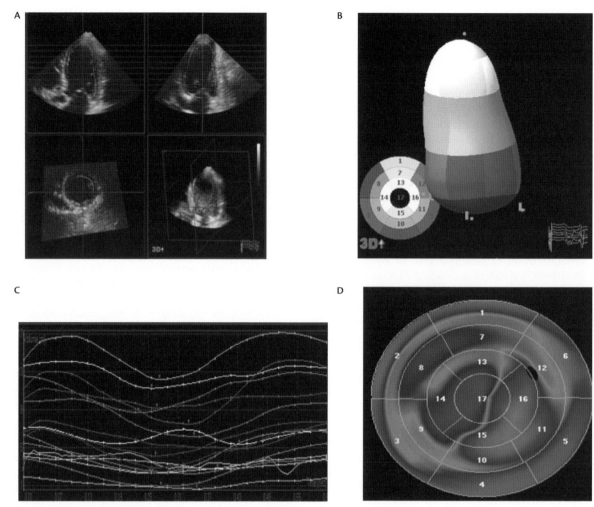

Fig. 58.3 A From a full-volume 3D dataset, an LV volume can be generated by automated tracking of the endocardial wall. **B** The LV model is divided into 17 segments. **C** From each of the 17 LV segments a time/volume curve is derived. **D** Time to peak minimal volume of the segments is presented in a bull's eye plot. Colour-coding allows quick visual identification of the area of latest mechanical activation. (See color plate section)

subsequent study involving 57 HF patients the systolic dyssynchrony index was significantly larger in patients who showed LV reverse remodelling at 6 months follow-up compared to non-responders (9.7% ± 3.6% vs 5.1% ± 1.8%, $p < 0.0001$)[40]. The technique is ambiguous for akinetic segments and is currently limited by low frame rates of 20–30 frames/s.

The PROSPECT study: predictors of response to CRT

The Predictors of Response to CRT (PROSPECT) study was an attempt to identify which of several previously published echocardiographic markers of dyssynchrony would forecast success of CRT using a prospective, multicentre approach. It was designed as a non-randomized observational study evaluating predefined baseline echocardiographic dyssynchrony parameters for their ability to predict clinical and echocardiographic response to CRT[41]. A total of 426 patients eligible for CRT according to the guidelines were included. The 6-month end-points included a clinical composite score and ≥ 15% reduction in LV end-systolic volume.

The echocardiographic dyssynchrony parameters comprised simple parameters such as SPWMD, aortic pre-ejection time interventricular dyssynchrony, and more complex parameters based on the evaluation of 2, 4, 6 or 12 LV segments using colour-coded TDI. Clinical improvement was observed in 69% of the population and echocardiographic improvement in 56%. The results demonstrated only a modest contribution of the included echocardiographic dyssynchrony parameters to predict response to CRT, with sensitivities ranging between 41% and 78% and specificities ranging between 31% and 74%.

Several methodological and procedural problems could explain these disappointing results[42]. An important confounding factor was the inclusion of less severe HF patients with LV ejection fraction > 35% and LV end-diastolic diameter < 65 mm. Consequently, reverse LV remodelling is less likely in these patients. A large percentage of echocardiographic data could not be analyzed reliably with feasibility ranging between 50% and 81%. Moreover interobserver variability of M-mode and TDI parameters was large. This underscores the need for standardization, better training and education. In addition, improvement in technology for the assessment of LV dyssynchrony is needed. Specifically in patients with ischemic cardiomyopathy M-mode and TDI often fail to provide optimal information on LV dyssynchrony. The septum is frequently a flat line on M-mode imaging and TDI provides only myocardial velocities, which does not permit differentiation between passive motion and active deformation. Deformation imaging techniques such as strain, including speckle tracking may be preferred in these cases. Also 3-dimensional techniques, taking into account dyssynchrony information of the entire LV, seem promising but further studies are needed. Other imaging modalities such as magnetic resonance imaging and nuclear imaging can also quantify dyssynchrony and underscore the value of mechanical dyssynchrony[43,44]. It has become clear that besides technological issues, pathophysiological issues – not included in the PROSPECT trail – are also influencing the result of CRT. Positioning the LV pacing lead in myocardium that contains scar tissue may reduce the effect of CRT[45]. Not only the location and transmurality of scar (Fig. 58.4) seem important but also the total amount of scar tissue in the LV. A higher scar burden limits the response to CRT[46]. The actual position of the LV pacing lead seems also important as some studies indicate that positioning the LV lead outside the echocardiographic area of latest mechanical activation resulted in poor response to CRT[47,48]. Positioning the LV pacing lead through an endocardial approach is limited by the anatomical variation of the coronary sinus tributaries. Pre-procedural noninvasive imaging of the cardiac veins using multi-slice computed tomography could be useful (Fig. 58.5). Preliminary data showed that poor venous anatomy can be encountered in patients with a previous myocardial infarction; in this case a surgical approach with epicardial LV lead placement may be preferred[49,50].

Conclusions and outlook

Evidence of 10 large trials and numerous small studies have demonstrated the benefit of CRT on HF symptoms, exercise capacity,

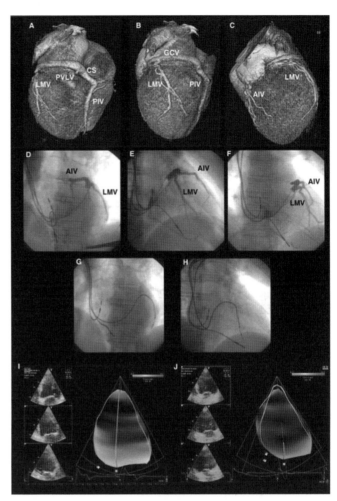

Fig. 58.5 Case example of an 85-year-old patient with idiopathic dilated cardiomyopathy, NYHA class III HF and wide QRS complex (157 ms, LBBB-configuration). MSCT shows a large left marginal vein with prominent side branches (A, B, C). These findings are confirmed by invasive venography (D, E, F). In the 3D LV dyssynchrony assessment with TSI (I), the late mechanical activation (yellow) is located in the lateral wall. The LV lead is positioned in the left marginal vein (G, H), resulting in synchronous activation of the LV, represented (green) on TSI, obtained immediately after CRT (J). In addition, a reduction of LV end-systolic volume from 191 to 153 ml was observed, with an increase in LV ejection fraction from 13% to 28%. [Reproduced, with permission, from Van de Veire NR, Marsan NR, Schuijf JD, *et al.* (2008) Noninvasive imaging of cardiac venous anatomy with 64-slice multi-slice computed tomography and noninvasive assessment of left ventricular dyssynchrony by 3-dimensional tissue synchronization imaging in patients with heart failure scheduled for cardiac resynchronization therapy. *Am J Cardiol* **101**:1023–1029.] (See color plate section.)

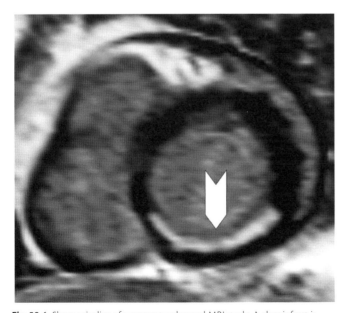

Fig. 58.4 Short-axis slice of a contrast-enhanced MRI study. A clear infarct is shown in the inferior wall (arrow, white tissue); the black tissue represents viable myocardium.

systolic LV function, HF hospitalization and mortality. A major issue is that if patients are selected according to current guidelines, 30% do not have a beneficial response. Mechanical dyssynchrony appears to be an important determinant for response to CRT as demonstrated by a multitude of small, single-centre studies. In a large observational study to identify responders to CRT, PROSPECT, echocardiographic dyssynchrony had only modest accuracy to predict response to CRT. Patient selection, technical issues and pathophysiological issues are significant confounding variables that need to be considered when interpreting the PROSPECT results. Better technology to evaluate dyssynchrony including 3-dimensional approaches and strain-based techniques merit further investigation, particularly in patients with an ischemic cardiomyopathy. There is a need for an integrated approach including assessment of extent and location of scar, extent and location of LV dyssynchrony and distribution of cardiac venous anatomy. Refinement in the technical aspects of data acquisition and analysis along with a greater understanding of pathophysiology will continue to add benefit to the care of CRT patients.

Few studies have tried to explain the mechanisms between the effects of biventricular pacing on the electrical system and the resulting mechanical resynchronization. Non-contact mapping catheter systems can record endocardial surface electrical potentials creating an electrical activation map and total activation time[51]. Non-contact mapping studies of LV endocardial activation have provided greater insights into ventricular dyssynchrony, LV activation patterns and response to CRT[52]. The system is able to identify regions of slow conduction which delay the spread of depolarisation over the LV endocardium[52]. Pacing outside regions of slow conduction can lead to additional improvements in acute haemodynamic improvements. Combined studies are needed in CRT candidates, using non-compact mapping to report on activation patterns and slow conduction and simultaneous advanced imaging techniques to correlate the electrical activation patterns with the mechanical activation patterns. Additionally, slow conduction zones should be compared with scar tissue as identified with imaging techniques. Finally it should be tested prospectively if pacing outside zones of slow conduction, specifically in patients with an ischemic cardiomyopathy, will improve the response rate to CRT.

References

1. McAlister FA, Ezekowitz J, Hooton N, et al. Cardiac resynchronization therapy for patients with left ventricular systolic dysfunction. A systematic review. JAMA 2007;**297**:2502–2514.

2. Epstein AE, DiMarco JP, Ellenbogen KA, et al, ACC/AHA/HRS 2008 Guidelines for device-based therapy of cardiac rhythm abnormalities: executive summary. A report of the American College of Cardiology/American Heart Association task force on practice guidelines (writing committee to revise the ACC/AHA/NASPE 2002 guideline update for implantation of cardiac pacemakers and antiarrhytmia devices). Developed in collaboration with the American Association for Thoracic Surgery and Society of Thoracic Surgeons. J Am Coll Cardiol 2008;**51**:2085–2105.

3. Kass DA. An epidemic of dyssynchrony. But what does it mean? J Am Coll Cardiol 2008;**51**:12–17.

4. Bax JJ, Abraham T, Barold SS, et al. Cardiac resynchronization therapy : part 1 – issues before device implantation. J Am Coll Cardiol 2005;**46**:2153–2167.

5. Butter C, Auricchio A, Stelbrink C, et al. Effect of resynchronization therapy stimulation site on the systolic function of heart failure patients. Circulation 2001;**104**:3026–3029.

6. Cazeau JG, Leclercq C, Lavergne T, et al. Effects of multisite biventricular pacing in patients with heart failure and intraventricular conduction delay. N Engl J Med 2001;**344**:873–880.

7. Auricchio A, Stellbrinck C, Sack S, et al. Long-term clinical effect of hemodynamically optimized cardiac resynchronization therapy in patients with heart failure and ventricular conduction delay. J Am Coll Cardiol 2002;**39**:2026–2033.

8. Abraham WT, Fisher WG, Smith AL, et al. Cardiac resynchronization in chronic heart failure. N Engl J Med 2002;**346**:1845–1853.

9. Young JB, Abraham WT, Smith AL, et al. Combined cardiac resynchronization and implantable cardioversion defibrillation in advanced chronic heart failure: the MIRACLE ICD trial. JAMA 2003;**289**:2685–2694.

10. Auricchio A, Stellbrinck C, Sack S, et al. Long-term clinical effect of cardiac resynchronization therapy in patients with heart failure and ventricular conduction delay. J Am Coll Cardiol 2003;**42**:2109–2116.

11. Higgings SL, Hummel JD, Niazi K, et al. Cardiac resynchronization therapy for the treatment of heart failure in patients with intraventricular conduction delay and malignant ventricular tachyarrhythmias. J Am Coll Cardiol 2003;**42**:454–459.

12. Bristow MR, Saxon LA, Boehmer J, et al. Cardiac-resynchronization therapy with or without an implantable defibrillator in advanced chronic heart failure. N Engl J Med 2004;**350**:2140–2450.

13. Cleland JG, Daubert JC, Erdmann E, et al. The effect of cardiac resynchronization on morbidity and mortality in heart failure. N Engl J Med 2005;**352**:1539–1549.

14. Linde C, Abraham WT, Gold MR, St John Sutton M, Ghio S, Daubert C; on behalf of the REVERSE Study Group. Randomized trial of cardiac resynchronization in mildly symptomatic heart failure patients and in asymptomatic patients with left ventricular dysfunction and previous heart failure symptoms. J Am Coll Cardiol 2008;**52**: 1834–1843.

15. Moss AJ, Hall WJ, Cannom DS, et al. Cardiac resynchronization therapy for the prevention of heart failure events. New Engl J Med 2009;**361**:1329–1338.

16. Rivero-Ayerza M, Theuns DAMJ, Garcia-Garcia HM, Boersma E, Simoons M, Jordaens LJ. Effects of cardiac resynchronization therapy on overall mortality and mode of death: a meta-analysis of randomized controlled trials. Eur Heart J 2006;**27**:2682–2688.

17. Vardas PE, Auricchio A, Blanc JJ, et al. Guidelines for cardiac pacing and cardiac resynchronization therapy: The Task Force for Cardiac Pacing and Cardiac Resynchronization Therapy of the European Society of Cardiology. Developed in collaboration with the European Heart Rhythm Association. Eur Heart J 2007;**28**:2256–2298.

18. Ypenburg C, Westenberg JJ, Bleeker GB, et al. Noninvasive imaging in cardiac resynchronization therapy – part 1: selection of patients. Pacing Clin Electrophysiol 2008;**31**:1475–1499.

19. Bleeker GB, Schalij MJ, Molhoek SG, et al. Relationship between QRS duration and left ventricular dyssynchrony in patients with end-stage heart failure. J Cardiovasc Electrophysiol 2004;**15**:544–549.

20. Ghios S, Constantin C, Klersy C, et al. Interventricular and intraventricular dyssynchrony are common in heart failure patients, regardless of QRS duration. Eur Heart J **25**:571–578.

21. Bordachar P, Lafitte S, Reuter S, et al. Echocardiographic parameters of ventricular dyssynchrony validation in patients with heart failure using sequential biventricular pacing. J Am Coll Cardiol 2004;**44**: 2157–2165.

22. Pitzalis MV, Lacoviello M, Romito R, et al. Cardiac resynchronization therapy tailored by echocardiographic evaluation of ventricular asynchrony. J Am Coll Cardiol 2002;**40**:1615–1622.

23. Marcus GM, Rose E, Viloria EM, et al. Septal to posterior wall motion delay fails to predict reverse remodeling or clinical improvement in patients undergoing cardiac resynchronization therapy. J Am Coll Cardiol 2005;**46**:2208–2214.

24. Bleeker GB, Schalij MJ, Boersma E, et al. Relative merits of M-mode echocardiography and tissue Doppler imaging for prediction of response to cardiac resynchronization therapy in patients with heart failure secondary to ischemic or idiopathic dilated carciomyopathy. Am J Cardiol 2007;**99**:68–74.

25. Penicka M, Bartunek J, De Bruyne B, et al. Improvement of left ventricular function after cardiac resynchronization is predicted by tissue Doppler imaging echocardiography. Circulation 2004;**109**: 978–983.

26. Hawkins NM, Petrie MC, Burgess MI, McMurray JJV. Selecting patients for cardiac resynchronization therapy. The fallacy of echocardiographic dyssynchrony. J Am Coll Cardiol 2009;**53**: 1944–1955.

27. Bax JJ, Marwick TH, Molhoek SG, *et al.* Left ventricular dyssunchrony predicts benefit of cardiac resynchronization therapy in patients with end-stage heart failure before pacemaker implantation. *Am J Cardiol* 2003;**92**:1238–1240.

28. Bax JJ, Bleeker GB, Marwick TH, *et al.* Left ventricular dyssynchrony predicts response and prognosis after cardiac resynchronization therapy. *J Am Coll Cardiol* 2004;**44**:1834–1840.

29. Yu CM, Fung WH, Ling H, *et al.* Predictors of left ventricular reverse remodeling after cardiac resynchronization therapy for heart failure secondary to idiopathic dilated or ischemic cardiomyopathy. *Am J Cardiol* 2003;**91**:684–688.

30. Yu CM, Gorcsan J III, Bleeker GB, *et al.* Usefulness of tissue Doppler velocity strain and strain dyssynchrony for predicting left ventricular reverse remodeling response after cardiac resynchronization therapy. *Am J Cardiol* 2007;**100**:1263–1270.

31. Gorcsan J III, Kanzaki H, Bazaz R, Dohi K, Schwartzman D. Usefulness of echocardiographic tissue synchronization imaging to predict acute response to cardiac resynchronization therapy. *Am J Cardiol* 2007;**93**:1178–1181.

32. Van de Veire NR, Bleeker G, De Sutter J, *et al.* Tissue synchronization imaging accurately measures left ventricular dyssynchrony and predicts response to cardiac resynchronization therapy. *Heart* 2007;**93**:1034–1039.

33. Yu CM, Zhang Q, Chan YS, *et al.* Tissue Doppler imaging is superior to displacement and strain mapping in predicting left ventricular reverse remodeling response after cardiac resynchronization therapy. *Heart* 2006;**92**:1452–1456.

34. Dohi K, Sufoletto MS, Schwartzman D, *et al.* Utility of echocardiographic radial strain imaging to quantify left ventricular dyssynchrony and predict acute response to cardiac resynchronization therapy. *Am J Cardiol* 2006;**96**:112–116.

35. Suffoletto MS, Dohi K, Cannesson M, *et al.* Novel speckle-tracking radial strain from routine black-and-white echocardiographic images to quantify dyssynchrony and predict response to cardiac resynchronization therapy. *Circulation* 2006;**113**:960–968.

36. Delgado V, Ypenburg C, van Bommel RJ, *et al.* Assessment of left ventricular dyssynchrony by speckle tracking strain imaging comparsion between longitudinal, circumferential, and radial strain in cardiac resynchronization therapy. *J Am Coll Cardiol* 2008;**51**:1944–1952.

37. Van de Veire NR, Bleeker GB, De Sutter J, *et al.* Tri-plane Tissue Doppler Imaging: a novel 3-dimensional imaging modality that predicts reverse left ventricular remodeling after Cardiac Resynchronization Therapy. *Heart* 2008;**94**:e9.

38. Kapetanakis S, Kearny MT, Siva A, Gall N, Cooklin M, Monaghan MJ. Real-time three-dimensional echocardiography: a novel technique to quantify global left ventricular mechanical dyssynchrony. *Circulation* 2005;**112**:992–1000.

39. Marsan NA, Bleeker GB, Ypenburg C, *et al.* Real-time three-dimensional echocardiography permits quantification of left ventricular mechanical dyssynchrony and predicts acute response to cardiac resynchronization therapy. *J Cardiovasc Electrophysiol* 2008;**19**:392–399.

40. Ajmone Marsan N, Bleeker GB, Ypenburg C, *et al.* Real-time three-dimesnional echocardiography as a novel approach to assess left ventricular and left atrium reverse remodeling and to predict response to cardiac resynchronization therapy. *Heart Rhytm* 2008;**5**:1257–1264.

41. Chung E, Leon AR, Tavazzi L, *et al.* Results of the Predictors of Response to CRT (PROSPECT) trial. *Circulation* 2008;**117**:2608–2616.

42. Bax JJ, Gorcsan J III. Echocardiography and noninvasive imaging in cardiac resynchronization therapy. Results of the PROSPECT Study in perspective. *J Am Coll Cardiol* 2009;**53**:1933–1941.

43. Boogers MM, Chen J, Bax JJ. Myocardial perfusion single photon emission computed tomography for the assessment of mechanical dyssynchrony. *Curr Opin Cardiol* 2008;**23**:431–439.

44. Helm RH, Lardo AC. Cardiac magnetic resonance assessment of mechanical dyssynchrony. *Curr Opin Cardiol* 2008;**23**:440–446.

45. Bleeker GB, Kaandorp TA, Lamb HJ, *et al.* Effect of posterolateral scar tissue on clinical and echocardiographic improvement after cardiac resynchronization therapy. *Circulation* 2005;**113**:969–976.

46. Ypenburg C, Roes SD, Bleeker GB, *et al.* Effect of total scar burden on contrast-enhanced magnetic resonance imaging on response to cardiac resynchronization therapy. *Am J Cardiol* 2007;**99**:657–660.

47. Murphy RT, Sigurdsson G, Mulamalla S, *et al.* Tissue synchronization imaging and optimal left ventricular pacing site in cardiac resynchronization therapy. *Am J Cardiol* 2007;**97**:1615–1621.

48. Becker M, Kramann R, Franke A, *et al.* Impact of left ventricular lead position in cardiac resynchronization therapy on left ventricular remodelling. *Eur Heart J* 2007;**28**:1211–1220.

49. Van de Veire NR, Schuijf JD, De Sutter J, *et al.* Non-invasive visualization of the cardiac venous system in coronary artery disease patients using 64-slice computed tomography. *J Am Coll Cardiol* 2006;**48**:1832–1838.

50. Van de Veire NR, Marsan NR, Schuijf JD, *et al.* Noninvasive imaging of cardiac venous anatomy with 64-slice multi-slice computed tomography and noninvasive assessment of left ventricular dyssynchrony by 3-dimensional tissue synchronization imaging in patients with heart failure scheduled for cardiac resynchronization therapy. *Am J Cardiol* 2008;**101**:1023–1029.

51. Schilling RJ, Peters NS, Davies DW. Mapping and ablation of ventricular tachycardia with the aid of a non-contact mapping system. *Heart* 1999;**81**:570–575.

52. Fung JWH, Chan JYS, Yip GWK, *et al.* Effect of left ventricular endocardial activation pattern on echocardiographic and clinical response to cardiac resynchronisation therapy. *Heart* 2007;**93**:423–427.

Mechano-electric coupling in patients treated with ventricular assist devices: insights from individual cases and clinical trials

Cesare M. Terracciano, Michael Ibrahim, Manoraj Navaratnarajah and Magdi H. Yacoub

Background

The last few decades have seen a substantial increase in the application of ventricular assist devices (VAD) in patients needing circulatory support. These devices act predominantly by mechanically unloading the heart, hence reducing its workload. A number of structural and functional changes to the myocardium have been reported after VAD therapy. These changes include effects on heart rhythm and ion transporter physiology, showing an electrophysiological response of the heart to mechanical unloading in patients. This is indicative of cardiac mechano-electric coupling (MEC). VAD are predominantly used for circulatory support in heart failure (HF) patients.

HF is a devastating disease with an estimated prevalence of 2.5% in the world population[1] and with increased incidence in the elderly. Children, particularly infants, are affected in large numbers by congenital cardiomyopathy and rheumatic heart disease[2], affecting an estimated 15 million patients in developing countries[3]. Arrhythmias are important clinical sequelae of HF and can account for a significant number of deaths[1]. Advances in the pharmacological treatment of HF have improved the outcome of this disease significantly, but there are still many patients who, despite optimal medical treatment, have a very poor prognosis, with mortality up to 80% at 1 year from diagnosis[4]. Cardiac transplantation is the most effective treatment for patients with refractory HF, but this option is often unavailable due to a shortage of donor hearts. Alternative therapeutic strategies are based on the use of non-pharmacological approaches. While some new treatments, such as gene and cell therapy, have been predominantly tested at the experimental level with few, controversial clinical trials[5], there is substantial clinical evidence that mechanical devices can be effective in the management and treatment of HF.

In this chapter we discuss VAD technology and describe its current clinical indications. We then provide evidence for the effects of VAD therapy on heart rhythm in patients and the associated risk factors for the development of ventricular arrhythmias. We finally discuss the evidence for ion transporter remodelling observed in patients and animal models after mechanical unloading.

Circulatory support: evolving technology

Mechanical devices for the treatment of HF can be classified into either VAD, i.e. mechanical pumps offering active circulatory support while unloading the ventricles (the subject of the present chapter), or cardiac support devices which offer passive containment of the dilated ventricles.

Substantial clinical experience exists with the use of VAD, with 20,000 VAD reportedly implanted to date and an implantation rate of 1,500 per year[6]. VAD technology has evolved significantly in the last few years, with the development of devices for internal placement with continuous flow and significantly improved power management. VAD can be classified as extracorporeal devices, percutaneous short-term devices and 'longer'-term assist devices[7]. Three generations of longer-term assist devices have been developed to date, differing in the type of flow and the degree of mechanical unloading provided. The first VAD generation consists of pulsatile devices that use pusher plates combined with inflow and outflow valves. These devices, such as the HeartMate® I and XVE (Thoratec Corporation, USA), offer a significant potential to unload the left ventricle and have a high blood pumping capacity (up to 10 L/min). However, first generation VAD are very large in size and can lead to important complications due to malfunctioning of the prosthetic valves. Second generation VAD are continuous-flow impeller pumps. One well-studied second generation device is the HeartMate® II (Thoratec Corporation, USA). Second generation VAD are smaller in size and quieter in operation, but their blood pumping capacity is not as high as that of pulsatile pumps. In addition, they require the use of full anticoagulant therapy. The third generation of VAD are also continuous pumps but use a mechanically or magnetically suspended rotor, removing the need for bearings, with consequently improved durability. Many third generation pumps, such as the DuraHeart® (Terumo Kabushiki Kaisha Shibuya-ku, Japan) and the HVAD® (HeartWare, Miramar, Florida, USA) devices, are currently the subject of phase I clinical trials[8]. Recent evidence, presented at the American Heart Association 2010 Scientific Sessions, suggests that these devices have effects on functional capacity, quality of life and safety profiles that are at least comparable to second generation VAD.

Among the CDS devices, the CorCap™ cardiac support device (Acorn Cardiovascular Inc, St Paul, Minnesota, USA)[9], a mesh surgically wrapped around the heart, has been studied recently in randomized clinical trials for HF (Acorn Randomized Clinical Trial)[10]. The CorCap™ cardiac support device has been shown to induce beneficial remodelling, particularly when associated with mitral valve repair[10]. However, a 3-year follow-up study of the Acorn randomized clinical trial showed that in 300 patients treated with the device there was no improvement in survival. The incidence of arrhythmias was not affected by this treatment, suggesting that passive containment does not affect electrical remodelling in patients[11]. As there is little clinical evidence of the effects of cardiac support device on heart rhythm (and, hence, MEC), the remainder of this chapter will focus on VAD.

VAD support: current applications

When first developed, VAD were principally used to rescue the circulation in patients with post-cardiotomy cardiogenic shock. Their use in this context is now rare, but VAD are still of significant interest for the acute management of haemodynamically unstable patients undergoing percutaneous interventions, or in postmyocardial infarction cardiogenic shock[12]. Randomized trials have failed so far to show additional benefits of the available percutaneous devices compared with intra-aortic balloon pumps[13], but this is likely to change due to improvements in device technology and more rigorous patient selection criteria[12].

Although rare, the use of VAD for the management of intractable ventricular arrhythmias represents an important example of how mechanical unloading can alter the electrical activity of the myocardium. Information regarding this application is sparse and somewhat anecdotal. There are a small number of documented cases in which VAD placement has been used to 'treat' intractable ventricular tachycardia/fibrillation (VT/VF)[14–16]. The rationale for this indication comes from the beneficial effects of cardiopulmonary bypass in intractable VF[16], ascribed to acute cardiac decompression and improved myocardial perfusion. In the few cases where VAD support was used to treat arrhythmias, mechanical unloading seemed to exhibit an antiarrhythmic effect in both the short and long term, possibly by ameliorating ventricular distension. This is in contrast to the acute pro-arrhythmic effects reported during VAD implantation (see below and Fig. 59.1), and more substantial clinical evidence is needed to consider VAD treatment among the available antiarrhythmic strategies.

The major application of VAD in both adult and paediatric populations involves their chronic use for the treatment of chronic HF. There are three major chronic indications for VAD therapy: bridge-to-transplantation, destination therapy and bridge-to-recovery[6].

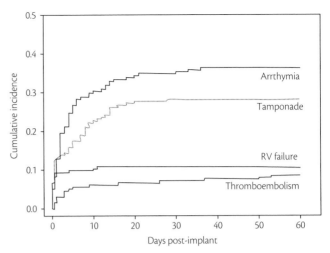

Fig. 59.1 Cumulative incidence of complications post-VAD implantation. Arrhythmia is a relatively common complication after mechanical unloading. The incidence of new arrhythmia is high during the early post-operative period, but there are no further arrhythmias beyond this. This may suggest an acute effect of mechanical unloading on ventricular arrhythmias. [Reproduced, with permission, from Genovese EA, Dew MA, Teuteberg JJ, *et al.* (2009) Incidence and patterns of adverse event onset during the first 60 days after ventricular assist device implantation. *Ann Thorac Surg* **88**:1162–1170]

Bridge-to-transplantation is by far the most common and successful application for the use of VAD, with significant evidence that VAD improve circulatory function and quality of life in patients awaiting cardiac transplantation[17] and bring about a normal or improved post-transplant outcome[18].

A large population of patients with contraindications to transplantation could benefit from VAD as **destination therapy**. In this modality VAD are implanted permanently to support the circulation. The evidence regarding this approach from clinical trials is controversial, particularly regarding the survival in the longer term[19], but the use of safer and more durable devices, as well as better patient selection, are likely to strengthen this VAD indication in the near future[7].

The third, and most contentious but exciting, application is the use of VAD as **bridge-to-recovery**. This modality is the use of VAD for the treatment of the underlying myocardial dysfunction. Bridge-to-recovery involves the temporary use of VAD, until the native myocardium has recovered sufficiently to allow VAD explantation without the need for cardiac transplantation. However, significant clinical recovery has been shown only in a small number of patients[20,21]. Strategies that involve the combination of VAD with specific pharmacological regimens are more promising. We have shown that VAD used in conjunction with pharmacological agents aimed at inducing reverse remodelling and preventing myocardial atrophy substantially increase the rate of clinical recovery[22,23], making this indication a plausible option. Future studies should also consider the use of VAD as a platform for myocardial regeneration using gene and cell therapy.

The improved coronary circulation and mechanical unloading brought about by VAD treatment have a number of effects on the myocardium, described below, which are collectively termed 'reverse remodelling'[24]. These changes may be crucial for the effects of VAD on heart rhythm observed in some clinical trials.

In the following section, the evidence that VAD treatment affects heart rhythm will be discussed.

VAD and MEC: evidence for effects on heart rhythm

Current knowledge of the effects of VAD on heart rhythm is limited, with much of the evidence originating from a small number of observational clinical case series[25–29]. The development of atrial arrhythmias after open cardiac surgery is a common but generally benign and easily treated phenomenon, with a similar incidence reported after VAD insertion (~30%)[28]. For this reason, this chapter focuses on the incidence of more sinister, haemodynamically significant and potentially life-threatening ventricular arrhythmias (VA).

The exact prevalence of VA after VAD implantation, their aetiology, clinical consequences and optimal therapy remain poorly defined. The incidence of post-operative VA, defined as VF, non-sustained VT or sustained VT, varies from 18%[26] to 43%[25]. This range has been established using data from two early small series ($n < 30$). Recently, two larger studies have suggested that the overall incidence is approximately 35%[28,30]. VAD-associated VA are clinically important: a mortality of 33% in the VA group versus 18% in the non-VA group has been reported, with mortality rising to as high as 54% when VA occurred in the first week[29]. A separate 100-patient study showed a similar trend with a 28% all-cause mortality in the VA group versus 14% in the non-VA group at 1 year after VAD implantation[30].

Risk factors for arrhythmia development

The pathogenesis of VA after mechanical unloading is not completely understood, and identification of positive predictors or modifiable risk factors has yielded inconsistent results. An ischaemic aetiology for the cardiomyopathy appears to be an independent positive predictor of post-operative VA in several studies[25–27,30], paralleling the elevated incidence seen in ischaemic cardiomyopathy during medically treated end-stage[31]. However, a recent 23-patient study specifically looking at the continuous flow device HeartMate II found no such relationship[32].

Non-use of post-operative beta blockade has also been identified to be a positive predictor of VA[27]. Systemic electrolyte abnormalities, e.g. potassium and magnesium alterations, have unsurprisingly displayed an arrhythmogenic predictive value, with a hazards ratio of 5.2 (CI 2.1–12.9, $p = 0.0004$)[27,30].

The influence of preoperative VA on post-VAD arrhythmogenesis is not clear, with some studies demonstrating a trend towards elevated risk[27,33] and others reporting a statistically significant rise in de novo monomorphic VT (MVT) post-VAD insertion. Indeed, the latter study suggested that after VAD insertion the development of new-onset MVT was 4.5 times more likely than the elimination of pre-existing MVT and found no definable relationship between incidence of pre- and post-VAD polymorphic VT/VF (PVT/VF)[30].

Factors promoting the development of MVT may differ from those promoting PVT in the post-VAD setting. Myocardial ischaemia, unstable haemodynamic state and intensive inotropic therapy may be more important in the development of PVT, while MVT development may be more dependent on the presence of either old or newly acquired myocardial scars, i.e. apical scarring at the cannula site[30]. This view is supported by the findings that reduced VAD output and haemodynamic instability are only correlated with PVT and not with MVT occurrence, and also that the majority of the frequent, de novo post-operative MVT originated from the apical cannulation site.

Effects of prolonged mechanical unloading on the incidence of ventricular arrhythmias

After an initially increased occurrence of VA in the first 30 days from implantation, the incidence of VA post-VAD insertion is greatly reduced, and by 60 days it is virtually eliminated (Fig. 59.1)[27,28,30]. Exact quantification of the longer-term VA incidence is limited by lack of electrocardiogram (ECG) monitoring after hospital discharge, with the majority of studies only detailing in-hospital events up to a maximum range of approximately 150 days. Re-admissions for treatment of symptomatic VA are documented, but the incidence of out of hospital, asymptomatic, self-terminating VA remains to be studied. The shortening of the QT interval observed in the late period after VAD insertion could contribute to VA reduction during prolonged treatment[33].

VAD support and electrical, structural and functional reverse remodelling

The chronically failing heart is characterized by a number of changes to its normal structural, functional and electrical phenotype. The advent of VAD has provided an opportunity to test the hypothesis that the removal of the pressure and/or volume overload in HF might cause a regression of the pathological remodelling process, a concept termed 'reverse remodelling'. Here we briefly introduce the evidence for structural, electrical and functional reverse remodelling of the myocardium after VAD support, and show how this is possibly linked to modifications in heart rhythm.

The regression of ventricular dilation and restoration of normal end-diastolic pressure–volume relationships in human patients treated with VAD has been widely noted[24,34–36]. Both chronic changes in ventricular structure and rapid changes in ventricular dimensions may play a role in altering the electrical activity of the heart. The mechanisms responsible for heart rhythm changes upon acute myocardial deformation are the subject of other chapters (see, for example, Chapter 45 for pro-arrhythmic and Chapter 50 for antiarrhythmic effects of acute mechanical stimulation). These reports prove, in principle, that rapid VAD-induced distortions in ventricular dimensions may alter the electrical activity of the heart. We have observed gross and rapidly changing distortions of the ventricular cavity during continuous VAD support[37]. Whether or not this is causally associated with alterations to the electrical activity of the heart is not clear (Fig. 59.2).

Ischaemia, the mismatch between the supply of blood and the demand for it, is a well-recognized risk factor for arrhythmia. Some investigators have suggested that VAD implantation can cause a reduction in myocardial blood flow[38], although we have not found this[39]. There are a number of theoretical mechanisms for VAD-induced ischaemia. Because VAD reduce the work of the heart, they might reduce coronary flow[40]. Further, in the case of pulsatile VAD that are not synchronized with the cardiac cycle, increased input pressure at the coronary arteries during the systolic phase, i.e. when intramyocardial pressure is also elevated, may

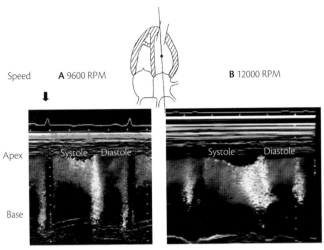

Fig. 59.2 Colour M-mode recording of the left ventricle showing continuous systolic and diastolic flow at the apex at a VAD-speed of 9,600 RPM (**A**) and 12,000 RPM (**B**). The continuous pump may result in discontinuous flow. The distortions in the ventricular wall induced by the VAD might alter a number of functional properties in the myocardium including the heart rhythm. The colour scale is a visual representation of the blood flow. Blue represents flow away from the probe and red represents flow towards the probe. RPM: rotations per minute. [Reproduced, with permission, from Henein M, Birks EJ, Tansley PD, Bowles CT, Yacoub MH (2002) Images in cardiovascular medicine. Temporal and spatial changes in left ventricular pattern of flow during continuous assist device "HeartMate II". *Circulation* **105**:2324–2325.] (See color plate section.)

limit the perfusion of the heart. However, even with reduced coronary flow, since the workload of the heart is profoundly reduced during mechanical unloading, it is unlikely that mismatch between blood supply and demand exists in the VAD-treated hearts.

Structural remodelling extends to the cytoskeletal level and the reported derangements of a number of structural proteins is normalized after chronic VAD support, e.g.[41,42]. Additionally, structural changes in response to VAD insertion are observed in a number of extracellular matrix constituents, cell signalling pathways and fibrosis levels, although the latter is controversial (see below).

Functional recovery is mediated by improvements in cellular function[43] as well as partly reversed metabolic derangements[44,45]. Improved function may be explained by the increased expression of a number of Ca^{2+} handling genes, known to be downregulated in HF, including sarco/endoplasmic reticulum Ca^{2+} ATPase 2a (SERCA2a), the ryanodine receptor (RyR) and the Na^+/Ca^{2+} exchanger (NCX)[46]. These and other functional improvements at the myocardial level can lead to such improved cardiac function that the VAD may be removed and the patient returned to reliance on his or her own heart[23]. While we have found some evidence that structural genes are associated with the probability of recovery[47], we have reported clear electrical changes which are unique to hearts that underwent reverse remodelling to recovery[48]. Specifically, while cardiomyocytes from patients whose hearts recovered (allowing explanation of the VAD) and those that did not (requiring transplantation) were structurally remodelled (e.g. 50% reduction in cell size), only the patients who recovered showed specific changes associated with the electrophysiology of the cardiomyocytes. These were (1) a reduction in action potential duration, (2) faster L-type Ca^{2+} current ($I_{Ca,L}$) inactivation, and (3) increased sarcoplasmic

reticulum (SR) Ca^{2+} content (Fig. 59.3). Thus the mechanical unloading of the left ventricle appears to have the potential of causing important electrical reverse remodelling effects which may be of consequence to the phenomenon of cardiac recovery.

Basic cellular mechanisms: mechanical unloading and electrical remodelling

As previously described, mechanical unloading of failing myocardium is associated with reverse electrical remodelling[49]. The mechanisms underlying this include (1) effects on the action potential; (2) effects on Ca^{2+} handling; (3) effects oncardiac conduction; and (4) effects on fibrosis, with possible arrhythmogenic effects.

Effects on the action potential

VAD insertion induces early and delayed electrical effects on the myocardium[49] which may be associated with arrhythmia in the early stages post-implantation[33]. We have seen an increased action potential duration (APD) after unloading (1 week) in experimental animals[50], which could explain the increased QT interval observed by Harding *et al.*[49]. In acute mechanical unloading during the first week, the increase in VA is associated with QTc prolongation[49], consistent with the finding that the majority of VA occur in the initial period after VAD insertion. The relationship between a decreasing afterload and increasing APD in myocardium is long established[51], as is a similar finding regarding QTc[52,53].

In the long term, the electrical remodelling that occurs in response to mechanical unloading results in a less arrhythmia-prone myocardium. These changes counteract the prolonged duration (and increased variability) of QTc associated with increased APD[49], both of which are linked to an elevated risk of arrhythmia and risk of sudden cardiac death in HF[54,55]. Using samples from post-VAD patients, taken at the time of transplantation or explantation of the VAD, it has been shown at the level of isolated cardiomyocytes that the VAD-induced reduction in QT interval was due to a reduction in APD. Indeed, we found that a reduction in APD was a characteristic of patients who responded to prolonged mechanical unloading by recovering[48]. Thus, the effects of prolonged unloading are opposite to the acute effects, with a biphasic response. While such a biphasic response is not always found (and probably depends on the patient cohort), it has been confirmed that prolonged mechanical unloading causes a decrease in the QRS interval and the QT interval[56].

Changes at the level of the action potential cannot fully explain the electrical changes, acute or prolonged. NCX upregulation, associated with rising intracellular sodium levels and greater predisposition to delayed after-depolarizations, has been widely associated with VA post-VAD[27,33,49,57–59]. Down-regulation of the gap junctional protein connexin 43 (Cx43) is associated with reductions in conduction velocity and a predisposition to VT[60,61], and it has been shown to occur in patients suffering from VA post-VAD[27]. In the same study, NCX upregulation and potassium channel Kv4.3 downregulation was noted in the VA group, a combination known to lengthen APD and predispose to arrhythmias[62,63]. Clearly, Ca^{2+} homeostasis plays a critical role in the response of the heart to mechanical unloading (as discussed in more detail in other chapters, e.g. Chapter 10), both in the pro-arrhythmic early phase and in the later less arrhythmogenic phase.

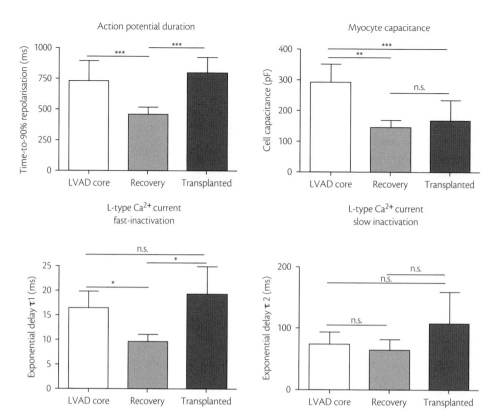

Fig. 59.3 Electrophysiological signature of clinical recovery in patients who underwent LVAD implantation. Electrophysiological parameters of myocytes isolated from myocardial tissue taken at time to LVAD insertion (LVAD core), at time of LVAD extraction (Recovery) and from hearts without recovery (Transplanted). Top left: action potential duration. Top right: cell capacitance. Bottom: fast (left) and slow (right) components of inactivation of Ca^{2+} current. $*p < 0.05$; $**p < 0.01$; $***p < 0.001$. n.s. not significant difference. [Reproduced, with permission, from Terracciano CM, Hardy J, Birks EJ, Khaghani A, Banner NR, Yacoub MH (2004) Clinical recovery from end-stage heart failure using left-ventricular assist device and pharmacological therapy correlates with increased sarcoplasmic reticulum calcium content but not with regression of cellular hypertrophy. *Circulation* **109**: 2263–2265.]

Effects on Ca^{2+} handling

For efficient contraction, the trigger Ca^{2+} influx via $I_{Ca,L}$ must be well coupled to the RyR in order for adequate SR Ca^{2+} to be released to activate the sarcomeres[64]. Among others [e.g.[65]] we have shown $I_{Ca,L}$ to be significantly reduced in human[66] and experimental models[67] of HF. We have shown that this derangement is corrected in experimental models by mechanical unloading alone, even within a period as short as 1 week[50]. In human patients, we found that, compared to the time of implantation, a shorter fast inactivation time of $I_{Ca,L}$ is positively correlated with recovery[48]. It is widely accepted that the SR becomes Ca^{2+}-depleted in HF[68]. VAD therapy can increase the SR Ca^{2+} content significantly compared to the time of implantation of the device. Indeed our results show that increased SR content is necessary for cardiac recovery[48]. Thus, long-term mechanical unloading of failing hearts has electrically beneficial reverse remodelling effects.

Other mediators of Ca^{2+} homeostasis also play an important, if less clear, role. It is widely believed that NCX expression and function rise in HF [e.g.[69]]. However, this is a controversial finding[70]. We have suggested that HF results in an increased expression of NCX which results, however, in production of poorly or inadequately functioning proteins. In our data, VAD support induced an increase in the level of NCX gene expression [compared to SERCA2a expression[71]], in contrast to some other reports[57]. Although we did not measure NCX protein in this study, NCX activity was increased in those patients who recovered on VAD support, but not in those who remained in need of cardiac transplantation. The other main competitor for cytoplasmic Ca^{2+} is

SERCA2a, which is also reported to be downregulated in HF[72]. Protein levels of SERCA2a were increased after VAD therapy, which could mediate the increase in SR Ca^{2+} seen after mechanical unloading[46].

Effects on cardiac conduction

Alterations to electrocardiographic markers of cardiac conduction have been noted after VAD insertion, but the underlying mechanisms are unknown and remain largely uninvestigated. A single report highlights changes in the expression of the gap junctional protein Cx43 in patients who have undergone VAD insertion, which may be partly explanatory[27]. Cx43 was downregulated in the hearts of patients who had VAD and who developed VA, whereas expression of Cx43 was unchanged in patients who did not display ventricular arrhythmias. There may be an underlying susceptibility to arrhythmia in some patients, whereby mechanical unloading causes downregulation of Cx43 (although cardiac cell culture work shows stretch-induced upregulation of Cx43; for more detail see Chapter 18).

Effects on fibrosis

It is known that the failing heart displays a higher than normal level of collagen, increasing ventricular stiffness and distorting chamber dimensions[4]. The presence of fibrotic patches of myocardium could be arrhythmogenic as it increases electrical heterogeneity which can set up re-entry circuits. However, the concept that VAD insertion induces fibrosis is controversial. A number of investigators have shown increased collagen[73–75] while others show reductions in collagen[76–78]. There are no studies correlating the level of fibrosis with the rate of arrhythmias in post-VAD patients, and partial contributions of cellular and a-cellular constituents of the cardiac connective tissue may form an exciting target for further research (for potential relevance of cardiac fibroblasts see Chapter 19).

Conclusions and outlook

VAD treatment is associated with an early increased risk of VA during the first few days/weeks after implantation. In the longer term, VA do not represent an important complication of VAD. VAD induce (at least partial) reverse pathological electrical remodelling in patients with severe HF. The degree of unloading and the type of flow provided by the different generations of VAD are important variables, and it is likely that future devices and improved associated medical treatment will offer significant improvements in reducing and managing arrhythmias in patients treated with VAD. The evidence discussed above indicates a clear electrophysiological response of the chronically unloaded myocardium, which represents an important and interesting example of MEC. Future research should focus on dissecting the mechanisms that underlie this response and how they might be better modulated to maximize the clinical efficacy of VAD.

References

1. American Heart Association. (2009) *Heart and Stroke Facts: 2006 Update*. www.americanheart.org.
2. Lipshultz SE, Sleeper LA, Towbin JA, et al. The incidence of pediatric cardiomyopathy in two regions of the United States. *N Engl J Med* 2003;**348**:1647–1655.
3. Mayosi BM. Contemporary trends in the epidemiology and management of cardiomyopathy and pericarditis in sub-Saharan Africa. *Heart* 2007;**93**:1176–1183.
4. Jessup M, Brozena S. Heart failure. *N Engl J Med* 2003;**348**:2007–2018.
5. Abdel-Latif A, Bolli R, Tleyjeh IM, et al. Adult bone marrow-derived cells for cardiac repair: a systematic review and meta-analysis. *Arch Intern Med* 2007;**167**:989–997.
6. Yacoub MH, Miller LW. Long-term left-ventricular-assist-device therapy is here to stay. *Nat Clin Pract Cardiovasc Med* 2008;**5**:60–61.
7. Terracciano CM, Miller L.W, Yacoub MH. Contemporary Use of Ventricular Assist Devices. *Ann Rev Med* 2010;**61**:1–31.
8. Morshuis M, El-Banayosy A, Arusoglu L, et al. European experience of DuraHeart magnetically levitated centrifugal left ventricular assist system. *Eur J Cardiothorac Surg* 2009;**35**:1020–1027.
9. Acker MA, Bolling S, Shemin R, et al. Mitral valve surgery in heart failure: insights from the Acorn Clinical Trial. *J Thorac Cardiovasc Surg* 2006;**132**:568–577.
10. Mann DL, Acker MA, Jessup M, Sabbah HN, Starling RC, Kubo SH. Clinical evaluation of the CorCap Cardiac Support Device in patients with dilated cardiomyopathy. *Ann Thorac Surg* 2007;**84**:1226–1235.
11. Mann DL, Taegtmeyer H. Dynamic regulation of the extracellular matrix after mechanical unloading of the failing human heart: recovering the missing link in left ventricular remodeling. *Circulation* 2001;**104**:1089–1091.
12. Henriques JP, de Mol BA. New percutaneous mechanical left ventricular support for acute MI: the AMC MACH program. *Nat Clin Pract Cardiovasc Med* 2008;**5**:62–63.
13. Cheng JM, den Uil CA, Hoeks SE, et al. Percutaneous left ventricular assist devices vs. intra-aortic balloon pump counterpulsation for treatment of cardiogenic shock: a meta-analysis of controlled trials. *Eur Heart J* 2009;**30**:2102–2108.
14. Kulick DM, Bolman RM, III, Salerno CT, Bank AJ, Park SJ. Management of recurrent ventricular tachycardia with ventricular assist device placement. *Ann Thorac Surg* 1998;**66**:571–573.
15. Maile S, Kunz M, Oechslin E, et al. Intractable ventricular tachycardia and bridging to heart transplantation with a non-pulsatile flow assist device in a patient with isolated left-ventricular non-compaction. *J Heart Lung Transplant* 2004;**23**:147–149.
16. Durand-Dubief A, Burri H, Chevalier P, Touboul P. Short-coupled variant of torsades de pointes with intractable ventricular fibrillation: lifesaving effect of cardiopulmonary bypass. *J Cardiovasc Electrophysiol* 2003;**14**:329.
17. Pagani FD, Miller LW, Russell SD, et al. Extended mechanical circulatory support with a continuous-flow rotary left ventricular assist device. *J Am Coll Cardiol* 2009;**54**:312–321.
18. Christiansen S, Klocke A, Autschbach R. Past, present, and future of long-term mechanical cardiac support in adults. *J Card Surg* 2008;**23**:664–676.
19. Rose EA, Gelijns AC, Moskowitz AJ, et al. Long-term mechanical left ventricular assistance for end-stage heart failure. *N Engl J Med* 2001;**345**:1435–1443.
20. Mancini DM, Beniaminovitz A, Levin H, et al. Low incidence of myocardial recovery after left ventricular assist device implantation in patients with chronic heart failure. *Circulation* 1998;**98**:2383–2389.
21. Maybaum S, Mancini D, Xydas S, et al. Cardiac improvement during mechanical circulatory support: a prospective multicenter study of the LVAD Working Group. *Circulation* 2007;**115**:2497–2505.
22. Yacoub MH, Birks EJ, Tansley P, Henien MY, Bowles CT. Bridge to recovery: the Harefield Approach. *J Cong Heart Failure Circ Support* 2001;**2**:27–30.
23. Birks EJ, Tansley PD, Hardy J, et al. Left ventricular assist device and drug therapy for the reversal of heart failure. *N Engl J Med* 2006;**355**:1873–1884.
24. Levin HR, Oz MC, Chen JM, Packer M, Rose EA, Burkhoff D. Reversal of chronic ventricular dilation in patients with end-stage cardiomyopathy by prolonged mechanical unloading. *Circulation* 1995;**91**:2717–2720.
25. Oz MC, Rose EA, Slater J, Kuiper JJ, Catanese KA, Levin HR. Malignant ventricular arrhythmias are well tolerated in patients receiving long-term left ventricular assist devices. *J Am Coll Cardiol* 1994;**24**:1688–1691.
26. Arai H, Swartz MT, Pennington DG, et al. Importance of ventricular arrhythmias in bridge patients with ventricular assist devices. *ASAIO Trans* 1991;**37**:M427–M428.
27. Refaat M, Chemaly E, Lebeche D, Gwathmey JK, Hajjar RJ. Ventricular arrhythmias after left ventricular assist device implantation. *Pacing Clin Electrophysiol* 2008;**31**:1246–1252.
28. Genovese EA, Dew MA, Teuteberg JJ, et al. Incidence and patterns of adverse event onset during the first 60 days after ventricular assist device implantation. *Ann Thorac Surg* 2009;**88**:1162–1170.
29. Bedi M, Kormos R, Winowich S, McNamara DM, Mathier MA, Murali S. Ventricular arrhythmias during left ventricular assist device support. *Am J Cardiol* 2007;**99**:1151–1153.
30. Ziv O, Dizon J, Thosani A, Naka Y, Magnano AR, Garan H. Effects of left ventricular assist device therapy on ventricular arrhythmias. *J Am Coll Cardiol* 2005;**45**:1428–1434.
31. Singh BN. Significance and control of cardiac arrhythmias in patients with congestive cardiac failure. *Heart Fail Rev* 2002;**7**:285–300.
32. Andersen M, Videbaek R, Boesgaard S, Sander K, Hansen PB, Gustafsson F. Incidence of ventricular arrhythmias in patients on long-term support with a continuous-flow assist device (HeartMate II). *J Heart Lung Transplant* 2009;**28**:733–735.
33. Harding JD, Piacentino V, III, Rothman S, Chambers S, Jessup M, Margulies KB. Prolonged repolarization after ventricular assist device support is associated with arrhythmias in humans with congestive heart failure. *J Card Fail* 2005;**11**:227–232.

34. Scheinin SA, Capek P, Radovancevic B, Duncan JM, McAllister HA, Jr., Frazier OH. The effect of prolonged left ventricular support on myocardial histopathology in patients with end-stage cardiomyopathy. *ASAIO J* 1992;**38**:M271–M274.

35. De JN, van Wichen DF, Schipper ME, Lahpor JR, Gmelig-Meyling FH, De Weger RA. Does unloading the heart by a left ventricular assist device result in sustained reversal of myocyte dysfunction in end-stage heart failure? *J Heart Lung Transplant* 2001;**20**:202.

36. Rivello HG, Meckert PC, Vigliano C, Favaloro R, Laguens RP. Cardiac myocyte nuclear size and ploidy status decrease after mechanical support. *Cardiovasc Pathol* 2001;**10**:53–57.

37. Henein M, Birks EJ, Tansley PD, Bowles CT, Yacoub MH. Images in cardiovascular medicine. Temporal and spatial changes in left ventricular pattern of flow during continuous assist device "HeartMate II". *Circulation* 2002;**105**:2324–2325.

38. Xydas S, Rosen RS, Ng C, *et al.* Mechanical unloading leads to echocardiographic, electrocardio-graphic, neurohormonal, and histologic recovery. *J Heart Lung Transplant* 2006;**25**:7–15.

39. Tansley P, Yacoub M, Rimoldi O, *et al.* Effect of left ventricular assist device combination therapy on myocardial blood flow in patients with end-stage dilated cardiomyopathy. *J Heart Lung Transplant* 2004;**23**:1283–1289.

40. Heusch G. Heart rate in the pathophysiology of coronary blood flow and myocardial ischaemia: benefit from selective bradycardic agents. *Br J Pharmacol* 2008;**153**:1589–1601.

41. Aquila LA, McCarthy PM, Smedira NG, Young JB, Moravec CS. Cytoskeletal structure and recovery in single human cardiac myocytes. *J Heart Lung Transplant* 2004;**23**:954–963.

42. De JN, Lahpor JR, van Wichen DF, *et al.* Similar left and right ventricular sarcomere structure after support with a left ventricular assist device suggests the utility of right ventricular biopsies to monitor left ventricular reverse remodeling. *Int J Cardiol* 2005;**98**:465–470.

43. Dipla K, Mattiello JA, Jeevanandam V, Houser SR, Margulies KB. Myocyte recovery after mechanical circulatory support in humans with end-stage heart failure. *Circulation* 1998;**97**:2316–2322.

44. Heerdt PM, Schlame M, Jehle R, Barbone A, Burkhoff D, Blanck TJ. Disease-specific remodeling of cardiac mitochondria after a left ventricular assist device. *Ann Thorac Surg* 2002;**73**:1216–1221.

45. Razeghi P, Myers TJ, Frazier OH, Taegtmeyer H. Reverse Remodeling of the Failing Human Heart with Mechanical Unloading. *Cardiology* 2002;**98**:167–174.

46. Heerdt PM, Holmes JW, Cai B, *et al.* Chronic unloading by left ventricular assist device reverses contractile dysfunction and alters gene expression in end-stage heart failure. *Circulation* 2000;**102**:2713–2719.

47. Hall JL, Birks EJ, Grindle S, *et al.* Molecular signature of recovery following combination left ventricular assist device (LVAD) support and pharmacologic therapy. *Eur Heart J* 2007;**28**:613–627.

48. Terracciano CM, Hardy J, Birks EJ, Khaghani A, Banner NR, Yacoub MH. Clinical recovery from end-stage heart failure using left-ventricular assist device and pharmacological therapy correlates with increased sarcoplasmic reticulum calcium content but not with regression of cellular hypertrophy. *Circulation* 2004;**109**:2263–2265.

49. Harding JD, Piacentino V, III, Gaughan JP, Houser SR, Margulies KB. Electrophysiological alterations after mechanical circulatory support in patients with advanced cardiac failure. *Circulation* 2001;**104**:1241–1247.

50. Soppa GK, Lee J, Stagg MA, *et al.* Role and possible mechanisms of clenbuterol in enhancing reverse remodelling during mechanical unloading in murine heart failure. *Cardiovasc Res* 2008;**77**:695–706.

51. Taggart P, Sutton PM, Treasure T, *et al.* Monophasic action potentials at discontinuation of cardiopulmonary bypass: evidence for contraction-excitation feedback in man. *Circulation* 1988;**77**:1266–1275.

52. Levine JH, Guarnieri T, Kadish AH, White RI, Calkins H, Kan JS. Changes in myocardial repolarization in patients undergoing balloon valvuloplasty for congenital pulmonary stenosis: evidence for contraction-excitation feedback in humans. *Circulation* 1988;**77**:70–77.

53. Lab MJ. Contraction-excitation feedback in myocardium. Physiological basis and clinical relevance. *Circ Res* 1982;**50**:757–766.

54. Grimm W, Steder U, Menz V, Hoffman J, Maisch B. QT dispersion and arrhythmic events in idiopathic dilated cardiomyopathy. *Am J Cardiol* 1996;**78**:458–461.

55. Okin PM, Devereux RB, Howard BV, Fabsitz RR, Lee ET, Welty TK. Assessment of QT interval and QT dispersion for prediction of all-cause and cardiovascular mortality in American Indians: The Strong Heart Study. *Circulation* 2000;**101**:61–66.

56. Xydas S, Kherani AR, Chang JS, *et al.* Beta-2 adrenergic stimulation attenuates left ventricular remodeling, decreases apoptosis, and improves calcium homeostasis in a rodent model of ischemic cardiomyopathy. *J Pharmacol Exp Ther* 2006;**317**:553–561.

57. Chaudhary KW, Rossman EI, Piacentino V, III, *et al.* Altered myocardial Ca^{2+} cycling after left ventricular assist device support in the failing human heart. *J Am Coll Cardiol* 2004;**44**:837–845.

58. Chen Y, Park S, Li Y, *et al.* Alterations of gene expression in failing myocardium following left ventricular assist device support. *Physiol Genomics* 2003;**14**:251–260.

59. Flesch M, Margulies KB, Mochmann HC, Engel D, Sivasubramanian N, Mann DL. Differential regulation of mitogen-activated protein kinases in the failing human heart in response to mechanical unloading. *Circulation* 2001;**104**:2273–2276.

60. Saez JC, Nairn AC, Czernik AJ, Fishman GI, Spray DC, Hertzberg EL. Phosphorylation of connexin43 and the regulation of neonatal rat cardiac myocyte gap junctions. *J Mol Cell Cardiol* 1997;**29**:2131–2145.

61. Poelzing S, Rosenbaum DS. Altered connexin43 expression produces arrhythmia substrate in heart failure. *Am J Physiol* 2004;**287**:H1762–H1770.

62. Lebeche D, Kaprielian R, Hajjar R. Modulation of action potential duration on myocyte hypertrophic pathways. *J Mol Cell Cardiol* 2006;**40**:725–735.

63. Lebeche D, Kaprielian R, del Monte F, *et al.* In vivo cardiac gene transfer of Kv4.3 abrogates the hypertrophic response in rats after aortic stenosis. *Circulation* 2004;**110**:3435–3443.

64. Bers DM. Cardiac excitation-contraction coupling. *Nature* 2002;**415**:198–205.

65. Chen X, Piacentino V, III, Furukawa S, Goldman B, Margulies KB, Houser SR. L-type Ca^{2+} channel density and regulation are altered in failing human ventricular myocytes and recover after support with mechanical assist devices. *Circ Res* 2002;**91**:517–524.

66. Terracciano CM, Harding SE, Adamson D, *et al.* Changes in sarcolemmal Ca entry and sarcoplasmic reticulum Ca content in ventricular myocytes from patients with end-stage heart failure following myocardial recovery after combined pharmacological and ventricular assist device therapy. *Eur Heart J* 2003;**24**:1329–1339.

67. Soppa GK, Lee J, Stagg MA, *et al.* Prolonged mechanical unloading reduces myofilament sensitivity to calcium and sarcoplasmic reticulum calcium uptake leading to contractile dysfunction. *J Heart Lung Transplant* 2008;**27**:882–889.

68. Lindner M, Erdmann E, Beuckelmann DJ. Calcium content of the sarcoplasmic reticulum in isolated ventricular myocytes from patients with terminal heart failure. *J Mol Cell Cardiol* 1998;**30**:743–749.

69. Pogwizd SM, Qi M, Yuan W, Samarel AM, Bers DM. Upregulation of Na^{+}/Ca^{2+} exchanger expression and function in an arrhythmogenic rabbit model of heart failure. *Circ Res* 1999;**85**:1009–1019.

70. Sipido KR, Volders PG, Vos MA, Verdonck F. Altered Na/Ca exchange activity in cardiac hypertrophy and heart failure: a new target for therapy? *Cardiovasc Res* 2002;**53**:782–805.

71. Terracciano CM, Koban MU, Soppa GK, *et al.* The role of the cardiac Na^{+}/Ca^{2+} exchanger in reverse remodeling: relevance for LVAD-recovery. *Ann N Y Acad Sci* 2007;**1099**:349–360.

72. Arai M, Alpert NR, MacLennan DH, Barton P, Periasamy M. Alterations in sarcoplasmic reticulum gene expression in human heart failure. A possible mechanism for alterations in systolic and diastolic properties of the failing myocardium. *Circ Res* 1993;**72**:463–469.

73. McCarthy PM, Savage RM, Fraser CD, *et al.* Hemodynamic and physiologic changes during support with an implantable left ventricular assist device. *J Thorac Cardiovasc Surg* 1995;**109**:409–417.

74. Nakatani S, McCarthy PM, Kottke-Marchant K, *et al.* Left ventricular echocardiographic and histologic changes: impact of chronic unloading by an implantable ventricular assist device. *J Am Coll Cardiol* 1996;**27**:894–901.

75. Li YY, Feng Y, McTiernan CF, *et al.* Downregulation of matrix metalloproteinases and reduction in collagen damage in the failing human heart after support with left ventricular assist devices. *Circulation* 2001;**104**:1147–1152.

76. Bruckner BA, Stetson SJ, Farmer JA, *et al.* The implications for cardiac recovery of left ventricular assist device support on myocardial collagen content. *Am J Surg* 2000;**180**:498–501.

77. Bruckner BA, Stetson SJ, Perez-Verdia A, *et al.* Regression of fibrosis and hypertrophy in failing myocardium following mechanical circulatory support. *J Heart Lung Transplant* 2001;**20**:457–464.

78. Wohlschlaeger J, Schmitz KJ, Schmid C, *et al.* Reverse remodeling following insertion of left ventricular assist devices (LVAD): a review of the morphological and molecular changes. *Cardiovasc Res* 2005;**68**:376–386.

SECTION 9

Novel directions in cardiac mechano-electric coupling

60. **Measuring strain of structural proteins *in vivo* in real time**   *431*
Fanjie Meng and Frederick Sachs

61. **Roles of cardiac SAC beyond mechano-electric coupling: stretch-enhanced force generation and muscular dystrophy**   *435*
David G. Allen and Marie L. Ward

62. **Distributions of myocyte stress, strain and work in normal and infarcted ventricles**   *442*
Elliot J. Howard and Jeffrey H. Omens

63. **Evolving concepts in measuring ventricular strain in canine and human hearts: non-invasive imaging**   *450*
Elisa E. Konofagou and Jean Provost

64. **Evolving concepts in measuring ventricular strain in the human heart: impedance measurements**   *456*
Douglas A. Hettrick

65. **Mechano-sensitive channel blockers: a new class of antiarrhythmic drugs?**   *462*
Ed White

Measuring strain of structural proteins *in vivo* in real time

Fanjie Meng and Frederick Sachs

Background

Mechanical forces change the shape of cells and molecules and confer motion to organs and organisms. At the cell and molecular level, these forces affect a vast range of physiological and pathological processes, including angiogenesis, osteogenesis, osteoporosis, muscle development, muscular dystrophy, aortic aneurysms and tumour growth[1,2]. Mechanical forces also affect embryonic differentiation, cell locomotion and auditory transduction[3-5]. One of the best understood mechanical sensing elements in cells are mechano-sensitive ion channels that transduce membrane tension into chemical and/or electrical signals[6,7]. Most mechanical stresses in cells are born by the extracellular matrix and the cytoskeleton where they are tightly linked to the biochemistry[8]. Molecular dynamics is the study of the interaction of forces with molecular structure [9]. Single molecule force spectroscopy *in vitro* has shown that external forces can unfold molecules in a predictable manner[10-12] and can expose cryptic hidden sites[13] that alter the biochemistry[14-16]. (Note: in what follows, 'stress' refers to force differentials and 'strain' to distance changes.)

Mechanical activity is obviously integral to the study of the heart, but histoanatomy and cell structure are too complex, anisotropic and heterogeneous (e.g. see Chapters 9 and 30) to allow a continuum analytic approach to calculating the details of mechanical stress–strain dynamics from the whole organ to the subcellular domain (see Chapters 34–36). Multiple mechanical stress–strain sensors are present in the cardiac cytoskeleton, notably the contractile system itself as well as the Z-disk and titin[17], but the distribution of stress between different proteins is not known, although the gradients of mechanical stress within cardiac tissue have been measured. Hess *et al.* combined two magnetic resonance imaging (MRI) techniques, displacement encoding with stimulated echoes (DENSE) and strain encoding (SENC), to formulate a three-dimensional (3D) strain map in a single slice of myocardium[18]. Ultrasound imaging has also been employed for strain estimation[19], while stress has been assessed using a needle probe equipped with strain gauges[20]. At the level of cells, however, their small size requires other techniques.

Cardiac cells have been stressed using cultured cardiomyocytes attached to elastic membranes, or single cells connected to probes such as carbon fibres[21,22], suction pipettes[23] or by application of shear stress (see Chapters 5 and 20). However, none of these methods can resolve the distribution of stress among the different proteins within the cell. To measure those stresses we need stress sensitive probes for particular proteins. Ideally these will also be sufficiently fast to allow us to measure how forces change during contraction and relaxation. With this goal in mind, we designed a series of FRET [Förster (or Fluorescence) Resonance Energy Transfer]-based force sensors that can be genetically inserted into different filamentous proteins[24].

FRET-based molecular force sensors

FRET is based on the following principle. A fluorescent donor molecule (D) is excited by absorption of a photon. If a fluorescent acceptor (A) is close by (~10–100 nm), energy absorbed by D can be transferred to A, which then emits a lower energy (red-shifted) photon. The value of the technique is that the D-to-A energy transfer is very sensitive to the distance between D and A[25,26]. The rate of energy transfer, k_T, is given by Equation(1):

$$k_T = \frac{1}{\tau_D}\left(\frac{R_0}{R}\right)^6 \tag{1}$$

where τ_D is the fluorescent life-time of the donor in the absence of the acceptor (typically in the range of nanoseconds) and R is the distance between D and A. R_0 is known as the Förster distance, at which half of the donor decay is due to non-radiative energy transfer from D to A. R_0 is mostly determined by the spectral overlap of D and A. We used the distance dependence of transfer to measure the strain in a molecular spring placed between a donor and an acceptor. According to Hooke's law:

$$F = -kx \tag{2}$$

where F is the applied force, k is the stiffness of the spring and x is the strain. If we know k and use the FRET value to calculate x, we can estimate the force.

Development and characterization of the force sensors

The original force sensor cassette, called stFRET, consisted of the green fluorescence protein (GFP) monomers Cerulean and Venus (both the plasmids were gifts from Dr David Piston)[27,28] linked by a stable α-helix[29] (Fig. 60.1). The linker structure can be changed to match the compliance of the host protein. The proper length of the linker for maximal strain sensitivity is $R = R_0$, and for Venus and Cerulean, R_0 is ~5 nm[30]. For characterization, the cassette was expressed in bacteria, extracted and purified. *In vitro* spectrometer measurements showed a robust energy transfer (Fig. 60.2A) which was stable from room temperature to > 80°C and in mild denaturing conditions. The linker could be approximated as a linear spring. We measured the strain sensitivity by pulling at the two ends of the cassette by attaching it to a distensible rubber membrane (Flexcell International, Hillsborough, North Carolina). Stretching the membrane[31] led to a decrease of energy transfer that was proportional to the strain, and this was reversible upon release[24] (Fig. 60.2B).

stFRET is compatible with multiple host proteins

We genetically incorporated stFRET into various cytoskeletal proteins including actinin, filamin, spectrin and myosin 2A and B. We then expressed the chimeric proteins in human embryonic kidney (HEK) cells, bovine aortic endothelial (BAEC) cells and 3T3 (3-day transfer, inoculum 3 x 10⁵ cells) fibroblasts. The distribution patterns of the chimeric proteins were indistinguishable from host proteins tagged by GFP (unpublished data). stFRET is also compatible with *in vivo* imaging. In *Caenorhabditis elegans* we labelled collagen-19[32] in three different positions along the chain, and generated transgenic worms. The mutant with the probe in the middle of the target showed similar striation patterns as collagen-19-GFP (Fig. 60.3)[24] and the worms behaved normally. The other two mutants had collagen distributions that were different from control, showing that placement of the probe within the host can affect function.

stFRET can detect constitutive molecular force *in vivo*

The reduced FRET efficiency in resting cells was indicative of the presence of resting tension (stress) in labelled proteins. This suggests

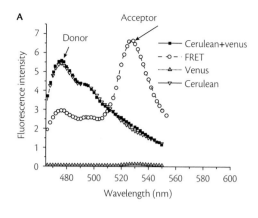

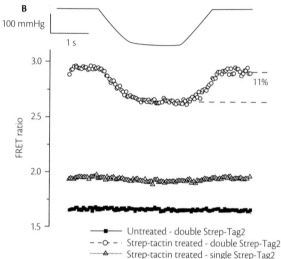

Fig. 60.2 A Emission spectra of stFRET, Cerulean and Venus monomers and Cerulean and Venus in 1:1 mixture. Excitation wavelength 433 nm. The spectrum of sstFRET is shown by the dashed line with circles, showing quenching of donor emission and enhancing of acceptor emission. **B** Demonstration of the strain sensitivity of stFRET. Each end of the stFRET probe was tagged with streptavidin (double Strep-Tag I), bound to the surface of a silicone rubber sheet that could be stretched. The black trace on the top shows the suction applied to the rubber sheet to distend it (Flexcell International, Hillsborogh, North Carolina) and the circle trace shows the FRET ratio. Controls with only one end attached show no response (triangle trace). Untreated rubber sheet had little protein attached to it and FRET ratio showed no response to stretch (square trace). [Reproduced, with permission, from Meng F, Suchyna TM, Sachs F (2008) A fluorescence energy transfer-based mechanical stress sensor for specific proteins in situ. *FEBS J* **275**:3072–3087.]

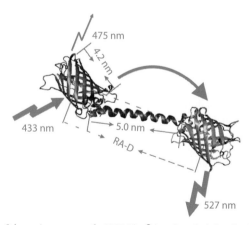

Fig. 60.1 Schematic structure of stFRET. The β-barrel on the left is the donor, Cerulean, and the one on the right is the acceptor, Venus. The height of the β-can structure is 4.2 nm. The helix linker has a nominal length of 5.0 nm. Incoming arrows indicate the excitation and outgoing ones the emission of photons, with the wavelength marked nearby and the width of the arrows proportional to the light intensity. R_{A-D} is the distance between donor and acceptor chromophores. [Reproduced, with permission, from Meng F, Suchyna TM, Sachs F (2008) A fluorescence energy transfer-based mechanical stress sensor for specific proteins in situ. *FEBS J* **275**:3072–3087.]

that the cell membrane, which is easily buckled under compression[33], is probably not under resting tension in agreement with laser trap studies[34]. However, there were gradients of stress in the cytoskeleton proteins of migrating cells. In migrating fibroblasts, the stress is low in actinin and filamin at the lagging edge where the focal adhesions are detached and high at the leading edge (Fig. 60.4)[35]. The stress in actinin and filamin could be released by trypsinizing the cells, causing them to separate from the coverslip. The presence of constitutive strain in these proteins suggests that modulation of stress is important for normal physiology.

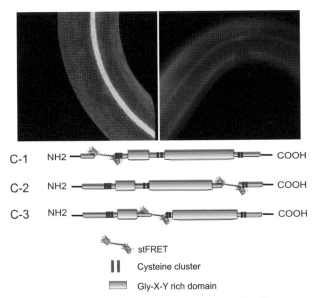

Fig. 60.3 Expression of labelled collagen in living *C. elegans*. Left: collagen-19-stFRET. Right: collagen-19-GFP (for control). Cartoons show three chimeric collagen-19 constructs, C-1, C-2 and C-3. Only C-3 displayed a fluorescence signature similar to terminally tagged GFP collagen-19. [Reproduced, with permission, from Meng F, Suchyna TM, Sachs F (2008) A fluorescence energy transfer-based mechanical stress sensor for specific proteins in situ. *FEBS J* **275**:3072–3087.]

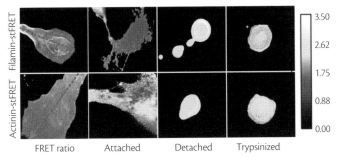

Fig. 60.4 stFRET detects resting strain in living cells. Dashed arrows in the left panels show the migrating directions. The cells show decreasing FRET (higher stress) at the front of the cell. Filamin and actinin in attached cells showed lower stress and local domains with stress gradients. Naturally rounded cells (Detached) and cells detached with trypsin (Trypsinized) displayed higher energy transfer as the stress in filamin and actinin was released. The FRET ratio calibration bar is given on the right. (See color plate section.)

Improving the sensor

Despite its sensitivity and linearity, the α-helix linker in stFRET may be too soft for monitoring the constitutive force in some cytoskeleton proteins. To study higher stress in proteins we developed another cassette where the α-helix was replaced by a spectrin repeat domain. Because spectrin repeats are conservative domains in the spectrin superfamily, the new sstFRET is expected to be suitable for proteins including actinin, spectrin and dystrophin.

In addition, to properly monitor strain (in order to deduce force) the sensor should be inserted near the middle of the host protein. However, given the 50–60 kDa molecular mass of the sensor, the tertiary structure of host proteins may be affected. A primary goal

is to reduce the size of the sensor. A recent variant of the sensor does not have a linker but uses the angle between the donor and acceptor dipole as the FRET variable. At rest, the new sensor generates approximately 80% energy transfer at parallel orientation of donor and acceptor, and mechanical forces that increase the angle between donor and acceptor reduce the energy transfer. Preliminary data show that external application of ~10 pN produces a two-fold change in FRET efficiency.

Finally, moving on from *C. elegans*, we are now creating transgenic mice with the probes inserted into various cytoskeletal and extracellular proteins, so that we can study the real-time biomechanics of specific proteins in mammalian tissues and cells.

Conclusions and outlook

Stress-sensitive probes provide novel tools to examine the distribution of cytoskeletal strain and stress within living cells, which allow one to assess changes in the internal and external mechanical environment on real time. Mature fluorescence microscopy technologies, notably multiphoton microscopy, will allow one to probe molecular mechanics in proteins deep inside living cells and tissues. This is a first step towards probing the stress and strain distribution in multiple structural proteins in a beating heart.

References

1. Wallace GQ, McNally EM. Mechanisms of muscle degeneration, regeneration, and repair in the muscular dystrophies. *Annu Rev Physiol* 2009;**71**:37–57.
2. Kumar S, Weaver VM. Mechanics, malignancy, and metastasis: the force journey of a tumor cell. *Cancer Metastasis Rev* 2009;**28**:113–127.
3. Huang S, Ingber DE. The structural and mechanical complexity of cell-growth control. *Nat Cell Biol* 1999;**1**:E131–E138.
4. Martin P, Parkhurst SM. Development. May the force be with you. *Science* 2003;**300**:63–65.
5. Avvisato CL, Yang X, Shah S, *et al.* Mechanical force modulates global gene expression and beta-catenin signaling in colon cancer cells. *J Cell Sci* 2007;**120**:2672–2682.
6. Sotomayor M, Schulten K. Molecular dynamics study of gating in the mechanosensitive channel of small conductance MscS. *Biophys J* 2004 ;**87**:3050–3065.
7. Sukharev S, Anishkin A. Mechanosensitive channels: what can we learn from 'simple' model systems? *Trends Neurosci* 2004;**27**:345–351.
8. Trepat X, Deng L, An SS, *et al.* Universal physical responses to stretch in the living cell. *Nature* 2007;**447**:592–595.
9. Zaman MH. Understanding the molecular basis for differential binding of integrins to collagen and gelatin. *Biophys J* 2007;**92**:L17–L19.
10. Carter NJ, Cross RA. Kinesin's moonwalk. *Curr Opin Cell Biol* 2006;**18**:61–67.
11. Walther KA, Brujic J, Li H, Fernandez JM. Sub-angstrom conformational changes of a single molecule captured by AFM variance analysis. *Biophys J* 2006;**90**:3806–3812.
12. Li H, Fernandez JM. Mechanical design of the first proximal Ig domain of human cardiac titin revealed by single molecule force spectroscopy. *J Mol Biol* 2003;**334**:75–86.
13. Johnson CP, Tanb HY, Carag C, Speicher DW, Discher DE. Forced unfolding of proteins within cells. *Science* 2007;**317**:663–666.
14. Discher DE, Mooney DJ, Zandstra PW. Growth factors, matrices, and forces combine and control stem cells. *Science* 2009;**324**: 1673–1677.
15. Min W, English BP, Luo G, Cherayil BJ, Kou SC, Xie XS. Fluctuating enzymes: lessons from single-molecule studies. *Acc Chem Res* 2005;**38**:923–931.

16. Forde NR, Izhaky D, Woodcock GR, Wuite GJ, Bustamante C. Using mechanical force to probe the mechanism of pausing and arrest during continuous elongation by Escherichia coli RNA polymerase. *Proc Natl Acad Sci USA* 2002;**99**:11682–11687.

17. Hoshijima M. Mechanical stress–strain sensors embedded in cardiac cytoskeleton: Z disk, titin, and associated structures. *Am J Physiol* 2006;**290**:H1313–H1325.

18. Hess AT, Zhong X, Spottiswoode BS, Epstein FH, Meintjes EM. Myocardial 3D strain calculation by combining cine displacement encoding with stimulated echoes (DENSE) and cine strain encoding (SENC) imaging. *Magn Reson Med* 2009;**62**:77–84.

19. Elen A, Choi HF, Loeckx D, *et al.* Three-dimensional cardiac strain estimation using spatio-temporal elastic registration of ultrasound images: a feasibility study. *IEEE Trans Med Imaging* 2008;**27**: 1580–1591.

20. Lunkenheimer PP, Redmann K, Florek J, *et al.* The forces generated within the musculature of the left ventricular wall. *Heart* 2004;**90**: 200–207.

21. Rana OR, Zobel C, Saygili E, *et al.* A simple device to apply equibiaxial strain to cells cultured on flexible membranes. *Am J Physiol* 2008;**294**:H532–H540.

22. Sugiura S, Yasuda S, Yamashita H, *et al.* Measurement of force developed by a single cardiac myocyte using novel carbon fibers. *Adv Exp Med Biol* 2003;**538**:381–386.

23. Zeng T, Bett GCL, Sachs F. Stretch-activated whole-cell currents in adult rat cardiac myoctes. *Am J Physiol* 2000;**278**:H548–H557.

24. Meng F, Suchyna TM, Sachs F. A fluorescence energy transfer-based mechanical stress sensor for specific proteins in situ. *FEBS J* 2008;**275**:3072–3087.

25. Förster T. Zwischenmolekulare Energiewanderung und Fluoreszenz. *Ann Physik* 1948;**6**:22.

26. Förster T. Fluoreszenz organischer Verbindungen. *Vandenhoek & Ruprecht Gottingen* 1951.

27. Qiao W, Mooney M, Bird AJ, Winge DR, Eide DJ. Zinc binding to a regulatory zinc-sensing domain monitored in vivo by using FRET. *Proc Natl Acad Sci USA* 2006;**103**:8674–8679.

28. Ha T, Rasnik I, Cheng W, *et al.* Initiation and re-initiation of DNA unwinding by the Escherichia coli Rep helicase. *Nature* 2002;**419**:638–641.

29. Chen C, Brock R, Luh F, *et al.* The solution structure of the active domain of CAP18--a lipopolysaccharide binding protein from rabbit leukocytes. *FEBS letters* 1995;**370**:46–52.

30. Patterson GH, Piston DW, Barisas BG. Förster distances between green fluorescent protein pairs. *Analytical biochemistry* 2000;**284**:438–440.

31. Besch SR, Suchyna T, Sachs F. High-speed pressure clamp. *Pflugers Arch* 2002;**445**:161–166.

32. Thein MC, McCormack G, Winter AD, Johnstone IL, Shoemaker CB, Page AP. Caenorhabditis elegans exoskeleton collagen COL-19: an adult-specific marker for collagen modification and assembly, and the analysis of organismal morphology. *Dev Dyn* 2003;**226**:523–539.

33. Honore E, Patel AJ, Chemin J, Suchyna T, Sachs F. Desensitization of mechano-gated K-2P channels. *Proc Natl Acad Sci USA* 2006;**103**: 6859–6864.

34. Sheetz MP, Dai J. Modulation of membrane dynamics and cell motility by membrane tension. *Trends Cell Biol* 1996;**6**:85–89.

35. Meng F, Suchyna T, Lasalovitch E, Gronostajski RM, Sachs F. Real time FRET based detection of mechanical stress in cytoskeletal and extracellular matrix proteins. *Cell Mol Bioeng* 2011; (in press: DOI:10.1007/s12195-010-0140-0).

Roles of cardiac SAC beyond mechano-electric coupling: stretch-enhanced force generation and muscular dystrophy

David G. Allen and Marie L. Ward

Background

Developed force in cardiac muscle increases in two phases following stretch: (1) a rapid component due to increased overlap of thick and thin filaments coupled to an increase in calcium sensitivity; and (2) a slow phase caused by increased calcium-activated force. We have proposed that increased calcium entry through a calcium-permeable stretch-activated channel is responsible for the slow phase. In this chapter we discuss candidate genes that may encode this stretch-activated channel, focusing on transient receptor potential channels TRPC1 & TRPC6, and the vanilloid transient receptor potential channel TRPV2. While stretch-activated channels (SAC) were first recognized by their increased activity when stretched in a patch pipette, this does not appear to be the dominant physiological pathway of activation. Instead complex pathways including integrins, angiotensin, nicotinamide adenine dinucleotide phosphate (NADPH) oxidase and reactive oxygen species (ROS) appear to be involved. SAC may also have roles in disease. For instance, SAC are over-active in skeletal muscle in Duchenne muscular dystrophy and appear to have a role in the calcium entry, which is a central pathological pathway of this disease. Cardiac muscle is also affected in Duchenne muscular dystrophy and SAC may have a role in the dilated cardiomyopathy which develops.

Slow force response to stretch

Stretch is an important regulator of cardiac function and an increase in ventricular end-diastolic volume, which increases the sarcomere length of ventricular muscle, increases the subsequent force of contraction[1,2]. Although these observations have been established for a century, the underlying cellular and molecular mechanisms remain incompletely understood. An early observa-tion by Parmley and Chuck (1973) was that the response to rapid stretch in isolated papillary muscles was an immediate increase in force, followed by a slower component[3]. This second, slower response to stretch, now commonly referred to as the 'slow force response' (SFR), suggested that activation of the heart is enhanced by stretch[3]. This was subsequently confirmed by the demonstration that the SFR is accompanied by a slow increase in the magnitude of the Ca^{2+} transients[4,5].

An example of the biphasic response to stretch is shown in Fig. 61.1 in which a mouse trabecula, loaded with fura-2, was subjected to a 2 min step increase in length. Immediately on stretching, the muscle isometric force was increased, with no change in the amplitude of the Ca^{2+} transient. Both force and Ca^{2+} then continued to increase following the stretch, i.e. the SFR. The immediate increase in force following a stretch is thought to be a consequence of increased filament overlap[6] and the increased myofibrillar Ca^{2+} sensitivity[7]. However, the mechanisms that produce the slow augmentation of the calcium transients are still being debated.

Cellular mechanisms that might underlie the SFR

Increased Ca^{2+} transients could arise if stretch induces additional trans-sarcolemmal Ca^{2+} influx, either associated with excitation–contraction (EC) coupling (for example, via a stretch-dependent increase in L-type Ca^{2+} channel entry) or by some other pathway that is continuously active throughout the stretch. Alternatively increased Na^+ influx could result in increased Ca^{2+} transients by promoting Na^+ efflux and Ca^{2+} influx on the Na^+/Ca^{2+} exchanger (NCX). Any of these mechanisms would increase the sarcoplasmic reticulum (SR) Ca^{2+} load and cause increased Ca^{2+} release with

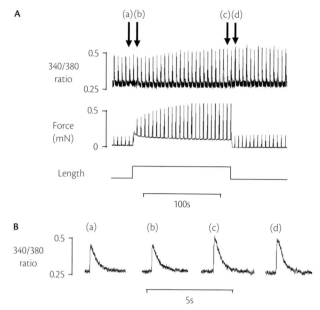

Fig. 61.1 The myocardial response to stretch. Simultaneous measurement of isometric force and $[Ca^{2+}]_i$ (fura-2) in a representative right ventricular trabecula isolated from mouse hearts subjected to a 2 min step increase in muscle length. **A** shows data before, during and after stretch. **B** shows individual Ca^{2+} transients from **A**, as labelled. [Modified, with permission, from Ward ML, Williams IA, Chu Y, Cooper PJ, Ju YK, Allen DG (2008) Stretch-activated channels in the heart: contributions to length-dependence and to cardiomyopathy. *Prog Biophys Mol Biol* **97**:232–249.].

each subsequent beat. Alternatively, transients might increase if stretch acted directly on the gating of the SR Ca^{2+} release channels, the ryanodine receptors (RyR), inducing greater Ca^{2+} release. For instance, it has been suggested that stretch enhances nitric oxide (NO) release, which increases Ca^{2+} spark frequency and triggers greater SR Ca^{2+} release in response to the action potential[8] (for review see[9]). Another possibility is that the activity of the cardiac Na^+/H^+ exchanger (NHE1) is increased by stretch[10] which would operate by initially increasing Na^+ influx (for review see[9]).

There is good evidence that the stretch-dependent increase in the Ca^{2+} transients is not due to an EC coupling-dependent mechanism. Isolated papillary muscles shortened only during diastole still exhibit the effect of shortening on the amplitude of the systolic Ca^{2+} transients[11]. Furthermore, a steady increase in intracellular Ca^{2+} concentration $([Ca^{2+}]_i)$ has also been reported in quiescent preparations when stretched[9,12]. Thus it seems clear that stretch increases resting $[Ca^{2+}]_i$ by a process that occurs in diastole and subsequently causes the increased systolic Ca^{2+} release.

Possible role of stretch-activated channels

SAC were discovered by Guharay and Sachs (1984) whilst patch-clamping skeletal muscle fibres[13]. Since then three families of SAC have been described in cardiac muscle: (1) K^+ selective channels (SAC_K)[14]; (2) anion or Cl^-selective channels (usually activated by cell volume changes, and hence called volume-activated channels; VAC_{Cl})[15]; and (3) non-specific cationic channels (SAC_{NS}) that allow entry of K^+, Na^+ and/or Ca^{2+} when open. Several studies have investigated a possible role for SAC_{NS} in the SFR[9,16].

Virtually all cell types have mechano-sensing abilities of one form or another, and it is becoming increasingly obvious that the

nature of the response is dependent on the mechanical signal applied. In studying the response to stretch in isolated cardiac muscle preparations such as papillary muscles, trabeculae and single myocytes, a linear stretch is commonly applied. Under these conditions, given that the volume of myocytes is constant, the cross-sectional area must fall, suggesting that the length of the t-tubules would become shorter. SAC located in the t-tubules might therefore behave very differently to those located on the external sarcolemma. However, the t-tubular system also contains interconnecting longitudinal tubules[17]. Thus it is likely that axial stretch could have differential effects on channels in the longitudinal t-tubules, the radial t-tubules and the external sarcolemma.

In contrast to linear stretch, various other types of stimuli have been used to activate SAC in isolated ventricular myocytes: (1) increase in cell volume by hypotonic solutions[18] or by cell inflation using positive pressure applied to a patch pipette[19]; (2) radial stretch as applied to magnetic beads fixed to the (external) sarcolemmal β-integrins by antibodies[15]; and (3) shear stress applied to an isolated cell by means of two tools attached to the upper surface while the lower surface is attached to the glass[20]. While each of these stimuli may provide some linear stretch of the outer cell membrane, they will also lead to stretching of the t-tubules so that, if SAC are located in the t-tubules, they will see a very different stimulus under these circumstances compared to linear stretch.

The current evidence for the involvement of SAC_{NS} in SFR is primarily pharmacological. We showed recently that in mouse trabeculae the established blockers of SAC_{NS} [gadolinium (Gd^{3+}), streptomycin and *Grammostola spatulata* mechano-toxin 4 (GsMTx-4)] were all capable of reducing the magnitude of SFR[9]. Gd^{3+} and streptomycin are non-selective and thus provide little information about the identity of SAC_{NS}. GsMTx-4 seems to be specific for SAC_{NS} but does not bind to a specific site on the channel because GsMTx-4 synthesized from D-amino acids (instead of the normal L-type) is equally effective at blocking SAC_{NS}[21]. This suggests that GsMTx-4 interferes with the interaction between the bilayer lipids and the channel protein rather than a stereo-specific binding site. Mechano-sensitive channels are particularly sensitive to the lipid–protein interaction and, consequently, GsMTx has been shown to block mechano-sensitive activity generated by a range of genes (TRPC1[22], TRPC6[20,23], TRPC5[24]). Thus the pharmacological evidence suggests that SAC_{NS} are involved in the SFR but do not identify the molecular identity of the channel.

Candidate genes for SAC

If SAC are a contributor to the SFR, then a criticial issue is their molecular identification and how they are activated during stretch. We first briefly review some possible molecular identities and then consider the possible activation pathways.

TRPC1

SAC_{NS} from frog oocytes have similar properties to mammalian SAC_{NS} and Maroto *et al.*[25] showed that the purified channel had a molecular weight of 80 kDa (similar to TRPC1) and bound the TRPC1 antibody. Maroto *et al.* also expressed human TRPC1 in both frog oocytes and COS cells and observed a tenfold increase in SAC_{NS} expression. Finally, they showed that antisense RNA to human TRPC1 reduced the expression of both endogenous oocyte SAC_{NS} and human TRPC1-expressed channels. Later, however, many of the same authors found that overexpression of TRPC1 in either COS or Chinese hamster ovary (CHO) cells did not reliably increase the endogenous SAC$_{NS}$ activity[26]. They also showed that, although TRPC1 was extensively expressed, the protein was mainly intracellular and did not show obvious membrane expression. This finding is in keeping with various earlier attempts to express TRPC1 in cell lines[27]. We recently expressed TRPC1 in C2 myoblasts (a skeletal muscle cell line) and observed that the expression was mainly intracellular[28]. However, when TRPC1 was co-expressed with caveolin-3 (Cav-3), some of the TRPC1 was expressed in the membrane, and Ca^{2+} influx could be stimulated by a known activator, H$_2$O$_2$. Thus our interpretation is that TRPC1 requires Cav-3 to assist its trafficking to the membrane, and when appropriately inserted in the membrane it can be activated by ROS in the same way as the endogenous SAC$_{NS}$ in *mdx* muscle[28].

TRPC6

Pressure activation of non-specific cation channels in a patch-clamp experiment has not been observed in adult ventricular muscle despite repeated attempts[29]. However, SAC have been observed by several groups when isolated myocytes are either stretched[29] or subject to shearing strain[20]. Dyachenko *et al.*[20] applied shear strain to isolated mouse ventricular cells and elicited robust currents similar to those caused by axial stretch of rat ventricular myocytes[29]. These currents have several components and are abolished by detubulation, suggesting that they arise from channels within the t-tubules. One current is a non-specific cation current (reversal potential ~−10 mV) activated by stretch and blocked by streptomycin and GsMTx-4 (I$_{SAC,NS}$). I$_{SAC,NS}$ was blocked by an antibody to TRPC6 applied intracellularly, but unaffected when the antibody was applied extracellularly. Immunohistochemistry showed TRPC6 to be located primarily in the t-tubules in ventricular myocytes. Thus a shearing-strain activated TRPC6, located in the t-tubules, may well contribute to the increased [Ca^{2+}]$_i$ which causes the SFR[20].

TRPV2

TRPV2 has been identified as an osmotically sensitive and stretch-sensitive Ca^{2+}-permeable channel in aortic vascular smooth muscle[30]. These authors also expressed TRPV2 in CHO cells and demonstrated that the channels caused Ca^{2+} influx when the cells were stretched. Previously this group had shown that an insulin-like growth factor-regulated channel, now thought to be TRPV2, was overexpressed in skeletal muscle of another mouse model of muscular dystrophy, the δ-sarcoglycan-deficient mouse. This channel appeared to be a source of Ca^{2+} entry and subsequent pathology in this mouse model[31]. This background led them to cross a dominant–negative mutant of TRPV2 with both the *mdx* mouse and the δ-sarcoglycan-deficient mouse [32]. This cross produced a greatly reduced dystrophic pathology and suggests that TRPV2 might be one important source of stretch-induced Ca^{2+} entry in normal muscles which is pathologically enhanced in muscular dystrophy.

Mechanism of activation of SAC$_{NS}$

In a patch-clamp experiment SAC$_{NS}$ is activated in 10–100 ms and channels turn off with a similar time-course when the pressure is removed[33,34]. However, in skeletal muscle subjected to a series of contractions in which the muscle is stretched (eccentric contractions), there is no detectable Ca^{2+} change at the moment of the stretch[35]; instead there is a rise in resting [Ca^{2+}]$_i$ which continues for 20 min and is blocked by pharmacological blockers of SAC$_{NS}$[33]. In this situation, the rise of [Ca^{2+}]$_i$ occurs at the control length and outlasts the stretching stimulus by many minutes, yet it is prevented by blockers of the SAC$_{NS}$. Thus the activation of SAC$_{NS}$ appears to occur by some indirect pathway.

Theoretically there are several classes of mechanisms by which SAC might be activated (for review see[36,37]):

1. Intrinsic bilayer forces: channels sit in the lipid bilayer and are potentially sensitive to the shape or curvature of the lipids surrounding them. The shape change can be generated by positive or negative pressure applied to a section of membrane sucked into a patch pipette, or by inserting lipids with different shapes into the bilayer or by the use of drugs which locate themselves at the protein–lipid interaction.

2. Tethered proteins: a mechanical connection to the channel whose stress changes can potentially alter the open state of a channel. The cell cytoskeleton is ubiquitous and makes numerous connections with proteins in cell membrane. Many channels have been shown to have their mechano-sensitivity altered by drugs which interfere with the cytoskeleton[13]. A recent study was able to activate a small group of channels by manipulating a phalloidin bead attached to the actin cytoskeleton[38].

3. Indirect activation by signalling pathways: while many mechano-sensitive channels were discovered by patch-clamp and direct pressure modulation of the curvature of the membrane, this is not necessarily the pathway by which they are normally activated. Figure 61.2 illustrates the signalling pathways reported for four mechano-sensitive cell functions.

The swelling-activated chloride current (Fig. 61.2, panel A) has been intensively studied and the isolated channel can be activated in an inside-out patch by negative pressure applied through a patch-clamp pipette[39]. However, the activation appears slow (5–10 s), suggesting that the pathway of activation is not direct. Detailed examination was made using magnetically induced movement of beads with antibodies to β1-integrin attached to the cell surface which could stimulate the current[15]. It is well known that stretch of ventricular myocytes can induce angiotensin release[40] and that this can activate NADPH oxidase[41]. Browe and Baumgarten used inhibitors to show that these elements were involved in the activation of VAC$_{Cl}$. They proposed that ROS stimulate the channel based on the observation that channels could be activated by exogenous H$_2$O$_2$[15].

Stretch-induced activation of the cardiac NHE1 shows many of the features of the VAC$_{Cl}$ pathway (Fig. 61.2, panel B)[42]. In this case intact papillary muscles were stretched and angiotensin receptor type II release was thought to stimulate NADPH oxidase, although evidence was provided that endothelin release may also contribute. ROS production was thought to activate extracellular signal-regulated kinase (ERK) 1/2 kinase and downstream P90 RS kinases and these are known to phosphorylate and activate NHE1[43]. Thus, in this case, the length-dependent signalling pathway activates a non-channel target.

The study by Dyachenko *et al.*[20] used shear strain to stimulate a current in ventricular myocytes (Fig. 61.2, panel C). They found

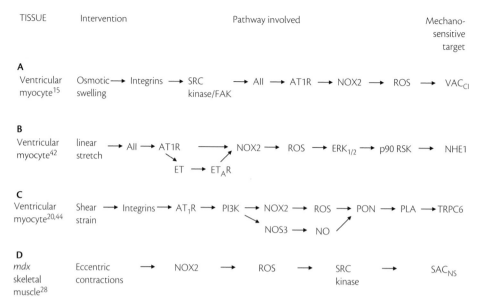

Fig. 61.2 Table showing mechano-sensitive targets activated indirectly in muscle. Src kinase, proto-oncogenic tyrosine kinase found in sarcoma; FAK, focal adhesion kinase; AII, angiotensin receptor type II; AT₁R, angiotensin type I receptor; NOX, NADPH oxidase; ET, endothelin; ETₐR, endothelin type A receptor; ERK, extracellular signal regulated kinase; RSK, ribosomal S6 kinase; PI3K, phosphoinositol 3 kinase; NOS, nitric oxide synthase; PON, peroxynitrite; PLA, phospholipase type A.

evidence that integrins invoked the activation of NADPH oxidase, although evidence of phosphatidylinositol-3,4,5-trisphosphate (PIP₃) kinase (PIP₃K) as an intermediary was obtained. They also proposed that NO synthase was activated and that reaction between superoxide and NO produced peroxynitrite[44]. This caused activity of phospholipases which generated amphipaths which change the curvature of the membrane and thereby activate TRPC6. An important feature of their study is that the current was blocked by the standard and non-specific SAC blocker Gd³⁺, by GsMTx-4, and also by intracellularly applied antibody against TRPC6. These studies provide strong evidence of the molecular identity of the channel.

Eccentric contractions of skeletal muscle elevate resting intracellular Ca²⁺ after a delay[35]. This increased [Ca²⁺]ᵢ (1) is an intermediary in the damage pathway[45], (2) is part of the hypertrophic pathway triggered by eccentric contractions[46], and (3) contributes to the severe stretch-induced damage observed in the *mdx* muscle[47]. There is pharmacological evidence that SAC_NS are the source of Ca²⁺ entry[33] and some evidence that TRPC1 is the candidate gene[28]. Gervasio *et al.* proposed that increased activity of NADPH oxidase produced ROS which were thought to activate sarcoma (Src) kinase, based on the observation that the elevated [Ca²⁺]ᵢ caused by H₂O₂ was prevented by the specific Src kinase inhibitor protein phosphatase 2 (PP2)[28].

The involvement of NADPH oxidase and ROS in all these pathways is striking and many of the discrepancies may arise simply because no investigation of the relevant pathway was made, e.g. Gervasio *et al.* did not test whether angiotensin receptor type II might have triggered the activity of NADPH oxidase. The data at present suggest that an elementary pathway activated by various forms of of stretch may act as an intermediary in a range of cell functions.

These data highlight the paradox that SAC were first discovered by their mechano-sensitivity within patch electrodes, but these same channels now appear to be activated by an indirect pathway in intact cells. This suggests that the features that make a channel mechano-sensitive are the same features that are targeted by the elementary stretch-activated signalling pathway. One possibility is that the end product of the signalling pathway is amphipathic molecules which insert into the channel–protein interface and modulate channel gating[44].

Evidence that TRPC1 is not involved in SFR

Previously, we characterized the SFR in isolated ventricular trabeculae from mouse hearts[9] and showed that the magnitude of the SFR after stretch was reduced by three different blockers of SAC. Since TRPC1 had been identified as a stretch-activated cation channel in vertebrate muscle[25], we used immunolabelling to confirm that TRPC1 was expressed in mouse ventricular tissue[9].

To further test the hypothesis that influx of Ca²⁺ and/or Na⁺ through TRPC1 channels was responsible for the increased Ca²⁺ transients during the SFR, TRPC1 −/− mice were compared with age-matched wild-type (WT) (TRPC1 +/+) controls (for details see[9]). The SFR was characterized by stretching trabeculae for 2 min. Figure 61.3A shows the SFR in representative trabeculae from WT and TRPC1 −/−. Figure 61.3B shows mean SFR data 1 min and 2 min after stretch. No difference in the magnitude of the SFR was found between TRPC1 −/− and WT groups. These data suggest that the SFR in mouse ventricular muscle is not dependent on influx of Ca²⁺ and/or Na⁺ through TRPC1. However, a difficulty in the interpretation of knock-out experiments is the possibility that, in the absence of one gene, other genes change their expression and function in a compensatory manner. This possibility could be addressed by means of acute knockdown of TRPC1.

Dilated cardiomyopathy in Duchenne muscular dystrophy

Duchenne muscular dystrophy (DMD) is a degenerative disease of muscle caused by the absence of the cytoskeletal protein dystrophin[48]. Skeletal muscle is affected early, leading to walking

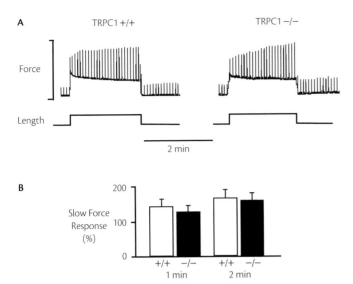

Fig. 61.3 Simultaneous measurement of isometric force and $[Ca^{2+}]_i$ (fura-2/AM) in representative right ventricular trabeculae isolated from TRPC1 WT (+/+) and TRPC1 knockout (KO) (−/−) hearts subjected to a 2 min step increase in muscle length. **A** Original recordings. **B** Mean ± SEM for $n = 4$ muscles per group. The amplitude of the SFR was unchanged in TRPC1 KO mice in comparison to WT at either 1 min or 2 min post-stretch.

difficulties in affected young boys and obligatory wheelchair use by the age of 8–12 years. The respiratory muscles are involved so that mechanical ventilation is increasingly required after the age of 15–20 years. While the skeletal muscle disease is most obvious, dystrophin is also absent from cardiac and smooth muscle[48]. The cardiac consequences are manifested as dilatation, replacement of normal myocardium by fat and fibrosis, and ECG abnormalities such as sinus tachycardia. Later in the disease progression, ventricular arrhythmias, reduced ejection fraction and frank heart failure may develop. Heart failure secondary to dilated cardiomyopathy is the cause of death in 20% of boys with DMD, but clinical evidence of cardiac involvement is present in 90% of patients[49].

While the primary cause of muscular dystrophy is the absence of dystrophin, multiple secondary effects occur and the details of how the pathology develops are uncertain. Dystrophin is a long cytoskeletal protein, attached at its C-terminus to a complex of proteins, known as the dystrophin-associated complex, located in the surface membrane. The N-terminus of dystrophin binds to the cytoskeletal actin so that dystrophin forms a mechanical link between the cytoskeleton / contractile machinery of the cell and the surface membrane (for diagram see[50]). The dystrophin-associated complex also binds to 'neuronal type' nitric oxide synthase (nNOS) and to Cav-3, the scaffolding protein of the caveolae. Cav-3 binds many proteins including TRPC1[28] and Src kinase[51]. In *mdx* and DMD muscle, dystrophin is absent and the dystrophin-associated proteins are reduced in expression[52], including nNOS[53]. However, Cav-3 displays increased expression and, concomitantly, caveolae show increased numbers and abnormal distribution[54]. Caveolae are a site at which many signalling pathways are regulated[55], raising the possibility that abnormal signalling in the caveolae contribute to the development of the disease. This view is reinforced by the fact that mutations in Cav-3 cause a mild form of

muscular dystrophy[56], and overexpression of Cav-3 leads to a severe form of muscular dystrophy[57].

Possible role of SAC_{NS} in DMD

Studies in skeletal muscle have shown that SAC_{NS} were more active both in *mdx* muscles[58] and in muscle biopsies from DMD patients[59]. This led to the hypothesis that SAC_{NS} were overactive and allowed excessive Ca^{2+} entry, which then triggered many aspects of the disease[60]. This hypothesis was supported by the observations that blockers of SAC_{NS} could prevent the stretch-induced increase in intracellular calcium and ameliorate many aspects of the disease[33]. Recent developments of this hypothesis have focused on the pathways by which the SAC_{NS} might be activated and suggest a complex pathway of activation involving Src kinase and TRPC1 which are held in close proximity by binding to Cav-3 in the caveolae[28].

Does a similar pathway operate in the heart? Globally the pathology is not dissimilar, with both cardiac and skeletal muscle showing a late loss of muscle mass, coupled with inflammation and fibrosis. However, as noted above, SAC_{NS} have not been found by patch-clamping in ventricular muscle[29] and the best defined SAC is that activated by shear stresses and encoded by TRPC6 in the t-tubules[20]. Interestingly, the activation pathway for TRPC6 in ventricular cells has some common elements with the activation pathway for SAC_{NS} in *mdx* muscle (see Fig. 61.2).

A potential link to SAC_{NS} in *mdx* ventricular myocytes has been suggested. Williams and Allen investigated Ca^{2+} regulation in *mdx* ventricular myocytes and found that the resting $[Ca^{2+}]_i$ was higher in *mdx* myocytes from old (9–12 month) animals compared to either young *mdx* or WT myocytes[61]. This elevated $[Ca^{2+}]_i$ could be lowered to normal levels by either streptomycin or GsMTx-4, suggesting that it was caused by a mechano-sensitive channel. In addition it was noted that TRPC1 showed a threefold increase in expression in aged *mdx* compared to aged WT and a fivefold increase in expression compared to young WT or *mdx*. In support of the possible role of ROS in activating the SAC_{NS}, it was shown that treatment with a ROS scavenger ameliorated many of the cardiac abnormalities associated with the disease[62]. These data suggest that mechano-sensitive channels may have a role in elevated $[Ca^{2+}]_i$ in the *mdx* heart and this is likely to be a pathogenic feature in the same manner as in skeletal muscle.

Conclusions and outlook

Although mechano-sensitive channels were originally identified by their response to mechanical deformation within a patch pipette, there is increasing evidence that their physiological and pathological pathways of activation can be different and involve complex signalling pathways. A common element to these pathways appears to be involvement of angiotensin release and receptors, the activation of NADPH oxidase and the use of various ROS as subsequent signalling molecules. The complexity and specificity of these pathways suggest they may provide therapeutic targets for those diseases in which mechano-sensitive channels play a part.

Acknowledgements

D.G. Allen is funded by a Program grant from the National Health and Medical Research Council of Australia. M.L. Ward gratefully acknowledges financial support from the Health Research Council of New Zealand and the Auckland Medical Research Foundation.

References

1. Frank O. Zur Dynamik des Herzmuskels. *Z Biol* 1895;**32**:370–447.

2. Patterson S, Starling EH. On the mechanical factors which determine the output of the ventricles. *J Physiol* 1914;**48**:357–379.

3. Parmley WW, Chuck L. Length-dependent changes in myocardial contractile state. *Am J Physiol* 1973;**224**:1195–1199.

4. Allen DG, Kurihara S. The effects of muscle length on intracellular calcium transients in mammalian cardiac muscle. *J Physiol* 1982;**327**:79–94.

5. Kentish JC, Wrzosek A. Changes in force and cytosolic Ca^{2+} concentration after length changes in isolated rat ventricular trabeculae. *J Physiol* 1998;**506**:431–444.

6. Gordon AM, Huxley AF, Julian FJ. The variation in isometric tension with sarcomere length in vertebrate muscle fibres. *J Physiol* 1966;**184**:170–192.

7. Hibberd MG, Jewell BR. Calcium- and length-dependent force production in rat ventricular muscle. *J Physiol* 1982;**329**:527–540.

8. Petroff MG, Kim SH, Pepe S, *et al.* Endogenous nitric oxide mechanisms mediate the stretch dependence of Ca^{2+} release in cardiomyocytes. *Nat Cell Biol* 2001;**3**:867–873.

9. Ward ML, Williams IA, Chu Y, Cooper PJ, Ju YK, Allen DG. Stretch-activated channels in the heart: contributions to length-dependence and to cardiomyopathy. *Prog Biophys Mol Biol* 2008; **97**:232–249.

10. Alvarez BV, Perez NG, Ennis IL, Camilion de Hurtado MC, Cingolani HE. Mechanisms underlying the increase in force and Ca^{2+} transient that follow stretch of cardiac muscle: a possible explanation of the Anrep effect. *Circ Res* 1999;**85**:716–722.

11. Allen DG, Nichols CG, Smith GL. The effects of changes in muscle length during diastole on the calcium transient in ferret ventricular muscle. *J Physiol* 1988;**406**:359–370.

12. Le Guennec JY, White E, Gannier F, Argibay JA, Garnier D. Stretch-induced increase of resting intracellular calcium concentration in single guinea-pig ventricular myocytes. *Exp Physiol* 1991;**76**:975–978.

13. Guharay F, Sachs F. Stretch-activated single ion channel currents in tissue-cultured embryonic chick skeletal muscle. *J Physiol* 1984;**352**:685–701.

14. Li XT, Dyachenko V, Zuzarte M, Putzke C, Preisig-Muller R, Isenberg G, *et al.* The stretch-activated potassium channel TREK-1 in rat cardiac ventricular muscle. *Cardiovasc Res* 2006;**69**:86–97.

15. Browe DM, Baumgarten CM. Angiotensin II (AT1) receptors and NADPH oxidase regulate Cl⁻ current elicited by beta1 integrin stretch in rabbit ventricular myocytes. *J Gen Physiol* 2004;**124**:273–287.

16. Calaghan S, White E. Activation of Na⁺-H⁺ exchange and stretch-activated channels underlies the slow inotropic response to stretch in myocytes and muscle from the rat heart. *J Physiol* 2004;**559**:205–214.

17. Soeller C, Cannell MB. Examination of the transverse tubular system in living cardiac rat myocytes by 2-photon microscopy and digital image-processing techniques. *Circ Res* 1999;**84**:266–275.

18. Tseng GN. Cell swelling increases membrane conductance of canine cardiac cells: evidence for a volume-sensitive Cl channel. *Am J Physiol* 1992;**262**:C1056–C1068.

19. Hagiwara N, Masuda H, Shoda M, Irisawa H. Stretch-activated anion currents of rabbit cardiac myocytes. *J Physiol* 1992;**456**:285–302.

20. Dyachenko V, Husse B, Rueckschloss U, Isenberg G. Mechanical deformation of ventricular myocytes modulates both TRPC6 and Kir2.3 channels. *Cell Calcium* 2009;**45**:38–54.

21. Suchyna TM, Tape SE, Koeppe RE, Andersen OS, Sachs F, Gottlieb PA. Bilayer-dependent inhibition of mechanosensitive channels by neuroactive peptide enantiomers. *Nature* 2004;**430**:235–240.

22. Bowman CL, Gottlieb PA, Suchyna TM, Murphy YK, Sachs F. Mechanosensitive ion channels and the peptide inhibitor GsMTx-4: history, properties, mechanisms and pharmacology. *Toxicon* 2007;**49**:249–270.

23. Spassova MA, Hewavitharana T, Xu W, Soboloff J, Gill DL. A common mechanism underlies stretch activation and receptor activation of TRPC6 channels. *Proc Natl Acad Sci USA* 2006;**103**:16586–16591.

24. Gomis A, Soriano S, Belmonte C, Viana F. Hypoosmotic- and pressure-induced membrane stretch activate TRPC5 channels. *J Physiol* 2008;**586**:5633–5649.

25. Maroto R, Raso A, Wood TG, Kurosky A, Martinac B, Hamill OP. TRPC1 forms the stretch-activated cation channel in vertebrate cells. *Nat Cell Biol* 2005;**7**:179–185.

26. Gottlieb P, Folgering J, Maroto R, *et al.* Revisiting TRPC1 and TRPC6 mechanosensitivity. *Pflugers Arch* 2008;**455**:1097–1103.

27. Beech DJ, Xu SZ, McHugh D, Flemming R. TRPC1 store-operated cationic channel subunit. *Cell Calcium* 2003;**33**:433–440.

28. Gervasio OL, Whitehead NP, Yeung EW, Phillips WD, Allen DG. TRPC1 binds to caveolin-3 and is regulated by Src kinase: role in Duchenne muscular dystrophy. *J Cell Sci* 2008;**121**:2246–2255.

29. Zeng T, Bett GC, Sachs F. Stretch-activated whole cell currents in adult rat cardiac myocytes. *Am J Physiol* 2000;**278**:H548–H557.

30. Muraki K, Iwata Y, Katanosaka Y, *et al.* TRPV2 is a component of osmotically sensitive cation channels in murine aortic myocytes. *Circ Res* 2003;**93**:829–838.

31. Iwata Y, Katanosaka Y, Arai Y, Komamura K, Miyatake K, Shigekawa M. A novel mechanism of myocyte degeneration involving the Ca^{2+}-permeable growth factor-regulated channel. *J Cell Biol* 2003;**161**: 957–967.

32. Iwata Y, Katanosaka Y, Arai Y, Shigekawa M, Wakabayashi S. Dominant-negative inhibition of Ca^{2+} influx via TRPV2 ameliorates muscular dystrophy in animal models. *Hum Mol Genet* 2009;**18**: 824–834.

33. Yeung EW, Whitehead NP, Suchyna TM, Gottlieb PA, Sachs F, Allen DG. Effects of stretch-activated channel blockers on $[Ca^{2+}]_i$ and muscle damage in the *mdx* mouse. *J Physiol* 2005;**562**:367–380.

34. Hamill OP. Twenty odd years of stretch-sensitive channels. *Pflugers Arch* 2006;**453**:333–351.

35. Balnave CD, Allen DG. Intracellular calcium and force in single mouse muscle fibres following repeated contractions with stretch. *J Physiol* 1995;**488**:25–336.

36. Kung C. A possible unifying principle for mechanosensation. *Nature* 2005;**436**:647–654.

37. Christensen AP, Corey DP. TRP channels in mechanosensation: direct or indirect activation? *Nat Rev Neurosci* 2007;**8**:510–521.

38. Hayakawa K, Tatsumi H, Sokabe M. Actin stress fibers transmit and focus force to activate mechanosensitive channels. *J Cell Sci* 2008;**121**:496–503.

39. Sato R, Koumi S. Characterization of the stretch-activated chloride channel in isolated human atrial myocytes. *J Membr Biol* 1998;**163**: 67–76.

40. Sadoshima J, Xu Y, Slayter HS, Izumo S. Autocrine release of angiotensin II mediates stretch-induced hypertrophy of cardiac myocytes in vitro. *Cell* 1993;**75**:977–984.

41. Griendling KK, Minieri CA, Ollerenshaw JD, Alexander RW. Angiotensin II stimulates NADH and NADPH oxidase activity in cultured vascular smooth muscle cells. *Circ Res* 1994;**74**:1141–1148.

42. Caldiz CI, Garciarena CD, Dulce RA, Novaretto LP, Yeves AM, Ennis IL, *et al.* Mitochondrial reactive oxygen species activate the slow force response to stretch in feline myocardium. *J Physiol* 2007;**584**:895–905.

43. Rothstein EC, Byron KL, Reed RE, Fliegel L, Lucchesi PA. $H_2O_2^-$ induced Ca^{2+} overload in NRVM involves ERK1/2 MAP kinases: role for an NHE-1-dependent pathway. *Am J Physiol* 2002;**283**: H598–H605.

44. Dyachenko V, Rueckschloss U, Isenberg G. Modulation of cardiac mechanosensitive ion channels involves superoxide, nitric oxide and peroxynitrite. *Cell Calcium* 2009;**45**:55–64.

45. Morgan DL, Allen DG. Early events in stretch-induced muscle damage. *J Appl Physiol* 1999;**87**:2007–2015.

46. Bassel-Duby R, Olson EN. Signaling pathways in skeletal muscle remodeling. *Annu Rev Biochem* 2006;**75**:19–37.

47. Allen DG, Whitehead NP, Yeung EW. Mechanisms of stretch-induced muscle damage in normal and dystrophic muscle: role of ionic changes. *J Physiol* 2005;**567**:723–735.

48. Emery AE, Muntoni F. *Duchenne Muscular Dystrophy*. 3 ed. Oxford University Press; 2003.

49. Finsterer J, Stollberger C. The heart in human dystrophinopathies. *Cardiology* 2003;**99**:1–19.

50. Allen DG, Gervasio OL, Yeung EW, Whitehead NP. Calcium and the damage pathways in muscular dystrophy. *Can J Physiol Pharmacol* 2010;**88**:83–91.

51. Li S, Couet J, Lisanti MP. Src tyrosine kinases, Galpha subunits, and H-Ras share a common membrane-anchored scaffolding protein, caveolin. Caveolin binding negatively regulates the auto-activation of Src tyrosine kinases. *J Biol Chem* 1996;**271**:29182–29190.

52. Ervasti JM, Campbell KP. Membrane Organization of the Dystrophin-Glycoprotein Complex. *Cell* 1991;**66**:1121–1131.

53. Froehner SC. Just say NO to muscle degeneration? *Trends Mol Med* 2002;**8**:51–53.

54. Shibuya S, Wakayama Y, Inoue M, Oniki H, Kominami E. Changes in the distribution and density of caveolin 3 molecules at the plasma membrane of mdx mouse skeletal muscles: a fracture-label electron microscopic study. *Neurosci Lett* 2002;**325**:171–174.

55. Parton RG, Simons K. The multiple faces of caveolae. *Nat Rev Mol Cell Biol* 2007;**8**:185–194.

56. Minetti C, Sotgia F, Bruno C, *et al.* Mutations in the caveolin-3 gene cause autosomal dominant limb-girdle muscular dystrophy. *Nat Genet* 1998;**18**:365–368.

57. Galbiati F, Volonte D, Chu JB, *et al.* Transgenic overexpression of caveolin-3 in skeletal muscle fibers induces a Duchenne-like muscular dystrophy phenotype. *Proc Natl Acad Sci USA* 2000;**97**:9689–9694.

58. Franco-Obregon A, Jr., Lansman JB. Mechanosensitive ion channels in skeletal muscle from normal and dystrophic mice. *J Physiol* 1994;**481**:299–309.

59. Vandebrouck C, Duport G, Cognard C, Raymond G. Cationic channels in normal and dystrophic human myotubes. *Neuromuscul Disord* 2001;**11**:72–79.

60. Gailly P. New aspects of calcium signaling in skeletal muscle cells: implications in Duchenne muscular dystrophy. *Biochim Biophys Acta* 2002;**1600**:38–44.

61. Williams IA, Allen DG. Intracellular calcium handling in ventricular myocytes from mdx mice. *Am J Physiol* 2007;**292**:H846–H855.

62. Williams IA, Allen DG. The role of reactive oxygen species in the hearts of dystrophin-deficient mdx mice. *Am J Physiol* 2007;**293**:H1969–H1977.

Distributions of myocyte stress, strain and work in normal and infarcted ventricles

Elliot J. Howard and Jeffrey H. Omens

Background

The ventricles of the heart are heterogeneous structures with regional variations in geometry, for example, wall thickness and curvature, as well as variations in cell-level architecture such as myocyte orientation and extracellular matrix structure. Regional heterogeneities are also found in myocyte function: cellular protein expression[1,2], ionic currents[3], electrophysiology properties[4], action potential morphology[5] and mechanical twitch[6] have been shown to vary with position in the wall of the left ventricle (LV). It is known that these cellular and structural heterogeneities are important determinants of normal and pathological cardiac function. The complex interaction of structural and cellular heterogeneities gives rise to variations in local myocyte mechanical function. The focus of this chapter is to describe the regional and transmural distributions in stress, strain and work in normal and infarcted ventricles as measured experimentally and predicted with a computational finite element model of canine cardiac electromechanics. Experimental data combined with computational simulations show highly heterogeneous distributions of mechanical function in the ventricles. In turn, such distributions in myocyte function contribute to mechanically induced heterogeneity of cardiac electrophysiology via mechano-electric coupling (MEC).

LV structure: arrangement of cardiomyocytes

The cardiac muscle cell or cardiomyocyte is a roughly cylindrical cell that forms attachments to neighbouring cells through gap junctions preferentially aligned with the long axis of the cells, as well as transverse connections via costameres and extracellular matrix attachments. The term 'fibre' is also used for cardiomyocytes; in particular we refer to the 'fibre direction' as the long axis of these elongated muscle cells, and fibre function will be a mechanical parameter associated with that direction. The cardiomyocytes of the LV are arranged in a helical fashion, with (sub-)epicardial cells oriented in a counterclockwise spiral and (sub-)endocardial cells in a clockwise spiral, viewed from apex to base. In the dog, epicardial myocytes are oriented roughly –60° from circumferential,

mid-wall myocytes are aligned at 0° and endocardial myocytes at 60°[7]. This transmural gradient in fibre direction has been shown to have functional implications. It was demonstrated in a numerical model that the distribution of stress and strain in the LV wall is sensitive to the spatial organization of the cardiomyocytes[8] and that their orientation serves to maximize the homogeneity of fibre stress during ejection[9]. At low ventricular volumes sarcomere lengths vary transmurally, and they are more uniformly distributed at higher volumes[10] due to cardiomyocyte orientation as well as residual stress[11]. There also exists a transmural distribution of myocyte diameter, with cells at the epicardium being larger than those near the endocardium[12]. The thinner wall and greater distensibility near the apex (compared to the base) gives rise to longer sarcomere lengths at the apex compared to the base[13].

There is a secondary level of myocardial structural organization. Cardiac myocytes are arranged into discrete muscle layers, termed myocardial laminae or sheets, which are roughly four to eight cells thick[14]. Spotnitz was the first to describe the existence of myocardial gaps or 'sliding planes' in the rat LV and proposed that these planes could give rise to large changes in wall thickness during systole[15]. Like myocyte orientation, sheet arrangement has been shown to vary regionally and transmurally throughout the LV. Through sheet extension and shearing, ventricular wall thickening is accomplished and can be as large as 40% at the endocardial layer[16].

In order to relate regional mechanical function to the orientation of cellular tissue components, a cardiac coordinate system can be defined to represent local circumferential, longitudinal and radial axes. By measuring mean fibre and sheet angles as a function of location, a local fibre–sheet coordinate system can be defined in terms of these angles in order to relate local stress and strain to the underlying anisotropic structure (Fig. 62.1).

Regional ventricular mechanics

The functional role of the heart is to convert metabolic energy into mechanical work in order to generate adequate pressure to eject blood throughout the body's circulation. In global terms one can describe cardiac function through the pressure–volume relationship,

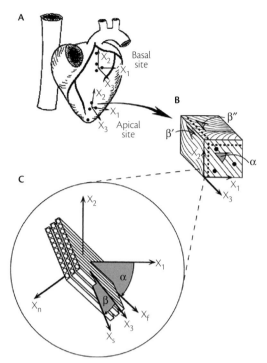

Fig. 62.1 Local fibre-sheet coordinates can be defined regionally on the LV. **A** Epicardial markers are used to define the cardiac coordinate system with local circumferential (X_1), longitudinal (X_2) and radial (X_3) directions. **B** Transmural wedge of tissue used to histologically define mean fibre (α) and sheet angle (β). **C** Local tissue architecture can be described by a rotation of the cardiac coordinates into the material axes of the fibre (X_f) and sheet (X_s) directions. [Reproduced, with permission, from Costa KD, Takayama Y, McCulloch AD, Covell JW (1999) Laminar fiber architecture and three-dimensional systolic mechanics in canine ventricular myocardium. *Am J Physiol* **276**:H595–H607.]

which gives insight into both the diastolic and systolic performance of the heart. However, measures of cavity pressure and volume cannot provide information about the local stress and strain dynamics within the cardiomyocytes or the extracellular matrix surrounding and attached to the myocytes. Therefore a regional description of cardiac function is needed in order to study the mechanics and mechanical interactions between the heart's cells and their extracellular environment. Measures of deformation such as engineering strain describe local changes in material length with respect to local coordinate axes, and typically this axis system is aligned with the local muscle cells. For example, shortening of the muscle cells (negative fibre strain) during systole allows the heart to contract and change its shape to eject blood. Conversely, during diastolic filling, the cardiac myocytes elongate (positive fibre strain) as the ventricular cavity volume increases. Thus it is important to define local mechanical function in terms of a coordinate system aligned with the cardiomyocytes.

Another regional measurement that is used to describe cardiac mechanics is stress. Stress in a material is defined as a force per unit area that acts upon a surface. The distribution of wall stress in the intact heart has a high functional relevance because it determines overall ventricular performance, coronary blood flow and oxygen demand and most likely mediates hypertrophy and remodelling[17]. Due to the large deformations accompanying the ventricular cycle

of contraction and relaxation, direct experimental measurements of stress are few and controversial. Rather than measuring stress directly to assess regional function, some measure of deformation (i.e. strain) is found experimentally, and then mathematical models are used to determine stress. Finite element (FE) models[18–20] have become state of the art for mathematical modelling of cardiac mechanics. FE models may include accurate measurements of geometry and muscle cell orientations, non-linear passive constitutive laws, active stress relationships and boundary conditions described as pressure or displacement constraints. These models show similar patterns of three-dimensional (3D) strain as measured experimentally and predict substantial regional heterogeneity of ventricular mechanics.

Material properties of the myocardium

Distributions of stress and strain in the heart are governed by the underlying 3D tissue structure, the boundary conditions of cavity pressure and volume and the material properties of the myocardium during passive (diastolic) and active (systolic) phases. Fibre and sheet anatomy can be measured histologically and pressures can be measured *in vivo*; however, quantifying the material properties of the myocardium requires extensive mechanical testing. The importance of understanding the mechanical properties of the myocardium can be illustrated in disease states in which cellular and extracellular remodelling occur and alter the mechanical environment.

The myocardium is a soft biological tissue that is anisotropic, meaning that the material properties are a function of direction. Theoretically, to fully express the material properties of the myocardium, a 3D analysis is required. In reality such tests are practically limited. Therefore the use of uniaxial and biaxial testing has become the norm for mechanical testing to determine the local material properties.

Uniaxial tests using papillary muscles and ventricular trabeculae can be used to define passive stress–strain relationships in the fibre direction. The main findings from these experiments are that the stress–strain relationships are non-linear and time-varying, and that the stiffness–stress relationships are linear. For example, the material properties of the rabbit papillary muscle were characterized by an exponential stress–strain relationship[21]. For a comprehensive review of uniaxial muscle mechanics the reader should consult the review by Mirsky and Parmley[22].

Due to the incompressibility of cardiac tissue, biaxial tests can be used to infer 3D material properties of myocardial tissue samples. Typically, isolated hearts are sectioned into rectangular slabs cut tangential to the epicardial surface, mounted onto a biaxial stretcher, and then stretched in two in-plane orthogonal directions. The data collected by Demer and Yin suggested that the passive myocardium is non-linear, anisotropic and regionally heterogenous[23]. Data from Humphrey *et al.*, collected in a single region of the canine LV, illustrated that the myocardium was stiffer in the fibre direction than in the cross-fibre direction[24].

Experimental measurements of fibre strain in normal and infarcted tissue

Due to the impracticality of directly measuring stress in the beating heart, regional myocardial function is typically measured with some type of deformation analysis, for example tissue strain or muscle cell stretch. While stretch represents a uniaxial length change of tissue (typically quantified as a stretch ratio), strain is classically used to describe the 3D deformation of a material. The relationship between the stretch ratio, λ_f, and a component of strain, E_{ff}, can be described as:

$$E_{ff} = \frac{1}{2}\left(\lambda_f^2 - 1\right);$$
$$\lambda_f = L/L_o$$

where L is deformed length, L_o is undeformed length and E_{ff} is the Lagrangian strain component. In this example, the subscript f of the strain and stretch ratio refers to the fibre direction/component. Experimentally, segment length changes have been assessed with various techniques, including ultrasonic piezoelectric crystals, and show substantial variations in function across the ventricle. The major findings from these studies were that fibre shortening increased from base to apex, and that endocardial shortening exceeded that of the epicardium[25]. Furthermore, mid-wall fibre shortening in the anterior wall exceeded that of the lateral and posterior walls[26]. 2D and 3D strains can be measured *in vivo* using implantable radiopaque markers. Waldman *et al.* used implantable markers to measure transmural distributions of cardiac strain[27]. Ashikaga and colleagues showed a significant transmural distribution in fibre strain throughout the cardiac cycle[28]. Wyman and colleagues used tagged magnetic resonance imaging (MRI) to measure regional distributions of fibre strain at the mid-wall and showed significant differences from apex to base and around the hoop axis of the heart, as shown in Fig. 62.2[29]. Specifically, fibre strain was highest in the anterior wall compared to the lateral, posterior and septal walls and increased from base to apex. Experimental measures have also shown that local ventricular electrical pacing results in remote areas of tissue that 'pre-stretch', i.e. lengthening

of late-activated tissue segments during the late diastolic and isovolumic contraction phases[30,31].

The effect of ischaemia on regional LV function has been assessed using ultrasonic gauges[32–34] which revealed fibre bulging or 'paradoxical segment lengthening' within the ischaemic tissue during systole. Normal fibre function was characterized by fibre shortening during the isovolumic contraction and ejection phases followed by relengthening during the isovolumic relaxation and early filling phases. During ischaemia, fibres within the ischaemic zone were stretched, indicated by positive strain, throughout systole. This stretching of the muscle cells was due to the reduced contractility of cells in the ischaemic region, in combination with active contraction and shortening of normal myocardium surrounding the ischaemic zone.

The diastolic material properties of the LV during normal and ischaemic conditions have also been studied. Biaxial testing of infarcted tissue revealed increases in circumferential and longitudinal stiffness for 1- to 2-week-old infarcts, along with increased stresses in the circumferential direction[34]. Using MRI tagging and computation modelling, Walker and colleagues showed that infarct stiffness increased nearly 15 times more than non-infarcted tissue in 22-week-old sheep infarcts[35]. Omens and co-workers demonstrated that the increased passive fibre stiffness was due to an increase in collagen fibres that ran parallel to the muscle fibre axis, as depicted in Fig. 62.3[36]. Despite the increase in overall ventricular compliance (Fig. 62.3C), the fibre stiffness was increased substantially in the infarcted hearts.

Redistribution of work during ischaemic heart disease

Abnormal strain and stress patterns for extended periods of time can alter cardiomyocyte physiology and lead to structural, mechanical and electrical remodelling. During ischaemia, the oxygen supply is less than the working demand of cardiomyocytes, typically due to a change in local blood supply following an obstruction in a coronary vessel. The ischaemic region is said to be akinetic, whereas the non-ischaemic region demonstrates 'hyperkinetic' functionality. This hyperkinesis is in part due to a compensatory adaptation of the non-ischaemic cardiomyocytes that increase their contractile function in response to the dysfunction in the non-contracting ischaemic region (see also Chapter 21). Therefore a result of ischaemia is a reduction of work in both the ischaemic and non-ischaemic regions. Lew demonstrated the effect of varying infarct size on non-ischaemic myocardial function[37]. As shown in Fig. 62.4, pressure–length segment loops reveal that with increasing infarct size, segment shortening increases in the non-ischaemic zone. The distribution of work can be inferred from the area of the pressure–length loops. Increasing infarct size reduced the amount of work done by the anterior and posterior walls. In the infarcted region (anterior wall) work was reduced to that of passive inflation (negative work) compared to that in the actively contracting (positive work) non-infarcted posterior wall.

Modelling ventricular mechanics in the healthy and infarcted heart

A finite element approach was used to model the regional electromechanics of a cardiac contraction in normal and infarcted canine

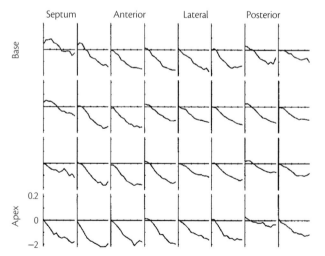

Fig. 62.2 MRI tagging reveals regional variation in fibre strain in the mid-wall of the LV. Vertical axis depicts fibre strain and horizontal axis depicts time. Time courses of fibre strain are shown for septum, anterior, lateral and posterior wall. [Reproduced, with permission, from Wyman BT, Hunter WC, Prinzen FW, McVeigh ER (1999) Mapping propagation of mechanical activation in the paced heart with MRI tagging. *Am J Physiol* **276**:H881–H891.]

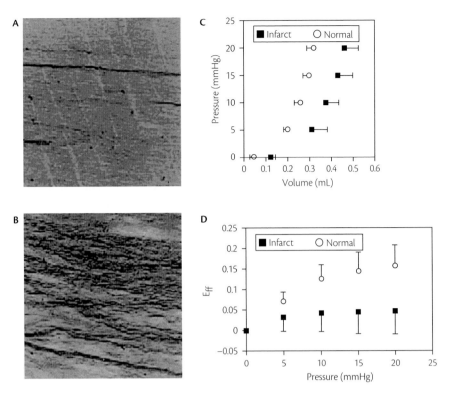

Fig. 62.3 Change in passive fibre stiffness after myocardial infarction due to increased collagen deposition and uncoiling. Collagen content for normal (**A**) and infarcted (**B**) tissue is shown to correlate with increased ventricle chamber compliance (**C**) and fibre stiffness (**D**). E_{ff} the Lagrangian strain component. [Reproduced, with permission, from Omens JH, Miller TR, Covell JW (1997) Relationship between passive tissue strain and collagen uncoiling during healing of infarcted myocardium. *Cardiovasc Res* **33**:351–358.]

ventricles. This model has been previously described by our group[20,38]. Briefly, realistic geometries of both right and left ventricles were fit in prolate-spheroidal coordinates by 48 (normal) and 60 (infarct) cubic Hermite elements. The normal heart had a cavity to wall volume ratio of 0.27, whereas dilated hearts with infarcts had a cavity to wall volume of 0.57. Realistic myofibre architecture was included in both models. In the infarcted region transmural fibre angle gradient, which represents that of collagen fibres, was larger than in non-infarcted tissue due to the thinner wall thickness in this region.

Passive mechanics were modelled using a transversely isotropic exponential constitutive law with parameters obtained from previous models[19], whereas the passive parameters of the infarct were scaled from experimental data[35]. Active mechanics were modelled using a modified Hill's equation that related tension along the myofibre long axis to intracellular calcium concentration. Model parameters for the normal heart were obtained from previous models[19]; in the infarcted region parameters were changed such that the peak force was 27% lower than non-infarcted healthy tissue and the force twitch duration was 17% longer[38].

The ventricles were coupled to a systemic and pulmonary circulation, each comprised of two windkessel compartments in series representing arterial and venous blood. Atria were incorporated as time-varying elastance models. The hearts were passively inflated to the end-diastolic pressure and were then activated to contract by prescribing a local activation time from which the myofibres began to develop tension at a delay of 8 ms from activation.

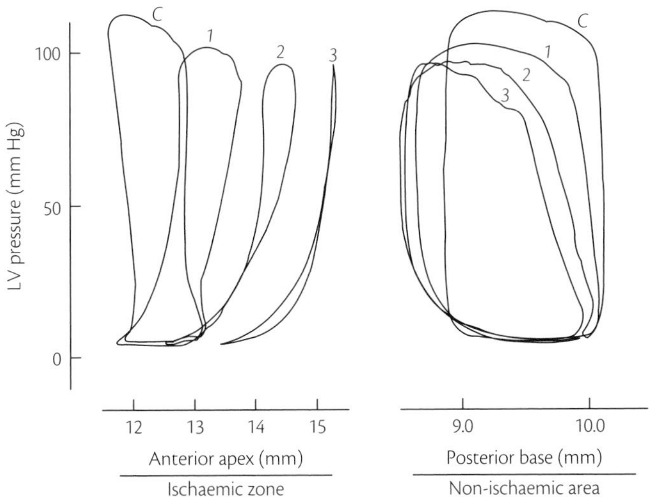

Distribution of fibre strain, stress and work in simulations of healthy ventricles

Model results shown below indicate marked differences in fibre mechanics at varying locations. Figure 62.5 shows the transmural distribution of fibre strain (in terms of stretch ratio), stress and work in the anterior wall of the normal LV at three distinct regions: base, equator and apex. Endocardial shortening (stretch ratio less than 1) during isovolumic contraction (IVC) and ejection was

Fig. 62.4 Pressure–segment length loops for ischaemic (left) and non-ischaemic (right) zones with varying infarct size. Control loops are denoted as C. Infarct size increases from 1 to 3. [Reproduced, with permission, from Lew WY (1987) Influence of ischemic zone size on nonischemic area function in the canine left ventricle. *Am J Physiol* **252**:H990–H997.]

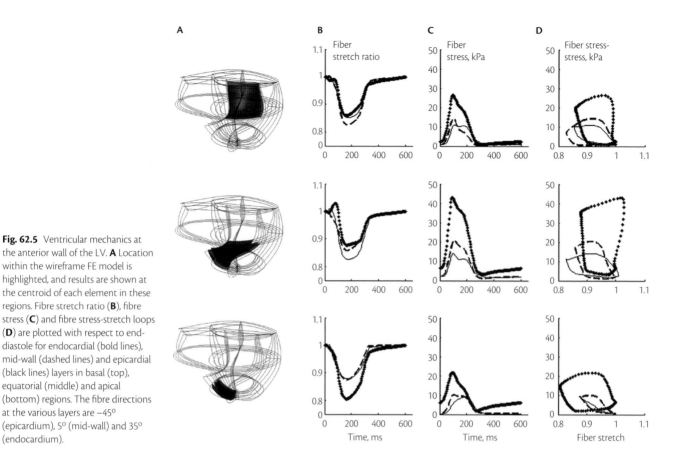

Fig. 62.5 Ventricular mechanics at the anterior wall of the LV. **A** Location within the wireframe FE model is highlighted, and results are shown at the centroid of each element in these regions. Fibre stretch ratio (**B**), fibre stress (**C**) and fibre stress-stretch loops (**D**) are plotted with respect to end-diastole for endocardial (bold lines), mid-wall (dashed lines) and epicardial (black lines) layers in basal (top), equatorial (middle) and apical (bottom) regions. The fibre directions at the various layers are −45° (epicardium), 5° (mid-wall) and 35° (endocardium).

greatest in the anterior apex compared to the base and equator, whereas peak fibre stress was highest for equatorial endocardial fibres and least at the anterior apex. In both the basal and apical regions, a transmural gradient in fibre stretch ratio is observed throughout the ejection phase, with epicardial strain being the least, followed by mid-wall and endocardial strain. At the equator endocardial fibres are stretched during IVC and shorten less than the epicardial fibres during systole. Between the different layers (endocardial, mid-wall and epicardial) external work (area within the stress–stretch loop) done by the fibres is highest at the endocardium. The higher tension for endocardial fibres at the equator results in larger work done at the equator. Mid-wall and epicardial work was similar for all three regions.

Figure 62.6 shows the corresponding stretch ratio, stress and work in the posterior basal, equatorial and apical regions. As in the anterior wall, endocardial shortening is highest at the apex and lowest at the base. Additionally in all three regions endocardial shortening exceeds epicardial shortening. Peak fibre stress is highest at the base and equatorial endocardial fibres. Marked transmural gradients are seen in the fibre stretch ratio, stress and work at all sites. Fibre work at the endocardium is similar at all three regions, whereas in the mid-wall fibre work was highest at the base and lowest at the apex.

Effect of LV anterior infarct on fibre strain, stress and work

The effect of an anterior infarct on LV function was simulated in the model. The anterior LV infarct occupied 21% of the total LV wall volume. Figure 62.7 shows the fibre stretch ratio, stress and work distributions for infarcted (top), border zone (middle) and remote regions (bottom). Stretch ratio was plotted for each layer (endocardial, mid-wall and epicardial) throughout the isovolumic phase and was referenced to zero LV cavity pressure. At end-diastole, endocardial fibres were stretched more than epicardial and mid-wall fibres in the infarcted and border zone regions. In the infarcted region, all layers were stretched during the isovolumic contraction phase, with endocardial fibres being stretched the most. In the border zone, endocardial fibres were stretched late during isovolumic contraction, whereas mid-wall and epicardial fibres began to shorten. Conversely, in tissue remote from the infarct, endocardial and mid-wall fibres began to shorten, while epicardial fibres lengthened near the end of IVC. Fibre stress was greatest for the endocardial fibres in all regions, followed by mid-wall and epicardial fibres. Compared to the normal fibre stress distributions shown in Figs 62.5 and 62.6, fibre stress in the infarcted and border zone regions at the endocardium was much

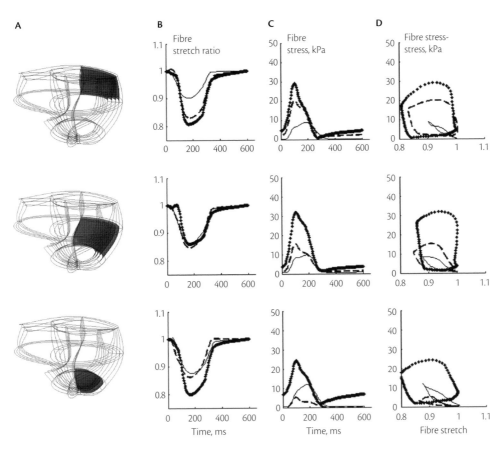

Fig. 62.6 Ventricular mechanics at the posterior wall of the LV. **A** Location within the wireframe FE model is highlighted, and results are shown at the centroid of each element in these regions. Fibre stretch ratio (**B**), fibre stress (**C**) and fibre stress-stretch loops (**D**) are plotted with respect to end-diastole for endocardial (bold lines), mid-wall (dashed lines) and epicardial (black lines) layers in basal (top), equatorial (middle) and apical (bottom) regions. The fibre directions at the various layers are −40° (epicardium), 2° (mid-wall) and 25° (endocardium).

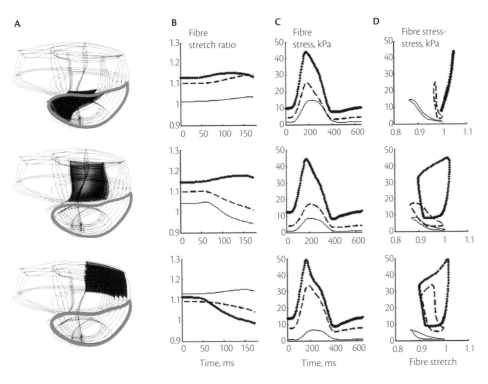

Fig. 62.7 Distribution of cardiac fibre stretch, stress and work in infarcted LV. Location within the wireframe FE model is shaded grey, and results are shown at the centroid of each element in these regions. The epicardial surface of the infarct region is outlined in red. Fibre stretch during the isovolumic contraction phase (**B**) fibre stress (**C**) and work (**D**) in infarcted (top), border zone (middle) and remote regions (bottom). Fibre stretch is referenced to zero cavity pressure, whereas fibre stress and work are referenced to end-diastole. Transmural distributions are shown for epicardial (black lines), mid-wall (dashed lines) and endocardial (bold lines) layers. The fibre directions at the various layers are −45° (epicardium), 5° (mid-wall) and 35° (endocardium).

higher at end-diastole and during IVC. Stress vs stretch ratio plots revealed that all myocytes in the infarcted region displayed akinetic behaviour as indicated by a purely passive stress vs stretch curve. This passive behaviour can also be described by paradoxical systolic stretching of the fibres due to contraction of the surrounding healthy myocardium. In the border zone and remote regions, external work was similar to that of the normal heart, with endocardial work being greatest and epicardial work being smallest.

Conclusions and outlook

In summary, assessments of cardiac function obtained experimentally and through the use of computational models reveal substantial regional variations in fibre stress, strain and work in normal hearts. These distributions are due to the complex structural arrangement of cardiac muscle cells within their extracellular environment, and the anisotropic material properties that depend on these structures. During ischaemic heart disease, scarring can occur and result in an infarct that alters the passive and active state of the myocardium. Experimental findings show that fibre shortening is replaced with paradoxical bulging in ischaemic regions during systole, which results in passive pressure–length loops characterized by negative external work. The passive properties of the chronic infarct scar are changed as well, observed as increased stiffness in the fibre direction and increased fibre stresses. The results obtained from our computation simulations illustrate the regional differences in fibre function in the normal heart. Fibre shortening is greatest at the apex compared to the base and is largest for endocardial compared to epicardial myocytes. The transmural distribution of fibre stress and work show that endocardial cells are subjected to higher stresses and perform greater work than do midwall and epicardial cells. Simulations of the effect of an anterior infarct on regional function demonstrate that in areas of infarction the cardiomyocytes are stretched throughout isovolumic contraction, contrary to the fibre shortening displayed by non-infarcted myocardium. Infarcted regions performed the least amount of external work, compared to border zone and remote tissue, thus illustrating the redistribution of work that accompanies ischaemic heart disease.

The altered mechanical state of the infarcted ventricle may have functional implications on cellular electrophysiology and MEC. The ability of cardiomyocytes to sense mechanical loading and the cell's functional response is discussed elsewhere in this book (see, in particular, Chapter 24). Abnormal stretching of the myocytes in infarcted and border zone regions may give rise to abnormal electrical activation and arrhythmias. Therefore, understanding the regional differences in myocyte function in normal and pathological states is a requirement for new insight relevant for diagnosis and treatment of many cardiac diseases[11].

Acknowledgements

The authors would like to thank Dr Roy Kerckhoffs for the use of his computational model of canine electromechanics to simulate normal and infarcted ventricular function.

References

1. Suurmeijer AJ, Clement S, Francesconi A, *et al.* Alpha-actin isoform distribution in normal and failing human heart: a morphological, morphometric, and biochemical study. *J Pathol* 2003;**199**:387–397.

2. Cazorla O, Freiburg A, Helmes M, *et al.* Differential expression of cardiac titin isoforms and modulation of cellular stiffness. *Circ Res* 2000;**86**:59–67.

3. Wolk R, Cobbe SM, Hicks MN, Kane KA. Functional, structural, and dynamic basis of electrical heterogeneity in healthy and diseased cardiac muscle: implications for arrhythmogenesis and anti-arrhythmic drug therapy. *Pharmacol Ther* 1999;**84**:207–231.

4. Sicouri S, Antzelevitch C. Electrophysiologic characteristics of M cells in the canine left ventricular free wall. *J Cardiovasc Electrophysiol* 1995;**6**:591–603.

5. Libbus I, Rosenbaum DS. Transmural action potential changes underlying ventricular electrical remodeling. *J Cardiovasc Electrophysiol* 2003;**14**:394–402.

6. Cordeiro JM, Greene L, Heilmann C, Antzelevitch D, Antzelevitch C. Transmural heterogeneity of calcium activity and mechanical function in the canine left ventricle. *Am J Physiol* 2004;**286**: H1471–H1479.

7. Streeter DD, Jr., Spotnitz HM, Patel DP, Ross J, Jr., Sonnenblick EH. Fiber orientation in the canine left ventricle during diastole and systole. *Circ Res* 1969;**24**:339–347.

8. Bovendeerd PH, Arts T, Huyghe JM, van Campen DH, Reneman RS. Dependence of local left ventricular wall mechanics on myocardial fiber orientation: a model study. *J Biomech* 1992;**25**:1129–1140.

9. Rijcken J, Bovendeerd PH, Schoofs AJ, van Campen DH, Arts T. Optimization of cardiac fiber orientation for homogeneous fiber strain during ejection. *Ann Biomed Eng* 1999;**27**:289–297.

10. Grimm AF, Lin HL, Grimm BR. Left ventricular free wall and intraventricular pressure-sarcomere length distributions. *Am J Physiol* 1980;**239**:H101–H107.

11. Rodriguez EK, Omens JH, Waldman LK, McCulloch AD. Effect of residual stress on transmural sarcomere length distributions in rat left ventricle. *Am J Physiol* 1993;**264**:H1048–H1056.

12. Hoshino T, Fujiwara H, Kawai C, Hamashima Y. Myocardial fiber diameter and regional distribution in the ventricular wall of normal adult hearts, hypertensive hearts and hearts with hypertrophic cardiomyopathy. *Circulation* 1983;**67**:1109–1116.

13. Laks MM, Morady F, Swan HJ. Canine Right and Left Ventricular Cell and Sarcomere Lengths after Banding the Pulmonary Artery. *Circ Res* 1969;**24**:705–710.

14. LeGrice IJ, Smaill BH, Chai LZ, Edgar SG, Gavin JB, Hunter PJ. Laminar structure of the heart: ventricular myocyte arrangement and connective tissue architecture in the dog. *Am J Physiol* 1995;**269**: H571–H582.

15. Spotnitz HM, Spotnitz WD, Cottrell TS, Spiro D, Sonnenblick EH. Cellular basis for volume related wall thickness changes in the rat left ventricle. *J Mol Cell Cardiol* 1974;**6**:317–331.

16. Covell JW. Tissue structure and ventricular wall mechanics. *Circulation* 2008;**118**:699–701.

17. McCulloch AD, Omens JH (1991) *Factors Affecting the Regional Mechanics of the Diastolic Heart. Theory of the Heart: Biomechanics, Biophysics and Nonlinear Dynamics of Cardiac Function.* Springer, New York, pp 87–119.

18. Nielsen PM, Le Grice IJ, Smaill BH, Hunter PJ. Mathematical model of geometry and fibrous structure of the heart. *Am J Physiol* 1991;**260**: H1365–H1378.

19. Guccione JM, Costa KD, McCulloch AD. Finite element stress analysis of left ventricular mechanics in the beating dog heart. *J Biomech* 1995;**28**:1167–1177.

20. Kerckhoffs RC, Neal ML, Gu Q, Bassingthwaighte JB, Omens JH, McCulloch AD. Coupling of a 3D finite element model of cardiac ventricular mechanics to lumped systems models of the systemic and pulmonic circulation. *Ann Biomed Eng* 2007;**35**: 1–18.

21. Pinto JG, Fung YC. Mechanical properties of the heart muscle in the passive state. *J Biomech* 1973;**6**:597–616.

22. Mirsky I, Parmley WW. Assessment of passive elastic stiffness for isolated heart muscle and the intact heart. *Circ Res* 1973;**33**:233–243.

23. Demer LL, Yin FC. Passive biaxial mechanical properties of isolated canine myocardium. *J Physiol* 1983;**339**:615–630.

24. Humphrey JD, Strumpf RK, Yin FC. Determination of a constitutive relation for passive myocardium: II. Parameter estimation. *J Biomech Eng* 1990;**112**:340–346.

25. LeWinter MM, Kent RS, Kroener JM, Carew TE, Covell JW. Regional differences in myocardial performance in the left ventricle of the dog. *Circ Res* 1975;**37**:191–199.

26. Lew WY, LeWinter MM. Regional comparison of midwall segment and area shortening in the canine left ventricle. *Circ Res* 1986;**58**: 678–691.

27. Waldman LK, Fung YC, Covell JW. Transmural myocardial deformation in the canine left ventricle. Normal in vivo three-dimensional finite strains. *Circ Res* 1985;**57**:152–163.

28. Ashikaga H, Omens JH, Ingels NB, Jr., Covell JW. Transmural mechanics at left ventricular epicardial pacing site. *Am J Physiol* 2004;**286**:H2401–H2407.

29. Wyman BT, Hunter WC, Prinzen FW, McVeigh ER Mapping propagation of mechanical activation in the paced heart with MRI tagging. *Am J Physiol* 1999;**276**:H881–H891.

30. Coppola BA, Covell JW, McCulloch AD, Omens JH. Asynchrony of ventricular activation affects magnitude and timing of fiber stretch in late-activated regions of the canine heart. *Am J Physiol* 2007;**293**: H754–H761.

31. Ashikaga H, van der Spoel TIG, Coppola BA, Omens JH. Transmural myocardial mechanics during isovolumic contraction. *JACC Cardiovasc Imaging* 2009;**2**:212–215.

32. Akaishi M, Weintraub WS, Schneider RM, Klein LW, Agarwal JB, Helfant RH. Analysis of systolic bulging. Mechanical characteristics of acutely ischemic myocardium in the conscious dog. *Circ Res* 1986;**58**:209–217.

33. Stirling MC, Choy M, McClanahan TB, Schott RJ, Gallagher KP. Effects of ischemia on epicardial segment shortening. *J Surg Res* 1991;**50**:30–39.

34. Gupta KB, Ratcliffe MB, Fallert MA, Edmunds LH, Jr., Bogen DK. Changes in passive mechanical stiffness of myocardial tissue with aneurysm formation. *Circulation* 1994;**89**:2315–2326.

35. Walker JC, Ratcliffe MB, Zhang P, *et al.* MRI-based finite-element analysis of left ventricular aneurysm. *Am J Physiol* 2005;**289**: H692–H700.

36. Omens JH, Miller TR, Covell JW. Relationship between passive tissue strain and collagen uncoiling during healing of infarcted myocardium. *Cardiovasc Res* 1997;**33**:351–358.

37. Lew WY. Influence of ischemic zone size on nonischemic area function in the canine left ventricle. *Am J Physiol* 1987;**252**:H990–H997.

38. Kerckhoffs RC, McCulloch AD, Omens JH, Mulligan LJ. Effects of biventricular pacing and scar size in a computational model of the failing heart with left bundle branch block. *Med Image Anal* 2009;**13**:362–369.

39. Costa KD, Takayama Y, McCulloch AD, Covell JW. Laminar fiber architecture and three-dimensional systolic mechanics in canine ventricular myocardium. *Am J Physiol* 1999;**276**:H595–H607.

Evolving concepts in measuring ventricular strain in canine and human hearts: non-invasive imaging

Elisa E. Konofagou and Jean Provost

Background

The study of cardiac mechano-electric coupling (MEC) in patients requires the ability to map *both* electrical *and* mechanical events in the human heart in a non-invasive manner, with sufficient spatio-temporal resolution, and with infrastructural investments that are compatible with the realities of day-to-day clinical practice. The significant challenges that arise in this context, and emerging solutions, are discussed in this chapter.

Imaging cardiac mechanics

Several techniques, such as X-ray, sonomicrometry, echocardiography and magnetic resonance imaging (MRI), have been developed and clinical systems have been manufactured in order to follow cardiac motion and deformation or strain. Invasive techniques usually require the implantation of a small number of beads directly into the myocardium. X-ray techniques use implanted metal beads that serve as 'markers', indicating how different cardiac structures move during a heartbeat[1]. Sonomicrometry systems rely on small (~1 mm) implanted ultrasound transducers emitting and receiving signals and thus giving their positions[2]. These methods usually offer high temporal resolution, but since the number of beads that can be implanted without significantly damaging the heart is limited, the resulting trade-off between spatial resolution and the size of the region of interest strongly limits studies.

Non-invasive approaches include imaging based on MRI and echocardiography. In MRI, myocardial tagging[3], harmonic phase (HARP)[4] and displacement encoding with stimulated echoes (DENSE)[5] imaging methods have been shown capable of estimating all principal components of the strain tensor. Efforts to improve spatial and temporal resolution have led to experimental setups allowing simultaneous imaging of strains and electrical activation in paced canines[6]. However, as of today, these methods are not routinely used in clinics despite the fact that MRI is becoming increasingly familiar to cardiologists. In addition, these techniques can be time consuming due to the large efforts required to segment the heart walls, and MRI is hindered in its myocardial applications due to safety restrictions in its patient population that may exclude children, pregnant women, and patients with old stents, pacemakers, claustrophobia, obesity and breath-holding issues. Echocardiography, on the other hand, remains the predominant imaging modality in 'everyday' diagnostic cardiology due to its real-time feedback, non-invasive application, low cost, high temporal resolution and multitude of complementary methods that can be used for a complete and accurate diagnosis. However, due to its associated low image quality, diagnosis is often subject to low inter- and intra-observer reproducibility. Ultrasound-based elasticity imaging is a relatively new field that deals with the estimation and imaging of mechanically related responses and properties for detection of pathological diseases, most notably cancer[7–9] and has thus emerged as an important field complementary to ultrasonic imaging. More recently, the focus of the elasticity imaging field has been steered towards cardiac applications[10–12]. This technique encompasses imaging of several kinds of mechanical functions, such as displacement, strain, strain rate, velocity, shear strain and rotation angle, which can highlight the mechanical properties of the myocardium and their changes in the presence of disease.

Ultrasound-based, high-resolution motion estimation can be achieved with time-shift-based or Doppler effect-based motion estimation techniques. For example, strain rate imaging and tissue Doppler imaging are mainly based on the use of the Doppler effect for measuring velocity and strain rate[13]. Drawbacks associated with the use of frequency domain techniques include low signal-to-noise ratio, poor resolution and aliasing. Time-shift-based methods based on the raw, radiofrequency ultrasound signals typically require more computational power, but provide higher accuracy[14] which increases with the imaging frame-rate. Therefore, recent efforts to improve quantitative myocardial elastography have led to a temporal resolution at the scale of the electrical propagation time[15], i.e. 2–3 ms per frame, and have since opened a new avenue towards real-time, non-invasive, high precision imaging of the cardiac conduction based on the intrinsic electro-mechanical coupling[16].

Imaging cardiac electrophysiology

Currently, no non-invasive electrical conduction mapping techniques of the heart are used diagnostically in the clinic. Although non-invasive approaches under development, such as electrocardiographic imaging (ECGI), have shown highly detailed three-dimensional (3D) images of the electrical activation sequence in humans[17,18], imaging cardiac electrophysiology remains a challenging problem. Magnetocardiography (MCG) is one of the most promising non-invasive mapping techniques that records magnetic fields generated by the electrical activity of the heart[19,20]. Despite it being a non-invasive and safe recording technique, in order to achieve the highest quality, the highly sensitive superconducting quantum interference device (SQUID) sensors used require measurements to be performed in optimally shielded areas. Currently, this involves a very costly and customized infrastructure that is non-existent in most hospitals worldwide and has thus confined MCG to physics laboratories instead of the clinic[19].

In the clinic, the available methods are catheter-based, costly and time-consuming. Even though they can provide maps of activation, they also require involved catheterization procedures, while being limited to the endocardium and the epicardium. Even in a laboratory setting, mapping the 3D electrical activation sequence of the heart *in vivo* remains a challenging problem[21]. While activation of the epicardium[6], the endocardium[22] or both[23] has been studied *in vivo* using electrode arrays, studies of the transmural activation are limited to *ex vivo* applications[24,25], to small regions of interest *in vivo*[26] or to small animals, e.g. the rabbit[18] and mouse[27].

As non-pharmacological treatments for arrhythmias, such as catheter ablation and cardiac resynchronization therapy (CRT), become increasingly popular because of the high failure rate, common proarrhythmic actions and toxicity associated with antiarrhythmic drugs[28], clinicians are in need of accurate, albeit still non-existing, non-invasive and direct measurement and mapping methods of the cardiac electrical activation sequence. Imaging the electro-mechanics of the heart, i.e. imaging the mechanical response immediately following the heart's electrical activation, can therefore become a valuable alternative.

Imaging the cardiac electro-mechanics

In conventional echocardiography, M-mode, tissue Doppler[29] and other methods offer the capability of assessing electro-mechanical dyssynchrony as an indication of arrhythmia and are used to monitor the performance of treatments such as CRT. M-mode echocardiography is often effective in examining intraventricular dyssynchrony[29]. For example, it is possible to compare the activation times of the posterior and septal walls by noting the times of peak contraction in the case of a left bundle branch block (LBBB). Under normal electro-mechanical coupling, a mechanical delay is a direct consequence of a delayed electrical activation – a chief symptom of LBBB. Although no single standard exists, a septal-to-posterior wall motion delay of > 130 ms has been suggested as a marker of intraventricular dyssynchrony[29]. Tissue Doppler is an ultrasound-based technique used to indirectly detect conduction abnormalities by identifying time delays at which peak displacement or strain rate occurs in distinct segments of the heart[29]. After treatment, these delays are used as indices to verify whether they were reduced to minimal or normal range values. In MRI, circumferential strains are imaged using MR tagging techniques and good agreement has been shown between the mechanical and electrical activation sequences when pacing from the right-ventricular wall[6,30].

Electro-mechanical wave imaging

Electro-mechanical wave imaging (EWI) is an entirely non-invasive, non-ionizing, ultrasound-based imaging method capable of mapping the electro-mechanical activation sequence of the myocardium along various echocardiographic planes *in vivo*. EWI[15,16,31–33] is capable of detecting and mapping the electro-mechanical contraction wave. The direction of propagation of this wave has already been shown to be dependent on the pacing origin in mice and dogs[16,34], hence suggesting that the EWI technology could be used to assess conduction properties of the myocardium.

By increasing the frame rate of standard echocardiography by up to sevenfold, EWI can map the small, transient deformations following similar propagation patterns to the electrical activation, i.e. the electro-mechanical wave (EW). The EW is a direct, tissue-level result of the cardiac excitation–contraction coupling[35]: the depolarization of a myocyte is followed by an uptake of calcium, which triggers contraction after the electro-mechanical delay. Since the deformations associated with the EW are small (< 0.25% interframe at 481 fps) and their propagation is fast (0.5–2.0 m/s), they are not usually detected or mapped with existing imaging modalities in the clinic such as standard echocardiography or MRI. EWI relies on radiofrequency (RF)-based cross-correlation methods, which provide higher accuracy as the frame rate increases. Since the only required equipment to perform EWI is a clinical ultrasound scanner[36], the application of EWI can be flexible and with a broad range, as it can be used at the doctor's office or the point of care, to identify patients at risk, inform on diseases in greater detail, or monitor and follow-up therapeutic interventions such as CRT and ablation.

EWI has been shown capable of non-invasively mapping the conduction wave during propagation. A high frame-rate (~500 fps), two-dimensional (2D) imaging modality was specifically developed[36] so that the transient cardiac motion resulting from the fast EW can be mapped in murine[32], canine[16,31] and human[36] left ventricles *in vivo*. This is achieved through electrocardiogram (ECG) gating (Fig. 63.1), or displacement matching[13], of small sectors on a clinically used, open-architecture ultrasound system for full-view, high frame-rate imaging. EWI may thus constitute a unique non-invasive technique for conduction mapping. It is important to note that the EWI technique is fundamentally different from conventional 'speckle tracking' methods, i.e. it aims at identifying transient myocardial effects and unveiling the propagation of the resulting EW. None of the available speckle tracking techniques is concerned with these types of effects or waves in the heart and might not optimally track them due to the lack of the precision of the methods used (most clinically available techniques are based on B-mode tracking for faster processing) and the

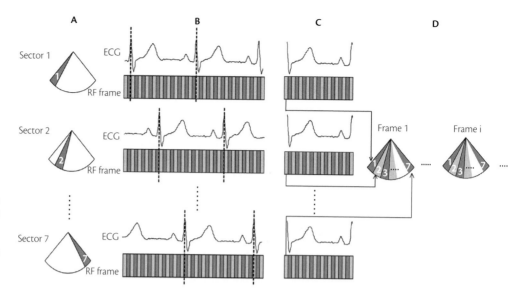

Fig. 63.1 The ECG-gated composite technique for high frame-rate, full-view ultrasound imaging. **A** Seven sectors at different angles are employed. **B** Seven ECG and RF signals are acquired in a continuous sequence during experiment. **C** One full cardiac cycle of ECG and RF frame signals is extracted. **D** Corresponding frames are recombined to generate full-view and high frame-rate ultrasound images.

required sensitivity and temporal resolution for depiction of transient phenomena. The existing speckle tracking techniques aim at determining the overall global motion of the myocardium (i.e. thickening or thinning) and determining the total myocardial contraction. EWI aims thus at overcoming the current limitations of echocardiography, i.e. lack of depiction of cardiac activation, and going beyond its existing applications in the clinic of merely depicting the mechanical function of the heart.

The EW onset in EWI is defined as the time at which the incremental strains, usually obtained by applying a gradient estimator to displacements estimated via RF-based cross-correlation, cross zero following the Q wave of the ECG. This definition can be interpreted as the time at which the heart muscle transitions from a relaxing state (e.g. radial thinning) to active contraction (e.g. radial thickening) and can be used to generate isochronal maps of activation in any echocardiographic plane.

EWI in canines *in vivo*

Open-chest canine hearts have been imaged using EWI during sinus rhythm, apical pacing and graded ischaemia and have been shown to be a good indicator of the electrical activation sequence and of the viability of the myocardium[16]. It should be noted that closed-chest hearts can also be imaged using EWI, but the studies in question entailed validation using invasive techniques (electrosonomicrometry) that required direct access to the myocardium. During sinus rhythm, the natural pacemaker, the sino-atrial node, located in the right atrium, activates the heart. Action potentials are generated spontaneously from there (at the P-wave) and travel through the atrio-ventricular node, the bundle of His (during the P–R segment) and finally the Purkinje fibre network and the ventricular myocardium (at the QRS complex). Since activation will originate from multiple locations following the Purkinje fibre network, complex activation patterns are expected when imaging the ventricles.

Figure 63.2a shows the isochrones of the EW propagation in a normal dog during sinus rhythm[16]. The EW was initiated at the mid-cavity segment in the septal and in the lateral walls, travelling

towards the apex and base. In the right-ventricular wall, the EW appeared on the endocardium near the apex a few milliseconds later and travelled towards the base.

During pacing from the apical region of the anterior-lateral wall[34], the pattern of propagation of the EW was entirely different (Fig. 63.2b). It was initiated from the pacing site and propagated towards the base. Contrary to sinus rhythm, where multiple, unconnected regions of early activation were observed, the EW originated from a single location.

The EW was also reproduced in an anatomically and biophysically accurate electro-mechanical simulation model[37] during various pacing schemes, and its isochrones were shown to be closely correlated with the electrical activation times[38].

As indicated in the section above (Electro-mechanical wave imaging), EWI can image the electro-mechanical response of the muscle at high temporal resolution, thereby producing ciné-loops during the EW propagation. An example of such a sequence that corresponds to the isochrones in Fig. 63.2b is shown in Fig. 63.2c–f.

To assess the performance of EWI in the detection of cardiac disease, the behaviour of the EW has been studied in the presence of graded ischaemia[16]. To generate graded ischaemia levels, the left-anterior descending (LAD) coronary artery flow was increasingly obstructed to full ligation by increments of 20% through external artery constriction, henceforth limiting the inflow of oxygenated blood and thus the contractility of the apical antero-septal myocardium. At each level of obstruction, EWI was performed and it was observed that the EW could not propagate through the ischaemic region. Therefore, to map the location of the ischaemic region, an image of the full extent of the EW can be used. Figure 63.3 depicts such maps and reliably shows the increasing size of the ischaemic region with the percentage of coronary flow obstruction.

EWI in human subjects

Since standard clinical echocardiography systems are used, EWI is also directly applicable to human subjects. Figure 63.4a–d shows the EW during normal sinus rhythm in a healthy human subject.

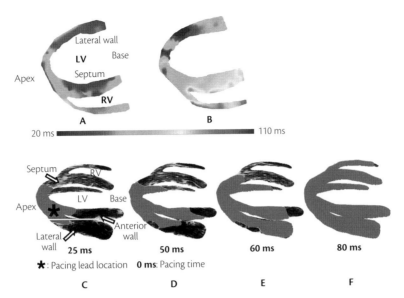

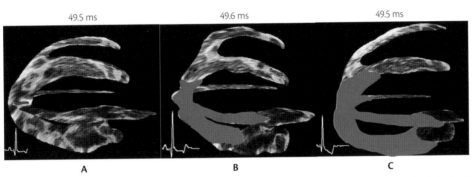

Fig. 63.2 Experimental canine heart EWI isochrones during (**A**) normal sinus rhythm and (**B**) apical pacing. In **A**, 0 ms is the onset of the QRS complex, and in **B** it is equivalent to the pacing stimulus application time. **C–F** Propagation of the EW (delineated in yellow) during pacing from the apical region of the antero-lateral wall in a normal canine heart. Propagation is initiated at the pacing lead location close to the apex and continues towards the base. (See color plate section.)

Fig. 63.3 Bi-plane (two-chamber and four-chamber) view of the same heart under different LAD coronary artery flow occlusion levels. Red, white and green arrows indicate the propagation of the EW in the septal, anterior and lateral wall, respectively. **A** Without any occlusion, i.e. normal coronary flow, radial thinning is visible up to regions where the axial direction of the ultrasound beam coincides with the longitudinal direction of the cardiac geometry, where shortening is expected (in blue). **B** At 60% flow occlusion, this behaviour is reversed in the presence of ischaemia: a region (delimited with a yellow line) containing radial thinning (blue) and longitudinal lengthening (red) is observed. **C** At complete occlusion this region increases in size. The ischaemia is visible in the anterior, posterior and lateral wall near the apex at 60% flow occlusion and in the anterior, posterior, lateral and septal wall at 100% flow occlusion. (See color plate section.)

Its propagation is initiated at the onset of the QRS complex at the mid-level of the interventricular septum (Fig. 63.4a,b). It then appears in the lateral wall, and then in the apical region of the right-ventricular wall (Fig. 63.4c). Approximately 60 ms after the onset of the QRS complex, both ventricles were activated, with the exception of the basal region of the lateral wall (Fig. 63.4d).

Conclusions and outlook

In this chapter, we introduced and described EWI that can non-invasively and directly map the conduction wave in the heart as well as identify the presence and progress of an abnormality. In the canine studies, the EW exhibited different patterns of propagation in the presence and at the site of mild and acute ischaemia. This supported the hypothesis that the waves imaged are closely linked to the electrical activation of the myocardium and its disruption in the presence of abnormalities. In human studies, the EW was depicted in a normal heart in both long-axis and short-axis

echocardiographic views. EWI could thus be used for both the detection and treatment monitoring of conduction-related pathologies.

The EW was compared with electrical activation patterns in the sinus rhythm case, by referring to the intramural electrical activation pathways previously described[24,39,40] for mammalian ventricles. According to Scher and Young[39], the earliest activity in dogs occurs at the region of the terminations of the left bundle on the mid-left septal endocardium at the mid-basal level, a few milliseconds before the QRS deflection. Activity on the right side of the septum occurs slightly later, again at the Purkinje terminals. During the first quarter of the QRS, most of the endocardial layer of the apical and mid-cavity region of the myocardium is depolarized. The activity then propagates from the endocardium to the epicardium, and towards both the apex and base. At the R-wave peak, only portions of the basal and lateral left ventricle and of the basal septum remain to be activated. Other studies performed later in swine, rats and humans[40] identified three points of early activation: (1) an area high on the anterior para-septal wall immediately below the

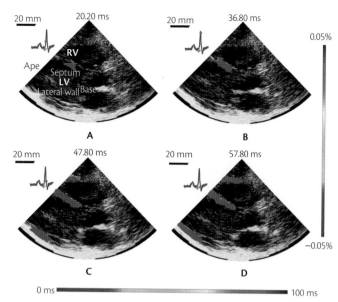

Fig. 63.4 Propagation of the EW (delineated in yellow) overlayed on the echocardiogram of a healthy human subject. The EW is initiated at the mid-septum (**A**) and propagates toward the apex (not shown) and the base (**B**). Activation of the lateral wall and right-ventricular wall follow approximately 10 ms later (**C**). **D** Propagation in the right-ventricular wall occurs from the apex to the base. The time shown denotes time lapsing after the onset of the QRS complex (green cross on the ECG; top left on images). Red denotes contraction (i.e. thickening). (See color plate section.)

mitral valve, (2) an area at half the distance from apex to base in the left side of the inter-ventricular septum, and (3) the posterior para-septal area at approximately one third of the distance from apex to base.

Those observations are in agreement with results obtained with EWI in both canines and humans, when considering that a delay of a few milliseconds [20–40 ms *in vivo*[26]] exists between the electrical and mechanical activation of the myocardium. In both canines and humans, the EW was initiated in the mid-cavity segment on the left side of the septum, and from the endocardium of the lateral wall near the base. It was also initiated from the posterior and anterior mid-cavity segments in the two-chamber view. In the right-ventricular wall, the wave was initiated later and travelled towards the base. Moreover, the basal wall regions remained inactivated even 60 ms after the onset of the Q-wave. This is also in agreement with previous reports[39] indicating that at the peak of the R-wave, basal regions are not electrically activated yet. Considering the electro-mechanical delay, it is then expected that the basal region will not contract before the onset of the isovolumic contraction phase occurs, in the vicinity of the R-wave peak, where the mechanical waves induced by the mitral valve closure do not allow a clear identification of the EW onset.

Current limitations of the methodology include angle dependence, which has been recently shown to be overcome using isochrones[41], and 2D imaging of a 3D propagation pattern. As a result, several artifacts may result on the images generated, especially at the level of the apex where the ultrasound beam is almost perpendicular to the direction of the myocardial motion. Those issues are expected to be resolved with the advent of 2D strain imaging[9] and 3D ultrasound RF signal availability at high frame rates. This will allow a full 3D depiction of the electro-mechanical function of the heart.

As a result, we expect that this technology will allow for simultaneous depiction of both mechanical and electrical activation sequences in the heart in human subjects in order to detect disease at its early onset, i.e. ischaemia at low coronary occlusion levels or arrhythmia with a single focus, in the ventricles or the atria. The advantages of this technique lie in the fact that it can provide such information regionally and non-invasively, something that is currently severely lacking in the clinic. Even though the electro-mechanical activity in one part of the muscle may affect that of its neighbouring regions, we believe that direct association between electrical and electro-mechanical patterns can be reliably made, especially based on what we have observed in simulations of the EW[41]. The main difference between the two would naturally be the delayed onset (by the electro-mechanical delay) of the electro-mechanical relative to the electrical patterns. Another advantage is that the MEC could also be unveiled by knowing both activities and relating the electrical to the mechanical one. The reciprocity between the two phenomena could thus be more thoroughly studied starting with simulations and confirming findings *in vivo*.

References

1. Waldman L, Fung Y, Covell J. Transmural myocardial deformation in the canine left ventricle. Normal in vivo three-dimensional finite strains. *Circ Res* 1985;**57**:152–163.
2. Ellis RM, Franklin DL, Rushmer RF. Left ventricular dimensions recorded by sonocardiometry. *Circ Res* 1956;**4**:684–688.
3. Pai V, Axel L. Advances in MRI tagging techniques for determining regional myocardial strain. *Curr Cardiol Rep* 2006;**8**:53–58.
4. Osman NF, Kerwin WS, McVeigh ER, Prince JL. Cardiac motion tracking using CINE harmonic phase (HARP) magnetic resonance imaging. *Magn Reson Med* 1999;**42**:1048–1060.
5. Aletras AH, Ding S, Balaban RS, Wen H. DENSE: displacement encoding with stimulated echoes in cardiac functional MRI. *J Magn Reson* 1999;**137**:247–252.
6. Faris OP, Evans FJ, Ennis DB, *et al.* Novel technique for cardiac electromechanical mapping with magnetic resonance imaging tagging and an epicardial electrode sock. *Ann Biomed Eng* 2003;**31**:430–440.
7. Parker KJ, Huang SR, Musulin RA, Lerner RM. Tissue response to mechanical vibrations for "sonoelasticity imaging". *Ultrasound Med Biol* 1990;**16**:241–246.
8. Ophir J, Céspedes I, Ponnekanti H, Yazdi Y, Li X. Elastography: a quantitative method for imaging the elasticity of biological tissues. *Ultrason Imaging* 1991;**13**:111–134.
9. O'Donnell M, Skovoroda A, Shapo B, Emelianov S. Internal displacement and strain imaging using ultrasonic speckle tracking. *IEEE Trans Ultrason Ferroelec Freq Control* 1994;**41**:314–325.
10. Heimdal A, Støylen A, Torp H, Skjærpe T. Real-time strain rate imaging of the left ventricle by ultrasound. *J Am Soc Echocardiography* 1998;**11**:1013–1019.
11. Konofagou EE, D'hooge J, Ophir J. Myocardial elastography – a feasibility study in vivo. *Ultrasound Med Biol* 2002;**28**:475–482.
12. D'hooge J, Konofagou EE, Jamal F, *et al.* Two-dimensional ultrasonic strain rate measurement of the human heart in vivo. *IEEE Trans Ultrason Ferroelec Freq Control* 2002;**49**:281–286.
13. D'hooge J, Heimdal A, Jamal F, *et al.* Regional strain and strain rate measurements by cardiac ultrasound: principles, implementation and limitations. *Eur J Echocardiogr* 2000;**1**:154–170.
14. Walker W, Trahey G. A fundamental limit on the performance of correlation based phase correction and flow estimation techniques. *IEEE Trans Ultrason Ferroelectr Freq Control* 1994;**41**:644–654.

15. Pernot M, Fujikura K, Fung-Kee-Fung SD, Konofagou EE. ECG-gated, Mechanical and electromechanical wave imaging of cardiovascular tissues in vivo. *Ultrasound Med Biol* 2007;**33**:1075–1085.

16. Provost J, Lee WN, Fujikura K, Konafagou EE. Electromechanical wave imaging of normal and ischemic hearts in vivo. *IEEE Trans Med Imag* 2010;**29**:625–635.

17. Ramanathan C, Ghanem RN, Jia P, Ryu K, Rudy Y. Noninvasive electrocardiographic imaging for cardiac electrophysiology and arrhythmia. *Nat Med* 2004;**10**:422–428.

18. Zhang X, Ramachandra I, Liu Z, Muneer B, Pogwizd SM, He B. Noninvasive three-dimensional electrocardiographic imaging of ventricular activation sequence. *Am J Physiol* 2005;**289**: H2724–H2732.

19. Strasburger JF, Cheulkar B, Wakai RT. Magnetocardiography for fetal arrhythmias. *Heart Rhythm* 2008;**5**:1073–1076.

20. Zhang S, Wang Y, Wang H, Jiang S, Xie X. Quantitative evaluation of signal integrity for magnetocardiography. *Phys Med Biol* 2009; **54**:4793–4802.

21. Nash MP, Pullan AJ. Challenges Facing Validation of Noninvasive Electrical Imaging of the Heart. *Ann Noninvasive Electrocardiol* 2005;**10**:73–82.

22. Schilling RJ, Peters NS, Davies DW. Simultaneous endocardial mapping in the human left ventricle using a noncontact catheter: comparison of contact and reconstructed electrograms during sinus rhythm. *Circulation* 1998;**98**:887–898.

23. Derakhchan K, Li D, Courtemanche M, Smith B, *et al.* Method for simultaneous epicardial and endocardial mapping of in vivo canine heart: application to atrial conduction properties and arrhythmia mechanisms. *J Cardiovasc Electrophysiol* 2001;**12**:548–555.

24. Durrer D, Van Dam RT, Freud GE, Janse MJ, Meijler FL, Arzbaecher RC. Total excitation of the isolated human heart. *Circulation* 1970;**41**: 899–912.

25. Sutherland DR, Ni Q, MacLeod RS, Lux RL, Punske BB. Experimental measures of ventricular activation and synchrony. *Pacing Clin Electrophysiol* 2008;**31**:1560–1570.

26. Ashikaga H, Coppola BA, Hopenfeld B, Leifer ES, McVeigh ER, Omens JH. Transmural dispersion of myofiber mechanics: implications for electrical heterogeneity in vivo. *J Am Coll Cardiol* 2007;**49**:909–916.

27. Hillman EMC, Bernus O, Pease E, Bouchard MB, Pertsov A. Depth-resolved optical imaging of transmural electrical propagation in perfused heart. *Opt Express* 2007;**15**:17827–17841.

28. The Cardiac Arrhythmia Suppression Trial (CAST) Investigators. Preliminary report: effect of encainide and flecainide on mortality in a randomized trial of arrhythmia suppression after myocardial infarction. *N Engl J Med* 1989;**321**:406–412.

29. Bax JJ, Poldermans D, Schuijf JD, Scholte AJ, Elhendy A, van der Wall EE. Imaging to differentiate between ischemic and nonischemic cardiomyopathy. *Heart Failure Clinics* 2006;**2**:205–214.

30. McVeigh E, Faris O, Ennis D, Helm P, Evans F. Electromechanical mapping with MRI tagging and epicardial sock electrodes. *J Electrocardiol* 2002;**35**(Suppl):61–64.

31. Pernot M, Konofagou EE (2005) Electromechanical imaging of the myocardium at normal and pathological states. In: Proceedings of IEEE International Ultrasonics Symposium, Rotterdam, pp. 1091–1094.

32. Konofagou EE, Luo J, Saluja D, Cervantes DO, Coromilas J, Fujikura K. Noninvasive electromechanical wave imaging and conduction-relevant velocity estimation in vivo. *Ultrasonics* 2010;**50**:208–215.

33. Konofagou EE, Luo J, Saluja D, Fujikura K, Cervantes D, Coromilas J (2007) Noninvasive electromechanical wave imaging and conduction velocity estimation in vivo. In: *Proceedings of IEEE International Ultrasonics Symposium*, New York, pp. 969–972.

34. Provost J, Gurev V, Trayanova N, Konofagou EE (2008) Characterization of wave origins in electromechanical wave imaging. In: Proceedings of the IEEE International Ultrasonics Symposium, Beijing.

35. Bers DM. Cardiac excitation–contraction coupling. *Nature* 2002; **415**:198–205.

36. Wang S, Lee W, Provost J, Luo J, Konofagou EE. A composite high-frame-rate system for clinical cardiovascular imaging. *IEEE Trans Ultrason Ferroelectr Freq Control* 2008;**55**:2221–2233.

37. Gurev V, Constantino J, Trayanova N. Transmural dyssynchrony of myofiber shortening is determined by depolarization sequence within myocardial layers. *Circulation* 2008;**118**:S349–S350.

38. Gurev V, Provost J, Konofagou EE, Trayanova N. In silico characterization of ventricular activation pattern by electromechanical wave imaging. *Heart Rhythm* 2009;**6**:S357.

39. Scher AM, Young AC. The pathway of ventricular depolarization in the dog. *Circ Res* 1956;**4**:461–469.

40. Sengupta PP, Tondato F, Khandheria BK, Belohlavek M, Jahangir A. Electromechanical activation sequence in normal heart. *Heart Fail Clin* 2008;**4**:303–314.

41. Provost J, Gurev V, Trayanova N, Konofagou EE. Mapping of cardiac electrical activation with electromechanical wave imaging: an in silico — in vivo reciprocity study. *Heart Rhythm* 2011 (in press).

Evolving concepts in measuring ventricular strain in the human heart: impedance measurements

Douglas A. Hettrick

Background

In order to investigate cardiac mechano-electric coupling in patients, quantification of both the passive and the active cardiac loading conditions is imperative. The ultimate haemodynamic sensor for an implantable device would provide information about multiple aspects of cardiovascular performance, including systolic function (the ability of the ventricle to generate pressure), diastolic function (the ability of the ventricle to fill), preload and afterload. Note that preload, an index of the strain or volume of the ventricle just prior to ejection, and afterload, the pressure and tension developed by the left ventricle (LV) to overcome the forces opposing ejection, are distinct physical entities with different units and methods of quantification. To this end, pressure–volume plane analysis combining direct LV pressure measurements with intra-cardiac impedance measurements is a well-known research tool to help quantify overall cardiovascular function[1–3]. This chapter reviews some applications of intra-thoracic impedance to track changes in vascular dimension or cardiac chamber volume.

Pressure–volume vs stress–strain

The pressure–volume loop has long been considered the scientific gold standard for evaluating cardiovascular function (Fig. 64.1). Pressure–volume plane analysis considers the major mechanical determinants of myocardial performance, including both mechanical stress and strain. Stress and strain are related through mechanical stiffness or elastance (elastance = stress/strain), the inverse of compliance. Thus, the pressure volume plane enables quantification of changes in myocardial elastance throughout the cardiac cycle[3].

Pressure measurements alone provide primarily an index of mechanical stress, or the force acting on the tissue. Conversely, fluoroscopically or echocardiographically derived indices of dimension such as ventricular diameter, end-diastolic volume (EDV), ejection fraction and dyssynchrony are primarily indices of strain, or the mechanical deformation of tissue in response to the applied stress. Thus, pure echo-based indices of chamber strain do not consider the associated stress or pressure that lead to the resultant strain. Indices of cardiovascular performance such as the time derivative of LV pressure (dP/dt), or cardiac output or stroke volume are highly dependent on chamber loading conditions. However, by combining stress and strain into a single evaluation

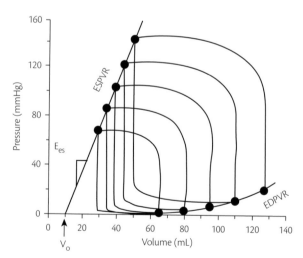

Fig. 64.1 Pressure –volume plane analysis. Acute changes to loading conditions allow determination of various indices of ventricular systolic and diastolic function including the linear end-systolic pressure –volume relationship (ESPVR) and its slope (maximal elastance E_{es}) as well as the non-linear end-diastolic pressure –volume relationship (EDPVR). Preload recruitable stroke work (PRSW) may also be determined from this relationship by plotting loop area (stroke work) as a function of end-diastolic volume. V_o, extrapolated zero-pressure volume. [Reproduced, with permission, from Burkhoff D, Mirsky I, Suga H (2005) Assessment of systolic and diastolic ventricular properties via pressure–volume analysis: a guide for clinical, translational, and basic researchers. *Am J Physiol* **289**:H501–H512.]

tool, pressure–volume plane analysis objectively quantifies all four major components of cardiovascular function, namely preload, afterload, systolic and diastolic function, independent of loading conditions (see Table 64.1).

Quantification of systolic function

Systolic function describes the ability of the ventricles to eject blood into the afterload or arterial system. On a cellular level, it describes the ability of the myocyte to develop force against a given afterload for any given initial stretch or preload. Many common clinical indices of cardiac performance are relative indices of systolic function. For example, cardiac index (or output), stroke volume, aortic velocity time integrals, ejection fraction, stroke work and dP/dt are all common clinical indices of cardiovascular performance. However, although clinically useful, these indices are all load dependent. This implies that a change in any of these indices may be due simply to changes in preload or afterload, and not necessarily to changes in actual systolic function. Therefore, ventricular systolic function is best described using load-independent indices such as the end-systolic pressure–volume relationship (ESPVR) or preload recruitable stroke work (PRSW). The ESPVR quantifies the maximum of the dynamic myocardial elastance. PRSW describes the constant ratio of the myocardial stroke work to the ventricular preload (Fig. 64.1).

Quantification of ventricular diastolic function

Likewise, 'diastolic function' is the ability of the LV to fill. The four key phases of diastole include active relaxation, passive or early filling, diastasis or reduced filling, and active filling resulting from atrial contraction. The rate and extent of active relaxation can be indicated by either the time constant of isovolumic relaxation (τ) or peak negative LV dP/dt. The later phases of LV chamber filling are completely described by the end-diastolic pressure–volume relationship (EDPVR) or passive ventricular stiffness. Delayed or incomplete relaxation, myocardial hypertrophy or other disease states can lead to pathological stiffening of the LV that limits filling and, hence, overall cardiovascular performance. Indeed, the LV EDPVR has been identified as the quintessential index of identifying

diastolic heart failure[2,4]. Likewise, Echo-Doppler derived indices of mitral valve blood flow velocity including peak early 'passive' (E) and late 'atrial contraction driven' (A) filling velocity and their resultant ratio (E/A) are commonly applied in the clinical environment to identify impaired LV filling. Monitoring pulmonary capillary wedge pressure alone cannot indicate true changes in passive LV stiffness or the EDPVR.

Quantification of preload

Preload is perhaps the most important parameter for monitoring heart failure patients and can be defined on a cellular scale as the length of the myocyte at the time of contraction. On a larger cardiac scale, it is defined as LVEDV. Estimates of LV filling pressure such as LV end-diastolic pressure, pulmonary capillary wedge pressure (PCWP) and left atrial pressure are all clinical surrogates of LV preload. However, none of these indices measures preload directly.

Quantification of afterload

Afterload is defined as the forces opposing ejection. Normally, this is primarily determined by the mechanical resistance and compliance of the arterial system. Other determinants of afterload include the mechanical status of the aortic outflow tract and the aortic valve. Hydraulic impedance mismatches in the arterial system due to discontinuities in the arterial wall compliance, vessel branching and vessel tapering can result in partial reflection of the pressure and flow waves back towards the ventricle. Thus, arterial wave reflections can also influence LV afterload. A useful index of afterload would be a key parameter to monitor arterial hypertension. LV or arterial systolic pressure and LV wall stress are indices of LV afterload. However, these primarily reflect arterial vascular tone and not necessarily compliance or wave reflection. To this end, aortic input impedance and its interpretation via various lumped parameter models such as the Windkessel model have been applied to the study of afterload[4,5]. In addition, the effective arterial elastance (E_A) is another index of LV afterload that considers both resistance and compliance of the arterial vasculature. E_A is defined as the ratio of LV end-systolic pressure to stroke volume and may be determined directly from the pressure–volume plane.

Conductance catheter for LV volume measurement

The conductance catheter technique enables continuous measurement of LV volume using multiple intra-cardiac impedance measurements and was first described by Jan Baan and colleagues in the early 1980s[6]. This method has been used extensively to assess global systolic and diastolic ventricular function. In many respects, the conductance catheter revolutionized the study of cardiovascular mechanics in both laboratory and clinical settings by making the study of ventricular pressure–volume relationships practical. The technique led to a renaissance of cardiac physiology by increasing the understanding of the effect of pharmacological agents, disease states, pacing therapies and other interventions on cardiovascular function[2,3]. Conductance catheter systems are available for both clinical and laboratory monitoring applications, including a miniature system capable of measuring LV volume and pressure

Table 64.1 Indices of cardiovascular function

Systolic function	Diastolic function
+dP/dt*	-dP/dt*
Stroke volume*	τ*
Aortic velocity*	E/A
Stroke work*	EDPVR (stiffness)
ESPVR	
PRSW	
Afterload	**Preload**
ESP	EDV
E_A	EDP

dP/dt, time derivative of LV pressure; ESPVR, slope of the end-systolic pressure–volume relationship; PRSW, slope of preload recruitable stroke work relationship; τ, time constant of isovolumic relaxation; E/A; ratio of early (E) to late (A) peak mitral flow velocity EDPVR, end-diastolic pressure–volume relationship ; ESP, end-systolic pressure; E_A, effective arterial elastance; EDV, end-diastolic volume; EDP, end-diastolic pressure; *, load-dependent indices.

in mice[7]. The conductance methodology is based on the parallel cylinder model:

$$V(t) = \left[\rho l^2 / \alpha R(t) \right] + V_C$$

where V is volume, t is time, ρ is blood resistivity, l is the segmental interelectrode distance and R is measured resistance. The slope correction term α accounts for non-uniformity of the electric field and the parallel conductance volume V_C results from current leakage beyond the LV chamber. The cylindrical model assumes that the volume of interest has a uniform cross-sectional area along its length. Therefore, the ventricular volume is subdivided into multiple segments determined by equipotential surfaces bounded by multiple sensing electrodes along the axis of the conductance catheter. When combined with an integrated pressure sensor, the conductance catheter can be used to measure real-time pressure–volume relationships within the ventricle, as in Fig. 64.1.

Intra-thoracic impedance monitoring

Besides providing potentially life-saving therapies, some implantable devices including pacemakers, implantable cardiac defibrillators (ICD) and cardiac resynchronization therapy (CRT) devices also contain detailed diagnostic information about the patient. These diagnostic indices include long-term trends of various parameters such as heart rate, heart rate variability, respiration trends, patient activity and atrial and ventricular tachyarrhythmia recurrence. Some experimental devices currently under investigation also measure intra-cardiac chamber pressure[8,9]. Intermittent monitoring of pulmonary fluid accumulation via intra-thoracic impedance monitoring has also been shown to be a clinically useful diagnostic tool that can identify patients at significant risk for worsening heart failure events with reasonable accuracy[10,11].

Within these devices, measurements are typically performed once per cardiac cycle using the device case (can) and the right ventricular (RV) defibrillation coil as electrodes in a bipolar configuration, or with some alternative electrode configuration. The measured 'daily impedance' values are processed post hoc to generate a daily 'reference impedance' using a propriety algorithm (for example, OptiVol, Medtronic, Minneapolis). The negative daily difference between the impedance and calculated reference impedance increments a daily 'fluid index' that can cross a pre-specified threshold.

Recently published investigations[12,13] have shown that sustained acute decreases in intra-thoracic impedance identify subjects at significantly higher prospective risk of heart failure hospitalization.

Figure 64.2 shows an interesting case example of how device-based intra-thoracic impedance monitoring could provide an index of increased strain. The patient is an 81-year-old female with a history of congestive heart failure including pulmonary hypertension, tricuspid valve regurgitation, atrial fibrillation and an enlarged RV. The implanted CRT device had been atypically placed subcutaneously on the right side. Figure 64.2A shows the observed gradual decrease in intra-thoracic impedance (daily impedance, bottom graph) and the corresponding increases in the fluid index (top graph) which were recorded over 1 year. Figure 64.2B shows a chest X-ray of the same subject taken in December 2008. No pulmonary oedema was observed on X-ray. As part of a clinical trial, a right heart catheterization was performed revealing a somewhat elevated pulmonary capillary wedge pressure (20 mmHg) and a high pulmonary arterial pressure (54/19 mmHg). Based on these clinical findings and patient history, the most probable cause for the gradually declining impedance was determined not to be pulmonary oedema, but rather gradual progressive dilation of the right heart chambers due to chronic pressure overload and

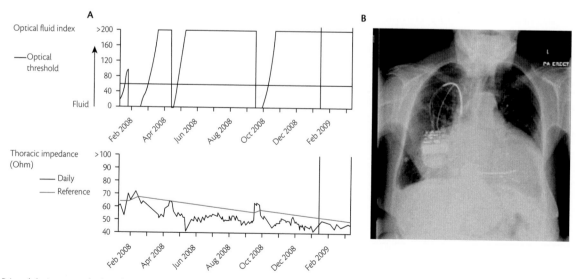

Fig. 64.2 A Printed device report for intrathoracic impedance monitoring feature for a patient with RV dilation. Top panel: fluid index derived from the difference between the daily and reference impedance. Bottom panel : raw device-measured daily impedance (dark line) and calculated reference impedance (grey line). The continuous gradual decline in daily impedance causes the fluid index to surpass a prespecified threshold (grey line in top panel). **B** Chest X-ray showing enlarged heart and system implant configuration. In this case it is likely that gradual dilation of the right and left atrium may have caused the steady declines in impedance (see text for details; data courtesy of Roy Small, MD, and Lisa Rathman, NP, The Heart Group, Lancaster, Pennsylvania).

valvular dysfunction. That is, the close proximity of the RV to the bipolar impedance monitoring system leveraging the device case and the intraventricular defibrillation electrode coil resulted in the intra-thoracic impedance measurement becoming quite sensitive to gradual increases in chamber size. Thus, this case provides anecdotal support for the hypothesis that intra-thoracic impedance measurement can track acute changes in cardiac chamber size and hence strain.

In addition, two recent studies including one animal[14] and one human[15] trial further explored the potential of multiple bipolar impedance vectors, including the LV epicardial leads, to improve the specificity of intra-thoracic impedance monitoring to predict major clinical heart failure events (Fig. 64.3). The later trial demonstrated strong linear correlations between serial changes in left ventricular end-diastolic volume (LVEDV), or preload, and changes in intra-thoracic impedance between the LV epicardial lead and the RV defibrillation coil in patients with implantable devices. Thus, the results of these trials further demonstrate the potential to monitor changes in ventricular strain directly using currently available impedance monitoring techniques.

Haemodynamic monitoring via continuous intra-thoracic impedance monitoring

The application of haemodynamic data derived from intra-thoracic impedance measurements made by implantable devices such as pacemakers and implantable defibrillators has been investigated for quite some time. As early as 1984, Salo and colleagues described a system of RV impedance measurements determined from a tripolar pacing electrode for use in both diagnostics and device control[16]. More recently, Stahl and colleagues demonstrated in a pig model of heart failure that changes of intra-cardiac impedance revealed haemodynamic deterioration as reflected by EDV and EDP[17].

The clinical utility of intra-thoracic impedance monitoring could be extended by performing continuous (i.e. high sampling

frequency) impedance measurements within a chamber of interest, such as the LV, in order to highlight haemodynamic changes within the cardiac cycle. Furthermore, the combination of a device-based impedance measurement with a device-based pressure measurement could result in a clinical tool to analyze cardiovascular function in a manner similar to the pressure–volume plane.

A recent clinical trial explored the potential clinical utility of simultaneous measurement of LV pressure and continuous intra-thoracic impedance from a variety of electrode positions in a group of 20 patients undergoing intra-venous ablation for atrial fibrillation[18]. Subjects under general anaesthesia were acutely instrumented with a traditional conductance catheter in the LV. Temporary standard multipolar electrophysiology catheters were positioned in the RV and LV epicardial free wall via the coronary sinus, respectively. The temporary catheters served as surrogates for permanent implantable system leads used commonly for cardiac resynchronization therapy. Following baseline measurements of traditional LV conductance volume (control), LV pressure and conductance measurements were repeated using the surrogate device electrode configuration. In some subjects, a transient occlusion of the inferior *vena cava* was performed using a balloon catheter to create a transient decrease in ventricular preload.

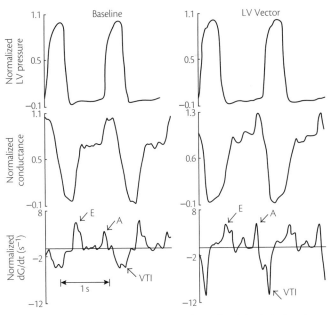

Fig. 64.4 Raw LV pressure (top), conductance (centre) and the derivative of conductance (dG/dt; bottom) using gold standard conductance catheter techniques (left) and pacemaker LV lead configuration (right). Since the raw conductance is proportional to LV volume, the derivative of the conductance signal is therefore proportional to mitral flow (during filling) and aortic flow during ejection. Note the presence of a distinct 'E' and 'A' wave in the derivative of both conductance signals. The negative portion of the dG/dt signal is likewise analogous to ejection velocity, similar to aortic velocity time integral (VTI) measurements. Thus, the raw LV vector conductance signal and its derivative may be used to derive important indices of both systolic and diastolic LV function. [Reproduced, with permission, from Hettrick D, Schwartzman D (2009) Human feasibility study of hemodynamic monitoring via continuous intrathoracic impedance monitoring. In: *Proceedings of IEEE EMBS 31st Annual International Conference*, Minneapolis, pp. 4611–4614, © IEEE.]

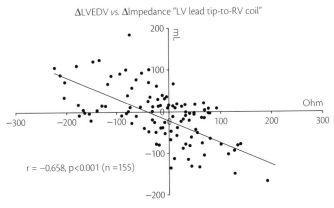

Fig. 64.3 High correlation between serial changes in left ventricular preload (LVEDV) and changes in intrathoracic impedance between the LV epicardial lead and the RV defibrillation coil in patients with implantable devices. [Reproduced, with permission, from Maines M, Landolina M, Lunati M, *et al.* on behalf of the Italian Clinical Service Optivol-CRT Group (2009) Intrathoracic and ventricular impedances are associated with changes in ventricular volume in patients receiving defibrillators for CRT. *Pacing Clin Electrophysiol* **33**:64–73.]

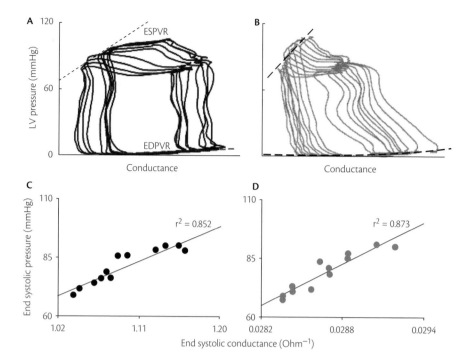

Fig. 64.5 **A** and **B** Raw pressure–conductance (volume) loops during transient IVC occlusion in one subject using gold standard conductance catheter (**A**) and LV vector (**B**). Dashed lines represent calculated ESPVR and EDPVR, respectively[19]. **C** and **D** ESPVR calculation for one representative subject using gold standard conductance catheter (**C**) and LV vector (**D**). Similar linear correlations indicate that impedance derived from common device electrode configurations could act as a surrogate for traditional conductance catheter measurements. [Reproduced, with permission, from Hettrick D, Schwartzman D (2009) Human feasibility study of hemodynamic monitoring via continuous intrathoracic impedance monitoring. In: *Proceedings of IEEE EMBS 31st Annual International Conference*, Minneapolis, pp. 4611–4614, © IEEE.]

Sample raw LV pressure, 'conductance catheter' and LV–RV vector conductance signals are shown in Figs 64.4 and 64.5 along with simultaneously recorded LV pressure. The morphometry of both waveforms is consistent with LV volume morphology including rapid filling, diastasis, atrial systole and LV contraction. The derivative of the conductance signal, an analogue of mitral and aortic valve flow, shows features consistent with early filling ('E' wave), atrial contraction ('A' wave) and aortic flow patterns.

Surrogate indices of LV function, including ESPVR, EDPVR and PRSW, were derived by combining real-time pressure and conductance. Figure 64.5 shows representative pressure conductance loops from one subject with inferior *Vena cava* (IVC) occlusion for both the conductance catheter technique and conductance measurements performed from the LV vector. Figure 64.5 also demonstrates the determination of the ESPVR for the subject depicted in Fig. 64.4. The high linear correlation values calculated indicate that it is feasible to calculate indices of cardiovascular function using conductance data derived from an implanted device electrode configuration common in CRT patients. Group linear correlations for all subjects for the ESPVR as well as for PRSW and EDPVR were also high and statistically similar to correlations derived from traditional conductance catheter analysis[18].

Conclusions and outlook

Conventional implantable device electrode configurations provide a robust continuous intra-cardiac haemodynamic signal that may be useful for quantifying cardiovascular function in both animal and human subjects. Alone, such a signal could be used to derive several important indices of LV systolic and diastolic function as well as LV preload. Furthermore, if combined with an analogue of LV pressure, quantification of all four components of cardiovascular function, namely systolic function, diastolic function, preload and afterload, may also be feasible. Thus, the stage is set for an implantable device that could chronically monitor an LV pressure–volume loop analogue in an implantable device using existing technology.

Besides haemodynamic monitoring, ventricular function parameters derived from intra-cardiac impedance measurements could also be used to 'close the loop' and provide feedback control for device therapies. Many key programmable device features could potentially be further automated based on changes in LV function, particularly strain. Some of these therapy parameters could include heart rate, pacing (stimulus) location, pacing mode (triggered versus inhibited) or delays (e.g. atrio–ventricular delay, left-to-right inter-ventricular delay). Pacing with a goal to minimize chamber size may also have benefits in terms of potentially reducing the occurrence of premature ventricular contractions and perhaps other ventricular tachyarrhythmias. Likewise, smaller chambers may require lower defibrillation energy thresholds, as described in Chapter 52.

References

1. Baan J, Jong TT, Kerkhof PL, *et al.* Continuous stroke volume and cardiac output from intra-ventricular dimensions obtained with impedance catheter. *Cardiovasc Res* 1981;**15**:328–334.
2. Lee WS, Nakayama M, Huang WP, *et al.* Assessment of left ventricular end-systolic elastance from aortic pressure–left ventricular volume relations. *Heart Vessels* 2002;**16**:99–104.
3. Burkhoff D, Mirsky I, Suga H. Assessment of systolic and diastolic ventricular properties via pressure–volume analysis: a guide for clinical, translational, and basic researchers. *Am J Physiol* 2005; **289**:H501–H512.

4. Nichols WW, Conti CR, Walker WE, Milnor WR. Input impedance of the systemic circulation in man. *Circ Res* 1977;**40**:451–458.

5. Westerhof N, Lankhaar JW, Westerhof BE. The arterial Windkessel. *Med Biol Eng Comp* 2009;**47**:131–141.

6. Baan J, VanDerVelde E, DeBruin H, *et al.* Continuous measurement of left ventricular volume in animals and humans by conductance catheter. *Circulation* 1984;**70**:812–823.

7. Segers P, Georgakopoulos D, Afanasyeva M, *et al.* Conductance catheter based assessment of arterial input impedance, arterial function, and ventricular-vascular interaction in mice. *Am J Physiol* 2005;**288**:H1157–H1164.

8. Zile MR, Bourge RC, Bennett TD, *et al.* Application of implantable hemodynamic monitoring in the management of patients with diastolic heart failure: a subgroup analysis of the COMPASS-HF trial. *J Card Fail* 2008;**14**:816–823.

9. Adamson PB, Conti JB, Smith AL, *et al.* Reducing events in patients with chronic heart failure (REDUCEhf) study design: continuous hemodynamic monitoring with an implantable defibrillator. *Clin Cardiol* 2007;**30**:567–575.

10. Yu CM, Wang L, Chau E, *et al.* Intrathoracic impedance monitoring in patients with heart failure: correlation with fluid status and feasibility of early warning preceding hospitalization. *Circulation* 2005;**112**: 841–848.

11. Vollmann D, Nägele H, Schauerte P, Wiegand U, Butter C, Zanotto G, Quesada A, Guthmann A, Hill MR, Lamp B. European InSync Sentry Observational Study Investigators. Clinical utility of intrathoracic impedance monitoring to alert patients with an implanted device of deteriorating chronic heart failure. *Eur Heart J* 2007;**28**:1835–1840.

12. Perego GB, Landolina M, Vergara G, Lunati M, Zanotto G, Pappone A, Lonardi G, Speca G, Iacopino S, Varbaro A, Sarkar S, Hettrick DA, Denaro A. Optivol-CRT Clinical Service Observational Group. Implantable CRT device diagnostics identify patients with increased risk for heart failure hospitalization. *J Interv Card Electrophysiol* 2008;**23**:235–242.

13. Small RS, Wickemeyer W, Germany R, *et al.* Changes in intrathoracic impedance are associated with subsequent risk of hospitalizations for acute decompensated heart failure: clinical utility of implanted device monitoring without a patient alert. *J Card Fail* 2009;**15**: 475–481.

14. Khoury DS, Naware M, Siou J, *et al.* Ambulatory monitoring of congestive heart failure by multiple bioelectric impedance vectors. *J Am Coll Cardiol* 2009;**53**:1075–1081.

15. Maines M, Landolina M, Lunati M, *et al.*; on behalf of the Italian Clinical Service Optivol-CRT Group. Intrathoracic and ventricular impedances are associated with changes in ventricular volume in patients receiving defibrillators for CRT. *Pacing Clin Electrophysiol* 2009;**33**:64–73.

16. Salo R, Pedersen B, Olive A, *et al.* Continuous ventricular volume assessment for diagnosis and pacemaker control. *Pacing Clin Electrophysiol* 1984;**7**:1267–1272.

17. Stahl C, Beierlein W, Walker T, *et al.* Intracardiac impedance monitors hemodynamic deterioration in a chronic heart failure pig model. *J Cardiovasc Electrophysiol* 2007;**18**:985–990.

18. Hettrick D, Schwartzman D. Human feasibility study of hemodynamic monitoring via continuous intrathoracic impedance monitoring. *Conf Proc IEEE Eng Med Biol Soc* 2009;**2009**:4611–4614.

Mechano-sensitive channel blockers: a new class of antiarrhythmic drugs?

Ed White

Background

The activation of mechano-sensitive ion channels (MSC) has been implicated in the generation of stretch-activated cardiac arrhythmias [e.g.[1]], which are reported to be more prevalent in diseased tissue[2]. MSC may also be involved in the remodelling process that occurs in response to chronic stress (e.g. hypertension) and strain (e.g. dilatation) overload. Thus the targeting of MSC would seem a valid goal for pharmacological intervention. However, it should also be noted that mechano-sensitivity is a property of most tissues[3] and that in the heart it is associated with the normal regulation of contractility, Ca^{2+} handling, electrical activity and physiological growth[4].

This chapter discusses some of the factors that need to be resolved if the targeting of MSC, as a therapeutic tool, is to be achieved. For example, if an effective pharmacological strategy is to be devised for MSC their identity, structure and mode of gating, in human cardiac tissue, must be understood. Readers are also referred to reviews[5,6] for further information on the pharmacology of MSC.

The identity of MSC

The structure of certain bacterial MSC has been solved[7–9], but this has led to the conclusion that there is no common MSC structure. The identity of MSC in the human heart is still uncertain. Excluding channels activated by changes in cell volume, there seems to be two major types of MSC in mammalian myocardium: channels that are non-specific with regard to the conduction of cations (MSC_{NS}) and those specific for K^+ (MSC_K). It is the role of MSC_{NS} in atrial and ventricular myocardium that has attracted most attention with respect to the modulation of electrical activity in the heart.

Recent evidence suggests that the transient receptor potential (canonical) channels (TRPC) are potentially MSC_{NS}. TRPC subunits consist of six trans-membrane domains with, putatively, four of these subunits making a functional channel in homo- or hetero-multimer format. TRPC are known to act as calcium entry pathways and there is also evidence from non-cardiac tissue that they

are mechano-sensitive[10]. Interest was initially focused upon TRPC1 as a vertebrate MSC_{NS}[11], but there is now evidence that TRPC6 may be responsible for MSC_{NS} in mouse myocytes[12]. TRPC expression in the heart may differ between species, and there are contrasting observations in the literature [compare[13,14] with[12]]. In the human heart TRPC5 and 6 have been reported[14]. Some evidence for the mechano-sensitivity of TRPC has come from expression systems and the interpretation of these results has been discussed by Gottlieb et al.[15].

The measurement of TRPC currents in native adult cardiac myocytes in the presence of physiological solutions is difficult and it is therefore difficult to judge whether their current–voltage relationship matches those of MSC_{NS}, which tend to be linear (e.g. see Fig. 65.2B later in this chapter). Therefore it is at present difficult to predict whether TRPC current would be capable of triggering arrhythmias.

There is stronger evidence to suggest that the MSC_K channels include members of the two-pore domain family of K^+ channels. These channels have four trans-membrane segments in each subunit. A functional channel is made from a dimer of subunits. In particular, weak inwardly rectifying two pore-domain K^+ channel (TWIK)-related K^+ channel (TREK-1) has been identified as an MSC_K in rat myocytes[16,17], but to date TREK-1 has not been found in the human heart. There is also evidence that the adenosine triphosphate (ATP)-sensitive K^+ channel (K_{ATP}) and the acetylcholine-activated K^+ channel (K_{ACh}) are mechano-sensitive[16].

Activation of MSC_K channels by mechanical stimulation would be expected to hyperpolarize the cell, stabilize the diastolic membrane potential and shorten the action potential duration. These effects are usually thought to be protective against arrhythmias, so the blockade of these channels may not be beneficial. However, glibenclamide, a blocker of K_{ATP} channels, was able to reduce the incidence of ventricular fibrillation induced by chest impact in a pig model of *Commotio cordis*[18]. It was suggested that the electrical effects created by K_{ATP} activation were not uniform and that dispersion of excitability and refractoriness were increased, increasing the chance of re-entrant arrhythmias developing.

Gating of MSC

The lipid bilayer has an effective pressure that varies with depth[10]. Mechanical stimulation increases the mean tension, and by Poisson's constant thins as it stretches. For bacterial MSC this tends to create a hydrophobic mismatch between the thickness of the channel protein and the inner and outer leaflets of the membrane (Fig. 65.1A). There is evidence from studies using bacterial MSC, in reconstituted bilayer experiments, that bilayer tension is sufficient to activate MSC[3,7,10].

However, the sarcolemma of the mammalian cardiac myocyte is much more complex than a simple bilayer and there is evidence[19] to support a tether model of activation, whereby force is sensed and transmitted to the MSC via the cytoskeleton and extracellular matrix (Fig. 65.1B). Disruption of the cytoskeleton, by agents such as cytochalasin D or colchicine, might therefore reduce channel activity via breakage of series elastic components, but cytoskeletal disruption could increase MSC activity due to a reduced parallel elasticity[20].

The role of the extracellular matrix is consistent with the modulation of MSC via mechanical manipulation of integrins[21] and it is possible that accessory proteins close to the MSC may be involved (Fig. 65.1C).

Finally there is accumulating evidence to suggest that mechanical stimulation may result in the activation of signalling pathways remote from the MSC, and that mechanically induced second messengers are responsible for the activation of MSC (Fig. 65.1D). Studies in cardiac muscle have implicated mechanically induced reactive oxygen and nitrogen species (ROS and RNS, respectively)[22,23]. Note that in a scenario as described in Fig. 65.1D, and in contrast to the mechanisms described in Fig. 65.1A–C, MSC are mechano-sensitive but not mechanically gated. The idea that mechanical stimulation triggers signalling pathways is well accepted for cardiac hypertrophy [e.g.[24]], but the potential for such a mechanism to activate MSC has been less appreciated. However, while second messengers are clearly not essential for the MSC phenotype, the role of amphipaths in modulation of MSC is well established[16].

The varied potential mechanisms of cardiac MSC gating have important implications for the design of pharmaceutical agents: (1) MSC need not be the site of action and (2) most of the potential sites of action described in Fig. 65.1 (e.g. the lipid bilayer and the cytoskeleton) are not specific to the MSC, i.e. their modulation is likely to have multiple ramifications. In addition, the generation of diffusible, mechanically activated, signalling compounds may affect channels other than the 'classic' MSC.

Agents used to modulate MSC

Gadolinium

Gadolinium (Gd^{3+}) is an agent that is commonly used to inhibit MSC_{NS}. In a situation such as a voltage clamp experiment, where the MSC_{NS} can be isolated by study design, Gd^{3+} has been shown to be a useful tool. Its mode of action seems to be via membrane surface charge screening and the alteration of bilayer properties[5,25,26]. In addition it has been shown to reduce stretch-activated arrhythmias [e.g.[27]].

However, Gd^{3+} also blocks numerous other cardiac ion channels in the same range of concentrations (1–10 μM) that it affects MSC_{NS}[6]. It is also chelated by anions such as phosphate and bicarbonate, which are present in physiological solutions[28]. Interestingly there is some evidence that this Gd^{3+} anion complex is still active against mechanically induced events[29]. Indeed in an alternative interpretation of the implications of Gd^{3+} chelation on its channel blocking properties, the Gd^{3+} anion complex has been deliberately chosen in preference to free Gd^{3+} in some studies[30]. The Gd^{3+} anion complex appears to be much less effective against certain types of ion channel, such as the L-type Ca^{2+} channel, than free Gd^{3+}, while retaining its mechano-sensitive effects[6]. It is possible that the Gd^{3+} anion complex can influence MSC via bilayer interactions[5].

Streptomycin

Streptomycin sulphate (Strep) is another experimental agent commonly used to block MSC. In millimolar concentrations Strep blocks Ca^{2+} and K^+ channels[31]. However, at 40 μM Strep inhibits MSC_{NS} currents in myocytes (Fig. 65.2). This concentration is equivalent to a peak serum level of 50 μg/ml after a standard intramuscular injection. We have found that 50 μM Strep has no effect on the action potential in unstretched cardiac myocytes, an indication

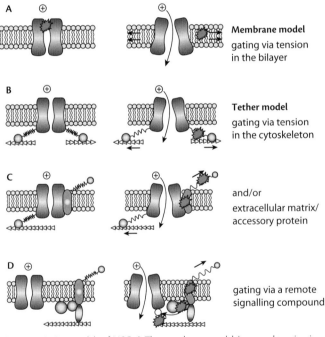

Fig. 65.1 Gating models of MSC. **A** The membrane model: increased tension in the lipid bilayer favours occupancy of the open state as a result of the open channel having a larger in-plane area and a contribution of hydrophobic mismatch. **B** The tether model: the MSC is gated by tension in the cytoskeleton linked to the channel and by (**C**) the extracellular matrix which keeps the channel from being pulled through the bilayer. Accessory proteins close to the channel may be involved. **D** Force may be transmitted remotely to the MSC and/or a signalling pathway is activated that results in an intracellular second messenger gating the channel. Possible sites of action for pharmacological agents are shown (flashes). It is apparent that MSC need not be the site of action of agents. [Modified, with permission, from Christensen AP, Corey DP (2007) TRP channels in mechanosensation: direct or indirect activation? *Nat Rev Neurosci* **8**:510–521.] (See color plate section.)

The membrane model
gating via tension in the bilayer

Tether model
gating via tension in the cytoskeleton

and/or
extracellular matrix/
accessory protein

gating via a remote
signalling compound

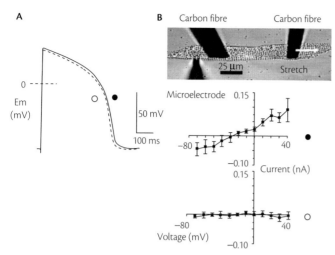

Fig. 65.2 Streptomycin blocks MSC$_{NS}$. **A** 50 μM streptomycin sulphate (dashed line) has no effect on the profile of the action potential in unstretched, single guinea pig ventricular myocytes. Em, membrane potential. **B** Axial stretch of these myocytes by 5–6% via attached carbon fibres (upper panel) induces a whole cell current consistent with the activation of non-selective cationic MSC (middle panel, solid circles); this current was not activated in the presence of 40 μM streptomycin (lower panel, open circles), suggesting that, in this preparation, streptomycin can be used to specifically block MSC$_{NS}$. [Reproduced, with permission, from Belus A, White E (2003) Streptomycin and intracellular calcium modulate the response of single guinea-pig ventricular myocytes to axial stretch. *J Physiol* **546**:501–509.]

that it is not affecting the ion channels that underlie the action potential.

Streptomycin has a +2 charge and is reported to act on MSC via partial occlusion of the channel pore[32]. It is able to inhibit stretch-activated arrhythmias in whole hearts at higher concentrations than those used in single myocytes [e.g.[33]] but is not effective in all preparations[34]. However, because of its ototoxicity and the undesirable aspects of chronic exposure to antibiotics, streptomycin is not a viable therapeutic agent.

GsMTx-4

Animal venoms are a useful source of agents to target ion channels. The Chilean tarantula (whose Latin name undergoes regular modification: *Grammostola spatulata / Phixotrichus spatulata / Grammostola rosea*) has venom that contains such agents. The raw venom has a potent blocking effect upon L-type Ca^{2+} channels. However, the group of Fred Sachs has isolated a peptide from the venom (GsMTx-4) that selectively blocks MSC$_{NS}$ channels [see[35] for a fuller version of the GsMTx-4 story]. At a concentration of 0.4 μM it has no effect on the action potential of rabbit ventricular myocytes[36] but at 0.17 μM was able to suppress the volume over-load-dependency of pacing-induced atrial fibrillation in the study by Bode *et al.*[1] (Fig. 65.3).

The cloned 34 residue peptide has an inhibitory cysteine knot motif (a common feature in animal venoms). It has a +5 charge and a hydrophobic domain. From its effects on the kinetics of MSC channels (both the D and L forms are effective at blocking MSC) it seems to bind not to the channel itself but to the membrane close to the channel, thus affecting its deformation by

mechanical stimuli[37,38]. Thus the peptide acts as an amphipath – an agent that, depending on its charge, inserts into the inner (if negatively charged) or outer (if positively charged) leaflet of the membrane, causing membrane deformation (convex or concave, respectively). Exactly why GsMTx-4 peptide is so specific, when the proposed mechanism of action is not, is not fully understood, but of all the agents used to investigate MSC it is the most promising in terms of a therapeutic agent. Indeed, there are many interesting questions to be answered, for example, what are the *in vivo* effects of GsMTx-4 in an animal arrhythmia model and is GsMTx-4 more effective upon arrhythmias associated with specific regions of the heart (see below)?

MSC$_{NS}$ and TRPC

Earlier in this chapter it was suggested that TRPC may be responsible for MSC$_{NS}$ currents. If this were the case one might expect there to be some evidence that the 'classic' MSC blockers are effective upon TRPC. Gd^{3+} has been used in TRPC studies, but the effects are variable[39,40]. Both streptomycin and raw tarantula venom have been reported to be ineffective upon TRPC1-mediated processes in smooth muscle[41]. However, TRPC6 antibodies have been shown to block MSC$_{NS}$ currents in mouse myocytes[12] and GsMTx-4 has been reported to block TRPC6 channels expressed in human embryonic kidney cell-line 293 (HEK293) cells[42]. Agents often used to block TRPC, e.g. 2-aminoethanoxydiphenyl borate (2-APB) and 1-[2-(4-methoxyphenyl)-2-[3-(4-methoxyphenyl)propoxy] ethyl-1H-imidazole hydrochloride (SKF96363) are thought to act via interaction with the channel, but are not specific to TRPC[39]. It has recently been suggested that a pyrazole compound, ethyl-1-(4-(2,3,3-trichloroacrylamide)phenyl)-5-trifluoro-methyl)-1H-pyrazole-4-carboxylate (Pyr3), may be selective for TRPC3 channels[43].

MSC and chronic mechanical overstimulation

Chronic mechanical stimulation is known to cause both structural and electrical remodelling. There is some evidence for the involvement of MSC in these events[24] but much less than the body of evidence linking MSC to the triggering of arrhythmias. It may be that the difficulty of experimentally extricating the role of MSC in complex signalling pathways has led to an underappreciation of their role, particularly if there are mechanically induced signalling compounds (see Fig. 65.1D) with multiple targets. Because studies have shown that MSC can inactivate in the presence of continual stimulation, MSC may be important in the initiation of remodelling, via modulation of intracellular Ca^{2+} and Na$^+$. However, a role for maintained activation of MSC in the presence of chronically increased mechanical stimuli is not impossible. Indeed persistent cation and anion currents, which are normally activated by cell swelling, have been reported in diseased hearts[44,45].

Much stronger evidence exists for major roles played by hypertrophic signalling pathways such as those associated with angiotensin II (AT-II)[24] and the downregulation of gene expression of K$^+$ channels responsible for currents such as the transient outward current (I$_{to}$). Thus the commonly observed prolongation of the action potential in diseased tissue is not thought to arise from the action of MSC.

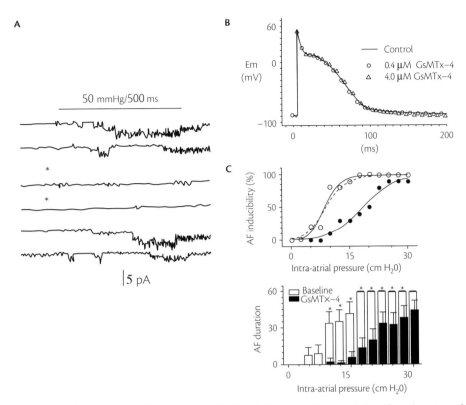

Fig. 65.3 Tarantula peptide GsMTx-4 blocks MSC$_{NS}$ and atrial arrhythmias. **A** GsMTx-4 (a 35 amino acid peptide isolated from the venom of the Chilean tarantula, *Grammostola spatulata/Phixotrichus spatulata/Grammostola rosea* or a cloned 34 amino acid peptide) blocks non-selective cationic MSC in rat astrocytes. Traces show pressure-induced MSC openings in the absence (two upper sweeps) and following wash (two lower sweeps) but not in the presence of ~2 μM GsMTx-4 (*, two middle sweeps). **B** GsMTx-4 has no effect upon the action potential of single rabbit ventricular myocytes at a concentration of 4 μM. **C** 170 nM GsMTx-4 reduces the probability of stretch-induced atrial fibrillation in rabbit hearts (upper panel, solid circles) and the duration of any induced fibrillation (lower panel, filled columns). [Part **A** reproduced, with permission, from Suchyna TM, Johnson JH, Hamer K, *et al.* (2000) Identification of a peptide toxin from *Grammostola spatulata* spider venom that blocks cation-selective stretch-activated channels. *J Gen Physiol* **115**:583–598. Part **B** reproduced, with permission from Elsevier, from Sachs F (2005) Stretch-activated channels in the heart. In: *Cardiac mechano-electric feedback and arrhythmias, from pipette to patient* (eds P Kohl, F Sachs, MR Franz). Elsevier Saunders, Philadelphia, pp. 2–10. Part **C** reproduced, with permission, from Bode F, Sachs F, Franz MR (2001) Tarantula peptide inhibits atrial fibrillation. *Nature* **409**:35–36.]

Although the above discussion suggests a minor role for MSC in dysfunctional modelling, several recent studies have implicated various TRPC in hypertrophic signalling [see[46] and especially[40]]. Hypertensive AT-II-induced hypertrophy and associated signalling pathways were largely suppressed in TRPC1 knockout mice or by angiotensin type 1 (AT-I) receptor blockade. Additionally electrophysiological data from adult mouse myocytes showed non-specific cation currents induced by pressure overload and attributed to TRPC1, and these currents were blocked by Gd^{3+} and suppressed in TRPC1 knockout mice. The authors suggest that mechanical stimulation of AT-I receptors[47] trigger signalling pathways that activate TRPC1 channels (i.e. via the mechanism described in Fig. 65.1D). This study provides evidence for the identity of the channels responsible for MSC$_{NS}$ (and by implication the generation of acute arrhythmias) and a role for MSC in the recognized signalling pathways responsible for structural remodelling induced by chronic mechanical overstimulation.

Conclusions and outlook

Mechanical stimuli are thought to affect the electrical activity of the heart via activation of MSC. Potential therapeutic goals are the suppression of mechanically induced arrhythmias and the prevention of structural and electrical remodelling. However, we have quite limited knowledge about the identity of human cardiac MSC and the details of the sensing and transduction of mechanical stimuli. In addition, the heart is highly heterogeneous[48] and it is likely that MSC blockade will be more effective in correcting some conditions than others. At present the literature does not allow a good comparison of the efficacy of agents upon mechanically induced events between the atria, pacemaker/conducting system and ventricles, for example.

Treatments currently in use that seek to improve the condition of diseased hearts by attenuating wall stress or volume overload and by inducing reverse remodelling (antihypertensives; diuretics; adrenergic blockers; vasodilators; left ventricular assist devices) may already be indirectly affecting the gating of MSC via the mechanisms described in Fig. 65.1. Mechanical stimulation triggers multiple signalling pathways and, in the context of the unknowns mentioned above, the specific targeting of particular MSC may not be an effective strategy. However, in this respect, the data described in Fig. 65.3B and the recent data presented by Seth *et al.*[40] are important. The former describes the ability of an agent (GsMTx-4) to decrease the level of mechanically modulated atrial fibrillation (atrial fibrillation is a common arrhythmia) at concentrations that do not affect the electrical activity of unstretched myocytes. This treatment is thought to affect MSC_{NS}. The latter study provides electrophysiological evidence that AT-II-induced hypertrophy is linked to the activity of TRPC1 channels. These investigations suggest that direct targeting of MSC could prove clinically rewarding.

References

1. Bode F, Sachs F, Franz MR. Tarantula peptide inhibits atrial fibrillation. *Nature* 2001;**409**:35–36.

2. Evans SJ, Levi AJ, Jones JV. Wall stress induced arrhythmia is enhanced by low potassium and early left ventricular hypertrophy in the working rat heart. *Cardiovasc Res* 1995;**29**:555–562.

3. Hamill OP, Martinac B. Molecular basis of mechanotransduction in living cells. *Physiol Rev* 2001;**81**:685–740.

4. Calaghan SC, White E. The role of calcium in the response of cardiac muscle to stretch. *Prog Biophys Mol Biol* 1999;**71**:59–90.

5. Hamill OP, McBride DW, Jr. The pharmacology of mechanogated membrane ion channels. *Pharmacol Rev* 1996;**48**:231–252.

6. White E. Mechanosensitive channels: therapeutic targets in the myocardium? *Curr Pharm Des* 2006;**12**:3645–3663.

7. Perozo E, Cortes DM, Sompornpisut P, Kloda A, Martinac B. Open channel structure of MscL and the gating mechanism of mechanosensitive channels. *Nature* 2002;**418**:942–948.

8. Bass RB, Strop P, Barclay M, Rees DC. Crystal structure of *Escherichia coli* MscS, a voltage-modulated and mechanosensitive channel. *Science* 2002;**298**:1582–1587.

9. Betanzos M, Chiang CS, Guy HR, Sukharev S. A large iris-like expansion of a mechanosensitive channel protein induced by membrane tension. *Nat Struct Biol* 2002;**9**:704–710.

10. Christensen AP, Corey DP. TRP channels in mechanosensation: direct or indirect activation? *Nat Rev Neurosci* 2007;**8**:510–521.

11. Maroto R, Raso A, Wood TG, Kurosky A, Martinac B, Hamill OP. TRPC1 forms the stretch-activated cation channel in vertebrate cells. *Nat Cell Biol* 2005;**7**:179–185.

12. Dyachenko V, Husse B, Rueckschloss U, Isenberg G. Mechanical deformation of ventricular myocytes modulates both TRPC6 and Kir2.3 channels. *Cell Calcium* 2009;**45**:38–54.

13. Ward ML, Williams IA, Chu Y, Cooper PJ, Ju YK, Allen DG. Stretch-activated channels in the heart: contributions to length-dependence and to cardiomyopathy. *Prog Biophys Mol Biol* 2008;**97**:232–249.

14. Vassort G, Alvarez J. Transient receptor potential: a large family of new channels of which several are involved in cardiac arrhythmia. *Can J Physiol Pharmacol* 2009;**87**:100–107.

15. Gottlieb P, Folgering J, Maroto R, *et al.* Revisiting TRPC1 and TRPC6 mechanosensitivity. *Pflugers Arch* 2007; **455**:1097–1103.

16. Patel AJ, Honore E. (2005) Potassium-selective cardiac mechanosensitive ion channels. In: *Cardiac mechano-electric feedback: and arrhythmias, from pipette to patient* (eds P Kohl, F Sachs, MR Franz). Elsevier Saunders; Philadelphia, p. 11–20.

17. Tan JH, Liu W, Saint DA. Differential expression of the mechanosensitive potassium channel TREK-1 in epicardial and endocardial myocytes in rat ventricle. *Exp Physiol* 2004;**89**:237–242.

18. Link MS, Wang PJ, Vanderbrink BA, Avelar E, Pandian NG, Maron BJ, *et al.* Selective activation of the K^+_{ATP} channel is a mechanism by which sudden death is produced by low-energy chest-wall impact (*Commotio cordis*). *Circulation* 1999 27;**100**:413–418.

19. Kamkin A, Kiseleva I, Isenberg G. Ion selectivity of stretch-activated cation currents in mouse ventricular myocytes. *Pflugers Arch* 2003;**446**:220–231.

20. Kim D. A mechanosensitive K^+ channel in heart cells. Activation by arachidonic acid. *J Gen Physiol* 1992;**100**:1021–1040.

21. Browe DM, Baumgarten CM. Stretch of beta 1 integrin activates an outwardly rectifying chloride current via FAK and Src in rabbit ventricular myocytes. *J Gen Physiol* 2003;**122**:689–702.

22. Browe DM, Baumgarten CM. Angiotensin II (AT1) receptors and NADPH oxidase regulate Cl- current elicited by beta1 integrin stretch in rabbit ventricular myocytes. *J Gen Physiol* 2004;**124**:273–287.

23. Dyachenko V, Rueckschloss U, Isenberg G. Modulation of cardiac mechanosensitive ion channels involves superoxide, nitric oxide and peroxynitrite. *Cell Calcium* 2009;**45**:55–64.

24. Sadoshima J, Izumo S. The cellular and molecular response of cardiac myocytes to mechanical stress. *Annu Rev Physiol* 1997;**59**:551–571.

25. Franco A, Jr., Winegar BD, Lansman JB. Open channel block by gadolinium ion of the stretch-inactivated ion channel in mdx myotubes. *Biophys J* 1991;**59**:1164–1170.

26. Yang XC, Sachs F. Block of stretch-activated ion channels in *Xenopus* oocytes by gadolinium and calcium ions. *Science* 1989;**243**:1068–1071.

27. Bode F, Katchman A, Woosley RL, Franz MR. Gadolinium decreases stretch-induced vulnerability to atrial fibrillation. *Circulation* 2000;**101**:2200–2205.

28. Caldwell RA, Clemo HF, Baumgarten CM. Using gadolinium to identify stretch-activated channels: technical considerations. *Am J Physiol* 1998;**275**:C619–C621.

29. Hansen DE, Borganelli M, Stacy GP, Jr., Taylor LK. Dose-dependent inhibition of stretch-induced arrhythmias by gadolinium in isolated canine ventricles. Evidence for a unique mode of antiarrhythmic action. *Circ Res* 1991;**69**:820–831.

30. Lamberts RR, Van Rijen MH, Sipkema P, Fransen P, Sys SU, Westerhof N. Increased coronary perfusion augments cardiac contractility in the rat through stretch-activated ion channels. *Am J Physiol* 2002;**282**: H1334–H1340.

31. Belus A, White E. Effects of streptomycin sulphate on I_{CaL}, I_{Kr} and I_{Ks} in guinea-pig ventricular myocytes. *Eur J Pharmacol* 2002;**445**: 171–178.

32. Winegar BD, Haws CM, Lansman JB. Subconductance block of single mechanosensitive ion channels in skeletal muscle fibers by aminoglycoside antibiotics. *J Gen Physiol* 1996;**107**:433–443.

33. Salmon AH, Mays JL, Dalton GR, Jones JV, Levi AJ. Effect of streptomycin on wall-stress-induced arrhythmias in the working rat heart. *Cardiovasc Res* 1997;**34**:493–503.

34. Cooper PJ, Kohl P. Species- and preparation-dependence of stretch effects on sino-atrial node pacemaking. *Ann N Y Acad Sci* 2005; **1047**:324–335.

35. Bowman CL, Gottlieb PA, Suchyna TM, Murphy YK, Sachs F. Mechanosensitive ion channels and the peptide inhibitor GsMTx-4: history, properties, mechanisms and pharmacology. *Toxicon* 2007;**49**:249–270.

36. Sachs F (2005) Stretch-activated channels in the heart. In: *Cardiac mechano-electric feedback and arrhythmias: from pipette to patient* (eds P Kohl, F Sachs, MR Franz). Elsevier Saunders, Philadelphia, pp. 2–10.

37. Ostrow KL, Mammoser A, Suchyna T, *et al.* cDNA sequence and in vitro folding of GsMTx4, a specific peptide inhibitor of mechanosensitive channels. *Toxicon* 2003;**42**:263–274.

38. Suchyna TM, Tape SE, Koeppe RE, Andersen OS, Sachs F, Gottlieb PA. Bilayer-dependent inhibition of mechanosensitive channels by neuroactive peptide enantiomers. *Nature* 2004;**430**:235–240.

39. Birnbaumer L. The TRPC class of ion channels: a critical review of their roles in slow, sustained increases in intracellular Ca^{2+} concentrations. *Annu Rev Pharmacol Toxicol* 2009;**49**:395–426.

40. Seth M, Zhang ZS, Mao L, *et al.* TRPC1 Channels are critical for hypertrophic signaling in the heart. *Circ Res* 2009;**105**:1023–1030.

41. Beech DJ, Muraki K, Flemming R. Non-selective cationic channels of smooth muscle and the mammalian homologues of Drosophila TRP. *J Physiol* 2004;**559**:685–706.

42. Spassova MA, Hewavitharana T, Xu W, Soboloff J, Gill DL. A common mechanism underlies stretch activation and receptor activation of TRPC6 channels. *Proc Natl Acad Sci USA* 2006;**103**:16586–16591.

43. Kiyonaka S, Kato K, Nishida M, *et al*. Selective and direct inhibition of TRPC3 channels underlies biological activities of a pyrazole compound. *Proc Natl Acad Sci USA* 2009;**106**:5400–5405.

44. Clemo HF, Stambler BS, Baumgarten CM. Persistent activation of a swelling-activated cation current in ventricular myocytes from dogs with tachycardia-induced congestive heart failure. *Circ Res* 1998;**83**:147–157.

45. Clemo HF, Stambler BS, Baumgarten CM. Swelling-activated chloride current is persistently activated in ventricular myocytes from dogs with tachycardia-induced congestive heart failure. *Circ Res* 1999;**84**:157–165.

46. Abramowitz J, Birnbaumer L. Physiology and pathophysiology of canonical transient receptor potential channels. *FASEB J* 2009;**23**:297–328.

47. Zou Y, Akazawa H, Qin Y, *et al*. Mechanical stress activates angiotensin II type 1 receptor without the involvement of angiotensin II. *Nat Cell Biol* 2004;**6**:499–506.

48. Stones R, Gilbert SH, Benoist D, White E. Inhomogeneity in the response to mechanical stimulation: Cardiac muscle function and gene expression. *Prog Biophys Mol Biol* 2008;**97**:268–281.

Index

A-kinase anchoring proteins 21, 22, 23, 337
ACE 178, 207–209, 298
    atrial fibrilliation 208, 302
    heart failure 209, 372
    inhibitors 208, 299, 307, 342, 398, 403, 404
        clinical trials 398-9
        for reducing sudden death 403
        remodelling 298
acetylcholine receptor, nicotinic 12
∝-actinin 70, 81, 89
action potential 4, 15, 43, 442
    monophasic 103, 105, 188, 218, 223, 269–70
        heart failure 341
        stretch-related electrophysiologic effects
            174–5
        U-wave 275
    pulmonary vein cells 110–1
    sino-atrial node (SAN) 95–6
    stretch-related effects 76–8
    VAD effects 423–4
action potential duration 28, 31, 104, 127, 168, 188–9,
    258–61, 269, 369, 423
    acute mechanical stimulation 291
    atrial stretch 291
    duplex formation 156–7
    haemodynamic unloading 369
    interaction with cycle length 270–1
        regional heterogeneity 270
        volume/pressure overload 315
    myocyte heterogeneity 220
    sacrolemmal ionic influx 76
    U-wave 275
    Valsalva manoeuvre 371–2
    volume loading 106, 269–70
    in whole heart 183–4
activation sequence 153–9
acute stretch 82, 104, 106, 369, 376
adherens
    cell-to-cell 132–4
    junctions 132–4, 229, 409
    see also gap junctions
adhesion kinase, focal see FAK
advanced life support (ALS) 364, 365
after-depolarization 105
    delayed 16, 105, 111, 117, 162, 253, 254, 255
        volume/pressure overload 315–6
    early 104, 111, 341

altered loading 272
    stretch pulse 105, 223
        triggered 177
afterload 103–5, 107, 155, 164, 181, 217, 246, 270,
    342, 372, 423, 457
age
    AF 168, 203, 397
    atrial remodelling 295
    commotio cordis 325
agkistrodon halys toxin (AgTx) 46
AKAP see A-kinase anchoring proteins
Akt 53, 84, 85
alamethicin 12
aldosterone antagonist 299, 342, 403
alternans 125–31
    electrophysiological 177
    heterogeneous 176–7
    stretch effects 173–9
    whole heart in vivo studies 173–4
4-aminopyridine 20, 23, 188
amiodarone 300, 301, 341
    derivatives 301
amphiphilic compound 15
amphipaths 11–2, 59, 77
    anionic 21, 22, 62
    arachidonic acid 62
    crenation 28
    cupping 28
    membrane modifiers 62–3
    MSC 463
    GsMTx-4 100
    TREK-1 21–2
ANDROMEDA study 301
angiogenesis 88
    fibroblasts 140
    mechanical forces 431
angiotensin converting enzyme see ACE
angiotensin II 31, 52, 77, 82, 134, 189, 207–8, 227–8,
    296, 300, 307, 310, 342, 399
    blocker 398
    inhibition 403
        stretch-activation 77–8
        Na⁺/H⁺ exchanger activation 77
    receptor 29, 82, 207–8
    receptor blocker 299, 310
    tissue chymase 208
angiotensin receptor antagonist 299, 398

animal models
    arrhythmias 227–33
    asynchronous activation 388
    atrial fibrillation 205–6
    canine heart 450–5
    commotio cordis 326, 327
    defibrillation efficacy 374
    Langendorff rabbit heart 168–9, 171,
        223–4, 286
    rat cell culture 144
anisotropy 71, 143, 146–8, 164, 181, 203, 208, 209,
    247, 252–3, 294, 296, 299, 376, 443
ankyrin-1 70
Anrep effect 74, 75, 81, 84
antiarrhythmics 300–1, 341–2
antifibrotics 300
antihypertensive therapy
    and atrial size 397
    sudden death prevention 228
anti-VEGF antibody 135
aortic occlusion 105
    and AP configuration 175
    MEC 175, 270
aortic stenosis 219, 228, 345
aortic stiffness 397–8
AP see action potential
apoptosis 193, 195, 402
    ICl_swell 28
    MEC 145
    mitochondria 37
arachidonic acid 15
    K_AA 20
    TREK-1 7, 19, 22
    TWIK 19, 28
arginine-glycine-aspartate peptides 81,
    135, 146
arrhythmias
    altered kinase function 228
    aortic occlusion 342
    atrial 110–16, 204–5
        see also atrial fibrillation; atrial flutter
    and Ca²⁺ leaks 228–9
    cardiopulmonary bypass 272
    commotio cordis 223–5, 259, 325
    haemodynamic unloading for 369–73
    hypertrophic cardiomyopathy 229
    intra-aortic balloon pump 372

arrhythmias (*Cont'd*)
  ischaemia 352–8
    in vivo and isolated hearts 352–3
    simulation studies 354–6
    substrate 353–4
    trigger 354
  mechanical stimulation for 160–5, 361–8
  murine models 227–33
  in non-uniform muscle 122
  stretch-induced 352–8
  postconditioning effect 195–6
  preconditioning effect 194
  sudden death 227–8, 352
  supraventricular tachycardia 290
  trigger events *see* arrhythmogenesis
  ventricular 105, 125
    tachy-arrhythmias *see* ventricular fibrillation;
      ventricular tachycardia
  VGC mutants 44–6
arrythmogenesis 110–4, 160, 195, 313–17
  alternans-mediated 125
  drugs 100–1, 462–6
  electrophysiological changes 314–16
  plakoglobin mutations 407–9
  right ventricular cardiomyopathy 228, 229, 407–11
  wall stress 184
assist device, *see* ventricular assist devices
asynchronous activation 387–8
  treatment *see* cardiac resynchronization therapy
asynchronous (VVI) pacing 290, 291, 396
asystole 362–3
atenolol 299, 397, 398
ATP-sensitive K⁺ channel 31, 88, 173, 194, 225, 261,
  277, 328, 462
atrial brady-cardiomyopathy 229–30
atrial dilation 46, 292, 318, 395
  in atrial fibrillation 111, 212–4
atrial effective refractory period 298
atrial fibrillation 110, 111, 168–72, 187, 302, 395–9
  aortic stiffness 397–8
  and atrial pressure overload 212–3, 396–7
  and body mass index 396, 397
  and dilatation 111, 204–5
    animal models 205–6
    cellular mechanisms 206–8
    promotion of 208–9
  drug effects 298–304
    antifibrotics 300
  feedback loops 203
  mechanisms underlying 302
  MEC 395–401
    clinical studies 398–9
  paroxysmal 110
  profibrillatory changes 395–6
  and pulmonary vein ectopy 212–15
  stretch effects 168–72
    conduction 169
    refractory period 171
  stretch-related 111, 168, 318–21
    vago-sympathetic input 320–1
  treatment 299–302
  ventricular contraction 236–7
atrial flutter 236–9
atrial natriuretic peptide 23, 27, 206, 228, 285
  heart failure 227–8
  stretch 23
  TREK-1 21

atrial remodelling 293–5, 298
  age effects 295
  electrical 298
  structural 206–8, 298–9
atrial repolarization-delaying agents 301–2
atrial septal defects 290, 293–5
atrio-ventricular (AV)
  block 103–4
  dyssynchrony 412
  node 96
  valves 238
atriopeptin *see* atrial natriuretic peptide
atropine 97, 361, 372
autonomic signalling in heart failure 336–7
axial stretch 98–9, 175–6, 436, 464

Bainbridge reflex 95
BAPTA-AM 29
β-blocker 178, 341, 403–4
  remodelling 403
  sudden death 403–4
bilayer-couple hypothesis 22–3
biological duplex 154
biventricular stimulation 404–5
bradykinin 194, 195, 208
Brugada syndrome 220, 328
bundle branch block
  left 189, 326, 387, 404, 451
  right 275
bypass, cardiopulmonary 371

Ca^{2+}
  binding by troponin C 118–19
  buffering 251
  channel 203
  in chronic stretch 376
  cycling 127–8
  duplex 118
  leaks 37, 228–9
  and left ventricular assist device 384–5
  length-dependent sensitivity in changes of 74–5
  overload 40
  preconditioning 194
  respiratory sinus arrhythmia 236
  sarcoplasmic reticulum release 36–9, 43, 52, 76,
    77, 96, 118, 126, 156, 190, 208, 228, 313, 334–5,
    384, 436
  in sinoatrial node 96
  sparks 16, 36–8, 436
  stretch response 74–80
  transient 75, 77, 127–8, 347–8, 435–6
  transmembrane potential coupling 125–7
  wave 40
    dynamic muscle stretch 122
    force maintenance 118–22
    force development/relaxation 122
    in non-uniform cardiac muscle 121–2
    stretch effects 122
Ca^{2+} blocker 341
CABG 195, 342
cadherin 11 140
E-cadherin 133
N-cadherin 132, 133, 135, 140, 146, 409
Caenorhabditis elegans 7, 19
calcineurin 228
  $ICl_{,swell}$ 29
calcium *see* Ca^{2+}

calmodulin 228
  defective binding 229
  -dependent kinase II *see* CaMK
  -dependent kinase IV *see* CaMK
calpains 59, 71
calsequestrin 229, 231
CaMK 228, 230
cAMP response element binding protein *see* CREB
cAMP responsive element modulator *see* CREM
candesartan 207, 399
canine heart model 450–5
captopril 397
cardiac assist devices *see* ventricular assist devices
cardiac catheterization 361, 451
cardiac hypertrophy *see* hypertrophic cardiomyopathy
cardiac mechano-sensitivity *see* mechano-sensitivity
cardiac memory 305, 306, 307, 308, 387, 388
cardiac myocyte *see* cardiomyocytes
cardiac resynchronization therapy 286, 342
  anti- and pro-arrhythmic effects 387–91
  clinical studies 387–8
  computer simulations 388–90
  efficacy and safety 412–3
  electrical remodelling 330–1
  implantable cardioverter-defibrillator 340,
    374, 387
  MEC 412–19
  PROSPECT study 416–17
cardiac support device *see* ventricular assist devices
cardiocutaneous syndrome 407–8
cardiomyocytes 66–73, 87–91
  adult cardiomyocytes 147
  AP duration 330
  assist device affecting 382
  contractile machinery 35
  coupling of, with fibroblasts 252, 258
  cytoskeleton 35
    filaments 66–7
    remodelling 88–9
  gap junctions 132–3
  integrin-mediated stretch signalling 81–2
  MEC 87–8
    diastolic/systolic effects 103–9
  membrane 35, 59–60
  mitochondria 37–8
  myofibrillogenesis 89–90
  pulmonary vein 111–2
  SAC in 35–41
  stretch-activated currents 111–2
  titin *see* titin
  VAC 27–34
  VGC 42–9
cardiomyopathy 133–4
  arrhythmogenic right ventricular 228,
    229, 407–11
  atrial brady-cardiomyopathy 229–30
  dilated 59, 67, 330, 404, 417
    in Duchenne muscular dystrophy 438–9
  hypertrophic *see* hypertrophic cardiomyopathy
  ischaemic 88, 382, 417
  left ventricular 204
    assist device 422
  right ventricular 133–4, 228, 229, 407–11
  ventricular fibrillation 340
cardiopulmonary bypass 371
CARE-HF study 387–8, 413–4
Carvajal syndrome 134, 407

catheter-tip-induced cardioversion 361
cation, polyvalent 62–3
caveolae 50–6, 59, 439
    morphology 50–1
    proteins in 52–3
    response to mechanical stimuli 53–4
    in stretch-sensing 50–6
    structure 50
    TEM 53–4
caveolin 51, 52, 54, 59, 439
cell culture 143–50
    future models 147–8
    MEC 145–7
    microenvironment 144–5
    vs. intact tissue 143–4
    vs. single cells 144
cell junctions
    adherens 132-4, 144, 229
    fascia adherens 132, 133
    gap junctions see gap junctions
cell swelling 27
cell volume-sensitive ion channels 27–34
    transducing cell volume 27
    volume activated, $I_{Cl,swell}$ 27–9
cell-cell adhesion 132–7
cell-cell coupling 133
    arrhythmogenesis 316
cell-matrix interactions 132, 144
chamber dilation 219
CHARM study 399
Chilean tarantula 100, 464–5
chloride channels 27–9
chlorpromazine 15
chronic asynchronous ventricular (VVI) pacing 291
chronic overload 206, 342
    remodelling in 403, 404
chronic pressur e overload 458
ciliates, mechano-transduction in 4
colchicine 66, 87, 220, 463
collagen 69, 88, 138, 140, 242
commotio cordis 160, 162, 163, 164, 165, 223–6,
    325–9, 352, 362, 378, 462
    animal models
        Langendorff rabbit heart 223–4, 327
        porcine 326
    arrhythmias 223–5, 259, 325
    cellular mechanisms 224–5
    epidemiology 325
    model systems 259–61
    pathological mechanisms 326–8
    prevention 326
    resuscitation 325
    right ventricular 218–9
    ventricular fibrillation 223
COMPANION study 187, 387, 413
computer simulations 388–90
conduction velocity 97, 108, 180–3
    gap junctions 134–5
    stretch effects 180–3
        in atrial tissue 169
        measurement during myocardial stretch 181
        regional wall stress/strain 181
        speed and path of conduction 180–1
    volume/pressure overload 316
congenital heart disease 111, 293–5
congestive heart failure 206–8, 235–6, 290, 293, 299,
    313, 321, 341, 372, 398

connexins 310
    and fibroblasts 140–1
    gap junctions 336
    stretch and expression of 134–5
connexin 40 134, 140
connexin 43 133, 140, 228, 230, 310, 408
connexin 45 96–7, 140
CONTAK-CD study 413
contractile function
    postconditioning effect 196
    preconditioning effect 193–4
contraction
    eccentric 437, 438
    entrant phase 153
    isovolumic 389
    left ventricular 153–4, 330, 404
contusio cordis 325, 327
cooperativity 74, 122
CorCap device 421
coronary artery bypass grafting see CABG
cortical cytoskeleton 59, 60
costameres 35, 59, 81
coughing, and cardioversion 361
CREATIVE-AF study 399
CREB 308, 310
CREM 230
crista terminalis 96, 97, 100, 252, 291, 293, 294, 295
cross-bridge 119–21
curvature
    epicardial 181
    membrane 15, 21, 27, 50, 62, 77
    wave front 181
cytochalasin-D 347, 463
cytoskeleton 11, 21, 35, 87
    filaments 66–7
    role of 87, 88
    see also membrane/cytoskeleton interface

daidzein 30
DAVID study 187
DCM see dilated cardiomyopathy
DDD pacing 291, 396
defibrillation
    efficacy 374–80
    extrinsic 375–6
    indirect 377
    intrinsic 376–7
    mechanisms 275–7
    preload changes 377
    upper limit of vulnerability 263–4, 375
    threshold
        heart failure 377–8
        left ventricular dilatation 374
        and mechanical deformation 262–4, 374
        ventricular fibrillation 378
delayed after-depolarization 16, 105, 111, 117, 162
    stretch-induced 253–5
    volume/pressure overload 315–16
density, channel 13
desmin 66, 89, 133
desmocollin 407
desmoglein 132, 407
desmoplakin 132, 135, 146, 229
desmosomes 132, 229, 407
    desmosomal diseases 133–4
diacylglycerol 22, 51, 78

diastolic
    Ca^{2+} levels 78
    compliance 282, 283
    sarcomere 36
    stimulation 161–2
    timing 104–5
diastolic depolarization 96, 213, 214, 346
    spontaneous 99
diastolic heart failure 70, 241
diastolic potential, maximum 95
dilated cardiomyopathy 67, 330, 417
    in Duchenne muscular dystrophy 438–9
    with left ventricular assist device 382
diltiazem 15, 397
dimethylamiloride (DMA) 32
discodin domain receptor (DDR) 2 140
displacement encoding 431, 450
dofetilide 300, 301, 341
dronedarone 301
Duchenne muscular dystrophy 438–9
duplex 154–9
dyssynchrony 412
    echocardiographic assessment 413–16
    in heart failure 330–1
    interventricular 412
    mechanical 412, 413
    pacing-induced 196
    see also cardiac resynchronization therapy
dystrophin 59, 61, 67, 438–9

early after-depolarization 104, 111, 296, 298, 301,
    315, 341, 382–4
ECG 451
    cardiac alternans 125, 126
    commotio cordis 223, 325, 326
    mechanical dyssynchrony 413–16
    prolonged AP duration 269
    QRS complex 306–7
        prolongation 404
    QT interval see QT interval
    surface 103
    T-wave 305
    U-wave 274–80
    ventricular electrical remodelling 188
ECM see extracellular matrix
effective refractory periood see refractory period
ejection fraction 219, 241
    left ventricular 244, 330
electric shocks, vulnerability to 262–4
electrical alternans see cardiac alternans
electrical remodelling 187–91, 305
    atrial 298, 299
    in atrial fibrillation 110
    ventricular 187–91, 305–12
electrocardiogram see ECG
electromechanical coupling see mechano-electric
    coupling
electrophysiological heterogeneity 177
end-diastolic pressure-volume relationship 422, 423
end-systolic pressure-volume relationship 456, 457
endothelial nitric oxide synthase (eNOS)
    53, 54, 83
endothelin-1 (ET-1) 77
enzyme, proteolytic 13, 139
epidermal growth factor receptor 29, 82
epimysium 139, 242
epinephrine 349, 361

eplerenone 342, 403
   see also aldosterone receptor blockers
ERK 70, 81, 437
   chronic atrial dilation 206–8
ERM proteins 59
ERP *see* effective refractory period
Escherichia coli 3, 4
esmolol 348, 350
Eukarya 4
eukaryotes 4
EURIDIS study 301
EWI *see* electro-mechanical wave imaging
excitation-contraction coupling 81, 87, 389
extracellular matrix (ECM) 47, 138
   collagen in 242
   components 138
   relationship of fibroblasts to 139–40
extracellular signal regulated kinase *see* ERK

F-actin 66–7
   and I_{K-ATP} 31
FAK 81, 134, 135, 208
FAK-related non-kinase 29
fascia adherens junction 132, 133
fibre strain/stress 247–8, 249
   healthy tissue 445–8
   infarcted tissue 443-4, 446–8
   negative 443
   positive 443
fibrillatory interval 290
fibroblasts 138–42
   ERK in 207
   growth factor 140
   mechano-sensitivity 258
   origin and distribution 138–9
   relationship to ECM 139–40
   role in MEC 140–1
fibrocytes 138, 139
fibronectin 88
   and myofibroblasts 139
fibrosis 88, 203, 242, 299, 324,
   cytoskeleton architecture 89
   heart failure 403
   mitral valve 205
   VAD effects 424–5
finite element models 245, 249, 443
flecainide 300
FN *see* fibronectin
focal adhesion kinase *see* FAK
force-sarcomere length relationship *see* FSLR
force-sarcomere velocity relationship *see* FSVR
Förster resonance energy transfer *see* FRET
Frank-Starling mechanism 71, 81, 103, 160,
   217, 284
   relation 70
FRET 431–3
   development and characterization 431–2
   Förster distance 431
   molecular force sensors 431–3
   stFRET 431–3
FSLR 74, 117
   effects in uniform/non-uniform muscle 128, 129
   mechanism underlying 118–19
FSVR 117
   cross-bridge dynamics 119–21
   effects in uniform/non-uniform muscle 128, 129
fusion of vesicles 14

G-protein coupled receptors 52, 82
   see also G_q protein-coupled receptors
gadolinium 77, 83, 100, 273, 300, 371, 463
   induction of atrial fibrillation 169, 171
   inhibition of conduction velocity 182
   inhibition of SAC 111, 195, 352–3
GAG *see* glycosamnioglycan
gap junctions 97, 180–1
   desmosomal diseases 133–4
   in heart failure 336
   interaction with mechanical junctions 133
   modulators 300
   molecular structure 132–3
   remodelling 132–7
   stretch effects 182
Gd^{3+} *see* gadolinium
genistein 12, 30
   and $I_{Cl,swell}$ 29
   and I_{Ks} 30
GISSI-AF study 299, 342
glibenclamide 20, 163, 225
global mechanical stimulation 164–5
glycosaminoglycans 140
Goldman-Hodgkin-Katz equation 20, 252
Golgi apparatus 138
   connexions 134
G_q protein-coupled receptors 52–3
GPCR *see* G-protein coupled receptors
Grammostola spatulata mechano-toxin 4 *see* GsMTx-4
green fluorescence protein 431
   see also stFRET
GsMTx-4 13, 14, 15–16, 43, 63, 83, 100–1, 164, 214,
   300
   induction of atrial fibrillation 169, 171
   reduction of slow force response 436
   as SAC blockers 464
   as SAC_{NS} blockers 184
GTPases 59, 146

haemodynamic
   loading
      and arrhythmogenesis 342
      and electrophysiological changes
   unloading
      arrhythmia termination 369–73
   ventricular arrhythmias 340–4
HCN (hyperpolarization-activated cyclic nucleotide-gated) channel 43
heart failure 129–30, 160, 204, 227, 241, 313–4,
   340–2
   autonomic signalling 336–7
   Ca^{2+} handling and arrhythmic risk 334–5
   cardiac mechanics 244–5
   chronic 207
   clinical studies 398–9
   congestive 235, 293, 313
   defibrillation in 377–8
   device therapy 381–5
   diastolic 70, 241, 457
   dyssynchronous 330–1
   hypertrophy 403
   K^+ channel remodelling 331–4
   mechano-electric coupling in 402–6
   models of 241–50
      murine 227–33
   myocardium
      fibre strain 247–8, 249

mechanical modelling 246
   structure 241–3
natriuretic peptide in 227–8
phosphatases in 228
remodelling in 134, 336
repolarization changes 330–9
respiratory sinus arrhythmia 235
right ventricular 217
sudden death 227–9, 313, 325
systolic 340, 398
tissue remodelling 247
treatment
   biventricular stimulation 404–5
   cardiac resynchronization therapy *see* cardiac resynchronization therapy
   left ventricular electrical activation 404–5
   mechanical support *see* ventricular assist devices
   non-pharmacological 342
   pharmacological 341–2
ventricular arrhythmias 272, 340–4
   haemodynamic load 342, 402
   mechanisms 340–1
   treatment 341–2
see also cardiomyopathy
heart rate 234
   and alternans 127–8
   Bainbridge reflex 95
   variability 173, 235
heart-transplant patients, respiratory sinus
   arrhythmia 235
HeartMate devices 421, 422, 423
heterogeneity 107, 127, 154–5, 220
   Ca^{2+} handling 128
   mechano-electric 164, 165
   regional 153, 154, 156, 165
   sarcomere 117–23
heterogeneous alternans 127
heterogeneous membrane 59
Hill coefficient 21, 74, 75
His-Purkinje network 187, 188, 336
   delayed repolarization 274–5
homogeneous membrane 57–9
hybrid duplex 154, 156
hydrochlorothiazide *see* antihypertensive therapy
hydrostatic pressure 13, 27, 145
3-hydroxy-3-methylglutaryl coenzyme A reductase
   inhibitors *see* statins
hypertension 111
   and atrial pressure overload 396–7
   clinical studies 398
   and diabetes mellitus 398
   pulmonary artery 219
hypertrophic cardiomyopathy 227–9
   gap junction remodelling 134
hypertrophy 134–5, 143, 190, 227, 308, 345
   compensatory myocardial 134
   fibroblasts 140–1
   mechanical overload 132

I-band 68–9, 70, 71
I_{Ca-L} 31
   CREB 310
I_{Ca-T} 31
ICD *see* implantable cardioverter-defibrillator
$I_{Cir,swell}$ 29
$I_{Cl,swell}$ 27–9, 34, 52, 54
I_{K-ACh} 31, 298, 462

$I_{K\text{-}ATP}$ 31
I_{Kr} 31, 308
I_{Ks} 30–1
ILCOR 364–5, 368
imaging 450–5
   cardiac electrophysiology 451
   cardiac mechanics 450–1
   electro-mechanical wave imaging 451–3
   pulsed-wave Doppler echocardiography 413–14
   tissue Doppler
      colour-coded 415
      pulsed-wave 414
      tissue synchronization imaging (TSI) 414, 415
immediate force response 74–5
impact
   chest wall 325–8
   extracorporal, as mechanical stimulation 363
impedance monitoring
   intra-thoracic 458–9
      haemodynamics 459–60
   ventricular strain 456–61
implantable cardioverter-defibrillator 340, 374, 387, 402
   see also cardiac resynchronization therapy
infarct size
   postconditioning 195
   preconditioning 193
InSync ICD study 387
intact tissue models 143–4
integrin 35, 77, 81–2, 190, 208, 410, 438
   β1 integrin 28, 410, 436, 437
   integrin-linked kinase 81
   signalling 81–2, 135
intercalated disc 35, 407–9
International Liaison Committee on Resuscitation
   (ILCOR) 364
intra-aortic balloon pump 372
intra-thoracic impedance monitoring 458–9
   haemodynamics 459–60
intra-thoracic pressure 234–5,
   termination of tachy-arrhythmias 361
   venous return 371
ion channels
   acid sensing 47
   in caveolae 52
   ligand-gated 11, 31
   mechano-sensitive 431, 462
   stretch-activated see SAC
   voltage-gated see voltage-gated channels
   volume-activated see VAC
   volume-sensitive 27–32
IP3 207, 228
ischaemia 23, 117, 173–8, 193–6
   and arrhythmias 352–8, 422–3
   bulging, ischaemic 163, 197, 448
   K^+ accumulation 174
   regional 175–7
ischaemic bulging 163
ischaemic cardiomyopathy 88
ischaemic preconditioning see preconditioning
isovolumic contraction 389
isovolumic relaxation 276–7

JAK/STAT pathway 134, 206, 207

K^+
   hypokalaemia 178
   in ischaemia 174

   in pathological myocardium 173–9
K^+ channels
   ATP-sensitive 88, 163, 176
   in heart failure 331–4
   ion-gated 31
   selective stretch activated channel 20, 161
   2P-type see K2P channels
   voltage-gated 46
      I_{Kr} 31
      I_{Ks} 30–1
      TREK-1 see TREK-1
K2P channels 7, 19
   TREK-1 19–26
KCNK7 19
Kir2.1 31, 333, 336
Kir3.1 31
Kir3.4 31
Kluyveromyces lactis 5
Kv channels 46
KvLQT1 333

L-NAME 36, 83
L-type Ca^{2+} current 334, 385
Langendorff rabbit heart model 168–9, 171, 286
   commotio cordis 223–4
lanthanides 14–15
Laplace's law 13, 21, 51
lateralization 189, 336
lattice spacing 70, 75
left atrium 169
   pulmonary vein junction 110, 213
left bundle branch block 103, 107, 326, 330, 388
left ventricular assist devices see ventricular assist
   devices
left ventricle 117
   activation sequence 153–4
   anterior infarct 446–8
   cardiomyocytes in 442
   defibrillation 374–6
   dilatation 246–7
   ejection fraction 402
   filling pressure 284–5
   hypertrophy 227–8
   improved electrical activation 404–5
   in left bundle branch block 388
   monophasic action potential recordings
      from 106
   pressure 104
   structure 442–3
   volume 402–3
      end-diastolic 281, 282, 285–7, 402
      end-systolic 402
      measurement 457–8
legislation on mechanical stimulation 364–5
LIFE study 299, 398
ligand-gated channels 31
lipid bilayer 13, 35, 42–3, 51, 100, 437, 462
load dependence of ventricular repolarization
   269–73
   atrium 271
   cycles of 269
   human studies of 269–70
   laboratory models of 269
   in pathology 272
   proarrhythmic effect of altered loading 272
   regional heteeogeneity in 270
loading, ventricular stretch 107, 108

long QT syndrome 274, 341, 347–8
   acquired 383–4
   LQT1 46
   LQT3 44–5
   ventricular wall abnormalities 348–50
losartan 82, 135
L-type Ca^{2+} 203
L-type Ca^{2+} current 256, 298, 307, 331, 334
L-type calcium channel 214, 228, 300, 346
LVADs see ventricular assist devices
lysophosphatidic acid 22
lysophospholipid, TREK-1 modulation by 23

M-band 66
M-mode echocardiography 414
MADIT-CRT study 405, 412, 413
MADIT-II study 187
MAP kinase 134, 206
   hypertrophy 70, 134, 206
   SAC_K/K_{AA} channel 20
matrix, extracellular (ECM) 47, 138
   collagen in 242
   components 138
   relationship of fibroblasts to 139–40
matrix metalloproteinases 138
   and atrial stretch 208
matrix protein synthesis 206
maximum diastolic potential 95, 236
maximum systolic potential 96, 236
MEA see microelectrode
MEC see mechano-electric coupling
mechanical deformation 262–4
mechanical heterogeneity 270, 345–51
mechanical stimulation 361–8
   arrhythmia termination 361–8
   during diastole 161–2
   during systole 162–4
   global 164–5
   regional 165
   spatial aspects 164–5
   temporal aspects 161–4
mechano-electric coupling 16, 42, 103, 342
   and arrhythmic mechanisms 177–8
   aortic stiffness 397–8
   atria 168–9, 252, 271, 299
   atrial fibrillation 203–11
   atrial flutter 238–9
   bidirectional 126
   and cardiac alternans 128–9
   cardiac muscle activation 153–9
   cardiac resynchronization therapy 412–19
   cardiomyocytes 87–8, 103–9
   cell culture 145–7
   clinical correlates 177–8
   clinical studies, atrial fibrillation 395–401
   experimental, and clinical conditions 177
   extrinsic 374
   fibroblasts in 138–42
   heart failure 402–6
   impaired 46
   intrinsic 374
   ischaemia 174, 175–7
      phase 1b arrhythmias 352–3
   right ventricle 217–22
   transgenic models 230–1
   and U-wave 275
   VAC 420–7

mechano-sensitive channels *see* SAC
mechano-transduction 3–8
membrane
  cardiomyocytes 35, 59–60
  costameric 59
  heterogeneous 59
  homogeneous 57–9
  modifiers 62–3
  specialized 59–60
membrane capacitance 61, 180
  stretch effects 182
membrane/cytoskeleton interface 22, 57–65
MERLIN-TIMI study 301
mexiletine 46, 348
microelectrode
  arrays (MEA) 145
  recording 97, 103, 145, 183, 275
microtubule buckling 89
MIRACLE study 187, 413
MIRACLE-ICD study 413
mitochondria 37–8
mitogen-activated protein kinase *see* MAPK
mitral regurgitation 292–3
  atrial fibrillation in 203–4
  atrial dilatation in 205–6
mitral stenosis 291–2
model systems
  animal models
    arrhythmias 227–33
    asynchronous activation 388
    atrial fibrillation 205–6
    canine heart 450–5
    commotio cordis 326, 327
    defibrillation efficacy 374
    Langendorff rabbit heart 168–9, 171, 223–4,
      286, 327
    neonatal rat cell culture 144
  atria 251–7
  cell culture 144, 147–8
  heart failure 241–50
  intact tissue 143–4
  precordial thump 365–6
  SAC 259
  single cell 144, 174
  ventricular arrhythmias 258–66
  ventricular mechanics 444–5
  ventricular myocardial band 154
  ventricular repolarization 269
monocrotaline (MCT) 219, 220
monophasic action potentials 103, 105, 175, 188, 218,
  223, 269–70
  atrial fibrillation 168
  stretch-related electrophysiological effects 103–6
  ventricular repolarization 218
muscle duplex 154–7
muscular dystrophy *see* Duchenne muscular
  dystrophy
MUSTIC-SR study 413
myocardial hypertrophy 134
myocardial stretch 180–4, 286
  effects of 183–4, 318–22
  measurement of 181
  path of 180
  potential interactions of 182
  regional wall stress and strain in 181
  speed of 180–1
myocardium

activation sequence 154–8
  1D models 157–8
  muscle duplex approach 154–7
  underlying mechanisms 158
  left ventricular assist device affecting 384
  in heart failure 241–9
  material properties 443
  regional stretch effect in 173–9
myocytes *see* cardiomyocytes
myofibrillogenesis 89–90
  premyofibrils 89
myofibroblasts 138–9
  smooth muscle actin 139
myofilaments, Ca^{2+} sensitivity 190

Na^+
  intracellular 75–6
    in heart failure 335–6
  voltage-gated fast current 180
Na^+ channels, voltage-gated 12, 42, 180
Na^+-Ca^{2+} exchanger 32, 298
  activation of 117
  reverse mode 112, 113, 114
  in slow force response 85–6, 435–6
Na^+-H^+ exchanger 32, 76, 77, 436
Na^+-K^+ exchanger 31–2
  in heart failure 336
NADPH oxidases 77
NAV channels 44–7
  1.5 channels 44–5, 46–7
  1.6 channels 46–7
Naxos disease 134, 407, 408
N-cadherin 132–3, 408, 409
necrosis 193, 229
  see also apoptosis
needle insertion, transthoracic 361
neonatal rat cell culture model 144, 146–7
nicotinic acetylcholine receptors 12
nifedipine 20, 310
nitrate therapy in heart failure 287
nitric oxide 52, 53, 82–5, 195, 236
  stretch-activated production 77
  stretch-activated release 436
nitric oxide synthase 53
  endothelial 53, 54, 83
    regulation of EC coupling 84–5
    stretch activation 83–4
Nkx.2.5 134
NMDA receptors 8, 12
non-invasing imaging *see* imaging
non-sarcolemmal SAC 35–41
  stretch responses 36–9
  see also SAC
non-selective cation channels 29–30, 83
  stretch-activated 99–100
  volume-activated 29, 30
NOS *see* nitric oxide synthase

ω-3 polyunsaturated fatty acids 208
Oryza 4
osmotic stress 13, 27, 31
osmotic swelling 27, 28–33, 97, 111
overload
  chronic 206, 342
    remodelling in 403, 404
  hypertrophy 132
oxidative stress 299

pacemaker currents 43–4
pacemaker electrophysiology 95–102
pacing 291
  dyssynchrony 196
  preconditioning 194–5
Paramecium 4
PATCH-CHF study 413
patch-clamp 3, 4, 437
  channel density 13
  SAC_K 20
peptide
  atrial natriuretic 111, 206, 227–8
  GsMTx-4 15, 100, 259, 464–5
  as membrane modifier 62–3
percutaneous coronary intervention (PCI) 196
pericardial pressure 282–3
pericardium 281–9
  clinical implications related to 286–7
  Frank-Starling law 284, 285, 287
  physiological implications related to 284–6
  transmural pressure 281–2
  ventricular interaction 282–4
pericytes 139, 140
perymysium 242–3
phosphatidic acid 22
phosphatidylinositol 3-kinase 77
phosphatidylinositol 4,5, bisphosphate 51
phospholamban 231, 334
phospholipase C 51, 77, 134, 207
phospholipase D 134
pirfenidone *see* antifibrotics
plakoglobin 132, 135, 146, 229
  in ARVC 407–11
  mutations 408–9
    effects on cellular biomechanics 410–11
  Naxos 410
plants 5, 6
  SAC 12
platelet-derived growth factor 206–7
polarity
  T-wave 187, 188, 275
  U-wave 275
polyunsaturated fatty acids 22–3, 342
polyvalent cations 62–3
postconditioning 193, 195–6
  stutter reperfusion 193
potassium *see* K^+
prazosin *see* antihypertensive therapy
preconditioning 193–5
  arrhythmias 194
  clinical data 195
  infarct size 193
  pacing/stretch-induced 194–5
  stunning and contractile function 193–4
precordial percussion 362
precordial thump 261–2, 361–4
  in cardioversion 362
    asystole 362
    clinical utility 363–4
    tachycardia 362–3
    ventricular fibrillation 363
  legal issues 364–5
    history 364
    procedural instructions 364–5
    recommendations 364
  mechanisms 365–6
premature beats 354, 356

premature ventricular contractions 161, 340, 398
pressure overload 313–17
   and AP duration 315
   arrhythmogenesis 313–17
   and atrial fibrillation 396–7
   and conduction velocity 316
   and delayed after-depolarizations 315–16
   Framingham studies 396
   and sinus node rhythm 314
pressure-volume loop 456–7, 460
   pulmonary artery occlusion 219
prokaryotes 3, 4
propranolol 97, 321
PROSPECT study 416–7
proteins
   Ca^{2+}-regulating 52
   GPB-binding 219
   Heatshock 70
   kinase A 134
     and arrhythmias 228
   kinase C 69, 77, 134, 146, 207
   melusin 84
   phosphatases 228
   syntrophin 59, 60
   tethered 437
proteoglycans 140, 164
   see also extracellular matrix
pulmonary veins 252
   in atrial fibrillation 110, 169
   ectopic activity 214
   ectopic electrical trigger activity 169
   ectopy 215
   left atrial junction 110, 213
   mechano-sensitivity 110–16
     arrhythmogenic role 112–13
   stretch-activated currents 111–12, 214, 215
   structure and function 213–14
pulsed-wave TDI 414
   see also imaging
pulsus alternans 173-4, 177
pumps/exchangers 31–2
   intra-aortic balloon 372
   Na^+-Ca^{2+} 32, 298
     activation by Ca^{2+} waves 117
     reverse mode 112, 113, 114
     in slow force response 85–6, 435–6
   Na^+-H^+ 32
     protein kinase activation 77
     ROS activation 77
     in slow force response 76, 436
   Na^+-K^+ 31–2
     in heart failure 336
   pusher plates 420
Purkinje fibres 96, 106, 275
   conduction velocity 181
   heart failure 336

QRS complex 125, 306–7
   heart failure 404–5
   in imaging 413, 414, 415, 417, 452
   resynchronization therapy 330
   T-wave 275
QT interval 269, 302, 341, 349, 382–5
   corrected 349
   long QT syndrome see long QT syndrome
   short QT syndrome 275–7
   U-wave 274, 275, 276–7

QTc interval 349
quinidine 20, 178

rafts 51, 58
RALES study 399
ranolazine 47, 301
   see also NAV channels
re-entrant rhythms, mechanical modulation 236–9
re-entrant waves 253–4
reactive oxygen species 29, 82, 435
   activation of Na^+-H^+ exchanger 77
   and apoptosis 193
reflex, Bainbridge 95
refractoriness
   atrial stretch 171
   ventricular stretch 180–6
refractory period 104, 106, 168, 177, 183–4, 203,
   259, 298
   absolute 395–6
   effective 104, 168, 269, 290
     and AP duration 183
     atrial 298
     shortening of 395
     stretch effects 183–4
     volume loading effect 270
regional heterogeneity 153, 154, 156, 165
regional ischaemia 175–7
relaxation 154
   isovolumic 154, 217, 218, 242–3
   sub-endocardial 345
   sub-epicardial 345
remodelling
   atrial 293–5, 298
   electrical 330–1
   gap junction 132–7
   reverse 382–5, 422–5
   structural 206–8, 298–9
   tissue 247
   ventricular 187–92, 305–12, 402
repolarization 223–5, 330–7
   dispersion of 106, 154, 155, 177, 310, 372
   of sinoatrial node pacemaker 97
   and T-wave 223, 327
   and U-wave 275
respiration, and atrial flutter 236–7, 238
respiratory sinus arrhythmia 95, 234–6
   exercise and heart failure 235–6
   heart-transplanted patients 235
   non-neural 234–6
restitution hypothesis 127
reverse remodelling 382–5, 422–5
REVERSE study 412, 413
RGD see arginine-glycine-aspartate peptides
rheumatic heart disease 291–2
right ventricular/ventricle 217–22
   arrhythmogenic cardiomyopathy 228, 229, 407–11
   commotio cordis see commotio cordis
   end-diastolic pressure 281
   failure 217
   heterogeneity 220
   monophasic action potential recording 218
   pressure-volume relationship 217, 218
   structure and function 217
riluzole 23, 47
ROS see reactive oxygen species
ryanodine receptor (RyR) 36, 78, 83, 122, 128, 228,
   252, 384

defective calmodulin binding 229
nitric oxide 53, 83

SAC 3–10, 12-13, 103-4, 106–7, 190, 220, 234–40
   acid sensing ion channels 47
   activation
     by atrial dilatation 111
     by membrane tension 60–2
     by superoxide 77–8
     intracellular Ca^{2+} effects 16
   amiloride 15
   in animal cells 6–8
   in arrhythmogenesis 341
   atria 251, 253–6
   atrial fibrillation 212–3
   bacteria 3-5
   blood pressure regulation 8
   candidate genes 436–8
   cation non-selective see SAC_{NS}
   channel density 13
   chronic mechanical overstimulation 464–5
   evolution of 3–10, 12
   ion channel 141
   see also ion channels
   identity of 462
   K^+ channels see SAC_K
   mechano-sensitivity 12–13, 103–4
   membrane/cytoskeleton interface 57–65
   modelling 259
   modulators 15, 42, 463–4
   non-sarcolemmal 35–41
   non-selective see SAC_{NS}
   patch measurements of 13
   pharmacology of 14–16
   pulmonary vein cells 110–16
   in slow force response 77, 436
   stimuli 13
   structure of 12
SAC_K 20, 161–5, 365–6, 436
SAC_{NS} 60, 99–100, 161, 164
   activation of 437–8
   in commotio cordis 327–8
   in Duchenne muscular dystrophy 439
   inhibition 182
     GsMTx-4 184
     streptomycin 163, 182, 184
   and TRPC 464
   see also SAC
SAFE-T study 300
sANK-1 see ankyrin-1
sarco/endoplasmic reticulum Ca^{2+}-ATPase pump see
   SERCA pump
sarcolemmal ionic influx 76–7
sarcomere length 117–24, 190
sarcoplasmic reticulum
   in heart failure 334–5
   protein dysfunction 228–9
   stretch response 36–8
second messengers
   in slow force response 77–8
   MSC activation 463
   stretch effects 81–6
     integrins 81–2
     membrane receptor-mediated 82
     nitric oxide 82–5
   TREK-1 modulation by 23
sentinel cells 139

SERCA pump 77
SERCA2a 127–8, 129, 146, 346
    in heart failure 334–5
    and LVAD support 384
SFR *see* slow force response
Shaker channels 12, 46, 47
short transient stretch 104–6
signal transduction 38, 134
    $I_{Cl,swell}$ 29
    integrins 81–2, 135
    titins 71
    ventricular electrical remodelling 189
signalosomes 50, 81, 84
    activation 27
sino-atrial node 95–7
    pacemaking
        architecture and conduction pathways of
            96–7
        Bainbridge reflex in 95
        electrophysiology of 95–6
        physiological stimuli in 95
        stimulation in 97–9
        stretch response in 98–100
    respiratory sinus arrhythmia 235, 236
sinus node
    dysfunction 295
    mechanical modulation 234–6
    volume/pressure overload 314
slow force response 75–8, 435
    cellular mechanisms 435–6
    inositol triphosphate, in slow 78
    Na$^+$-Ca^{2+} exchanger in 75–6
    SAC in 77, 436
    sarcolemmal ionic influx 76
    SR Ca^{2+} release 77
    second messenger systems 77–8
    TRPC1 in 438
sodium *see* Na$^+$
SOLVD study 399
sotalol 300, 301, 341
spatial heterogeneity 157
spatio-temporal periodicity 318
spectraplakin family 59
spectrin 59, 89
spironolactone 208, 342
spontaneous focal discharges 319–21
SR *see* sarcoplasmic reticulum
statins 208, 299
stFRET 431–3
    compatibility with multiple host proteins 432
    molecular force detection 432–3
    see also FRET
STOP H2 study 398
strain 306, 345
    circumferential 309
    regional wall, determinants of 181
streptomycin 15, 100, 163, 182, 214, 224–5, 327,
    436, 463–4
stretch-activated channel *see* SAC
stimulation
    adrenergic 113, 135
    mechanical 361–8 *see also* mechanical stimulation
    sino-atrial node 97–9
Stokes-Adams attack 362
stress 345, 352, 376
    contractile 246
    wall *see* wall stress

stress-strain loop 446–7
stretch
    acute 82, 104, 106, 369, 376
    atrial 111, 168–72
        conduction path affected by 180–2
        refractory period affected by 183
    and Ca^{2+} waves 122
    chronic, Ca^{2+} in 206
    cardiac alternans 173–9
    cardiac muscle response 74–80
    conduction velocity 180–3
        measurement during myocardial stretch 181
        regional wall stress/strain 181
        speed and path of conduction 180–1
    diastolic 36
    electrophysiological effects of 104–6
    ERP 183–4
    long-term adaptation 70–1
    membrane capacitance 182
    pathological myocardium 173–9
    preconditioning by 194–5
    regional 121, 277
    systolic 174, 388
    U wave 274
    ventricular 107, 108, 168, 180–6
stretch response
    cardiac muscle 74–80
    connexin channels in 38–9
    non-sarcolemmal SAC 36–9
    sino-atrial node 98–9
    slow force *see* slow force response
stretch-activated ion channels *see* SAC
stretch-induced depolarization 169
stretch-induced preconditioning 194–5
stretch-sensing 50–1
structural proteins, strain measurement 431–4
structural remodelling 206–8, 298–9
    atrial fibrillation 203
    with cardiac assist device 385
    in chronic stretch 206
    JAK/STAT pathway 206
    postconditioning effect 196
    preconditioning effect 193–4
substrate
    defibrillation effect 376–7
    ischaemic arrhythmias 353–4
sudden death 227–8, 229
    cardiac death 125, 402
        commotio cordis see commotio cordis
        diagnostic markers 404
        and left ventricular ejection fraction 402
        and left ventricular volume 402–3
        and prevention of ventricular
            remodelling 403–4
        from ventricular arrhythmia 352
        unexpected nocturnal death syndrome 44
superior vena cava 96, 252
superoxide, activation of SAC current 77–8
support device *see* ventricular assist devices
supraventricular tachycardia 290
    Valsalva manoeuvre 371
sustained stretch 106, 108, 168, 259, 272
systole 103, 161
    maximum systolic potential 96
    mechanical stimulation during 162–4
    tethering 103
    timing 104–5

systolic function 457
systolic stretch 174, 388

T-tubule 13–4, 46–7, 59–60, 67, 305, 436, 437
T-wave
    alternans 340–1
    origin of 305
    T-wave memory 187, 190
tachycardia
    atrial *see* atrial fibrillation; atrial flutter
    cardiac mechanical stimulation for 361, 362–3
    supraventricular 291, 301
    termination
        by intrathoracic pressure increase 361
        by precordial thump 362–3
    ventricular *see* ventricular fibrillation; ventricular
        tachycardia
talin 59, 81, 89
TASK1 20
TASK3 20
TDI *see* imaging
TEM *see* transmission electron microscopy
tetraethylammonium 20, 23
tetrodotoxin 15, 20, 97
TGF-β 134–5, 146
    TGF-β3 407
Timothy syndrome 48
TIMP 208
tissue inhibitor of metalloproteinase *see* TIMP
tissue slices 147–8
titin 66, 67–8, 242
    length-dependent activation 70
    long-term adaptation to stretch 70–1
    passive tension response 68–70
    restoring tension response 69
    signalling pathways 71
TOK-1 channel 19
torsades de pointes 162, 300, 315, 340, 345–51, 384
    long QT syndrome *see* long QT syndrome
    mechanical heterogeneity 345–6
    prevention 348
    triggers for 347–8
TRAAK 7, 19, 63
trans-thoracic needle insertion 361
transducing cell volume *see* cell volume
transforming growth factor-β *see* TGF-β
transient dilation 272
transient outward current I_{to} 228, 251, 298, 464
transient receptor potential channels *see* TRP channels
transmembrane potential Ca^{2+} coupling 125–7
transmembrane pressure 13
transmission electron microscopy, caveolae 53–4
transmural pressure 281–2
    pressure difference 281
TREK1 7, 8, 19–26, 462
    carboxy terminal domain 21
    and cardiac function 23–4
    expression 20–1
    mechano-activation 21–2
    modulation of 22–3
    pharmacology 23
    temperature sensitivity 22
    voltage dependency 21
TREK2 7
TREK3 7
troponin
    Ca^{2+} affinity 75

C, Ca^{2+} binding and FSLR 118–19
TRP channels 5, 7–8, 47, 50, 52, 60, 220
  G_q protein-coupled receptors 52–3
  and SAC_{NS} currents 464
  TRPA 7, 8
  TRPC1 436–7, 438, 462
  TRPC6 77–8, 437, 462
  TRPM 7
    in mechano-transduction 8
  TRPML 7
  TRPP 7
    in autosomal dominant polycystic kidney
      disease 8
  TRPV 7
    as heat thermosensors 8
  TRPV2 437
TSI see imaging
tubulin 87, 219
TWIK channels 7, 19, 28

U-wave 274–80
  characteristics of 274
  hypotheses for origin of 274–5
    delayed repolarization of His-Purkinje
      system 274–5
    delayed repolarization of mid-myocardial
      layers 275
    MEC 275
  I_{K1} as modulator of 278, 279
  intracellular Ca^{2+} dynamics 277–8
  and isovolumic relaxation 277
  in short QT syndrome 275–7
  and T-wave 274
  ventricular repolarization 275
unexpected nocturnal death syndrome 44
VAC 11, 12, 161
  in cardiomyocytes 27–34
    I_{Ca-L} 31
    I_{Ca-T} 31
    $I_{Cl,swell}$ 27–9
    non-selective cation 29–30

VAD see ventricular assist devices
Val-HeFT study 399
Valsalva manoeuvre 160, 238, 272, 286
  and arrhythmia termination 361, 371–2
vascular endothelial growth factor see VEGF
vasodilation 23
vasodilator-stimulated phosphoprotein 84
VEGF 134–5, 140
venae cavae 95, 97
venous return 95, 99, 160, 234, 284
  intrathoracic pressure 371
  as stretch trigger 295
ventricle
  end-diastolic pressure-volume relationship of
    422, 457
  filling 95
  left see left ventricular/ventricle
  MEC 258–66
  myocardium 241–3
  right see right ventricular/ventricle
  stretch effects 107, 108, 168, 180–6
ventricular arrhythmia
  aortic occlusion 342

heart failure 340–4, 402
  initiation of 313–17
  intra-aortic balloon pump 372
  and left ventricular assist device 381–2
  mathematical models 258–66
  mechanical stimulation
    spatial aspects 164–5
    temporal aspects 161–4
  premature ventricular contractions 161, 340
  risk factors 422
  and sudden cardiac death 352
  torsades de pointes 162, 300, 315, 340
  see also ventricular fibrillation; ventricular
    tachycardia
  volume and pressure overload in 313–6
ventricular assist devices 381–6, 420–7
  acquired long QT syndrome 383–4
  applications 421–2
  Ca^{2+} cycling 384–5
  effects of
    action potential 423–4
    Ca^{2+} handling 424
    cardiac conduction 424
    fibrosis 424–5
    heart rhythm 422
  electrophysiological alterations 382–3
  HeartMate devices 421, 422, 423
  HVAD device 421
  incidence of ventricular arrhythmias 381–2
  L-type Ca^{2+} current 385
  MEC 420–7
  ventricular remodelling 422–3
ventricular fibrillation 125, 258, 272, 340
  chest blow-induced see commotio cordis
  dilation 374
  defibrillation threshold 378
  precordial thump for 363
  prolonged 376, 378
  stretch-related 321
ventricular interaction 282–4
  clinical implications 286–7
  physiological implications 284–6
ventricular mechanics 245–6
  normal and infarcted heart 444–5
  regional 442–3
  see also cardiac mechanics
ventricular remodelling 402
  electrical 187-92, 305-12
    Rosenbaum, Mauricio 187, 188
  ionic changes 188–9
  long-term 308–11
  mechano-electrical feedback 189–90
  pathophysiological consequences 187
  prevention of 403–4
  short-term 306–8
  signalling mechanisms 189
  VAC 422–3
ventricular repolarization
  human studies 269–79
  interaction with cycle length 270–1
  laboratory models 269
  load dependence 269–73
  pathology 272
  proarrhythmic effect of altered loading 272
  regional heterogeneity 270

ventricular strain 450–5
  impedance monitoring 456–61
    afterload 457
    left ventricular volume 457–8
    preload 457
    pressure-volume vs stress-strain 456–7
    systolic function 457
    ventricular diastolic function 457
    see also cardiac mechanics; ventricular
      mechanics
ventricular tachycardia 160–7, 258, 272, 301, 340
  decay into fibrillation 262
  in heart failure 272
  termination by percordial thump 261–2
  see also ventricular fibrillation
ventricular tissue 241–2
verapamil 169, 184, 214, 348–50
vernakalant 301, 302
VGC see voltage-gated channels
vimentin 140
vinculin 59, 81
voltage clamp 13
voltage sensor toxins 43–4
  GsMTx4 13, 14, 15–6, 43
voltage-gated channels
  Ca^{2+} 12
    I_{Ca-L} 31
    I_{Ca-T} 31
  K^+ 12
    I_{Kr} 31
    I_{Ks} 30–1
    TREK-1 21
  and lipid bilayer 42–3
  Na^+ 12
  stretch modulation 42–9
    arrhythmia-inducing mutants 44–6
    Cav channels 48
    Kv channels 46
    and myocardial physiology 43
    Nav1.5 vs Nav1.6 channels 46–7
    pacemaker channels 48
    study of 43–4
    swelling effects 30–1
volume overload 70, 293–4, 395
  defibrillation 376–7
  ventricular arrhythmogenesis 160, 313–7
    AP duration 314–6
volume-activated channels see VAC
VVI pacing see asynchronous pacing

wall stress/strain 181, 219, 356, 403, 433
  regional, determinants of 181
wavelength 300
wedge pressure, pulmonary capillary 457–8
Wnt1 134
Wolff-Parkinson-White syndrome 188, 388
Women's Health Study 397

XIP 32
X-ray diffraction 70, 75
yeasts 4–5

Z-disk 66, 68, 70
Z-line 51, 53, 89
Zyxin 84